# DEMENTIA

## Handbook & Resource Guide

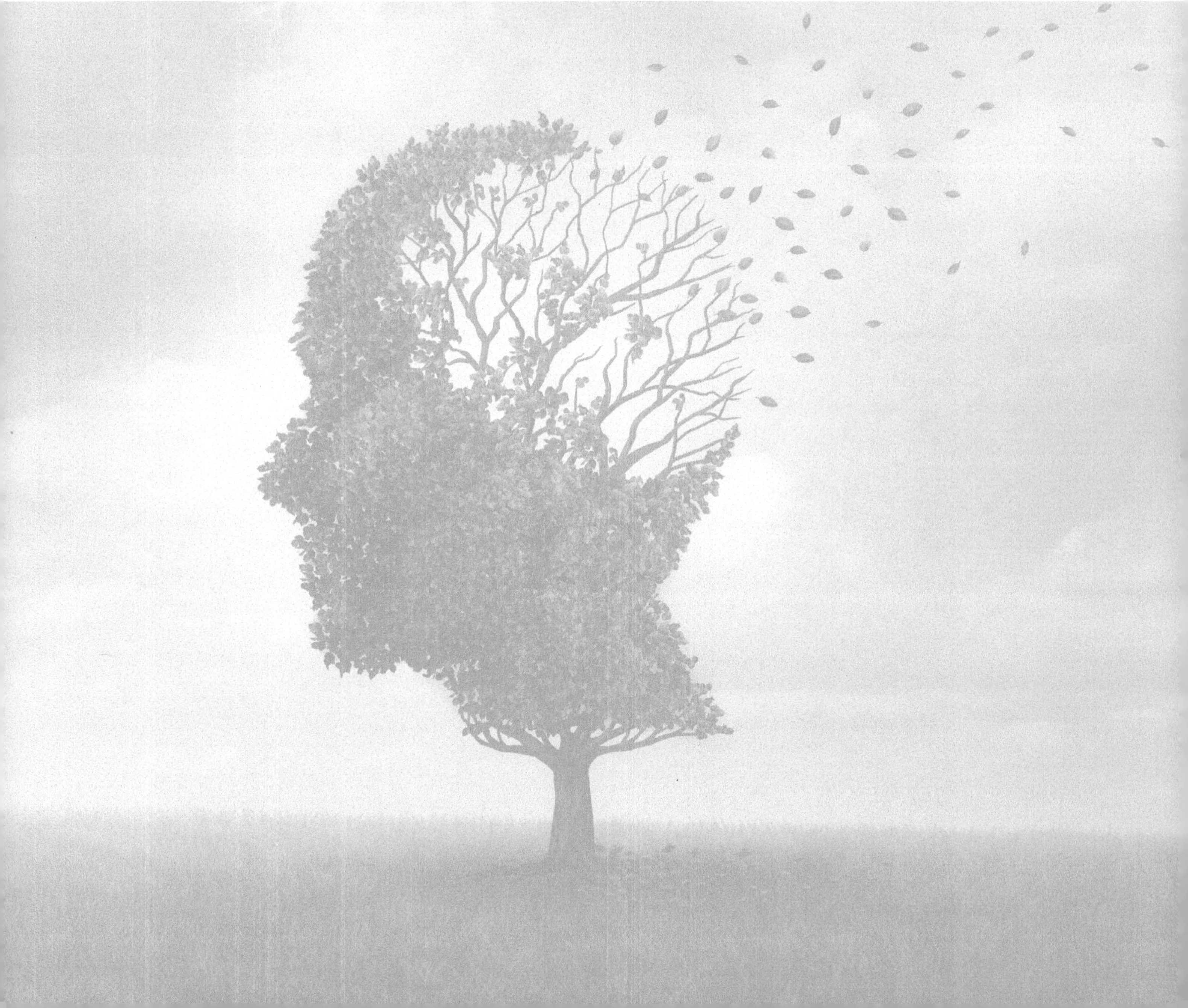

*First Edition*

# DEMENTIA

## Handbook & Resource Guide

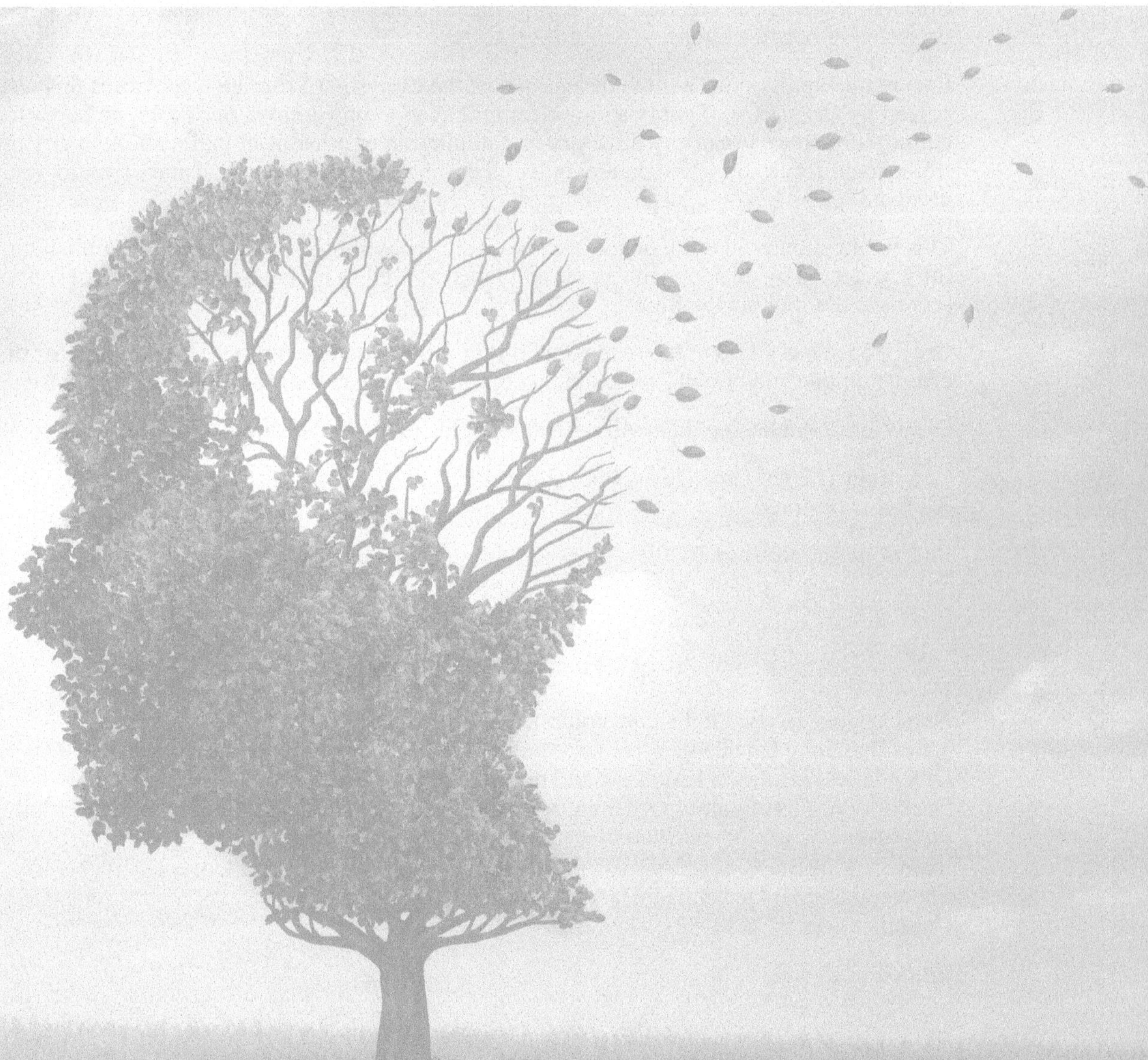

GREY HOUSE PUBLISHING

PRESIDENT: Richard Gottlieb
PUBLISHER: Leslie Mackenzie
EDITORIAL DIRECTOR: Laura Mars
PRODUCTION MANAGER: Kristen Hayes
MARKETING DIRECTOR: Jessica Moody

Grey House Publishing, Inc.
4919 Route 22
Amenia, NY 12501
518.789.8700
Fax: 845.373.6390
www.greyhouse.com
books@greyhouse.com



First edition published 2020

Publisher's Cataloging-In-Publication Data
(Prepared by The Donohue Group, Inc.)

Names: Grey House Publishing, compiler.
Title: Dementia handbook & resource guide / [compiled by Grey House Publishing].
Other Titles: Dementia handbook and resource guide
Description: First Edition. | Amenia, NY : Grey House Publishing, 2020. | Includes bibliographical references.
Identifiers: ISBN 9781642654707 (softcover) 9781637003886 (hardcover)
Subjects: LCSH: Dementia—Handbooks, manuals, etc.
Classification: LCC RC521 .D46 2020 | DDC 616.83—dc23

Printed in Canada

# Table of Contents

## Section Three: Appendixes

# Publisher's Note

Grey House Publishing is excited to announce a new work—*Dementia Handbook & Resource Guide*—taking its place alongside our long-standing consumer health titles on such topics as mental health, older Americans, chronic illness, pediatric disorders, people with disabilities, and learning disabilities.

This comprehensive work comes at a time when a new case of dementia is being diagnosed, worldwide, every three seconds, according to the World Health Organization. Today, about 50 million people suffer from dementia. That number is expected to reach 82 million in 2030 and 152 million by 2050. *Dementia Handbook & Resource Guide* combines valuable educational information for patients, families, and caregivers. It offers statistics, both nationally and state by state, as well as discussions about treatment and outcomes. In addition, it offers details on 23 different types of dementia and conditions that can cause, or affect, dementia from Aging to Wernicke-Korsakoff syndrome.

## Arrangement

### Introduction

Following this Publisher's Note is an excerpt from *Dementia Reimagined* by Tia Powell, MD, described by Steve Silberman, *New York Times* bestselling author, as "A brave, sobering, and profoundly humane book about one of the most serious challenges we face both as individuals and as a society." Dr. Powell's introduction, reprinted here, is a moving combination of medicine and memoir that addresses the challenges she faced as her grandmother, then her mother, were diagnosed with dementia.

### Section One: Studies & Statistics About Dementia

This robust, colorful section of more than 300 pages includes a number of detailed reports from The Alzheimer's Association, the World Health Organization, and the Centers for Disease Control. They cover attitudes toward dementia, a global action plan, prevalence, costs, care giving, and state statistics. These reports include:

- World Alzheimer's Report 2019: Attitudes to Dementia
- Dementia: Public Health Priority
- Global Action Plan
- 2020 Alzheimer's Disease Facts & Figures
- Facts & Figures of Alzheimer's
- State of the States

### Section Two: Types of Dementia

This section comprises 23 chapters, each covering a different type of dementia or health condition that can cause, relate to, or effect dementia. Chapters cover Alzheimer's disease, brain tumors and injuries, drug & alcohol misuse, Huntington's disease, dementia with Lewy bodies, Parkinson's disease, vascular dementia, environmental causes, and more. Each chapter begins with a concise description of the specific condition and goes on to include a variety of resources for patients, their families and caregivers. Specific categories include; National Agencies & Associations; State Agencies & Associations; Foundations & Research Centers; Support Groups & Hotlines; Magazines; and Websites.

This section ends with a list of medications that have been used or are currently used to treat symptoms of dementia and related conditions.

### Section Three: Appendixes

- **Mediagraphy** includes a wide variety of films, TV programs, books of fiction, plays and music that deal with the subject of dementia. Each of the nearly 80 listings are annotated to help support specific interests of the reader.
- **Glossary** includes more than 100 terms that are both included in this work and ones that the reader might come across in his or her own research of dementia and related disorders.
- **Entry Index** lists all directory entries alphabetically.
- **Geographic Index** organizes listings alphabetically by state.

In addition to the print directory, *Dementia Handbook & Resource Guide* includes two years of free online access to G.O.L.D., Grey House OnLine Databases. This gives you immediate access to the most valuable in-depth information on the many causes of this neuro-cognitive disorder, early warning signs, diagnosis, treatment options, advice for caretakers, preventative therapy, and support. G.O.L.D. also offers easy-to-use keyword searches, organization type and subject searches, hotlinks to web sites and emails, and so much more. Call 800-562-2139 for a free trial or visit http://gold.greyhouse.com for more information.

# De-'Men-Sha: An Introduction

An Excerpt from *Dementia Reimagined: Building A Life Of Joy And Dignity From Beginning To End*
by Tia Powell, MD

...

Here is the thing: Dementia lasts for years. Most of that time, people with dementia retain the skills, memories, and passions that allow joy and inclusion in the larger social world, if we would but let them in.

A family story started me thinking about dementia some years ago. On an autumn day, two women sit together on a sunny screen porch in Washington, DC. They look alike; they are mother and daughter. Silver-haired and tiny, neither is quite five feet tall. One is in her sixties, one in her nineties. The younger woman radiates energy, bustling about, always the good daughter. She has managed to get the frail, mute older woman settled in a comfortable chair to enjoy the mild and lovely day. She arranges a rainbow-colored afghan, crocheted many years ago by the older woman, tucking it in around her. "There, Mother!" She beams."How is that?" The older woman struggles to speak, which she has not done for months. The daughter waits. The silence is tremendous. The older woman produces a single word, a word that must stand for all she cannot say. Her eyes are fierce with effort. She whispers, "Lousy."

That was my grandmother's last word, spoken some months before she died of dementia, and long before my mother herself developed the dementia whose consequences would kill her.[1] I didn't know it at the time, but when my mother told me this story, it triggered a change in the way I understood dementia, a change that is ongoing. Like other serious diseases, dementia affects not only the person with the illness but all those whose lives touch hers.

My family has certainly felt the sting of dementia. I am a physician, but medical training never prepared me to address the challenges of dementia that I faced as a daughter and granddaughter. Having dementia or seeing a loved one suffer from it can be lousy, as my grandmother said. Millions of people across the globe can attest to that. But dementia isn't always lousy. Bad aspects can't be eliminated, but they can be diminished and compressed, making the experience *less* lousy for everyone.

My formal education in dementia started in medical school, though what we learned on the topic then, in the 1980s, was not enormously useful. We studied the different types, based on the initial symptoms or the type of brain pathology. Since there were essentially no treatments, the focus was on taxonomy rather than assistance. We were like eighteenth-century biologists, identifying different species of snails or butterflies, with no plan other than description. I learned about SDAT, or senile dementia of the Alzheimer type, about organic brain syndrome. Many of those categories have subsequently been renamed, redefined, combined, or eliminated altogether.

We also learned the basics of brain anatomy. In our first year, a professor projected a slide of a fleshy blob the size of a big shrimp and asked the class to identify it. I am not sure any of us got the answer—I certainly did not. The blob turned out to be the hippocampus; we each have two of these, resting on either side of and near the base of the brain. The name in Latin suggests they look like sea horses, but I never saw the family resemblance. I was taught that the hippocampus is crucial in the work of remembering. That much remains true, though plenty else I was taught is now out-of-date. Of course, that happens throughout medicine. Our current knowledge of cancer, of cystic fibrosis, of HIV provides a radically different and better understanding than was available decades ago. Still, even relative to other fields in medicine, our knowledge about how the brain works, what happens in neurons and brain networks—and how they break down—has exploded in the last twenty-five years.

But it is not only the technical, scientific understanding of dementia that is rapidly shifting. The most important change is our notion of where it sits in the arena of medical problems. A few decades ago, dementia was relegated to the back rows. There was nothing much to do about it, but more crucially, what would be the point? It was something that happened to old people and a few unlucky others. Surely it would make more sense to attack diseases that, if eradicated, would yield the survivors years of healthy life. If you fix something that affects only ninety-year-olds, your patient has a correspondingly brief life expectancy.

Medicine's view of dementia has undergone radical revision. Importantly, there are many more older people than there used to be, and since the risk increases with age, cognitive impairment is a concern for them all. Today there are more than 5 million people in the United States with dementia. That number will continue to grow as the population ages; in the United States, 10, 000 baby boomers turn sixty-five every day. By the time a person reaches eighty-five, the chances of having dementia approach 40 percent.[2] Because of the cost of care, it is also one of our most expensive diseases, more than either cancer or heart disease. Dementia costs us about $200 billion yearly, a figure that includes both formal payment for care and an extraordinary amount of unpaid care.[3]

And here is more bad news: There is no effective cure or prevention, and none likely to arrive in the immediate future. That is one reason why dementia is the disease Americans fear most.[4] Recent major research trials can fairly be described as a series of unfortunate failures. It takes a new drug roughly twelve years to go from inspiration through testing in FDA-approved trials to market. Only a tiny percent of drugs successfully complete this process, either because most don't work or because they have side effects that make their risks greater than the benefits. With no *cure* in sight, our research efforts need to incorporate how to *care* for those who have and will develop dementia. Vile cannot neglect the millions whose comfort should be supported through better palliative treatment.

Medicine is a hierarchical field, and one that clings to a sense of masculinity, whether appropriate or not. Years ago, my two young children were waiting in line at summer camp. Two middle school boys in front of them were wearing towels over their swimsuits. One boy said to the other, "Dude, your towel is pink!" The other boy, flustered, answered, "Dude! It's *faded red!*" The answer: "Dude, it's pink." "DUDE—

FADED RED!" The second boy felt his manliness under attack, and was willing to deny reality to defend himself.

Medicine essentially makes the same denial. It sees itself as manly, offering heroic cures. But a great deal of what medicine offers patients is care—incremental, accommodating, feminine (if you stick with the outmoded metaphor). Yet medicine is too embarrassed to admit this. Care seems soft and unscientific; we'd prefer to hand out swashbuckling cure.

It could have gone another way. Medicine could have taken seriously the Hippocratic instruction to cure sometimes, treat often, comfort always. The dream of cure can push care to the lowest rung of the medical ladder. But though we have yet to find cures for many illnesses, including dementia, defining cure as success means viewing care as failure. For dementia in particular, we must do better. Setting up cure as the only goal, especially when it is linked to saving money, is bound to fail. We do not need science *or* compassion, but always both. We should fund science to try to dent the trajectory of dementia, and we must also care for those who are incurably ill today. We need care *and* cure.

• • •

Our view of dementia is changing, but it needs to change more. How we treat others, particularly vulnerable others, is part of what defines us as a society. When we hide demented elders because they look or act strange, when we fail to provide caring ways and places to live with dementia, we fail in important responsibilities. And yet people struggle with how to meet their obligations and find little guidance available. Should I lie to my father to get him to take medication? To get him to move out of the house where he has lived for decades but is no longer safe? Can we prevent those with cognitive impairment from driving, and if we do, how will we improve public transportation to better accommodate elders?

At one point in my life, I thought I knew something about dementia because I could recognize its symptoms and identify a hippocampus. But even as a doctor, I was not prepared when my mother developed the disease. I did not understand the options. I had to learn along with my siblings what sort of care she might need at any given stage and try to get that for her. I don't think we made terrible mistakes, but we made some. Our choices were difficult and the consequences were impossible to know in advance.

Dementia experts note a number of factors that make dementia care, especially at the end of life, both poor in quality and costly without benefit. When I think back over my mother's treatment, I see markers of less than ideal care: barriers to pain control, unhelpful transitions from hospital to nursing home to emergency room. Her journey through dementia was typical in many ways. It illustrates just how far we are from a system that respects those with dementia and their families. All across the country, families are facing similar choices, and they are struggling to find the right thing to do.

My mother was lucky in many ways. She grew up in a big Irish Catholic family in the suburbs of Washington, DC. She was bookish and shy. She always excelled in school, skipping a grade and finishing college first in her class. She married a good man who had gone to the same parochial school. (A 1935 issue of the church bulletin celebrated the children with highest marks in each grade, listing my father in eighth grade and my mother in fourth.) She had six healthy babies, now six healthy adults. She possessed a mysterious, renewable personal energy source. She marshaled her troops through homework, dog walking, piano lessons, sports practices, and rehearsals for school plays, and then she painted the furniture and fixed the toilets.

Not everything was easy. The late sixties were hard for a good Catholic woman, a time when teenage boys had long hair like Neanderthals and teenage girls went without bras like you-know-whats. They used bad language and questioned authority. My mother was bewildered. She embarked on a graduate degree in women's studies to see if she could figure out what was happening. She read, among others, Shulamith Firestone, who advocated the abolition of pregnancy and the nuclear family. My mother was appalled. But gradually things calmed down. Her children grew up and made better choices in hairstyles and lingerie. They got jobs, they married; chaos no longer reigned.

Decades rolled by. My mother's dementia came on gradually and late in life. By her mid-seventies, she had noticeable lapses in memory. My father was still alive, and together they made a reasonably functional team, living most of the year in Florida. My father had cancer, and he remained mentally sharp though increasingly weak. In contrast, as my mother's cognitive skills steadily declined, a lifetime of physical activity kept her spry. She could ride her bike in their gated retirement community, since the circular trails always led back to her own apartment. When they set out for the grocery store, my mother would drive. My father would tell her where to turn, where to park. He would lean on the grocery cart and she would bird-dog items as he directed. Sometimes he had to stay anxiously with the cart while she brought the car around, but generally they got through their daily life without major mishaps.

But then their system began to fail. As my father became weaker, he couldn't always accompany my mother. Her cognitive deficits progressed. She got lost on her way to a doctor's appointment; she arrived very late and beside herself with anxiety. She was badly shaken for days after. Things were falling apart. It was time to change, but my parents were angry with us for suggesting as much. We were frightened. We couldn't keep them safe more than a thousand miles away from their closest child. All six of us lobbied hard, in unison, for a parental return to Maryland, where they had raised us; still had an apartment, doctors, and friends; and where two of my siblings still lived.

With some resistance and much assistance, my parents moved back. My father got sicker. He enrolled in home hospice, and after a time, he succumbed to cancer. A home health aide had moved in during my father's final illness, and she stayed on after his death to care for my mother. Things did not go well. My mother was grieving and her symptoms got worse. Once she ended up around the corner from my sister's house in downtown DC and asked a stranger planting tulips if my sister lived near there. My mother couldn't remember her daughter's married name, but the neighbor figured it out and pointed her in the right direction. The neighbor also ratted her out to my sister. We started to worry about her driving and finally got her to stop. She was extremely angry about giving up the keys. Hostile negotiations earned her a new nickname: the THWP, or Tiny Hibernian Warrior Princess.

My mother became paranoid. She lost small objects and blamed the aide. She began to stockpile pencils, since she believed the aide was hiding them to prevent her working on the crossword puzzle. Pencils were under the mattress, in the drawers, in the bathroom. In her prime, my mother cooked Thanksgiving dinner for twenty-five people with the tactical skill of a general going into battle. Now she was a risk in the kitchen, forgetting a pot on the stove or saving leftovers until they were blue and furry. Medication management became a problem. Knowing her memory was faulty, my rule-loving mother made an index card and taped it to her bathroom mirror. It said, "Take your medicines." And she did, over and over, until she became delirious from overdosing. Under protest, the index card was removed.

She had very little to do all day. Hours crawled by. My always active mother had no chores, no tasks to structure her lifelong productivity. The aide wanted to watch television; my mother didn't. They were not happy together. My sister found activity groups that helped a bit but didn't solve the problem. In one moment of comic relief, my Catholic mother went with my sister to the basement of a local synagogue that sponsored activities for those with dementia. My mother looked around at the nice ladies with Jewish names. She smiled tentatively. She spoke slowly, confiding to the ladies, "Some of my best friends . . . are synagogues." Laugh out loud or crawl out of the room? My sister was torn. But they took her revelation in stride and went on with bingo. Over time, my mother's theories about the pencils grew more elaborate, and the atmosphere at home grew more strained. Something had to give.

It came as a surprise to me that staying in one's home is not always the best option. For my mother, home had become a prison. My sister took her to visit an assisted living facility connected with a parish church and parochial school. My mother loved seeing the school kids trooping by. She would have more to do, people to talk to. She could dine with a group of silver-haired ladies each night, at a sweet round table with a tablecloth and a flower in the middle. She could bring some of her furniture, enough to fill her single room. She had few regrets leaving behind her apartment, her last independent dwelling. She was a great walker, even then, and could easily walk more than a mile. She enjoyed strolling around her new neighborhood, always accompanied, looking at the school, the old trees, the vegetable gardens.

Assisted living had its ups and downs. My mother flunked having dinner with the first group she was assigned to, since she introduced herself to everyone at every meal. They complained and she went to a different group, more obviously impaired. The staff was not unkind, but they were busy. My mother always preferred baths to showers—she loved nothing better than a relaxing "soaky bath." Although there was a bathtub available, it meant a worker standing by to make sure she was okay. It was easier for the staff if my mother showered in her own bathroom. Baths became a pleasure she would have to do without. This is what you can lose in moving to an institution, even one that tries to be friendly: They evolve to match the needs of those who run the place. What is fun or pleasing for residents may not make the top of anyone else's list.

• • •

Things rolled along for a year or so, until the next crisis. My mother had trouble breathing and went by ambulance to the hospital. A physician called me from the emergency-room and asked whether they should try to resuscitate her heart if it stopped. I asked if she showed signs that her heart was likely to stop. He said no. I asked if he knew why she was short of breath, causing her trip to the hospital. He said no. I observed there was no way to know if her unidentified condition was easily treatable. He agreed. I said that her family would be happy to discuss resuscitation status when the need arose, but his call seemed premature. I wanted to know what the initial tests showed and what her doctors thought the matter was. He seemed a bit embarrassed. This too for me was a revelation. To this young doctor, my mother was an old woman with dementia and therefore not someone who should receive an ordinary evaluation for a common medical problem. How was he to know how we saw her, as someone who enjoyed her life, walked miles a week, had no particular physical ailments, and was a force of nature? Was he out of line? Or was I now one of those unrealistic family members who demand unhelpful treatment, increasing burdens and bringing no benefit?

The hospitalization was scary. My mother went to the ICU with an unusual blood disorder with the ominous name thrombotic thrombocytopenic purpura. I stayed overnight; she became increasingly confused and agitated, constantly trying to get out of bed and remove her tubes. I slept on and off, holding her hand, with my head on our hands to make sure she didn't sneak away. Late that night she had a seizure. A grand mal seizure is terrifying to watch, even when you have seen one before. Watching your mother have one is not an experience I recommend.

She returned to the assisted living facility, weaker and more cognitively impaired; she soon ricocheted back to the hospital. Now she had clots blocking the main arteries to her lungs, a consequence of her blood disease. We opted for a simple procedure, the insertion of a filter to keep clots from reaching the brain and causing a stroke. A kind physician who looked like a middle schooler came to her room and drew all over the whiteboard to explain the procedure. Since she was recovering from delirium—an acute state of confusion common in critically ill elderly people—and was suffering from dementia, it is entirely a fiction that she provided informed consent. Nonetheless, Doogie Howser said the appropriate words, and she smiled and signed the paper. No harm done. I was her surrogate decision-maker and thought the procedure was appropriate; I didn't insist on signing the form. But in hospitals all over the country, patients with limited understanding are agreeing to procedures that may not be in their best interest. Later that day, my mother proudly pointed out the doctor's diagram. There were lots of big loopy arrows that looked like the long ears of a basset hound. She told me the picture showed she'd given birth to a puppy and that was why she needed to stay in the hospital. I told her gently that she had a problem with blood clots. She looked put out. We went back to discussing events from her childhood. Her procedure went forward without a hitch.

This hospital stay marked the turning point from healthy demented person to a frail elder at risk for falling, both literally and metaphorically. My mother had almost never entered a hospital except to have babies, and now she'd had two serious admissions in short order. An enthusiastic walker just months before, she could no longer get from bed to chair. Never tall, she had become minuscule, a feisty leprechaun who might almost rest in the palm of your hand. She went to a rehab facility, where I came upon her working away like a terrier on the upper-arm bike, pedaling for all the world. Her arms and legs grew stronger, but her cognition did not. This is typical for a person with dementia. A frail brain at baseline makes it easier for a serious illness to harm cognition further. And that sparked the next transition. She was no longer welcome in her assisted living facility. She would need a skilled nursing facility.

My siblings who lived in Washington took on the lion's share of checking out nursing homes. Some were pretty to look at but seemed cold. Some were too far to visit regularly. One was small and attractive enough, but visitors were welcome only during a few hours daily, and upon arrival were kept in a windowless antechamber for what seemed like a long time. This lack of transparency gave the impression that things going on inside should not be seen, and that was a deal-breaker.

My father had been a successful attorney; they had saved so that my mother had funds to pay for nursing home care. But until we started looking, I had no idea the costs were so staggering. If you look up the average cost of a nursing home, you may find estimates of roughly $85,000 per year, but that is a deceptive number that typically reflects the rate that Medicaid pays. If you don't qualify for Medicaid or live in a higher-cost area—Anchorage, Alaska, is especially expensive—you may face annual costs nearly twice that amount.[5] A surprising number of people are under the impression that Medicare pays for long-term care. It does not. For those without assets, Medicaid will cover costs, though not every nursing home welcomes the lower Medicaid fees. People in the middle, with some assets but not enough to cover the crushing financial burden of long-term care, can "spend down" their assets until they qualify for Medicaid. There will be no inheritance for the family, and a surviving spouse may be in financial trouble, too. My mother's costs were covered by savings, but this level of expense is not feasible for most Americans. We lack an adequate national plan to cover the costs of care for the millions who will develop dementia in the coming decades. What I l earned in medical school and in my training as a psychiatrist never prepared me for this.

My mother went to a memory care facility with a pleasant living and dining area, and a little garden you could see from the main rooms. Inexorably, she became weaker and more impaired. She could not walk independently. She could no longer dress or bathe or use the toilet. She could feed herself, but with substantial help and increasing difficulty. This is severe dementia, approaching the end stage of a fatal illness. She spoke less often, though she would beam at family members who came to visit. Once, as I spooned pudding into her mouth, I recalled feeding my children when they were small and thought about my mother feeding me. It felt both elemental and very sad.

My mother was happier than when she was less demented. She no longer elaborated complex paranoid theories about people hiding her pencils; she didn't have the bandwidth. She was content to be cared for and was mostly cheerful. But then she started to have odd spells in which she'd stare into space, shaking and speechless. She was evaluated for strokes and seizures, but nothing turned up. After one of these episodes, back in the ER again, a monitor showed heart block—the electrical system that controls the heartbeat was failing, causing ominous pauses. An excellent problem, for there is a solution. My mother needed a pacemaker.[6]

But not so fast. My grandmother had lived for twelve years with a pacemaker, and her own six children deeply regretted ever agreeing to it. My grandmother's dementia culminated in bed-bound immobility and muteness, and an apparent lack of joy. My mother had told us never to give her a pacemaker, and her siblings all felt the same. As far as advance directives went, my mother had done everything right. She formed an educated opinion about a specific treatment in a specific context and expressed that opinion in unambiguous terms on more than one occasion. She had a child who is a physician and bioethicist and appointed that child as a health care proxy.

Nonetheless, along came the cardiologist. He told my siblings that "no one is allowed to die of heart block." Also, no palliative care could be offered, since any symptom would come without warning and would be untreatable. He claimed that her death from heart block would feel like drowning." He also noted that most cardiologists would refuse to turn off a pacemaker. He would consider doing so only if all six siblings agreed in writing. Not only could we lose the option of ceasing treatment if the cardiologist moved or changed his mind, but this last condition of unanimity was a way to override my mother's selection of a health care agent. Our family would be required to maintain her pacemaker if any one of us wanted it.

Even today I am angry at this doctor. Instead of helping, he made things worse. He was not able to say, "Think of this medical problem as one among many. How will what we do with her heart fit in with the overall goals of her care?" He didn't mean to be unkind. But doctors too often shrink their responsibilities to fit the size of their expertise. For older patients, who are likely to have many things going wrong at once, this is a disaster. He saw only a tree and missed the forest of my mother's serious medical problems.

My mother, though reluctant to comment, ventured: "Whatever the doctor thinks is best." Should we stay with her earlier wishes or go with her current passive neutrality? We had agonizing and anxious conversations, laced with dark humor. My brother said, "Whatever else happens, I am telling you right now I don't want a pacemaker." There was a brief silence. Then several of us spoke at once: "Oh, you are definitely getting a pacemaker!" "You'll get one if I have to put it in myself!" I'm heading over there *right now.*"

We were joking, yet we were deadly serious. Most of my siblings thought it was a terrible mistake to consider a pacemaker, even if my mother did not currently object, but we were not unanimous. I felt I should be able to get the pacemaker shut down later, though I knew this could be a real challenge; the doctor had as much as said he would refuse. Surely all my training should allow me to provide this small service for my mother. Ambivalently, I agreed to the procedure, promising to find a way to have it turned off when the time came.

Some days later, the cardiologist showed up at my mother's bedside, shower cap on his head. Two of my siblings were there with her. "What are you doing here?" asked my mother. "I've come to take you for a pacemaker." "I don't want a pacemaker. You doctors do too much stuff to old people." My siblings asked my mother the same question in as many ways as they could. "Do you understand you might not live as long without the pacer?" "Yes. I've lived a good long time." And so forth. The pacemaker was canceled.

My mother was placed in hospice care at the nursing home so she would not be subjected to ER visits with every episode of heart block. The episodes would last for a few seconds with a complete loss of consciousness, leaving no memory behind. She had no fear ahead of time, no pain during, no memory after. She did not suffer, in sharp contrast to the cardiologist's prediction.

Then late one night my mother developed a slow heart rate, sweating, and shortness of breath. Hospice care at the nursing home was well intentioned but poorly organized. These clinicians should have had on hand the morphine and perhaps oxygen my mother would need, and they did not. No supplies could get there until the next morning, many hours away and likely after her time was out. My brother rushed to her side. She was transferred to the emergency room one last time, where she received the necessary oxygen and morphine, though lying on an uncomfortable gurney and not in her bed. She should have been spared this last, wholly unnecessary transition. She slept a good deal of the time. And then she was done. My mother did not die of dementia, as her mother had. She died *with* dementia, but *of* heart disease.

If my mother had received that pacemaker, she might have lived longer to die of dementia, just as she had not wanted. Medical technology comes attached to an engine that propels it toward patients. Unlike the vast majority of older people in America, she had six adult children to help her and we still stumbled our way along, trying our best, making mistakes. Yet she was one of the lucky ones. My family learned the hard way about caring for someone with dementia. We faced hard choices large and small, about what care we want for ourselves and how we ought to treat others.

**Notes:**


1. Tia Powell, "Voice: Cognitive Impairment and Medical Decision Making," *Journal of Clinical Ethics* 16.4 (2005): 303–13.
2. *2017 Alzheimer's Disease Facts and Figures.* Alzheimer's Association, 2017. alz.org/documents_custom/2017-facts-and-figures.pdf.
3. Michael D. Hurd et al., "Monetary Costs of Dementia in the United States." *New England Journal of Medicine* 368.14 (2013) 1326–34.
4. Ibid.
5. John Hancock, 2016 Cost of Care Survey; Long Term Care Insurance. ubsnet.com/assets/Uploads/Newspdf/2016-LTC-Cost-of-Care-Survey-Results.pdf.
6. Tia Powell, "Life Imitates Work." *JAMA* 305.6 (2011): 542–43.

# STUDIES & STATISTICS ABOUT DEMENTIA

This first section of *Dementia Handbook & Resource Guide* includes the most current research regarding dementia, with data from The Alzheimer's Association International, The World Health Organization, and the Centers for Disease Control. Totaling more than 300 pages, Studies & Statistics comprises three detailed reports and three summaries with easy to understand graphics. The entire section is printed in color with dozens of graphs, charts and maps to help visualize the data.

The three large reports all start with a detailed table of contents to help you maneuver through the large amount of information that each contains.

Alzheimer's Disease International

*The global voice on dementia*

# World Alzheimer Report 2019

## Attitudes to dementia

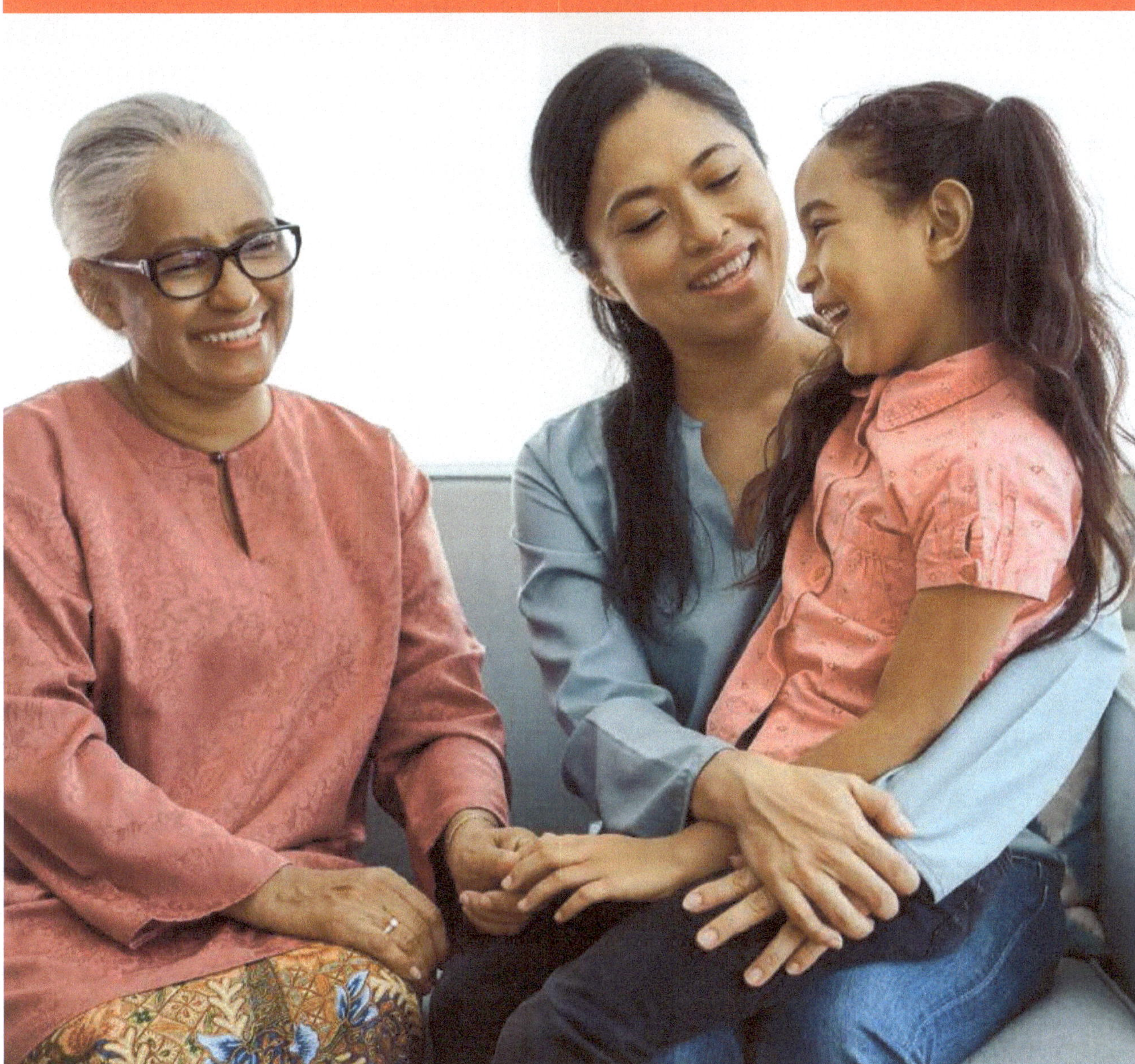

**Author:** Alzheimer's Disease International

**Contributors:**
We would like to thank the large number of contributors involved in this world report, including the survey translators, from 32 countries, without whom this would not have been possible.

The views expressed in the essays, case studies and programmes to reduce stigma are those of the authors.

**Attitudes to dementia survey:** London School of Economics and Political Science: Dr Sara Evans-Lacko, Jem Bhatt, Asst Professor Adelina Comas-Herrera, Dr Francesco D'Amico, Dr Nicolas Farina, Sophie Gaber, Prof Martin Knapp, Maximilian Salcher-Konrad, Madeleine Stevens, Emma Wilson.

**Expert essays, case studies, and programmes to reduce stigma:** (Alphabetical order)

Dementia Australia
Sue Baker
Prof Sube Banerjee
Dr Linda Barclay
Dr Anna Brorsson
Dr Zoe Cashin
Su-Yuan Chan
Asst Prof Adelina Comas-Herrera
Olivier Constant
Prof Colm Cunningham
Dr Stephanie Daley
Walter Dawson
Dr Nicolas Farina
Rosa Ma Farrés
Prof Cleusa Ferri
Sophie N. Gaber
Nouha Ben Gaied
Dr Serge Gauthier
Dale Goldhawk
Howard Gordon
Dr Nori Graham
Dr Wendy Grosvenor
Birgit Heuchemer
Jayme Hill
Berrie Holtzhausen
Prof Kristen Jacklin
Shiva Krishnamurthy
Pippa Kelly
Maryna Lehmann
Asst Prof Christopher Lind
Christine Maddocks
Victor Madrigal-Borloz
Dr Fabiana da Mata
Prof Elaine Mateus
Dr Etuini Ma'u
Andre Mauritz
Pare Meha
Sarah-Jane Meyer
Princess Nouf bint Muhammad
María Cecilia López Murga
Dr Christine Musyimi
Elizabeth Mutunga
Prof David Ndetei
Prof John Oetzel
Dr Deborah Oliveira
Prof JB Orange
Guadalupe Ponce Ozuna
Jim Pearson
Silvia Perel-Levin
Dr Jaewon Phee
Karen Pitawanakwat
Mario Possenti
Rangimahora Reddy
Glenn Rees
Prof Nicolas Rüsch
Dr Hamed Al Sinawi
DY Suharya
Ruth Stone
Kate Swaffer
LiYu Tang
Sarah Tilsed
Lawrence H Yang
Jessica Young

**Translators:** (Alphabetical order)

ARDSI (Alzheimer's and Related disorders Society of India)
Alzheimer's South Africa
Muriel Rason Andriamaro
Bulga Bulganchimeg
Susanne van den Buuse
Sophie Gaber
Konstantinos Gkikas
Major Gopalakrishnan
Stefania Ilinca
Sebastien Kabacinski
Faraneh Kaboli
Nancy Kalaba
Joost Martens
Prof Elaine Mateus
Nilanjana Maulik
Elizabeth Mutunga
Tuan Nguyen
Meera Pattabiraman
Katarzyna Pogorzelska
Mario Possenti
Anastasia Psoma
Aditya Putra
Thankane Raditapole
Narendhar Ramasamy
Isabelle Salameh
Susanna Saxl
Alexandra Shchetkina
Dr Hamed AL Sinawi
LiYu Tang
Petra du Toit
Huali Wang
Noriyo Washizu
Peach Wattana
Jackie Wong

Published by Alzheimer's Disease International (ADI), London.

September 2019.



**Suggested citation:**
Alzheimer's Disease International. 2019. *World Alzheimer Report 2019: Attitudes to dementia.* London: Alzheimer's Disease International.

Design: David O'Connor – www.daviddesigns.co.uk

Due to the diverse nature and number of contributors to this report several key phrases are used interchangeably, including:
Carers / caregivers / care providers / care partners
Healthcare practitioners / healthcare providers / healthcare professionals

Alzheimer's Disease International

*The global voice on dementia*

# World Alzheimer Report 2019

## Attitudes to dementia

# Partners & donors

**ADI would like to thank our corporate partners and donors:**

Anonymous Foundation

Helen Daniels Bader Fund, A Bader Philanthropy

Biogen

Boehringer-Ingelheim

Janssen

Lundbeck International Neuroscience Foundation

Roche

Otsuka America Pharmaceutical, Inc.

Mary Oakley Foundation

The Van Otterloo Family Foundation

# Contents

CHAPTER 4

**Case studies:**

Alzheimer's Disease International
The global voice on dementia

# ADI Global survey on **attitudes to dementia**

## Almost 70,000 respondents from 155 countries

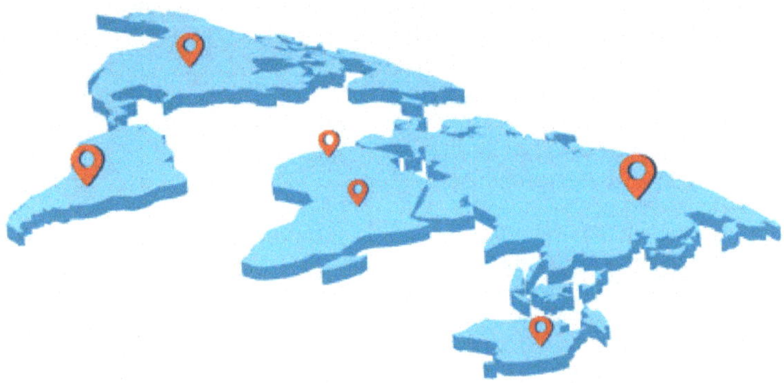

2 in 3 people think that dementia is caused by normal ageing

1 in 4 people think that there is nothing we can do to prevent dementia

95% of the general public think they could develop dementia at some point in their lifetime

Just under 40% of the general public think that there are adequate community services in place for people living with dementia and carers

54% of respondents think lifestyle factors play a part in developing dementia

91% of respondents say that people should not hide the fact they have dementia

**Men are more likely to hold stigmatising views about dementia than women**
*Although they were more likely to let a relative with dementia move in with them*

## Attitudes of healthcare practitioners to dementia

62% of healthcare practitioners still believe that dementia is part of normal ageing

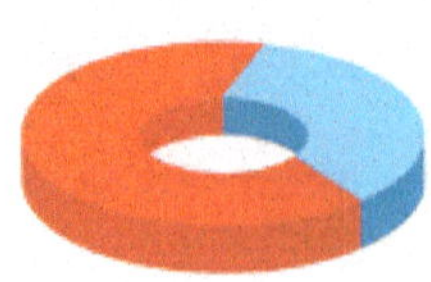

Around 40% of the public think healthcare practitioners ignore people with dementia

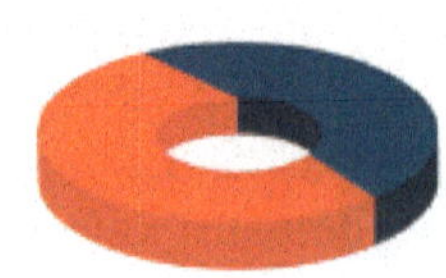

"My neurologist ignored my presence when my diagnosis was discussed with my husband."

"Neurologist diagnosed me with Alzheimer's at 56, telling me to go home and get my final affairs in order and wait until my premature death."

"They sometimes talk to my wife about things like I'm not even there, but I'm sitting right there."

"Many healthcare practitioners often do not believe I have dementia - which is abusive and offensive. But, also, they then talk over me, about me, and never to me..."

## Experiences of carers

Over 50% of dementia carers expressed positive sentiments about their role

Over 50% of dementia carers said their health suffered as a result of their caring responsibilities

35% of carers globally have hidden the diagnosis of a person with dementia

Over 60% of dementia carers said their social life suffered as a result of their caring responsibilities

## Dementia: not a laughing matter?

63% of respondents living with dementia in South-East Asia said their dementia symptoms were joked about by others

67% of respondents living with dementia in Africa said their dementia symptoms were joked about by others

**Carers of people with dementia said:**

"So-called Alzheimer's humour does much more than annoy and hurt those who work hard to make life better for the 50 million plus people in the world living with dementia. It trivialises the disease."

**People with dementia said:**

"It is 100% offensive, and inexcusable to joke about my symptoms (unless it is me joking about it)."

"When others who also have a dementia diagnosis joke this is just an expression that we are able to maintain a sense of humour and is a great stress reliever."

"Laughter is good for the soul and if you can laugh about your circumstances it can reduce anxiety. So we laugh from time to time when something incoherent comes out of my mouth."

## Dementia, intimacy and relationships

Between 35% in high income and 57% in low and lower-middle income countries reported being treated unfairly in dating or intimate relationships

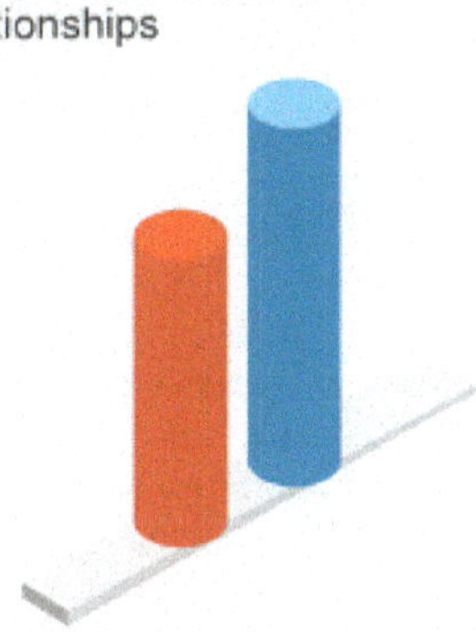

**People with dementia said:**

"To be honest, NO ONE wants to date a 58-year-old guy with Alzheimer's."

"I call it the friendship divorce. I have lost a fair amount of people in my life that at one time considered friends."

"... my wife and I divorced due to my Alzheimer's... her decision."

"I don't date at all now. As soon as I mention I have dementia, they presume the worst... My last boyfriend wanted to hide me away and I spoke openly about my dementia. Hence why that relationship didn't work... "

www.alz.co.uk/worldreport2019

# Foreword

**Paola Barbarino, CEO**

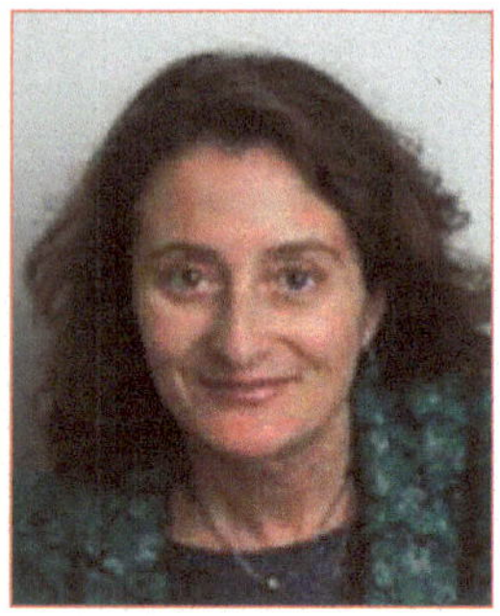

Time to roll our sleeves up (again, and again!)

I cannot express enough pride at being able to introduce this year's World Alzheimer Report on global attitudes to dementia. This report belongs to all the 70,000 of you who replied to our survey, so first of all, **thank you**.

When you look back at our international movement, which started in 1984, you see how a group of committed and energetic doctors and of professional and family carers, decided they had had enough of Alzheimer's being hidden in society and that the time was right to bring the disease to the attention of governments, politicians and the public at large.

Behind the foundation of an International Non-Governmental Organisation like ADI there is always the feeling that things could be much better and a sense that if we campaign strongly enough, if our voice is loud enough, we **will** be heard, and things **will** change.

At times I wonder why we did not start sooner. Alzheimer's disease was first described in 1906 but ADI was only founded in 1984. If we look at the Union for International Cancer Control (UICC), which is the equivalent of ADI, that was founded in 1933, about 50 years before us. The UICC is now a multimillion-pound organisation and the driving force behind cancer de-stigmatisation.

We, on the other hand, are running 50 years behind and still have a mountain to climb. In the words of one of our survey respondents:

*"Shunned by hundreds in my home town. People would sooner have stage 4 breast cancer than my diagnosis. (They) couldn't look me in the eye."*

Today people march together against cancer and support each other through cancer. We all talk about it as the last frontier. We talk of battles and of survivors. We appropriate a military language which, whilst not quite suitable to the people going through the disease (who can resent the idea of having to fight the inevitable), it certainly works from an awareness raising perspective. It also gives people a sense that they can be proactive and not just passive victims of the disease.

If society feels that they play a positive role then they will demand a solution. Last year's World Alzheimer Report[1] – which focused on research – stated unequivocally that for every 12 studies on cancer there is only one on neurocognitive disorders (not just on Alzheimer's disease!). This is the size of the research gap - but there still isn't enough funding in Alzheimer's and dementia research - despite civil society's collective efforts.

Going back to the genesis of this report, one of my biggest challenges, as I stepped into my role at ADI, was my Board and my members' desire to see a decrease in stigma and heightened awareness. The thinking was that if we manage to raise awareness, then we will have a more determined grassroots movement. People will understand that Alzheimer's is a disease, not just old age, and ask their governments to acknowledge that we have a crisis on our hands. This in turn could mean the creation of dedicated services for those going through the disease and for their carers, for better diagnostic and post-diagnostic support, as well as an increased focus on finding a disease-modifying treatment. In short, all the actions described in the World Health Organization (WHO) Global action plan on dementia[2], which we fought so hard for but that is so difficult to implement.

ADI already runs World Alzheimer's Day and Month awareness campaigns, which get a lot of traction in the public and in the press, and it publishes the World Alzheimer Report, which is possibly the most quoted and trusted source of information on Alzheimer's and dementia globally. But, for all this output, there isn't a corresponding measurement that can tell us how well we are doing at changing attitudes to dementia, and not just globally but nationally and locally.

In Alzheimer's and dementia there has undoubtedly been a great increase in awareness in higher income countries - certainly in the last 10 years - pretty much since ADI promoted the global figures on prevalence and incidence of the disease for the first time[3-4]. However, in low- and middle- income countries there are still reports of stigma felt by people with dementia and by carers – I need only recount the appalling stories of physical restriction and murder in Africa, as reported by our members there.

Even in high income countries (and this really comes into sharp focus in the survey) the general public, healthcare professionals, our members and other advocacy organisations report widespread shortages of services as well as noticeable differences in service provision between rural areas and urban areas. Also, despite high-profile awareness campaigns people still delay seeking out help, advice and support when they first start to worry about their memory or that of a family member. If this was a physical or visible ailment, how much more quickly would people react?

Back in 2018 however, our problem was that because much of this evidence was anecdotal, we did not know how we could measure whether these issues were sporadic or consistent throughout the world, or peculiar to a particular region; whether some issues were real for everyone or just perceptions; and, crucially, whether anything was getting better as a result of our advocacy efforts.

This report was borne out of a resounding need to establish a strong baseline so we could start measuring whether we really are doing better and making a difference once and for all. But we did not want to focus just on those countries where there are resources and means of taking action. In the spirit of solidarity and love that is the bedrock of ADI, we wanted to know more about those countries where there is little or nothing.

A prior survey on stigma by ADI in 2012[5] had 2,500 participants. A laudable effort (and a first) but statistically a very low sample to consider it as a strong baseline for global attitudes. Looking at other diseases and how they had addressed stigma was also interesting and frankly a bit disheartening. I remember some of my early conversations about HIV/AIDS and cancer with professionals who had been working in those areas at the time of greatest stigma, and almost everyone pointed out that the real change in attitudes (both from the point of view of people seeking a diagnosis and from the point of view of the general public acknowledging the disease) had happened when a drug-based treatment and a cure started appearing on the horizon. Well, we still don't have a cure and have had no treatment breakthrough for almost 20 years for Alzheimer's and dementia. We are yet to have that light at the end of the tunnel, but this is not a good reason to let go and do nothing.

As the Dementia Friendly Community[6-7] movement has demonstrated, time and time again, there is so much we can do to make life for those who have dementia and their carers immensely better by making them feel supported, loved and understood by our society and wherever possible by empowering them in every aspect of dementia activity, including advocacy. This makes a marked contrast to feeling shunned, hidden or ashamed, as in the quote above.

Indeed, the word love is something that comes out strongly from one of this report's essays, the one focusing on Canada's First Nation's attitudes to dementia:

*"... Reminds us that the person with dementia, who is being cared for, is in need of a lot of love. He urges the use of 'loved one' to refer to the person with dementia so that we remember that they are loved. He shared that using the words 'loved one' serves as a reminder of how care providers should be treating and respecting the person with dementia".*

Ironically, and sadly, the enormous swelling of population with the disease is on our side. When people ask me what I do for a living, and we start a conversation, it's rare they don't have a case in the family, wherever I am in the world.

When we commissioned this ambitious survey, we asked several universities and I am delighted that the London School of Economics and Political Science (LSE) was enthusiastic to pick up the gauntlet. They share our vision and our passion and as the numbers for our survey went up and up, there was a shared sense of joy undeterred by the enormity of the analytical task ahead.

I should not underestimate the size of the challenge faced by ADI and its members and partners in distributing the survey globally to so many different audiences. Nobody had ever attempted such a large survey in this field, and we were not sure whether we would have the capacity to mobilise our network to a whole new level.

A smidgen under 70,000 people later we can say that we certainly did! But it did take a huge amount of work on the part of everyone involved and I would particularly like to thank Australia, Brazil, Canada, China, India, Indonesia, Italy, Mexico, the Netherlands, New Zealand, TADA Chinese Taipei, Vietnam, the UK and USA who really went for it and helped us drive the numbers up globally. This survey, and its dataset, will now form part of the freely available shared resources we can use from now on to measure our performance on attitudes and hopefully make stigma a thing of the past – in all countries. It is our intention to repeat this research process after 5 years.

I know if you have picked this up that you will read the report in detail and I don't want to pre-empt it, but I leave you with a few thoughts.

- **Almost 80% of the general public are concerned about developing dementia at some point and 1 in 4 people think that there is nothing we can do to prevent dementia.** Clearly the messages on the importance of risk reduction highlighted recently by a WHO report are not getting through.[8] People don't know what to do. We need to do more to spread this message at every level.
- **35% of carers across the world said that they have hidden the diagnosis of dementia of a family member from at least 1 person**. Our next target will be to get to 0%.
- **75% carers globally say "I am often stressed between caring and meeting other responsibilities" even whilst expressing positive sentiments about their role and over 50% of carers said their health suffered as a result of their caring responsibilities.** Are we doing enough for carers? Obviously not. Help and support for carers should be a fundamental lynchpin of any national dementia plan and we will continue to advocate towards it and empower our members to do so at national level. In the report it is clear that even in high income countries, most categories of survey respondents felt there were not enough services available.

- **Health Care Professionals in lower income countries were most positive about their willingness to work with a colleague with dementia. However, the public (most of whom will not work in a health setting) were least willing to work with a colleague with dementia.** We need to change that, and we will work in the next few years both on the issue of the rights for carers in the workplace and the issue of disability rights for people living with dementia.
- **Almost 62% of healthcare providers worldwide think that dementia is part of normal aging.** Our message that dementia is NOT part of normal aging but a disease, is loud and clear, but is clearly not getting through. We must work much harder at this with all our members.
- I see a worrying trend developing with **36% of all respondents saying they would seek help on the internet**. There is so much unreliable information over the web, and it is an area with exponential growth, so we do need to be proactive and create trusted repositories of real information. We give the example with our website where all resources are freely available and so do our members.
- And last but not least around **40% of the general public think doctors and nurses ignore people with dementia** – time for primary healthcare practitioners to look closely at their practice and for governments to increase dementia training.

In the enthusiasm to include the views and voices of the people with dementia we must never forget the family carers. This extract of the Mexican essay is a sobering reminder of that:

*"After about ten days I made the decision that I was going to take my husband who has dementia to the federal highway and I was going to throw myself under the wheels of a trailer, the biggest one I saw pass by, together with my husband, because I was not going to be able to bear everything that was coming. I woke up that day very early with my decision taken, to clean the house and leave everything ready, so they could hold vigil over us afterwards that day."*

It is a relief that the person in this stark story lived to tell the tale, but these stories are happening all over the world and we must do something to stop this. It is terrible that a human being should contemplate suicide because they cannot cope caring for another human being by themselves. Respite and care must be made available globally, it is a matter of social justice.

As you have gathered from above, alongside the survey results you will read expert essays and case studies that highlight the scope and scale of the global challenge and the often spirited and galvanising response from people, like us, trying to affect change. Amongst many topics we look at:

- the double stigma attached to both age and dementia
- the challenges experienced by some indigenous populations around the world
- stigma in marginalised or lesser heard from communities including prison settings, people with learning disabilities and the LGBTQ community
- the media's role in helping raise awareness or exacerbating stigma
- the history and influence of working groups of people living with dementia and carers
- a philosophical question about the introduction and evolution of dementia friendly communities

I would like to thank the founders of ADI and the hundreds of thousands of you who work so hard day in day out on all aspects of the disease. You are doing so much, but we need to do more. This is just the beginning.

Ultimately, reality is not what governments tell us it is, it is not what experts like us tell us it is; reality is what people on the ground are feeling. Reality is what people feel every morning when they wake up and every night when they go to sleep. We must never forget that, and this is why this World Alzheimer Report is for all of you.

## References


1 Patterson, C. 2018. *World Alzheimer Report 2018: The state of the art of dementia research; New frontiers*. London: Alzheimer's Disease International.

2 World Health Organization. *Global action plan on the public health response to dementia 2017–2025*. Geneva: World Health Organization; 2017. Licence: CC BY-NC-SA 3.0. online: <https://apps.who.int/iris/bitstream/handle/10665/259615/9789241513487-eng.pdf?sequence=1> Last accessed 20 August 2019.

3 Alzheimer's Disease International. 2009. *World Alzheimer Report 2009: The Global Prevalence of Dementia*. London: Alzheimer's Disease International.

4 Prince, M., Wimo, Guerchet, M., Ali, , G-C, Wu, Y-T., Prina, M. 2015. *World Alzheimer Report 2015: The Global Impact of Dementia. An Analysis of Prevalence, Incidence, Cost and Trends*. London. Alzheimer's Disease International.

5 Batsch, N. L., Mittelman, M. S. 2012. *World Alzheimer Report 2012: Overcoming the Stigma of Dementia*. London: Alzheimer's Disease International.

6 Alzheimer's Disease International. 2016. *Dementia Friendly Communities: Key Principals* (1st Edition) online: <https://www.alz.co.uk/dementia-friendly-communities/principles> Last accessed 20 August 2019.

7 Alzheimer's Disease International. 2017. *Dementia Friendly Communities: Global developments* (2nd Edition) online: <https://www.alz.co.uk/adi/pdf/dfc-developments.pdf> Last accessed 19 August 2019.

8 World Health Organisation 2019. *Risk reduction of cognitive decline and dementia: WHO guidelines*. Geneva: World Health Organization; 2019.

# Executive summary

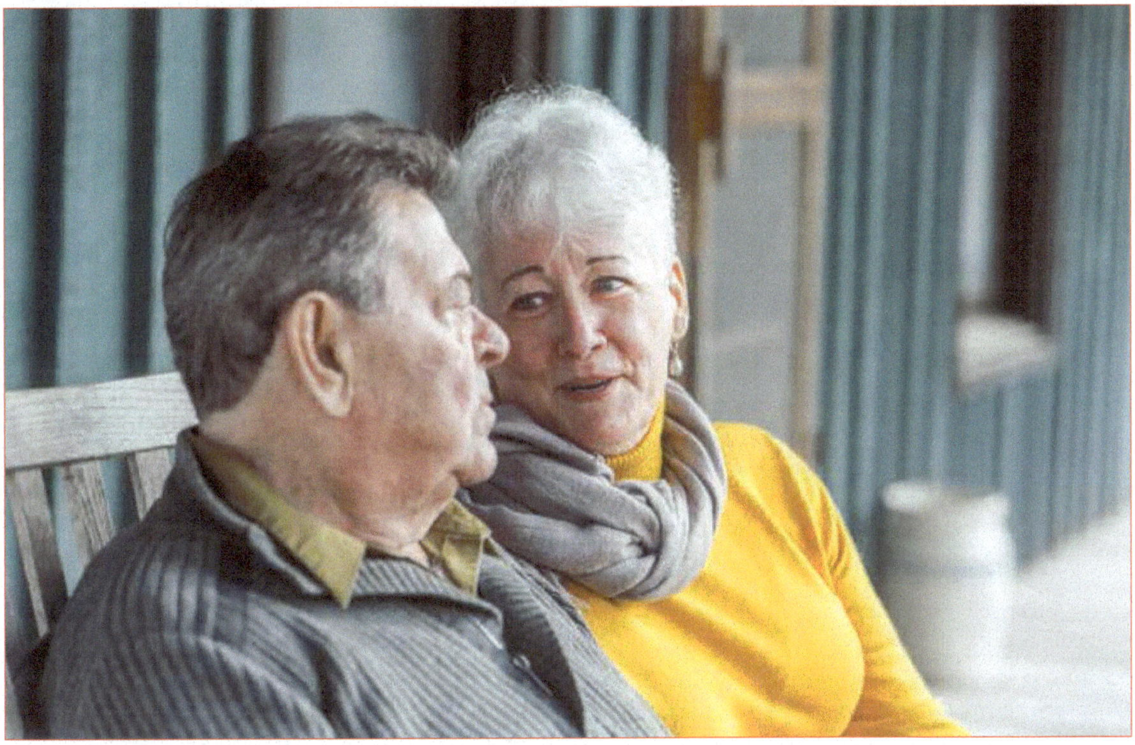

In 2019 ADI estimates that there are over 50 million people living with dementia globally, a figure set to increase to 152 million by 2050. Someone develops dementia every three seconds and the current annual cost of dementia is estimated at US $1trillion, a figure set to double by 2030.

In the World Alzheimer Report 2012 *'Overcoming the stigma of dementia'* we explored the nature of dementia related stigma. The core of the report focussed on the results of a survey of 2,500 people; people living with dementia and carers, in a limited number of countries around the world. The report helped define dementia related stigma and offered recommendations to tackle it, alongside a series of case studies and practices aimed at stigma reduction.

In this 2019 World Alzheimer Report, we revisit attitudes to dementia and stigma to better understand the role they play and to set a baseline against which we can gauge future changes. This report details the scale of the challenge we face where attitudes to dementia, and specifically stigma, are still a major barrier to people seeking out information, help, advice, support and even a diagnosis; preventing or delaying people from putting plans in place; progressing to a stage of acceptance and being able to adjust to live with dementia. Stigma may be overt; in some countries it is still associated with witchcraft resulting in people being restrained and isolated. Or it can be more subtle; even in countries with national dementia plans and profile awareness campaigns, many people still delay seeking help when they first become aware that something is wrong.

## The 2019 World Report:

At the core of the 2019 report are the results of a global survey, commissioned by ADI and undertaken by the London School of Economics and Political Science (LSE). Almost 70,000 people globally engaged with the survey, making it the biggest of its kind ever undertaken.

LSE developed the survey to target four key groups, (1) people living with dementia, (2) carers, (3) healthcare practitioners and (4) the general public, with analysis being provided in three categories: knowledge, attitudes and behaviour. In the survey analysis we highlight the behavioural element first, giving prominence to the voices and experiences of people living with dementia as direct assessment of actual behaviour is central to discrimination and is the closest representation of the true impact of stigma on people living with dementia.

The report also poses the question *"what is stigma?"*, looking to define dementia related stigma and to better understand the component parts based on power, stereotypes, prejudice and discrimination. Then, through a series of expert essays, case studies and programmes, the report sheds light on the nature and complexity of attitudes and stigma; it looks to other sectors for guidance and inspiration; showcases examples of the different challenges and responses at global, regional, national and local levels; and offers some examples of programmes developed to improve awareness and to tackle stigma.

## Key findings

### Knowledge

- 95% of the public think they will develop dementia in their lifetime
- 78% are concerned about developing dementia at some point
- 1 in 4 people think that there is nothing you can do about dementia
- 2 out of 3 think dementia is caused by normal ageing
- 62% of healthcare practitioners think that dementia is a normal part of ageing
- 82% of people would take a genetic test to learn about their risk
- 54% of respondents think that lifestyle factors play a part in developing dementia
- Just under 40% of the general public think that there are adequate community services for people living with dementia and for carers
- Just under 70% of the general public think there are adequate competent physicians for the diagnosis and treatment of dementia

Two years into the WHO Global action plan on dementia, 35 years into the life of ADI, and longer for many associations around the world, should we be surprised at these findings? There is evidently underlying fear in global populations about developing dementia - 78% expressing concern – and some media portraying dementia as the most feared illness. Journalist Pippa Kelly, in this report, articulates that *"Stigma stems from fear. Fear breeds silence, which in turn perpetuates ignorance and misunderstanding".*

A key reason for developing this survey and establishing a baseline for future review is to help us understand the scale of the challenge in informing and educating the 2/3rds of people who still think that dementia is a normal part of ageing, rather than a neurodegenerative disease and a leading cause of death; in some countries the leading cause of death.

Perhaps an even bigger challenge, and more worrying, is the staggering 62% of healthcare practitioners that think dementia is a normal part of ageing.

With an increasing focus on risk reduction research and messaging, and in the continued absence of a disease modifying treatment, we now have a clear understanding of how important people think that lifestyle factors are. The stark finding of this survey reveals that currently just over 50% of people think that lifestyle factors are influential. These figures form a baseline from which we can measure the impact of future global risk reduction efforts.

### Behaviour

- Over 85% of respondents living with dementia stated that their opinion had not been taken seriously
- Around 40% of the general public think doctors and nurses ignore people with dementia
- 67% of people living with dementia in Africa, and 63% in South East Asia, said their dementia symptoms were joked about by others
- Between 35% in high income countries and 57% in low-middle income countries reported being treated unfairly in dating and intimate relationships
- Around 30% of people in Europe are willing to have a person with dementia move in with them, rising to 62% in South East Asia and 71% in the Eastern Mediterranean region

We wanted to better understand the stigma and discrimination experienced by people living with dementia, and particularly, what kinds of treatment they felt were unfair and the outcomes associated with these negative experiences. Unfair treatment can be experienced in many ways – at home, in the community, even in healthcare settings – and include things like being denied choice, being ignored, unfair treatment in dating and intimate relationships, lack of privacy, joking about dementia, and of particular interest, inappropriate treatment by healthcare practitioners.

Respondents reported feeling "avoided", "ignored" and "ostracized" in their social life due to having dementia where many of them "no longer get invited to social gatherings". Poignantly, one respondent captures this with:

*"I call it the friendship divorce. I have lost a fair amount of people in my life that at one time considered friends".*

Half of the respondents living with dementia from lower-middle income countries reported that they had experienced their rights or responsibilities taken away from them unfairly.

Over 85% of respondents living with dementia stated that their opinion had not been taken seriously. One respondent reported being told *"your opinion no longer matters"*.

Unfair treatment by health or medical staff is an area of concern, as are the attitudes of some healthcare practitioners – with around 40% of the general public thinking doctors and nurses ignore people with dementia. *"My neurologist ignored my presence when my diagnosis was discussed with my husband"*.

Joking and humour around dementia is a very sensitive subject. Respondents in the African region (66.7%) and South-East Asia (62.5%) reported the highest prevalence of their dementia being joked about. However, this is a tricky area, humour can be therapeutic, but it is often permission based. The challenge is evidently how difficult it is to judge appropriateness. *"It is 100% offensive and inexcusable to joke about my symptoms, unless it is me joking about it!"*

## Attitudes

- 91% of respondents say that people should not hide the fact they have dementia and the vast majority of carers never hide the person with dementia
- However, around 20% of respondents would keep their own dementia a secret when meeting people
- Concealment of dementia varied regionally - with the general public in Europe (25.7%) and the Americas (24.5%) reporting they would keep their dementia a secret. Healthcare practitioners also reported higher levels of concealment in Europe (19%) and the Americas (17.4%)
- Respondents stating they would hide their dementia when meeting people was highest in Russia (66.7%), Poland (57.9%), and Puerto Rico (51.1%),
- 45% of people living in South-East Asia and 48% of healthcare practitioners in the region feel that people with dementia are dangerous.
- 60% of people felt it was important to remove responsibilities of people living with dementia

Dating and intimate relationships are another sensitive area. Respondents with dementia reported unfair treatment in relationships, the highest figures in low / lower middle-income countries (57.1%) and upper-middle countries (50%). "*To be honest, NO ONE wants to date a 58-year old guy with Alzheimer's"*.

A very high proportion believe that people should not hide the fact that they have dementia, supported by a high number of people (80%) agreeing that people with dementia can participate in a variety of activities. Attitudes to concealment, however, varied regionally – in Europe and the Americas around 25% saying they would keep their dementia a secret, with Healthcare practitioners also reporting higher levels of concealment in Europe (19%) and the Americas (17.4%).

Concealment and secrecy are key examples of stigma surrounding dementia and some specific country level figures warrant attention – with people in Russia (66.7%), Poland (57.9%), Puerto Rico (51.1%) saying they would hide their dementia when meeting people.

In relation to attitudes and views around danger 45% of people living in South-East Asia, and 48% of healthcare practitioners, think that people with dementia are dangerous, however, this is interesting considering relatively high proportions of people living in the South-East Asia region are willing to have a family member living with dementia to move in with them.

Around 60% of people felt it was important to remove responsibilities of people living with dementia which is interesting in the context that many of the experiences of discrimination reported by people living with dementia pertain to loss of status and loss of roles.

Around 40% of the general public think that healthcare practitioners (physicians and nurses) ignore people with dementia (38% in high-income, 49% in upper-middle income and 32.5% in low/lower middle-income countries).

Ironically, respondents had a vastly more negative opinion of the behaviours of others than about their own behaviour. Both healthcare practitioners and the general public believe that other people are likely to engage in stigmatising behaviours.

## Carers

- Majority of carers expressed positive sentiments about their caring role
- 52% of carers said their health had suffered
- 49% of carers said their work had suffered
- 62% of carers said their social life had suffered
- Over 35% of carers globally have hidden the diagnosis of a person with dementia

Although just over half of carers expressed positive sentiments about their caring role, and found it fulfilling, 52% of carers said their health, 49% their work and 62% their social life suffered because of their caring responsibilities. This raises key questions about formal support services for carers and brings into perspective the importance of a resilient response to action area 5 of the WHO Global action plan on dementia. Attitudes to caring vary by region, by socio-economic grouping and by culture and expectation.

The extent to which work is affected by the provision of care may be influenced not only by the amount of care that is provided and the support available to the carers, but also by differences in the propensity for women (who are most likely to be carers) and older people to work, and by policies to support the employment of people with caring responsibilities.

## Recommendations

Stigma and knowledge issues around dementia are evidently still major barriers, not only to people seeking out more information, advice, support and a diagnosis but also in the basic understanding of Alzheimer's disease and related dementias as a medical conditions, that require treatment, support, even rehabilitation. By default, stigma thus also impacts negatively on research and research participation as we strive for a disease modifying treatment breakthrough.

Therefore, it is essential to take action, to improve awareness, to help dispel lingering myths around dementia and ultimately aim to reduce or even eradicate stigma.

### Recommendations

1. Targeted public health awareness campaigns
2. Promotion of timely diagnosis and better post diagnostic support
3. Global evolution of dementia friends programmes and dementia friendly/inclusive communities - with people living with dementia and carers at the heart of their design, implementation and evaluation
4. Increased public advocacy of people living with dementia – amplifying the voice of lived experience
5. Increase advocacy focused on carers experiences – whilst improving the understanding of first-hand experience
6. Specialised education about dementia-related stigma and person-centred care practice for healthcare practitioners
7. Call for local governments to increase the funding, range and quality of community services for people living with dementia
8. Changes to public policy relating to employment, health and insurance for both people living with dementia and their carers
9. Full adoption of a rights-based approach to dementia including full compliance with the Convention of Rights of Persons with Disabilities (CRPD)
10. Increase funded research – for both a disease-modifying drug as well as further understanding of stigma. We know from other high stigma illnesses, including cancer and HIV-AIDS, that medical treatment breakthroughs can be a catalyst to stigma reduction – and we also need to better understand the complex role stigma plays throughout society in order to tackle it and change hearts and minds.

CHAPTER 1

# What is stigma?

**Contributors:** Jessica Young, Flinders University and Western University, Professor JB Orange, Western University, and Associate Professor Christopher Lind, Flinders University

*"Diagnosis has changed our world forever. Our lives become limited by the stigma we face in the world around us. It's like we have a target painted on our foreheads shouting out 'dementing' for all the world to see. People become awkward in our presence, are unsure of our behaviour, and our world becomes circumscribed by the stigma of our illness".* Christine Bryden, Dementia Activist[1]

For persons living with dementia, full and equitable engagement in everyday life activities often is compromised by the stigma associated with dementia[2&3]. But what is *stigma* exactly? Here we introduce the concept of stigma and describe its relationship to the concepts of 'stereotype', 'prejudice', 'discrimination' and 'power'. We provide context for later discussions of stigma in this report and form a foundation for initial recommendations to reduce dementia-related stigma.

The word 'stigma' originates from Greek language, meaning a 'mark' or 'brand'. In the social sciences, the term 'stigma' refers to marked differences from what is 'normal' for a group of people, and to negative emotional and/or behavioural responses to those differences. Sociologist Erving Goffman[4] has been influential in our understanding of stigma as a social phenomenon. Goffman described stigma as the marginalisation of persons in response to traits they exhibit, such as ethnicity, religious beliefs, physical disability, skin scarring, or 'weaknesses' of character (e.g., represented by imprisonment or addiction). He showed how being 'marked' with any of these traits could have negative consequences in a given social context.

## Four key components

Contemporary stigma research adds clarity to our understanding of what stigma is, what outcomes it creates, and who it affects. This research advances our understanding of how people labelled as somehow abnormal (i.e., those being stigmatised) experience their everyday lives. Recently, researchers, clinicians, policy makers, care providers and persons living with dementia have used the concept of stigma to explain how *dementia* often is seen as a socially undesired trait, leading to discrimination, social isolation, and disenfranchisement.

There are many contemporary models of stigma[5-7]. One model[8], which has proven particularly useful in understanding dementia-related stigma[9-11], identifies four critical components essential for stigma to have its effect: *power, stereotypes, prejudice,* and *discrimination*. 'Stigma' is said to occur when persons with relative social, economic, or political power internalise generalised negative beliefs (stereotypes) which then manifest as negative emotional responses (prejudice) and negative behavioural responses (discrimination). Below we describe each component in greater detail and consider how each contributes to dementia-related stigma.

## Component 1: Power

Stigma is dependent on social, economic, or political *power*[8]. The type and severity of stigma can differ depending on who holds relative power over another[7]. For example, persons living with dementia may form stereotypes of medical professionals, yet often lack the power to discriminate against them (e.g., they may lack the social, economic or political resources required to exclude that individual from decision-making about their care).

### Examples of stereotypes

All persons living with dementia are:

- a burden to family,
- a burden on the healthcare system,
- delirious,
- hopeless,
- incapable of speaking for themselves,
- incompetent,
- invariably old,
- on a path to inevitable death,
- unable to contribute to society,
- unaware of their abilities or limitations,
- unreliable, and
- untrustworthy.

**Figure 1.** Dementia-related stereotypes [13-18]

## Component 2: Stereotypes

*Stereotypes* refer to the generalised beliefs, often negative, about what it means to have a certain trait. According to common dementia stereotypes, having dementia is an inherently negative experience (see Figure

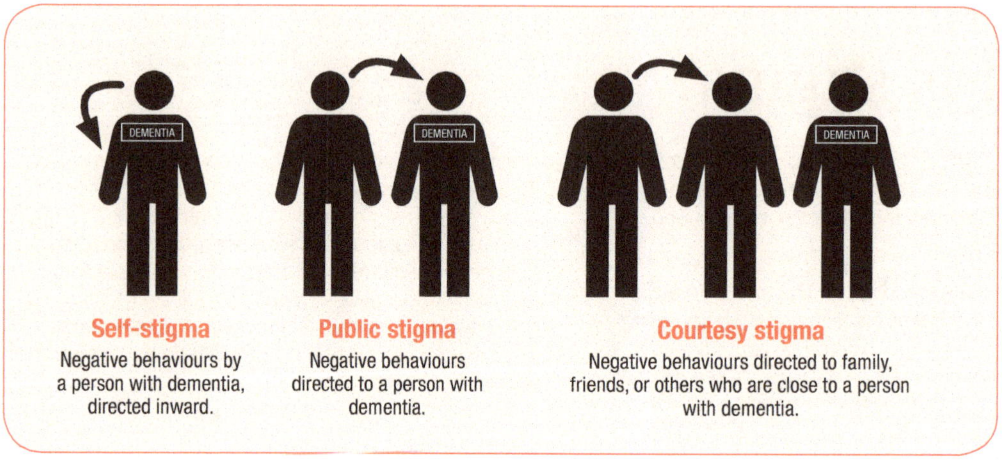


**Figure 2.** Three types of stigma [2,23]

1). Stereotypes are powerful because they are created and perpetuated in many different ways[11]. They:

1 are perpetuated through the language used to talk about persons living with dementia (e.g., by referring to them as "'demented' 'sufferers', 'subjects', 'victims', and 'not all there'"[12]);

2 are perpetuated through the prevailing medical model of dementia, which portrays dementia as an inexorable decline in all aspects of human functioning including loss of personhood and self;

3 are compounded with other stereotypes (such as stereotypes about older adults or about persons who are institutionalised); and

4 are shaped by cultural beliefs about the cause of dementia (e.g., karma, lack of religious or spiritual adherence).

## Component 3: Prejudice

*Prejudice* refers to the uptake of stereotypes and negative emotional reactions to those stereotypes. Adopting these stereotypes often is subconscious but can have real, significant impacts on our emotions and behaviours. Within the context of dementia, negative emotional reactions most often include *fear*, *shame*, *revulsion* or *disgust*[19-21]. The severity of prejudice is shaped by age, gender, profession, ethnicity, culture and understandings of dementia prognosis, among other factors[22].

## Component 4: Discrimination

*Discrimination* refers to negative behavioural responses to prejudice[8]. These responses include behaviours such as avoiding, ignoring, or actively excluding persons living with dementia. At the most extreme, discrimination may result in the denial of basic human rights including, for example: the choice of where to live, deciding what and when to eat, and access to medical care.

## Who does stigma affect?

It is important to note that: (1) both persons *with* dementia and persons *without* dementia can exhibit discriminatory behaviours, and (2) discriminatory behaviours can be directed toward the person living with dementia or to persons close to them. To demonstrate these two points, a useful distinction can be drawn among three types of stigma: *self-stigma*, *public stigma*, and *courtesy stigma* (See Figure 2).

In the context of *self-stigma*, stereotypes and prejudice may lead to discrimination of persons living with dementia, with many possible negative outcomes. These include a person living with dementia being reluctant to seek help, presenting late to health services, disbelieving the diagnosis, and/or social isolation caused by avoidance of, or total withdrawal from, interactions with others[2,24,16].

In the context of *public stigma*, persons living with dementia may experience discrimination in the form of: loss of quality social interactions, social roles, and relationships; exclusion from decision-making; delayed or withheld disclosure of dementia diagnosis[25,26]; and limited or delayed referral to dementia-appropriate services or treatment[27,28].

In the context of *courtesy stigma*, also known as 'stigma by association', stereotypes and prejudice lead to discrimination of persons close to an individual with dementia[29]. Courtesy stigma is expressed in the form of social isolation or exclusion of family members or friends of persons living with dementia[13,30], or by staring at or by talking about formal caregivers and friends behind their backs[31], for example.

## Reducing stigma

There are many approaches to reducing dementia-related stigma, but limited evidence for or consensus about which are the most effective[22,23]. To date, the most promising approaches to reducing stigma include:

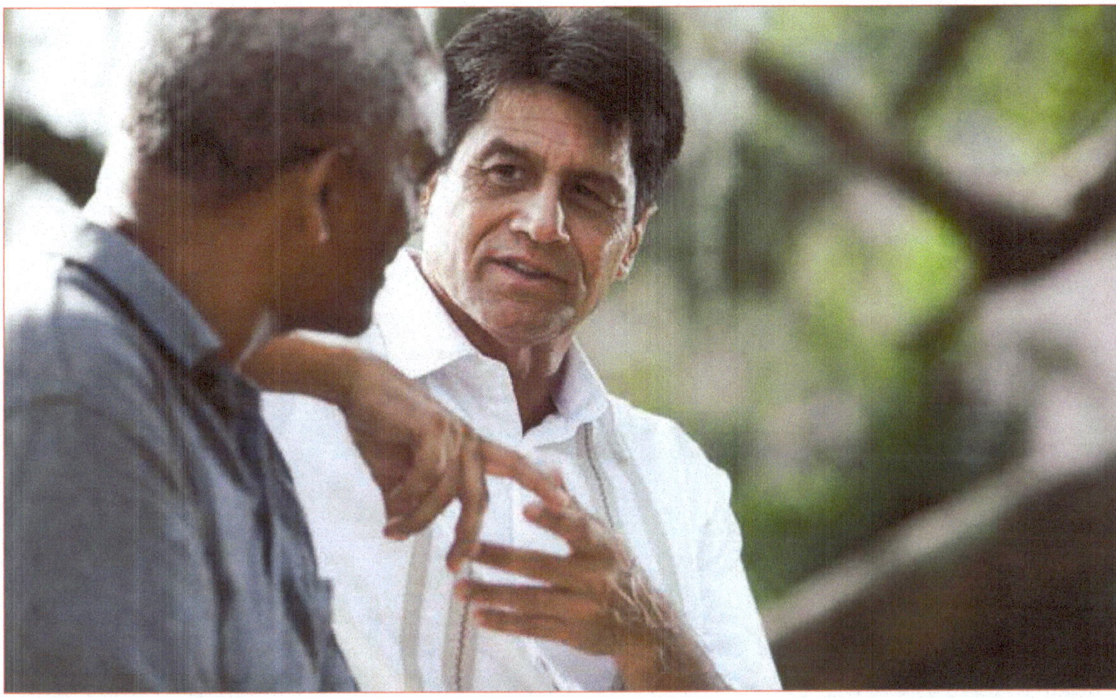

1 Specialised education about dementia-related stigma[32,33].

2 Social contact with persons living with dementia[34,35,36].

3 Targetted public health awareness / messaging / education[37], through:

  - public advocacy by persons living with dementia[38];
  - arts-based approaches, such as musical performance by persons living with dementia[39]; and
  - short film[40,41], for example.

4 Changes to public policy (e.g., relating to employment, health insurance)[42].

We also suggest that interventions aimed at any of the four components described above (i.e., power, stereotype, prejudice or discrimination) may break the cycle of stigma. For example, combatting dementia-related stigma may involve:

- challenging negative stereotypes, assisted by increased awareness of specific stereotypes and of the ways they are perpetuated;
- challenging prejudices and attitudes by exposing where these come from (i.e., from stereotypes);
- mediating behavioural enactment of prejudices (discrimination); and/or
- acknowledging and adjusting power imbalances, achieved by promoting active involvement of persons living with dementia in research, advocacy, and care.

Only when active measures are taken to reduce stigma can we begin to uphold for persons with dementia the human right to full and equitable engagement in, and access to, meaningful activities of everyday life.

## References


1 Bryden, C.2015. *Nothing about us, without us!: 20 years of dementia advocacy*, Jessica Kingsley Publishers, London, UK, p. 40.

2 Ashworth, R 2017. 'Perceptions of stigma among people affected by early- and late-onset Alzheimer's disease', *Journal of Health Psychology* Epub ahead of print. Available at: https://doi.org/10.1177/1359105317720818 Last accessed: 7 August 2019.

3 Lion, KM, Szczesniak, D, Bulinska, K, Evans, SB, Evans, SC, Saibene, FL, d'Arma, A, Farina, E, Brooker, DJ, Chattat, R, Meiland, FJM, Droes, RM & Rymaszewska, J 2019. 'Do people with dementia and mild cognitive impairments experience stigma? A cross-cultural investigation between Italy, Poland and the UK', *Aging and Mental Health* Epub ahead of print. Available at: https://doi.org/10.1080/13607863.2019.1577799 Last accessed: 7 August 2019.

4 Goffman, E 1963. *Stigma: Notes on the management of spoiled identity*, Simon and Schuster, New York, NY.

5 Corrigan, PW 2000. 'Mental health stigma as social attribution: Implications for research methods and attitude change', *Clinical Psychology: Science and Practice*, 7(1) 48-67.

6 Link, BG, Cullen, FT, Struening, E, Shrout, PE & Dohrenwend, BP 1989. 'A modified labeling theory approach to mental disorders: An empirical assessment', *American Sociological Review*, 54 (3), 400-23.

7 Link, BG & Phelan, JC 2001. 'Conceptualising stigma', *Annual Review of Sociology*, vol. 27, 363-85.

8 Rüsch, N, Angermeyer, MC & Corrigan, PW 2005. 'Mental illnes s stigma: Concepts, consequences, and initiatives to reduce stigma', *European Psychiatry*, 20(8), 529-39.

9 Blay, SL & Peluso, ETP 2010. 'Public stigma: The community's tolerance of alzheimer disease', *American Journal of Geriatric Psychiatry*, 18 (2), 163-171.

10 Gove, D, Small, N, Downs, M & Vernooij-Dassen, M 2017. 'General practitioners' perceptions of the stigma of dementia and the role of reciprocity', *Dementia*, 16 (7), 948-64.

11 Young, JA, Lind, C, Orange, JB & Savundranayagam, MY 2019. 'Expanding current understandings of epistemic injustice and dementia: Learning from stigma theory', *Journal of Aging Studies*, 48 (76-84).

12 Swaffer, K 2014. 'Dementia: Stigma, language, and dementia-friendly', *Dementia*, 13(6): p. 709-16.

13 AboJabel, H & Werner, P 2016, 'Exploring family stigma among caregivers of persons with Alzheimer's disease: The experiences of Israeli-Arab caregivers', *Dementia*, 18(1): p. 391-408.

14 Ballenger, JF 2017, 'Framing confusion: Dementia, society, and history', *AMA Journal of Ethics*, 19(7): p. 713-719.

15 Beard, RL 2017, 'Dementia and the privilege of growing old', *Dementia*, 16(6): p. 685-688.

16 Stites, SD, Rubright, JD & Karlawish, J 2018, 'What features of stigma do the public most commonly attribute to Alzheimer's disease dementia? Results of a survey of the U.S. general public', *Alzheimers and Dementia*, 14(7): p. 925-32.

17 Werner, P & Doron, I 2017, 'Alzheimer's disease and the law: Positive and negative consequences of structural stigma and labeling in the legal system', *Aging and Mental Health*, 21(11): p. 1206-13.

18 Werner, P, AboJabel, H, Reuveni, Y & Prilutzki, D 2017, 'Stigmatic beliefs toward a person with Alzheimer's disease among high-school students: Does majority–minority status make a difference?', *Educational Gerontology*, 43(12): p. 609-18.

19 Behuniak, SM 2011, 'The living dead? The construction of people with Alzheimer's disease as zombies', *Ageing and Society*, 31(1): p. 70-92.

20 Casado, BL, Hong, M & Lee, SE 2018, 'Attitudes toward Alzheimer's care-seeking among Korean americans: Effects of knowledge, stigma, and subjective norm', *Gerontologist*, 58(2): p. e25-e34.

21 Lopez, RP, Rose, KM, Kenney, L, Sanborn, V & Davis, JD 2019, 'Managing shame: A grounded theory of how stigma manifests in families living with dementia', *Journal of the American Psychiatric Nurses Association* Epub ahead of print. Available at: https://doi.org/10.1177/1078390319832965 Last accessed: 7 August 2019.

22 Herrmann, LK, Welter, E, Leverenz, JB, Lerner, A, Udelson, N, Kanetsky, C & Sajatovic, M 2018, 'A systematic review of Alzheimer's disease and dementia stigma research: How might we move the stigma dial?', *American Journal of Geriatric Psychiatry*, 26(3): p. 316-331.

23 Werner, P 2014, 'Stigma and Alzheimer's disease: A systematic review of evidence, theory, and methods', in PW Corrigan (ed), *The stigma of disease and disability: Understanding causes and overcoming injustices*, p. 223-244. American Psychological Association, Washington, DC.

24 Livingston, G, Baio, G, Sommerlad, A, de Lusignan, S, Poulimenos, S, Morris, S, Rait, G & Hoe, J 2017, 'Effectiveness of an intervention to facilitate prompt referral to memory clinics in the United Kingdom: Cluster randomised controlled trial', *PLoS Medicine*, 14(3): p. e1002252.

25 Low, LF, McGrath, M, Swaffer, K & Brodaty, H 2018, 'Communicating a diagnosis of dementia: A systematic mixed studies review of attitudes and practices of health practitioners', *Dementia* Epub ahead of print. Available at: https://doi.org/10.1177/1471301218761911 Last accessed: 7 August 2019.

26 O'Connor, D, Mann, J & Wiersma, E 2018, 'Stigma, discrimination and agency: Diagnostic disclosure as an everyday practice shaping social citizenship', *Journal of Aging Studies*, 44: p. 45-51.

27 Johnson, R, Harkins, K, Cary, M, Sankar, P & Karlawish, J 2015, 'The relative contributions of disease label and disease prognosis to Alzheimer's stigma: A vignette-based experiment', *Social Science & Medicine*, 143: p. 117-27.

28 Mukadam, N & Livingston, G 2012, 'Reducing the stigma associated with dementia: Approaches and goals', *Aging Health*, 8(4): p. 377-86.

29 Werner, P & AboJabel, H 2019, 'Who internalizes courtesy stigma and how? A study among Israeli Arab family caregivers of persons with dementia', *Aging and Mental Health* Epub ahead of print. Available at: https://doi.org/10.1080/13607863.2019.1584790 Last accessed: 7 August 2019.

30 Greenwood, N, Mezey, G & Smith, R 2018, 'Social exclusion in adult informal carers: A systematic narrative review of the experiences of informal carers of people with dementia and mental illness', *Maturitas*, 112: p. 39-45.

31 Werner, P & Hess, A 2016, 'Examining courtesy stigma among foreign health care workers caring for persons with Alzheimer's diseas: A focus group study', *Home Health Care Services Quarterly*, 35(2): p. 69-85.

32 Herrmann, LK, Udelson, N, Kanetsky, C, Liu, H, Cassidy, K, Welter, E & Sajatovic, M 2018, 'A new curriculum to address dementia-related stigma: Preliminary experience with Alzheimer's Association staff', *Dementia* Epub ahead of print. Available at: https://doi.org/10.1177/1471301217752706 Last accessed: 7 August 2019.

33 Kim, S, Werner, P, Richardson, A & Anstey, KJ 2019, 'Dementia Stigma Reduction (DESeRvE): Study protocol for a randomized controlled trial of an online intervention program to reduce dementia-related public stigma', *Contemporary Clinical Trials Communications*, 14, art. 100351.

34 Cheston, R, Hancock, J & White, P 2018, 'Does personal experience of dementia change attitudes? The Bristol and South Gloucestershire survey of dementia attitudes', *Dementia* Epub ahead of print. Available at: https://doi.org/10.1177/1471301217752707 Last accessed: 7 August 2019.

35 Goldman, JS & Trommer, AE 2019, 'A qualitative study of the impact of a dementia experiential learning project on pre-medical students: A friend for Rachel', *BMC Medical Education*, 19:127.

36 Kane, A, Murphy, C & Kelly, M 2018, 'Assessing implicit and explicit dementia stigma in young adults and care-workers', *Dementia* Epub ahead of print. Available at: https://doi.org/10.1177/1471301218804727 Last accessed: 7 August 2019.

37 Lawlor, B 2018, 'The local and global imperative to raise public awareness and knowledge about dementia', *Arquivos de Neuro-Psiquiatria*, 76(11): p. 729-30.

38 Phillipson, L, Hall, D, Cridland, E, Fleming, R, Brennan-Horley, C, Guggisberg, N, Frost, D & Hasan, H 2018, 'Involvement of people with dementia in raising awareness and changing attitudes in a dementia friendly community pilot project', *Dementia* Epub ahead of print. Available at: https://doi.org/10.1177/1471301218754455 Last accessed: 7 August 2019.

39 Reynolds, L, Poyner, C, Innes, A & Hambidge, S 2017, ''The stigma attached isn't true of real life': Challenging public perception of dementia through a participatory approach involving people with dementia (Innovative Practice)', *Dementia*, 16(2): p. 219-25.

40 Hand, MD 2019, 'Every three seconds: A review of an innovative documentary on research and stigma surrounding dementia across the globe', *Journal of Gerontological Social Work*, 62(3): p. 369-373.

41 Prins, M, Veerbeek, M, Willemse, BM & Pot, AM 2019, 'Use and impact of the Alzheimer Experience: a free online media production to raise public awareness and enhance knowledge and understanding of dementia', *Aging and Mental Health* Epub ahead of print. Available at: https://doi.org/10.1080/13607863.2019.1579781 Last accessed: 7 August 2019.

42 Stites, SD, Johnson, R, Harkins, K, Sankar, P, Xie, D & Karlawish, J 2018, 'Identifiable characteristics and potentially malleable beliefs predict stigmatizing attributions toward persons with Alzheimer's disease dementia: Results of a survey of the U.S. general public', *Health Communication*, 33(3): p. 264-73.

CHAPTER 2

# Attitudes to dementia survey results

**London School of Economics and Political Science.**

**Contributors:** Dr Sara Evans-Lacko, Jem Bhatt, Asst Prof Adelina Comas-Herrera, Dr Francesco D'Amico, Dr Nicolas Farina, Sophie Gaber, Prof Martin Knapp, Maximilian Salcher-Konrad, Madeleine Stevens, Emma Wilson

## Attitudes to dementia survey results

This section of the report summarises the findings from the largest ever global survey of people living with dementia, carers[(i)], healthcare practitioners and the general public. A more detailed, technical report will be made available online. We aimed to understand stigma-related knowledge, attitudes and behaviours around dementia and to understand how stigma affects people living with dementia. The consequences of stigma are often described as being as important as the condition itself. At the individual level, stigma can undermine life goals, reduce participation in meaningful life activities and lower levels of well-being and quality of life. At the societal level, structural stigma and discrimination can influence levels of funding allocated to care and support. Currently, there is very little information about how stigma manifests in relation to people with dementia and how this may vary around the world. A better understanding of knowledge, attitudes and behaviour towards people with dementia and how these link with consequences for people living with dementia could help us to understand where we might focus our efforts to reduce stigma in order to improve the lives of people living with dementia and their families.

Almost 70,000 people from 155 countries and territories[(ii)] engaged with the survey and this chapter summarises findings from 60,860 complete responses to questions on stigma-related knowledge, attitudes and behaviour in relation to people living with dementia. Some survey questions were asked among all respondents while others were tailored for a particular group (for example carers). This enabled us to compare findings across groups but also understand the specific experiences of certain groups. We generally categorise our findings in two ways: (1) by WHO Region (geographical location) and (2) by World Bank income groups (see Appendix 1). These categories capture broad cultural and economic variations in relation to stigma towards people living with dementia. In addition, we provide a break-down of selected questions by countries with more than 100 respondents.

(i) Throughout the survey analysis the word 'carers' also refers to caregivers and care partners.

(ii) Throughout the report, the word 'countries' also refers to countries and territories/regions together.

Further information on the study methodology including the survey development, data collection and analysis are described in detail in the methodology section (See Methodology Section page 61).

## Survey findings

We present survey findings according to three areas which contribute to stigma: (1) knowledge (problems of ignorance and misinformation), (2) attitudes (problems of prejudice) and (3) behaviour (problems of discrimination, e.g. social exclusion)[1]. In this report, we highlight the behavioural element first, as direct assessment of actual behaviour is central to discrimination and is the closest representation of the true impact of stigma on people living with dementia. Additionally, stigma surveys tend to focus on knowledge and/or awareness, assuming that these are linked with discrimination; however, it is essential that we assess true behaviour and experiences from the perspective of people living with dementia in order to validate these links[2]. Additionally, this gives prominence to the voices and reported experiences of people living with dementia so that we can understand the main areas in relation to which they feel society treats them unfairly as this should be the focus of any anti-stigma effort.

## Behaviour

### Experiences among people living with dementia

We wanted to understand the stigma and discrimination experienced by people living with dementia, in particular what kinds of treatment they felt were unfair and the outcomes associated with these negative experiences. In terms of outcomes, we looked at quality of life, life satisfaction, well-being and self-esteem, hypothesising that individuals experiencing greater levels of stigma and discrimination might have worse outcomes.

### Unfair treatment experienced by people living with dementia

Unfair treatment can be felt across many life domains such as being treated unfairly in hospitals or by family members, having jokes made about one's dementia symptoms or being denied the opportunity to do things by others because of a diagnosis of dementia. We present the reported prevalence of unfair treatment by respondents living with dementia according to different types of life domains and compare these responses across World Bank income groups and across WHO regions in Figures 1-2. Alongside each domain, we contextualise participant responses with quotes from

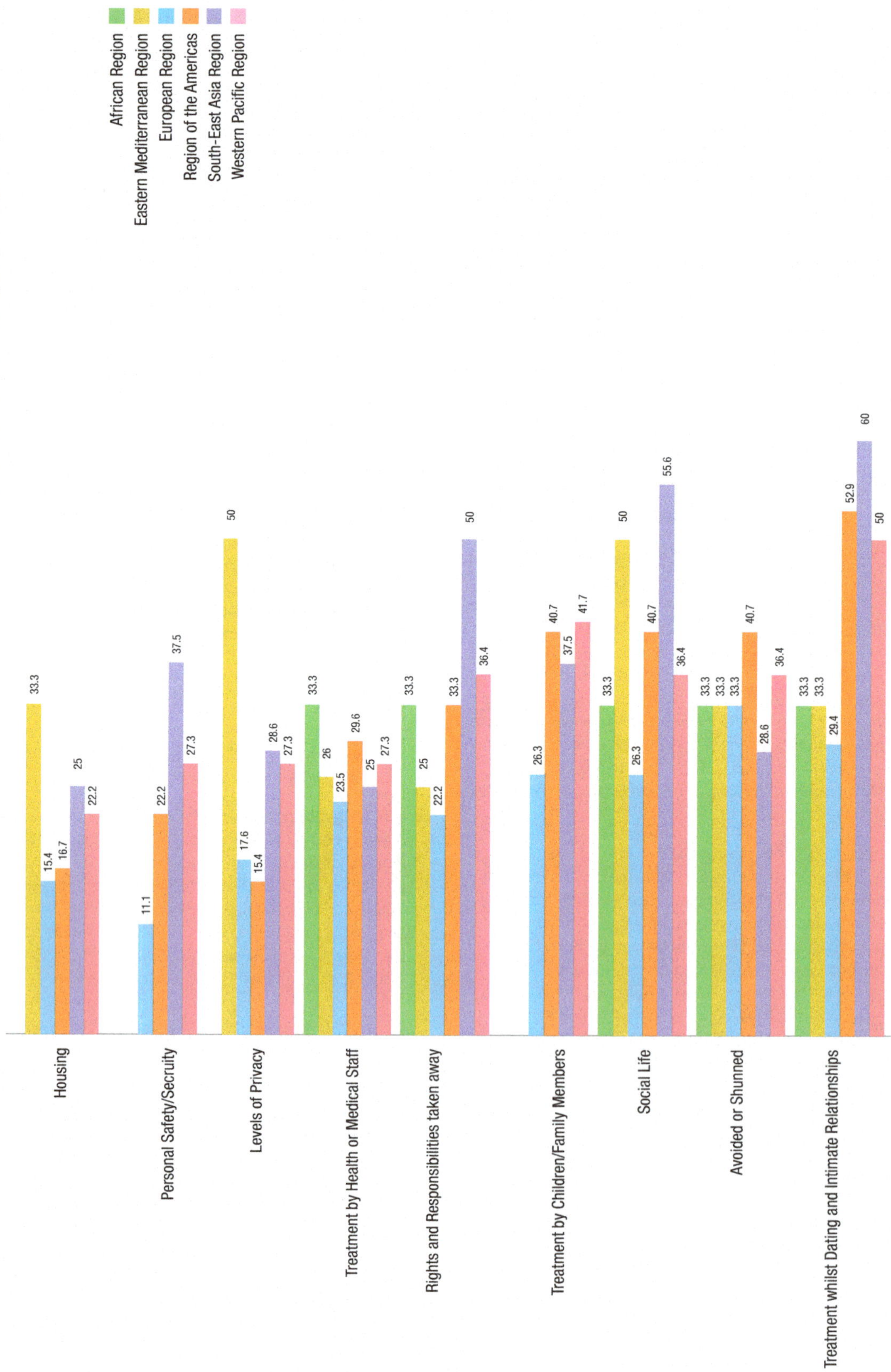


**Figure 1.** Domains in which respondents living with dementia have experienced unfair treatment across world regions (% of respondents)

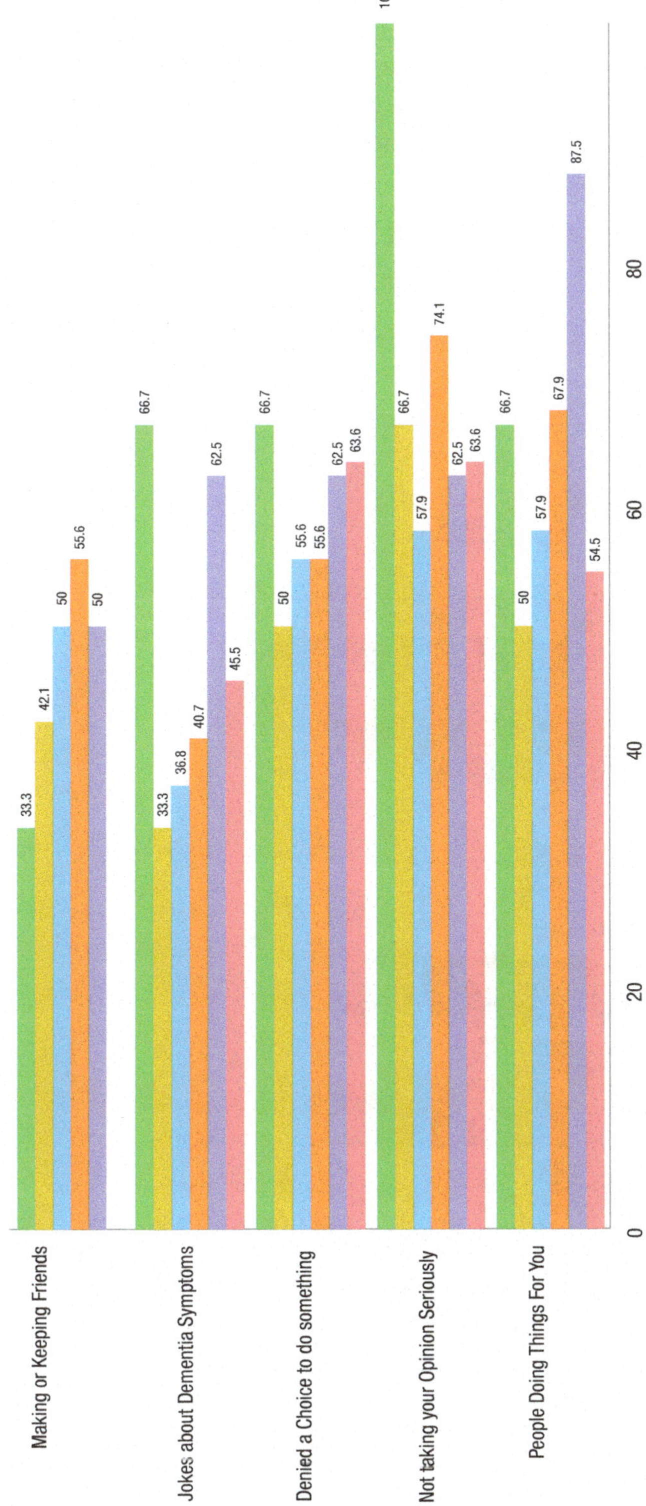
Making or Keeping Friends
33.3
42.1
50
55.6
50
Jokes about Dementia Symptoms
66.7
33.3
36.8
40.7
62.5
45.5
Denied a Choice to do something
66.7
50
55.6
55.6
62.5
63.6
Not taking your Opinion Seriously
100
66.7
57.9
74.1
62.5
63.6
People Doing Things For You
66.7
50
57.9
67.9
87.5
54.5
0
20
40
60
80

**Figure 2.** Domains of unfair treatment experienced by people living with dementia by World Bank income category (% of respondents)

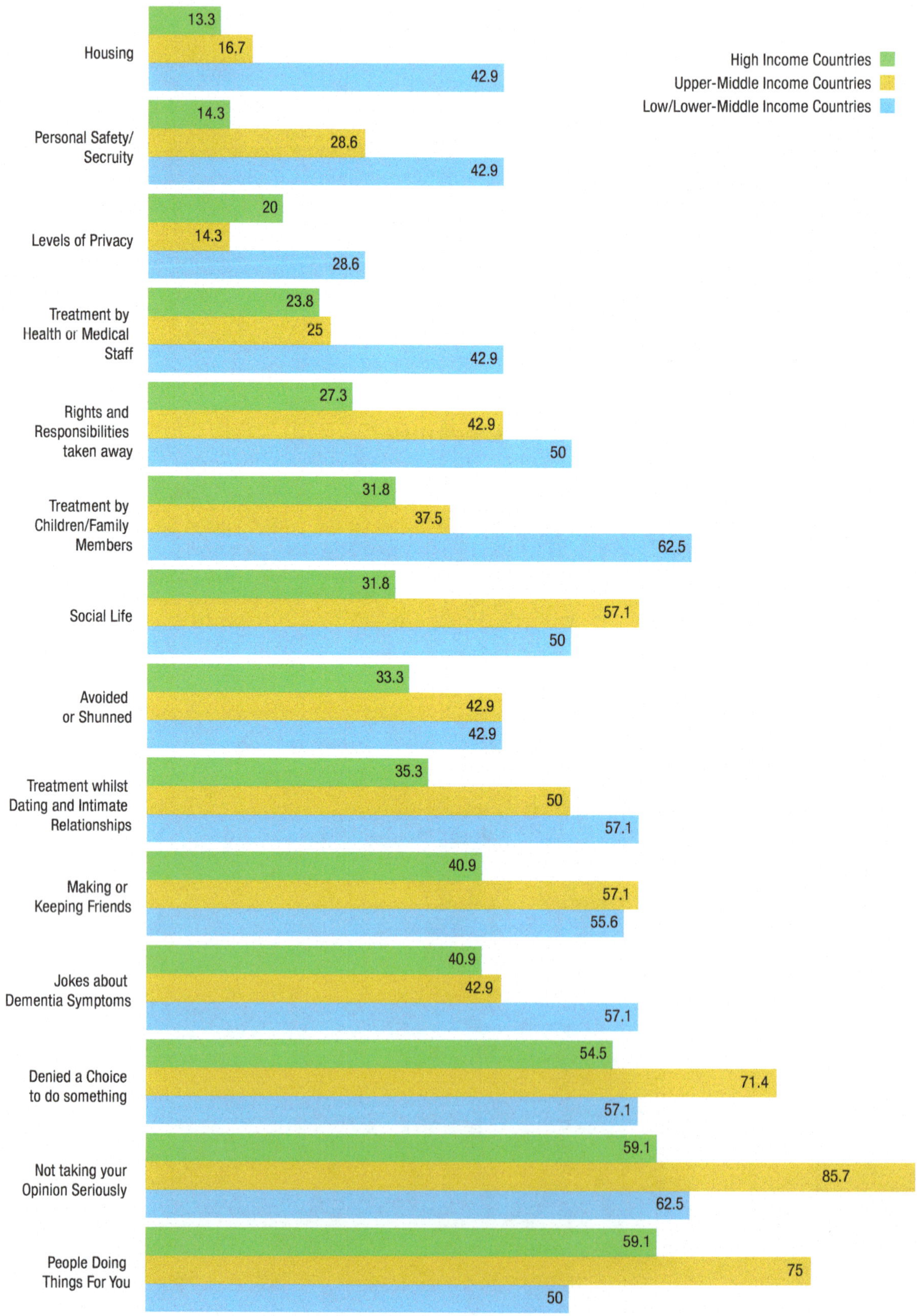

individuals living with dementia who have experienced being treated unfairly across different global regions.

## Global comparisons of unfair treatment according to life domain and / or experience

### Social life

When asked about being treated unfairly in social life, such as being excluded from socialising, hobbies or attending events, respondents living with dementia in high (38.1%), upper-middle (57.1%) and low/lower-middle income (50%) countries reported experiencing this form of unfair treatment because of their dementia and this was highest in upper-middle income countries (see Figure 2). Respondents reported feeling "avoided", "ignored" and "ostracized" in their social life due to having dementia where many of them *"no longer get invited to social gatherings"* (71 year old female from the United States (US)).

### Being avoided or shunned

A further 42.9% of respondents living with dementia in upper and low/lower-middle income countries experienced being avoided or shunned, whereas this was lower in high-income countries (33.3%). The greatest experience of avoidance or shunning was in the Region of the Americas (40.7%, see Figure 1).

### Personal safety and security

Respondents in low/lower-middle (42.9%) income countries experienced the greatest amount of unfair treatment in personal safety and security compared to respondents in high (14.3%) and upper-middle (28.6%) income countries. Respondents living with dementia said they had been *"pushed and verbally abused"* (66 year old male from the US) and *"emotionally abused"* (62 year old female from the US).

### Privacy

When asked have you been treated unfairly in your levels of privacy? Respondents living with dementia in low/lower-middle (28.6%), high (20%) and upper-middle (14.3%) income countries all reported this form of unfair treatment. For example, one respondent said, *"I know my health records have been shared without my consent"* (60 year old female from Australia). Another respondent spoke of a lack privacy across many different situations: *"I have 3 caretakers. One of them will open packages I get in the mail, even after I have asked her not to. It is impossible for me to have a private phone call and privacy with visitors. They usually go into my doctor visits, so I have no privacy there"* (75 year old female from the US).

### Housing

When respondents living with dementia were asked have you been treated unfairly in housing? those living in lower-middle income countries reported the greatest amount of unfair treatment (42.9%, see Figure 2). However, respondents from high (13.3%) and upper-middle (16.7%) income countries had also had this experience, saying things such as *"when the place reference to housing knew I had dementia they showed me the door… I was not welcome"* (73 year old female from the United Kingdom (UK)).

### Dementia symptoms being joked about by others

Fifty-seven percent of respondents living with dementia in low/lower-middle income countries reported that their dementia symptoms were joked about by others. This form of unfair treatment was also experienced by respondents living with dementia in high (40.9%) and upper-middle (42.9%) income countries. Respondents in the African (66.7%) and South-East Asia Regions (62.5%) reported the highest prevalence of their dementia being joked about often by others (see Figure 1).

### Having responsibilities taken away unfairly

Half of the respondents living with dementia from lower-middle income countries reported that they had experienced their rights or responsibilities taken away from them unfairly (see Figure 2), this was also experienced in high (27.3%) and upper-middle (42.9%) income countries. For example, one respondent said their *"spouse wants to do most of the work around the house, because she doesn't want me to get tired"* (57 year old female from the US), and one *"I feel I have little say in making a decision to move house"* (67 year old female from the UK).

### Been told you couldn't do something that you still thought you could do

When asked about being told that they couldn't do something that they still thought they could do because of their dementia, respondents living with dementia in upper-middle (71.4%), high (54.5%) and low/lower-middle (57.1%) income countries all experienced this form of unfair treatment with the greatest regional prevalence being in the African (66.7%), Western Pacific (63.6%) and South-East Asia (62.5%) regions of the world (see Figure 1).

### People do things for you that you could do yourself

When asked about whether people do things for you that you could do yourself because they know you have dementia, respondents living with dementia in upper-middle income countries (75%) reported higher rates of others doing things for them, in comparison to high-income (59.1%) and low/lower-middle income (50%) countries (see Figure 2). The highest prevalence of others doing things for respondents living with dementia that they can do themselves was in the South-East Asian region (87.5%). It may be possible that in some cultures doing things that people can do for themselves corresponds to a wish to show deference, particularly towards older people.

### People do not take your opinions seriously because of your dementia

To the question, Because of your dementia have some people not taken your opinions seriously?, 85.7% of respondents living with dementia in upper-middle income countries reported that some people have not taken their opinion seriously, and this was also commonly reported in low/lower-middle (62.5%) and high (59.1%) income countries (see Figure 2). Respondents reported being told *"but you have dementia, so what would you know"* (60 year old female from Australia) and *"your opinion no longer matters"* (60 year old male from the US).

### Unfair treatment by health or medical staff

Unfair treatment by health or medical staff was most commonly reported by people living in low/lower-middle income countries (42.9%) compared to high (23.8%) or upper-middle income countries (25%, see Figure 2). The highest prevalence being in the Africa region (33.3%) and in the region of the Americas (29.6%). Respondents living with dementia in the African region said *"my neurologist ignored my presence when my diagnosis was discussed with my husband"* (59 year old female from South Africa) and *"they tell me that I am not sick but too old"* (86 year old male from Zambia). Respondents living with dementia in the region of the Americas said *"my primary care doctor said to my face, too bad that euthanasia is illegal here"* (65 year old female from the US) and *"doctors don't talk to you but your caregiver"* (60 year old male from the US).

### Dating or intimate relationships

To the question Have you been treated unfairly in dating or intimate relationships, respondents living with dementia in low/lower-middle income countries reported the greatest prevalence (57.1%), compared to upper-middle (50%) and high (35.3%) income countries (see Figure 2). Respondents have reported difficulties and negative experiences while dating: *"As soon as I mention I have dementia, they presume the worst. I walk with a stick and that doesn't help either. My last boyfriend wanted to hide me away and I spoke openly about my dementia. Hence why that relationship didn't work"* (49 year old female from the UK).

### Making or keeping friends

When asked about being treated unfairly in making or keeping friends because of dementia, respondents from upper-middle (57.1%) income countries reported the greatest prevalence compared to high (40.9%) and low/lower-middle (55.6%) income countries (see Figure 2). Respondents living with dementia in the Americas reported the highest prevalence of unfair treatment when making or keeping friends (55.6%). Respondents added, *"People tend to run when they learn you have dementia"* (60 year old male from the US), or *"cannot cope with the different me"* (69 year old male from Australia). Respondents from the South-East Asia region said *"others are not able to comprehend the out of situation behaviour"* (62 year old male from India) and *"some friends do not talk or share information with me"* (64 year old female from Thailand).

### Treated unfairly by children or family

Being treated unfairly by children or other family members was most prevalent in low/lower-middle (62.5%) income countries rather than in high (31.8%) or upper middle (37.5%) income countries. Unfair treatment by children or family members was greatest in the Western Pacific region (41.7%) and the region of the Americas (40.7%). Respondents from Western Pacific regions said: *"my parents, siblings and many other family members have completely abandoned me"* (60 year old female from Australia) and *"I was excluded by over half of them. Told I was attention seeking"* (66 year old female from Australia). Respondents in the region of the Americas said: *"I have just one sister. Thinks I am making it all up"* (60 year old female from Canada) and *"My suggestions or comments are sometimes ignored"* (77 year old male from the US).

## Key themes

Key areas of participation relevant to people with dementia in all cultures and countries include social relationships and interactions with healthcare staff. These interactions represent meaningful relationships where many people reported being treated unfairly. Respondents articulated different ways in which they felt they were treated unfairly because of their dementia in social life including: no longer being invited out, being ostracised, losing contact with previous contacts, feeling they could no longer contribute and a lack of support to make interactions accessible. (See Figures 3-4, Tables 1-3)

**Table 1.** Respondent examples of being treated unfairly in social life because of dementia, categorised by theme

| Themes | Respondent examples |
|---|---|
| **Accessibility** | I rely on people to get me places, they often forget me or they are too busy – 59, female, United Kingdom |
| | They control what they think I can do. They say they will take me for a drive and then make excuses that they can't – 57, female, United Kingdom |
| | Having to always use a walker (rollator type) causes me to miss out on socialising and attending events. I can't even go to the movies now. Just recently missed out on attending a good concert which my son and daughter-in-law attended. They did not even try to include me. That hurt me – 75, female, United States |
| | I was not able to attend an event because I didn't have a caregiver to accompany me. I live by myself and don't need one yet – 65, female, United States |
| | Sometimes I am not included. Also because of physical disabilities (as an effect of the dementia) accessibility at a given venue makes it impossible for me to attend – 56, female, United Kingdom |
| **'Feel I can no longer contribute'** | Feel I can no longer contribute – 68, female, Europe |
| | To a family reunion because there are people who get annoyed or feel uncomfortable – 46, female, Panama |
| | I exclude myself, because I can't keep up – 58, male, the Netherlands |
| **Loss of contact** | Some work colleagues do not contact me any longer – 63, female, Finland |
| | Fewer people call to socialize – 58, female, United States |
| | After going to a social function with friends, those friends have all but disappeared – 56, female, United States |
| | Old friends do not call – 72, male, United States |
| **Not being invited** | Sometimes friends don't ask me to shindigs as often as they used to, because I don't drive anymore. That hurt to start with, not so much now – 49, female, United Kingdom |
| | Except for a couple of very close friends I no longer get invited to anything – 57, female, United States |
| | I'm no longer invited to do things with my friends. If I do something, it's usually by myself or with my ex-wife. I have very few close friends now – 58, male, United States |
| | Too many to tell. My daughter have me babysit while they go out with her in-laws. I'm never invited. My son's present girlfriend would not have me in their home. I am no longer allowed visitation with my five year old grandson who were her most of the time from birth to three and a half. The new girlfriend is in charge – 64, female, United States |
| | Not invited to family birthdays which hurt. Slowly changing but both my husband and I weren't on the invitations anymore – 66, female, Australia |
| | I am excluded from social get-togethers with in-laws or friends – 57, female, Suriname |
| **'You are ostracized'** | People treated me like a freak in our church meals. Neighbours avoid me – 69, female, United States |
| | Kicked out of book club – 69, female, United States |
| | I used to be active in a club, but now I am a non person – male, United States |
| | I used to volunteer in helping immigrants learn English until they found out I had dementia – 60, female, Canada |
| | First time at new resident clubhouse lunch function, after being accepted previously at their board meeting, they shunned my effort to help volunteer to prepare & serve the meal as they previously stated I would be helping – 77, female, United States |
| | They treat me like I don't exist. They move away from me. I feel alone – 65, female, Argentina |
| | The organizer denied a person living with dementia participation in the care training session and stopped sending the information about the session – 55, male, Japan |

**Figure 3.** Social life and family relationships. Themes based on textual responses of people living with dementia when asked 'Have you been treated unfairly in your social life? (for example, being excluded from socialising, hobbies, attending events, leisure activities)'

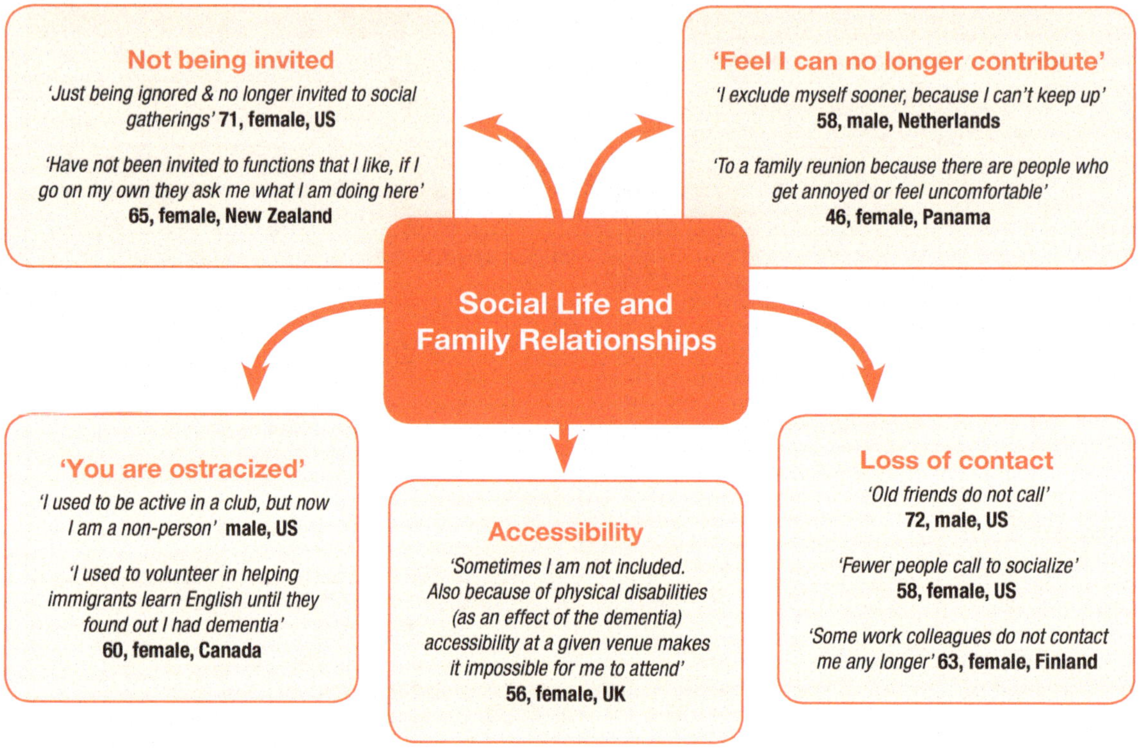


**Figure 4.** Unfair treatment within healthcare. Themes based on textual responses of people living with dementia when asked 'Have you been treated unfairly health or medical staff? (for example, did a health care professional suggest that you disengage from daily activities or social situation)'

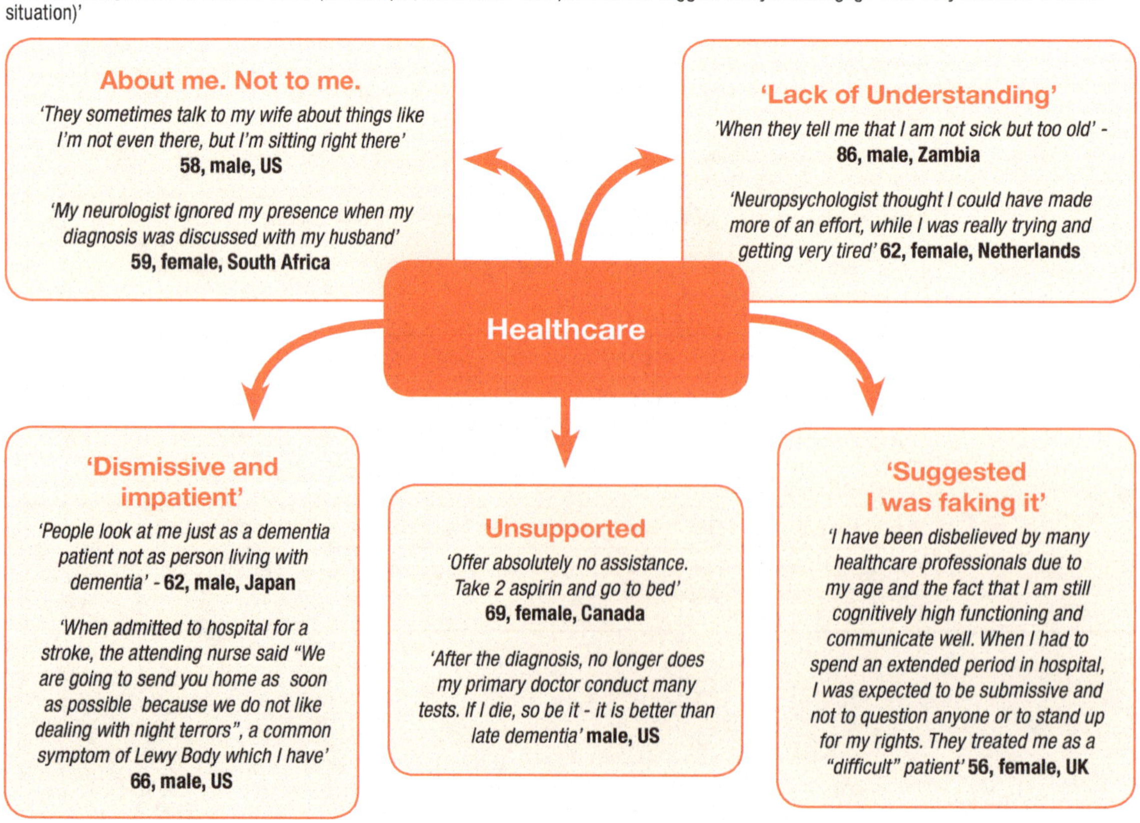

**Table 2.** Respondent examples of being treated unfairly in healthcare because of dementia, categorised by theme

| Themes | Respondent examples |
|---|---|
| **About me. Not to me.** | They sometimes talk to my wife about things like I'm not even there, but I'm sitting right there – 58, male, United States |
| | My neurologist ignored my presence when my diagnosis was discussed with my husband – 59, female, South Africa |
| | Being talked about not being talked too I sometimes feel invisible in a room I think a lot of health care officials need to retrain in dementia awareness skills – 56, male, United Kingdom |
| | Case manager who just wants to arrange things instead of talking about the difficulties I'm dealing with – 68, female, Netherlands |
| **Dismissive and impatient** | I was advised I should no longer scuba dive without any reason other than I have dementia. Not any specific symptom to drive this decision and I am in very early stage of disease – 57, female, United States |
| | One medical provider advised me to stop my social engagements because I am old – 70, male, Canada |
| | Doctor advised me not to cook anymore, not to drive. And some doctors totally ignored me and talked to my daughter in law only – 76, male, Malaysia |
| | My doctor told me that I shouldn't be able to continue with my voluntary activities – female, Australia |
| | Primary care doctor said to my face, "too bad that euthanasia is illegal here" – 65, female, United States |
| | Neurologist diagnosed me with Alzheimer's at 56, telling me to go home and get my final affairs in order and to wait until my premature death – 60, male, United States |
| **Lack of Understanding** | People including health professional ignoring what I am saying – 86, male, Zambia |
| | When admitted to hospital for a stroke, the attending nurse said, "We are going to send you home as soon as possible because we do not like dealing with night terrors", a common symptom of Lewy Body dementia which I have – 66, male, United States |
| | People look at me just as a dementia patient not as person living with dementia – 62, male, Japan |
| | The bluntness of the first neurologist and his diagnosis - without any additional examination – 78, male, Netherlands |
| | Not spending enough time, only showing me once how to use a gadget to read diabetes readings. I need shown a few times for me to remember how to use it – 73, female, New Zealand |
| **'Suggested I was faking it'** | While I was in hospital a nurse was moaning about a noisy patient with dementia - made me feel like what are they saying about me – 70, female, United Kingdom |
| | A primary care doctor told me that I wanted to be sick! – 69, female, United States |
| | When they tell me that I am not sick but too old – 86, male, Zambia |
| | Neuropsychologist thought I could have made more of an effort, while I was really trying and getting very tired – 62, female, Netherlands |
| | Suggested I was faking it – female, United Kingdom |
| **Unsupported** | Not in the ways you have asked for examples of, but many HCPs (healthcare professionals) often do not believe I have dementia - which is abusive and offensive. But, also, they then talk over me, about me, and never to me, if an inpatient, due to me having dementia. Very ironic indeed, and who's the level of IGNORANCE about dementia in HCPs – 60, female, Australia |
| | I have been disbelieved by many healthcare professionals due to my age and the fact that I am still cognitively high functioning and communicate well. When I had to spend an extended period in hospital I was expected to be submissive and not to question anyone or to stand up for my rights. They treated me as a "difficult" patient – 56, female, United Kingdom |
| | I am finding that health care professionals do not listen to me, or know how to ask the questions that I can answer...and they always say - who told you have this...and then discredit the diagnosis or say they don't believe that is the problem...when I try to explain the level of life change I have recently experienced, they blow me off – 56, female, United States |
| | One Doctor refused to believe what I said, implying I was making it up – 73, female, United Kingdom |
| | Some of my doctors don't pay much attention to what I tell them, and therefore they are unable to help me. I am now looking for a 3rd GI specialist, because the first 2 did nothing for me and both just dismissed me without treatment or relief of symptoms – 75, female, United States |

**Table 3.** Examples of unfair treatment reported by people living with dementia according to life domain

| Domain of unfair treatment | Quote from respondents living with dementia |
|---|---|
| **People doing things for you that you could do yourself because they know you have dementia** | My partner has taken over all our finances - I think I could manage some of the – 63, female, South Africa<br><br>Sometime people try to speak for me, but I insist I am still able to do this – 56, female, United Kingdom<br><br>People mean well, but I am not an invalid. My family can be like that hence why I live alone. If I offer to help when I go to their house they don't often let me – 49, female, United Kingdom<br><br>Giving a shower to the persons with dementia instead of assist and let them shower themselves because they don't have time and have to go to work – 50, female, Thailand<br><br>Spouse reminds me of things that I can remember on my own, i.e. Don't forget your keys. Do you have your phone? All in voice that sounds like she is reminding a child – 57, female, United States<br><br>A close friend sometimes finishes my sentence as I take time to find my words. I am in very early stage and aphasia is my major problem – 75, female, United States<br><br>A lot of things I feel I may still be able to do others do for me in the name of helping – 62, female, United States<br><br>Always volunteering to do stuff not wanted by me. Tiresome – 60, female, Malaysia<br><br>I was excluded from the rotating duty of the neighbourhood association – 87, female, Japan |
| **Not taking your opinion seriously because of your dementia** | Sometimes in open conversations in groups of friends, I feel my opinion is "sidelined" – 63, female, South Africa<br><br>They simply think I am dumb. Especially since I look 10+ years younger than my age – 48, female, Uganda<br><br>Some people have the impression that should be less vocal in my opinions. When speaking to carers (of others) in order to spread awareness of the dementia experience I have been shouted down and told I don't understand the situation, even though I have also been a carer for a family member with dementia – 56, female, United Kingdom<br><br>It's as if invisible, if I ask my husband to do something, he totally ignores it causing arguments all the time – 57, female, United Kingdom<br><br>I love a good debate. I have a debating back ground throughout my life. I remember attempting a debate with someone on a topic of interest to me. Her reply was you are very argumentative. That is the dementia talking – 61, male, Canada<br><br>People just don't listen when I talk – 69, female, United States<br><br>I have even been told, "but you have dementia, so what would you know!" – 60, female, Australia |
| **Denied a choice to do something that you still thought you could because of your dementia** | I can't do anything anymore without asking someone, but no one cares if I want to do it or not. People seem to forget, I'm still a real person with real feelings and very real emotions – 59, female, United Kingdom<br><br>Volunteering for Alzheimer's Association ESAG requires me to have a travel partner even for local events where I am the better of us at navigating. No exceptions just because I have Alzheimer's. I was also denied access to an Alzheimer's seminar because I have the disease and when insisted and raised the Americans with Disabilities Act, was allowed to attend but only if I didn't tell anyone I had dementia. This was a well-known hospital providing this seminar – 57, female, United States<br><br>Taking away carrying credit cards, cash – 81, male, United States<br><br>I still live on my own. I feel doctors are rushing to convince me to go into a care facility. I'd rather have discussions on how I can live on my own longer and what, if any, services are available to prolong my independence – 69, male, United States<br><br>Driving, finances, and especially payments for consulting or other usually funded advice from ALL Alzheimer's advocacy organisations. Curiously, organisations outside of the dementia sector have NO problem paying me for advice, consulting or appropriate disability support - it has been exclusively the dementia sector which has systematically denied me this, and I have had to fully or partially self-fund to even have a voice or be included – 60, female, Australia<br><br>Taking away my car key; disconnect my house gas supply and drive away my car and said thieves stole it after I refused to close the gate – 76, male, Malaysia |

| Domain of unfair treatment | Quote from respondents living with dementia |
|---|---|
| **People joke about your dementia symptoms** | They call me names – 55, female, Zambia<br>I put humour in my own situation to let other people feel comfortable – 56, female, South Africa<br>My grandchildren mock me that my decisions are not sound – 86, male, Zambia<br>Becoming a joke / joked about – 69, male, Indonesia<br>Bullying, speaking about dementia as a funny joke – 40, female, Thailand<br>I have been told, "Well my memory is better than yours!" or "Don't forget to wear the same type of shoes" – 57, female, United states<br>You can't remember anything! – 70, female, United States<br>How long before you become fully demented – 60, female, Canada<br>When I make a mistake they just say oh it's a senior moment but they don't really know that I have dementia because I haven't told them – 80, female, United States<br>It is 100% offensive, and inexcusable to joke about my symptoms (unless it is me joking about it). It also means I will not engage with these people afterwards. Asking people not to joke about us, always means they take offense, rather than accept they may be offending or upsetting us – 60, female, Australia<br>My child said that I looked like an alpaca when I dribbled saliva – 53, female, Japan<br>People said that I did not look like someone with dementia – 58, male, Japan |
| **Treated unfairly in making or keeping friends because of your dementia** | They tend to visit less often avoid visits – 74, female, South Africa<br>Forgetting their names or when to meet...makes them think I do it intentionally – 48, female, Uganda<br>With some friends they became distant on finding out about my diagnosis. I am not always included in the plans of friends I have kept and I put this down to my diagnosis – 56, female, United Kingdom<br>My siblings don't talk to me or ask how I am anymore – 62, male, United Kingdom<br>Barred from my Sister's house because they said I have used abusive and obscene language – 70, male, Canada<br>People tend to run when they learn you have dementia – 60, male, United States<br>When I make statements that are out of character some friends and family have taken it personally and stopped talking to me – 58, female, United States<br>I feel isolated – 65, female, Argentina<br>Many have told me they are not at all interested in "the dementia journey" – 60, female, Australia<br>Some friends don't like to talk to me because I repeat – 87, female, Singapore<br>I have a few people say don't talk to her she has no idea what she is talking about – 65, female, New Zealand<br>Some people cannot cope with the different me – 69, male, Australia |
| **Avoided or shunned by people who know that you have dementia** | Because they think that they cannot cope up to their standard of thinking – 55, female, Zambia<br>They avoid socialize – 74, female, South Africa<br>Close friend doesn't call at all anymore – 60, male, United states<br>In my faith community, avoiding me – 66, male, United States<br>No one comes to my house but one neighbour (who wants my furniture when I am moved away) and my adult children visit rarely - when they come they avoid me most of the time and go out to have fun. My in-laws posture was always like backing away from dangerous animal. My mother in law harassed and insulted me and threatened to call police on me for telling her to back off – 69, female, United States |

| Domain of unfair treatment | Quote from respondents living with dementia |
|---|---|
| **Treated unfairly by your children or other family members** | My children are more distant and are not acknowledging my condition, refusing to talk about it – 56, female, United Kingdom |
| | I have a daughter who has distanced her and her family since I was diagnosed – 55, female, United Kingdom |
| | Not being included in conversations. I stopped attending family gatherings for the last 9 years since diagnosis – 70, male, Canada |
| | Too much expected of me sometimes. Irritation that I don't remember things – 70, female, United States |
| | Family frustrated, angry, and in denial themselves – 69, female, Canada |
| | Children sometimes seem to dismiss my decisions regarding my future – 79 female, United States |
| | [being told] "You're a crazy mother" – 52, female, Brazil |
| | Excluded by over half of them. Told I was attention seeking, they didn't believe I had dementia. It was easier to believe the wrong diagnosis of hypomanic depression late onset bi/ polar schizophrenia. These aren't terminal diseases. Just didn't want it for me as not familial Dementia – 66, female, Australia |
| | My daughter insists that I should go for day care, my daughter in law took photos of the pots I have burnt and told me to look at what I have done – 76, male, Malaysia |
| | I am blamed for my mistakes due to my disease as if it were laziness - Japan |
| | People don't expect anything from me because I have dementia – 53, female, Japan |
| | My child dislikes me because I am slow and cannot clearly articulate my question – 65, male, China |
| | Since they cannot tolerate my behaviours, they do not want to contact me – 58, male, Chinese Taipei |
| **Rights and Responsibilities unfairly taken away from you because of your dementia** | The right to work and at times to think for myself – 63, male, UK |
| | My wife handles all finances even though I think I am capable – 79, male, Canada |
| | We are buying a second home. My wife assumes roles she is unfamiliar with because she fears (justifiably) I am incompetent – 77, male, United States |
| | Forced to apologize for my behavior – 67, female, United States |
| | Mother brother and sister cheated me out of large share of inheritance – 69, female, United States |
| | Rating at work was decreased – 59, female, United States |
| **Treated unfairly in your levels of privacy because of your dementia** | In hospital, psychiatric doctor did not give me my medical records – 60, female, Czech Republic |
| | Hospital lack of dementia protocols – 67, male, United States |
| | I have 3 caretakers. One of them will open packages I get in the mail, even after I have asked her not to. It is impossible for me to have a private phone call and privacy with visitors. They usually go into my doctor visits, so I have no privacy there – female, United States |
| | Financial info, asking neighbours about me without telling me – 69, female, United States |
| | I know my health records have been shared without my consent... and I have also felt the need to share them to prevent public defamation of the possibility of me faking dementia – 60, female, Australia |
| | Hospital moving from bed to bed. Manager does not understand dementia – total lack of training – 68, female, Europe |

| Domain of unfair treatment | Quote from respondents living with dementia |
|---|---|
| **Treated unfairly in your personal safety and security because of your dementia** | People harangue me cos I get things wrong or say something they don't like – 62, male, United Kingdom<br><br>I have been verbalized in the past by people not understanding about my dementia. Like people saying that my dementia is "Gods punishment to me for something I have done in my life" And other things like that – 49, female, United Kingdom<br><br>I feel that my husband will do something, get rid of something for example and when I approach him about it, he will say it never existed or it's all in my head, he will say I don't know what you're talking about or I'm starting an argument which normally happens – 57, female, United Kingdom<br><br>Elder verbal abuse by the society – 50, female, India<br><br>In the face of some crisis, as I have mild cognitive impairment.... my oldest son threw me on the floor – 55, female, Argentina<br><br>At first my kids would yell and so would my partner. He seemed to know I was weaker – 60, female, United States<br><br>Don't ask her as she has lost it – 65, female, New Zealand<br><br>Husband speaks badly. Children do not take into account what I say – 65, female, Argentina<br><br>Verbal abuse ... the maid my daughter employed. Physical abuse ... the nursing home nurse restraining me to my bed by tying me to the bed railing as they said I kept removing my diapers and mess up the bed and floor with urine and shit – 76, male, Malaysia |
| **Treated unfairly in housing because of your dementia** | When the place knew I had dementia they showed me the door and was told I was not welcome – 76, female, United Kingdom<br><br>I have lived in the country[side] for many years and after diagnosis I have been put in a town – 58, female, Ireland<br><br>Wants to live in his/her own home, but live in the kid's home instead – 68, female, Indonesia<br><br>Moving into independent senior facility when I mentioned I had short term memory loss I was told I'd have to be in a dependent section by their rules. I had to get a Dr.'s letter stating I was competent – 77, female, United States |

## Impact of stigma on intimate relationships among people living with dementia

Feeling loved and intimacy is considered an essential part of interpersonal relationships. Whilst an intimate relationship could imply sexual activity, conceptually an intimate relationship fulfils the desire for closeness and warmth from another person. The need for intimate relationships exists across cultures. Dementia may, however, negatively impact the maintenance of these relationships and could also impede the formation of new ones (e.g. dating).

As mentioned earlier, in the survey, people with dementia from low/lower-middle income countries more frequently reported that they had been treated unfairly in dating or intimate relationships (57.1%) compared to upper-middle-income countries (50%), and high-income countries (35.3%). Irrespective of region, the responses were quite variable.

Open text responses commonly described how the person with dementia felt they were treated differently within their existing intimate relationships. This included feelings that they are being ignored, others being less attentive to what they say, or even neglected.

*"In conversations when sharing my opinions. They are often ignored or put down."* (Female, 60, Canada).

*"There is no longer an equal dialogue with my partner"* (Female, 54, Netherlands)

*"Since they (friends) realized that I have dementia, they are not so intimate with me."* (Male, 58, Vietnam)

Generally, respondents did not openly report changes to sexual habits, and were more likely to discuss changes to sleeping arrangements (e.g. sleeping in separate beds). However, some did report a reduction in sexual contact, which resulted in conflict.

*"My husband does not understand my mood. He thinks that I do not want to have relations for other reason and is angry."* (Female, 65, Argentina)

In some cases, the diagnosis of dementia appeared to lead to a breakdown in the intimate relationship. It was not always clear the reason for this breakdown, though it was not always due to the partner leaving the person with dementia.

*".... my wife and I divorced due to my Alzheimer's ... her decision."* (US)

*"my husband would yell at me, refused to comfort my panic, refused to help me more. He also threatened me and I divorced him"* (Female, 69, US)

Respondents also described that dementia prevented the formation of new intimate relationships, through dating. Respondents either were self-stigmatizing in the belief that others would not want to date someone with dementia or had previous negative and stigmatizing experiences whilst dating in the past.

*"To be honest, NO ONE wants to date a 58-year-old guy with Alzheimer's."* (Male, 58, US)

*"I haven't dated in years. Had my confidence blown out of the water towards this. I met a nurse...on our second date I mentioned I had Alzheimer's. Thought I should get that out of the way. She said, 'I have met some losers in my time but you take the cake'. I asked why she said that. She said, 'everyone knows anyone with dementia should be locked up' and went on to say that I couldn't have dementia. I asked her why? She said, 'because you make sense when you talk.'"* (Male, 61, Canada)

*"I don't date at all now. As soon as I mention I have dementia, they presume the worse. I walk with a stick and that doesn't help either. My last boyfriend wanted to hide me away and I spoke openly about my dementia. Hence why that relationship didn't work. That was in 2016."* (Female, 49, UK)

## Concealing the diagnosis and life satisfaction

When asked about how comfortable they feel talking about their dementia, for example, telling others you have a dementia diagnosis and how it affects you, 14.1% of respondents living with dementia reported being 'not at all' comfortable when talking to a friend and 13% when talking to a family member. The highest rates of discomfort were felt in upper-middle income countries. Just under one- third of respondents living with dementia agreed that when meeting people for the first time I try to keep my dementia a secret, with higher rates of secrecy found in respondents who were from high-income and low/lower-middle income countries. Nonetheless, a significant majority of respondents living with dementia (86.3%) think that people should not hide their diagnosis.

Further analysis suggested that higher levels of secrecy were related to a greater experience of unfair treatment and negative quality of life factors such as loneliness, frustration and anger. Whereas being comfortable in disclosing to others was associated with higher levels of self-esteem and positive quality of life factors such as happiness, hopefulness and content. When respondents were asked How often in the past month did you feel satisfied with your life? 23.5% of people living with dementia reported they were at most satisfied 'about once or twice' in the last month. Respondents in low/lower-middle (55.5%) and upper-middle reported being satisfied less often than respondents in high-income countries.

## Behaviour among the general public, healthcare practitioners and carers

In addition to experiences of people living with dementia highlighting the unfair treatment that they face, understanding behaviours of the general public, healthcare practitioners and carers can help us understand the context in which people live.

## Intended behaviour in relation to allowing a person with dementia to move in

- As well as specific attitudes towards people living with dementia, the question of whether people would allow a person with dementia to move in with them, may reflect other cultural differences, as in some regions of the world multigenerational households are much more common than in others. When looking by World Bank income group, 40.6% of the general public living in high-income countries were willing or extremely willing to allow a person living with dementia to move in with them, compared to 58.4% of upper- and 64.1% low/lower-middle income countries (see Figure 5A).
- When looking at WHO Regions, those living in the Eastern Mediterranean (71.1%) and South East Asia (62%) were mostly likely to agree to have a person with dementia move in with them while those living in Europe were least likely to agree (30.6%) (see Figure 5B).

## Beliefs about secrecy and disclosure of dementia

- On the whole, attitudes strongly support openness about dementia, with 91% of respondents saying that people should not hide the fact that they have dementia.
- However, around 20% of respondents would keep their own dementia a secret when meeting people. Only a small proportion of respondents (4.2%) would advise a close relative to keep their dementia a secret from everyone. This figure was higher for male than for female respondents (see section below on gender differences, page 50)
- Individuals living in high-income countries were most likely to say they would make an effort to keep their dementia a secret when meeting people (24.2%) compared to those living in low or lower-middle income countries (18.8%). A preference for secrecy was more common among the general public compared to healthcare practitioners, where 16.2% of those living in high-income and 10.9% of those living in low or lower-middle income countries agreed with the statement (see Figure 6A).

**Figure 5A.** Willingness to have a person with dementia move in with them among the general public by World Bank income group

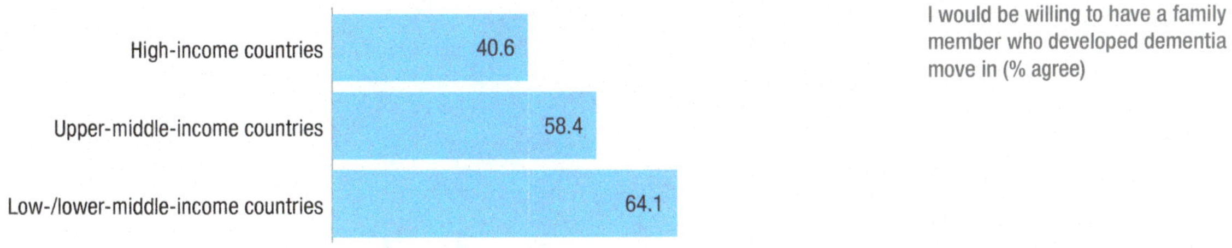


**Figure 5B.** Willingness to have a person with dementia move in with them among the general public by WHO Region

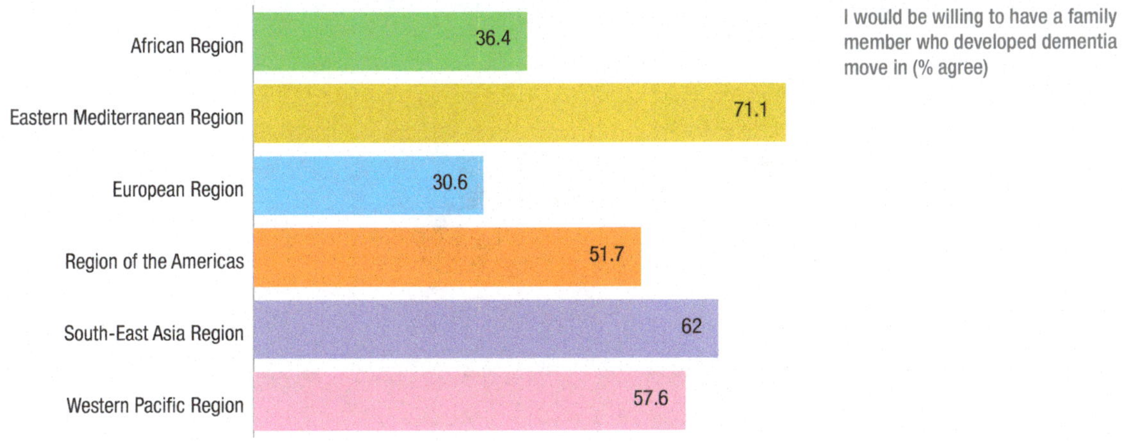


**Figure 6A.** Intended secrecy and concealment of dementia among healthcare practitioners and the general public by World Bank income group

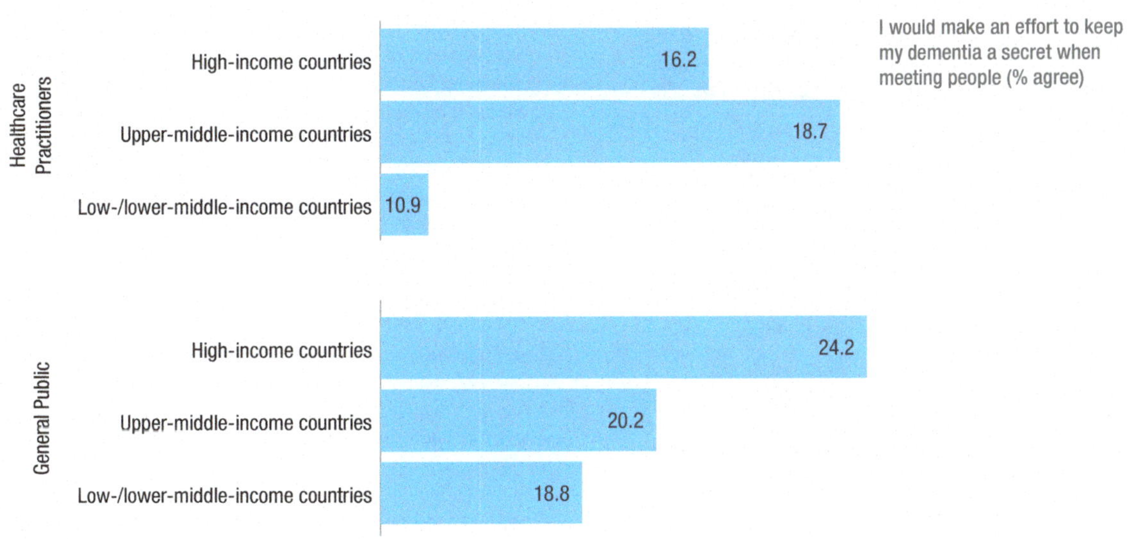

**Figure 6B.** Intended secrecy and concealment of dementia among healthcare practitioners and the general public by WHO Region

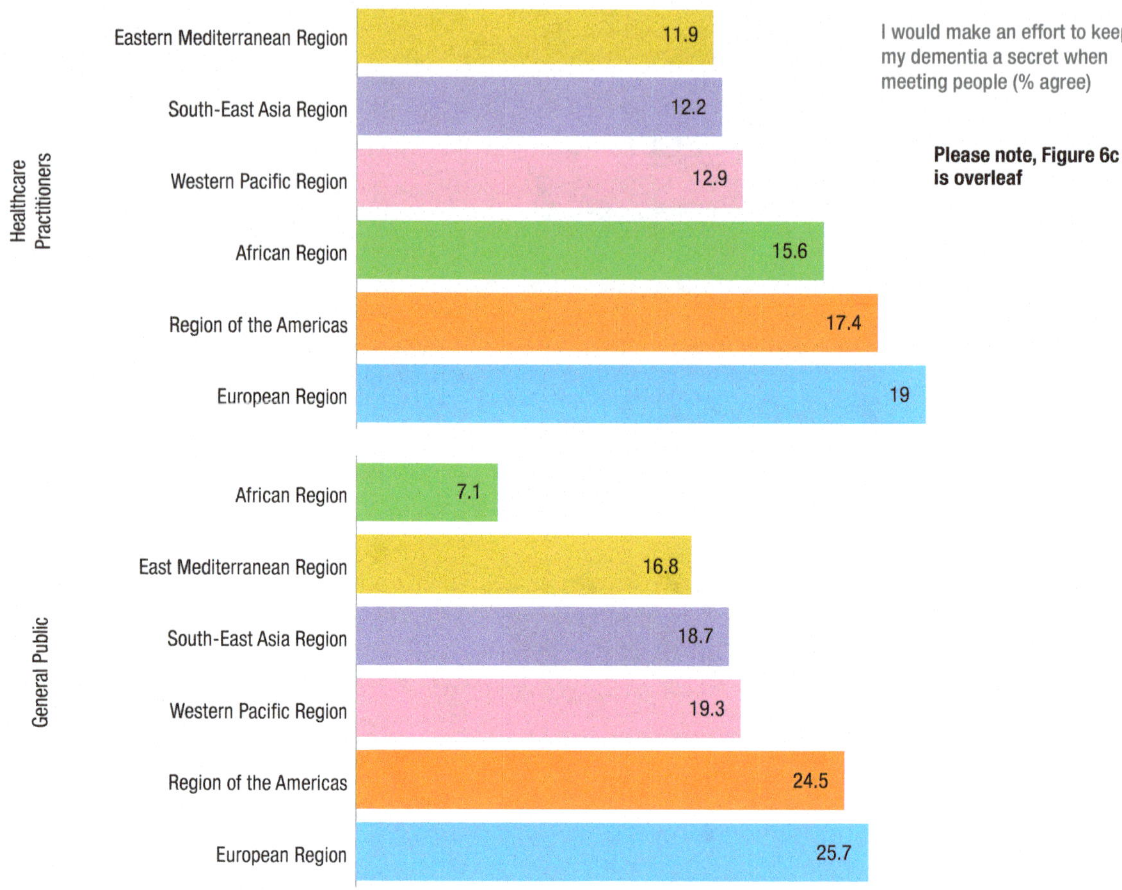


**Please note, Figure 6c is overleaf**

- Concealment of dementia varied regionally, with roughly a quarter of the general public in Europe (25.7%) and the Americas (24.5%) reporting they would keep their dementia a secret when meeting others compared, for example, to only 7% in Africa. Healthcare practitioners also reported higher levels of concealment in Europe (19%) and the Americas (17.4%) compared to other regions (see Figure 6B).
- Among countries/territories with more than 100 respondents, the countries with the highest proportion of respondents stating they would hide their dementia when meeting people were: Russia (66.7%), Poland (57.9%), Puerto Rico (51.1%), and Romania (36.7%), and the countries with the lowest proportion were: Iran (2.3%), Portugal (2.6%), Kenya (2.7%) and Singapore (3.4%) (see Figure 6C)
- Although a minority of respondents preferred secrecy, nearly a quarter of carers reported keeping a low profile while with the person they care for, and 37.3% report cutting down their contacts with friends and relatives, although this may be due to the other aspects of their caring role.

## Comparing own personal attitudes with perceptions of the general public

Respondents have a vastly more negative opinion of the behaviours of others than they do about their own behaviour. Both healthcare practitioners and the general public believe that other people are likely to engage in stigmatising behaviours. The general public responded, however, that they themselves were unlikely to engage in these behaviours. For example, 4.4% of the general public agreed that if someone they knew developed dementia they felt there would be no point in talking to people living with dementia, while 29.8% thought that others would behave in this way.

## Intended sources of support

Respondents were asked about where they would seek help if they were concerned they had early signs of dementia. They could choose as many options as they wished and were also given the option of providing a free text entry.

- Healthcare practitioner was the most commonly chosen source of support, selected by 87% of respondents, followed by a partner and a family member.

- Most of those who said they would seek help from a healthcare practitioner would also seek help from a family member or spouse, with only 18% saying they would seek help from a healthcare practitioner but not a spouse, family member or friend.
- 36% of people answered they would seek help online/internet.
- Although the vast majority of respondents answering this question would seek help, 1% replied that they would not seek help from any source.

## Carers experiences and behaviours

Just over half of the carers who answered the questionnaire expressed positive sentiments about their caring role and found it fulfilling. However, providing care is also challenging; particularly if lack of support from formal services or other family members or the wider community results in negative impacts for the carers.

We found that 52% of carers said their health, 49% their work and 62% their social life suffered because of their caring responsibilities.

## Impact on health of providing care to people with dementia

Carers in low/lower-middle income countries were more likely to answer that their health had been impacted by providing care (55.0%), compared to 49.9% of carers in high income countries. The highest proportion of carers reporting that caring had affected their health were those living the Eastern Mediterranean region at 64.9%, whereas the lowest was in the European region, 47.5%. These differences would be consistent with a relationship between the availability of formal services and the impact of providing care the health of carers.

## Impact on work of providing care to people living with dementia

People living in upper-middle income countries reported the highest rates of their work having been impacted by their caring role (52.8%), compared to 47.9% in high income countries and 44.1% in low/lower-middle income countries. The extent to which work is affected by the provision of care may be influenced not only by the amount of care that is provided and the support available to the carers, but also by differences in the propensity for women (who are most likely to be carers)

**Figure 7A.** Carers report of the impact of caring on their health, by World Bank income group

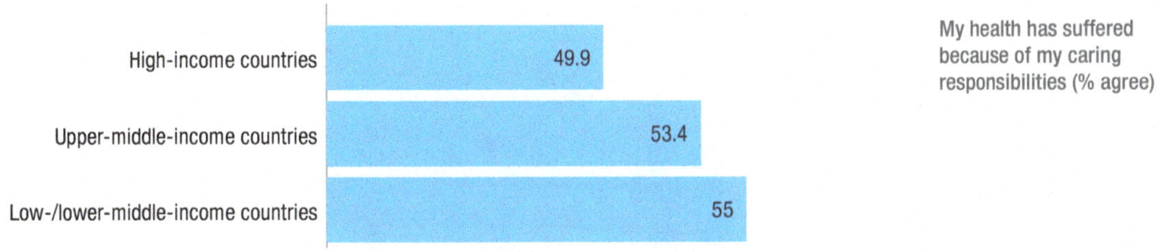


**Figure 7B.** Carers report of the impact of caring on their health, by WHO Region

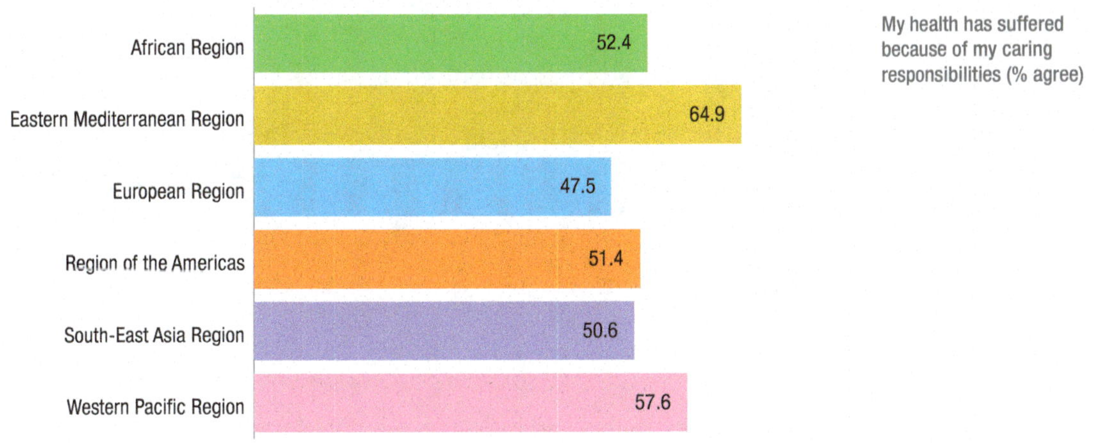

**Figure 6C.** Intended secrecy and concealment of dementia among healthcare practitioners and the general public by country

*Note: Croatia, Norway, and the Philippines were excluded due to low sample size (n<100) for this particular item/ target group*

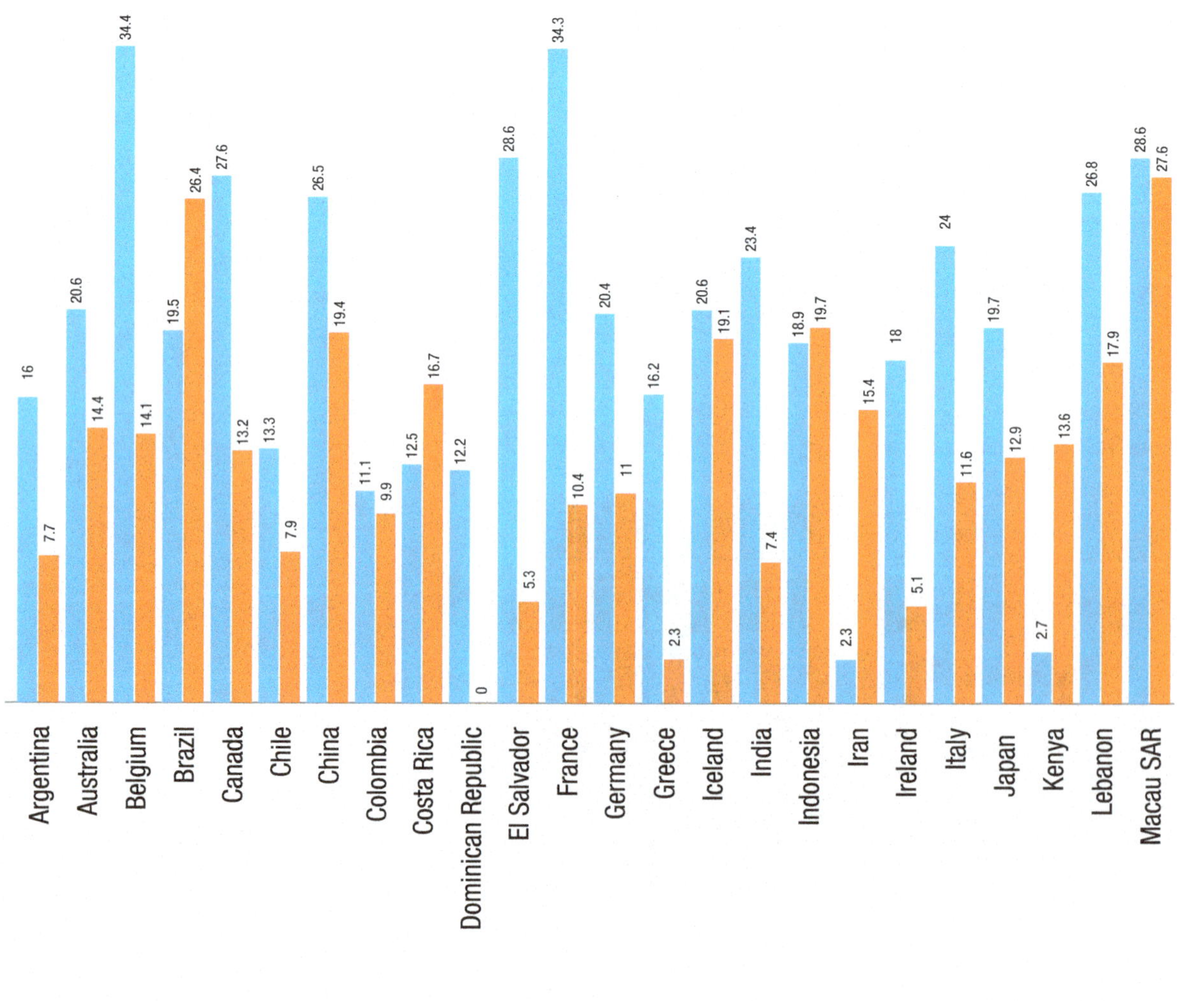

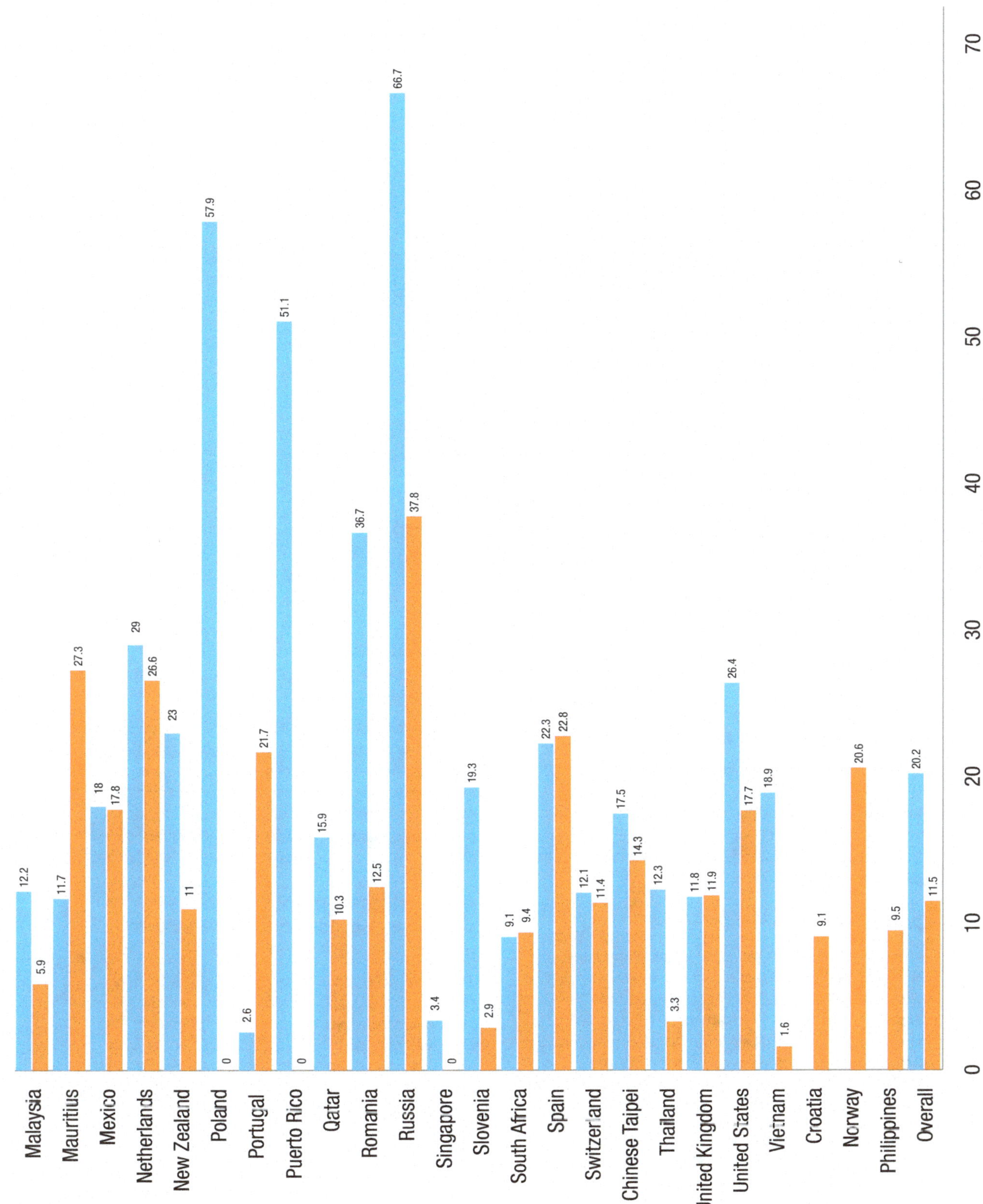
Malaysia
12.2
5.9
Mauritius
11.7
27.3
Mexico
18
17.8
Netherlands
29
26.6
New Zealand
23
11
Poland
57.9
0
Portugal
2.6
21.7
Puerto Rico
51.1
0
Qatar
15.9
10.3
Romania
36.7
12.5
Russia
66.7
37.8
Singapore
3.4
0
Slovenia
19.3
2.9
South Africa
9.1
9.4
Spain
22.3
22.8
Switzerland
12.1
11.4
Chinese Taipei
17.5
14.3
Thailand
12.3
3.3
United Kingdom
11.8
11.9
United States
26.4
17.7
Vietnam
18.9
1.6
Croatia
9.1
Norway
20.6
Philippines
9.5
Overall
20.2
11.5
0
10
20
30
40
50
60
70

**Figure 8A.** Carers report of caring impact on work, by World Bank income group

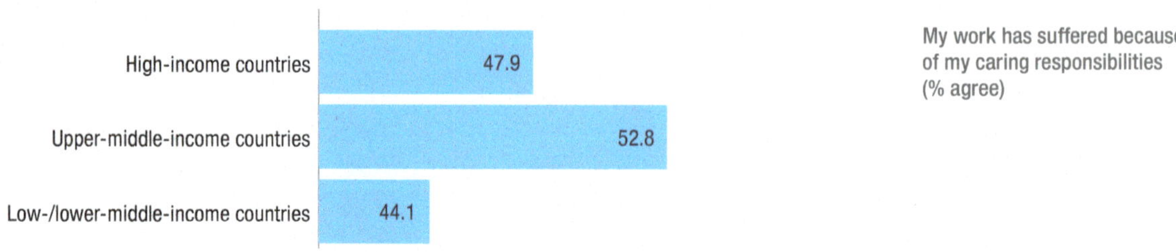


**Figure 8B.** Carers report of caring impact on work, by WHO Region

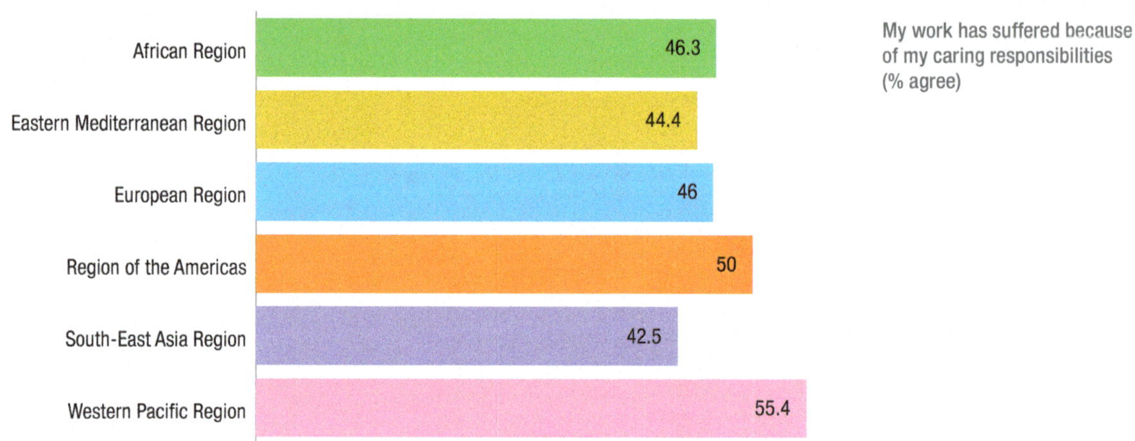


and older people to work, and by policies to support the employment of people with caring responsibilities.

## Impact of providing care to people with dementia on social life

More than half of all carers reported that their social life had been affected by their role, the highest rates were found in upper-middle countries (64.6%) and in the African region (69.0%) and the lowest in low/lower-middle income countries (55.9%) and in the South-East Asia region (49%).

## Carers' views on disclosure

Carers were asked in a separate question about the extent to which they hide the person they care for with dementia. The vast majority of carers never hide the person with dementia. There are some differences by geographical region but only small numbers responding to this question in some areas. Carers in South East Asia (16.3%) and the African Region (7.1%) are most likely to hide the person with dementia.

Carers were also asked whether they had ever concealed the diagnosis of the person they care for with dementia. 35% of carers said they had concealed the diagnosis of the person they cared for with dementia from at least one person.

## Perceptions about health and care resources for people with dementia and carers

The availability of services for people with dementia may be affected by structural stigma, meaning that, because of stigma, people with dementia are disadvantaged by the health and care systems. While our survey did not set out to analyse this, it did include questions on the perceptions about the availability and adequacy of health and care resources for people with dementia and carers.

## Adequate community services for people living with dementia and for carers

Just under 40% of the general public (37.8% in high-income, 37.3% in upper-middle income and 34.7% in low/lower middle-income countries) thought that there were adequate community services for people living with dementia and for carers. Healthcare practitioners and carers were slightly more likely to think there were adequate community services than the general public. There are interesting differences between countries (or territories) that do not always seem to correspond to what would be expected in terms of income levels, or levels of public spending on health and long-term care services. For example, over 50% of all three groups of

**Figure 9A.** Carers report of caring impact on social life, by World Bank income group

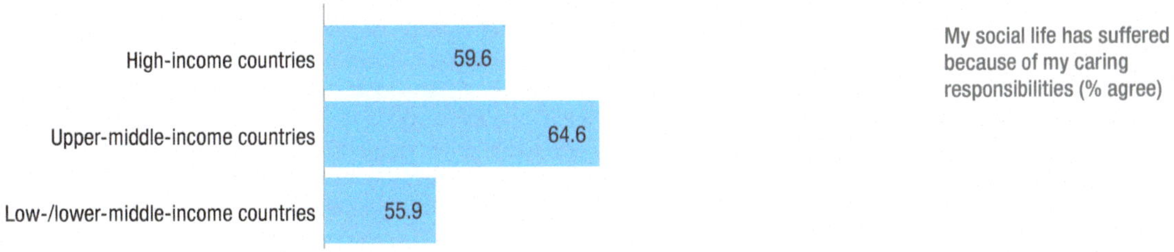


**Figure 9B.** Carers report of caring impact on social life, by WHO Region

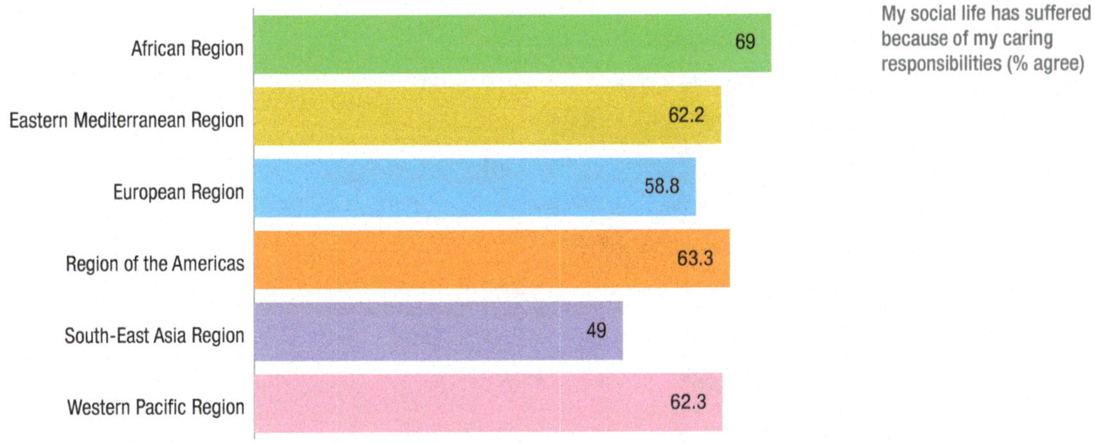


**Figure 10A.** Carers agreement they 'would hide the person I care for when out of the home', by World Bank income group (% agree)

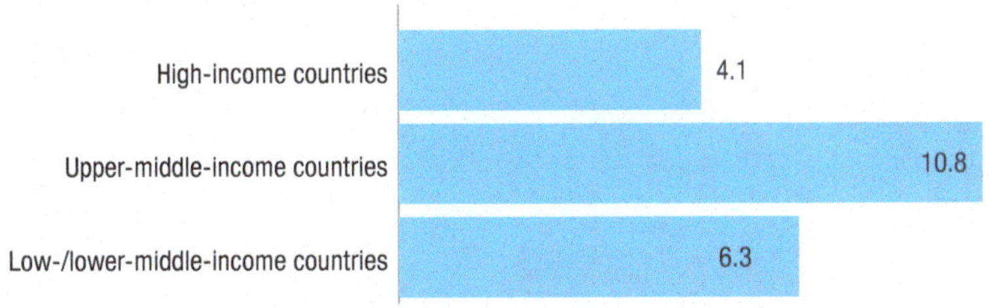


**Figure 10B.** Carers agreement they 'would hide the person I care for when out of the home', by WHO Region (% agree)

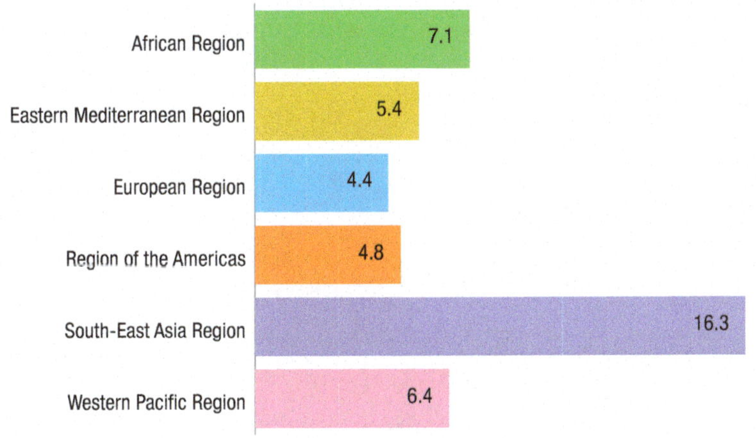

respondents (general public, healthcare practitioners and carers) in China, Germany, Macau, Chinese Taipei and Vietnam thought that there are adequate services. Additionally, 50% or more of the general public also thinks there are adequate services in Chile, Iceland, Singapore, Spain and Switzerland. There are some countries (Indonesia, the Netherlands and Slovenia) where over 50% of the carers and the healthcare practitioners also think there are adequate services.

## Enough competent physicians for the diagnosis and treatment of dementia

Just under 70% of the general public (71.6% in high-income, 69.9% in upper-middle income and 63.7% in low/lower middle-income countries) thought that there were enough competent physicians for the diagnosis and treatment of dementia. These rates were highest in the European and Western Pacific regions (76% in both) and lowest in the Eastern Mediterranean (44.7%) and Africa (42.9%). There were striking differences between countries too and, remarkably, in the United Kingdom (where there is a strong policy emphasis on increasing diagnostic rates), only 38.8% of carers and 53.3% of

**Figure 11A.** Agreement that there are adequate community services for people living with dementia, by World Bank income group (% agree)

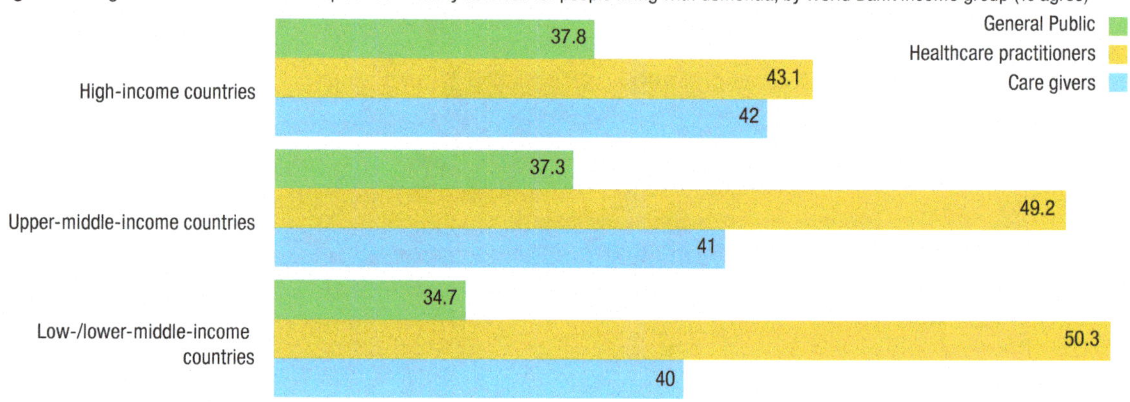


**Figure 11B.** Agreement that there are adequate community services for people living with dementia, by WHO Region (% agree)

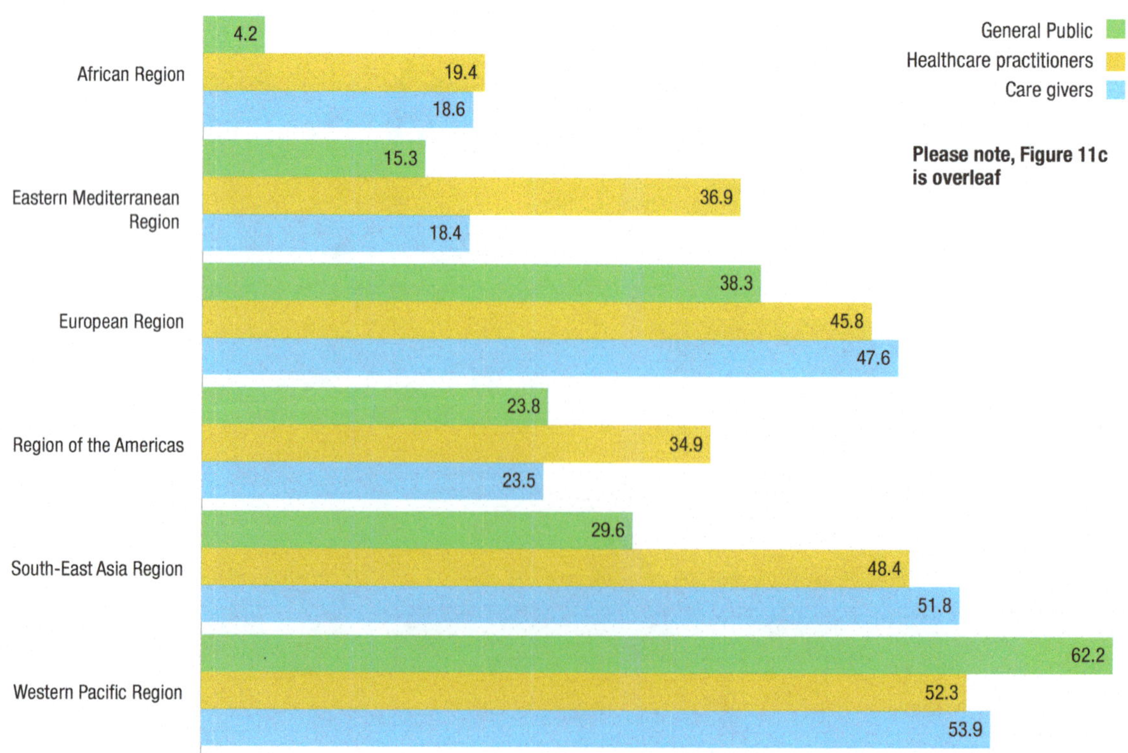


**Please note, Figure 11c is overleaf**

**Figure 12A.** Agreement that there are competent healthcare practitioners for the diagnosis and treatment of people living with dementia, by World Bank income group (% agree)

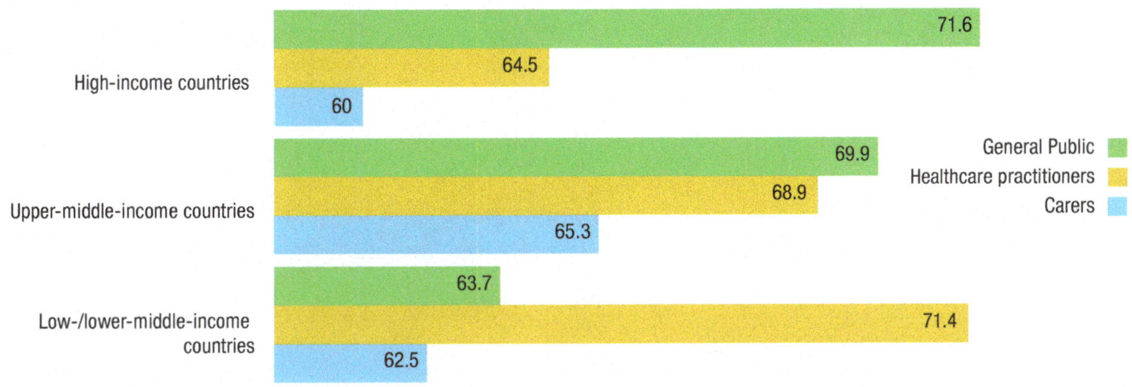


**Figure 12B.** Agreement that there are competent healthcare practitioners for the diagnosis and treatment of people living with dementia, by WHO Region (% agree)

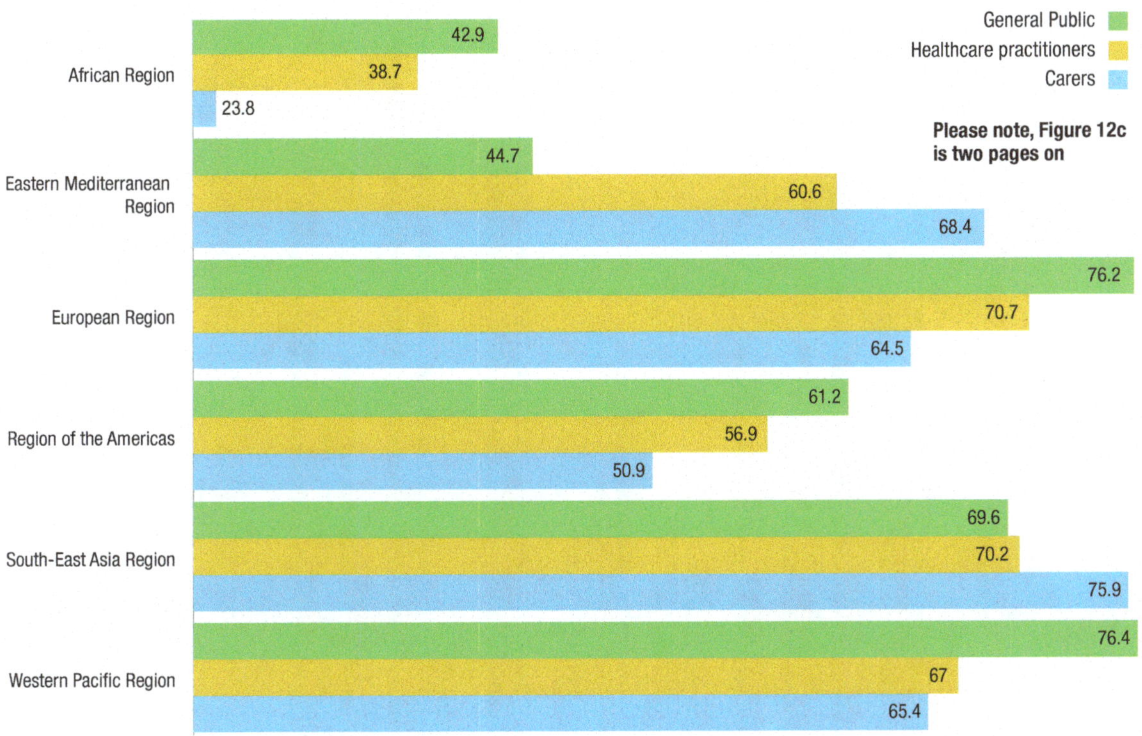


**Please note, Figure 12c is two pages on**

healthcare practitioners thought there enough competent physicians. Other countries might have elevated views of healthcare professionals, because they have limited first-hand experience of them.

## Healthcare practitioners (physicians and nurses) ignoring people with dementia

Around 40% of the general public think that healthcare practitioners (physicians and nurses) ignore people with dementia (38% in high-income, 49% in upper-middle income and 32.5% in low/lower middle-income countries). Similarly, as per the question about competence, the highest rates of thinking that healthcare practitioners ignore people with dementia were in the Eastern Mediterranean and the African regions (59% and 55.7% respectively, among the general public) and lowest in Europe (29.2%). However, there were high rates of concern (among the general public) about healthcare practitioners ignoring people with dementia in some European countries (59.3% in Iceland, 57.8% in

**Figure 11C.** Agreement that there are adequate community services for people living with dementia, by country (% agree)

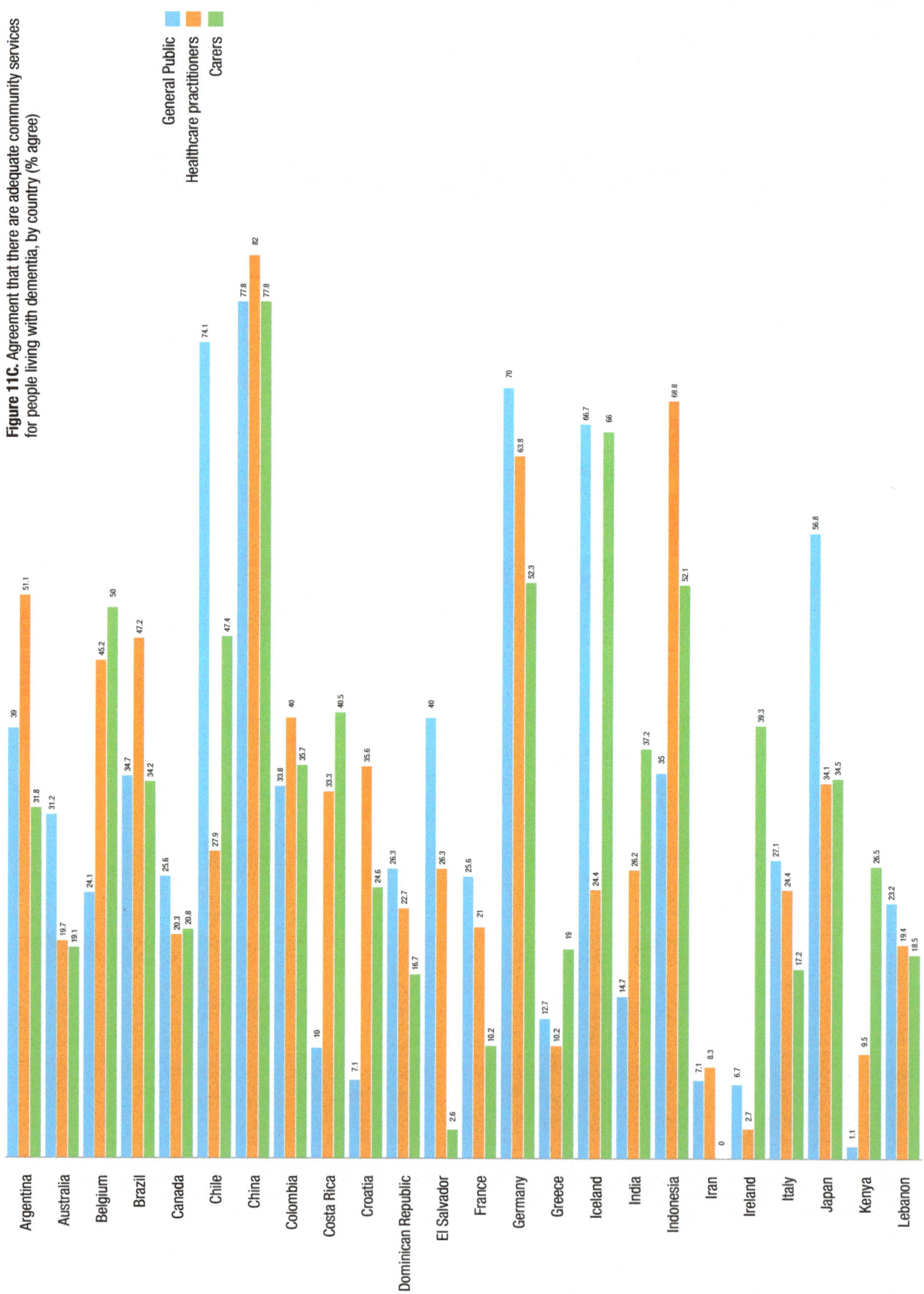

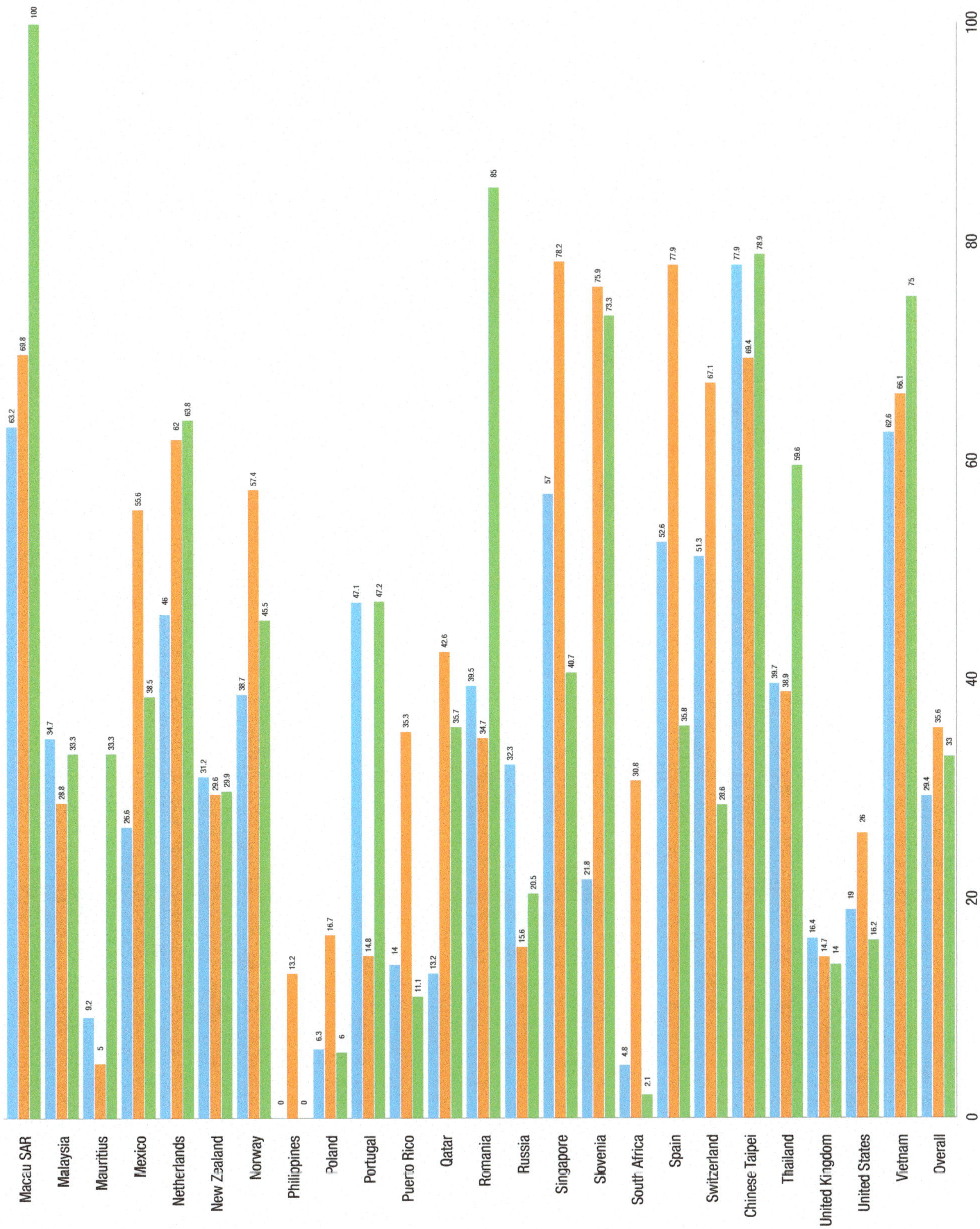
Macau SAR
Malaysia
Mauritius
Mexico
Netherlands
New Zealand
Norway
Philippines
Poland
Portugal
Puerto Rico
Qatar
Romania
Russia
Singapore
Slovenia
South Africa
Spain
Switzerland
Chinese Taipei
Thailand
United Kingdom
United States
Vietnam
Overall
0
20
40
60
80
100

**Figure 12C.** Agreement that there are competent healthcare practitioners for the diagnosis and treatment people living with dementia, by country (% agree)

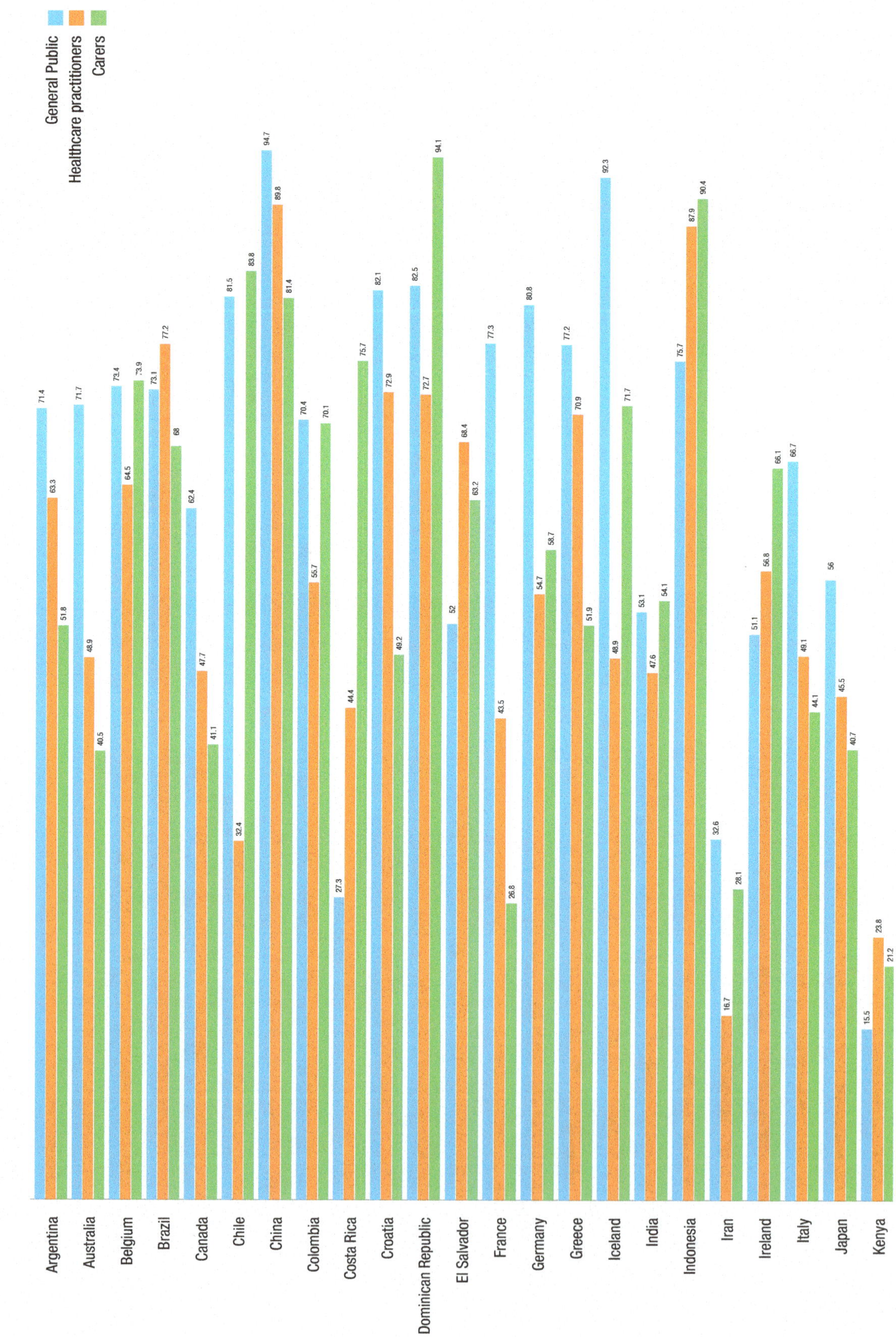

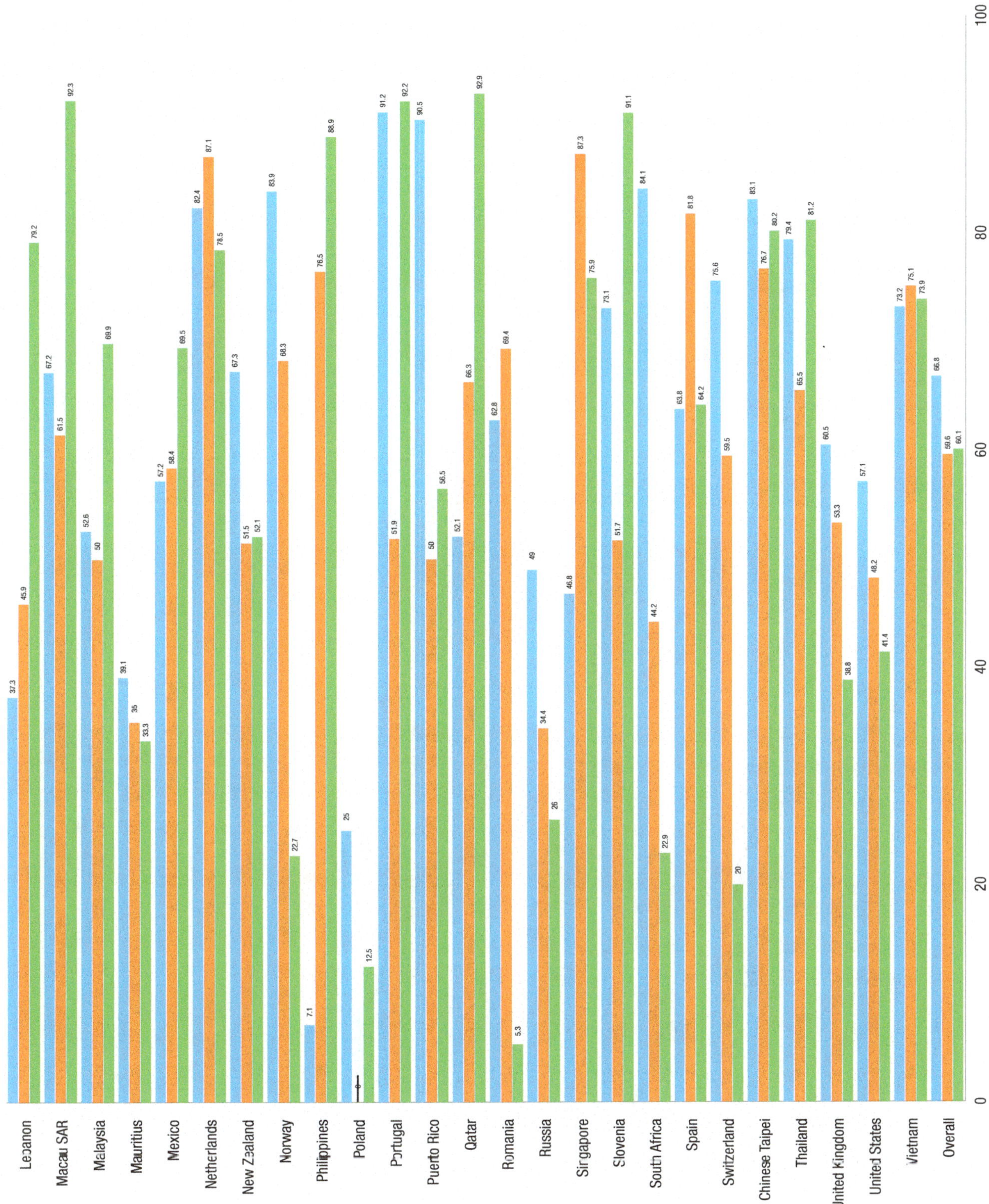
Lebanon 37.3 45.9 79.2
Macau SAR 67.2 61.5 92.3
Malaysia 52.6 50 69.9
Mauritius 39.1 35 33.3
Mexico 57.2 58.4 69.5
Netherlands 82.4 87.1 78.5
New Zealand 67.3 51.5 52.1
Norway 83.9 68.3 22.7
Philippines 7.1 76.5 88.9
Poland 25 0 12.5
Portugal 91.2 51.9 92.2
Puerto Rico 90.5 50 56.5
Qatar 52.1 66.3 92.9
Romania 62.8 69.4 5.3
Russia 49 34.4 26
Singapore 46.8 87.3 75.9
Slovenia 73.1 51.7 91.1
South Africa 84.1 44.2 22.9
Spain 63.8 81.8 64.2
Switzerland 75.6 59.5 20
Chinese Taipei 83.1 76.7 80.2
Thailand 79.4 65.5 81.2
United Kingdom 60.5 53.3 38.8
United States 57.1 48.2 41.4
Vietnam 73.2 75.1 73.9
Overall 66.8 59.6 60.1
0
20
40
60
80
100

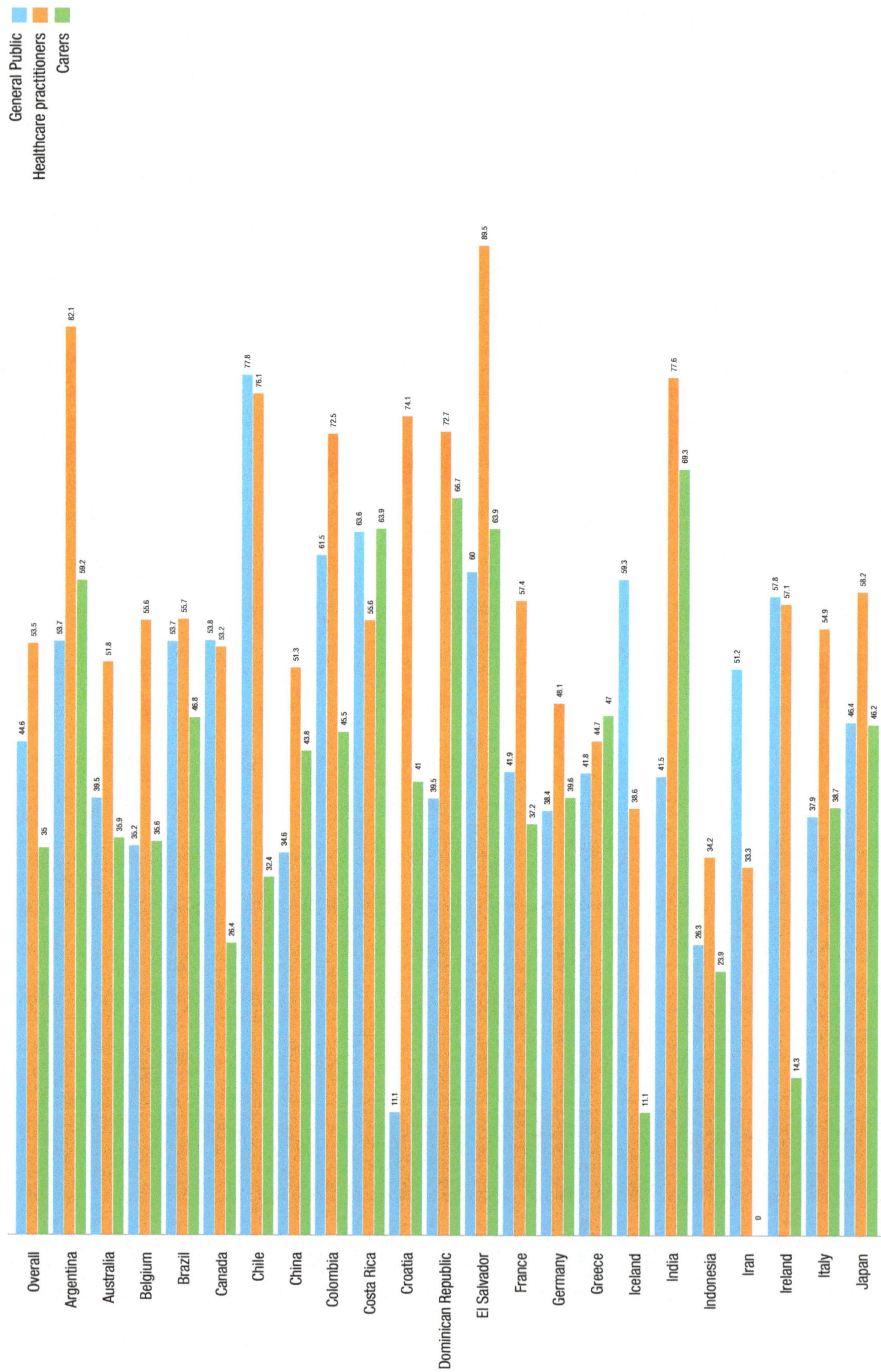


**Figure 13A.** Agreement that healthcare practitioners ignore the person living with dementia, by country (% agree)

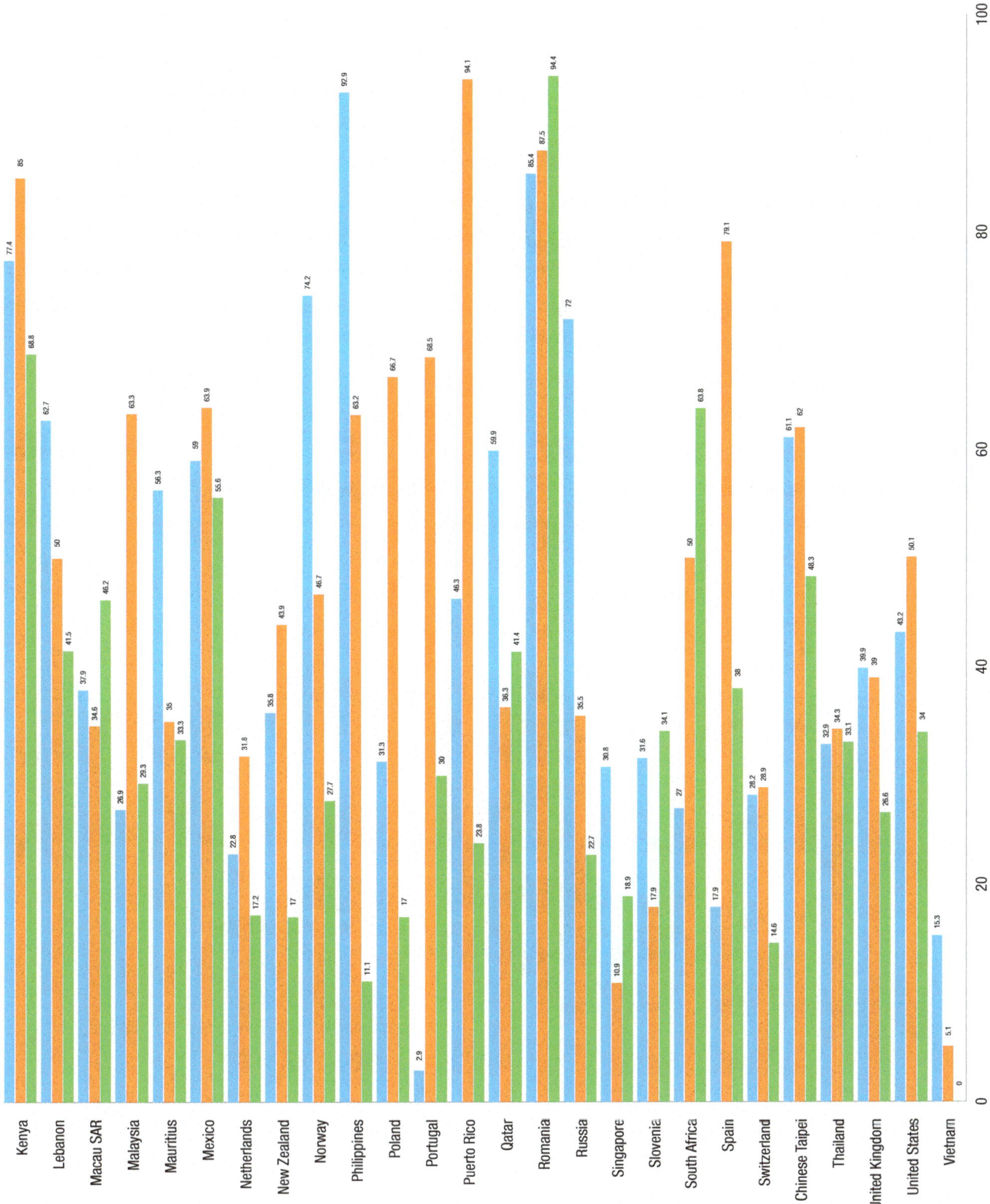
Kenya
Lebanon
Macau SAR
Malaysia
Mauritius
Mexico
Netherlands
New Zealand
Norway
Philippines
Poland
Portugal
Puerto Rico
Qatar
Romania
Russia
Singapore
Slovenia
South Africa
Spain
Switzerland
Chinese Taipei
Thailand
United Kingdom
United States
Vietnam
0
20
40
60
80
100

**Figure 13B.** Agreement that healthcare practitioners ignore the person living with dementia, by World Bank income group (% agree)

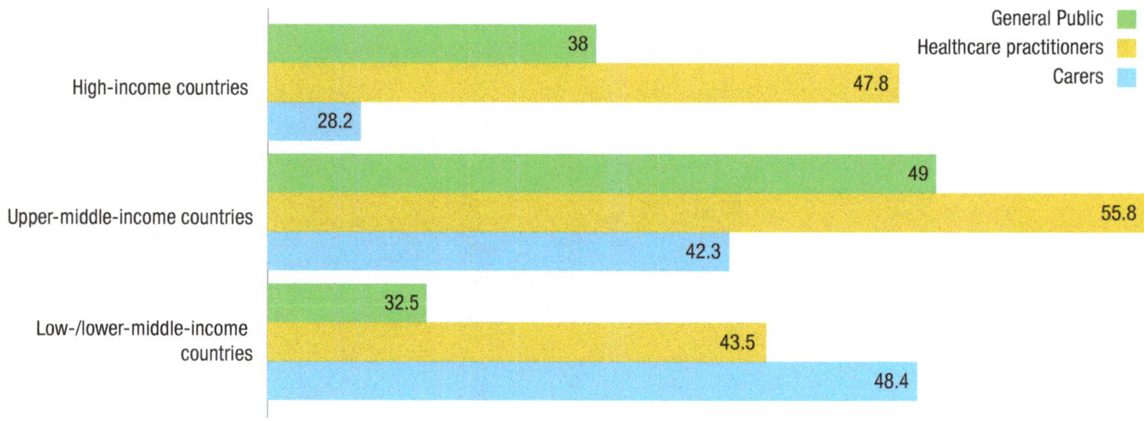


**Figure 13C.** Agreement that healthcare practitioners ignore the person living with dementia, by WHO Region (% agree)

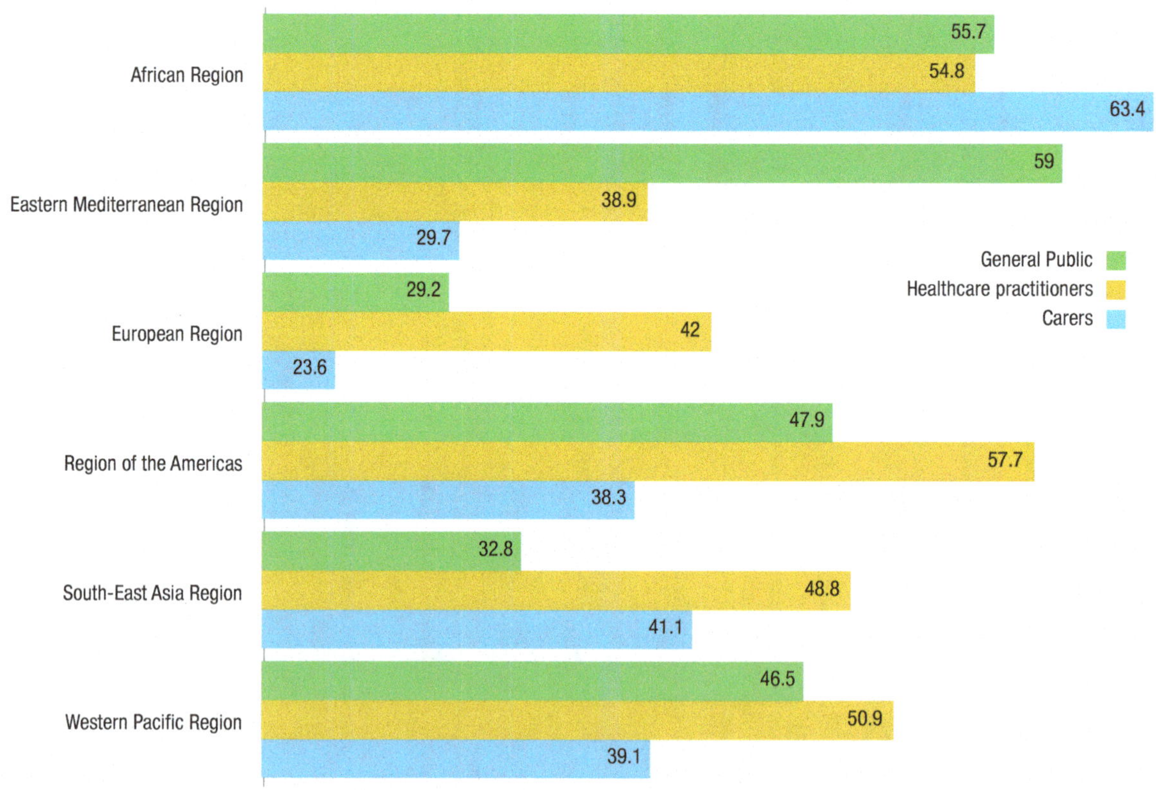


Ireland, 74.2% in Norway, 85.4% in Romania and 72% in Russia).

- The respondents who identified as healthcare practitioners were slightly more critical of their colleagues, with 47.8% in high-income, 55.8% in upper-middle income and 43.5% in low/lower-middle countries responding that healthcare practitioners ignore people with dementia.
- 33% of people think that if they had dementia, they would not be listened to by healthcare practitioners.

## Gender differences

The majority of survey respondents (nearly 80%) were women. (See description of survey respondents, page 63). Looking at the differences[iii] in responses between male and female respondents, male

(iii) We controlled for age, education, knowing someone with dementia, country.

**Figure 14.** Percentage of women and men agreeing with each statement – all statements represent responses from the general public except for the first one which refers to carers only
**Indicates statistical significance*

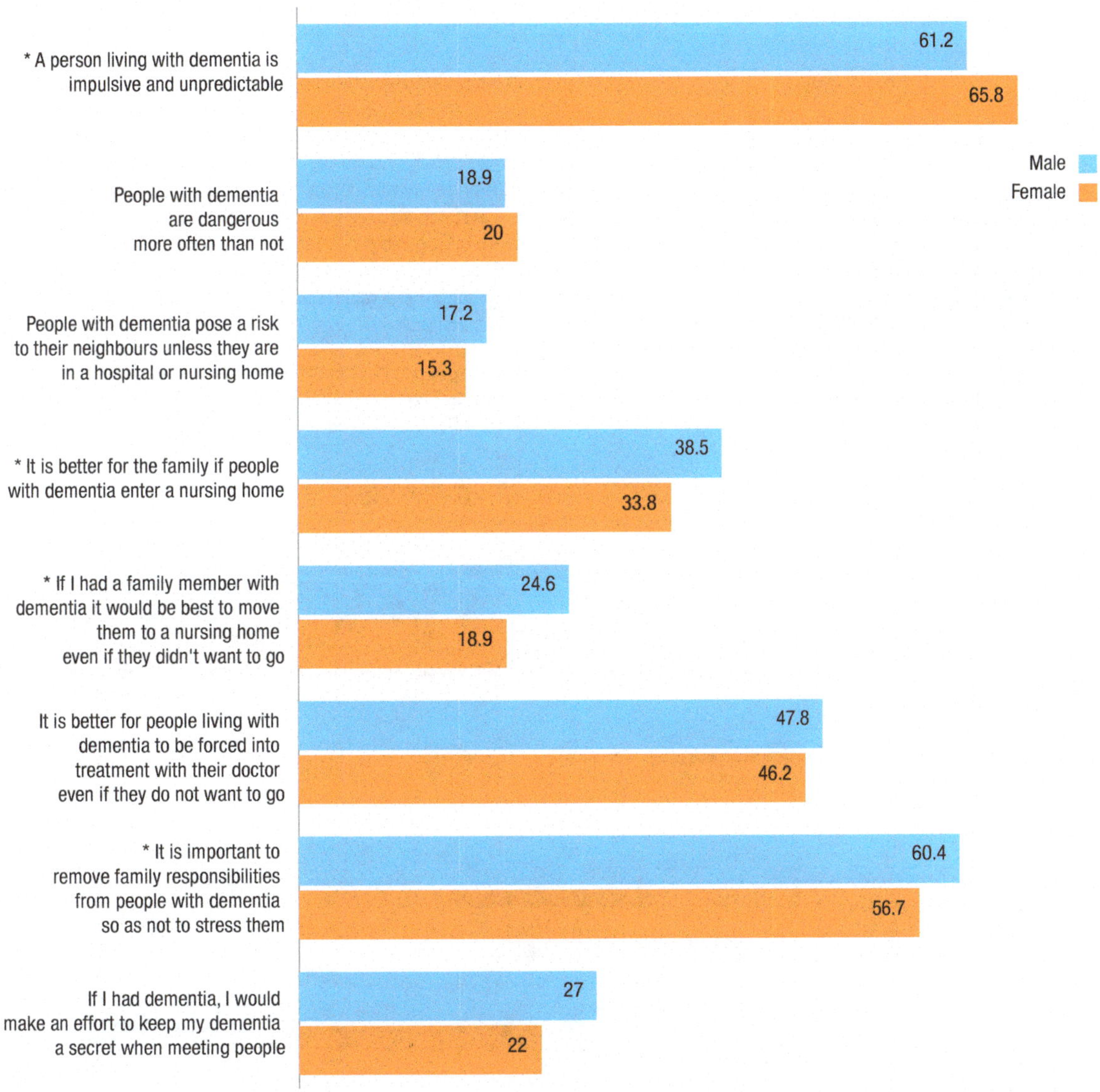


respondents tended to be somewhat more stigmatising in their views of people living with dementia compared to female respondents. Males were more likely to think that people living with dementia were impulsive or unpredictable, that it is better for the family if the person is in a nursing home and that they should be forced into a home or forced to accept treatment. They are more likely to think family responsibilities should be removed from someone with dementia so as not to stress them, and they are more likely to want to keep dementia a secret (see Figure 14). Males are also less likely to be stressed by their caring and other responsibilities. It is possible, particularly given the suggestion above, that male respondents are less likely to be the sole or primary carer[iv].

Males are less likely to say they would seek help from a healthcare practitioner if they thought they might have dementia. Males are, in fact, less likely to seek support from any of the alternative sources offered by the questionnaire (friend, family member, online/internet, healthcare practitioner or other) with one exception. Men are markedly more likely to seek help from their partner than are women. 75.5% of male respondents would seek help from their partner compared to only

(iv) Differences statistically significant at the P<.001 level.

**Figure 15.** Percentage of respondents agreeing that they are 'often stressed between caring and meeting other responsibilities', by gender*
**Indicates statistical significance*

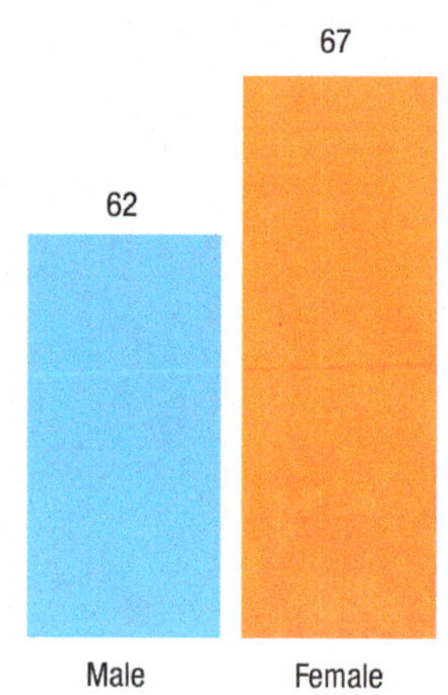


62.1% of women. People answering these questions were members of the public who have not identified as carers on the questionnaire. It may be that women are more likely than men to be acting as gatekeepers to informal and formal health and social care networks. Unfortunately, we do not have information on the marital status of respondents, so we don't know if this is due to a greater proportion of single female respondents. Given that our sample is skewed towards older ages, we looked to see if this finding held true at younger ages (when people would be less likely to be widowed). The difference remains large for under-60s (67% versus 74%) but is much smaller for under-50s (68% versus 72%). While it's possible this reflects something about marital status, it could also be that younger respondents have different gender relations which affect their answers to this question.

There was not much variation in healthcare practitioner attitudes towards people living with dementia according to gender. However, male healthcare practitioners were

**Figure 16.** Healthcare provider attitudes towards dementia, by gender (% agree)
**Indicates statistical significance*

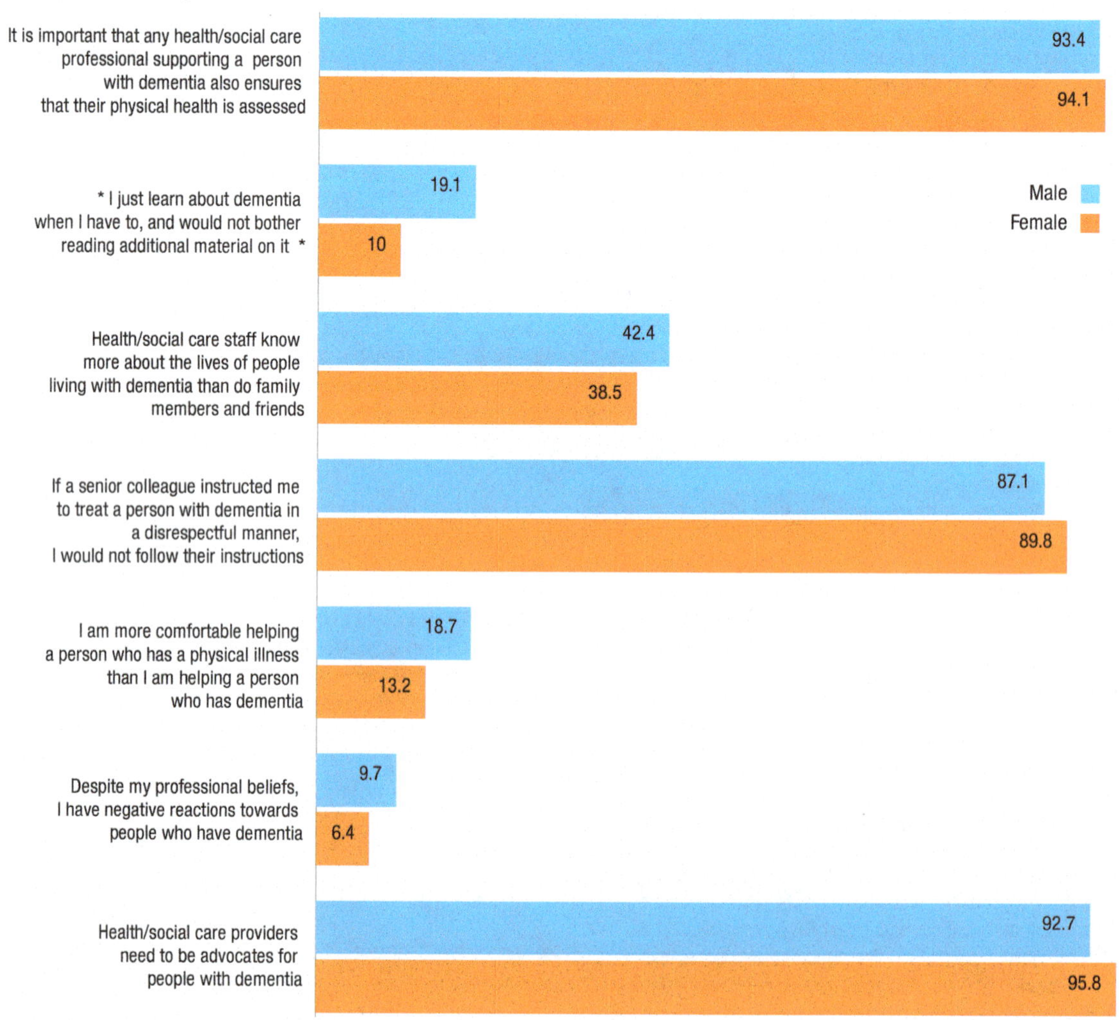

**Figure 17.** Agreement among the general public that 'I would take a genetic profiling test to learn whether I am at risk of developing dementia', by country (% agree)

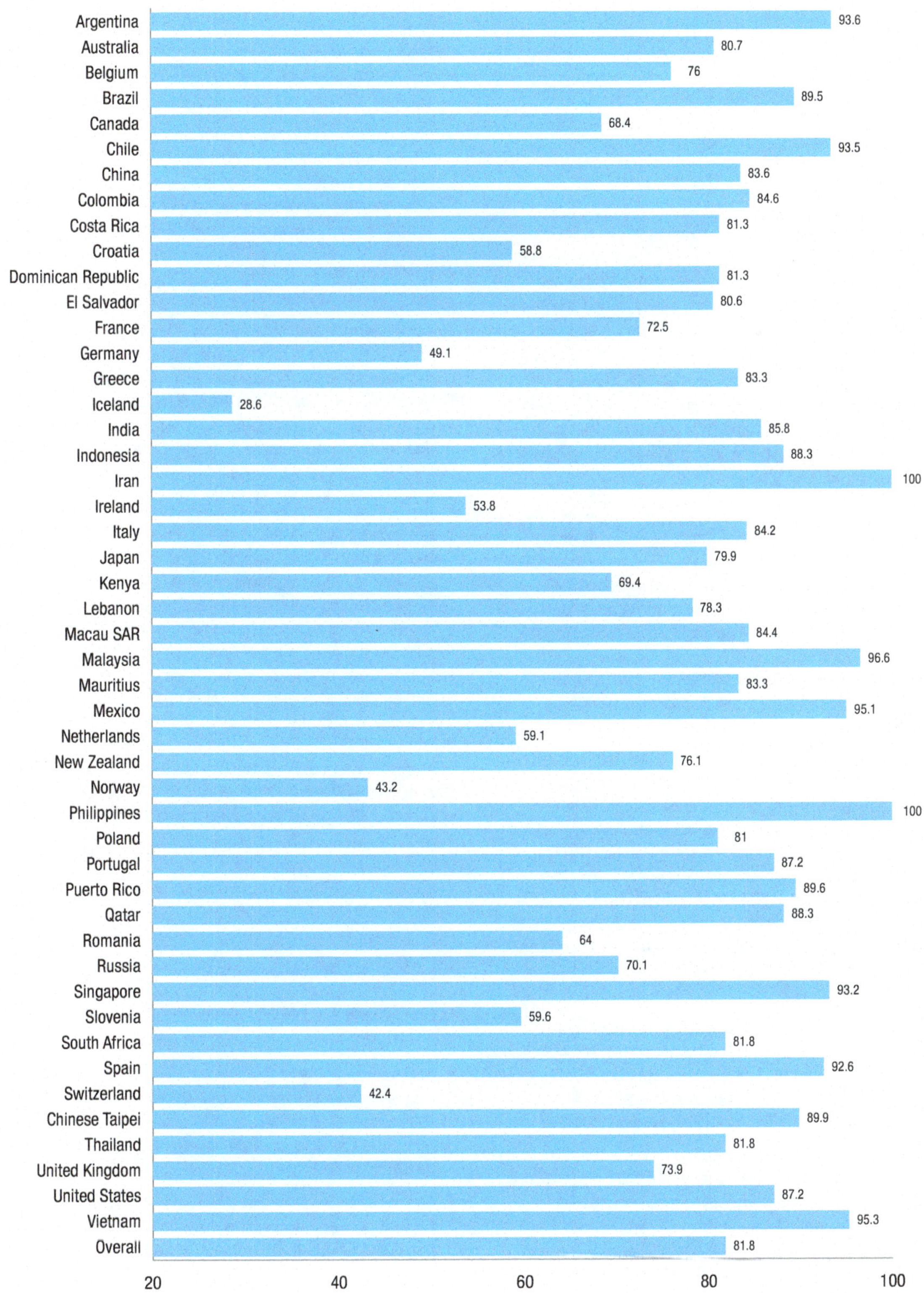

more likely to say they would just learn about dementia when they have to and would not bother reading additional material on it (19.1% vs. 10.0%). 18.7% of male healthcare practitioners said they agreed to feeling more comfortable helping a person who has a physical illness than helping a person who has dementia.

## Attitudes

### Personal risk

The vast majority of the general public think they could develop dementia at some point in their lifetime (95.2%) and are concerned about developing dementia at some point (78.2%). Although there are currently no disease modifying treatments for dementia, over two-thirds of respondents (81.8%) would take a genetic profiling test to learn whether they are at risk.

### Attitudes among the general public and healthcare practitioners about people living with dementia by country income groups and regions

When comparing attitudes about people living with dementia it is important to note that, because in many parts of the world there are low rates of diagnosis, it is likely that those who are known to have dementia in areas with low diagnostic rates are at more advanced stages. This may shape the perceptions of respondents.

- All regions had over 80% agreement that people living with dementia can participate in a variety of activities.
- Overall, the people living in South-East Asia were most likely to think that people with dementia are dangerous: 45.4% of respondents said 'people living with dementia are dangerous more often than not', compared to 25.7% in the Western Pacific, 17.2% in Africa, 14.6% in Americas, 15% in the European region, and 13.9% in the Eastern Mediterranean. This is interesting considering relatively high proportions of people living in the South-East Asia region are willing to have a family member living with dementia to move in with them.
- Views among healthcare practitioners showed a similar trend and agreement that people living with dementia are dangerous: by WHO Region: South-East Asia (48.1%), Eastern Mediterranean (31%), Western Pacific (18.4%) European Region (10.5%), Americas (8.9%).
- When answering whether they agreed 'a person living with dementia is impulsive and unpredictable' by WHO Region: African Region (70.5%), South-East Asia (70.1%), Europe (68.8%), Eastern Mediterranean Region (64.5%), Americas (62%), Western Pacific Region (49.5%).
- The majority of respondents felt it was important to remove responsibilities of people living with dementia as it might stress them. Agreement tended to be lower among carers (47.5%) compared to the general public (60%). In terms of region, those among the general public in the African region had the highest agreement (72.1%) followed by Europe (71.2%), Eastern Mediterranean Region (57.1%), Western Pacific Region (54.8%), Americas (46.6%) and South-East Asia (38.1%).
- This is interesting given that many of the experiences of discrimination reported by people living with dementia pertain to loss of status and loss of roles (See section below on experiences of discrimination among people living with dementia).

### Attitudes about treatment for people living with dementia

Results suggest that people living in high income countries are more likely to agree that people living with dementia should be moved into a nursing home even if they don't want to go (25%). This is higher than those living in upper middle-income (14.6%) or low / lower-middle income countries (8.6%). Respondents were also more likely to force someone living with dementia to a nursing home if it was not a member of their family.

When looking at the WHO Regions, the European Region had the highest proportion of respondents agreeing that 'If I had a family member with dementia it would be best to move them into a nursing home even if they didn't want to go (27.5%) compared to Western Pacific Region (22.7%), the Americas (17.5%), Africa (16.3%), Eastern Mediterranean Region (11.4%), South-East Asia (11.2%). There are important differences, worldwide, in both the availability of nursing homes and cultural and religious beliefs that may influence these attitudes. It is interesting that people living in South-East Asia had the lowest number agreeing that people living with dementia should be moved into a nursing home even if they didn't want to go and that they should have responsibilities removed from them; however, they had the highest feelings of fear because people living with dementia are dangerous.

## Knowledge

### Knowledge and causal attribution of dementia

- The vast majority of the general public think that dementia has biological roots, for example agreeing that dementia is in part a brain disease (93.7%), that it is due to a head or brain injury (71.3%) or is due to APOE[v] (87.5%)
- Significantly fewer respondents think that lifestyle factors play any part in the development of dementia, for example due to an unhealthy lifestyle (54.5%) or lack of family support (26%)

(v) Apolipoprotein e (APOE) is a gene which is associated with a higher risk of developing Alzheimer's disease.

**Figure 18A.** Attitudes among the general public towards people living with dementia by World Bank income group (% agree)

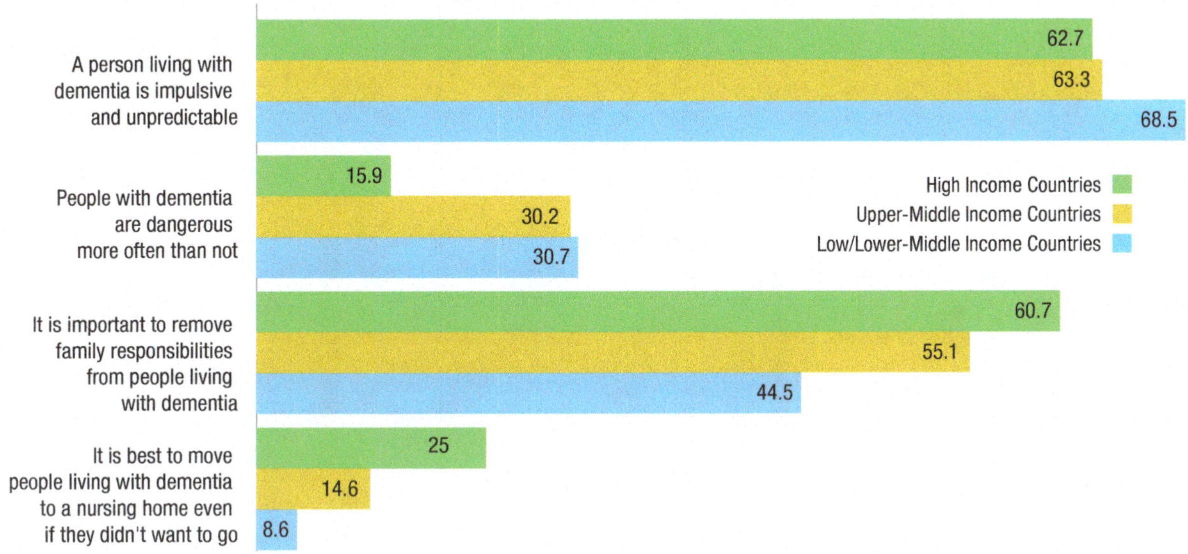


**Figure 18B.** Attitudes among healthcare practitioners towards people living with dementia by World Bank income group (% agree)

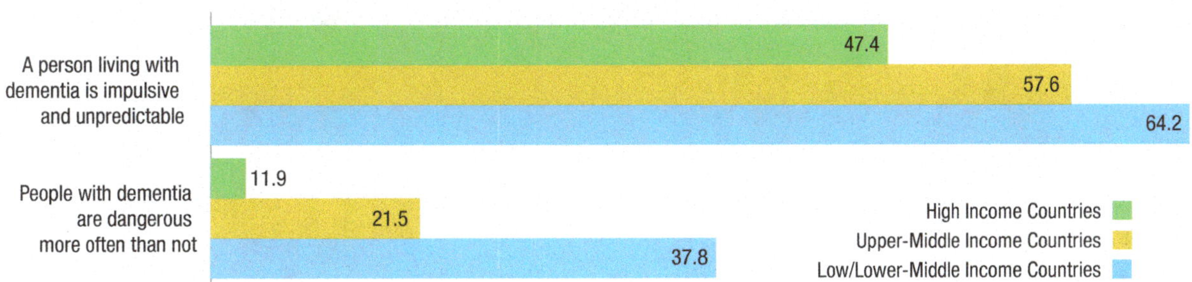


- More than two-thirds of respondents still feel that dementia is caused by normal ageing (70.1%). This is an important result considering global awareness raising efforts which position dementia as not being a natural part of ageing, and this area is explored further in the expert essays and case studies later in the report.
- More than one-fifth of people think that dementia is a result of external forces like bad luck (21.7 %), God's will (8.7%) or witchcraft (1.9%). Witchcraft and being "bewitched" are considered in a number of the report case studies, looking at how such beliefs impact on seeking out information, advice, treatment and support.
- Carers (60.6%) were less likely than the general public to agree that dementia is part of normal aging. Although less likely than the general public, almost 62% of healthcare practitioners that responded to the survey feel that dementia is part of normal ageing. This opens up for discussion the need for increased levels of awareness and training amongst healthcare practitioners and perhaps the figure is exacerbated by the fact there have been no disease modifying treatment breakthroughs for over 15 years and the current medical treatments available have limited long-term effectiveness.

## Knowledge of treatment and risk factors

- The vast majority of the general public think that it is useful to receive a formal diagnosis (88.1%).
- The vast majority of respondents from the general public also think that people living with dementia can enjoy life (87%) and that there are things we can do to improve the lives of people with dementia (90%). For example, most people think that a person with dementia's situation is likely to improve with social support (79.3%) and that people with a healthy lifestyle have a lower risk of dementia (64.3%).
- However, almost half think that a person with dementia's memory will never improve even with medical treatment (47.9%).
- About a quarter (25.2%) think that there is nothing

**Figure 18C.** Attitudes among the general public towards people living with dementia by WHO Region (% agree)

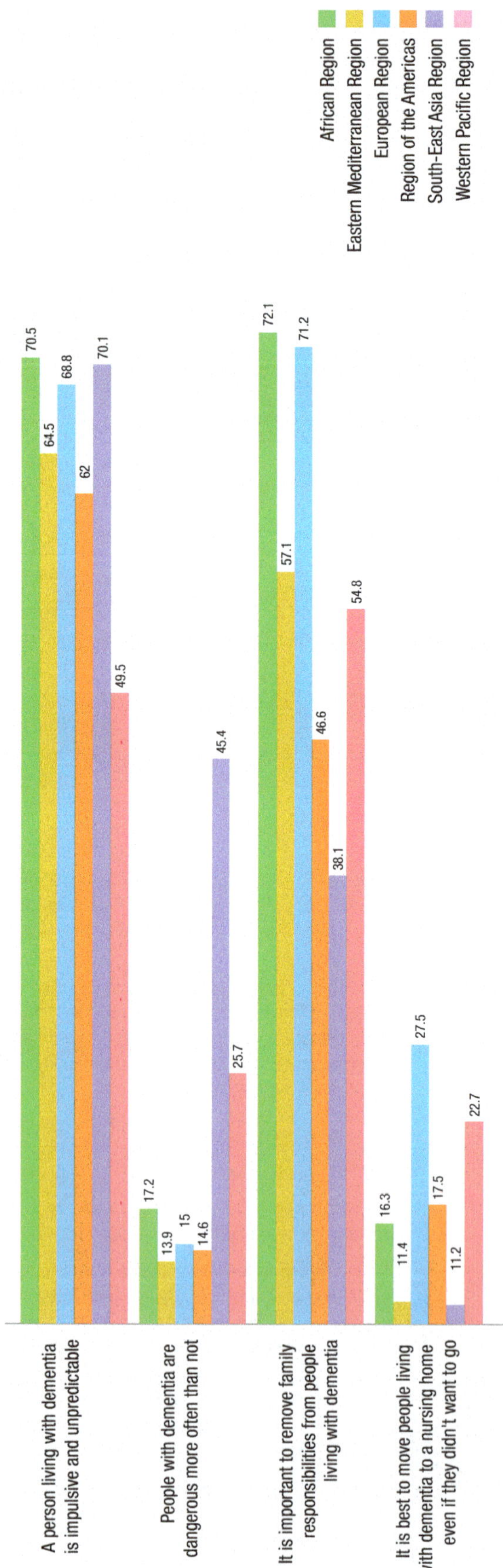


**Figure 19.** Attitudes among healthcare practitioners towards people living with dementia by WHO Region (% agree)

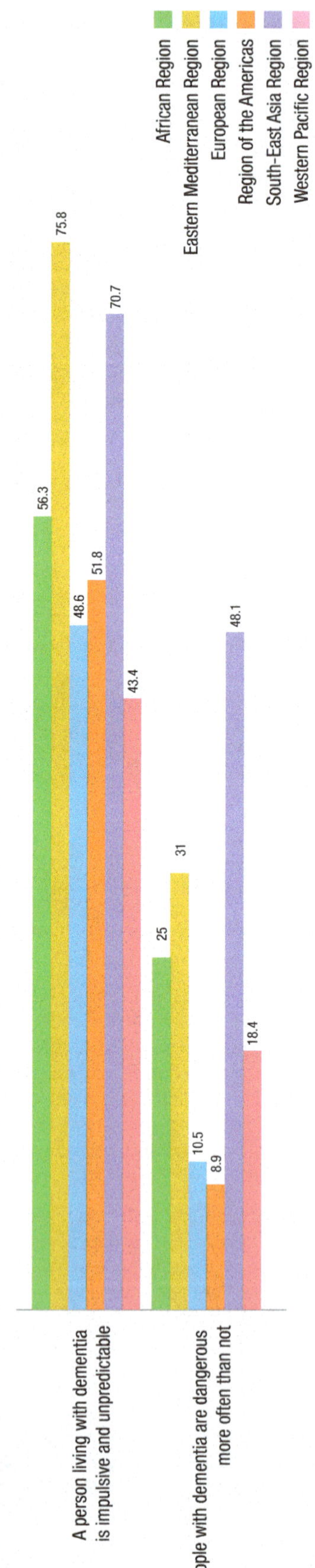

**Figure 20.** Agreement among the general public that people with dementia are perceived as dangerous, by country (% agree)

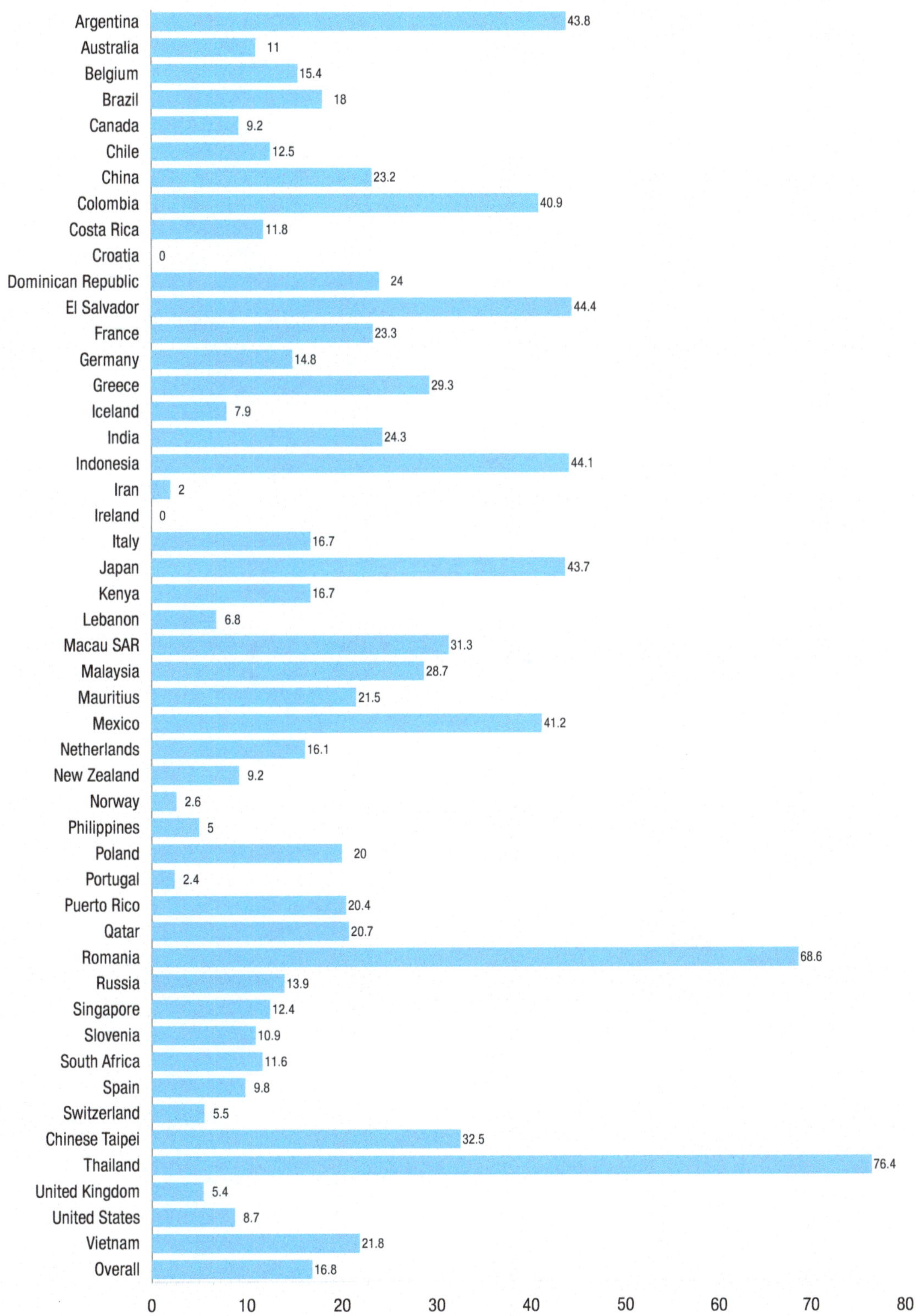

**Figure 21.** Agreement among healthcare practitioners that people with dementia are perceived as dangerous, by country (% agree)

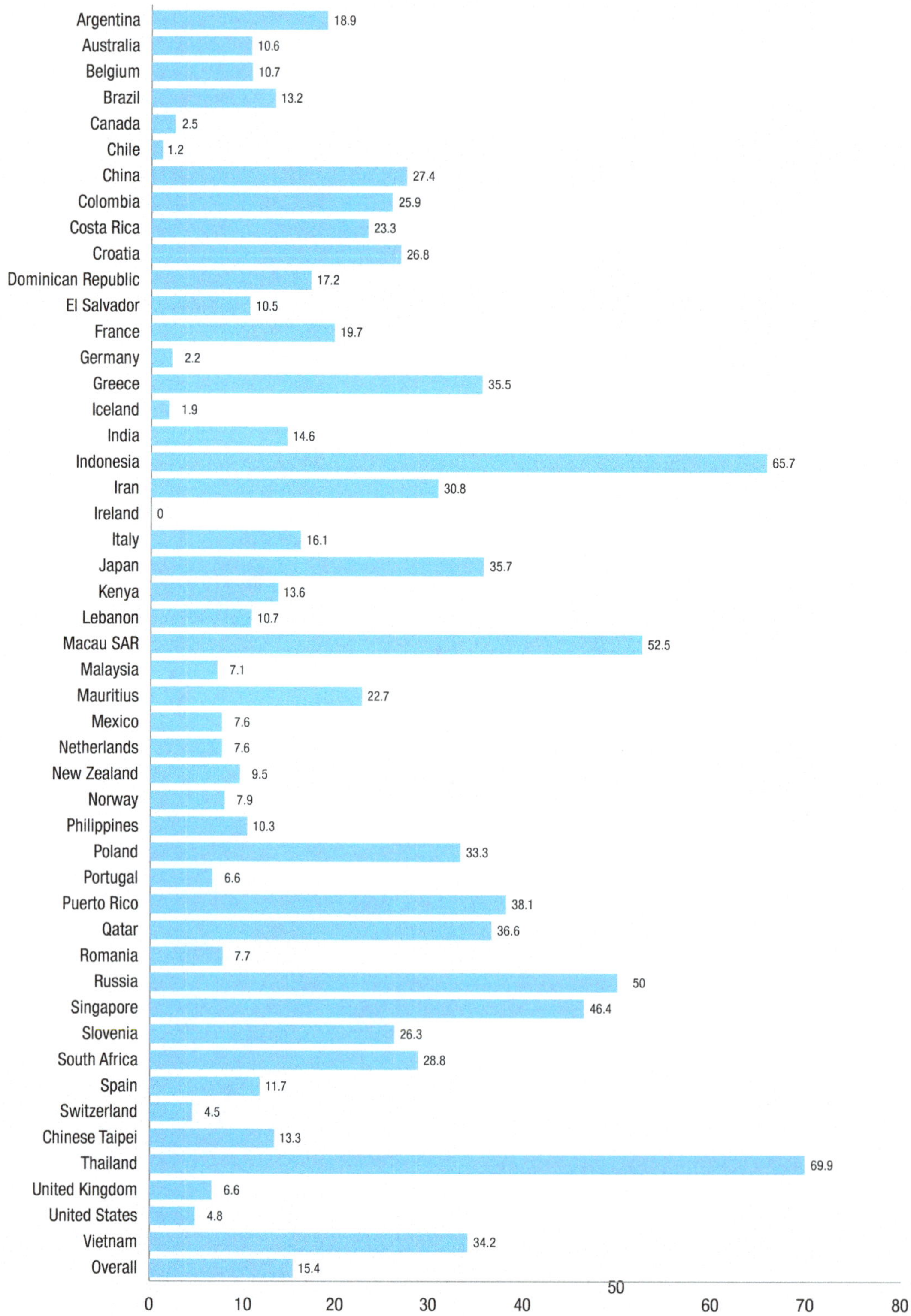

**Figure 22.** Agreement among the general public that people living with dementia are impulsive and unpredictable, by country (% agree)

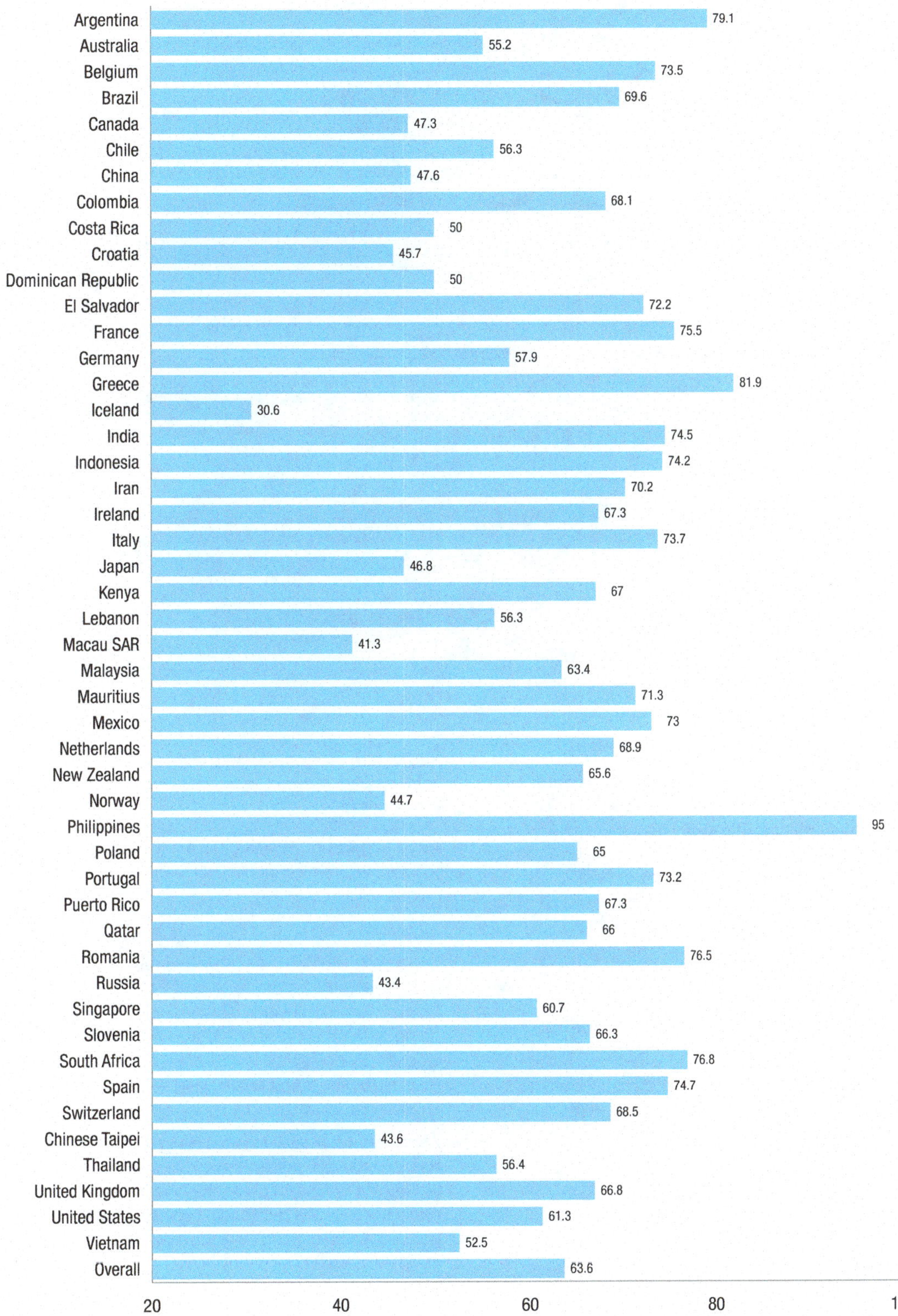

**Figure 23.** People living with dementia are / the person I care for is a good source of knowledge (% agree)

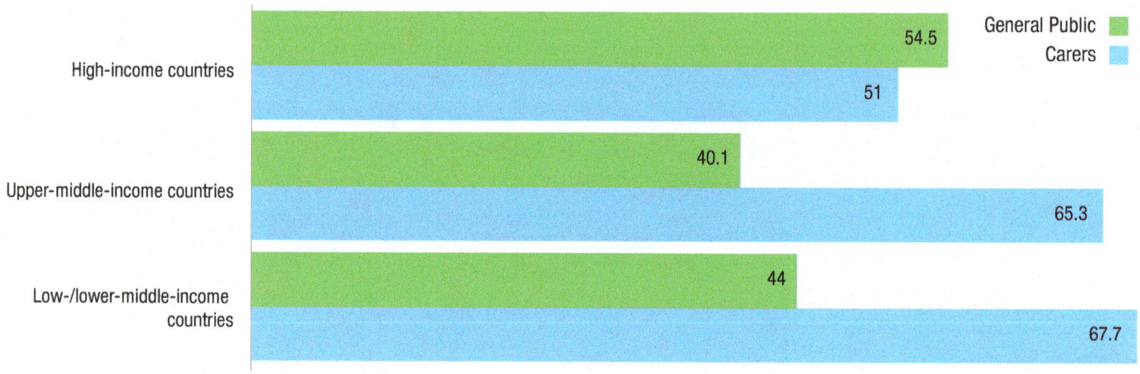
General Public
Carers
High-income countries
54.5
51
Upper-middle-income countries
40.1
65.3
Low-/lower-middle-income countries
44
67.7

**Figure 24.** People living with dementia / the person I care for can pass on valued traditions (% agree)

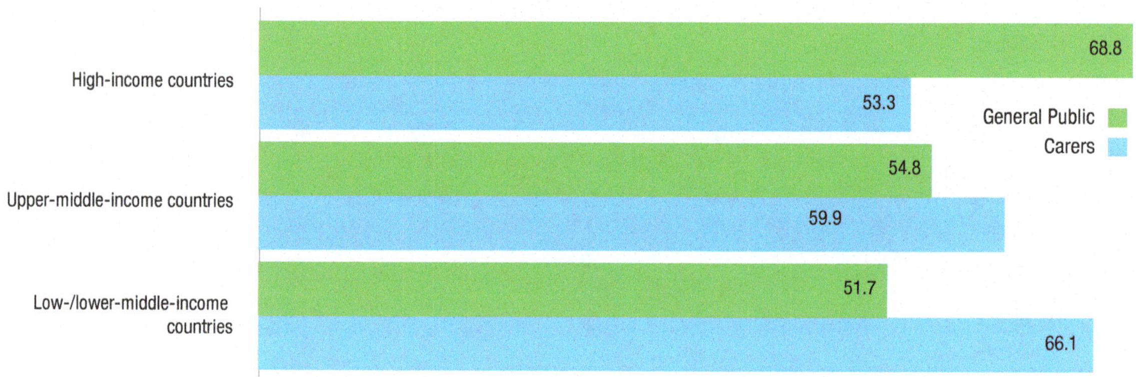
High-income countries
68.8
53.3
General Public
Carers
Upper-middle-income countries
54.8
59.9
Low-/lower-middle-income countries
51.7
66.1

we can do to prevent dementia. This presents an important opportunity for public health interventions as there are actions we can take to reduce the risk of developing dementia. The WHO dementia risk reduction guidelines published in 2019 strongly recommend public health interventions to help people cease smoking, increase physical activity, treat high blood pressure and manage diabetes. It also recommended interventions to manage cholesterol, hearing loss, depression, weight and diet, as well as interventions that reduce harmful drinking, enable social activity and provide cognitive training.

## Consequences of stigma and discrimination for people living with dementia

As we collected data from people living with dementia, this provided an opportunity to directly link public views of people living with dementia to experiences of people living with dementia. As respondents came from a number of diverse countries, this allowed us to examine whether living in a country with a higher level of stigma was associated with lower wellbeing, quality of life, concealment of dementia and reported experienced stigma among people living with dementia. We also looked at how individual factors (age, gender and education) were related to outcomes for people living with dementia.

Findings suggest public attitudes and behaviour are associated with consequences for people living with dementia.

- At the individual level females living with dementia and those with university education had higher levels of wellbeing. At the country level, those living in a country where the public felt more embarrassed going out with a friend or relative with dementia or where the public felt it is important to remove family responsibilities from people living with dementia had lower levels of wellbeing.
- At the individual level females living with dementia had lower levels of self-esteem. At the country level, individuals living with dementia who resided in a country where the public felt more embarrassed going out with a friend or relative with dementia had lower self-esteem.
- At the individual level females living with dementia were less likely to conceal their dementia. At the country level, those living with dementia who resided

in a country where healthcare practitioner felt as comfortable talking to a person with dementia as talking to a person with physical illness, were also less likely to conceal their dementia.

- At the individual level females living with dementia reported experiencing greater impact of stigma, while those with university education reported less impact. At a country level those living in a country where the public felt it is important to remove family responsibilities from people living with dementia reported lower levels of stigma impact.

### Quotations provided by people living with dementia

Respondents living with dementia were given the opportunity to write about their experiences of interacting with others in society. Many quotes illustrate discrimination and feelings of having been pushed out by friends or avoided. Several respondents refer to being discriminated against, or excluded, by their own family:

*I call it the friendship divorce. I have lost a fair amount of people in my life that at one time considered friends.*

*Many have told me they are not at all interested in 'the dementia journey'*

*People avoid you because they're not sure what to say.*

*Shunned by hundreds in my home town. People would sooner have stage 4 breast cancer than my diagnosis. Couldn't look me in the eye*

*A limited number of long time friends have shied away since my diagnosis. They will send Birthday, Christmas cards but no phone calls or offers to get together.*

Comments reveal perceived discomfort of others, or sweeping assumptions about capabilities:

*Some friends don't like to talk to me because I repeat*

*I have a few people say don't talk to her she has no idea what she is talking about*

*A friend thought I could not cope with things and felt I should not be out of the house. We had words over it and we really haven't spoken much since. I think I have found my true friends and that's all I need.*

People experience low levels of tolerance for some behaviours:

*When I make statements that are out of character some friends and family have taken it personally and stopped talking to me.*

Additional comments and quotations can be found in the extended, technical version of this report.

## Methodology

### Overall Methodology

These findings come from a survey of almost 70,000 individuals from 155 countries or territories. 66% of participants completed the survey in a non-English language.

The aim of the survey was to understand people's stigma-related knowledge, attitudes and experiences in relation to people living with dementia and questions were tailored to capture overarching knowledge, attitudes, behaviours and experiences. Respondents were asked to self-identify among four groups: people living with dementia, their family and/or carers, healthcare practitioners and the general public. Tailoring and dividing the survey into four target groups enabled us to compare findings across groups but also understand the specific experiences of certain groups.

In this report, we describe and discuss the results at a global and sometimes regional level, with some country level comparisons. More country level data and comparison can be found in the online technical report and appendix. We chose to group countries according to two methodologies: (1) by WHO Region (i.e., geographical locations) and (2) by World Bank income groups. By using these two categories, we aimed to capture cultural and economic differences. In addition, selected questions are presented by individual countries with at least 100 respondents.

### How we developed the stigma survey questions

We selected several questions for each of the four target groups based on previous surveys and a review of the academic literature (research papers). We conceptualised stigma as covering three domains: (1) knowledge and causal attribution of dementia, (2) attitudes and beliefs about people living with dementia and (3) behaviour towards persons living with dementia and their carers.

Targeting these key domains, we developed tailored questionnaires for the four groups of respondents. We aimed for overlap in questions between these four groups where possible, but also included questions specific to each group.

The questionnaires were developed through a rapid review of previous work on stigma in dementia. Based on relevant studies, we first identified constructs which were reported as important for people living with dementia or their carers. For qualitative studies, these were themes that emerged as key aspects of stigma experiences or knowledge, attitudes or beliefs reported as important among study participants (e.g. patronising behaviour by family members of people living with dementia). For quantitative studies, these would typically represent any knowledge, attitudes or behaviour which were significantly associated with quality of life, functioning or well-being outcomes among people with dementia or their carers or key stigma outcomes (for example, proportion of people living with dementia experiencing stigma). In parallel, we reviewed the literature for stigma related dementia items, including all items from studies included in a recently published systematic review of the literature[3]. We also adapted items related to the stigma of mental illness from a recent global survey which incorporated a comprehensive review of stigma items and domains to people living with dementia [4]. All identified items were then mapped onto the identified constructs and further categorised into the three stigma domains (knowledge and attribution; attitudes and beliefs; behaviour). For each construct, we then reviewed all items and selected those deemed most appropriate and reliable.

We aimed to develop questionnaires for each of the four target groups with a completion time of approximately 10-15 minutes and were not able to include all items. The constructs were therefore reviewed by stigma experts and representatives from Alzheimer's associations in order to identify those that should be prioritised in our survey.

## What other questions did we ask?

Participants were informed that this survey was looking to understand what they knew and thought about dementia; the survey was not described to participants as a survey on stigma.

To examine differences across regions and personal characteristics, we also collected information on: gender, age, highest level of education, country/territory of residence, area of residence (e.g. urban or rural), membership of a minority group and employment status.

## Ensuring the survey was understandable

The survey questions were reviewed and tested by several stakeholders, including people living with dementia, NGO representatives and expert researchers, before being launched to the wider public in April 2019. This was to ensure that the questions captured relevant topics from the perspective of people living with dementia and that the questions were clear and comprehensible. We also contacted world experts in the field of stigma research to ensure that the questions were theoretically and conceptually relevant. All questions were optional and participants were told they did not have to answer anything they did not wish to.

We allowed for a proxy respondent, something used by 80 people living with dementia. We were also keen to enable survey respondents to write about their own experiences and provided opportunities to write longer answers in a text box.

## How we translated the survey

One of our aims was to make the survey as accessible as possible. For this reason, the survey was translated into 32 different languages, and most of the translations were done by volunteers and staff of ADI member organisations. To ensure that translations were comparable across languages, we requested all sites to follow WHO guidelines [5]. Specifically, this comprised three stages: (1) forward-translation, (2) back-translation and (3) focus group 'concept checking'. The forward-translation required the translator to have his/her local language as their first language, with English as his/her second language. Any disputed items would be discussed with their study team. For the back-translation stage, when possible a different translator, whose first language was English and second language was the local language, would back-translate the document back into English. The study team was then asked to compare the new and original English versions, highlighting and resolving any differences in translation.

## How we collected the data

The survey was 10-15 minutes in length, with questions tailored for each of the four groups: people living with dementia, their family and/or carers, healthcare practitioner and the general public. Most questions were multiple choice, with very few open-ended responses. The survey was delivered in a flexible format, either: (1) self-completed online or (2) in person via a mobile device with a volunteer. If needed, paper forms could be used and the survey data later entered into the app by volunteers.

## The online survey

Most respondents completed the anonymous online survey using a web-based platform called Qualtrics. The online survey was an effective way to distribute the survey across the world, in the limited time frame which was available. For example, groups of people with dementia and their carers who are active on discussion boards, social media sites, and online in general helped to promote the survey. The survey was available to visitors of the ADI website and the survey link was emailed to contacts within the field of Alzheimer's and dementia, social care organisations, support groups, charities and faith-based organisations, all across the world.

Although online recruitment poses the risk of only including people with computers, the more highly educated and the most active members of the dementia community, the information from this survey provides valuable insights into the issues related to stigma and how this impacts the lives of people living with dementia, their families and society as a whole. We also tried to compensate for this risk by undertaking some data collection in more rural areas or with harder-to-reach populations using a mobile-based platform called Mobenzi, where data collection took place in-person.

## The in-person survey

The survey was also distributed by health and community workers in some rural regions and places without internet access using Mobenzi, enabling people to complete the survey on a smartphone or tablet. A total of 29 responses were collected in-person. Mobenzi is a survey tool administered via mobile devices that can be used off-line, thus enabling data collection in areas without internet access. Once surveys are completed and an internet connection is available, the data are uploaded to an online survey management platform. The survey questions and response options used in-person (via Mobenzi) were identical to those used in the online survey (via Qualtrics).

Some of the ADI member organisations facilitated access to the online survey to people without access to internet at their own offices and events.

## Recruitment strategy

Capturing the views of each target group required a different recruitment strategy. Generally, we aimed to achieve good representation across gender, age, socioeconomic group and urbanicity. We also wanted to make a considered effort in capturing the voices of individuals in rural areas.

We ran webinars for several of the ADI member organisations (in English and Spanish) and suggested two strategies to encourage diversity in our study population: (1) snowball sampling for the online survey and (2) targeted recruitment for the survey delivered by Mobenzi by volunteers in the community.

Using the snowball sampling technique, our contacts were encouraged to identify people with good social networks to complete the survey. Each person was asked to identify 3-4 additional individuals who could complete the survey. Contacts were then asked to further distribute the link to 3-4 further constituents and the social networks within their countries. Healthcare practitioners and members of the public who saw the survey link online could also raise awareness by sharing the link among their networks.

For the in-person survey, it was important to identify venues associated with the target characteristics (e.g., different types of shopping centres – some which attract young people, and some which attract persons of an older age). It was also important to explain to target groups why the survey was important and should be completed. For example, when asking healthcare practitioner to complete the survey, it was important to explain the reasons for the survey in a clear and concise manner, using key statistics to stress the importance and urgency of tho topic matter.

## Data security and consent

Participants were informed that their responses would be anonymous. They were also informed that survey data would be stored securely and did not include any personal identifiers. All data has been treated as confidential and kept on secure networks which are password protected. The Mobenzi app uses a secure format that complies with GDPR privacy legislation. Data storage, backup and recovery practices to eliminate data loss events are built into the app. All participants provided consent.

## How we analysed the data

Because our sample was a convenience sample, we performed a series of adjustments to allow for comparisons across countries and country groups. First, we developed survey weights which account for sample selection. Weights were developed to match characteristics of the sample recruited to the nationally representative characteristics in each country according to gender, age and educational level and were used in all analyses. Responses with weights greater than 20 were excluded (less than 0.2% of the sample) were excluded due to their non-representativeness [6]. For country comparisons, we also performed a pooled estimation technique (the meta-proportion command which is available in the statistical programme Stata) to compare across countries with at least 100 participants [7].

## Description of survey respondents

Of the almost 70,000 people who engaged with the survey 60,889 answered at least one question on stigma related knowledge, attitudes and beliefs in relation to dementia. This included 1,446 people living with dementia (2.4%), 18,377 carers for a person living with dementia (30.2%), 14,124 healthcare practitioners (23.2%) and 26,913 members of the general public (44.2%).

Respondents came from 155 countries or semi-autonomous regions/territories and answered the survey in one of 32 different languages. Responses were aggregated by World Bank income category and World Health Organisation (WHO) geographical region. The majority of participants resided in high-income countries (74.7%). Individuals from low-income and lower-middle-income economies represented 0.4% and 7.2% of respondents, respectively. The remaining 17.7% resided in upper-middle income countries. Because of the small numbers of respondents from low income countries, we combined respondents from low and lower middle-income countries, creating three World Bank categories. In relation to WHO Region, most respondents were from the European Region (42.4%), Region of the Americas (25.7%) and the Western Pacific Region (19.1%). A lower proportion of respondents came from the African Region (1.7%), Eastern Mediterranean Region (2.4%) and South-East Asia Region (5.7%).

Our recruitment resulted in a large and diverse sample; however, respondents over-represented females and individuals with university education: more females (78.8%) than males (21.2%) completed the survey and

68.8% of respondents had completed college/university or post-graduate studies. We developed survey weights to adjust for imbalances in relation to age, gender and education using nationally representative figures for each country.

**Table 4.** Characteristics of survey respondents by key group

| | People living with dementia (n = 1,446) | | | | | | Carers (n = 18,377) | | | | | |
|---|---|---|---|---|---|---|---|---|---|---|---|---|
| Gender | Female | | Male | | Unspecified | | Female | | Male | | Unspecified | |
| | 67.7% | | 30.8% | | 0.3% | | 82.4% | | 16.9% | | 0.1% | |
| Education | Secondary school or below | | Vocational training | | University degree or above | | Secondary school or below | | Vocational training | | University degree or above | |
| | 30.8% | | 11.5% | | 54.9% | | 24.1% | | 14% | | 60.1% | |
| Age | Aged 18-39 | Aged 40-52 | | Aged 53-65 | Aged 66-98 | | Aged 18-39 | Aged 40-52 | | Aged 53-65 | Aged 66-98 | |
| | NA | 17.5% | | 30% | 39.1% | | 9% | 24.7% | | 39.9% | 23.6% | |
| World Bank Income Group | Low income | Lower middle income | | Upper-middle income | High income | | Low income | Lower middle income | | Upper-middle income | High income | |
| | 0.5% | 8.9% | | 15.6% | 70.3% | | 0.3% | 3.1% | | 15.7% | 78% | |
| WHO Region | A | EM | E | RA | SEA | WP | A | EM | E | RA | SEA | WP |
| | 2.3% | 1.9% | 44.5% | 28.2% | 4.6% | 14% | 1.3% | 1.2% | 49.5% | 26.9% | 3.2% | 15.1% |

*Note.* **WHO** Regions: (A) African Region; (EM) Eastern Mediterranean Region; (E) European Region; (RA) Region of the Americas; (SEA) South-East Asia Region; (WP) Western Pacific Region.

Sample represent those who answered at least one stigma question (N = 60,860).
Not all participants shared their demographic information. Missing values are not reported on the table and explain why not all values total 100%.

| | Healthcare Practitioners (n = 14,124) | | | | | | General Public (n = 26,913) | | | | | |
|---|---|---|---|---|---|---|---|---|---|---|---|---|
| Gender | Female | Male | Unspecified | | | | Female | Male | Unspecified | | | |
| | 82% | 17.4% | 0.1% | | | | 74.1% | 25% | 0.2% | | | |
| Education | Secondary school or below | Vocational training | University degree or above | | | | Secondary school or below | Vocational training | University degree or above | | | |
| | 5.6% | 12.2% | 80.8% | | | | 21.3% | 10.6% | 66.5% | | | |
| Age | Aged 18-39 | Aged 40-52 | Aged 53-65 | Aged 66-98 | | | Aged 18-39 | Aged 40-52 | Aged 53-65 | Aged 66-98 | | |
| | 34% | 27.7% | 28.8% | 6.6% | | | 20.1% | 18.4% | 29.1% | 28.8% | | |
| World Bank Income Group | Low income | Lower middle income | Upper-middle income | High income | | | Low income | Lower middle income | Upper-middle income | High income | | |
| | 0.5% | 10.3% | 16.8% | 69.8% | | | 0.4% | 8.3% | 12.6% | 75.1% | | |
| WHO Region | A | EM | E | RA | SEA | WP | A | EM | E | RA | SEA | WP |
| | 1.6% | 4% | 36.1% | 22.4% | 7.8% | 25.8% | 2% | 2.4% | 40.8% | 26.5% | 6.4% | 18.7% |

## References


1 Thornicroft G, Rose D, Kassam A, Sartorius N. 2007. 'Stigma: ignorance, prejudice or discrimination?' Br J Psychiatry 190: 192–93.

2 Evans-Lacko S, Brohan E, Mojtabai, R*, Thornicroft G* 2012. 'Association between public views of mental illness and self-stigma among individuals with mental illness in 14 European countries. Psychological Medicine' 42(8):1741-1752.

3 Nguyen T, L. X. 2018. 'Understanding public-stigma and self-stigma in the context of dementia: A systematic review of the global literature.' Dementia 0, 1–34 (2018).

4 Pescosolido, Bernice A. Medina TR, Martin JK, L. S. 2013. 'The "Backbone" of Stigma: Identifying the Global Core of Public Prejudice Associated With Mental Illness.' Am. J. Public Health 103, 853–860 (2013.)

5 WHO (2014). Process of translation and adaptation of instruments. WHO. https://www.who.int/substance_abuse/research_tools/translation/en/ Last accessed 30 August 2019.

6 Lavallée, P. & Beaumont, J.-F. (2015), 'Why We Should Put Some Weight on Weights. Survey Insights: Methods from the Field, Weighting: Practical Issues and 'How to' Approach,' Invited article, Retrieved from https://surveyinsights.org/?p=6255 Last accessed 30 August 2019.

7 Nyaga VN, Arbyn M, Aerts M. 2014. 'Metaprop: a Stata command to perform meta-analysis of binomial data.' Archives of Public Health volume 72.

# Appendix 1

**Map 1.** World Health Organisation (WHO) Regions

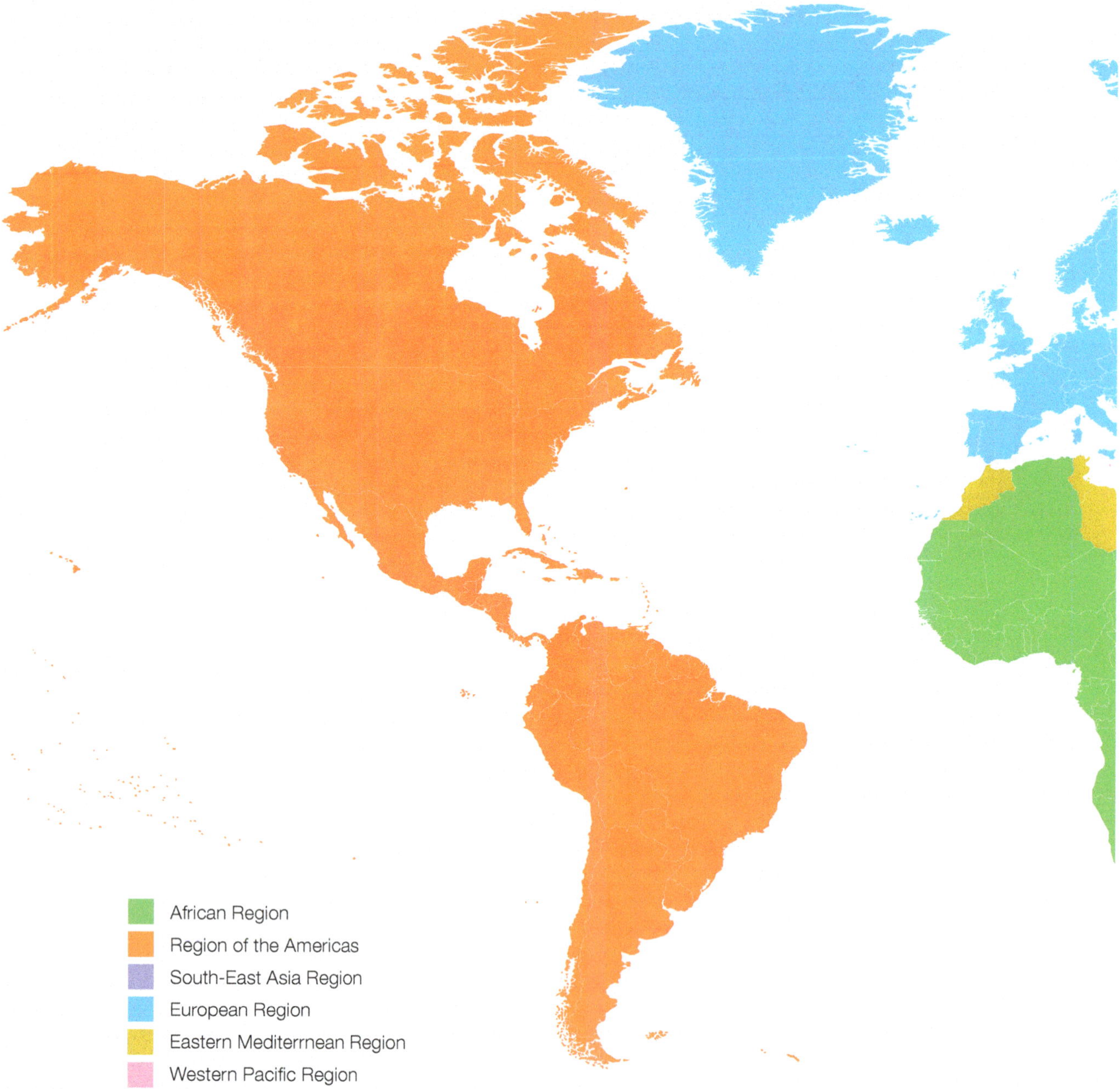


Reproduced with kind permission from the World Health Organisation

WHO Regional Offices - map
https://www.who.int/about/who-we-are/regional-offices

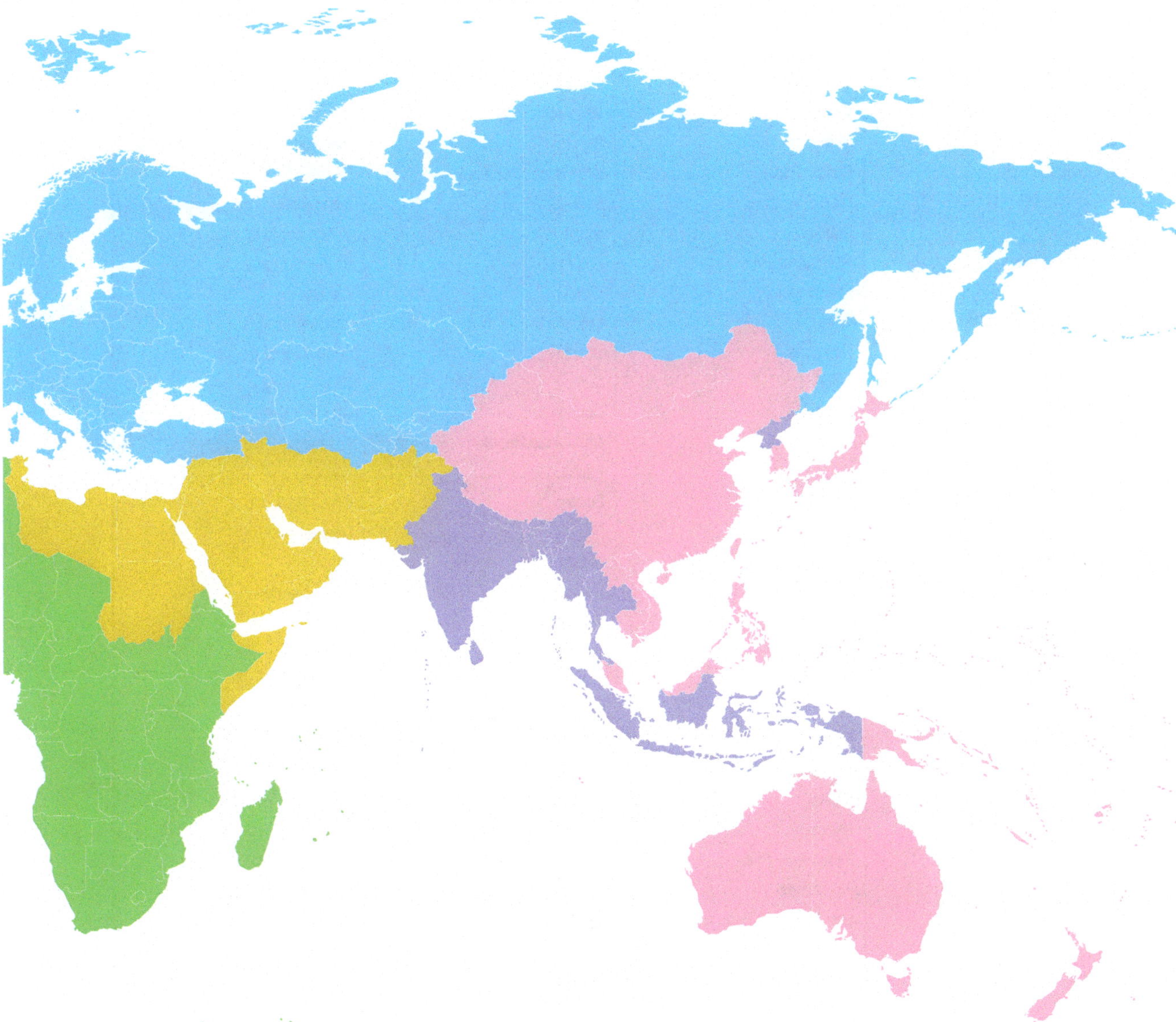

**Chart 1.** World Bank Income Groups 2019-2020

| Lower Income Countries | Lower Middle Income Countries | Upper Middle Income Countries | High Income Countries |
|---|---|---|---|
| Afghanistan | Angola | Albania | Andorra |
| Benin | Bangladesh | Algeria | Antigua and Barbuda |
| Burkina Faso | Bhutan | American Samoa | Aruba |
| Burundi | Bolivia | Argentina | Australia |
| Central African Republic | Cabo Verde | Armenia | Austria |
| Chad | Cambodia | Azerbaijan | Bahamas, The |
| Congo, Dem. Rep. of | Cameroon | Belarus | Bahrain |
| Eritrea | Comoros | Belize | Barbados |
| Ethiopia | Congo, Rep. | Bosnia and Herzegovina | Belgium |
| Gambia, The | Côte d'Ivoire | Botswana | Bermuda |
| Guinea | Djibouti | Brazll | British Virgin Islands |
| Guinea-Bissau | Egypt, Arab Rep. | Bulgaria | Brunei Darussalam |
| Haiti | El Salvador | China | Canada |
| Korea, Dem. People's Rep | Ghana | Colombia | Cayman Islands |
| Liberia | Honduras | Costa Rica | Channel Islands |
| Madagascar | India | Cuba | Chile |
| Malawi | Indonesia | Dominica | Croatia |
| Mali | Kenya | Dominican Republic | Curaçao |
| Mozambique | Kiribati | Equatorial Guinea | Cyprus |
| Nepal | Kyrgyz Republic | Ecuador | Czech Republic |
| Niger | Lao PDR | Fiji | Denmark |
| Rwanda | Lesotho | Gabon | Estonia |
| Sierra Leone | Mauritania | Georgia | Faroe Islands |
| Somalia | Micronesia, Fed. Sts | Grenada | Finland |
| South Sudan | Moldova | Guatemala | France |
| Syrian Arab Republic | Mongolia | Guyana | French Polynesia |
| Tajikistan | Morocco | Iran, Islamic Rep | Germany |
| Tanzania | Myanmar | Iraq | Gibraltar |
| Togo | Nicaragua | Jamaica | Greece |
| Uganda | Nigeria | Jordan | Greenland |
| Yemen, Rep. | Pakistan | Kazakhstan | Guam |
| | Papua New Guinea | Kosovo | Hong Kong SAR, China |
| | Philippines | Lebanon | Hungary |
| | Sao Tome and Principe | Libya | Iceland |
| | Senegal | Macedonia | Ireland |
| | Solomon Islands | Malaysia | Isle of Man |
| | Sudan | Maldives | Israel |
| | Swaziland | Marshall Islands | Italy |
| | Timor-Leste | Mauritius | Japan |
| | Tunisia | Mexico | Korea, Rep |
| | Ukraine | Montenegro | Kuwait |
| | Uzbekistan | Namibia | Latvia |
| | Vanuatu | Nauru | Liechtenstein |
| | Vietnam | Paraguay | Lithuania |
| | West Bank and Gaza | Peru | Luxembourg |
| | Zambia | Romania | Macao SAR, China |
| | Zimbabwe | Russia Federation | Malta |

| Lower Income Countries | Lower Middle Income Countries | Upper Middle Income Countries | High Income Countries |
|---|---|---|---|
| | | Samoa | Monaco |
| | | Serbia | Netherlands |
| | | Sri Lanka | New Caledonia |
| | | South Africa | New Zealand |
| | | St Lucia | Northern Mariana Islands |
| | | St Vincent and the Grenadines | Norway |
| | | Suriname | Oman |
| | | Thailand | Palau |
| | | Tonga | Panama |
| | | Turkey | Poland |
| | | Turkmenistan | Portugal |
| | | Tuvalu | Puerto Rico |
| | | Venezuela, RB | Qatar |
| | | | San Marino |
| | | | Saudi Arabia |
| | | | Seychelles |
| | | | Singapore |
| | | | Sit Maarten (Dutch part) |
| | | | Slovak Republic |
| | | | Slovenia |
| | | | Spain |
| | | | St Kitts and Nevis |
| | | | St. Martin (French part) |
| | | | Sweden |
| | | | Switzerland |
| | | | Chinese Taipei |
| | | | Trinidad and Tobago |
| | | | Turks and Caicos Islands |
| | | | United Arab Emirates |
| | | | United Kingdom |
| | | | United States |
| | | | Uruguay |
| | | | Virgin Islands (US) |

# Appendix 2[(vi)]

**Forest plots(vii)** for country comparisons(viii)

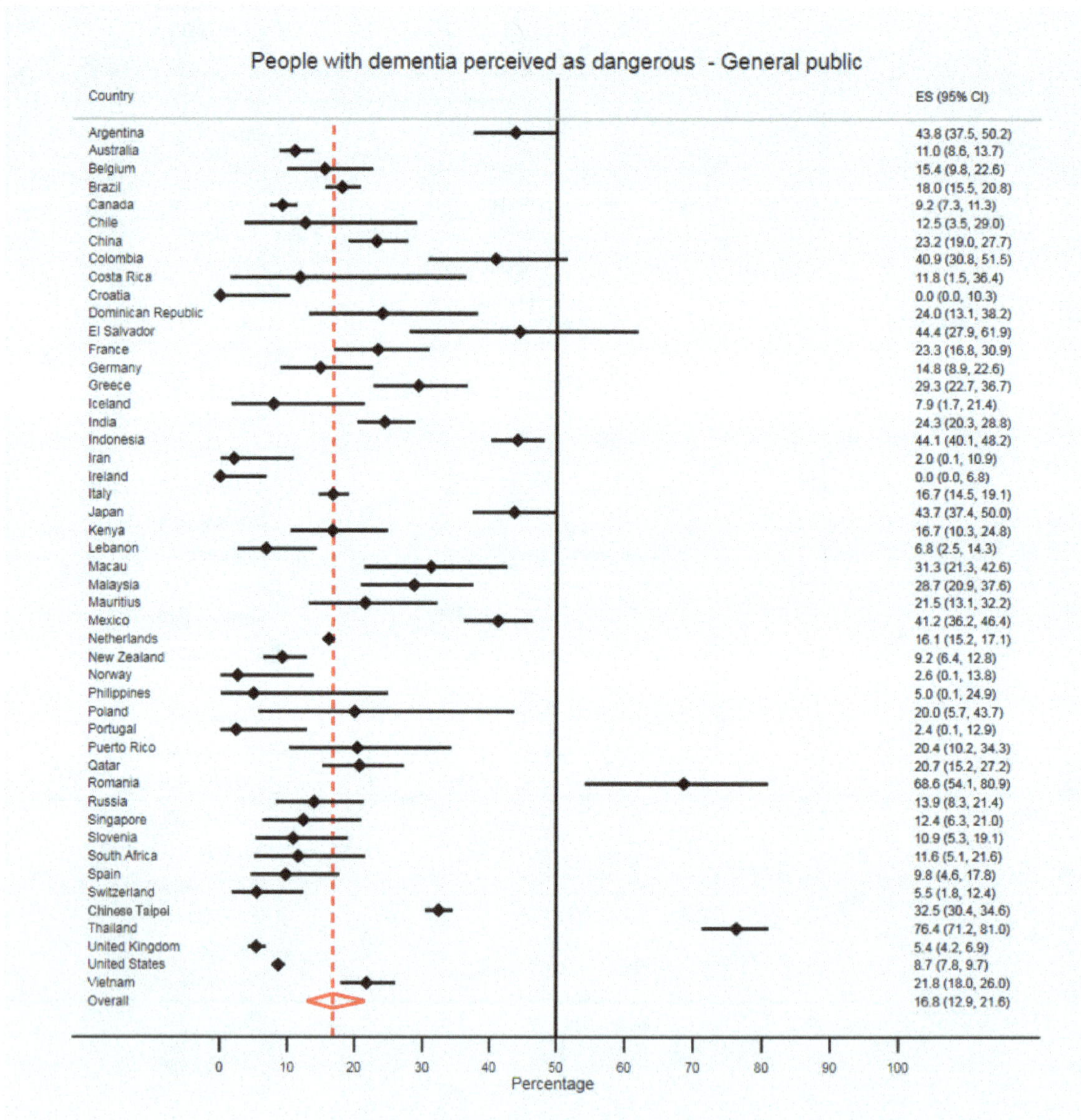


(vi) HCP refers to healthcare practitioners and PWD refers to people living with dementia.

(vii) Note: The forest plots summarise the responses for each group. The best estimate of the response is represented by the box and the horizontal line represents the 95% confidence interval. Those groups with a greater number of participants / respondents have a narrower confidence interval and a smaller line.

(viii) All analyses incorporated survey weights as described in the methodology section.

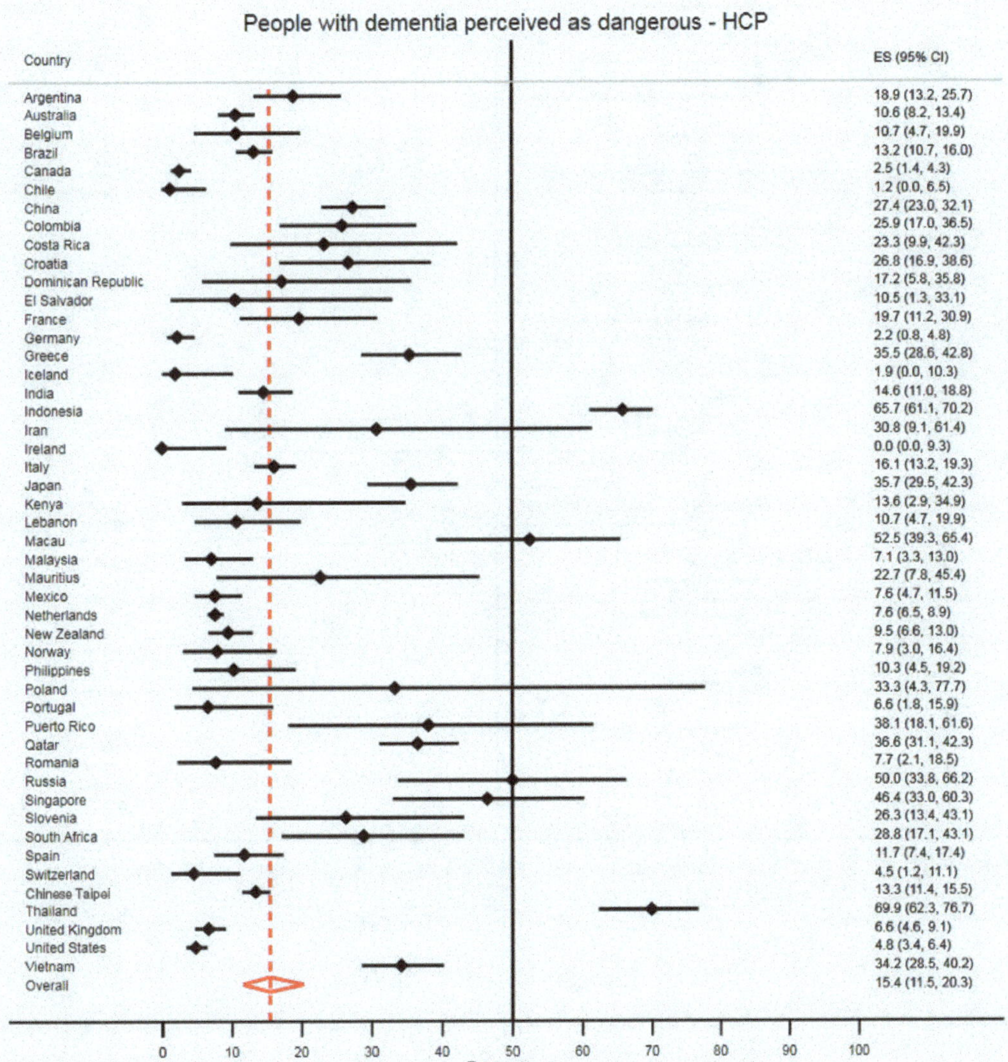
People with dementia perceived as dangerous - HCP
Country
ES (95% CI)
Argentina 18.9 (13.2, 25.7)
Australia 10.6 (8.2, 13.4)
Belgium 10.7 (4.7, 19.9)
Brazil 13.2 (10.7, 16.0)
Canada 2.5 (1.4, 4.3)
Chile 1.2 (0.0, 6.5)
China 27.4 (23.0, 32.1)
Colombia 25.9 (17.0, 36.5)
Costa Rica 23.3 (9.9, 42.3)
Croatia 26.8 (16.9, 38.6)
Dominican Republic 17.2 (5.8, 35.8)
El Salvador 10.5 (1.3, 33.1)
France 19.7 (11.2, 30.9)
Germany 2.2 (0.8, 4.8)
Greece 35.5 (28.6, 42.8)
Iceland 1.9 (0.0, 10.3)
India 14.6 (11.0, 18.8)
Indonesia 65.7 (61.1, 70.2)
Iran 30.8 (9.1, 61.4)
Ireland 0.0 (0.0, 9.3)
Italy 16.1 (13.2, 19.3)
Japan 35.7 (29.5, 42.3)
Kenya 13.6 (2.9, 34.9)
Lebanon 10.7 (4.7, 19.9)
Macau 52.5 (39.3, 65.4)
Malaysia 7.1 (3.3, 13.0)
Mauritius 22.7 (7.8, 45.4)
Mexico 7.6 (4.7, 11.5)
Netherlands 7.6 (6.5, 8.9)
New Zealand 9.5 (6.6, 13.0)
Norway 7.9 (3.0, 16.4)
Philippines 10.3 (4.5, 19.2)
Poland 33.3 (4.3, 77.7)
Portugal 6.6 (1.8, 15.9)
Puerto Rico 38.1 (18.1, 61.6)
Qatar 36.6 (31.1, 42.3)
Romania 7.7 (2.1, 18.5)
Russia 50.0 (33.8, 66.2)
Singapore 46.4 (33.0, 60.3)
Slovenia 26.3 (13.4, 43.1)
South Africa 28.8 (17.1, 43.1)
Spain 11.7 (7.4, 17.4)
Switzerland 4.5 (1.2, 11.1)
Chinese Taipei 13.3 (11.4, 15.5)
Thailand 69.9 (62.3, 76.7)
United Kingdom 6.6 (4.6, 9.1)
United States 4.8 (3.4, 6.4)
Vietnam 34.2 (28.5, 40.2)
Overall 15.4 (11.5, 20.3)
0 10 20 30 40 50 60 70 80 90 100
Percentage

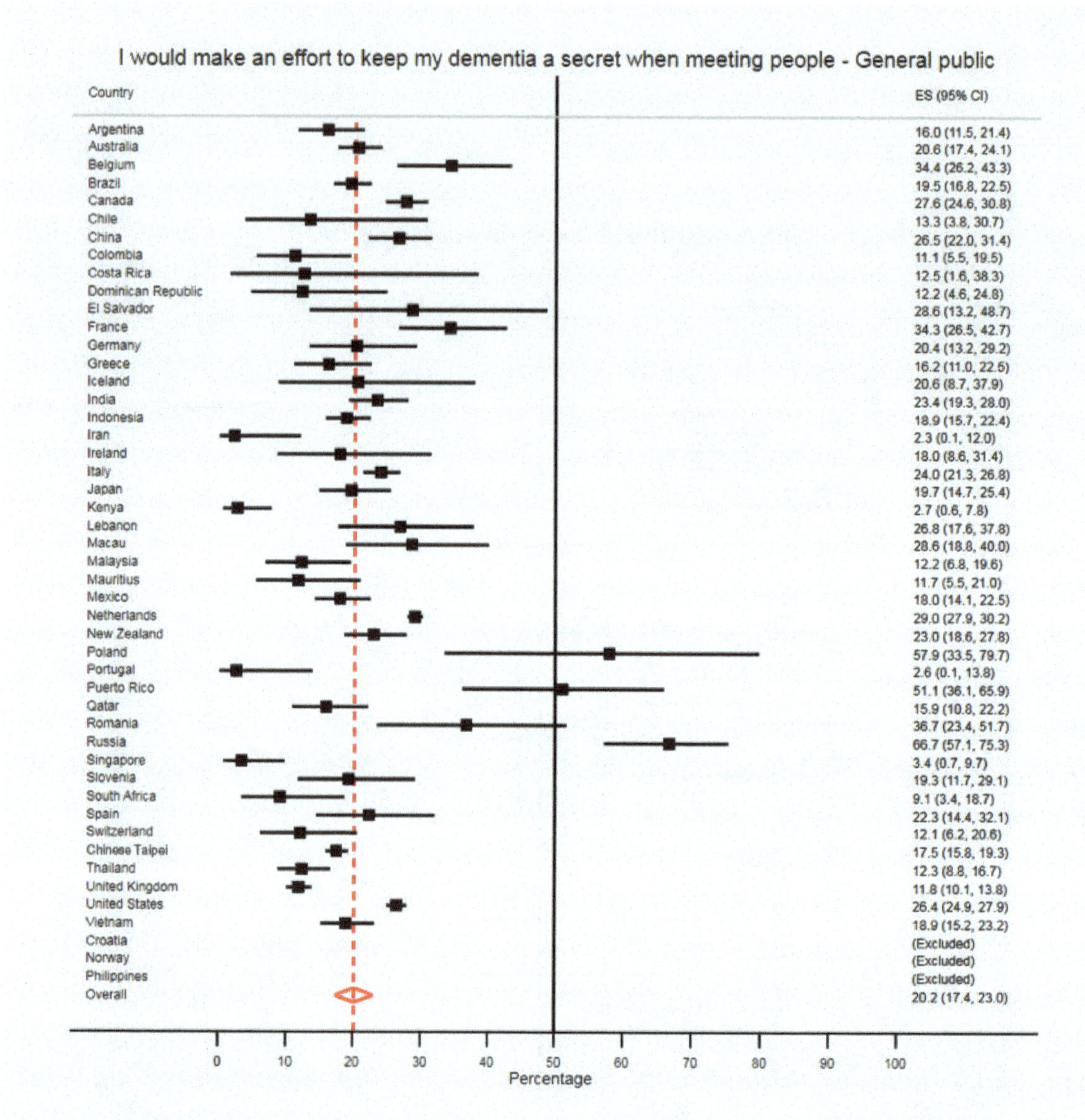
I would make an effort to keep my dementia a secret when meeting people - General public
Country
ES (95% CI)
Argentina 16.0 (11.5, 21.4)
Australia 20.6 (17.4, 24.1)
Belgium 34.4 (26.2, 43.3)
Brazil 19.5 (16.8, 22.5)
Canada 27.6 (24.6, 30.8)
Chile 13.3 (3.8, 30.7)
China 26.5 (22.0, 31.4)
Colombia 11.1 (5.5, 19.5)
Costa Rica 12.5 (1.6, 38.3)
Dominican Republic 12.2 (4.6, 24.8)
El Salvador 28.6 (13.2, 48.7)
France 34.3 (26.5, 42.7)
Germany 20.4 (13.2, 29.2)
Greece 16.2 (11.0, 22.5)
Iceland 20.6 (8.7, 37.9)
India 23.4 (19.3, 28.0)
Indonesia 18.9 (15.7, 22.4)
Iran 2.3 (0.1, 12.0)
Ireland 18.0 (8.6, 31.4)
Italy 24.0 (21.3, 26.8)
Japan 19.7 (14.7, 25.4)
Kenya 2.7 (0.6, 7.8)
Lebanon 26.8 (17.6, 37.8)
Macau 28.6 (18.8, 40.0)
Malaysia 12.2 (6.8, 19.6)
Mauritius 11.7 (5.5, 21.0)
Mexico 18.0 (14.1, 22.5)
Netherlands 29.0 (27.9, 30.2)
New Zealand 23.0 (18.6, 27.8)
Poland 57.9 (33.5, 79.7)
Portugal 2.6 (0.1, 13.8)
Puerto Rico 51.1 (36.1, 65.9)
Qatar 15.9 (10.8, 22.2)
Romania 36.7 (23.4, 51.7)
Russia 66.7 (57.1, 75.3)
Singapore 3.4 (0.7, 9.7)
Slovenia 19.3 (11.7, 29.1)
South Africa 9.1 (3.4, 18.7)
Spain 22.3 (14.4, 32.1)
Switzerland 12.1 (6.2, 20.6)
Chinese Taipei 17.5 (15.8, 19.3)
Thailand 12.3 (8.8, 16.7)
United Kingdom 11.8 (10.1, 13.8)
United States 26.4 (24.9, 27.9)
Vietnam 18.9 (15.2, 23.2)
Croatia (Excluded)
Norway (Excluded)
Philippines (Excluded)
Overall 20.2 (17.4, 23.0)
0 10 20 30 40 50 60 70 80 90 100
Percentage

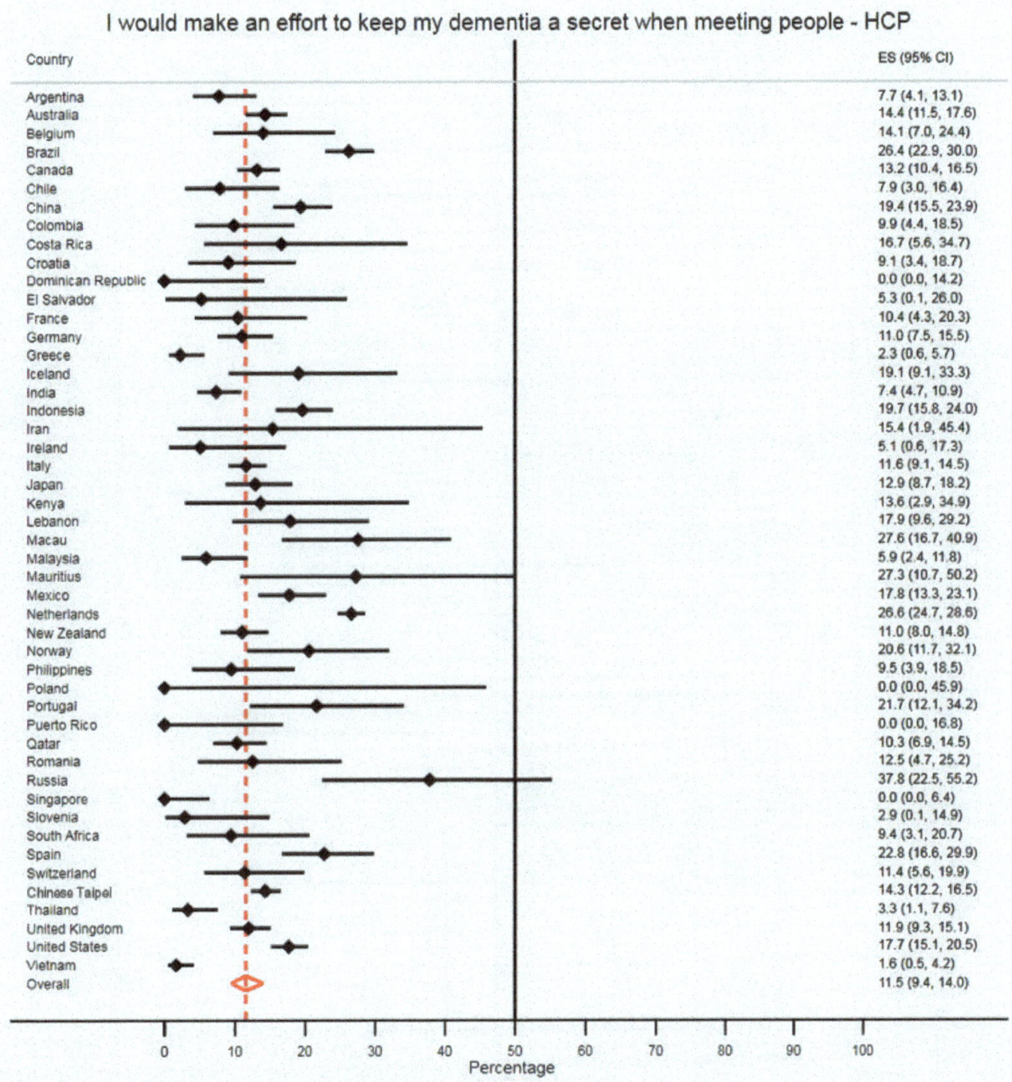
I would make an effort to keep my dementia a secret when meeting people - HCP
Country
ES (95% CI)
Argentina 7.7 (4.1, 13.1)
Australia 14.4 (11.5, 17.6)
Belgium 14.1 (7.0, 24.4)
Brazil 26.4 (22.9, 30.0)
Canada 13.2 (10.4, 16.5)
Chile 7.9 (3.0, 16.4)
China 19.4 (15.5, 23.9)
Colombia 9.9 (4.4, 18.5)
Costa Rica 16.7 (5.6, 34.7)
Croatia 9.1 (3.4, 18.7)
Dominican Republic 0.0 (0.0, 14.2)
El Salvador 5.3 (0.1, 26.0)
France 10.4 (4.3, 20.3)
Germany 11.0 (7.5, 15.5)
Greece 2.3 (0.6, 5.7)
Iceland 19.1 (9.1, 33.3)
India 7.4 (4.7, 10.9)
Indonesia 19.7 (15.8, 24.0)
Iran 15.4 (1.9, 45.4)
Ireland 5.1 (0.6, 17.3)
Italy 11.6 (9.1, 14.5)
Japan 12.9 (8.7, 18.2)
Kenya 13.6 (2.9, 34.9)
Lebanon 17.9 (9.6, 29.2)
Macau 27.6 (16.7, 40.9)
Malaysia 5.9 (2.4, 11.8)
Mauritius 27.3 (10.7, 50.2)
Mexico 17.8 (13.3, 23.1)
Netherlands 26.6 (24.7, 28.6)
New Zealand 11.0 (8.0, 14.8)
Norway 20.6 (11.7, 32.1)
Philippines 9.5 (3.9, 18.5)
Poland 0.0 (0.0, 45.9)
Portugal 21.7 (12.1, 34.2)
Puerto Rico 0.0 (0.0, 16.8)
Qatar 10.3 (6.9, 14.5)
Romania 12.5 (4.7, 25.2)
Russia 37.8 (22.5, 55.2)
Singapore 0.0 (0.0, 6.4)
Slovenia 2.9 (0.1, 14.9)
South Africa 9.4 (3.1, 20.7)
Spain 22.8 (16.6, 29.9)
Switzerland 11.4 (5.6, 19.9)
Chinese Taipei 14.3 (12.2, 16.5)
Thailand 3.3 (1.1, 7.6)
United Kingdom 11.9 (9.3, 15.1)
United States 17.7 (15.1, 20.5)
Vietnam 1.6 (0.5, 4.2)
Overall 11.5 (9.4, 14.0)
0 10 20 30 40 50 60 70 80 90 100
Percentage

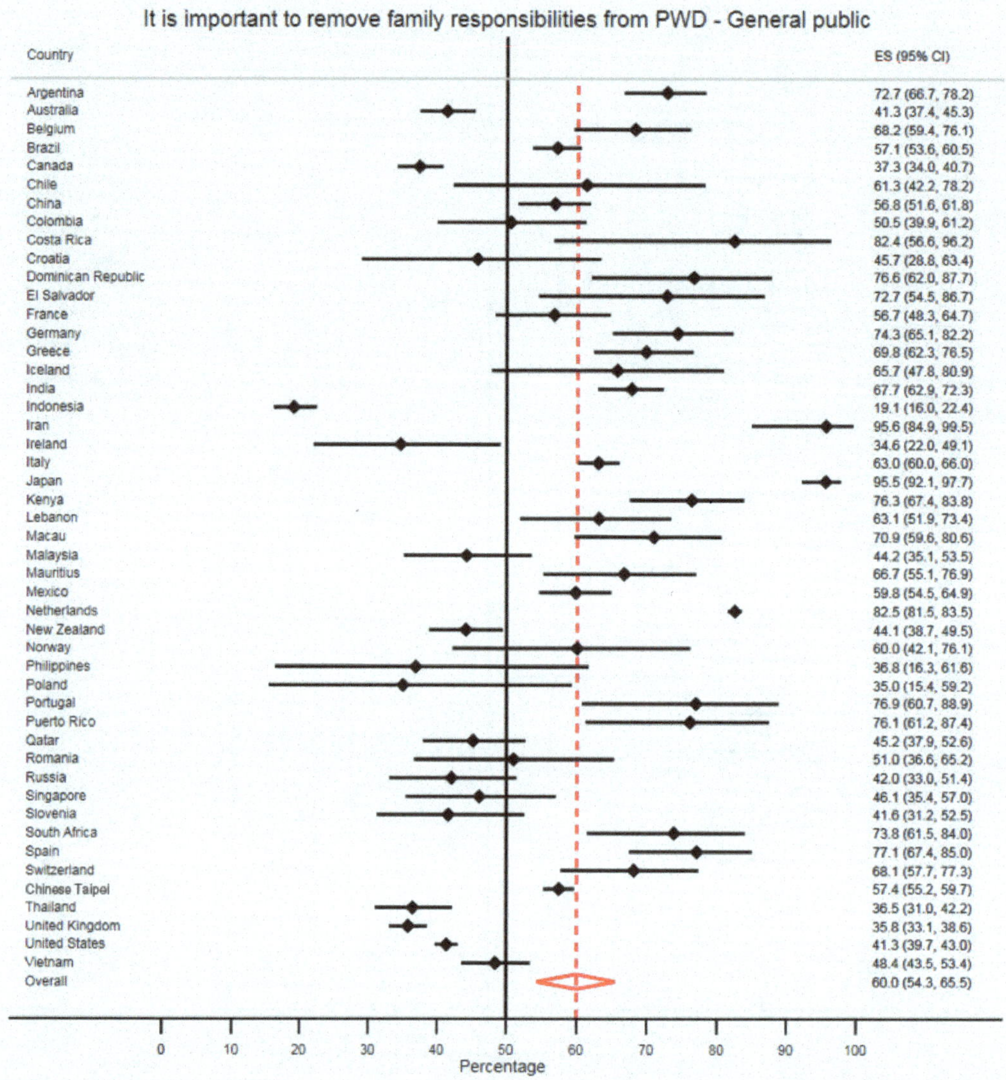
It is important to remove family responsibilities from PWD - General public
Country
ES (95% CI)
Argentina 72.7 (66.7, 78.2)
Australia 41.3 (37.4, 45.3)
Belgium 68.2 (59.4, 76.1)
Brazil 57.1 (53.6, 60.5)
Canada 37.3 (34.0, 40.7)
Chile 61.3 (42.2, 78.2)
China 56.8 (51.6, 61.8)
Colombia 50.5 (39.9, 61.2)
Costa Rica 82.4 (56.6, 96.2)
Croatia 45.7 (28.8, 63.4)
Dominican Republic 76.6 (62.0, 87.7)
El Salvador 72.7 (54.5, 86.7)
France 56.7 (48.3, 64.7)
Germany 74.3 (65.1, 82.2)
Greece 69.8 (62.3, 76.5)
Iceland 65.7 (47.8, 80.9)
India 67.7 (62.9, 72.3)
Indonesia 19.1 (16.0, 22.4)
Iran 95.6 (84.9, 99.5)
Ireland 34.6 (22.0, 49.1)
Italy 63.0 (60.0, 66.0)
Japan 95.5 (92.1, 97.7)
Kenya 76.3 (67.4, 83.8)
Lebanon 63.1 (51.9, 73.4)
Macau 70.9 (59.6, 80.6)
Malaysia 44.2 (35.1, 53.5)
Mauritius 66.7 (55.1, 76.9)
Mexico 59.8 (54.5, 64.9)
Netherlands 82.5 (81.5, 83.5)
New Zealand 44.1 (38.7, 49.5)
Norway 60.0 (42.1, 76.1)
Philippines 36.8 (16.3, 61.6)
Poland 35.0 (15.4, 59.2)
Portugal 76.9 (60.7, 88.9)
Puerto Rico 76.1 (61.2, 87.4)
Qatar 45.2 (37.9, 52.6)
Romania 51.0 (36.6, 65.2)
Russia 42.0 (33.0, 51.4)
Singapore 46.1 (35.4, 57.0)
Slovenia 41.6 (31.2, 52.5)
South Africa 73.8 (61.5, 84.0)
Spain 77.1 (67.4, 85.0)
Switzerland 68.1 (57.7, 77.3)
Chinese Taipei 57.4 (55.2, 59.7)
Thailand 36.5 (31.0, 42.2)
United Kingdom 35.8 (33.1, 38.6)
United States 41.3 (39.7, 43.0)
Vietnam 48.4 (43.5, 53.4)
Overall 60.0 (54.3, 65.5)
0 10 20 30 40 50 60 70 80 90 100
Percentage

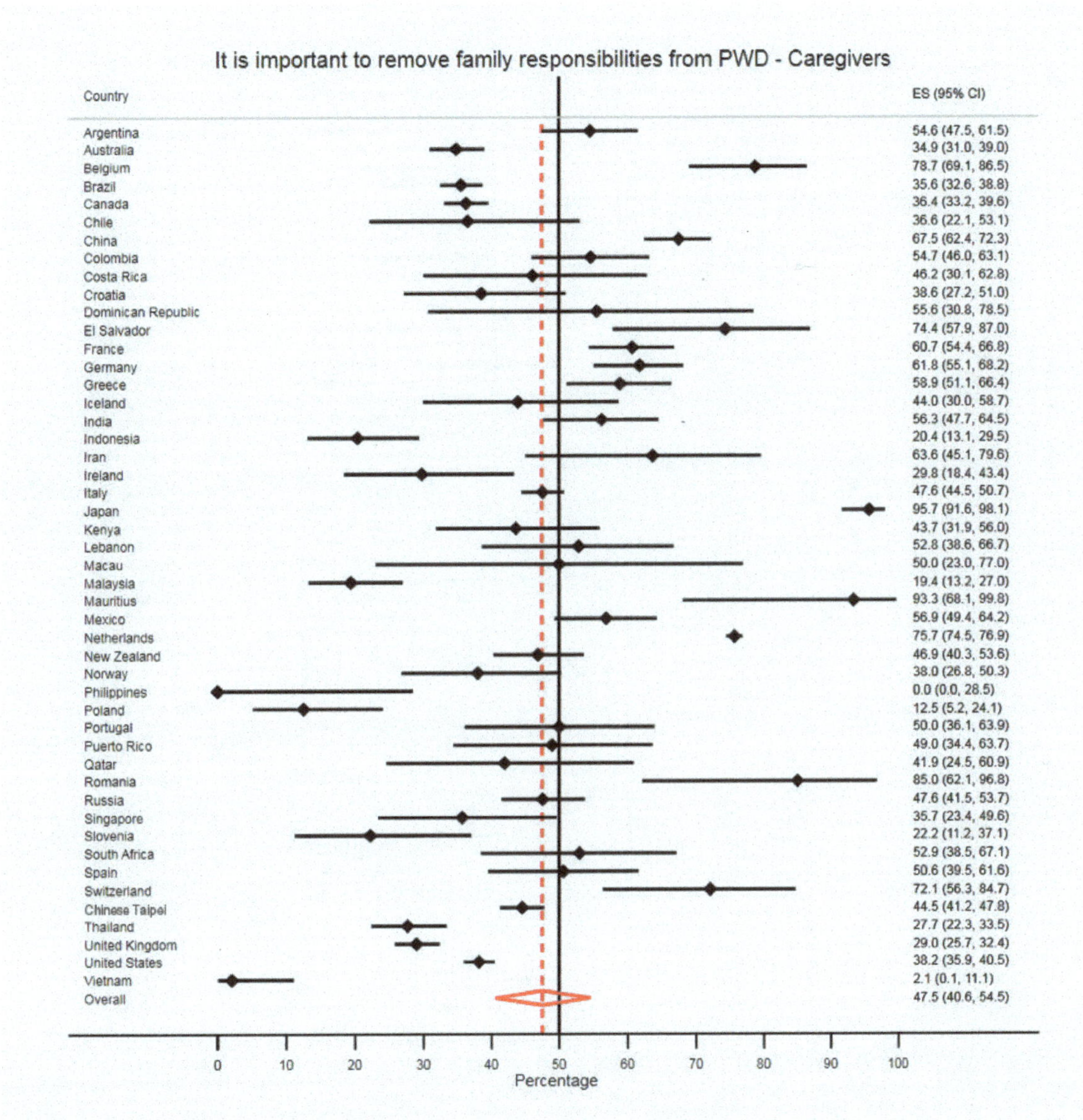
It is important to remove family responsibilities from PWD - Caregivers
Country
ES (95% CI)
Argentina
54.6 (47.5, 61.5)
Australia
34.9 (31.0, 39.0)
Belgium
78.7 (69.1, 86.5)
Brazil
35.6 (32.6, 38.8)
Canada
36.4 (33.2, 39.6)
Chile
36.6 (22.1, 53.1)
China
67.5 (62.4, 72.3)
Colombia
54.7 (46.0, 63.1)
Costa Rica
46.2 (30.1, 62.8)
Croatia
38.6 (27.2, 51.0)
Dominican Republic
55.6 (30.8, 78.5)
El Salvador
74.4 (57.9, 87.0)
France
60.7 (54.4, 66.8)
Germany
61.8 (55.1, 68.2)
Greece
58.9 (51.1, 66.4)
Iceland
44.0 (30.0, 58.7)
India
56.3 (47.7, 64.5)
Indonesia
20.4 (13.1, 29.5)
Iran
63.6 (45.1, 79.6)
Ireland
29.8 (18.4, 43.4)
Italy
47.6 (44.5, 50.7)
Japan
95.7 (91.6, 98.1)
Kenya
43.7 (31.9, 56.0)
Lebanon
52.8 (38.6, 66.7)
Macau
50.0 (23.0, 77.0)
Malaysia
19.4 (13.2, 27.0)
Mauritius
93.3 (68.1, 99.8)
Mexico
56.9 (49.4, 64.2)
Netherlands
75.7 (74.5, 76.9)
New Zealand
46.9 (40.3, 53.6)
Norway
38.0 (26.8, 50.3)
Philippines
0.0 (0.0, 28.5)
Poland
12.5 (5.2, 24.1)
Portugal
50.0 (36.1, 63.9)
Puerto Rico
49.0 (34.4, 63.7)
Qatar
41.9 (24.5, 60.9)
Romania
85.0 (62.1, 96.8)
Russia
47.6 (41.5, 53.7)
Singapore
35.7 (23.4, 49.6)
Slovenia
22.2 (11.2, 37.1)
South Africa
52.9 (38.5, 67.1)
Spain
50.6 (39.5, 61.6)
Switzerland
72.1 (56.3, 84.7)
Chinese Taipei
44.5 (41.2, 47.8)
Thailand
27.7 (22.3, 33.5)
United Kingdom
29.0 (25.7, 32.4)
United States
38.2 (35.9, 40.5)
Vietnam
2.1 (0.1, 11.1)
Overall
47.5 (40.6, 54.5)
0
10
20
30
40
50
60
70
80
90
100
Percentage

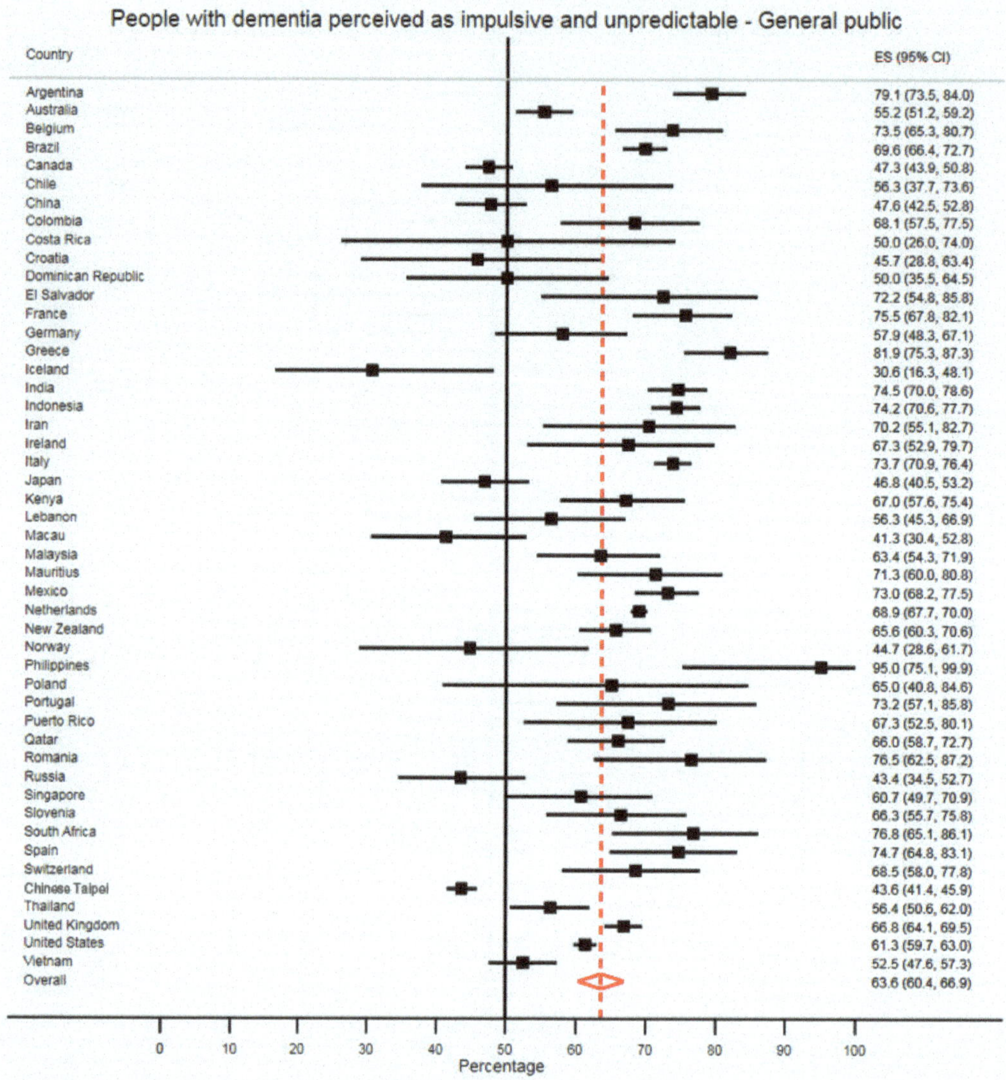

People with dementia perceived as impulsive and unpredictable - General public
Country
ES (95% CI)
Argentina 79.1 (73.5, 84.0)
Australia 55.2 (51.2, 59.2)
Belgium 73.5 (65.3, 80.7)
Brazil 69.6 (66.4, 72.7)
Canada 47.3 (43.9, 50.8)
Chile 56.3 (37.7, 73.6)
China 47.6 (42.5, 52.8)
Colombia 68.1 (57.5, 77.5)
Costa Rica 50.0 (26.0, 74.0)
Croatia 45.7 (28.8, 63.4)
Dominican Republic 50.0 (35.5, 64.5)
El Salvador 72.2 (54.8, 85.8)
France 75.5 (67.8, 82.1)
Germany 57.9 (48.3, 67.1)
Greece 81.9 (75.3, 87.3)
Iceland 30.6 (16.3, 48.1)
India 74.5 (70.0, 78.6)
Indonesia 74.2 (70.6, 77.7)
Iran 70.2 (55.1, 82.7)
Ireland 67.3 (52.9, 79.7)
Italy 73.7 (70.9, 76.4)
Japan 46.8 (40.5, 53.2)
Kenya 67.0 (57.6, 75.4)
Lebanon 56.3 (45.3, 66.9)
Macau 41.3 (30.4, 52.8)
Malaysia 63.4 (54.3, 71.9)
Mauritius 71.3 (60.0, 80.8)
Mexico 73.0 (68.2, 77.5)
Netherlands 68.9 (67.7, 70.0)
New Zealand 65.6 (60.3, 70.6)
Norway 44.7 (28.6, 61.7)
Philippines 95.0 (75.1, 99.9)
Poland 65.0 (40.8, 84.6)
Portugal 73.2 (57.1, 85.8)
Puerto Rico 67.3 (52.5, 80.1)
Qatar 66.0 (58.7, 72.7)
Romania 76.5 (62.5, 87.2)
Russia 43.4 (34.5, 52.7)
Singapore 60.7 (49.7, 70.9)
Slovenia 66.3 (55.7, 75.8)
South Africa 76.8 (65.1, 86.1)
Spain 74.7 (64.8, 83.1)
Switzerland 68.5 (58.0, 77.8)
Chinese Taipei 43.6 (41.4, 45.9)
Thailand 56.4 (50.6, 62.0)
United Kingdom 66.8 (64.1, 69.5)
United States 61.3 (59.7, 63.0)
Vietnam 52.5 (47.6, 57.3)
Overall 63.6 (60.4, 66.9)
0
10
20
30
40
50
60
70
80
90
100
Percentage

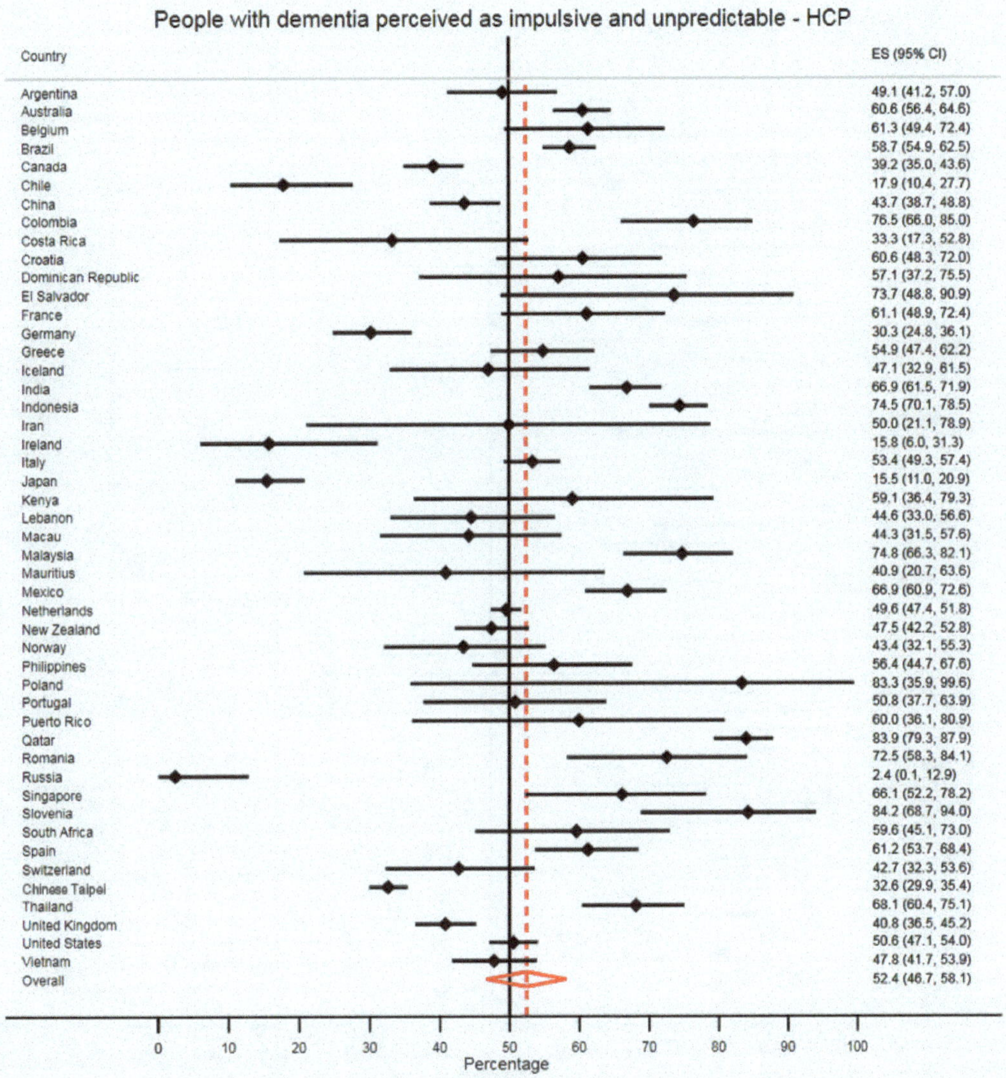
People with dementia perceived as impulsive and unpredictable - HCP
Country
ES (95% CI)
Argentina 49.1 (41.2, 57.0)
Australia 60.6 (56.4, 64.6)
Belgium 61.3 (49.4, 72.4)
Brazil 58.7 (54.9, 62.5)
Canada 39.2 (35.0, 43.6)
Chile 17.9 (10.4, 27.7)
China 43.7 (38.7, 48.8)
Colombia 76.5 (66.0, 85.0)
Costa Rica 33.3 (17.3, 52.8)
Croatia 60.6 (48.3, 72.0)
Dominican Republic 57.1 (37.2, 75.5)
El Salvador 73.7 (48.8, 90.9)
France 61.1 (48.9, 72.4)
Germany 30.3 (24.8, 36.1)
Greece 54.9 (47.4, 62.2)
Iceland 47.1 (32.9, 61.5)
India 66.9 (61.5, 71.9)
Indonesia 74.5 (70.1, 78.5)
Iran 50.0 (21.1, 78.9)
Ireland 15.8 (6.0, 31.3)
Italy 53.4 (49.3, 57.4)
Japan 15.5 (11.0, 20.9)
Kenya 59.1 (36.4, 79.3)
Lebanon 44.6 (33.0, 56.6)
Macau 44.3 (31.5, 57.6)
Malaysia 74.8 (66.3, 82.1)
Mauritius 40.9 (20.7, 63.6)
Mexico 66.9 (60.9, 72.6)
Netherlands 49.6 (47.4, 51.8)
New Zealand 47.5 (42.2, 52.8)
Norway 43.4 (32.1, 55.3)
Philippines 56.4 (44.7, 67.6)
Poland 83.3 (35.9, 99.6)
Portugal 50.8 (37.7, 63.9)
Puerto Rico 60.0 (36.1, 80.9)
Qatar 83.9 (79.3, 87.9)
Romania 72.5 (58.3, 84.1)
Russia 2.4 (0.1, 12.9)
Singapore 66.1 (52.2, 78.2)
Slovenia 84.2 (68.7, 94.0)
South Africa 59.6 (45.1, 73.0)
Spain 61.2 (53.7, 68.4)
Switzerland 42.7 (32.3, 53.6)
Chinese Taipei 32.6 (29.9, 35.4)
Thailand 68.1 (60.4, 75.1)
United Kingdom 40.8 (36.5, 45.2)
United States 50.6 (47.1, 54.0)
Vietnam 47.8 (41.7, 53.9)
Overall 52.4 (46.7, 58.1)
0 10 20 30 40 50 60 70 80 90 100
Percentage

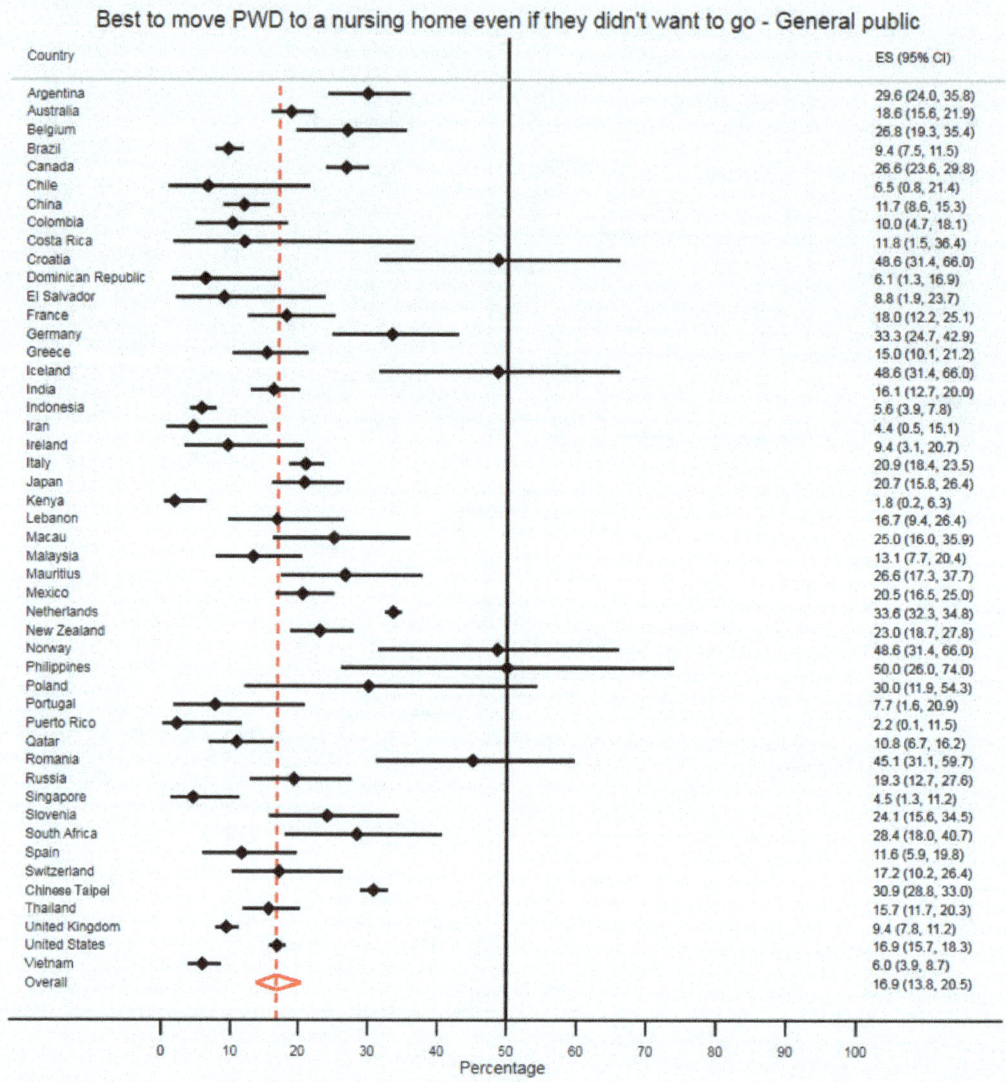
Best to move PWD to a nursing home even if they didn't want to go - General public
Country
ES (95% CI)
Argentina 29.6 (24.0, 35.8)
Australia 18.6 (15.6, 21.9)
Belgium 26.8 (19.3, 35.4)
Brazil 9.4 (7.5, 11.5)
Canada 26.6 (23.6, 29.8)
Chile 6.5 (0.8, 21.4)
China 11.7 (8.6, 15.3)
Colombia 10.0 (4.7, 18.1)
Costa Rica 11.8 (1.5, 36.4)
Croatia 48.6 (31.4, 66.0)
Dominican Republic 6.1 (1.3, 16.9)
El Salvador 8.8 (1.9, 23.7)
France 18.0 (12.2, 25.1)
Germany 33.3 (24.7, 42.9)
Greece 15.0 (10.1, 21.2)
Iceland 48.6 (31.4, 66.0)
India 16.1 (12.7, 20.0)
Indonesia 5.6 (3.9, 7.8)
Iran 4.4 (0.5, 15.1)
Ireland 9.4 (3.1, 20.7)
Italy 20.9 (18.4, 23.5)
Japan 20.7 (15.8, 26.4)
Kenya 1.8 (0.2, 6.3)
Lebanon 16.7 (9.4, 26.4)
Macau 25.0 (16.0, 35.9)
Malaysia 13.1 (7.7, 20.4)
Mauritius 26.6 (17.3, 37.7)
Mexico 20.5 (16.5, 25.0)
Netherlands 33.6 (32.3, 34.8)
New Zealand 23.0 (18.7, 27.8)
Norway 48.6 (31.4, 66.0)
Philippines 50.0 (26.0, 74.0)
Poland 30.0 (11.9, 54.3)
Portugal 7.7 (1.6, 20.9)
Puerto Rico 2.2 (0.1, 11.5)
Qatar 10.8 (6.7, 16.2)
Romania 45.1 (31.1, 59.7)
Russia 19.3 (12.7, 27.6)
Singapore 4.5 (1.3, 11.2)
Slovenia 24.1 (15.6, 34.5)
South Africa 28.4 (18.0, 40.7)
Spain 11.6 (5.9, 19.8)
Switzerland 17.2 (10.2, 26.4)
Chinese Taipei 30.9 (28.8, 33.0)
Thailand 15.7 (11.7, 20.3)
United Kingdom 9.4 (7.8, 11.2)
United States 16.9 (15.7, 18.3)
Vietnam 6.0 (3.9, 8.7)
Overall 16.9 (13.8, 20.5)
0
10
20
30
40
50
60
70
80
90
100
Percentage

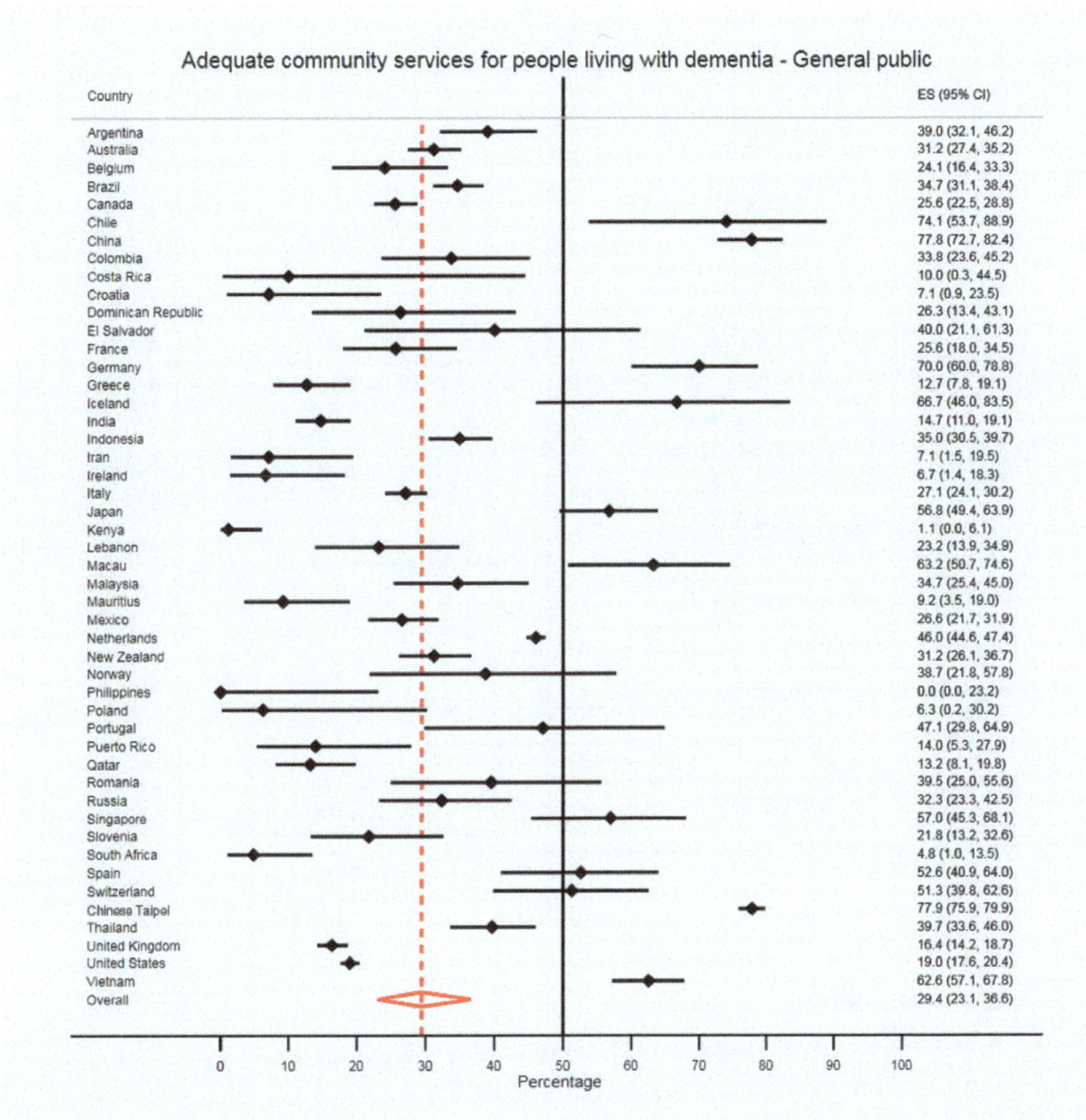
Adequate community services for people living with dementia - General public
Country
ES (95% CI)
Argentina 39.0 (32.1, 46.2)
Australia 31.2 (27.4, 35.2)
Belgium 24.1 (16.4, 33.3)
Brazil 34.7 (31.1, 38.4)
Canada 25.6 (22.5, 28.8)
Chile 74.1 (53.7, 88.9)
China 77.8 (72.7, 82.4)
Colombia 33.8 (23.6, 45.2)
Costa Rica 10.0 (0.3, 44.5)
Croatia 7.1 (0.9, 23.5)
Dominican Republic 26.3 (13.4, 43.1)
El Salvador 40.0 (21.1, 61.3)
France 25.6 (18.0, 34.5)
Germany 70.0 (60.0, 78.8)
Greece 12.7 (7.8, 19.1)
Iceland 66.7 (46.0, 83.5)
India 14.7 (11.0, 19.1)
Indonesia 35.0 (30.5, 39.7)
Iran 7.1 (1.5, 19.5)
Ireland 6.7 (1.4, 18.3)
Italy 27.1 (24.1, 30.2)
Japan 56.8 (49.4, 63.9)
Kenya 1.1 (0.0, 6.1)
Lebanon 23.2 (13.9, 34.9)
Macau 63.2 (50.7, 74.6)
Malaysia 34.7 (25.4, 45.0)
Mauritius 9.2 (3.5, 19.0)
Mexico 26.6 (21.7, 31.9)
Netherlands 46.0 (44.6, 47.4)
New Zealand 31.2 (26.1, 36.7)
Norway 38.7 (21.8, 57.8)
Philippines 0.0 (0.0, 23.2)
Poland 6.3 (0.2, 30.2)
Portugal 47.1 (29.8, 64.9)
Puerto Rico 14.0 (5.3, 27.9)
Qatar 13.2 (8.1, 19.8)
Romania 39.5 (25.0, 55.6)
Russia 32.3 (23.3, 42.5)
Singapore 57.0 (45.3, 68.1)
Slovenia 21.8 (13.2, 32.6)
South Africa 4.8 (1.0, 13.5)
Spain 52.6 (40.9, 64.0)
Switzerland 51.3 (39.8, 62.6)
Chinese Taipei 77.9 (75.9, 79.9)
Thailand 39.7 (33.6, 46.0)
United Kingdom 16.4 (14.2, 18.7)
United States 19.0 (17.6, 20.4)
Vietnam 62.6 (57.1, 67.8)
Overall 29.4 (23.1, 36.6)
0 10 20 30 40 50 60 70 80 90 100
Percentage

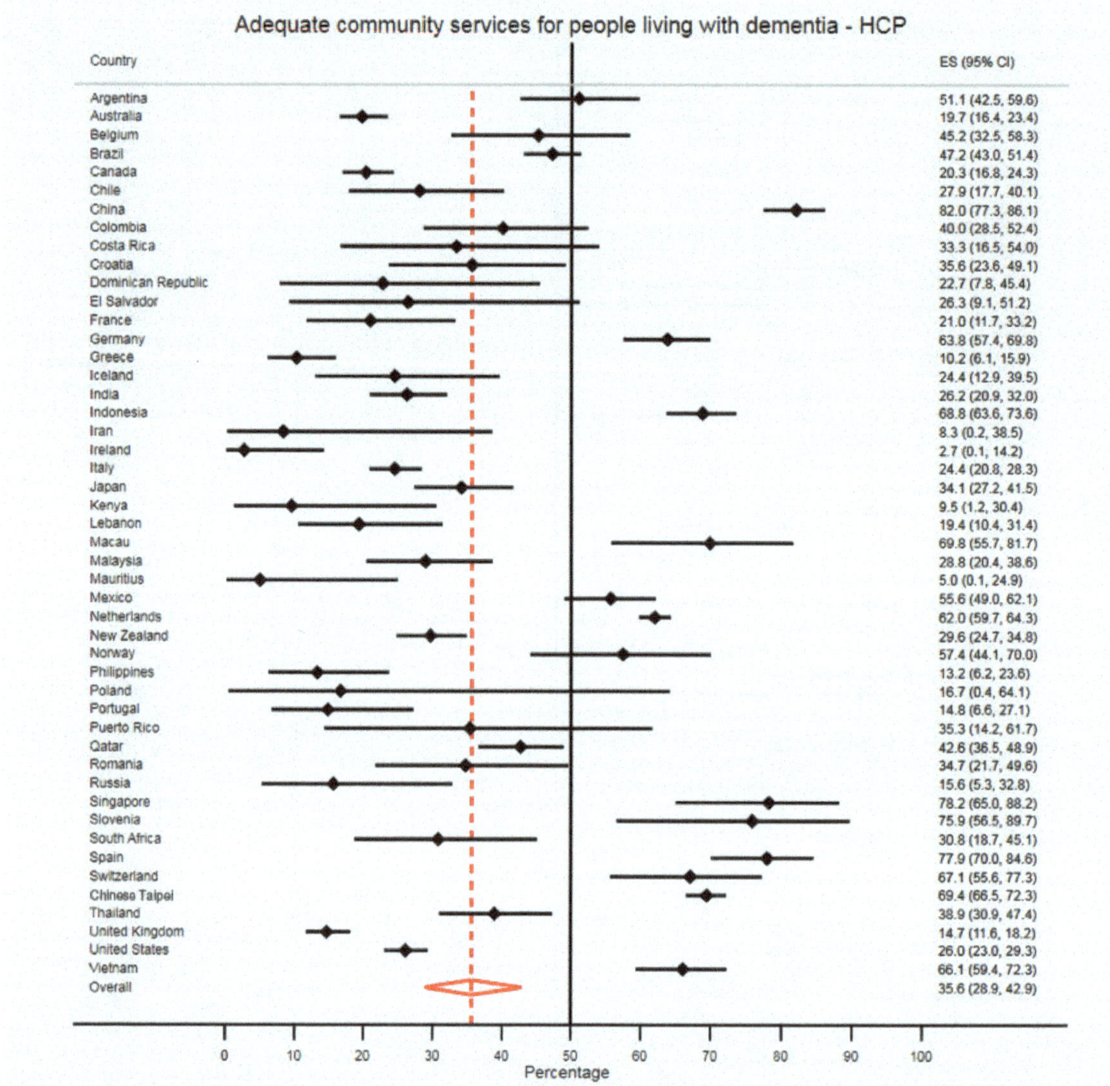
Adequate community services for people living with dementia - HCP
Country
ES (95% CI)
Argentina 51.1 (42.5, 59.6)
Australia 19.7 (16.4, 23.4)
Belgium 45.2 (32.5, 58.3)
Brazil 47.2 (43.0, 51.4)
Canada 20.3 (16.8, 24.3)
Chile 27.9 (17.7, 40.1)
China 82.0 (77.3, 86.1)
Colombia 40.0 (28.5, 52.4)
Costa Rica 33.3 (16.5, 54.0)
Croatia 35.6 (23.6, 49.1)
Dominican Republic 22.7 (7.8, 45.4)
El Salvador 26.3 (9.1, 51.2)
France 21.0 (11.7, 33.2)
Germany 63.8 (57.4, 69.8)
Greece 10.2 (6.1, 15.9)
Iceland 24.4 (12.9, 39.5)
India 26.2 (20.9, 32.0)
Indonesia 68.8 (63.6, 73.6)
Iran 8.3 (0.2, 38.5)
Ireland 2.7 (0.1, 14.2)
Italy 24.4 (20.8, 28.3)
Japan 34.1 (27.2, 41.5)
Kenya 9.5 (1.2, 30.4)
Lebanon 19.4 (10.4, 31.4)
Macau 69.8 (55.7, 81.7)
Malaysia 28.8 (20.4, 38.6)
Mauritius 5.0 (0.1, 24.9)
Mexico 55.6 (49.0, 62.1)
Netherlands 62.0 (59.7, 64.3)
New Zealand 29.6 (24.7, 34.8)
Norway 57.4 (44.1, 70.0)
Philippines 13.2 (6.2, 23.6)
Poland 16.7 (0.4, 64.1)
Portugal 14.8 (6.6, 27.1)
Puerto Rico 35.3 (14.2, 61.7)
Qatar 42.6 (36.5, 48.9)
Romania 34.7 (21.7, 49.6)
Russia 15.6 (5.3, 32.8)
Singapore 78.2 (65.0, 88.2)
Slovenia 75.9 (56.5, 89.7)
South Africa 30.8 (18.7, 45.1)
Spain 77.9 (70.0, 84.6)
Switzerland 67.1 (55.6, 77.3)
Chinese Taipei 69.4 (66.5, 72.3)
Thailand 38.9 (30.9, 47.4)
United Kingdom 14.7 (11.6, 18.2)
United States 26.0 (23.0, 29.3)
Vietnam 66.1 (59.4, 72.3)
Overall 35.6 (28.9, 42.9)
0 10 20 30 40 50 60 70 80 90 100
Percentage

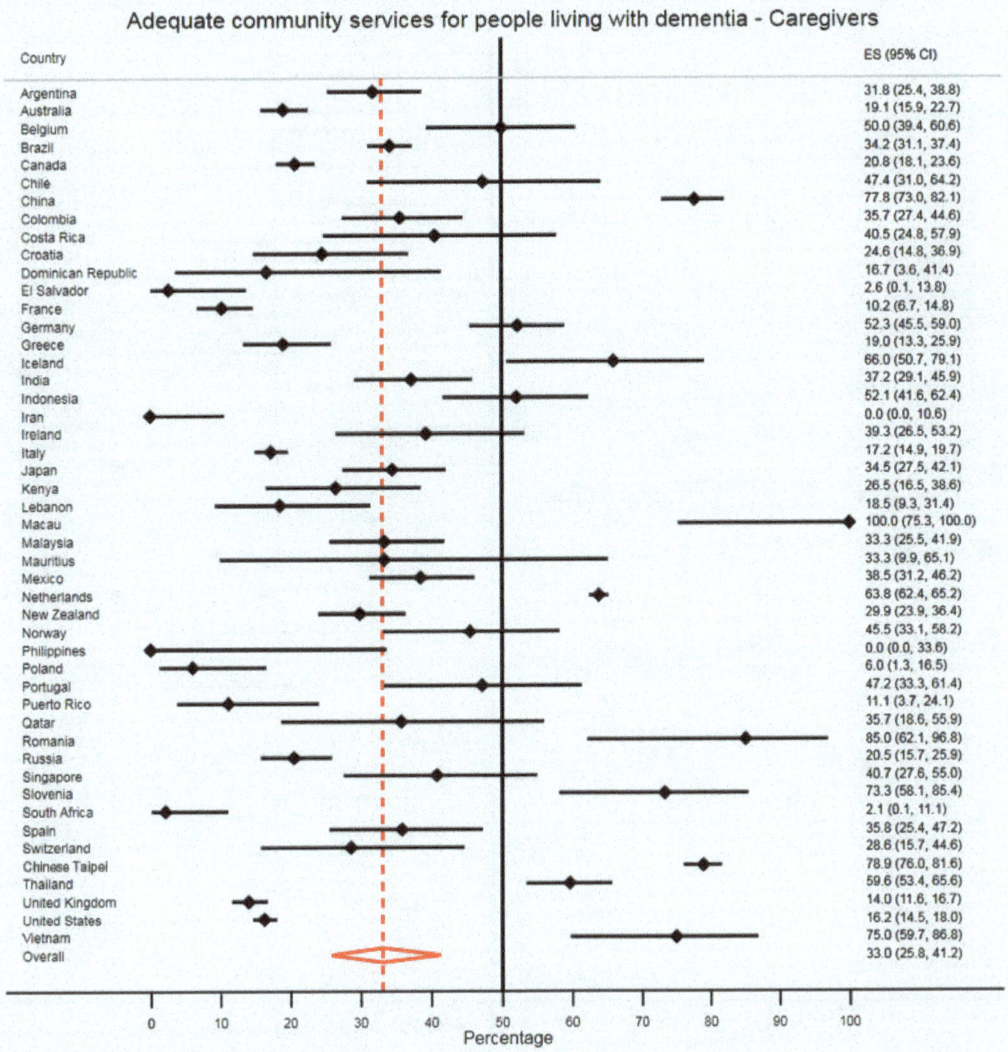
Adequate community services for people living with dementia - Caregivers
Country
ES (95% CI)
Argentina 31.8 (25.4, 38.8)
Australia 19.1 (15.9, 22.7)
Belgium 50.0 (39.4, 60.6)
Brazil 34.2 (31.1, 37.4)
Canada 20.8 (18.1, 23.6)
Chile 47.4 (31.0, 64.2)
China 77.8 (73.0, 82.1)
Colombia 35.7 (27.4, 44.6)
Costa Rica 40.5 (24.8, 57.9)
Croatia 24.6 (14.8, 36.9)
Dominican Republic 16.7 (3.6, 41.4)
El Salvador 2.6 (0.1, 13.8)
France 10.2 (6.7, 14.8)
Germany 52.3 (45.5, 59.0)
Greece 19.0 (13.3, 25.9)
Iceland 66.0 (50.7, 79.1)
India 37.2 (29.1, 45.9)
Indonesia 52.1 (41.6, 62.4)
Iran 0.0 (0.0, 10.6)
Ireland 39.3 (26.5, 53.2)
Italy 17.2 (14.9, 19.7)
Japan 34.5 (27.5, 42.1)
Kenya 26.5 (16.5, 38.6)
Lebanon 18.5 (9.3, 31.4)
Macau 100.0 (75.3, 100.0)
Malaysia 33.3 (25.5, 41.9)
Mauritius 33.3 (9.9, 65.1)
Mexico 38.5 (31.2, 46.2)
Netherlands 63.8 (62.4, 65.2)
New Zealand 29.9 (23.9, 36.4)
Norway 45.5 (33.1, 58.2)
Philippines 0.0 (0.0, 33.6)
Poland 6.0 (1.3, 16.5)
Portugal 47.2 (33.3, 61.4)
Puerto Rico 11.1 (3.7, 24.1)
Qatar 35.7 (18.6, 55.9)
Romania 85.0 (62.1, 96.8)
Russia 20.5 (15.7, 25.9)
Singapore 40.7 (27.6, 55.0)
Slovenia 73.3 (58.1, 85.4)
South Africa 2.1 (0.1, 11.1)
Spain 35.8 (25.4, 47.2)
Switzerland 28.6 (15.7, 44.6)
Chinese Taipei 78.9 (76.0, 81.6)
Thailand 59.6 (53.4, 65.6)
United Kingdom 14.0 (11.6, 16.7)
United States 16.2 (14.5, 18.0)
Vietnam 75.0 (59.7, 86.8)
Overall 33.0 (25.8, 41.2)
0 10 20 30 40 50 60 70 80 90 100
Percentage

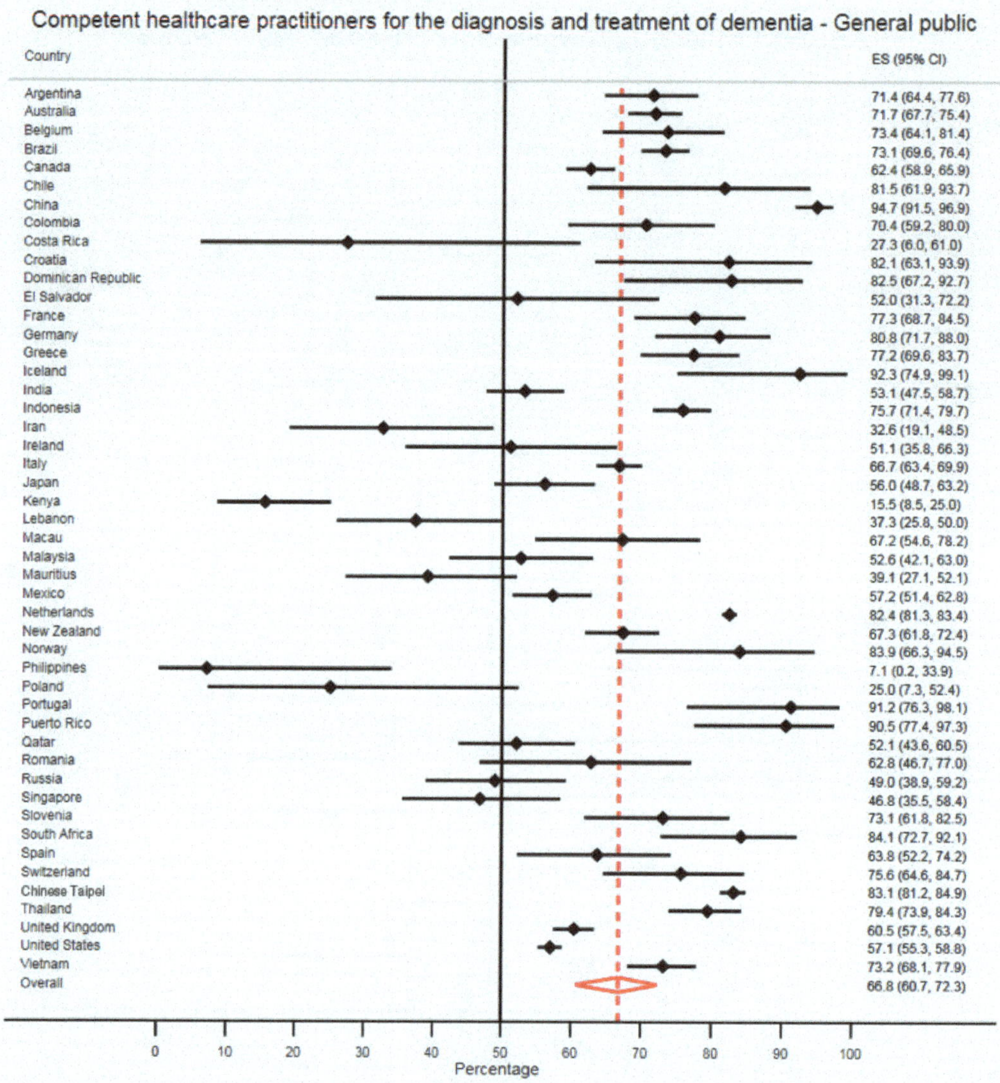
Competent healthcare practitioners for the diagnosis and treatment of dementia - General public
Country
ES (95% CI)
Argentina 71.4 (64.4, 77.6)
Australia 71.7 (67.7, 75.4)
Belgium 73.4 (64.1, 81.4)
Brazil 73.1 (69.6, 76.4)
Canada 62.4 (58.9, 65.9)
Chile 81.5 (61.9, 93.7)
China 94.7 (91.5, 96.9)
Colombia 70.4 (59.2, 80.0)
Costa Rica 27.3 (6.0, 61.0)
Croatia 82.1 (63.1, 93.9)
Dominican Republic 82.5 (67.2, 92.7)
El Salvador 52.0 (31.3, 72.2)
France 77.3 (68.7, 84.5)
Germany 80.8 (71.7, 88.0)
Greece 77.2 (69.6, 83.7)
Iceland 92.3 (74.9, 99.1)
India 53.1 (47.5, 58.7)
Indonesia 75.7 (71.4, 79.7)
Iran 32.6 (19.1, 48.5)
Ireland 51.1 (35.8, 66.3)
Italy 66.7 (63.4, 69.9)
Japan 56.0 (48.7, 63.2)
Kenya 15.5 (8.5, 25.0)
Lebanon 37.3 (25.8, 50.0)
Macau 67.2 (54.6, 78.2)
Malaysia 52.6 (42.1, 63.0)
Mauritius 39.1 (27.1, 52.1)
Mexico 57.2 (51.4, 62.8)
Netherlands 82.4 (81.3, 83.4)
New Zealand 67.3 (61.8, 72.4)
Norway 83.9 (66.3, 94.5)
Philippines 7.1 (0.2, 33.9)
Poland 25.0 (7.3, 52.4)
Portugal 91.2 (76.3, 98.1)
Puerto Rico 90.5 (77.4, 97.3)
Qatar 52.1 (43.6, 60.5)
Romania 62.8 (46.7, 77.0)
Russia 49.0 (38.9, 59.2)
Singapore 46.8 (35.5, 58.4)
Slovenia 73.1 (61.8, 82.5)
South Africa 84.1 (72.7, 92.1)
Spain 63.8 (52.2, 74.2)
Switzerland 75.6 (64.6, 84.7)
Chinese Taipei 83.1 (81.2, 84.9)
Thailand 79.4 (73.9, 84.3)
United Kingdom 60.5 (57.5, 63.4)
United States 57.1 (55.3, 58.8)
Vietnam 73.2 (68.1, 77.9)
Overall 66.8 (60.7, 72.3)
0 10 20 30 40 50 60 70 80 90 100
Percentage

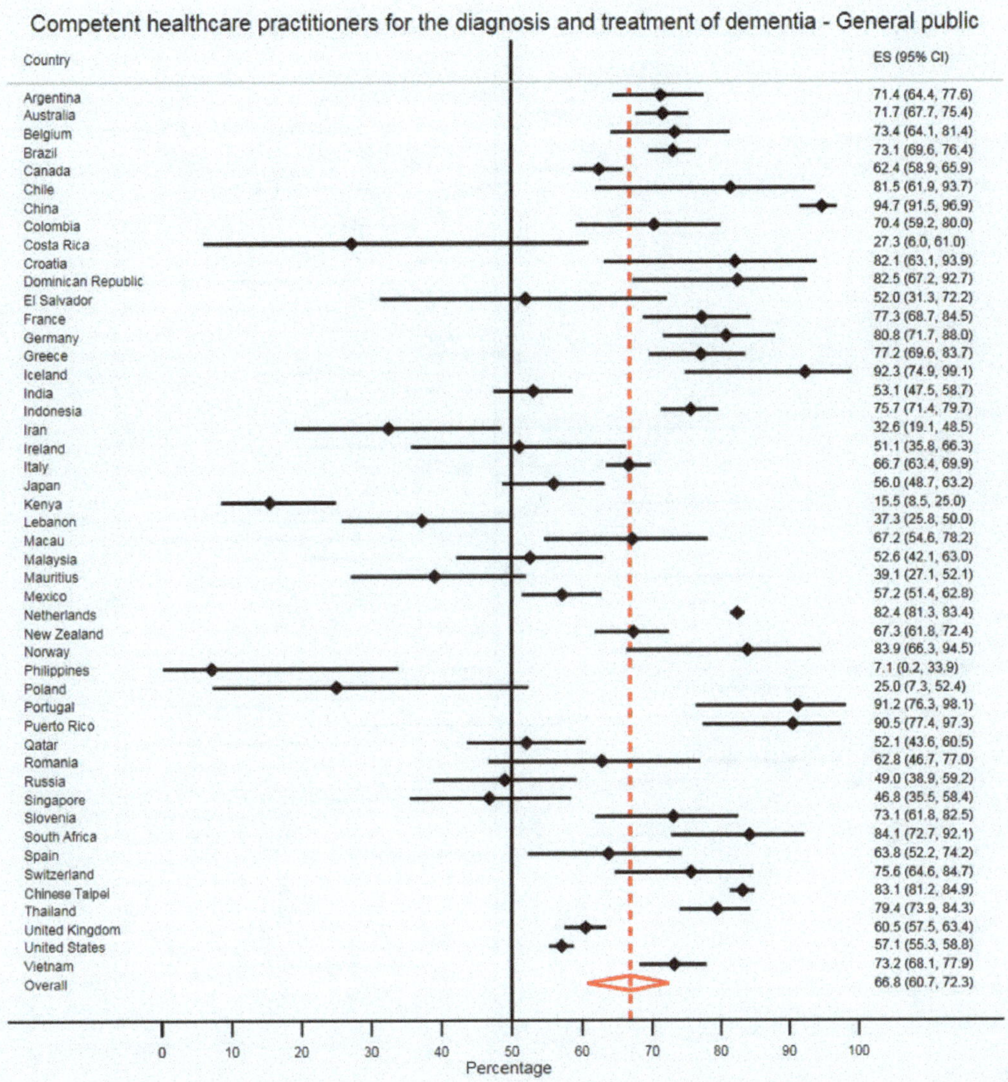
Competent healthcare practitioners for the diagnosis and treatment of dementia - General public
Country
ES (95% CI)
Argentina 71.4 (64.4, 77.6)
Australia 71.7 (67.7, 75.4)
Belgium 73.4 (64.1, 81.4)
Brazil 73.1 (69.6, 76.4)
Canada 62.4 (58.9, 65.9)
Chile 81.5 (61.9, 93.7)
China 94.7 (91.5, 96.9)
Colombia 70.4 (59.2, 80.0)
Costa Rica 27.3 (6.0, 61.0)
Croatia 82.1 (63.1, 93.9)
Dominican Republic 82.5 (67.2, 92.7)
El Salvador 52.0 (31.3, 72.2)
France 77.3 (68.7, 84.5)
Germany 80.8 (71.7, 88.0)
Greece 77.2 (69.6, 83.7)
Iceland 92.3 (74.9, 99.1)
India 53.1 (47.5, 58.7)
Indonesia 75.7 (71.4, 79.7)
Iran 32.6 (19.1, 48.5)
Ireland 51.1 (35.8, 66.3)
Italy 66.7 (63.4, 69.9)
Japan 56.0 (48.7, 63.2)
Kenya 15.5 (8.5, 25.0)
Lebanon 37.3 (25.8, 50.0)
Macau 67.2 (54.6, 78.2)
Malaysia 52.6 (42.1, 63.0)
Mauritius 39.1 (27.1, 52.1)
Mexico 57.2 (51.4, 62.8)
Netherlands 82.4 (81.3, 83.4)
New Zealand 67.3 (61.8, 72.4)
Norway 83.9 (66.3, 94.5)
Philippines 7.1 (0.2, 33.9)
Poland 25.0 (7.3, 52.4)
Portugal 91.2 (76.3, 98.1)
Puerto Rico 90.5 (77.4, 97.3)
Qatar 52.1 (43.6, 60.5)
Romania 62.8 (46.7, 77.0)
Russia 49.0 (38.9, 59.2)
Singapore 46.8 (35.5, 58.4)
Slovenia 73.1 (61.8, 82.5)
South Africa 84.1 (72.7, 92.1)
Spain 63.8 (52.2, 74.2)
Switzerland 75.6 (64.6, 84.7)
Chinese Taipei 83.1 (81.2, 84.9)
Thailand 79.4 (73.9, 84.3)
United Kingdom 60.5 (57.5, 63.4)
United States 57.1 (55.3, 58.8)
Vietnam 73.2 (68.1, 77.9)
Overall 66.8 (60.7, 72.3)
0 10 20 30 40 50 60 70 80 90 100
Percentage

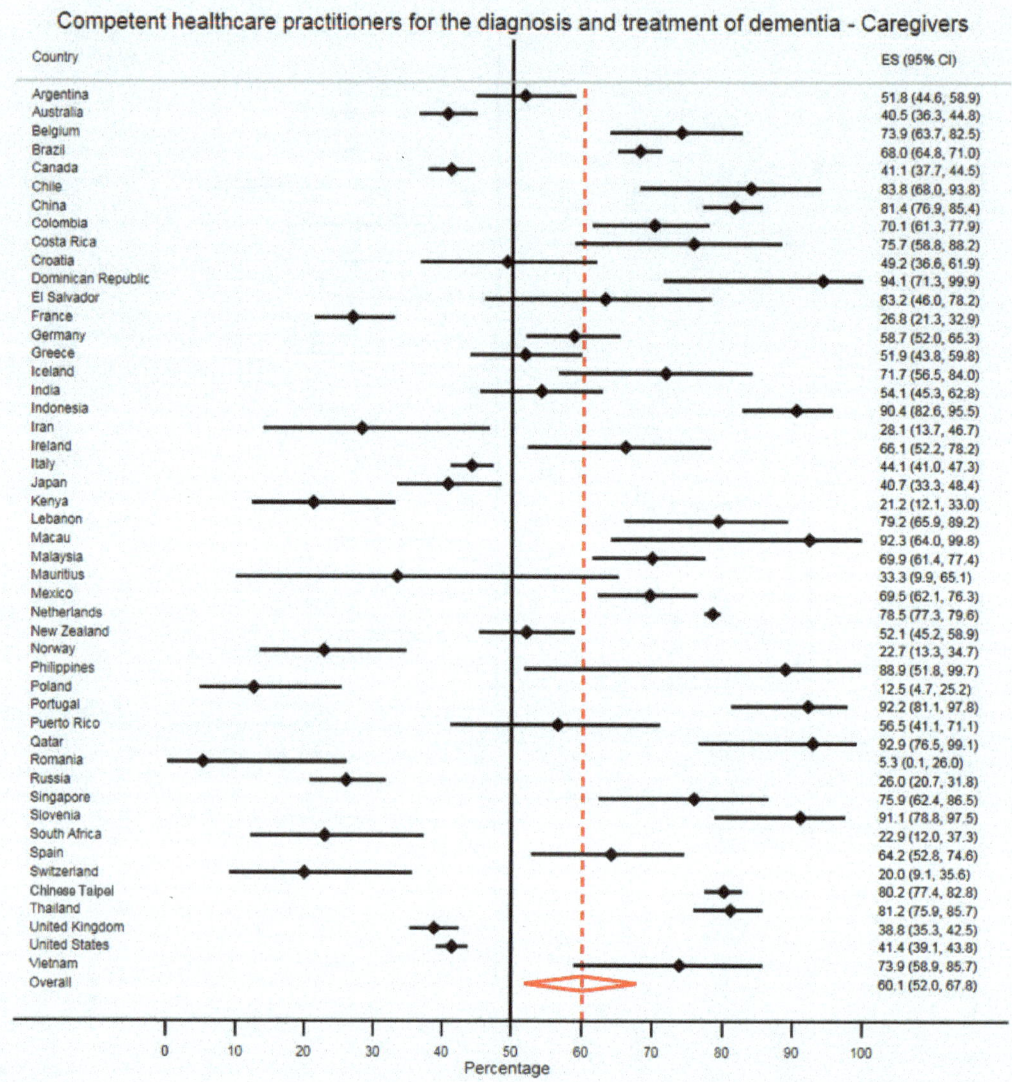
Competent healthcare practitioners for the diagnosis and treatment of dementia - Caregivers
Country
ES (95% CI)
Argentina 51.8 (44.6, 58.9)
Australia 40.5 (36.3, 44.8)
Belgium 73.9 (63.7, 82.5)
Brazil 68.0 (64.8, 71.0)
Canada 41.1 (37.7, 44.5)
Chile 83.8 (68.0, 93.8)
China 81.4 (76.9, 85.4)
Colombia 70.1 (61.3, 77.9)
Costa Rica 75.7 (58.8, 88.2)
Croatia 49.2 (36.6, 61.9)
Dominican Republic 94.1 (71.3, 99.9)
El Salvador 63.2 (46.0, 78.2)
France 26.8 (21.3, 32.9)
Germany 58.7 (52.0, 65.3)
Greece 51.9 (43.8, 59.8)
Iceland 71.7 (56.5, 84.0)
India 54.1 (45.3, 62.8)
Indonesia 90.4 (82.6, 95.5)
Iran 28.1 (13.7, 46.7)
Ireland 66.1 (52.2, 78.2)
Italy 44.1 (41.0, 47.3)
Japan 40.7 (33.3, 48.4)
Kenya 21.2 (12.1, 33.0)
Lebanon 79.2 (65.9, 89.2)
Macau 92.3 (64.0, 99.8)
Malaysia 69.9 (61.4, 77.4)
Mauritius 33.3 (9.9, 65.1)
Mexico 69.5 (62.1, 76.3)
Netherlands 78.5 (77.3, 79.6)
New Zealand 52.1 (45.2, 58.9)
Norway 22.7 (13.3, 34.7)
Philippines 88.9 (51.8, 99.7)
Poland 12.5 (4.7, 25.2)
Portugal 92.2 (81.1, 97.8)
Puerto Rico 56.5 (41.1, 71.1)
Qatar 92.9 (76.5, 99.1)
Romania 5.3 (0.1, 26.0)
Russia 26.0 (20.7, 31.8)
Singapore 75.9 (62.4, 86.5)
Slovenia 91.1 (78.8, 97.5)
South Africa 22.9 (12.0, 37.3)
Spain 64.2 (52.8, 74.6)
Switzerland 20.0 (9.1, 35.6)
Chinese Taipei 80.2 (77.4, 82.8)
Thailand 81.2 (75.9, 85.7)
United Kingdom 38.8 (35.3, 42.5)
United States 41.4 (39.1, 43.8)
Vietnam 73.9 (58.9, 85.7)
Overall 60.1 (52.0, 67.8)
0 10 20 30 40 50 60 70 80 90 100
Percentage

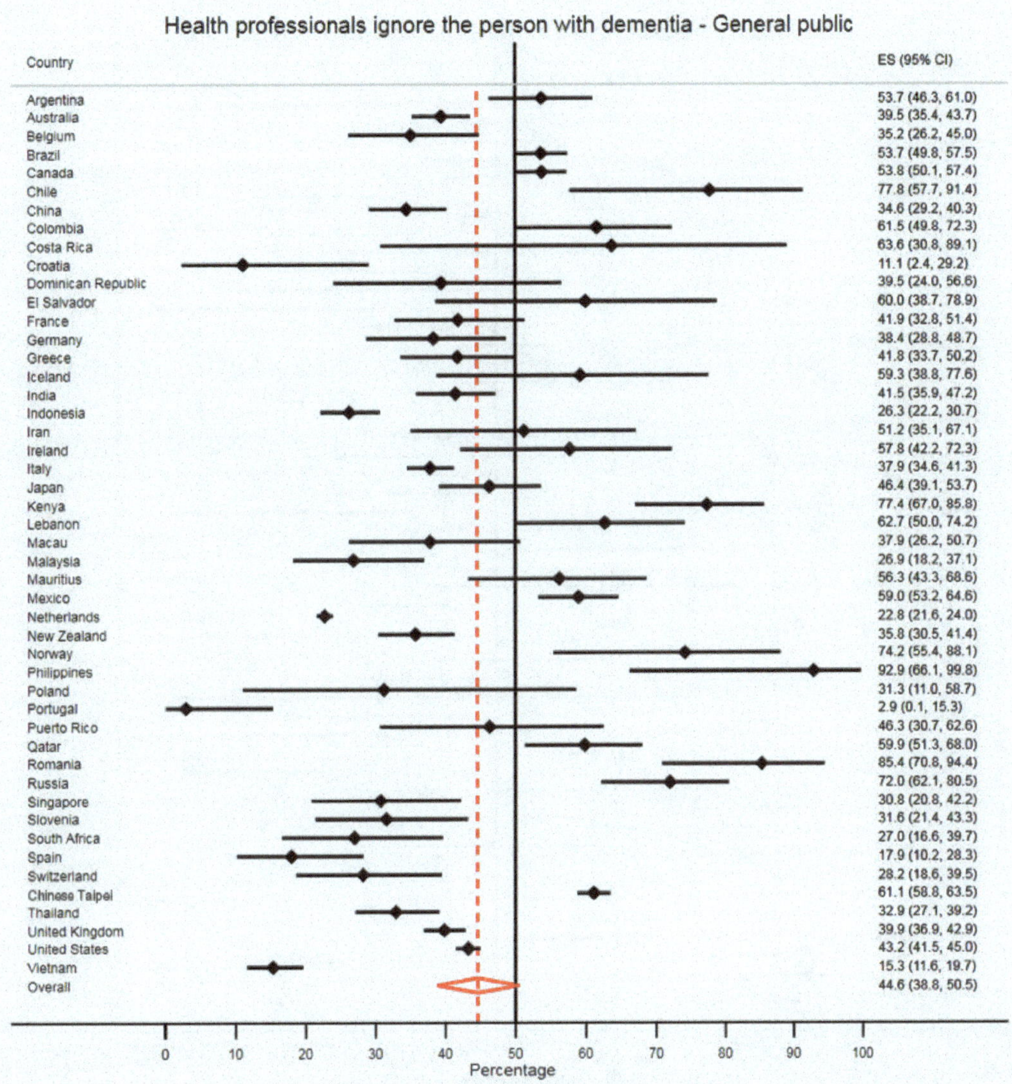
Health professionals ignore the person with dementia - General public
Country
ES (95% CI)
Argentina 53.7 (46.3, 61.0)
Australia 39.5 (35.4, 43.7)
Belgium 35.2 (26.2, 45.0)
Brazil 53.7 (49.8, 57.5)
Canada 53.8 (50.1, 57.4)
Chile 77.8 (57.7, 91.4)
China 34.6 (29.2, 40.3)
Colombia 61.5 (49.8, 72.3)
Costa Rica 63.6 (30.8, 89.1)
Croatia 11.1 (2.4, 29.2)
Dominican Republic 39.5 (24.0, 56.6)
El Salvador 60.0 (38.7, 78.9)
France 41.9 (32.8, 51.4)
Germany 38.4 (28.8, 48.7)
Greece 41.8 (33.7, 50.2)
Iceland 59.3 (38.8, 77.6)
India 41.5 (35.9, 47.2)
Indonesia 26.3 (22.2, 30.7)
Iran 51.2 (35.1, 67.1)
Ireland 57.8 (42.2, 72.3)
Italy 37.9 (34.6, 41.3)
Japan 46.4 (39.1, 53.7)
Kenya 77.4 (67.0, 85.8)
Lebanon 62.7 (50.0, 74.2)
Macau 37.9 (26.2, 50.7)
Malaysia 26.9 (18.2, 37.1)
Mauritius 56.3 (43.3, 68.6)
Mexico 59.0 (53.2, 64.6)
Netherlands 22.8 (21.6, 24.0)
New Zealand 35.8 (30.5, 41.4)
Norway 74.2 (55.4, 88.1)
Philippines 92.9 (66.1, 99.8)
Poland 31.3 (11.0, 58.7)
Portugal 2.9 (0.1, 15.3)
Puerto Rico 46.3 (30.7, 62.6)
Qatar 59.9 (51.3, 68.0)
Romania 85.4 (70.8, 94.4)
Russia 72.0 (62.1, 80.5)
Singapore 30.8 (20.8, 42.2)
Slovenia 31.6 (21.4, 43.3)
South Africa 27.0 (16.6, 39.7)
Spain 17.9 (10.2, 28.3)
Switzerland 28.2 (18.6, 39.5)
Chinese Taipei 61.1 (58.8, 63.5)
Thailand 32.9 (27.1, 39.2)
United Kingdom 39.9 (36.9, 42.9)
United States 43.2 (41.5, 45.0)
Vietnam 15.3 (11.6, 19.7)
Overall 44.6 (38.8, 50.5)
0 10 20 30 40 50 60 70 80 90 100
Percentage

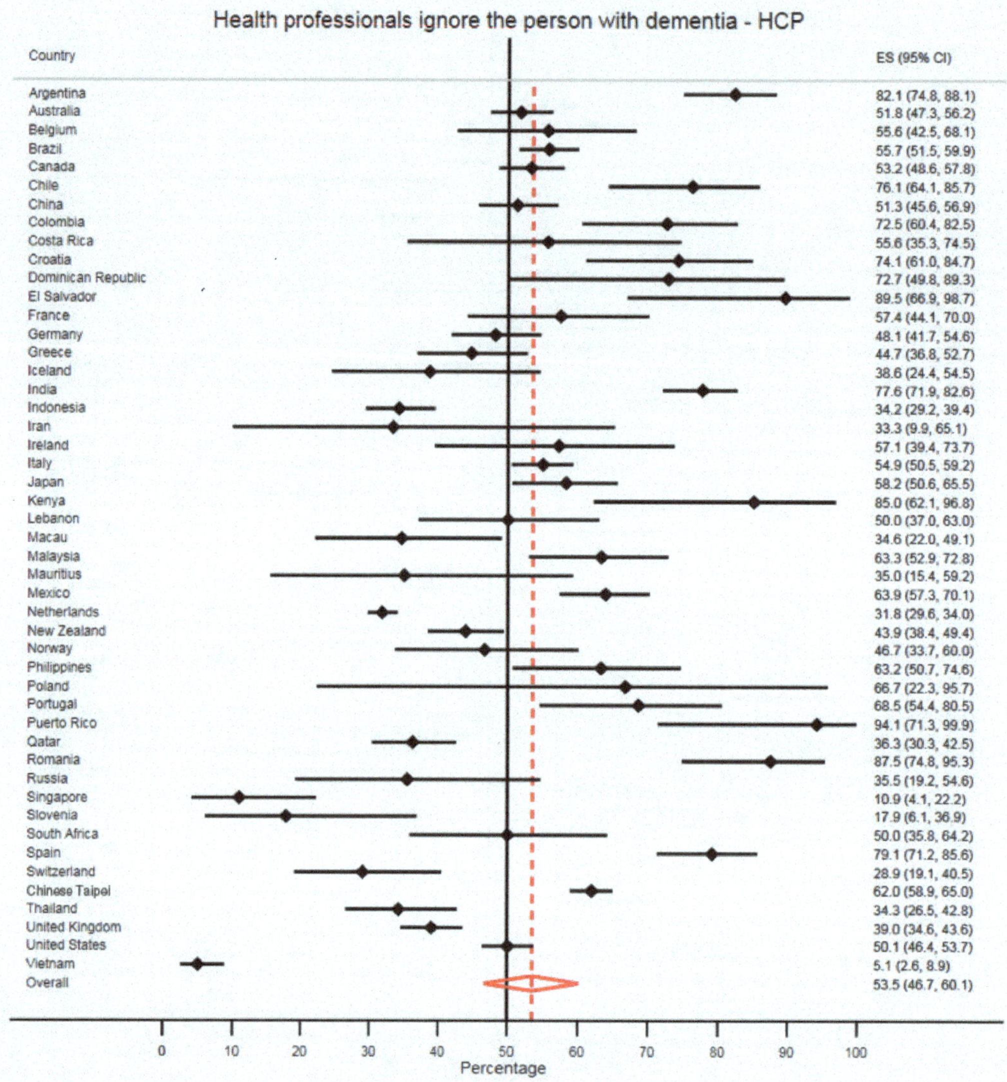
Health professionals ignore the person with dementia - HCP
Country
ES (95% CI)
Argentina 82.1 (74.8, 88.1)
Australia 51.8 (47.3, 56.2)
Belgium 55.6 (42.5, 68.1)
Brazil 55.7 (51.5, 59.9)
Canada 53.2 (48.6, 57.8)
Chile 76.1 (64.1, 85.7)
China 51.3 (45.6, 56.9)
Colombia 72.5 (60.4, 82.5)
Costa Rica 55.6 (35.3, 74.5)
Croatia 74.1 (61.0, 84.7)
Dominican Republic 72.7 (49.8, 89.3)
El Salvador 89.5 (66.9, 98.7)
France 57.4 (44.1, 70.0)
Germany 48.1 (41.7, 54.6)
Greece 44.7 (36.8, 52.7)
Iceland 38.6 (24.4, 54.5)
India 77.6 (71.9, 82.6)
Indonesia 34.2 (29.2, 39.4)
Iran 33.3 (9.9, 65.1)
Ireland 57.1 (39.4, 73.7)
Italy 54.9 (50.5, 59.2)
Japan 58.2 (50.6, 65.5)
Kenya 85.0 (62.1, 96.8)
Lebanon 50.0 (37.0, 63.0)
Macau 34.6 (22.0, 49.1)
Malaysia 63.3 (52.9, 72.8)
Mauritius 35.0 (15.4, 59.2)
Mexico 63.9 (57.3, 70.1)
Netherlands 31.8 (29.6, 34.0)
New Zealand 43.9 (38.4, 49.4)
Norway 46.7 (33.7, 60.0)
Philippines 63.2 (50.7, 74.6)
Poland 66.7 (22.3, 95.7)
Portugal 68.5 (54.4, 80.5)
Puerto Rico 94.1 (71.3, 99.9)
Qatar 36.3 (30.3, 42.5)
Romania 87.5 (74.8, 95.3)
Russia 35.5 (19.2, 54.6)
Singapore 10.9 (4.1, 22.2)
Slovenia 17.9 (6.1, 36.9)
South Africa 50.0 (35.8, 64.2)
Spain 79.1 (71.2, 85.6)
Switzerland 28.9 (19.1, 40.5)
Chinese Taipei 62.0 (58.9, 65.0)
Thailand 34.3 (26.5, 42.8)
United Kingdom 39.0 (34.6, 43.6)
United States 50.1 (46.4, 53.7)
Vietnam 5.1 (2.6, 8.9)
Overall 53.5 (46.7, 60.1)
0 10 20 30 40 50 60 70 80 90 100
Percentage

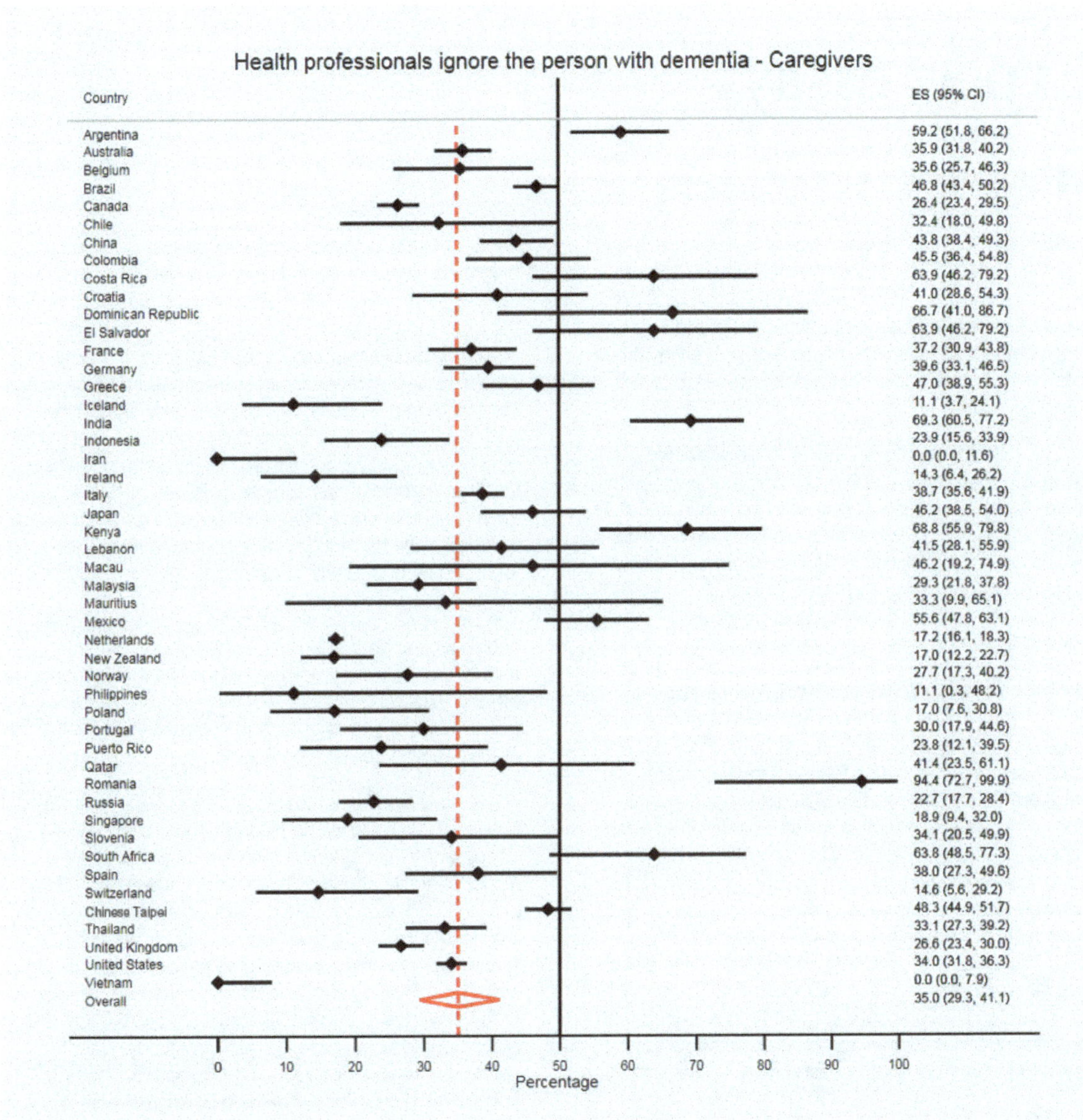
Health professionals ignore the person with dementia - Caregivers
Country
ES (95% CI)
Argentina 59.2 (51.8, 66.2)
Australia 35.9 (31.8, 40.2)
Belgium 35.6 (25.7, 46.3)
Brazil 46.8 (43.4, 50.2)
Canada 26.4 (23.4, 29.5)
Chile 32.4 (18.0, 49.8)
China 43.8 (38.4, 49.3)
Colombia 45.5 (36.4, 54.8)
Costa Rica 63.9 (46.2, 79.2)
Croatia 41.0 (28.6, 54.3)
Dominican Republic 66.7 (41.0, 86.7)
El Salvador 63.9 (46.2, 79.2)
France 37.2 (30.9, 43.8)
Germany 39.6 (33.1, 46.5)
Greece 47.0 (38.9, 55.3)
Iceland 11.1 (3.7, 24.1)
India 69.3 (60.5, 77.2)
Indonesia 23.9 (15.6, 33.9)
Iran 0.0 (0.0, 11.6)
Ireland 14.3 (6.4, 26.2)
Italy 38.7 (35.6, 41.9)
Japan 46.2 (38.5, 54.0)
Kenya 68.8 (55.9, 79.8)
Lebanon 41.5 (28.1, 55.9)
Macau 46.2 (19.2, 74.9)
Malaysia 29.3 (21.8, 37.8)
Mauritius 33.3 (9.9, 65.1)
Mexico 55.6 (47.8, 63.1)
Netherlands 17.2 (16.1, 18.3)
New Zealand 17.0 (12.2, 22.7)
Norway 27.7 (17.3, 40.2)
Philippines 11.1 (0.3, 48.2)
Poland 17.0 (7.6, 30.8)
Portugal 30.0 (17.9, 44.6)
Puerto Rico 23.8 (12.1, 39.5)
Qatar 41.4 (23.5, 61.1)
Romania 94.4 (72.7, 99.9)
Russia 22.7 (17.7, 28.4)
Singapore 18.9 (9.4, 32.0)
Slovenia 34.1 (20.5, 49.9)
South Africa 63.8 (48.5, 77.3)
Spain 38.0 (27.3, 49.6)
Switzerland 14.6 (5.6, 29.2)
Chinese Taipei 48.3 (44.9, 51.7)
Thailand 33.1 (27.3, 39.2)
United Kingdom 26.6 (23.4, 30.0)
United States 34.0 (31.8, 36.3)
Vietnam 0.0 (0.0, 7.9)
Overall 35.0 (29.3, 41.1)
0
10
20
30
40
50
60
70
80
90
100
Percentage

CHAPTER 3

# Expert essays

## 3.1 Stigma: a personal view 7 years on

**Contributor:** Dr Nori Graham. Honorary Vice President of ADI and a Vice President of the Alzheimer's Society (England), previous chair of each organisation; Honorary Fellow of the Royal College of Psychiatrists and Emeritus Consultant in the Psychiatry of Old Age at the Royal Free Hospital; honorary doctorate for public services to the Open University.

In 2012, I wrote a personal view on stigma that was included in the World Alzheimer Report that year.[1] In that article I wrote about how people with dementia and their carers suffered twice over from the shameful way they were regarded. The public turns away from old people and it prefers not to know about people with dementia. To be old and to have dementia is to be double stigmatised.

I described how my professional experience and my involvement with the voluntary sector had informed my view on stigma and how it might be overcome. I concluded with two suggestions for improvement. First there was a need to establish, to a much greater degree, high quality, effective services for the diagnosis and management of people with dementia and other mental illnesses, and their carers. Second, national Alzheimer associations were needed worldwide 'to raise awareness, put pressure on governments to achieve policy changes, provide quality information, bring people with dementia and their families together to talk and share problems, and encourage well-known people with dementia and their families to go public to show that they, at least, are not afraid or ashamed.'

***You can talk about your glaucoma, deafness, arthritis, heart bypasses, cancers, even depression and Parkinson's disease, but admitting to dementia is a step too far***

Since that time, there have been many significant improvements in our field. According to official numbers, certainly in the UK, the number of people receiving a diagnosis has increased so that over half living with symptoms receive a diagnosis. I have a concern that the drive for diagnosis has led to some people with non-progressive mild cognitive impairment rather than dementia being inappropriately diagnosed, but doubtless the overall impact has been positive. However, in low- and middle-income countries the numbers diagnosed remain very low. When I visited St. Petersburg, I was told that dementia was 'almost invisible' in Russia. In India I was told that only one in ten receives a diagnosis. In Africa it seems that, in many countries, dementia is regarded as due to witchcraft.

The Dementia Friends programme to raise awareness and reduce stigma started in Japan about 7 years ago. It is now well-established in the UK and in many other countries. It has started to impact on people's understanding of dementia and awareness and will reduce stigma perhaps on a very significant scale.

There have been other improvements on the international scene. In 2017 the World Health Organisation (WHO) adopted the Global action plan on the public health response to dementia.[2] There is now a target for 75% of Member States to have developed a dementia action plan by 2025. This is a very ambitious target, but ADI is encouraging and supporting its national members to work with governments and policy makers to achieve it. ADI now has 100 national member associations and federations which, in itself, is a huge step forward in raising awareness and reducing stigma amongst the general public, professionals and policy makers.

As far as improvement in services is concerned, there has been change for the better, but management after diagnosis remains a postcode lottery, at least in the UK. There are areas where the post diagnostic care is excellent with 'dementia wellbeing teams' liaising with GP (general practitioner) practices and offering ongoing support. But too often support after diagnosis is non-existent. One strongly positive development is that the 2018 National Institute for Health and Care Excellence (NICE) Guidelines recommend that every person with a diagnosis should have a named clinical person to contact.[3] Another positive development is the Alzheimer's Society (UK) pilot programme, Connect, which will link by telephone everyone with a diagnosis of dementia with a named person.

But it is still not widely acknowledged that a diagnosis of dementia is the start of usually many years of a slowly deteriorating mental and physical disorder with unpredictable challenges for all involved. Every country needs a skilled workforce properly paid for the job to help care for people in their own home and in care homes. We train teachers to teach our children. We need to train a workforce to take care of our older people with dementia. This is simply not happening in the UK or anywhere. The establishment of such a workforce would go some way to eliminate stigma.

Over the last seven years I've taken on several additional roles in the field. I have become a dementia specialist adviser to one of the largest care home companies in the UK, Care UK. In line with some other similar companies it has now fully acknowledged that the majority of its residents have some degree of dementia. Comprehensive training in dementia care is being carried out by staff from Worcester University together with lead staff in Care UK. As part of my role in the company, I deliver talks on 'understanding dementia' to people living in the community. These are free discussion events bringing me in close touch with the challenges people are facing.

For the last five years I have chaired the advisory group of a large research programme (IDEAL) looking at the meaning of living well with dementia by recording the experiences of people living with dementia and their carers after diagnosis.[(i)] On the advisory group, as well as professionals, there are people living with dementia and their carers.

In addition, on behalf of ADI, I have become a member of the advisory group for the research programme STRiDE (Strengthening responses to dementia in developing countries).[(ii)] This research aims to examine the way dementia is regarded, diagnosed and managed in a number of low- and middle-income countries. The group recently met in Cape Town where I was able to take an active part in our regional meeting of African National Associations.

Finally, and very sadly, my personal experience of dementia has vastly increased over the last seven years. Some of my closest friends are now living with a progressive dementia. My husband and I see them regularly, invite them to our home with or without their partners to give their partners a break. We have them to stay with us on holiday. I see them all at close quarters. I have to say I am often shocked, deeply taken aback by their attitudes to dementia and for the time it takes for them to accept the diagnosis. These are all people who are intelligent, well read and highly educated. Yet they simply cannot admit to significant memory problems either that they have themselves or that the person they are living with has. This is partly, but perhaps only partly, because they think dementia is a shameful condition. You can talk about your glaucoma, deafness, arthritis, heart bypasses, cancers, even depression and Parkinson's disease, but admitting to dementia is a step too far. Apart from stigma, this is partly because of accompanying radical physical and personality changes in the person with dementia. It is also partly because we do not have effective treatments but then this is also true for many of the conditions I have just mentioned.

One issue of which this personal experience with friends has taught me is what a difference it makes to carers if they can call on paid or voluntary help that is individually tailored to their needs. Of course, a national work force would help in providing a source of such help, but often it is not so much training as the right sort of personality and previous experience that seems most important.

Let me finish on an even more personal note. In 2012 I was a woman of (not to be too specific!) a certain age. My age is now even more certain. My chances of experiencing dementia have gone up. If I do develop dementia, I have numerous advantages over many others with that condition. I have professional knowledge about it and ready access to local excellent services. I have a family and many friends who would be supportive and helpful. I can afford good care. I would feel no shame at having the condition. And yet … and yet I still dread getting it. Of course, I know all about the fact that one can still lead a good life even if one has the condition. But the loss of all my lovely memories, the experience of confusion when I could not find my way about anymore, the humiliation of having to rely on others for my personal care, all these I dread. Let us not exaggerate the effect that overcoming the disadvantages that stigma brings with it. The complete removal of stigma which, of course I fervently desire, would result in a better life for those with dementia and their carers but it would remain an unutterably distressing condition. It has become even clearer over the past seven years that anything that can meaningfully be called a cure is still many years away. Roll on effective prevention!

(i) Find out more: http://www.idealproject.org.uk/

(ii) Find out more: https://www.stride-dementia.org/

## References


1 Alzheimer's Disease International, 2012. World Alzheimer Report 2012: Overcoming the stigma of dementia online: < https://www.alz.co.uk/research/WorldAlzheimerReport2012.pdf> Last accessed 20 August 2019.

2 World Health Organization. Global action plan on the public health response to dementia 2017–2025. Geneva: World Health Organization; 2017. Licence: CC BY-NC-SA 3.0. online: <https://apps.who.int/iris/bitstream/handle/10665/259615/9789241513487-eng.pdf?sequence=1> Last accessed 19 August 2019.

3 National Institute for Health and Care Excellence. 2018. NICE guideline NG97 *Dementia: assessment, management and support for people living with dementia and their carers* online: <https://www.nice.org.uk/guidance/ng97/chapter/Recommendations> Last accessed 20 August 2019.

## 3.2 Stigma, dementia and age

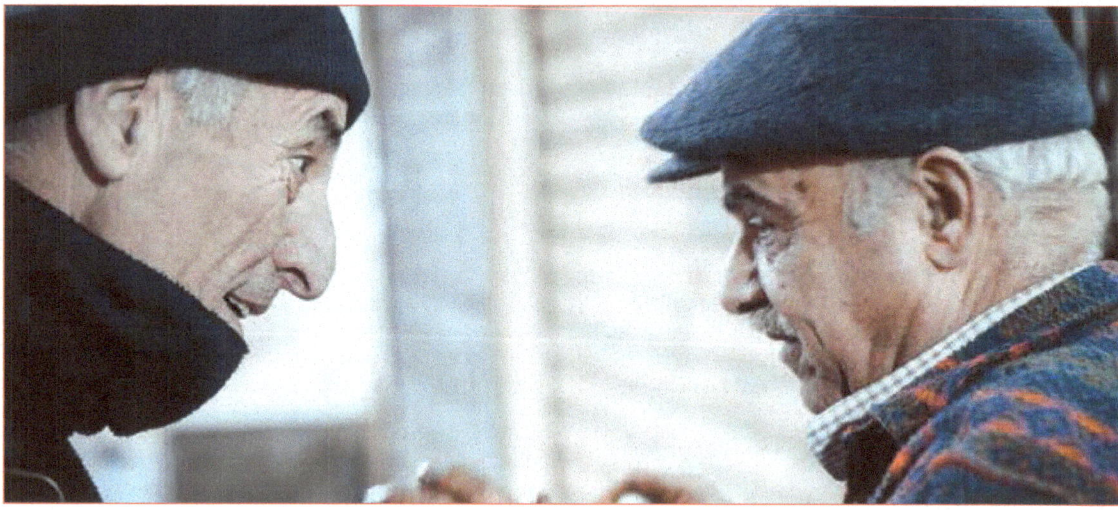

**Contributor:** Silvia Perel-Levin, International Longevity Centre Global Alliance (ILC GA) representative to the UN, Geneva; Chair, Geneva NGO Committee on Ageing

Dementia is not an inevitable result of ageing. However, as the risk of getting dementia greatly increases with age, people living with dementia are likely to experience a "double stigma". Because age is the major risk factor in developing dementia, those with the condition often experience the effects of dementia stigma in addition to the broader ageism older people encounter and the distinction between the two types of stigma often becomes blurred.[1]

We all age. That is a fact of life. More and more women and men live very long lives. However, everyone seems to want to live longer but only in good health and without getting older. Growing old does not mean that we cannot do the things we like doing. In fact, we can. There is evidence to support that many people over 60 are able to function in the same way as many people in their 20s or 30s. Therefore, the assumption that old age equals natural and inevitable decline is not totally accurate and has hidden preventable inequalities in the quality of life of older people.[2]

Despite the fact that older persons are able to function in multiple ways, we seem to require permission from society, our families or close ones in order to do the things we value, or indeed do them in hiding because we are either largely invisible, or would be looked at as a curious specimen, considered "demented" and too often be stripped of our rights. Prejudice and assumptions rule our lives. We are forced to retire, or to give up many of our routine activities simply because either we reached a certain age or because we were diagnosed with an "age-related" disease, regardless of what a person can or wants to do. No other disability acquired at younger "working age" would be treated in such a discriminatory fashion.

When a person has dementia, the condition takes over as the main descriptor of who they are. The stigma cancels the individual's personality or personal history. Care systems focus on the dementia rather than the needs of the individual. Inadequate medication management, and misinterpretation of symptoms mean that many people are receiving poorer services. This is in addition to the broader ageism in the healthcare system, which can also lead to reduced access to services. Old age is perceived as a synonym of frailty and cognitive decline and we are all put in the same bag, as if we were all the same.

*Old age is perceived as a synonym of frailty and cognitive decline and we are all put in the same bag, as if we were all the same.*

Ageist attitudes, combined with the stigma of the disease, will also have a detrimental impact on training and the development of practice amongst professionals and care staff. These attitudes contribute to the persistent and defeatist pessimism that characterize services for older people, especially those with dementia.[3]

People with dementia are likely to live with other medical conditions, many of which could be preventable and are often undiagnosed. People with dementia are not treated the same way as people without dementia.[4]

Ageism and the discrimination against individuals or groups, on the basis of their age, are the root cause of the multiple challenges that older persons face in all aspects of life. Ageist attitudes lead to lower quality of life, lack of access to preventive, adequate health care or rehabilitation services, and to abusive practices, such as refused or undignified treatment.

***When a person has dementia, the condition takes over as the main descriptor of who they are. The stigma cancels the individual's personality or personal history. Care systems focus on the dementia rather than the needs of the individual.***

Pension schemes are inadequate, as they are not conceived to cover care-related needs, but for the loss of work-related income. In fact, only one in four people over 65 in low and middle-income countries receives a pension at all (UN 2018). Abuse, including social isolation, neglect, physical restraints, disrespect for individual choices, being deprived of day-to-day decisions, of liberty, of privacy or of palliative care can be a reality for older persons both at home or in an institution. This abuse is mostly hidden and tolerated with lack of legislation or regular monitoring or adequate protection standards.

Older persons worldwide experience discrimination and the violation of their human rights at family, community, institutional and societal levels. Older persons with disabilities, their loved ones and caregivers, face numerous barriers. There are big inequalities between older persons who need support in their daily activities compared with younger persons with disabilities. Older persons are rarely consulted in decision-making processes meaning that their specific situation remains largely unknown and unaddressed.

Despite the fact that most international human rights treaties apply in principle to people of all ages, specific reference to older persons is rare, including in the United Nations Convention on the Rights of Persons with Disabilities (CRPD). Concerns are often expressed about possible conflicting messages and a perception of lack of cooperation between the movement for the rights of older persons and the disability movement, for example on issues of accessibility or legal capacity.

Often, older persons may not want to be identified as having a disability, despite having significant difficulties in functioning, because they may consider their level of functioning appropriate for their age. Should they be considered persons with disabilities because they encounter the same barriers even if they do not see themselves as having a disability? Persons with early onset dementia or another disability may not want to be identified as old. Should a person consider herself or himself old simply because society has put an arbitrary age or other characteristic to limit their activities and entitlements?

Human Rights are indivisible, interdependent and interrelated. Denying rights to one is like denying them to everybody. Denying one right is like denying them all. We all are human rights holders, whatever our gender, race, ability, health or any other status. The rights of persons with dementia need to be looked at with a perspective of disability, gender and age. After all, we are all ageing. It is crucial to ensure a human rights-based approach to dementia beyond the narrow medicalisation of the issue. People living with dementia have the right to participate in society and those who violate their human rights should be held accountable.

The United Nations Open-Ended Working Group on Ageing (OEWG), for the purpose of strengthening the protection of the human rights of older persons, was established by the UN General Assembly in 2010. An international convention on the rights of older persons will provide a definitive, universal position that age discrimination is morally and legally unacceptable.

## References

1 Evans S. C, 2018 in Ayalon L, Tesch-Römer, C (eds.), 'Contemporary Perspectives on Ageism' International Perspectives on Aging 19.

2 Venkatapuram et al. 2017. Bulletin of the World Health Organization 95:791-792 online: < https://www.who.int/bulletin/volumes/95/11/16-187609/en/> Last accessed 20 August 2019.

3 Milne, A. 2010. 'The 'D' word: Reflections on the relationship between stigma, discrimination and dementia' Journal of Mental Health 19:3, 227-233.

4 Scrutton, J and Brancati, C. U. 2016. Dementia and comorbidities; Ensuring parity of care ILC UK online: <https://ilcuk.org.uk/wp-content/uploads/2018/10/Dementia-and-Comorbidities-Ensuring-Parity-of-Care.pdf> Last accessed 20 August 2019.

## Further reading

Global Alliance for the Rights of Older People (GAROP): https://www.rightsofolderpeople.org

UN, 2018 Report on the World Social Situation: https://www.un.org/development/desa/dspd/report-on-the-world-social-situation-rwss-social-policy-and-development-division/2018-2.html

UN Open-ended Working Group on Ageing: https://social.un.org/ageing-working-group/

## 3.3 Thinking more deeply about dementia friendliness

**Contributors:** Dr Linda Barclay, Philosopher at Monash University, Australia specialising in disability and justice. Glenn Rees, Chair, Alzheimer's Disease International

The priority of every Alzheimer's association this century has been to achieve a greater awareness and understanding of dementia - a natural response to the negativity and myths that have been associated with dementia for centuries. There has been an assumption that greater understanding and awareness are key to tackling stigma.

A more positive way of talking about dementia has been made possible by many new insights over the last two decades. The legacy of Tom Kitwood (author and founder of the Bradford Dementia Group), and knowing that good dementia care is person-centred and based on the needs of the individual rather than the task or the organisation are examples; along with the improved evidence base for dementia reduction; the knowledge that the pathology of dementia develops in the brain decades before symptoms appear, meaning that timely diagnosis and disease modifying treatments may delay onset; and that Alzheimer's medications have resulted in changed attitudes of doctors towards treating the symptoms of dementia.

There has also been recognition of providing guidance on the language used around dementia - avoiding terms like 'dementia sufferers' - and in some countries a new word for dementia has been introduced to remove previous contemptuous connotations.

The thinking has been broadened beyond awareness under the banner of dementia friendly.[1&2] It has taken multiple forms through:

- Social support: Memory cafes where people with dementia often meet, with informal carers and the wider community; volunteer programmes in community gardens, activity programmes to enable the person to continue their interests
- Greater public awareness: exemplified by the 'dementia friends' programmes in Japan, South Korea and the United Kingdom which provide basic dementia awareness training in the community
- Inclusive communities: setting up an alliance in the community involving local government, people with dementia and their families, and health services to identify ways in which the community could be made more dementia inclusive
- Better quality health and dementia services: increasing the capacity of the workforce to be dementia friendly by training staff in health services and identifying them as dementia friends
- Improving the physical environment: whether in private homes or residential facilities, public spaces or government buildings

These developments are recognised in action area 2 of the WHO Global dementia action plan on the public health response to dementia 2017-2025 in Dementia Awareness and friendliness.[3] The rationale for action in the Global action plan is that "Increasing public awareness, acceptance and understanding of dementia and making the societal environment dementia friendly will enable people with dementia to participate in the community and maximise their autonomy through improved social participation". The Global action plan goes onto state "A dementia friendly society possesses an accessible community environment that optimises opportunities for health, participation and security for all people, in order to ensure quality of life and dignity for people with dementia, their carers and families."

The question is how far can we rely on awareness and dementia friendliness alone to achieve a reduction in stigma and improve quality of life for people with dementia?

### Quality of life

To reflect on the impact of dementia-friendly programmes it is necessary to think about what a good quality of life for a person with dementia might consist of. Some of the main elements that are widely recognised to contribute to quality of life are the following:[4]

*Well-being.* Being content, happy, feeling safe, experiencing pleasure and joy, having a sense of self-worth and purpose can all enhance a person's quality of life. Conversely, suffering pain, distress, fear, loneliness and humiliation can all detract from the quality of one's life.

We also rely on more objective measures in quality of life assessments. Health outcomes, income and quality housing, to name just a few, are often taken to be reliable indicators of some aspects of quality of life. Very poor health, poverty, insecure or poor-quality housing can all negatively impact quality of life.

*Autonomy/Independence.* It is hard to overstate the prominence of respect for individual autonomy or decision-making in health care contexts over the last 50 years. In cases where the necessity of substituted decision making or guardianship had been assumed, the emphasis has shifted to supported decision-making where possible, or a reliance on advance directives. Such options prioritise the values and preferences of the person affected as much as possible and assumes that doing so is at the heart of promoting a good life for each individual.

*Equality.* Along with autonomy, the value of equality has been equally prominent in discussions of quality of life and in medical ethics. Equality usually refers to our equal worth: despite all the differences between people – in their cognitive or physical capacities, in their ethnicity, religion, gender or sexual orientation, in their age or level of wealth and so on – we are all of equal worth. It is widely recognised that people who are routinely treated with disrespect, as inferiors, have reduced quality of life.

## The impact of awareness and dementia friendliness

How effectively are dementia-friendly programmes likely to promote well-being, autonomy and equality?

People on the receiving end of stigmatised attitudes and behaviour and the related social isolation are more likely to suffer a range of poor health outcomes and have reduced capacity to secure important needs, such a health, personal care and other support services. For people with dementia this starts with under diagnosis and failure to provide post diagnostic support which both stigmatises and increases the difficulty of accessing services that respond to their individual needs and builds on their capacities. It continues with frequent physical and medical abuse in institutional care.

***Information and knowledge about dementia are needed because the ignorance around dementia results in discrimination, loss of rights and perpetuates negative beliefs towards those affected by the disease. But in all countries stigma and social exclusion is rarely just the result of ignorance. Social structures also play a part and need to be addressed by governments through legal protections and services.***

Insofar as awareness and dementia friendliness can play a role in reducing stigma and facilitating inclusion, they can obviously promote well-being. It is likely that people who experience positive and warm relationships and are active in their communities are more likely to report feeling satisfied with their lives, to have a sense of self-esteem and purpose, and are less likely to suffer various forms of neglect. Training and education for informal carers and paid staff will also help. So, dementia friendly projects that focus on inclusion, social engagement that enables the person with dementia to continue their interests, and mentoring that enables voluntary and paid employment will have practical benefits.

Low income countries have generally not experienced the positive changes in the way dementia is talked about in high income countries. The stigma of dementia is great because of ignorance around dementia, other pressing health priorities, poor health infrastructure and cultural and spiritual factors. There is a need for information and knowledge about dementia among carers, care workers, healers and the community, in recognition of the fact that a lack of understanding of the condition fuels fear and discrimination and perpetuates negative beliefs towards those affected by the disease. In these countries stakeholder groups will require a better understanding of dementia and to adopt approaches that respond to the cultural understanding of dementia and beliefs about the causality of the condition.[5]

However, in all countries stigma and social exclusion is rarely just a result of ignorance. This concern is closely related to a deeper issue which can be provocatively presented as a question: how many of the difficulties confronting people with dementia are just "in the head"? In other words, to what extent does the stigma and exclusion experienced by people with dementia stem from ignorance and bad attitudes, as opposed to stemming from broader social *structures*?

The impact of social structures on stigma is arguably pervasive and insidious. For example, a diagnosis of dementia maybe used to exclude individuals from some forms of care e.g. rehabilitation and palliative care. Conversely, the absence of a diagnosis or post diagnostic support, for the majority of those with dementia, denies them access to health services. When people are excluded from the workforce, or do not receive the right resources to maintain their independence, then the effect can be that stigma around dementia is reinforced. When people do not receive adequate assistance to live in decent housing with high-quality support services, or when their own choices and decisions are not respected, then stigma is at play. And discrimination extends beyond services to research, where the priority for dementia research is clearly less than second best to what has been invested in cancer and HIV/AIDS.

In other words, we need to be modest in our expectations about how much awareness and dementia friendliness on their own can do to tackle stigma and social avoidance. In the light of serious under investment in medical research and treatment, housing and support services, and without legislative action to improve accessibility and address discrimination, stigma will persist, because it is reinforced daily.

## The disability rights movement

We have much to learn here from the disability rights movement. The disability community prefers to talk about disability *rights*, rather than disability friendliness, an older and largely abandoned phrase. Resources, accessibility and protection from discrimination are fundamental entitlements, enshrined in the Convention on the Rights of Persons with Disabilities (CRPD), now ratified by the vast majority of the world's countries. Their delivery is not an act of friendliness (or kindness): it is a fundamental right owed to all members of the community. Failure to secure them is now described as a failure to respect the rights of people with disability, a failure to treat them as equals and respect their dignity. The blind philosopher Adam Cureton has dubbed it 'offensive beneficence' when a person's rights are offered as an act of charity, kindness or generosity.[6]

In addition, people with disability also remind us that however well intentioned, action that does not aim at supporting their capacities to make their own decisions and manage their own lives, can do more harm than good. We can seek to be welcoming, helpful and friendly to people with disabilities, yet they may experience it as paternalistic or even condescending. Most people with disability want their relationships with others to be directed by their own views about what their needs are, as much as is possible, and based on recognising them as capable. Anything less, however well-intentioned, it is often said, is to fail to treat them as equals.

While the CPRD includes dementia, and much has been made of the need to normalise dementia and refer to it as a disability, the language and emphasis of dementia-friendliness is quite different to what is widely preferred in the disability rights movement. In that movement, reference to 'special needs' and 'assistance' has been replaced with 'human rights', 'fairness' and 'opportunity'. When disability advocates talk about 'normalising' disability, part of what they mean to do is reject assumptions that disability is a 'deficiency' or even a 'disease', but instead a normal part of human variation.[7]

As advocates for people with dementia, do we want to also deny that dementia is a disease, or deny that it is often experienced as a very negative development in a person's life? Would borrowing this view from the disability rights movement do justice to the experience of people with dementia and their loved ones? There is a need for careful reflection on exactly how and why dementia advocacy can be part of the broader disability rights movement.

## Conclusion

Awareness and dementia friendliness have a role to play in changing the way we think about dementia and achieve practical change to make societies more inclusive of people with dementia. But there is a risk that generalised notions of awareness and dementia friendliness may distract from the most important factors in ensuring a good quality of life for people with dementia and their loved ones – namely, resources and protections of various kinds: investment in diagnostic and health care resources and research, adequate income, housing, and high-quality support services, accessible environments and legal protection from discrimination, to name just a few. We should never underestimate the tendency of governments everywhere to support and prioritise solutions that shift focus away from their own responsibilities and demand less of them in terms of resources and legislative action.

Finally, we should be thinking more deeply about the relationship between dementia advocacy and the disability rights movement.

## References


1 Alzheimer's Disease International. 2016. Dementia Friendly Communities: Key Principals (1st Edition) online: <https://www.alz.co.uk/dementia-friendly-communities/principles> Last accessed 19 August 2019.

2 Alzheimer's Disease International. 2017. Dementia Friendly Communities: Global developments (2nd Edition) online: <https://www.alz.co.uk/adi/pdf/dfc-developments.pdf> Last accessed 19 August 2019.

3 World Health Organization. Global action plan on the public health response to dementia 2017–2025. Geneva: World Health Organization; 2017. Licence: CC BY-NC-SA 3.0. online: <https://apps.who.int/iris/bitstream/handle/10665/259615/9789241513487-eng.pdf?sequence=1> Last accessed 19 August 2019.

4 Routledge Handbook of the Philosophy of Well-Being (First edition) London: Routledge; 2015.

5 Alzheimer's Disease International. 2017. Dementia in Sub-Saharan Africa online: <https://www.alz.co.uk/research/dementia-in-africa> Last accessed 19 August 2019.

6 Cureton, A. 2016. 'Offensive Beneficence' Journal of the American Philosophical Association 2(1) online: < https://www.cambridge.org/core/journals/journal-of-the-american-philosophical-association/article/offensive-beneficence/7CCBCE6ACE96D26CA4FF3ABB0C46E11C> Last accessed 19 August 2019.

7 Barclay, L. Disability with Dignity. Human Rights, Justice and Equal Respect. London: Routledge; 2019.

## 3.4 The role of the media: Help or hinderance?

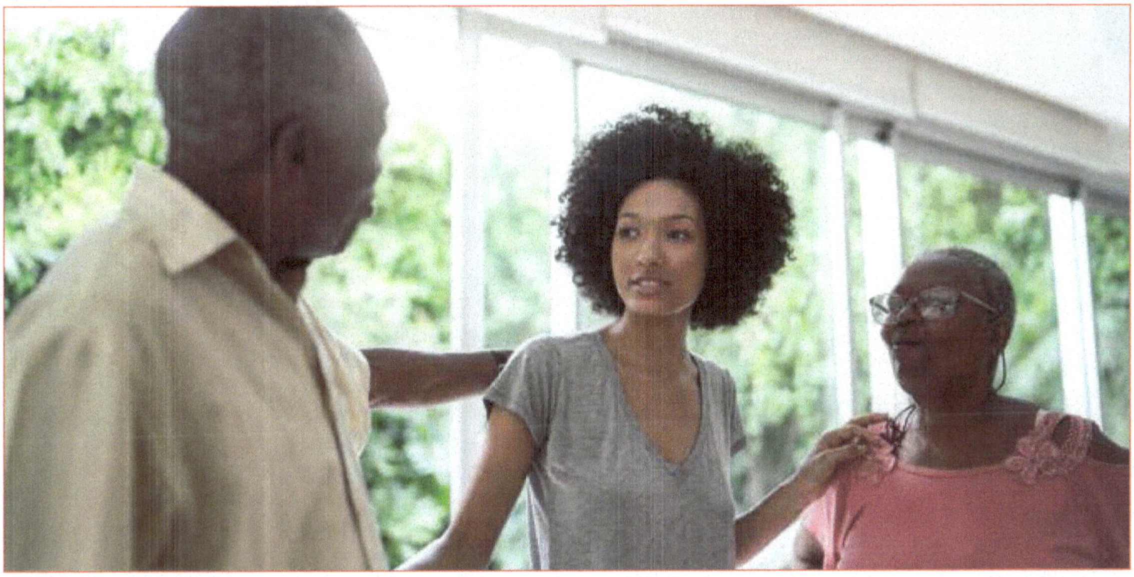

**Contributor:** Pippa Kelly, UK. Journalist, dementia blogger, public speaker.

Since Julie Austen's husband David was diagnosed with Alzheimer's disease three years ago her younger brother hasn't talked to her. Her mother and sister-in-law keep asking when David, 66, will get better.

The 59-year-old East Sussex woman believes her relatives' response to David's condition stems from lack of understanding. *"I don't know if it's the result of ignorance or because they don't know what to say".* Either way, Julie and her husband have become very isolated.

Such an extreme example of stigma might seem rare in the 21st century but it isn't restricted to uninformed members of the public. Stephen Atkinson-Jones' 89-year-old mother Audrey has Alzheimer's and shares her flat in Bexhill-on-Sea with a live-in carer.

This January, Audrey was admitted to hospital with an impacted bowel and various infections. Stephen says the green leaf mounted above Audrey's bed to show she had dementia was ignored and when he asked why she wasn't being given a CT scan the consultant told him there was no point as *"something was going to get her anyway."* His mother would poison herself, Stephen was told, by vomiting her own faeces.

Stephen is convinced that this extraordinary lack of care was due, not to hospital failings, but the preconceived idea that Audrey wasn't worth treating because of her dementia.

It's not uncommon to hear stories such as Audrey's in the media. In the last five to ten years dementia campaigners have gained a voice – I say this with authority because (as well as being a journalist) I am one. Where injustice and stigma lurk, we speak out against it.

Stigma stems from fear. Fear breeds silence, which in turn perpetuates ignorance and misunderstanding. The key to killing off stigma lies in communication, of which we members of the media are, like it or not, the most skilled operators. So, how well are we professionals doing with this, what can we do better and what can organisations such as Alzheimer's Disease International do to help us?

The first thing to remember is that the media's role is not to combat stigma or disseminate messages from dementia organisations, it's to attract readers, viewers and listeners. But the media and dementia sectors can benefit each other. The media need powerful, newsworthy human-interest stories and it's up to those in the dementia community to understand what these are and provide them, quickly and accurately.

One of the biggest sellers of newspapers – for which read, "What the public really want to hear about and are prepared to part with their money for" – are celebrities. Which is why any dementia story with a famous name will make the news – in the UK think of Terry Pratchett (author), Prunella Scales (actor), David Baddiel (comedian and author). Celebrities make great news copy because the public relate to them – they think (bizarrely) that they know them.

Once a condition such as dementia is given a human face, your attitude towards it changes. Gone is the stigma and fear: mum may be behaving in an unusual way, she may be incontinent or unable to speak properly, but she's my mum. Barbara Windsor (UK actor) may have dementia but she's still "Babs" from countless Carry On films and latterly the Queen Vic (from the UK Soap

EastEnders). These well-known, familiar faces bring home to us what dementia is. Use them. They show us that this frightening condition (it's the one that over 55s fear most) doesn't strike others, it strikes us.

---

***Stigma stems from fear. Fear breeds silence, which in turn perpetuates ignorance and misunderstanding.***

---

This sense of togetherness plays an important role in reducing stigma. Once dementia affected my mother I wanted to find out about it, in both human and practical terms, whereas before I'd turned away from it, metaphorically crossed the road away from it (a move guaranteed to breed stigma).

Which calls into question the merit of initiatives such as the Dementia Friends scheme and Dementia Friendly communities and shops. Is it helpful to compartmentalise those with dementia? I believe we're still in the early stages of informing people and changing perceptions, we're still raising awareness. To this end, public campaigns with clear and simple messages work.

The key is to build on these first steps, to ensure people understand that being dementia friendly means more than sticking a green leaf above a hospital bed, then ignoring it. It means appreciating that someone with dementia may not be able to identify the coins in their pocket, need more time at the till, have a problem with their balance or sight, may have a better memory in some respects than you or me – and it means respecting the brilliance with which those same people still sing, identify a little-known shrub or whittle a piece of wood.

In terms of the media, it means seeking out case studies that show – to the very best advantage – all of the above. When a Sainsbury's (a supermarket) in north London found different ways to keep employing a woman with dementia, it made it into all the national newspapers and onto national TV. It was a first-class human-interest story with which everyone connected. These stories are out there – find them, ensure you have the consent of everyone involved and feed them to the media.

An even more successful method of banishing stigma via the media is through the soft power of culture. Virtually every radio and TV soap opera contains a dementia storyline. When well executed, popular entertainment programmes such as the BBC's Our Dementia Choir (fronted by a celebrity with a personal interest in the subject) powerfully yet subtly convey to their several million viewers various stigma-busting messages.

UK dementia campaigners often tell journalists to use the phrase "people living with dementia" instead of "dementia sufferers" and avoid dramatic descriptions such as "a tsunami of dementia" in order to combat stigma. I understand the logic, but would you rather a national newspaper or TV station covered a story to raise awareness of young onset dementia using the phrase "dementia sufferers" or didn't cover it at all?

Compared to the relatively nuanced stigma encountered here in the UK, those living with dementia in other parts of the world face open hostility – in the black Caribbean they are sometimes viewed as possessing evil spirits. In recent years an elderly woman with dementia was found chained in a hut in the Kunene region of Namibia; she'd been kept there for twenty years for being a witch. On the other hand, unlike many minority ethnic communities, where elders are respected, British society tends to devalue old age, producing a double jeopardy of stigma.

I'm often told, "Dementia's where cancer was 30 to 40 years ago". Is it? A major breakthrough in reducing stigma around the Big C (as it was then referred to in hushed tones) occurred in 1965 when Richard Dimbleby, the "voice of the nation", announced on national television that he had testicular cancer. This wasn't 30 but 54 years ago.

In the first piece I wrote about my mother in 2006 I described her, in a national newspaper, as demented. She was my mum; I didn't do so to cause offence but out of ignorance. It could be argued a) my use of ill-chosen language fuelled stigma or b) my article in itself raised awareness.

Either way, I know better now and would never use the word. Like other people, we in the media are learning and adapting as the subject of dementia looms larger in everyone's lives. Our powerful role in changing public perceptions of dementia is, like stigma itself, complicated.

## 3.5 Stigma in 2019; you must be joking!

**Contributor:** Dale Goldhawk, Vice Chair, Alzheimer's Disease International & veteran advocacy journalist.

It's odd but I have always felt a warm place in my heart for Alzheimer's disease. It might seem strange that love could ever be found anywhere near dementia. Alzheimer's is a cruel disease. It gradually erases memory, personality and the ability to function. Then, after years of decline, Alzheimer's disease leads to death.

But the love is there. It's found in the attitudes and actions of the people in the Alzheimer family. The often unsinkable nature of those living with dementia; the courageous heroes who care for them; the tireless and devoted advocates, champions, doctors and scientists who fight for effective treatments and a cure.

Just spend a little time with the devoted staff and volunteers at Alzheimer's Disease International's associations and federations in 100 countries around the world. They care deeply. They're working hard to make a difference.

And yet, our own human nature often fights against progress and awareness when we encounter dementia. You probably know people who fear it, view it with distaste, avoid it whenever possible, are uneasy with unusual behaviour and uncertain about how to react themselves.

Stigma. The Oxford Dictionary has a stark definition, calling it "a mark of disgrace associated with a circumstance, quality or person."

Stigma is often accompanied by another, greater attack against our dignity, against our inherent humanity. And that's discrimination; the unjust or prejudicial treatment of different groups of people. Discrimination, in fact, violates the law in many countries; the United Nations Convention on the Rights of Persons with Disabilities has declared that people with disabilities (including those living with dementia) must enjoy all human rights and fundamental freedoms.

My father died of Alzheimer's disease after a seven-year-long, downward journey into dementia. My mother died after a sudden heart attack; her good health badly damaged by the stress of caregiving.

Stigma closed the door on Mom and Dad. Friends stopped dropping by to visit. There were hardly any calls inquiring about Dad's condition. It was as if he were already dead.

Back then, I often encountered the heartless insensitivity of Alzheimer related jokes. When I explained to friends and acquaintances that I was volunteering for the Alzheimer Society of Canada, the reaction was often an Alzheimer's related joke. I don't think there was any malice in it. They just forgot how deeply words can hurt. They really didn't know what to say.

In the beginning I got angry. *"Not funny,"* I would say. *"There's nothing funny about cancer and not much humour in heart disease."* In later years, I offered a more reasoned reaction hoping for a teachable moment. I seldom got one. None of the people who ever tried to crack an Alzheimer's related joke with me knew anything about dementia. Perhaps that lack of knowledge produced the feeble attempt at humour.

I still remember vividly the day Mom and I took Dad to the long-term care home where he would live, since Mom could no longer care for him at home. It was a heart-breaking decision that always kept Mom (and me and my brother and sisters) close to tears. Dad was distressed. He didn't want to go.

As we pushed his wheelchair up the front walk into the home, Dad turned and looked up at Mom and said: *"you did this to me, didn't you."*

No. Nothing funny there.

So-called Alzheimer's humour does much more than annoy and hurt those who work hard to make life better for the 50 million plus people in the world living with dementia. It trivialises the disease. Worse, humour is often used as a weapon today. If you can laugh at somebody, they lose credibility. They can't be taken seriously. So, what if every 3 seconds in the world somebody develops dementia. If dementia is somehow funny, stigma has a place to grow. The sense of urgency about dementia starts to fade.

The good news is that Alzheimer's jokes are not nearly as prevalent as they once were. The attempted humour is disappearing as awareness of dementia in its most common form, Alzheimer's disease, is growing. I have seen it in my years in broadcasting, where I have often raised dementia issues in my radio and television open line programmes. In earlier years, people had trouble even pronouncing the word 'Alzheimer' but gradually people learned from listening. They started telling their own stories on television and radio, stories of how their families and loved ones cared for, and still loved those living with dementia. There were stories about how those with dementia were still able to find a little peace and quality of life. After a while, the stories about dementia families just became stories about families.

But stigma remains a tough customer. Even today when I tell people I'm involved with Alzheimer's Disease International I usually get a polite but strained reaction, occasionally a raised eyebrow and few, if any, questions about the work my colleagues and I do. It was never like that when I worked as a volunteer to help children with physical disabilities. Everybody felt comfortable asking questions. It was familiar territory. Someday soon I hope the Alzheimer's family will move securely into that neighbourhood.

## 3.6 Alzheimer's disease, stigma and disclosure

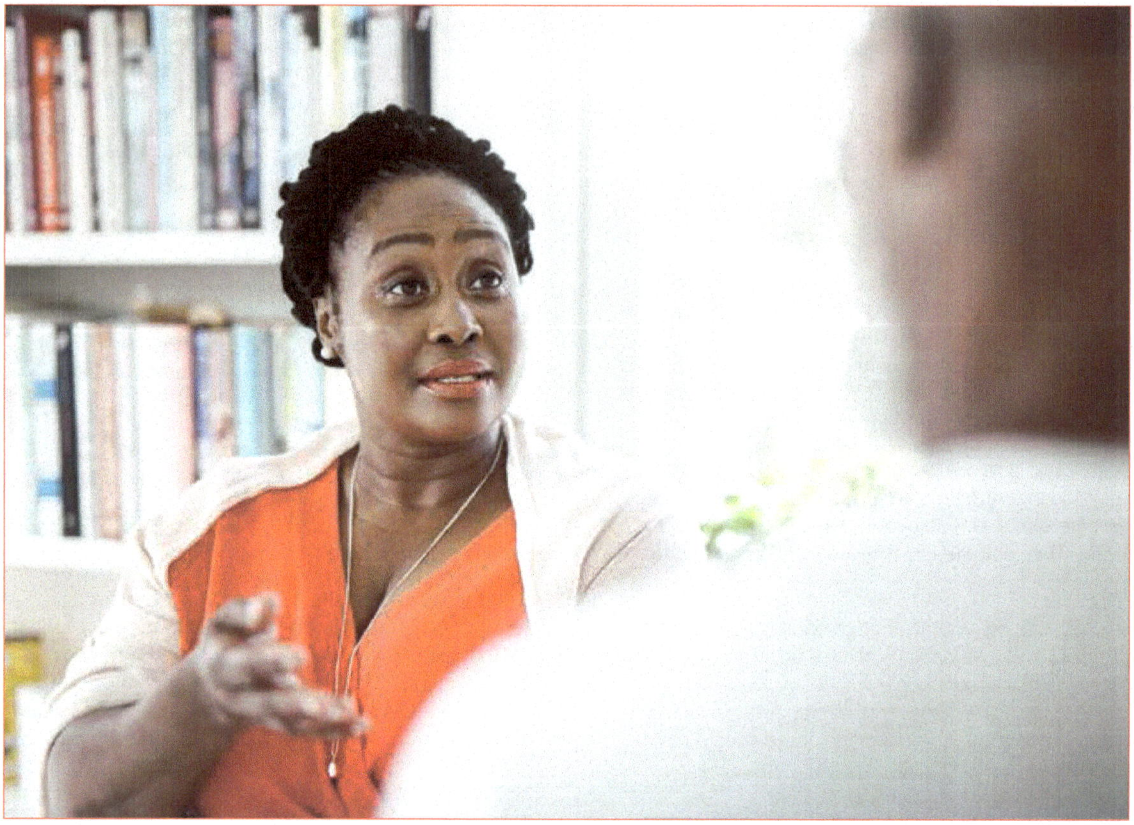

**Contributor:** Prof Nicolas Rüsch, Ulm University and BKH Günzburg, Germany

People with mental illness as well as individuals with Alzheimer's disease struggle with two kinds of problems. On the one hand, they have to cope with the symptoms and disabilities of their disorder such as anxiety or memory problems. On the other hand, they struggle with the stigma associated with these disorders. Stigma can be a heavier burden than the disease itself. One reason that stigma has such a big impact is that it comes in three forms: public, self and structural. Public stigma occurs when members of the general public endorse negative stereotypes ('This person with dementia is contagious, I'll stay away from her'), often leading to social exclusion or discrimination in work or private settings. If people with dementia agree with negative stereotypes and turn them against themselves, this is referred to as self-stigma ('Because I have dementia, I cannot decide anything'). Self-stigma is often associated with shame, social withdrawal and secrecy. Structural stigma refers to rules and regulations, for example in health or social care settings, that disadvantage people with the disorder. Here I briefly summarise a few themes from recent research on stigma and disclosure. Colleagues such as Perla Werner, from the University of Haifa in Israel, and many others have done ground breaking research on stigma and dementia, and their work offers more thorough orientation than this brief outline[1].

Attitudes to dementia and to ageing in general have varied a lot throughout history and across cultures. The Roman philosopher and politician Cicero provides an early example in his 44 BC book 'Cato the Elder on Old Age' in which he refutes various negative views of old age and ageing. Modern approaches to dementia have been very diverse too: Alois Alzheimer thought of it as a brain disorder, while others emphasised psychosocial factors that contribute to dementia because a lack of social support for people with dementia increases their disability[2]. Recent research has produced solid evidence of widespread stigma and discrimination currently associated with Alzheimer's disease and dementia in general[1].

The media also play a role. In terms of social media, a study found that dementia is an object of ridicule on Twitter[3]. News media often use catastrophic metaphors of dementia as a wave, flood, monster, enemy or the plague of our century[4]. It is not hard to imagine how this leads to reactions such as fear and avoidance. Probably the most malicious of these metaphors is the one of people with Alzheimer's disease as zombies because it dehumanises individuals[5]. We should respond by stating the obvious: people with Alzheimer's disease are first and foremost human beings with feelings and dignity.

Given these popular images, general population surveys unsurprisingly reveal ambivalent attitudes towards people with Alzheimer's disease: On the one hand members of the general public report empathy and willingness to help, on the other hand they show anxiety and avoidance[6]. Negative attitudes shape help-seeking behaviours because they are associated with more scepticism about screening for dementia, making early intervention more difficult[7].

How do people with Alzheimer's disease react to stigma? Many, along with their carers and relatives, struggle with shame and self-stigma. Many people with Alzheimer's disease are also aware of public stigma and therefore hesitate to disclose their condition. *"It's a strange life when you 'come out' – people get embarrassed, lower their voices and get lost for words"*, wrote the novelist Terry Pratchett after he was diagnosed[1]. As for people with other mental disorders, disclosure decisions are often complex and personal and depend on the person and the environment. Both disclosure and non-disclosure have pros and cons. Disclosure carries the risk of being labelled and discriminated against; but it also facilitates help-seeking, social support and authentic exchange with others. On the other hand, non-disclosure can protect against discrimination, but may lead to social isolation, the stress and fear to be 'found out' and can be a barrier to seeking care and support.

Disclosure is not an all-or-nothing decision, but people can learn to reveal certain things to certain people. They will likely want to tell more to a close friend than to a neighbour, and more to a trusted healthcare professional than to a person in the supermarket. Navigating the continuum between varying degrees of disclosure for different addressees, people with Alzheimer's disease can learn to make strategic choices of what to disclose to whom. The decision is not whether to disclose or not to disclose, but to find the right choice and level of disclosure, if any, for each context, after weighing pros and cons. This is a continuing process as people can and will learn from previous experiences of (non-) disclosure. It is helpful if people with Alzheimer's disease and their carers discuss disclosure decisions together. Patrick W. Corrigan and his colleagues in Chicago developed "Honest, Open, Proud" (HOP; www.hopprogram.org) as a peer-run group programme that supports people with mental illness in such disclosure decisions. It is HOP's aim to empower people to make their own decisions and to enable them to tell their stories safely, if they decide to do so. As disclosure and non-disclosure are one way to cope with public and self-stigma, HOP has the potential to reduce self-stigma. A couple of evaluations of the HOP programme have shown reductions in self-stigma and other positive effects among participants[8]. HOP has been adapted for a range of target groups, and Jem Bhatt, University College London (UCL), and her colleagues in London are currently working on a version for people with dementia.

Based on self-confident disclosure decisions, people will gain confidence whether, how, and when to tell their story. This can be an important part of their recovery – or, in other words, of their living as well as possible with dementia. First-person narratives of people with Alzheimer's disease, available online or in books, about their lives with the disease are also one of the best ways to reduce public stigma. Through these stories, members of the general public can learn about the perspectives of people with Alzheimer's disease and reflect on their views and stereotypes. For people with Alzheimer's disease, telling their story can be an act of self-affirmation and resistance against the disease and the associated stigma. Such stories may describe disability and loss, but also coping, as an opportunity for growth and for refocusing on important things in life[9]. Many stories show acceptance and gratitude for one's life. Telling one's story can evolve into art: there are moving poetry collections of people with Alzheimer's disease and other dementias online (e.g., www.alzpoetry.com/read-me). Participation in and experience of art for people with Alzheimer's disease can be found in museums, theatres and other cultural institutions. Along with media education and other targeted anti-stigma efforts, these kinds of grass-roots programmes may be the best way to counter stigma and empower people with Alzheimer's disease[10]. As stigma contributes to the burden of Alzheimer's disease and other types of dementia, programmes of this kind should be evaluated and, if successful, more widely implemented.

## References


1 Werner P 2014. Stigma and Alzheimer's disease: A systematic review of evidence, theory, and methods. In: Corrigan PW (Ed.) The stigma of disease and disability: Understanding causes and overcoming injustices. American Psychological Association, Washington, 223–244.

2 Ballenger JF 2017. ‚Framing confusion: Dementia, society, and history.' *AMA J Ethics* 19(7):713–719.

3 Oscar N, Fox PA, Croucher R et al. 2017. ‚Machine learning, sentiment analysis, and tweets: An examination of Alzheimer's disease stigma on Twitter.' *J Gerontol B Psychol Sci Soc Sci* 72(5):742–751.

4 Zeilig H 2014. ‚Dementia as a cultural metaphor.' *Gerontologist* 54(2):258–267.

5 Behuniak SM 2011 ‚The living dead? The construction of people with Alzheimer's disease as zombies.' *Ageing & Society* 31(1):70–92.

6 von dem Knesebeck O, Angermeyer MC, Ludecke D et al. 2014. ‚Emotional reactions toward people with dementia: Results of a population survey from Germany.' *Int. Psychogeriatr.* 26(3):435–441.

7 Martin S, Kelly S, Khan A et al. 2015. ‚Attitudes and preferences towards screening for dementia: a systematic review of the literature.' *BMC Geriatr* 15:66.

8 Mulfinger N, Müller S, Böge I et al. 2018. ‚Honest, Open, Proud for adolescents with mental illness: Pilot randomized controlled trial.' *Journal of Child Psychology & Psychiatry* 59(6):684–691.

9 O'Connor D, Mann J, Wiersma E 2018. ‚Stigma, discrimination and agency: Diagnostic disclosure as an everyday practice shaping social citizenship.' *J Aging Stud.* 44:45–51.

10 Bienvenu B, Hanna G 2017. ‚Arts participation: Counterbalancing forces to the social stigma of a dementia diagnosis.' *AMA J Ethics* 19(7):704–712.

## 3.7 The costs of dementia: advocacy, media and stigma

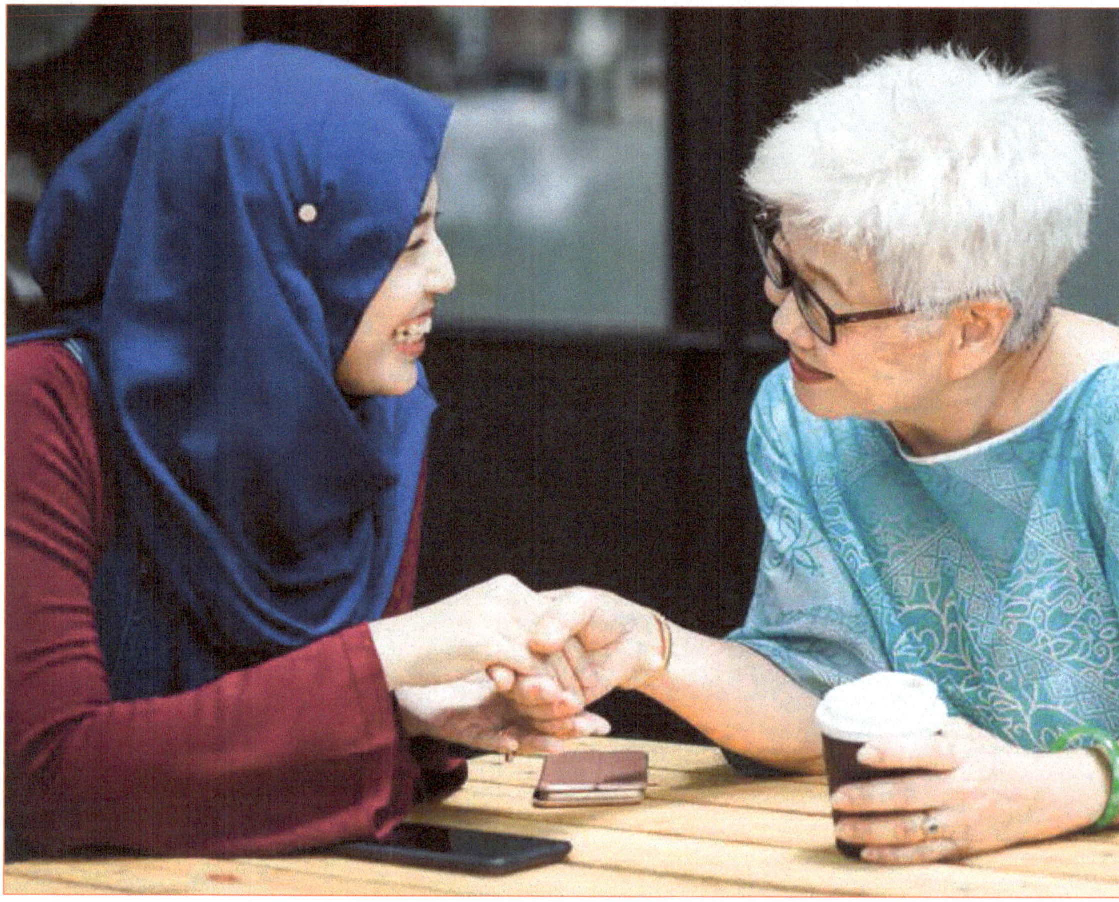

**Contributor:** Adelina Comas-Herrera, Assistant Professorial Research Fellow, London School of Economics and Political Science

The costs of dementia to society are very large and have been estimated to have reached 1 trillion dollars globally in 2019[1]. The scale of these costs is widely used for advocacy, in order to argue for a public health policy response, and also to make the case for increased public and private funding on research to find a disease-modifying treatment.

In some cases, to create a sense urgency, campaigners present dementia as an "economic catastrophe", suggesting that the costs of dementia are unsustainable. However, it is important to clarify that stating that because the costs of dementia care are high, they are not sustainable, involves an intellectual short cut. It takes a leap from the research finding that the costs are large and will be even larger in the future, to the conclusion that this will be unsustainable. The assessment of the sustainability of costs is different than their simple calculation: it requires consideration of a wider range of economic, fiscal, political and public factors. In fact, it may be that the current levels of public funding for the care, treatment and support of people living with dementia in many countries is unsustainably low (as compared to the size of the economy, the fiscal capacity of the country and the values of its citizens).

And how is this relevant to stigma? Campaigns that emphasize dementia as an "economic catastrophe" may be contributing to public, private and structural stigma (see Prof Nicolas Rüsch's essay in this volume). With regards to public stigma, most academic studies that have looked at how dementia is represented in the media and popular culture report on the frequent use of metaphors that invoke natural disasters (such as "rising tides", "silent tsunami"), the language of war or weaponry ("time-bomb"), comparisons to infectious diseases ("silent epidemic")[2,3,4]. This is often coupled by language emphasizing "financial imperatives": "burden, weight, crisis", suggesting that the societal and economic costs of dementia cannot be managed[2,4].

The language of burden and crisis is often coupled with one of blame, in a "panic-blame" framework (as identified by Peel[3]), which may contribute to private stigma. The "blame" part of the messaging comes from presenting findings around risk reduction in ways that over-emphasize individual responsibility, implying that those who go on to develop dementia are to blame for not having "behaved well". In fact, the evidence suggests, that at most, only a quarter of the risk of developing dementia can be attributable to modifiable factors[5].

While the argument that "the costs of dementia are so large that unless we find a cure, dementia will bankrupt us" may work well in terms of persuading donors and policymakers to support biomedical research, there is a danger that it may also contribute to structural stigma, by suggesting that our health and social care systems cannot do anything about addressing the challenges posed by dementia. There have long been concerns that advocacy campaigns that use cost of dementia studies to promote the idea that dementia is an economic catastrophe could be hampering the development of policies to address the care, treatment and support of people who are currently living with dementia and their carers[6,7,8].

In fact, other than highlighting the economic importance of dementia, the real value of cost of dementia studies (that are based on individual level data) lies in what they tell us about what the main cost components are (e.g. inpatient health care, primary care, medicines, social care, unpaid care), who bears the costs (health or social care system, families), who has access to services and what the reasons are for cost variability[9,10]. A more nuanced understanding of how we are currently spending on dementia can help us better prepare for a future when more of us will be living with dementia.

We know, for example, that the models of dementia health care predominant in high-income countries are very reliant on the role of specialist care, but in most countries there are already shortages of dementia specialists, usually neurologists, old-age psychiatrists and geriatricians[11]. The World Alzheimer Report 2016 explored evidence-based alternative models of dementia health care based on primary care and specially trained health workers that could potentially be expanded to deliver similar quality of care to larger numbers of people and a lower cost per person covered[12]. We also know that there are cost-effective dementia care, treatment and support interventions that could be more widely adopted.

Addressing public, private and structural stigma surrounding dementia requires a concerted effort. Dementia advocacy organisations face a difficult balance between communicating the importance and urgency of policy action on dementia while at the same time ensuring that the language and messaging they are using is not hampering their own efforts to reduce the stigma associated with dementia.

## References


1 Wimo, A., Guerchet, M., Ali, G.-C., Wu, Y.-T., Prina, A. M., Winblad, B., … Prince, M. 2017. 'The worldwide costs of dementia 2015 and comparisons with 2010.' Alzheimer's & Dementia : The Journal of the Alzheimer's Association, 13(1), 1–7. https://doi.org/10.1016/j.jalz.2016.07.150 Last accessed 30 August 2019.

2 Burke, L. 2017. 'Imagining a future without dementia: fictions of regeneration and the crises of work and sustainability.' *Palgrave Communications*, 3(52), 1–9. https://doi.org/10.1057/s41599-017-0051-y Last accessed 30 August 2019.

3 Peel, E. 2014. "The living death of Alzheimer's" versus "Take a walk to keep dementia at bay": representations of dementia in print media and carer discourse. *Sociology of Health & Illness*, 36(6), 885–901. https://doi.org/10.1111/1467-9566.12122 Last accessed 30 August 2019.

4 Zeilig, H. 2014. Dementia As a Cultural Metaphor. *The Gerontologist*, 54(2), 258–267. https://doi.org/10.1093/geront/gns203 Last accessed 30 August 2019.

5 Norton, S., Matthews, F. E., Barnes, D. E., Yaffe, K., & Brayne, C. 2014. Potential for primary prevention of Alzheimer's disease: An analysis of population-based data. *The Lancet Neurology*, 13(8), 788–794.

6 Binstock, R. H., Post, S. G., & Whitehouse, P. J. 1992. *Dementia and aging : ethics, values, and policy choices*. Johns Hopkins University Press.

7 Blank, R. H. 2019. *Social & Public Policy of Alzheimer's Disease in the United States*. Singapore: Springer Singapore. https://doi.org/10.1007/978-981-13-0656-3. Last accessed 30 August 2019.

8 Manthorpe, J., & Iliffe, S. 2016. *The dialectics of dementia*. London. Retrieved from https://www.kcl.ac.uk/sspp/policy-institute/publications/The-dialectics-of-dementia.pdf

9 Byford, S., Togerson, D. J., & Raftery, J. 2000. Economic Note: Cost of illness studies. BMJ, 320(7245), 1335. https://doi.org/doi: 10.1136/bmj.320.7245.1335.

10 Tarricone, R. 2006. Cost-of-illness analysis: What room in health economics? *Health Policy*, 77(1), 51–63. https://doi.org/10.1016/J.HEALTHPOL.2005.07.016 Last accessed 30 August 2019.

11 Hlávka, J. P., Mattke, S., & Liu, J. L. 2018. *Assessing the Preparedness of the Health Care System Infrastructure in Six European Countries for an Alzheimer's Treatment*. Retrieved from https://www.rand.org/content/dam/rand/pubs/research_reports/RR2500/RR2503/RAND_RR2503.pdf Last accessed 30 August 2019.

12 Prince, M., Comas-Herrera, A., Knapp, M., Guerchet, M., & Karagiannidou, M. (2016). *World Alzheimer Report 2016: Improving healthcare for people living with dementia. Coverage, quality and costs now and in the future*. London. Retrieved from https://www.alz.co.uk/research/world-report-2016 Last accessed 30 August 2019.

## 3.8 Women as carers: gender considerations and stigma in dementia care

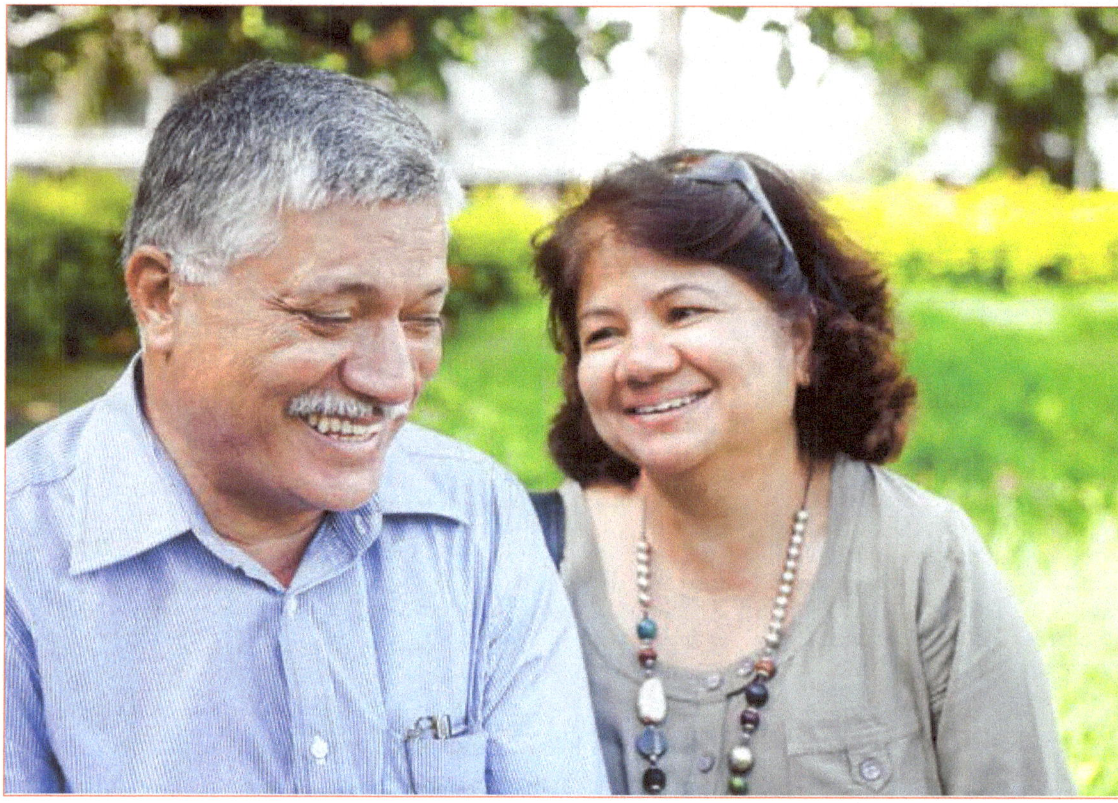

**Contributor:** Dr Nicolas Farina, PhD, MSc, BSc, Research Fellow in Dementia, Centre for Dementia Studies, Brighton & Sussex Medical School.

Dementia has a profound impact on those close to the person with dementia, particularly the family and family carers. Whilst some family members may find meaning in their new caring role, family carers often experience worsening physical and mental health, poorer quality of life and increased financial burden as a result of providing dementia care[1]. Gender is an area of importance in relation to dementia care, and whilst a report by Alzheimer's Disease International has previously reviewed in depth the experiences and impact of women as carers[2], it is still commonly overlooked. Female carers are likely to experience greater social restriction, and experience higher levels of burden and depression when compared to male carers[3-5]. Whilst there are many potential explanations for these gender differences (e.g. different coping strategies between men and women)[6], the route to which women specifically become carers for someone with dementia is an important determinant of negative outcomes.

Between 60% and 70% of all family carers of people with dementia are women[7]. Female spouses, daughters and daughters-in-law are more likely to take on the caring role compared to their male counterparts. The extent to which this occurs by choice is unclear, though the preference for women to take on the role as a family carer appears to stem from deep rooted gender norms. There is the common myth that women are better carers[8], and whilst there are certain personality traits that may support such notions (i.e. nurturance)[9], there is no conclusive evidence that women make better carers than men. Societal messages often dictate that caring behaviours are linked to being female, and therefore can create the expectation that women should fulfil this role when such as situation arises. These societal messages can also lead to external pressure, making women feel guilty if they choose not to adopt the carer role. Importantly, women are expected to become carers even if they do not have sufficient knowledge, or without sufficient preparation to become a carer[6]. Conversely, there is little societal pressure for men to become carers, in fact, there may be more societal and cultural pressures acting on men not to become carers. Globally there are many examples of the view that men should be masculine (e.g. machismo in Latin America), which nurturing and caring behaviours do not conform to.

Gender norms and societal pressures can also lead to men and women adopting different caring responsibilities[10]. Personal care (e.g. dressing, bathing) is seen as difficult irrespective of gender, though male carers report greater difficultly or discomfort in completing these tasks; it is therefore it unsurprising that women are more likely to take on these roles. Men on the other hand are more likely to focus necessary tasks, separating their emotions from the caring role. As such, men may adopt a more pragmatic approach to caring, and be more willing to access external resources to support the person with dementia. Whilst it is difficult to quantify the exact value of different care provision by family members, care should be holistic and should meet all the needs of the person with dementia.

*Irrespective of whether it is illness or childcare related, societal messages ultimately lead women to become the de facto carer in many situations. For some women this means adopting multiple carer roles, typically of their parent and a child. This "sandwich generation" are at greater risk of poorer physical and mental health, with also having a significant impact on free-time and finances.*

The influence of societal and gender norms in women adopting the caring role are even more difficult once we consider the complexities of family dynamics and other cultural pressures. For example, within Pakistan there is the view that it is the children's responsibility or privilege to provide care for their parents if they develop an illness such as dementia[11]. Whilst this responsibility may traditionally fall to the son, gender and cultural norms can lead to the daughter-in-law becoming the primary carer. In such scenarios this can lead to additional stress and resentment, as the daughter-in-law may not want to provide, or be capable of providing adequate care. Not providing individuals a choice to be a carer leads to reluctance, which results in a deterioration in the relationship between the person with dementia and the carer, and reduced quality of care. Importantly, the hierarchy in the household may mean that the head of the house (typically male), may prevent women from speaking out, which might lead to familial strain.

Irrespective of whether it is illness or childcare related, societal messages ultimately lead women to become the de facto carer in many situations. For some women this means adopting multiple carer roles, typically of their parent and a child. This "sandwich generation" are at greater risk of poorer physical and mental health, with also having a significant impact on free-time and finances[12]. A better understanding is needed of the routes by which women become dementia carers and how these pathways impact their health and wellbeing. Due to variation of cultural and societal norms and access to paid care, this is likely to differ between countries. However, the best quality of care comes from choice, both from the perspective of the person receiving care but also from the person providing it. There is no "one size fits all" approach, and women cannot (and should not) shoulder the responsibility for providing care for family members with dementia.

## References


1 Pinquart, M., Sörensen, S. 2003. 'Differences between caregivers and noncaregivers in psychological health and physical health: a meta-analysis' *Psychol Aging* 18(2):250.

2 Erol R, Brooker D, Peel E 2015. *Women and Dementia: A global research review*, London: Alzheimer's Disease International.

3 Sharma, N., Chakrabarti, S., Grover, S. 2016. 'Gender differences in caregiving among family - caregivers of people with mental illnesses' *World J Psychiatry* 6(1):7–17.

4 Akpınar, B., Küçükgüçlü, Ö., Yener, G. 2011. 'Effects of Gender on Burden Among Caregivers of Alzheimer's Patients' *J Nurs Scholarsh* 43(3):248–54.

5 Pillemer, S., Davis, J., Tremont G. 2018. 'Gender effects on components of burden and depression among dementia caregivers' *Aging Ment Health* 22(9):1156–61.

6 Papastavrou, E., Kalokerinou, A., Papacostas, SS., Tsangari, H., Sourtzi, P. 2007. 'Caring for a relative with dementia: family caregiver burden' *J Adv Nurs* 58(5):446–57.

7 Alzheimer's Research UK. Women and Dementia: A Marginalised Majority. London, England: Alzheimer's Research UK online: < https://www.alzheimersresearchuk.org/wp-content/uploads/2015/03/Women-and-Dementia-A-Marginalised-Majority1.pdf> Last accessed 20 August 2019.

8 Pruchno, RA., Smyer, MA, Smyer, PMA. 2007. Challenges of an Aging Society: Ethical Dilemmas, Political Issues *JHU Press*, p. 474.

9 Hyde, JS. 2014. 'Gender similarities and differences' *Annu Rev Psychol* 65:373–398.

10 Friedemann, M-L., Buckwalter, KC. 2014. 'Family Caregiver Role and Burden Related to Gender and Family Relationships' *J Fam Nurs* 20(3):313–36.

11 Zaidi, A., Willis, R., Farina, N., Balouch S, Jafri H, Ahmed I, et al. 2019. 'Understanding, Beliefs and Treatment of Dementia in Pakistan: Final Report'. London: Age International.

12 DeRigne, L., Ferrante, S. 2012. 'The sandwich generation: A review of the literature' *Fla Public Health Rev* 9(1):12.

## 3.9 "What Matters Most"; Conceptualizing cultural aspects of stigma of Alzheimer's disease and other dementias.

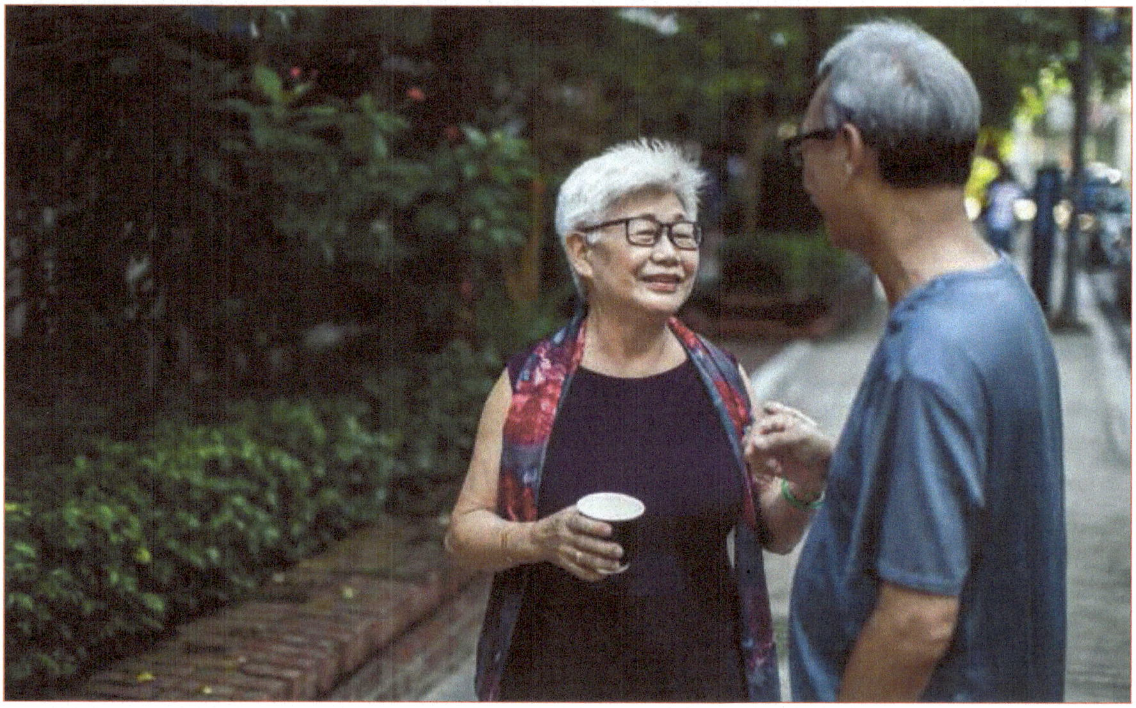

**Contributor:** Lawrence H Yang, Department of Social and Behavioral Sciences, New York University; Department of Epidemiology, Columbia University

Stigma is likely to be experienced differently across distinct sociocultural contexts, as stigma may be shaped by culturally patterned responses to dementia-related changes in cognition, behavioural symptoms, and/or disability. In its severe stages, Alzheimer's disease leads to diminished memory and behavioural impairments that signify loss of autonomy and sense of self, which violates fundamental Western European-American cultural values of self-control, productivity, and independence.[1-3] Yet stigma elicited by loss of these individual capacities may be further shaped in both positive and negative ways by culturally-salient factors, including normative expectations regarding the ageing process, labelling of illness, etiological beliefs, and the sociocultural experience and responses to the person and family.[4] To identify cultural features of stigma related to various illness conditions, including Alzheimer's disease, a theory has been articulated which emphasises how culture specific mechanisms shape stigma.[5,6] This theory, which conceptualises stigma in relation to "what matters most" for a cultural group, holds great promise for stigma related to Alzheimer's disease. To engage in activities that "matter most", or the interactions that define "full status" within a cultural setting, is to recognise an individual as having "full personhood" within a cultural group. Culture may thus act in varying ways to protect against, or to exacerbate stigma due to Alzheimer's disease, as this condition takes place within the context of actors (including the affected elder, family carers, and community members) striving to enact the activities that determine "what matters most" (or "personhood") within a cultural context.

The Chinese example is instructive to illustrate how the "what matters most" framework might be applied to a specific cultural group. As noted above, Alzheimer's disease leads to compromised memory, behavioural impairments, loss of productivity and ultimately loss of independence, which threatens one's claim as an "autonomous being" across settings.[1] On the one hand, traditional Chinese beliefs of normalized and expected changes accompanying ageing, i.e. that elders are like a "machine with worn-down parts", signal the inevitability of decline and may help to mitigate any stigma due to dementia-related deterioration[4,7]. Yet occurring in tandem with these normative cultural beliefs, Confucian influences, which are common in South and East Asia (e.g. China, Vietnam), dictate that parents and children are duty-bound to provide for one another. Parents first raise children; children in turn are obligated to producing offspring to perpetuate the lineage, supplying financial support throughout the lifetime, and performing rituals to ensure that support is continued into the next life.[8] The immersion into "an eternal chain of filial children" and enacting these obligations within a system of total economic, social, and spiritual support reflects "what matters most" for many traditional Chinese or Vietnamese groups; when the onset of Alzheimer's disease is seen to violate these core cultural engagements, stigma's effects may be compounded beyond the individual's core loss of autonomy.[9] Due to unpredictable and bizarre seeming behaviours, community members may first misattribute etiological beliefs of Alzheimer's disease to a condition of severe mental health, thus implicating moral failure on the family's part. Such misattributions to severe mental illness may provide a partial explanation for why respondents to the ADI survey in the South-East Asian region endorsed that people with dementia were dangerous (45-48% - the highest among world regions) as well as impulsive and unpredictable (70% - second highest among world regions). Further, having an elder family member who is seen as severe mental illness may be viewed by community members as a sign that either current or past family members neglected to honour filial obligations (i.e., violated "what matters most").

Of further consequence, due to the elder's loss of autonomy and inability to fulfil their demands of social reciprocity within the family, compounding any stigma of Alzheimer's disease is the experience of severe loss of status as the former head of the household's social structure to someone who is incapable of living independently (e.g., being seen to require care like a child[4]). As Alzheimer's disease symptoms progress in severity, diminished participation in (and acceptance from) the affected elder's social exchange network of close social others (i.e. exclusion from "guanxi") further signals a loss of personhood. With growing perceptions of incompetence in myriad life domains, family members may decrease efforts to communicate with the affected elder, and the elder may be excluded from highly valued social activities, including family visits or events.[4] This loss of moral standing from the community's perspective may be manifested as "loss of face" among family members, in that public exhibitions of abnormal behaviours (e.g. "confused speech elicit shame among family carers"). The "diminished personhood" associated with stigma, in addition to augmenting exclusion of the elder with dementia, leads to efforts to conceal the condition by family to preserve "face"[8]; e.g. carer respondents from the South-East Asian region were the most likely (33%) among world regions to hide the person with dementia when they were out of the home or in the home. This concealment in turn has substantial effects on family carers' attempts to obtain much-needed social support from others.

Yet despite this near-complete loss of social status (or "di wei"; i.e. respect or political power) within the home due to the symptoms of dementia, the adult children's obligation to enact "what matters most" (i.e. providing material and social support throughout, and oftentimes beyond, the lifetime) remains intact. The existence of these core lived values may thus limit the extent to which the family may ultimately reject or relegate care of affected elders to professional services provided by non-kin; e.g. carer respondents from the South-East Asian region were the least likely (11%) among world regions to endorse moving a family member with dementia into a nursing home even if they were unwilling, and were also least likely (4%) among regions to be "not at all willing" to have a family member with dementia move in with them. That is, while stigma may unfold to diminish the affected elder's standing from both the family and community members' perspectives, the obligations of family members to fulfil these core lived engagements consequently shields many elders from being rejected or abandoned. Consequently, when considering stigma of Alzheimer's disease in cross-cultural settings, stigma may be experienced not just at the level of the affected individual or family, but may also be strongly shaped by the broader cultural directives that the individual, family, and community members at large are seeking to fulfil. We direct attention to the possibility that in many contexts, understanding stigma of the affected elder and bolstering support for family carers could be facilitated by considering the core, culturally-defined activities that are most prized by actors within a cultural setting. Following prior findings, ascertaining "what matters most" may not only elucidate how the most harmful effects of stigma affect life domains in affected elders, but what cultural engagements might offer protection against local forms of stigma[10]. We intend for this analysis to spur future research regarding how cultural processes shape experiences of stigma of Alzheimer's disease and other dementias and the capacity of family members to provide effective caregiving in this[11] and other cross-cultural groups.

## References:

1 Behuniak, SM. 2011. 'The living dead? The construction of people with Alzheimer's disease as zombies' *Ageing & Society* 31(1): 70-92.

2 Kontos, PC. 2003. '"The painterly hand": embodied consciousness and Alzheimer's disease' *Journal of Aging Studies 17(2): 151-170.*

3 Luborsky, M. R. 1994. 'The cultural adversity of physical disability: Erosion of the full adult personhood' *Journal of Aging Studies, 8: 239–253.*

4 Liu, D., Hinton, L., Tran, C., Hinton, D., Barker, J.C. 2008. 'Reexamining the Relationships Among Dementia, Stigma, and Aging in Immigrant Chinese and Vietnamese Family Caregivers *Journal of Cross Cultural Gerontology* 23: 283–299.

5 Yang, L.H., Kleinman, A., Link, B.G., Phelan, J.C., Lee, S., Good, B. 2007. 'Culture and Stigma: Adding Moral Experience to Stigma Theory' *Social Science and Medicine* 64(7): 1524-1535.

6 Yang, L.H., Purdie-Vaughns, V., Kotabe, H., Link, B., Saw, A., Wong, G., Phelan, J. 2013. 'Culture, Threat, and Mental Illness Stigma: Identifying Culture-Specific Threat among Chinese American groups' *Social Science and Medicine* 88: 56-67.

7 Hinton, L., Fox, F., & Levkoff, S. 1999. 'Exploring the relationships among aging, ethnicity, and family dementia caregiving' *Culture, Medicine and Psychiatry 23:* 403–413.

8 Yang, L.H., Kleinman, A. 2008. ''Face' and the Embodiment of Stigma: Schizophrenia and AIDS in China' *Social Science and Medicine 67(3):* 398-408.

9 Stafford, C. 1995. *The roads of Chinese childhood: Learning and identification* in Angang Cambridge, UK: Cambridge University Press, p. 86.

10 Yang, L.H., Chen, F., Sia, KJ, Lam, J.J., Lam, K, Ngo, H., Lee, S., Kleinman, A., Good, B. 2014. '"What matters most:" a cultural mechanism moderating structural vulnerability and moral experience of mental illness stigma' *Social Science and Medicine* (special issue on Structural Stigma) 103: 84-93.

11 Chen, Z., Yang, X., Song, Y., Song, B., Zhang, Y., Liu, J., Wang, Q., Yu, J. 2017. 'Challenges of Dementia Care in China' *Geriatrics* 2(7).

## 3.10 Alzheimer's disease in the lived experience of Lesbian, Gay, Bisexual, Trans and Gender Diverse (LGBT) persons

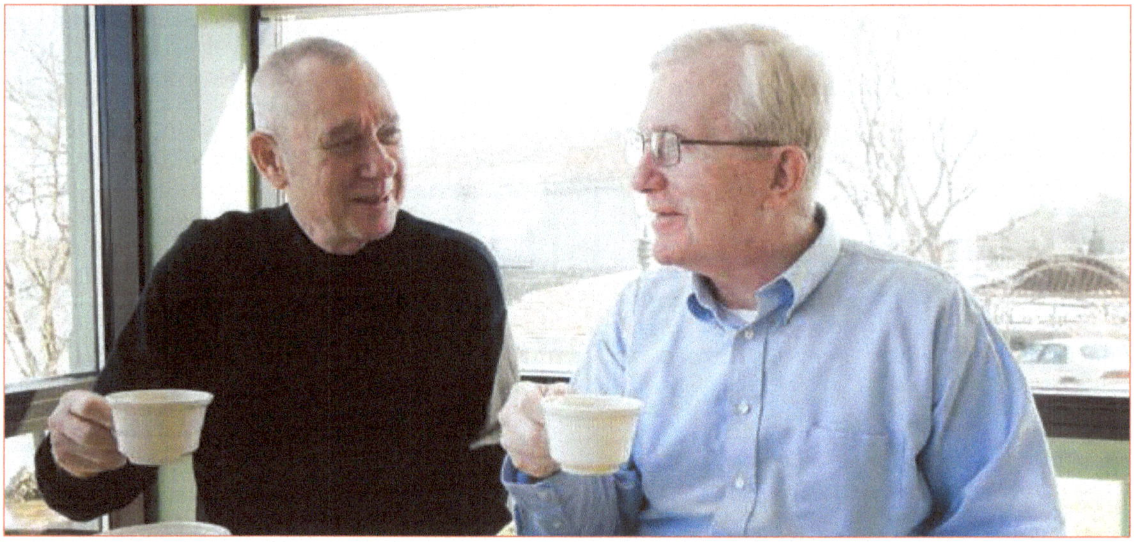

**Contributor:** Victor Madrigal-Borloz. Senior Visiting Researcher at the Harvard Law School Human Rights Program and United Nations Independent Expert on protection from violence and discrimination based on sexual orientation and gender identity.

As United Nations Independent Expert on protection from Violence and Discrimination based on Sexual Orientation and Gender Identity, the international community has asked me to raise awareness about the multiple, intersecting and aggravated forms of violence and discrimination that are perpetrated against persons every day, around the world, on the basis of their sexual orientation or gender identity, and to work to identify their root causes. In that connection, I am deeply intrigued by temporal intersectionality. All aspects of life are impacted by the passage of time, and just as a person's needs in relation to health, education, housing, employment and family relations mutate as she ages, the particular concerns of lesbian, gay, bisexual, trans and other gender diverse persons also evolve and change.

Intersectionality of LGTB concerns and the challenges raised by Alzheimer disease creates a space of great vulnerability and potential disempowerment owing to stigma and discrimination, but also to the disproportionate impact of certain predictors, in relation to which the little information that exists in a handful of countries of the global north paints a deeply worrisome picture: a survey carried out in Britain in 2010 reported that LGB older persons are less likely to see their biological family frequently; they are also more likely to drink alcohol, take drugs, and have a history of poor mental health, and to have been diagnosed with depression. All of these have been identified as risk factors for cognitive decline and dementia. The same can be said of HIV/AIDS –which, as is well documented, impacts disproportionately the key populations of men who have sex with men and trans women.

In their 2018 study, Frederiksen-Golden et al identify barriers to care and health such as those as particularly significant in that space, and added factors placing LGBT population at higher risk of developing Alzheimer's disease and of suffering disproportionate impact when living with it: the historical context (i.e. the pathologizing environments under which the LGBT older persons of today lived their whole lives) and unique family structures determining that older LGBT persons are more likely to be childless and live alone[1]. J.D. Flatt et al refer to studies that document 50% of LGBT older persons reporting subjective cognitive decline, with higher rates among ethnic or national minorities[2]. Members of the community describe additional challenges in bereavement, including a lack of acknowledgement of loss, legal complications and the exclusion of non-legally recognized family as part of the unit of care. LGBT couples who live in secrecy because of stigma, discrimination or even criminalization may be forcibly outed when they are in need of care, with care givers invading their privacy – either at home or in care or assisted living settings.

This problematic could be qualified as an exacerbated space in the larger context of the human rights concerns of older persons who self-identify as LGTB, the segment of the population which is rapidly growing: some researchers estimate that by 2060 it will reach 20 million in the United States of America alone. This makes my findings as to the prospects for their quality of life all the more disturbing. This year I reported to the UN General Assembly[3] that while I have received consistent information suggesting that LGTB older persons are under extreme risk, created by social isolation and discrimination, research and data on the root causes of these lived realities, and, most importantly, the dynamics to reverse them, is extremely scarce.

For older LGTB persons, unsurmountable barriers to access to health care are created by limited availability of and support for caregivers and higher rates of certain chronic illnesses which are compounded with stigma and discrimination. As a result, it is a general finding that LGBT persons do not perceive housing and support services for older persons as offering safe or welcoming accommodation and support; for example, it is reported that sometimes family and care staff refuse to affirm the gender identity of older trans and gender diverse persons and force them to live in denial of their orientation or according to the gender assigned at birth. This scenario is further complexed by the very nature, or characteristics of Alzheimer's disease and other dementias, involving memory loss and the potential implications and fears this could entail for LGBT persons.

In certain contexts, discrimination in employment will mean that LGBT individuals contribute less to pension schemes and therefore have less income later in life, on top of which individuals might not be (and in most of the world are not) eligible to pension entitlements of same-sex partners. This leaves them unable to pay their rent or mortgage and leads to evictions and homelessness. LGBT persons might not be able to legally leave property to a surviving partner and surviving partners might not be able to remain in public housing following a partner's death. While end-of-life considerations, affect all persons, I have received information about particular expressions of discrimination that include partners not being consulted and not being given decision-making power and affectation of survivor benefits including pensions and social security payments.

A particular feature of the lives of older LGBT persons is characterised as a disproportionate caregiving burden, as they are more likely to be acting as caregivers for loved ones and friends, with an estimated 27% providing caregiving assistance[1]. This factor bears particular significance: in most of the world, LGBT persons providing care for a loved one will not be recognised any decision-making rights when their loved ones live with declining cognitive abilities. Even when they do, historical discrimination and trauma play a significant role in underlying fears and anguish: in a 2019 submission to my Mandate, Ireland noted that older LGBT individuals are often fearful that their end-of-life and after-death wishes will not be respected by other family members, a situation that is exacerbated when States limit the legal recognition of certain family configurations.

To this situation, already critical, must be added the reality that in vast parts of the world, diversity in sexual orientation and gender identity remain deeply affected by stigma, violence, and criminalisation. As of mid-2019, 69 countries still criminalise homosexuality with punishments that oftentimes include imprisonment for years or decades and, in some cases, effective implementation of the death penalty. Dozens of countries criminalise lesbianism and/or gender diversity or maintain legislation with disproportionate criminalising impact on that basis. Even where criminalisation has been wiped off the books or never existed, social stigma remains the source for extreme violence that has been extensively documented by my Mandate. While research and data on the lived realities of older LGBT persons living with Alzheimer's disease is simply non-existent in most of these contexts, the logical presumption is that the risk factors identified before are exacerbated, and my working theory is that many of these older persons live for years under the violence and discrimination that comes with losing their ability to ascertain their sexual orientation and gender identity[i] [4]. From a human rights perspective, this is directly contrary to the full enjoyment of autonomy. As my colleague, the United Nations Independent Expert on the enjoyment of all human rights by older persons has identified, this right includes "not only the right to equal recognition before the law, legal capacity, dignity, self-determination, empowerment and decision-making, but also the right to choose where to live, the right to work, the right to vote and to the right to participate actively in all spheres of society"[5]. Among many other reasons, this is why I have called for a world free of criminalisation of sexual orientation and gender identity by 2030, and for the adoption of effective anti-discrimination legislation and public policies.

Awareness of lived realities of communities and populations of aging LGBT persons who live with Alzheimer's disease, as well as their needs in relation to care and support is, within this context, a task that cannot be postponed.

## References


1 Frederiksen-Goldsen K I, Jen S, Bryan A E B, and Goldsen, J 2018. 'Cognitive Impairment, Alzheimer's Disease and Other Dementias in the lives of Lesbian, Gay, Bisexual and Transgender (LGBT) Older Adults and their Caregivers: Needs and Competencies'. *Journal of Applied Gerontology*, Vol. 37(5) doi 10.1177/0733464816672047.

2 Flatt J D, Johnson J K, Karpiak S E, Seidel L., Larson B, Brennan-Ing M. 2018. 'Correlates of Subjective Cognitive Decline in Lesbian, Gay, Bisexual and Transgender Older Adults'. *Journal of Alzheimer Disease* 64 doi 10.3233/JAD-171061.

3 Madrigal-Borloz V, 2019. 'Protection against violence and discrimination based on sexual orientation and gender identity'. Report to the UN General Assembly, Seventy-fourth session Item 72 (b) of the preliminary list, A/74/181. Retrieved from https://undocs.org/en/A/74/181

4 Yarns B, Abrams J, Meeks T, Sewell D. 2016. The Mental Health of Older LGBT Adults. Current Psychiatry Reports 18:60 doi 10.1007/s11920-016-0697-y.

5 United Nations Human Rights Council, 30th Session of the Human Rights Council: Reports. A/HRC/30/43, par. 45 Retrieved from https://www.ohchr.org/EN/HRBodies/HRC/RegularSessions/Session30/Pages/ListReports.aspx Last accessed 3 September 2019.


(i) Even in environments in which legal protection is solid it is reported that "research with LGBT caregivers of individuals living with dementia identifies loss of an LGBT identity in response to the lack of cultural competence of health care service providers as a current unfortunate occurrence.

CHAPTER 4

# Case studies

## 4.1 Stigma and negative attitudes towards people with dementia still pervade: the importance of working together

**Contributor:** Kate Swaffer, Chair, CEO & Co-founder Dementia Alliance International

Dementia Alliance International (DAI), was launched in 2014 by eight people all diagnosed with dementia, from the USA, Canada and Australia, due to the need for international collaboration between people with dementia. The goal was to increase equal inclusion, change attitudes, and reduce stigma. DAI still seeks to represent members, now in 49 countries, and is an organisation whose goals are to provide advocacy and support of, and for people diagnosed with any type of dementia, and global campaigning for human rights and access to the Convention on the Rights of People with Disabilities (CRPD) at organisations including the United Nations and the World Health Organisation. All services for DAI members, including membership, are free.

Many members still report they receive few if any services or support elsewhere, as most support is for care partners.

There has been an increasing emergence of self-advocacy and Dementia Working (or Advisory) Groups (DWGs) globally. In spite of this, DAI founders felt when it was launched, and still believe that by collaborating globally we will eventually have a stronger impact on policy and services.

In 2000, Christine Bryden and a group of international self-advocates founded the first online self-advocacy group, Dementia Advocacy and Support Network International (DASNI), although membership was not limited to people with dementia. Then, in 2002, James McKillop and others founded the Scottish Dementia Working Group (SDWG), the first national group dedicated to the voices of people with dementia, funded by the Scottish Government and supported by Alzheimer Scotland. It took many years for more groups like this to materialise, and there are now a growing number of DWGs that are local, regional or national in demographic. The late Peter Ashley and a group of UK self-advocates were part of the first DWG in the UK, which existed for only a few years, and were instrumental in the development and implementation of the English National Dementia Strategy and the Prime Minister's Challenge on Dementia. The Alzheimer's Society again funds a Dementia Working Group, which came about after a meeting of DAI members and their CEO Jeremy Hughes, planned to initially discuss setting up a DAI Chapter in the UK. Subsequently the 3 Nations Dementia Working Group (3NDWG) covering England, Wales and Northern Ireland was established in May 2017.

It is also important to note there is a continuing emergence of self-advocates in countries primarily due to the work of DAI and some of the DWGs, as well as ADI members who are now determined to empower and enable the inclusion of people with dementia in their own countries.

The current known National, Regional or Local Dementia Working Groups include:

**2000:** Dementia Advocacy Support Network International (DASNI)

**2002:** Scottish Dementia Working Group (SDWG)

**2006**: Alzheimer's America Early-Stage Advisory Group (EAG)

**2012:** Highlands Dementia Working Group, Scotland (HDWG)

**2012:** European People with Dementia Working Group (EUPDWG)

**2013:** Dementia Australia Dementia Advisory Committee (DADAC)

**2013:** Irish Dementia Working Group (IDWG)

**2014:** Japan Dementia Working Group (JDWG)

**2014:** Southern (Kiama) Dementia Advisory Group, Australia (DAG's)

**2014:** New Zealand Dementia Advisory Committee (NZDAC)

**2015:** Ontario Dementia Advisory Group, Canada (ODAG)

**2016:** Dementia Advocacy Awareness Team, Australia (DAAT)

**2017:** 3 Nations Dementia Working Group (3NDWG)

**2019:** Finnish Memory Working Group

**2019:** Flemish Working Group for People with Dementia

**2019:** Icelandic Working Group of People with Dementia (IWGPWD)

**2019:** Dementia Advisory Group in Chinese Taipei

As an invited keynote speaker to the World Health Organisation (WHO) First Ministerial Conference on Dementia in March 2015, representing DAI, I made the following three demands:

1 That we have human rights to a more ethical pathway of care

2 Being treated with the same human rights as everyone else, under the Disability Discrimination Acts and CRPD

3 That research does not only focus on a cure, but also on care

These three demands were included in the Final Call to Action, and since then, there has been a snowball effect, and people with dementia are demanding human rights all around the world. These three demands also inspired a long-time disability expert and advocate, and DAI member, Professor Peter Mittler to become actively involved in supporting DAI. Peter is an Emeritus Professor of Special Needs Education, University of Manchester, UK. He is a former President of Inclusion International, and was a UN Consultant on disability and education, although has since retired.

The CRPD is relevant to persons with dementia because it defines persons with disabilities by saying *'persons with disabilities include those who have long-term physical, mental, intellectual or sensory impairments which in interaction with various barriers may hinder their full and effective participation in society on an equal basis with others.'*

Regardless of dementia falling within the definition of 'disability' within domestic and international law, people with dementia continue to face a number of challenges to have their rights respected. Often, many of the stakeholders and policy makers do not even see the need for those of us advocating for our rights to be included and the stigma and misperceptions about our potential to continue to contribute abound. This is partly due to the fact that symptoms of dementia are often 'hidden' or 'invisible' disabilities, until progression into old age.

Yet, in spite of the increasing numbers of DWGs and individuals with dementia speaking out, the misperceptions of people with dementia continue.

A persistent view is that we go straight to late stage dementia upon diagnosis, and should be unable to function well, if at all. It is certainly not yet seen as the norm for people with dementia to be living positively, which is likely due to ignorance, negative attitudes about people with dementia, as well as stigma, and the pervasive 20th Century views of dementia.

The task of speaking out against people causing us harm is complicated (and sometimes precluded) by the fact that many of them are well-intentioned, medical staff, service providers, advocacy organisation and close friends or family who are also often our care partners, but who may be ignorant, unwilling or unable to take the time to find out about our wishes and needs. Although we are grateful for the support of family and friends, we have sometimes been demonized for needing them. We have also been demonized for not needing them, and for daring to live positively with dementia, and the misguided under-estimations of our potential continues to create oppressive and humiliating barriers to our full engagement in society.

That younger people are more likely to be self-advocates does not mean they should not have a voice, nor does it mean they represent older persons in the later stages of dementia. It simply means they are less likely to accept the stigma, are often diagnosed much earlier in the disease process, and are therefore more functional for a longer period of time than was once expected for people with dementia.

Now that the WHO Global action plan on the public health response to dementia 2017-2025 [1] has been adopted, human rights must be included in all dementia services, as well as national dementia plans and strategies. This not only means receiving a timely diagnosis, it means receiving rehabilitation and disability support at the time of diagnosis.

Borrowed from the disability community, one of our mottos is also Nothing about us without us, and we are asking governments and civil society for human rights in dementia care which includes us at every level, and includes proactive cognitive and physical rehabilitation, access to a timely diagnosis, and risk reduction and prevention strategies, and equal access to proactive disAbility support immediately following a diagnosis.

Many people with dementia are now advocating for the phasing out all institutional care, the cessation of segregation in locked dementia units, and for all health care staff to be fully competent in dementia as well as disability. We want 'Inclusive Communities' that provide us with the same access as all others with disabilities, aligned to the CRPD. Hence, many people with dementia are also now questioning whether Dementia Friendly Communities and Dementia Villages are in fact, further segregating us, and unintentionally increasing the stigma and sense of 'otherness', rather than supporting us to be included in our community on an equal basis.

Changing attitudes towards dementia is a key element in reducing stigma, but even changing the attitudes of people in developed countries continues to be a challenge, and we believe will take a novel approach; the time is now for people with dementia to work together, rather than under the influence of their national associations.

People with dementia look forward to the day when we no longer have to be defined by our disease or our disabilities, and we are all treated equally.

## References

1 World Health Organization. 2017. *Global action plan on the public health response to dementia 2017–2025*. Geneva: World Health Organization.

## 4.2 A young person makes a difference – but have things changed?

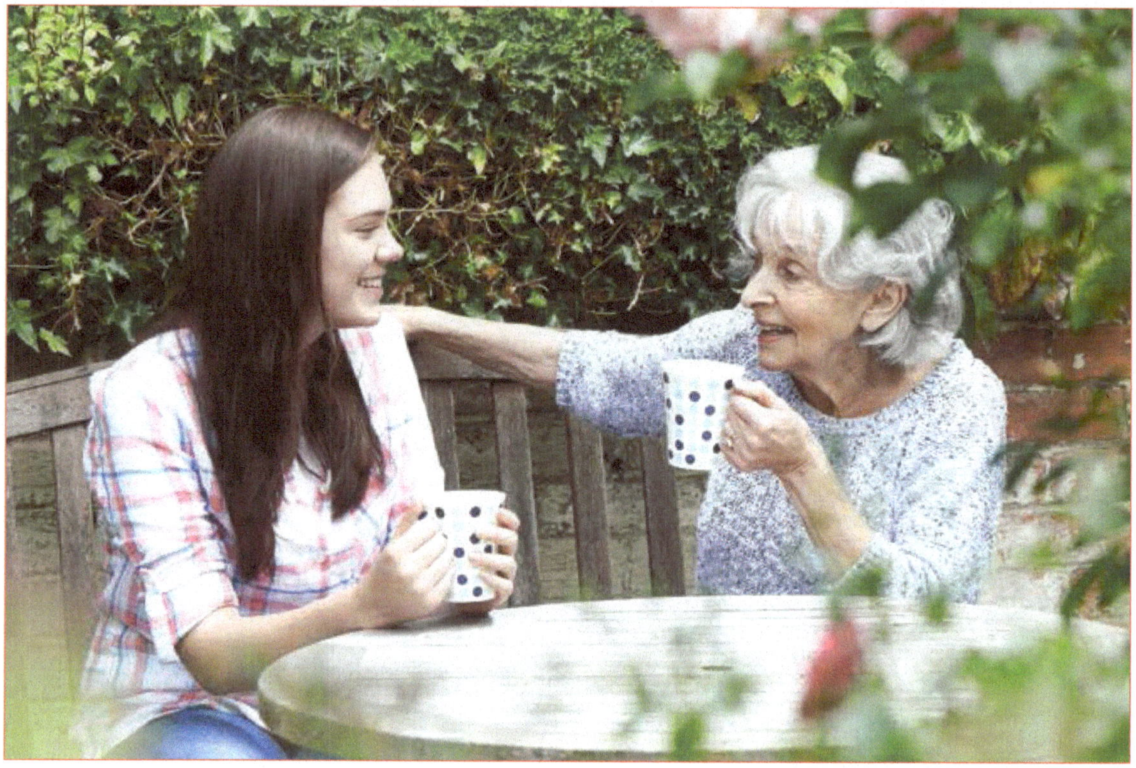

**Contributor:** Dr Walter Dawson, Atlantic Fellow for Equity in Brain Health at Global Brain Health Institute, University of California, San Francisco

My father received a diagnosis of Alzheimer's disease when I was eight years old. At this young age, I was confronted with the need to be a care partner for my father – an unusual role for a child. I was also confronted with the many challenges of the dementia care system in the United States, particularly for families like mine living in rural communities of low socio-economic status. At the time (in the early 1990s), my family lived in a very rural part of the State of Oregon, where very limited services and supports were available for someone like my father.

Watching my father slowly lose his ability to be a parent was incredibly difficult. His behavior was often hard for me, as a child, to understand. Why did he wander and become lost in familiar places? Why was he so anxious, especially at night when his anxiety made it impossible to sleep? Ultimately, my father, whose love of words and language were his defining characteristics, lost his ability to speak.

My mother and I made the difficult choice to place my father in a memory care community when we no longer felt we could safely care for him ourselves. The day I realized my father would never return home remains one of the hardest in my life.

While my father began to receive the care he needed, his care was prohibitively expensive. Within just a few months, we spent all of our savings, including anything that had been set aside for my future college education. Thankfully, my father became eligible for Medicaid, the public program that provides health care and long-term services and supports to low-income individuals and families in the United States.

Even though I was only a child, I knew the loss of our financial stability so that my father could be safe and properly cared for was not right. I knew my father and other people like him deserved better. I also knew I wanted to do something to help.

One day, I noticed my mother writing a letter and I asked her what she was doing. She responded that she was writing to our local Member of Congress about how impossibly expensive my father's care was. I thought that I could write a letter, too. I thought that if only people with power and influence heard our story then change would happen.

People did listen to our story. The unusualness of a child advocating for his father was a powerful image. Camera crews from the major news networks soon arrived at our door (in the middle of rural Oregon). It was not long before I found myself traveling to Washington, DC to testify before the United States Senate about my family's experiences caring for my father and the need to create a better system of care. I remain one of the youngest persons in US history to ever testify before the Congress on any issue, let alone Alzheimer's disease and dementia.

*People did listen to our story. The unusualness of a child advocating for his father was a powerful image. Camera crews from the major news networks soon arrived at our door (in the middle of rural Oregon). It was not long before I found myself traveling to Washington, DC to testify before the United States Senate about my family's experiences caring for my father and the need to create a better system of care*

I learned an important lesson from my early advocacy efforts: that one person can have an impact. I also learned that when we join forces and work together we become more powerful advocates for change. These experiences continue to guide and inform my professional work in public policy and dementia today. My research and policy work focus on improving the way dementia care is financed, by expanding access to publicly funded long-term services and supports. My research also seeks to demonstrate the role that wider screening for cognitive impairment can play in getting people living with dementia (and their family care partners) the support they need. This is particularly important for people who lack access to formal medical care due to cost or other systemic barriers as well as those living in rural areas where medical care is simply too far away.

## Stigma as a barrier to accessing care

In reflecting on those early days and the work I do today, the impact of the stigma that surrounds dementia continues to stand out as an obstacle that must be overcome. Stigma is one of the biggest barriers to better public policy, access to care, and ultimately a treatment for dementia. The stigma of dementia takes many forms and looks different across cultures, communities, and countries. We have made great progress in building awareness and in overcoming some of the stigma that surrounds dementia. Yet, we still have a long way to go.

Alzheimer's disease and other related dementias were not well understood in the early 1990s when my father lived with dementia. As an immigrant, my father was already treated differently by people within our community, but that difference became truly pronounced after his diagnosis of Alzheimer's. Family and friends often did not understand and withdrew. Physicians told us nothing could be done and it did not really matter if he had Alzheimer's or some other form of dementia – the trajectory and outcome would largely be the same. Often, people living with dementia and their families never receive a formal diagnosis. I consider my family lucky that we at least received that.

Stigma in the US plays a role in impeding a more robust and equitable financing system for care of people living with dementia. The stigma surrounding dementia serves as a barrier to getting dementia care onto the political and policy agenda in many societies and communities – a necessary, yet insufficient component of better policies and public programs. Disrupting the wider societal stigma will help policymakers and advocates advance better public polices for people living with dementia.

Access to care is for far too many people the biggest issue they face in their journey with dementia. As the prevalence of dementia increases around the world, how to finance long-term services and supports and provide social care must be a priority of all governments. Without a more coordinated system in place, individuals and families will continue to slip through the cracks.

## Stigma, cognitive screening and detection

A more robust dementia care system would include earlier and wider screening for cognitive impairment. Earlier and wider screening for cognitive impairment is needed in order to provide better dementia care. In countries like the United States and in Western Europe, it is estimated that as much as 50 percent of all people living with dementia never receive a formal diagnosis[1-2] In other countries, such as China and India, this lack of diagnosis is much higher, perhaps as high as 70-90 percent.[3-4] Stigma along with economic factors are significant barriers to wider screening for cognitive impairment and detection of dementia.

Some may say that in the absence of a cure or disease-modifying treatment there is little point in wider cognitive screening to detect dementia. Further, some say that without a cure or disease-modifying treatment, wider screening may actually be harmful. In other words, wider screening and detection can amplify the negative effects of stigma without offering anything to improve the lived experience of a person living with dementia.

> *"Let us be clear: cognitive screening can help promote better disease management and provides an opportunity for care planning to take place, including legal and financial planning. This does not replace the need for a treatment, but it is the best way to reduce the burden of dementia for individuals, families and ultimately the public and private systems that provide and finance care."*

This viewpoint overlooks the vital role that better disease management and care planning can play in the experiences of people living with dementia and their care partners. Let us be clear: cognitive screening can help promote better disease management and provides an opportunity for care planning to take place, including legal and financial planning. This does not replace the need for a treatment, but it is the best way to reduce the burden of dementia for individuals, families and ultimately the public and private systems that provide and finance care.

## Treatment and stigma

As we move closer to the day when we have a disease-modifying treatment for Alzheimer's disease and other related dementias, the need to overcome the barriers of stigma and the financial costs associated with the condition become more urgent. Once a treatment is available, stigma will remain a barrier to people seeking out treatment. The costs of the treatment may also prevent people from accessing it. We must ensure that any new treatment is widely accessible, that people know it is available, and that they are not afraid to seek it out.

Again, wider screening and detection will help both in identifying people who would benefit from a treatment as well as by further de-stigmatizing dementia care. But we must continue to raise awareness that dementia is not a normal part of aging, that dementia care management and care planning can help improve the lived experiences of people, and that wider access to treatment is needed to create more equitable dementia care systems.

## References

1 Amjad, H., Roth, D., Sheehan, O., Lyketsos, C., Wolff, J., & Samus, Q. 2018. 'Underdiagnosis of Dementia: An Observational Study of Patterns in Diagnosis and Awareness in US Older Adults' *Journal of General Internal Medicine 33(7): 1131–1138.*

2 Connolly, A., Gaehl, E., Martin, H., Morris, J., & Purandare, N. 2011. 'Underdiagnosis of dementia in primary care: variations in the observed prevalence and comparisons to the expected prevalence' *Aging Mental Health* 15(8):978-984.

3 Chen, R., Hu, Z., Chen, R., Ma, Y., Zhang, D., & Wilson, K. 2013. 'Determinants for undetected dementia and late-life depression' *British Journal of Psychiatry* 203(3):203-208.

4 Dias, A., & Patel, V. 2009. 'Closing the Treatment Gap for Dementia in India' *Indian Journal of Psychiatry* 51 Suppl 1: S93–S97.

## 4.3 The circle of life; Indigenous knowledge about dementia in Canada

**Contributors:** Prof Kristen Jacklin, Ph.D, Professor, Medical Anthropology, University of Minnesota Medical School Duluth and Karen Pitawanakwat, a member of the Wikwemikong Unceded Reserve, Onatario, Canada, Registered Nurse and Community Researcher for NAANDWECHIGE-GAMIG Wikwemikong Health Centre

We have been involved in dementia research with Indigenous communities for over 10 years. Our work on this topic began in 2007 when Indigenous community leadership from health centres across Ontario, Canada, began noticing more cases of dementia in their communities. Through discussions with key stakeholders, it was quickly realised that the dementia care needs of Indigenous people were distinct and required deep understanding of Indigenous culture, language and experience to be met effectively. Importantly, it was clear, very early on, that Indigenous knowledge concerning dementia was at odds with biomedical understandings and this was leading to culturally unsafe dementia care. The experience of dementia in Indigenous communities was gentler and showed a greater acceptance of the illness and its symptoms. These early discussions with communities sparked for us a long-term commitment to community-based research aimed at understanding experiences of dementia in Indigenous populations with the aim of translating these research findings into information that can help communities and providers plan and respond to Indigenous dementia care needs in culturally appropriate ways.

Our research on this topic in Canada has revealed many commonalities concerning experiences with dementia across diverse Indigenous peoples. We have been gifted with stories from Elders, Knowledge Keepers, people with dementia, their caregivers and formal care providers. This research, coupled with a handful of other such studies in Canada, allows us to cautiously put forward a collective narrative of the dementia experience for Indigenous peoples in Canada. Cautiously, because we must recognise that although we have uncovered common experiences and beliefs, the cultures, languages and experiences of Indigenous peoples in North America are diverse. We also must recognise that the well-being of Indigenous people in Canada has been severely undermined by colonialism, contemporary structural violence, and the resulting intergenerational trauma. Varying impacts of colonialism also contribute to diversity in experiences.

What has been shared with us suggests that Indigenous people understand dementia as something that some people get when they get old. It is thought to be normal, natural and part of the 'circle of life' or 'coming full circle'. This understanding is rooted in Indigenous knowledge frameworks and cultural teachings; that is to say, this is not a simplified understanding of a complex disease; to the contrary, the perspective is formed on the basis of Indigenous science, spirituality and culture. The cultural framework that leads to an understanding of dementia as part of the circle of life also leads to a greater acceptance of the illness. In this regard the behaviours associated with Alzheimer's and dementia, especially in the later stages, are understood in relation to Indigenous teachings. Some brief examples follow:

*'Memory loss' is a concept at odds with Indigenous teachings.* When memories cannot be accessed they are described as 'buried' or 'covered' and are inaccessible to the person at that time. This understanding allows the person's identity, roles, and knowledge to remain with them, never lost, but covered for the time being. Memories that are covered might be brought to the surface again by sounds, smells, or other stimuli. This is particularly the case with important, cherished childhood memories.

***...it was clear, very early on, that Indigenous knowledge concerning dementia was at odds with biomedical understandings and this was leading to culturally unsafe dementia care***

**A person experiencing a vision is thought to be in a moment where they are closer to the Creator and to the 'other side'**. During this experience they may be in discussion with relations who have passed and may be receiving important teachings. It is important to have these experiences and for the teachings to be transferred. *"Elders with dementiaare in a time of preparation to leave this physical earth. When the Elder with dementia is not making sense in conversation or talking about another place or time, that is not being experienced by all those listening, their spirit is actually travelling and amongst their next life (after life experiences/on the other side). These experiences are verbally passed on in stories and not considered hallucinations but a real part of what we know as the circle of life."* – Anishinaabe Expert Language Group Manitoulin Island, Ontario Canada.

**Experiences of 'child like' behaviours are also expected and described as such.** Cultural understandings of the life cycle accept that in older age one may return to a child stage where they will behave like children and need more care like children. *"The older people, they always refer to that term of going back into their childhood, but they use the Anishnawbe word for that, and that term is 'keewayabinoocheeaway'. That's returning back to childhood."* (Indigenous Older Adult, Thunder Bay, ON). There is no concern around 'infantilising' individuals or compromising 'personhood', rather there is an acceptance that helps all involved understand what is happening and what is needed.

Cultural values and teachings also underlie Indigenous care giving practices. We have found that although there are usually one or two primary family carers, there can be many carers for a person with dementia in the community: friends, neighbours, family, and formal providers. The Indigenous teaching concerning the value of 'Love' is paramount to care. We have received many teachings from Elder Jerry Otowadjiwan, Wikwemikong Unceded Territory, who reminds us that the person with dementia, who is being cared for, is in need of a lot of love. He urges the use of 'loved one' to refer to the person with dementia so that we remember that they are loved. He shared that using the words 'loved one' serves as a reminder of how care providers should be treating and respecting the person with dementia.

***Dementia is thought to be normal, natural and part of the 'circle of life' or 'coming full circle***

We also want to emphasise that the collective narrative includes an understanding that more people are experiencing dementia now than in the past and that some people are getting dementia at an early age. This experience has led to a complementary narrative that understands that dementia is sometimes brought on by injury, trauma, and/or other diseases and medications that cause you to be out of balance. Colonialism, and the resulting changes in lifeways and disconnection from land, is considered the cause of this phenomenon. A small number of studies have been conducted that confirm the original community concern that rates of dementia are increasing in Indigenous populations. While more evidence is needed what has been published suggests rates of dementia are higher in First Nations in Canada when compared to non-First Nation populations, rising more quickly and occurring at younger ages.[1]. Yet despite this intersection with western perspectives, core Indigenous values prevail and for the most part in our experience, dementia is not stigmatised.

Our ethnographic research on dementia in Indigenous contexts has resulted in a series of tools and guides describing dementia and the dementia journey from Indigenous perspectives, as well as guidelines for appropriate services and care. More details on what we have summarised are available from www.i-caare.ca/factsheets and www.i-caare.ca/practicetools. As we have shared the work of our team over the years it has been clear to us that non-Indigenous care providers, both formal and informal, have a deep appreciation for Indigenous views on dementia. Many have commented on how much mainstream (biomedical) services have to learn from Indigenous teachings. We hope that what we have shared provokes thoughtful discussion on what we can learn and what we can do better.

## References

1 Jacklin, K., Walker, J., Shawande, M. 2013. 'The emergence of dementia as a health concern among First Nations populations in Alberta, Canada' *The Canadian Journal of Public Health* 104(1) online: https://pdfs.semanticscholar.org/8fcf/2edb97bb733aa0b1bb4abc39eed98e5feda3.pdf Last accessed 19 August 2019.

## 4.4 Dementia discrimination, even by the language we use, a view from Québec, Canada

**Contributor:** Nouha Ben Gaied, PhD, director research and development quality of services Federation of Quebec Alzheimer Societies

Wherever you live around the globe, you are likely to have heard of the word "dementia" in English. Dementia being the umbrella term that embraces several neurodegenerative diseases such as Alzheimer's disease, fronto-temporal dementia or Lewy body dementia and define the final stage of cognitive decline. The word dementia is also widely used by people with lived experience, carers, healthcare professionals as well as the media. The broad usage of the word dementia has even led one the biggest Alzheimer association, Alzheimer's Australia to take the move in 2017 and change their brand to become Dementia Australia, to be more inclusive of all people living with a neurodegenerative illness who face different symptoms but who share a universal journey. A dozen other organizations have also included the word dementia in their name, leaving aside the word "Alzheimer".

Can we think of a similar change in Canada? A country that is officially bilingual and where the French is predominately used in the Province of Quebec? The situation is indeed rather different and complex when we look at the meaning of the word 'démence' in French. Even though the word démence refers to a medical term, it has been very much associated, since the end of the 19th century, with craziness, losing one's mind and mental health issue such as schizophrenia. A definition of the word démence, in the Petit Robert dictionary, mentions alienation, delirium, wandering, madness and unconsciousness and refers to a progressive and irreversible decline of mental and psychical activities. All these definitions refer rather to psychiatric disorder rather than a neurodegeneration decline and contribute therefore into the stigmatisation of people with Alzheimer's disease and related illnesses as well as their carers.

In 2013 a major change happened in the DSM-V (Diagnostic and Statistical Manual of Mental Disorders) with the replacement of the word "démence" by "troubles neurodégénératifs" as well as the introduction of diagnostic criteria for both mild and major neurodegenerative decline.[1] But did this major change impact those who live with the disease and their carers? Did it change the way we see dementia among French speaking societies and finally, did healthcare professionals actually replace the word démence in their practice?

To answer some of these questions, the Alzheimer Society of Canada shared the results of a large survey during the Alzheimer's awareness month in January 2018.[2] The results showed that 8 out of 10 Canadian anglophones were familiar with the word "dementia" as a medical term that refers to Alzheimer's disease or a related illness. A similar result was also observed among francophone Canadians (7 out of 10) indicating that dementia is rather a neutral word that can widely be used. It was very striking, however, to see that 54% of francophones Canadians consider the word "démence" as offensive and disparaging compared to only 16% anglophone Canadians. A large number of francophone Canadians still relate to démence with a negative connotation and a pejorative word to be used. Finally, when francophone Canadians were asked whether they prefer to use the word "maladie neurodégénérative" rather than "démence", a large majority (between 76% and 87%) responded yes. This final answer should raise awareness among healthcare professionals for the need to change the medical terms they use when providing a diagnosis.

When a person receives a diagnosis of démence, it's their whole world that seems to fall apart. That's what Murielle, a person living with dementia, experienced 3 years ago when her family doctor announced the word "démence" during a long-awaited appointment. *"I'm not demented! When I received the diagnosis, people around me had the impression that I'm not 'normal' anymore, I can't take decisions or have a normal conversation with my loved one, I lost my self-esteem and I was hiding. I didn't speak about it for a long time because I was afraid of how others will look at me or talk to me. I felt isolated and couldn't seek help".*

Démence is not just a word with a negative connotation, it can have broader consequences. Fifty percent of people who receive a diagnosis are already at a mild or moderate stage of the disease making pharmacological intervention ineffective and thus preventing any significant improvement. The fear of the stigma they know they will face, once referred to as a person with dementia, contributes to enhancing the feeling of denial and fear as well as the stress and isolation, instead of them looking and asking for much needed help.

A lot of hard work has been put forward to provide support, counselling, education and activities to dissipate stigma, based on a better understanding of the disease, but mainly to allow people with lived experience to consider a life that is worth living. Let's not allow a single word to jeopardise all these efforts.

### References

1 American Psychiatric Association. 2013. *Diagnostic and Statistical Manual of Mental Disorders* (5th Edition: DSM-5) ISBN 978-0-89042-554-1.

2 Survey Léger, Alzheimer Society of Canada, 2018 online: https://alzheimer.ca/sites/default/files/2018-01/Awareness2018-en.pdf Last accessed 20 August 2019.

## 4.5 Stigma in Brazil: The narrative of a person with young-onset dementia

**Contributors:** Prof Cleusa Ferri, Federal University of Sao Paolo (UNIFESP), Prof Elaine Mateus, Brazilian Federation of Alzheimer´s Associations (FEBRAZ), Dr Deborah Oliveira, UNIFESP, Dr Fabiana da Mata, UNIFESP

My name is Andrea, I am 56 years old and married, with four children, and I was diagnosed with Alzheimer´s disease eight months ago. My mother has Alzheimer's and so do her two sisters, but I had never imagined that this would happen to me. And then suddenly, I started to forget things, to forget my friends´ names, and the things I had to do. I also misplaced objects that I would find days later. I felt frustrated, got mad at myself many times, and wondered what was going wrong with me. At first, my husband Eduardo was angry too. He also could not understand what was going on. After the diagnosis and the beginning of the treatment, I felt less stressed. Now I go out by myself and drive in the neighbourhood. I am going to start swimming classes and I want to go back to my English lessons. I am slowly getting back on my feet. It is never going to be the same again, but I want to get involved with different things.

Shortly after the diagnosis, I realised things would change. Eduardo would not allow me to go to places I am not familiar with anymore. I used to walk by myself all over the city. Now, whenever I need to go to a distant place, he drives me. My routine is kept to a minimum. I do not use my cell phone as often, but my closest friends still remember me and invite me to parties. The last time I went to their party, I noticed them whispering in groups and I felt it was about me and my illness. I also quit my job as a dentist because I felt embarrassed many times for not doing the reports I was supposed to do. Despite having supportive colleagues, it was overwhelming.

Andrea was interviewed in her own house by a member of the Brazilian Federation of Alzheimer's Disease (FEBRAZ) and she was happy to maintain her real identity in this report. Andrea's brief narrative shows how much anger and frustration the symptoms were for her and her family before they knew she had dementia. Soon after the diagnosis, however, she started to relax and was slowly able to cope. At first, the dementia symptoms made Andrea become self-judgmental – and felt judged by others. However, when the diagnosis was revealed, she began to be able to cope better with the symptoms and to be more self-accepting.

Andrea was fortunate to have an early diagnosis. This is rare in Brazil as the majority of people with dementia are either not diagnosed (around 77% of the older population) or have their diagnosis only in the late stages of the condition. The fact that Andrea had good access to healthcare and that she is a health professional herself might have helped her get diagnosed sooner and to plan a strategy for a smoother transition into her new reality. Often, most people living in poverty in Brazil would not have such rapid access to a diagnosis. It is also common for people in Brazil to believe that dementia only affects older people, which may explain why the diagnosis of dementia came as a shock to Andrea at the age of 56, even though she has several family members with dementia. It is common for such stereotypes to hinder middle-aged and older adults in Brazil from seeking help when their first dementia symptoms appear. This also reflects a common belief in Brazil that dementia is inevitable in later life, which may hinder the prevention of modifiable risk factors for some dementias.

The diagnosis brought some stigmatising experiences to Andrea, who was kept from going outside on her own as her family feared for her safety. Not only were there small changes in her routine, but also in her social circle. Andrea knows that dementia will change her and anticipates that her friends might leave her in the future due to her illness. Despite her good socioeconomic position, Andrea is very likely to experience the feeling of isolation most people living with dementia and their carers experience as the disease progresses. Social stigmatisation is commonly reported by people with dementia. Very often, it is difficult to know whether the relationship with friends and relatives wane over time because most of them lack knowledge to cope with the challenges of the disease or whether people with dementia are slowly drawn from social interactions due to the fear of possible negative reactions to their symptoms. Hopelessness, anxiety, uneasiness and a sense of awkwardness are all embedded in discriminatory practices.

In many ways, the early stages of the condition allow individuals to keep up with their daily lives. Dementia became a disabling and isolating experience for Andrea at first, but a few months after the diagnosis, she is starting to enjoy her life again through new hobbies and experiences. However, not all people with dementia in Brazil are included in everyday life. The most common barriers are stigma and financial issues, both preventing access to services and resources. The more advanced the stage of the dementia, the harder to engage the individual.

Negative associations about people who have dementia in Brazil is pervasive. Even among more educated people, the lack of understanding about what dementia is permeates personal and professional relationships. Andrea realises that she has been exposed to shame and discriminatory experiences in her workplace since diagnosis, which has led her to quit her job, but she is slowly becoming more empowered and is feeling able to cope.

## 4.6 Stigma and response to dementia in Guatemala's indigenous populations

**Contributor:** María Cecilia López Murga, Executive, Association Grupo Ermita, Alzheimer de Guatemala

Our mission in the Association Grupo Ermita is to offer support, counselling, education, information and care to people living with dementia, family members, careers, health professionals and the general public about the care of patients with Alzheimer's and of the elderly, for a better and healthy quality of life in that segment of the population.

The indigenous population of Guatemala constitutes 41% of the total population of the country.

The largest indigenous population group in the country is the Maya, as it represents 39.3% of the total population and is made up of 22 linguistic communities: achi, akateko, awakateko, chalchiteko, ch'orti', chuj, itza', ixil, jakalteco or popti', kaqchikel, k'iche', mam, mopan, poqomam, poqomchi', q'anjob'al, q'eqchi', sakapulteko, sipakapense, tektiteko, tz'utujil and uspanteko. 28% of the Mayan population belong to the Mayan K'iche linguistic community, 19.3% to Maya Q'eqchi', 18.9% to Maya Kaqchikel and 14% to Maya Mam. Garifuna and Xinca represent only 1.7% of the population.[1].

In Guatemala, indigenous people have a conception of health and disease that is different from that of the non-indigenous population groups. Disease is not based solely on pathologies or biological aspects that denote some imbalance, but also considers social, environmental and spiritual factors.

Indigenous people have their traditions and customs, which are very deep rooted.

When Alzheimer's disease or some other type of dementia occurs in an indigenous family, it is taken with a lot of fear and superstition.

Any consultation at our Association normally only occurs when the disease is already very advanced and cognitive, neurological and physical deterioration is already severe.

We attended the case of a person of Kaqchikel descent, a 78-year-old married woman, mother of 13 children. When she was around 65, according to the family, she began experiencing very "strange" changes. At one time they thought it was witchcraft and visited the sorcerer of the region who was treating her for about five years, yet the problem continued to get worse. It reached such a point that on four occasions she was lost in the community for more than three days at a time. The last time she was lost, they found her 225 kilometres from the village of her origin.

At the time they visited our medical consultation, the husband told us about the extreme changes that his wife went through, and how in order to cure her and to prevent her from getting angry with everyone and getting violent, or from leaving the house, they locked her in the last room of the house and kept her there until she fell asleep and calmed down.

*We were also visited by the 13 children who were very worried about their mother's situation, since she was the one in charge of controlling everything in the house, but when this strange situation started, she had disregarded everything that had to be done at home and everything turned into chaos. They even thought that because of witchcraft she had gone crazy and that there was nothing left to do*

We were also visited by the 13 children who were very worried about their mother's situation since she was the one in charge of controlling everything in the house, but when this strange situation started, she had disregarded everything that had to be done at home and everything turned into chaos. They even thought that because of witchcraft she had gone crazy and that there was nothing left to do.

We could not communicate at all with the lady herself because she only spoke the Kaqchikel language. Although she had spoken some Spanish, with the advance of the disease she had already totally forgotten it.

The biggest challenge we had in the Association was to explain to the husband and children about Alzheimer's disease and its process. Thankfully the information was very well received and with the help of the doctor a pharmacological treatment could be given, and the family could be taught how best to treat the lady to give her quality of life.

This is the most significant case we have had. There are others, but now people from several communities in Guatemala are taking part in our diploma course, which is increasing knowledge and awareness.

For the Association it is a great challenge because we have reached very few people from the indigenous population. We hope soon to be able to have more presence in our indigenous communities.

Our National Alzheimer's Congress in 2019 will be held in the south-western region of the Country, in Quetzaltenango, to be able to provide training to professionals, family members and caregivers.

## References

1 Verdugo, L. (n.d.). *Atlas sociolingüístico de pueblos indígenas en América Latina*. Bollivia: Unicef y FUNPROEIB Andes, p. 855. online:_ https://www.unicef.org/honduras/tomo_1_atlas.pdf Last accessed 19 August 2019.

## 4.7 From despair to the courage to cope; a carer's story, Guerruro, Mexico.

**Contributor:** Guadalupe Ponce Ozuna, Psychologist and President of the Guerrero Alzheimer Foundation and Rosa Ma Farrés, G.S. Federación Mexicana de Alzheimer y Enfermedades Similares A.C.

The State of Guerrero has 3,533,251 living in poverty and 825,214 in extreme poverty.[1] Poverty is extremely painful when talking about indigenous peoples and communities, because it is a key indicator of less development, including food insufficiency, lack of public services and education, as well as health issues. The poorest municipality in Mexico is located in the high mountain of the State of Guerrero where levels of poverty are comparable to some African countries, such as Mali and Malawi.[2]

The basis of social organisation lies in the nuclear family and the extended family. In these communities, spontaneous groups of solidary support or "hands-in-return" emerge between relatives and friends, to support issues and activities such as marriages, christenings, crop cultivation or housing construction.

Men marry at an average age of 17 and women of 15. In some cases, it is the parents who choose the partner for their child.

The following testimony was written by Psychologist Guadalupe Ponce Ozuna in 2008, who has a support group in the city of Acapulco, Guerrero, about a 52-year-old woman (her age at the time Guadalupe met her) whose 55-year-old husband had dementia. In her village there is only a small health centre, attended from time to time by a General Practitioner (GP) and there is a nurse who sometimes attends, which is why the woman had to go first to Acapulco and then to Mexico City looking for someone to explain why her husband was behaving so strangely.

"When my husband began to get lost in our town, with people returning him home, because we all know each other, I realised that something was happening with him. I talked with his family, they told me that I had bewitched him with something that I gave him to drink. I was sure I had not done such a barbarity and I just told them that God and I knew that I would not do something like that. He started shouting and asking me who I was and then telling me I must be his mother; he would call me many names except for my own, which he had completely forgotten. I started taking him to the health centre, to the hospital in my town and they told me that it had to be a very rare disease, since he was 55 years old and they did not understand why he behaved that way. They told me that I should take him to Mexico City to the Fray Bernardino Hospital, where they would relieve him and so I sold my little house, since it was all I had, to have money to travel with him, as there was no treatment for my husband locally.

"I went to different hospitals and nobody told me anything. I was recommended to see a psychiatrist in Acapulco who was good, and he told me your husband has Alzheimer's and he is not going to be cured, don't spend any more money, go back to your home, and he gave me a description of what was waiting for me with my husband. I returned, very sad, to live with my daughter and that night I did not sleep, thinking about what the doctor had told me; that he was not going to know anything anymore about his life. And how I was going to manage, if I had no home to live with him in, and had to live with my daughter, who was married and so I felt sorry for her husband.

***After about ten days I made the decision that I was going to take him to the federal highway and I was going to throw myself under the wheels of a trailer – the biggest one I saw pass by – together with my husband, because I was not going to be able to bear everything that was coming. I woke up that day very early with my decision taken, to clean the house and leave everything ready, so they could hold vigil over us afterwards that day.***

"After about ten days I made the decision that I was going to take him to the federal highway and I was going to throw myself under the wheels of a trailer – the biggest one I saw pass by – together with my husband, because I was not going to be able to bear everything that was coming. I woke up that day very early with my decision taken, to clean the house and leave everything ready, so they could hold vigil over us afterwards that day.

"When I was cleaning the house the TV was on and a journalist asked a woman in the street what she would want from the people who were watching her, and the woman told him to just ask them to buy the tamales and atole (maize cakes and maize drink) she was selling, to have money to feed her sick husband and her disabled son. He told her again, many people are seeing you on TV, ask them for what you need - and she answered 'nothing for me, I only want them to buy my tamales and my atole so I can feed my sick husband and my disabled son'. At that moment I thought, 'What a coward am I? That woman is 65 years old, I am 52 and how it is possible that I do not have the courage to fight for my husband?' I kneeled down in the middle of the house and I asked God for forgiveness for what I was thinking to do, and I swore that I would take care of him as long as necessary. And here I am! Now he goes to the toilet by himself. I have diabetes and hypertension. I do not sleep. I worry a lot because I have to work to feed him - and he eats a lot because he keeps on being hungry."

## Psychologist Guadalupe Ponce Ozuna

The diagnosis was given to the wife in the year 2000, two years after her husband began to have the symptoms. The husband with Alzheimer's lived about ten more years, dying in 2010, by which point the wife was left in poor health; her toe about to be amputated but they managed to save it. She was hospitalized for 15 days. Today she has a hearing disability because of a traffic accident but continues fighting. A woman of solidarity; philanthropic, kind, a beautiful woman in all aspects.

We share this story in the training courses that we give in the different regions and municipalities of Guerrero, to doctors, nurses, social workers, psychologists, to create awareness and sensitivity towards people who have this type of disease. It's a real story that has a lot of impact.

## References

1 National Institute of Statistics and Geography (INEGI) (Mexico). 2015. online: http://www.inegi.org.mx Last accessed 20 August 2019.

2 United Nations Development Programme. 2011. 'Equipo del Informe sobre Desarrollo Humano México 2011' online: http://hdr.undp.org/sites/default/files/nhdr_mexico_2011.pdf Last accessed 20 August 2019.

## 4.8 Stigma and dementia care in Kenya; Strengthening Responses to Dementia in Developing Countries (STRiDE) Project

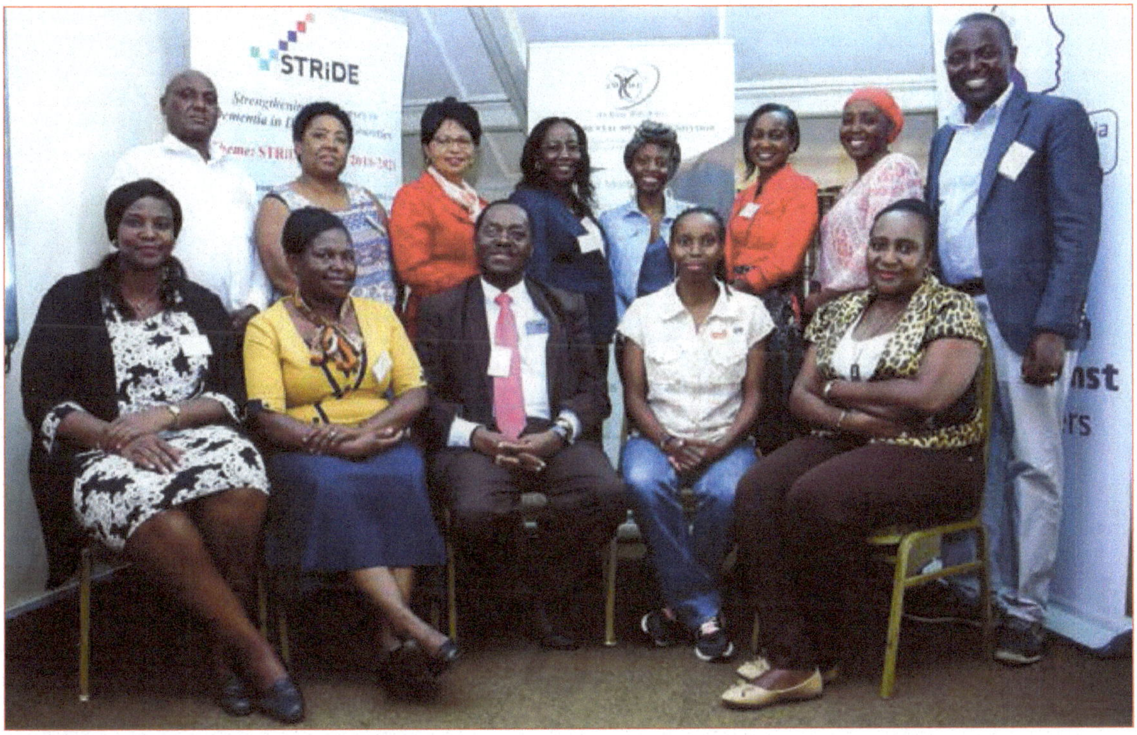


**Members of the STRiDE - Kenya National Advisory Group**

**Contributors:** Christine Musyimi, Africa Mental Health Research and Training Foundation (AMHRTF), Elizabeth Mutunga, Alzheimer's and Dementia Organization Kenya, and Prof David Ndetei, Senior Researcher AMHRTF

Dementia knowledge in Kenya is still at the nascent stages and many people associate the condition with normal ageing, witchcraft, or that one has done something wrong to the gods and is thus being punished. Creating awareness of the condition through media, churches, home visits and support groups has been one way of opening up the conversations as dementia is close to a taboo topic in Kenya.

These conversations have been instrumental in empowering carers and enabling others to understand what carers are dealing with. Most carers have stated that a lot of people do not visit their homes anymore as they are scared of contracting the disease that their loved ones have. Others have offered to bring prayers to the family to exorcise demons. Due to this, most carers suffer from self-stigma. They will not speak out publicly of what their loved ones are going though. Others will go to great lengths to hide their loved ones from the public as they do not know how best to handle them and they feel by hiding them it is the best for their loved ones.

Most carers have confessed to having gone through the five stages of grief developed by Elizabeth Kuber Ross namely: Denial, Anger, Bargaining, Depression and Acceptance[1]. In a support group run by Alzheimer's and Dementia Organization Kenya (ADOK), one month carers share they are at a point of acceptance, and the next month they are back to being angry. We allow them the space to be themselves as they are in a safe place at the support group, where they are not judged, nor are they stigmatised. But out "in the real world" they may not have the same luxury and often opt to hide their feelings and put on a brave face so that they are not judged.

Self-stigma is an issue that ADOK continues to address during the support group meetings to constantly empower the carers and to ensure they speak out without fear and without worrying about what the people around them think. The joy of seeing them take steps to overcome their stigma is exhilarating. They are becoming the mouthpieces to fight for the rights of their loved ones - be it on family issues, care by doctors or any other issues that touch on the welfare of their loved ones. This is key as it ensures that the people living with dementia are getting quality care from all angles and they are living a life of dignity each day.

Dementia detection and management is still not a priority in most primary care settings in Kenya. It is often considered a secondary condition with detection in inpatients rather than the point of contact at the outpatient clinic. In one of the rural counties in Kenya – and perhaps in most counties – health care workers do not routinely screen for dementia. Different cadres of mental health professionals approach management in different ways. For instance, psychologists, social workers and psychiatric nurses rely on diagnosis made by a medical doctor. Oftentimes, psychologists speak to the carers because they only receive the person with dementia at an advanced stage, making it difficult for the practitioner to have a conversation directly.

***...carers have stated that a lot of people do not visit their homes anymore as they are scared of contracting the disease... Others have offered to bring prayers to the family to exorcise demons.***

In the communities, dementia is viewed from the following perspectives;

1 It does not require medical attention since it is a waste of time unless there is evidence of a physical condition i.e. it is less treatable than physical conditions with poor prognosis.

2 It is associated with "something that one's ancestors did not do or a curse". For example a clinician in a rural hospital explained *"There was a patient who developed dementia at an old age (around 65 years) and this person was rich, so the community will start saying that this person was engaged in devil worshiping and that is the reason he is developing dementia symptoms."*

3 It is considered as a consequence of not associating with other community members at a time when one was employed i.e. before retirement. In one of the ethnic groups (Kamba), this is referred to as previously *"thinking high"*, an origin of the local idiom of dementia *(Thing'ai)* which is popular among the Kamba people. However, this local term *(Thing'ai)* is considered derogatory but is often understood by the community members. Some of the members take offense if the word is used for them after revealing some early signs of dementia such as forgetfulness and poor judgement.

4 Persons with dementia cannot be left alone or live independently.

Despite these beliefs, there is little or no literature around dementia specific stigma in Kenya. The misconceptions by the community members linked to stigma and lack of detection of dementia at the early stage are already barriers to accessing care and a hindrance to creating awareness of dementia. A hospital health care worker states *"Most of our health workers are not really well equipped with information on diagnosis and management of dementia."*

It is also important to note that stigma does not only affect persons with dementia but also family members or carers. With these community perceptions, carers resort to self-exclusion from communities to avoid;

1 Questions like "what happened to your relative?"

2 Blank stares at the person with dementia or carer

3 Intentional exclusion from social interaction for the person with dementia and carer by community members

4 Mockery statements from community members

The Strengthening Responses to Dementia in Developing Countries (STRiDE) Project, run in collaboration with ADI and London School of Economics and Political Science (LSE), funded by UK Research and Innovation's Global Challenges Research Fund, is attempting to address these barriers, by;

1 Reducing stigma by increasing understanding and awareness of dementia among healthcare professionals and community members and reduce delays in seeking help via healthcare professionals' increased capacity to identify and treat people. This will be feasible with the help of an anti-stigma toolkit for implementation in Kenya by the Africa Mental Health Research and Training Foundation (AMHRTF) and ADOK.

2 Providing recommendations for development of a national dementia Plan that incorporates the rights of people with dementia.

Dementia care in Kenya is clearly undergoing great change. Although stigma remains a key issue, programs such as ADOK and STRiDE are breaking down barriers and creating greater awareness – not only within the health sector, but more importantly, for people living with dementia and their families. This is clearly a country to watch – and one that is making great strides.

## References

1 E. Kübler-Ross and D. Kessler. 2009. "The Five Stages of Grief," in Library of CongressCatalogin in Publication Data (Ed.), On grief and grieving, 7–30.

## 4.9 The stigma of dementia - a personal story from South Africa

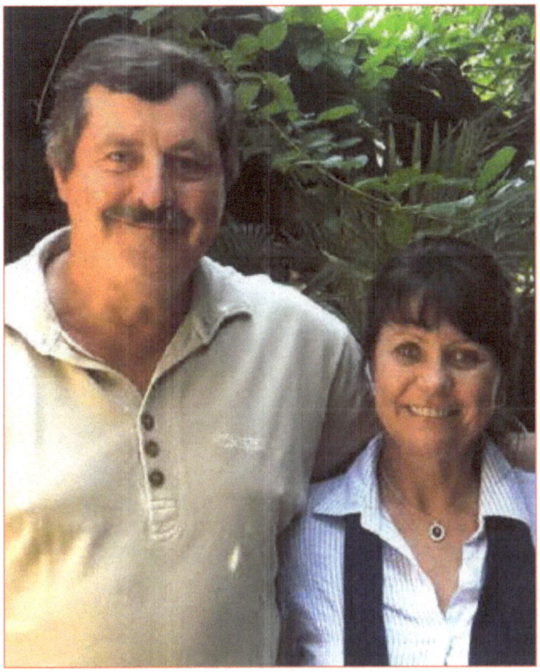

**Andre and Maryna**

**Contributors:** Maryna Lehmann and Andre Mauritz, as told to Sarah-Jane Meyer, freelance journalist

### Maryna's story

Like most people, if I thought of it at all, I considered dementia to be an ailment experienced by elderly people and I vaguely knew that it caused a loss of memory. I certainly never dreamt it would be my destiny – after all, no one in my family had ever had dementia.

What a shock it was when I was diagnosed with Alzheimer's disease. I was just 56 – far too young, I believed – and it felt as if I had been stripped of my identity. As an academic in agriculture, my passion was mentoring a new generation of farmers that would feed the nation, and my mind was my identity. I know there was so much more I could have contributed.

In 2017, when I was diagnosed, I experienced the reality that dementia – especially young onset dementia – can be grossly unrecognised and underdiagnosed. For some time, I had experienced numerous problems carrying out the daily tasks that I had previously taken in my stride. Multiplication sums, marking test papers and explaining formulas in class were often beyond me. I frequently forgot to attend meetings and on occasion had difficulty completing sentences when presenting lectures. I became extremely anxious, which led to more difficulties and I made an appointment to see my family doctor.

He told me I was too young to have dementia and put my difficulties down to work stress. This made sense at the time, as I had been under enormous pressure at work for the past few years. This was the result of the number of students more than doubling – from 25 to 60 – while the number of lecturers was halved. Instead of four lecturers overseeing 25 students, there were two of us managing 60 students. We were doing our best to cope under extremely difficult conditions.

I tried advocating to have more lecturers appointed to lessen the workload, but the University authorities were unsympathetic and, only after pressure from the trade union, the best they could do was to allocate funds for appointing an additional lecturer for a few months.

This step didn't do much to alleviate the extreme workload, and after another two years I had a complete breakdown. In that time my difficulties included:

- Losing my way while driving in the town I had lived in for more than ten years.
- Being stuck at a green traffic light, quite incapable of moving on.
- Being unable to perform calculations – formerly a regular part of my daily work.
- Inability to complete sentences while lecturing.
- Inability to recall students' names, even those I had worked with for several years.
- Inability to follow discussions in meetings.

Seriously worried, I went to a second doctor who referred me to a neurologist for further investigation. This is when I experienced the first instance of stigma. At the first consultation and throughout the various tests, the neurologist spoke to me quite normally. But, after the CT scan that showed my frontal lobe had started shrinking, she spoke only to my husband, Andre, who had been with me throughout the consultations. I had suddenly become a non-person, no longer to be considered when discussing matters of importance that affected me personally.

I also found that many of my former colleagues started avoiding me once they heard that I had Alzheimer's. This is possibly because they weren't quite sure how to treat me, and didn't know what to say to me. Many people are uncomfortable around those who are 'different' from themselves, so they find it easier to stay away.

Our children have been enormously supportive, though. We discussed the situation with them once we had the diagnosis and explained that they should treat me just as they always have. We still laugh and joke in the same way as before, and this is heartening.

Our friends and neighbours, too, have been encouraging and continue to visit just as they did previously.

After the diagnosis, Andre and I started the lengthy process of arranging my early retirement due to Alzheimer's disease. Without him I would have been completely lost. The intricacies of financial issues and dealing with the authorities, completing the necessary forms and all the formalities were quite beyond me.

Fortunately, that is all behind us now, and after his recent retirement we are looking forward to a life that still has much to offer. We are extremely fortunate in being financially secure, not wealthy, but we have enough for our present and future needs.

***Seriously worried, I went to a second doctor who referred me to a neurologist for further investigation. This is when I experienced the first instance of stigma. At the first consultation and throughout the various tests, the neurologist spoke to me quite normally. But, after the CT scan that showed my frontal lobe had started shrinking, she spoke only to my husband, Andre, who had been with me throughout the consultations***

So much is lost when Alzheimer's strikes, and it is crucial that effective treatments and preventative measures are found to combat this condition – for the present age group and for the generations to come.

## Andre's story

My first thought when Maryna was diagnosed with Alzheimer's disease was that I had to try and protect her from everything.

Of course, this was an over-reaction, but to be expected under the circumstances. After all, this is the woman I love, my soul mate.

She also happens to be a strong-minded person and has always been very independent. She was hurting, but over the past few years she has let me know that she is still in control of her faculties and doesn't want me to do everything for her. She can, and does, do most things for herself, including driving to the shops on her own on occasion.

We have found that one of the most important factors in dealing with Alzheimer's is communication. Because the person with Alzheimer's isn't always able to communicate their needs and wishes as clearly as they would like, those living with and caring for them need to hone their own listening skills.

I have deliberately developed the habit of never interrupting Maryna when she is talking, because I know she might forget what she started saying. Losing your train of thought happens to most of us at some time, but when you have dementia it leads to anxiety. You can't help wondering if you are deteriorating, and this only makes you more anxious.

There is a general lack of knowledge and understanding of Alzheimer's disease and it would be enormously satisfying and rewarding to be able to help change this. This is especially the case in countries like South Africa, our home country, where many poor people are affected by the condition and don't have adequate resources for dealing with it.

One of the startling facts uncovered during our dementia journey was that unlike cancer or heart disease, Alzheimer's disease is not considered to be a 'dreaded disease' so it is not covered under insurance policies. Anyone who has been affected by any form of dementia will testify to the devastating consequences of the condition, and this sorely needs to be addressed.

## 4.10 Stigma and dementia in sub-Saharan Africa: a Namibian experience

**Contributor:** Berrie Holtzhausen, CEO Alzheimer's Dementia Namibia

### Introduction

In sub-Saharan Africa there is not enough data about dementia, which has a direct impact in the quality of information available. Whereas it's clear that raising awareness and increasing education will help break down the walls of stigma in Africa, it's also important to understand the cultural context and beliefs that can influence this stigma.

Belief in witchcraft, HIV-AIDS, perceptions about western medicine and un-enforced laws, are key causes of stigma towards people living with dementia in Africa. This stigma leads to the perception in communities that it is okay to discriminate against people living with dementia. Many are perceived to be witches and are ostracised, isolated, chained-up with very little food and water and sometimes killed.

Although there is a commonality about dementia all over the globe, the situation in sub-Saharan Africa is unique; dementia needs to be demystified in order to reduce stigma against people living with dementia.

### The belief in witchcraft and stigma

In sub-Saharan Africa, many people use traditional means (witchcraft) to seek explanations for misfortune, illness or death. The fact is that the belief in witchcraft is common and is thus one of the main reasons why stigma against people living with dementia is so prevalent in the region.

In the Journal of Clinical Nursing, Professor Ingrid Hanssen, Registered Nurse and Doctor in Political Science, and Flora Mkhonto, Registered Nurse, introduce the reader to the consequences of perceiving people with dementia as witches, a common belief in sub-Saharan Africa.[1] They also demonstrate how lack of understanding about dementia being a disease, creates psychological distress and lack of care for people living with dementia.

An American University study by Boris Gershman, notes that *"...witchcraft beliefs can have a direct adverse effect on interpersonal relations via two main channels: by fostering the fear of bewitchment and by spreading the fear of witchcraft accusations, potentially entailing severe sanctions, from destruction of property to ostracism and even ritual killing."*[2]

In the 2016 documentary film, the African Witchfinder, the reality of believing in witchcraft and the stigma regarding people living with dementia in rural Namibia, is depicted very clearly.[3]

Witchcraft beliefs breed anxiety, uncertainty, suspicion and mistrust. They are fuelled by fear, jealousy and dreams.

This creates the perfect storm for stigma in a society that still accepts the belief in witchcraft as a part of its culture. Many sub-Saharan African countries have a law called: Witchcraft Suppression Law, however, there has been a reluctance to enforce it as it is often regarded as a discriminatory law.

### Namibia

According to the Chairperson of The Law Reform and Development Committee (LRDC), the Law is outdated, discriminatory and accusatory: *"A consolidated and contemporary law must be developed, that balances individual rights of freedom of persons, with the harm associated with witchcraft, thus, it became a criminal offence for African people to use their traditional conventional means to seek explanations for misfortune, illness or death."*[4]

Alzheimer's Dementia Namibia responded as follows: *"The weapons in the fight against stigma and discrimination of dementia are: awareness, education, the Constitution of Namibia and the Witchcraft Suppression Law. Laws never will, and can't change culture but laws do change behaviour and changed behaviour can change the stigma and discrimination in cultures."*

If LRDC believes that it is necessary to redesign the Witchcraft Suppression Law in order to be more in line with the Constitution of Namibia, and to be a more contemporary law, Alzheimer's Dementia Namibia will be the first to help - for the sake of many people in Namibia who are living with dementia and are not free; not because of a disease but because of the stigma and discrimination surrounding them.

### South Africa

On 23 March 2010, the Minister of Justice and Constitutional Development approved a South African Law Reform Commission project to review Witchcraft Legislation.[5]

One of the Commission's projects, the review of Witchcraft Legislation, supported the constitutional guarantee of freedom of religion and protected vulnerable groups. It was mostly women advanced in age that were persecuted as witches by communities holding traditional beliefs. These innocent victims were vulnerable to a double degree: as women and as older persons.[6]

This project was put on hold because the Traditional Healers council and New Paganists opposed it.

Witchcraft related stigma will never be stopped if the gross human rights violations against people living with dementia, perceived to be witches and wizards, are not exposed as unacceptable.

> ***Witchcraft beliefs breed anxiety, uncertainty, suspicion and mistrust and witchcraft beliefs are fuelled by fear, jealousy and dreams. This is the perfect storm for stigma in a society***

## HIV-AIDS

Out of the 34 million HIV-positive people worldwide, with roughly 23.8 million living in the continent of Africa. Sixty-nine percent live in sub-Saharan Africa. Ninety-one percent of the world's HIV-positive children live in Africa.[7]

HIV dementia is a common cause of dementia in African nations. AIDS Dementia Complex (ADC) is more common than Alzheimer's disease in Namibia, South Africa, Uganda, Kenya, Tanzania, Nigeria, Gabon, and Togo. So, an underestimation of dementia numbers in many African nations could be due to the Alzheimer-centric view of dementia (Professor William Hu).

Some of the side effects of treatments also exacerbate beliefs and issues around witchcraft. One medication called EFV 600mg (Efavirenz) describes side effects as: *"Changes in the shape or location of body fat, especially in your arms, legs, face, neck, breasts and waist" and "...serious mental health problems, unusual dreams and seizures..."*. These side-effects, especially for men developing breasts, are often interpreted as a person either being a witch or being bewitched.

## Access to medication and person-centred care

The fight against stigma in sub-Saharan Africa can't be won without access to correct medication and properly trained physicians and medical professionals, focusing on some important facts, namely:

- The belief in witchcraft is real
- Firmly establishing that dementia is not part of normal ageing but a terminal disease
- The very specific link between HIV-AIDS and dementia in Africa
- Discussing the cause of the disease and the diagnosis in detail with patients and their carers is vital
- Explaining what the physician wants to achieve with the medication (e.g. suppression of the viral load, managing high blood pressure, high blood sugar etc.)
- Explaining and being transparent about possible side effects: establishing the benefit of the medication over the side effects or the danger of side effects and that these need to be reported and discussed immediately with the physician. Plus giving people clear examples of how side effects have been misunderstood as signs of witchcraft

In order to better support members, Alzheimer's Dementia Namibia is in the process of employing a Registered Nurse with 11 years of experience in screening, awareness and education of people living with HIV-AIDS.

According to him, *"Combination HIV medication can cause a lot of side effects, most of them are psychotic in nature and psychosis is seen as one of the key signs of being a witch. Identified side effects include hallucinations, violence, removal of clothes, talking to yourself, slurred speech, being withdrawn, drowsiness, irritability, constant headaches, loss of memory. This has misled a lot of health professionals because they did not, and still do not recognise these symptoms as side effects of the medication. We admit these people living with dementia and put them on anti-psychotic medication".*

This was brought to the attention of the Ministry of Health, and from 2019 new guidelines were implemented so that anyone developing psychosis, as a side effect of Efavirenz, is switched to another anti-retroviral drug. This is now happening in Namibia and also in Zimbabwe. The previous dosage of Efavirenz has now also been reviewed, reducing it from 600 to 400 milligrams.

## Conclusion

The stigma and misunderstanding surrounding dementia in sub-Saharan Africa are a devastating reality for individuals living with the condition.

No nation can be free before everyone is free. People living with dementia are not free, not because of a disease such as Alzheimer's or HIV-AIDS related dementia, but because of the stigma and discrimination against people living with dementia.

The challenges of stigma in sub-Saharan Africa regarding dementia diseases ask for a holistic approach of the origin, role and place in the belief of witchcraft, western medicine, the way western medicine is being practiced, the relationship between western and traditional medicine, judiciary (common law and the traditional law, and human rights balance with every country's constitution.

## References


1 Mkhonto, F. and Hanssen, I. 2017. 'When people with dementia are perceived as witches. Consequences for patients and nurse education in South Africa' *Journal of Clinical Nursing* 27(1-2) online: https://onlinelibrary.wiley.com/doi/abs/10.1111/jocn.13909 Last accessed 19 August 2019.

2 Gershman, B. 2015. 'Witchcraft Beliefs and the Erosion of Social Capital: Evidence from Sub-Saharan Africa and Beyond' *Journal of Development Economics* 120 online: https://pdfs.semanticscholar.org/6ef4/41f0162e5e2e60b899d580cc3822725918ac.pdf Last accessed 19 August 2019.

3 African Witchfinder. ©2016 Heehaw Ltd. online: http://www.africanwitchfinder.com/ Last accessed 19 August 2019.

4 The Namibian. 2019. 'Call to revise witchcraft suppression law' online: https://www.namibian.com.na/185323/archive-read/Call-to-revise-witchcraft-suppression-law Last accessed 19 August 2019.

5 KLRC Blog. 2017. 'Justification For Review Of Witchcraft Act, Cap 67' *Kenya Law Reform Commission (KLRC)* online: http://www.klrc.go.ke/index.php/klrc-blog/518-justification-for-review-of-witchcraft-act-cap-67 Last accessed 19 August 2019.

6 South African Law Reform Commission. 2011. 'Thirty Eighth Annual Report 2010/2011' online: http://www.justice.gov.za/salrc/anr/2010-2011-anr.pdf Last accessed 19 August 2019.

7 DoSomething.org. 2019. '11 facts about HIV in Africa' online: https://www.dosomething.org/us/facts/11-facts-about-hiv-africa Last accessed 19 August 2019.

## 4.11 A carer's perspective: My life with my father Joel Mbithuka Kasimu

**Contributor:** Elizabeth Mutunga, CEO & Founder Alzheimer's & Dementia Organisation Kenya

My father's name was Joel Mbithuka Kasimu. He was a senior police officer with the rank of Officer Commanding Station (OCS) and a very well-dressed individual who loved his family immensely. Although he was a busy man, he took time each evening to read to me and these story books helped develop my language and imagination. Being the first born, in sharing these powerful stories, he made me believe I could be anything I wanted to be.

In 1984, when I was only 9 years old, my Dad went into a diabetic coma. It was frightening to see my hero unable to do much for himself. In 1985, he had to retire early due to medical reasons. This made him really sad, as he loved wearing his uniform and he also missed not being able to serve the community. In 1989, we lost a sister, and this added to my Dad's sadness. The reason I am giving this background is to illustrate how far back the issues started. In 1992, my Dad moved the family from a four-bedroom house to a five roomed house. He then started selling the car in parts; the tyres separately from the rest of the vehicle. This was shocking to us. He then became violent which was totally out of character. This created a rift in the family as he was always looking for an opportunity to fight with us. I soon had to go and look for work to provide for the family.

It wasn't until 2007 that I heard the word dementia. I was shocked when we were informed that there was no cure. This was almost 15 years after fighting with Dad and not understanding what the issue was. A lot of people in Africa in the 1990's believed that dementia was a disease of the West and thus Africans could not get it. My father came from a community where people believed if there were issues happening to you and they could not be explained it was because you had been bewitched; you must have done something bad to the gods and thus you were being punished. As he was elderly, others believed it was a normal part of ageing. Due to the stigma of the disease, a lot of people would not visit our homestead for fear of the same disease affecting them.

This prompted me to look for a support group to plug into so I could understand more about the condition - but there was none. This pushed me to start a group, which ran till 2009, when my Dad rested. The journey with dementia was gruesome and I did not want anything to do with it anymore and so packed away that part of life and moved on.

In 2013, I received five phone calls from different individuals who had been referred to me, or who had read my story, as I used writing as a way of dealing with the pain I went through with my Dad's illness. I was initially quite angry when I received all these calls as I had made a pact with God and myself that I would never do anything or come close to this condition again. The people calling were so persistent that I decided to have one meeting where we could decide way forward. We never turned back since then and the support group still runs today. We have invited experts to come to speak to caregivers during the monthly meetings and educate them on the condition. This has changed their perceptions on dementia.

As caregivers one of the things we have worked on is creating awareness about dementia. We have used both print and digital media and awareness in the church to combat stigma and the misbeliefs surrounding the condition. Initially, when we started creating awareness, we would have to make many calls for even one radio or television station to interview us but now it is them calling us, and that is a great shift.

Referrals from neurologists have also helped Alzheimer's and Dementia Organisation Kenya (ADOK) in that we are now able to support more people. Involvement by the Ministry of Health in all their Technical Working Groups has helped in pushing forward the agenda of ensuring that we are moving towards having a national dementia plan in Kenya and policies to cater for people living with dementia and their carers.

There are a lot of studies now being carried out in Kenya as there is very little data on dementia and even the Government needs to recognise it is a huge burden to the carers; financially, emotionally and spiritually. Kenya is also part of STRiDE (Strengthening responses to dementia in developing countries) and this has been beneficial as we have more interactions with the Ministry of Health and so, for anything on dementia, ADOK is the go-to organisation. In 2017 Kenya also held our first conference in partnership with ADI and this was an eye opener to how big the problem of stigma really is. I remember most people were shocked to know that there was an Alzheimer's association in Kenya.

The issue of stigma is still rife especially in some areas in Kenya, but this is changing as more people are calling ADOK to ask where to start. If they have seen a doctor, then they are directed to attend our support group. By meeting other people going through the same thing, it helps with acceptance. People are then more confident to speak out and this reduces self-stigma. Self-stigma is the greatest hinderance to dealing with dementia and once this is dealt with, it will have a ripple effect on the issue of stigma in general.

## 4.12 Fighting stigma in the Middle East. Who speaks on behalf of people with Alzheimer's and dementia?

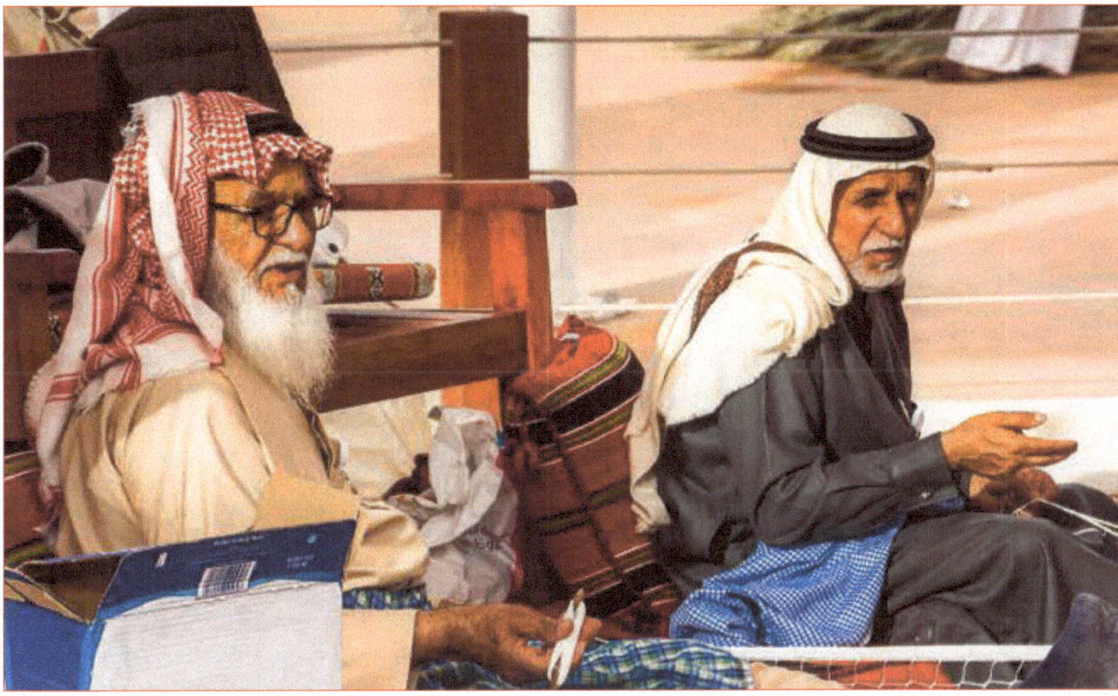

**Contributor:** Princess Nouf bint Muhammad, acting CEO of the King Khalid Foundation

My first encounter with Alzheimer's, that then curious disease with a strange sounding name, came many years ago when most of what we knew of such mental health issues was "senile dementia", which seemed inevitable, yet you prayed and hoped your elderly relatives, and eventually yourself, would escape its ravages.

What was it, what did it mean, how did it differ from other forms of dementia; all questions still unknown to many of us at the time; talked about quietly, and only between family members. Visits were limited to a smaller and smaller number of people, not as result of the anxiety it might cause, but to preserve the dignity of the person living with dementia. Sons and daughters wanted to protect their loved one as they lost their ability to communicate, to judge situations, and conduct themselves in the manner that suited their age and social standing, as family patriarch or matriarch.

As family awareness of the disease increases, and we know more about how it starts, how it affects the mind, and that it could start much earlier on in life, the stigma is reducing. Understanding the different stages, and that it is a medical condition and not a natural progression of old age, has helped family members cope better, and has reduced the embarrassment that they felt for themselves, as well as their diagnosed family member.

Unfortunately, that is only one source of stigma reduced and others remain.

Stigma associated with diseases and mental disorders manifest through a series of interconnected factors such as the spread of misinformation, lack of awareness, and prejudice that leads to discrimination. The fear of tackling cultural taboos and the systemic lag in public provision of education, health and social services are among the culprits as well. As I have been privileged with chairing the board of the Saudi ADHD (Attention Deficit Hyperactivity Disorder) Society (Ishraq), I have also seen the dangerous side effects of stigma, against what are considered mental health disorders. Many of the families were often resistant to accepting diagnosis and seeking assistance out of fear of the stigma they and their children might face. I believe this also happens to people living with Alzheimer's disease and other dementias, their carers and families. Moreover, unfortunately, limiting their options to seek care and support, accept diagnosis, and take advantage of the coping mechanisms that can be available to them.

Arab societies assign larger roles to extended families and greater social connections. We consider values of respect and dignity for the elderly as a duty and source of pride. This leads some families to avoid reaching out to healthcare professionals, carers or professional social services to help relieve the burden of their ill loved ones or the responsibilities associated with taking care of them. Families are intimidated by the stigma of care homes, which might be perceived as abandonment. Another disincentive to families seeking care is the damaged reputation of public social care institutions for the elderly and the perceived poor quality of the services they provide. Due to those factors, the stereotype about older age and dementia pushed people living with it to stay in the shadows. For that, the role of raising awareness of the disease and advocating for the rights of people living with it and their families serves as important solutions to those problems.

***Many of the families were often resistant to accepting diagnosis and seeking assistance out of fear of the stigma they and their children might face***

In addition to awareness, one of the important ways we can fight stigma is by making affordable, high quality governmental and non-governmental health and social services available to people with dementia. They should also be mindful of the needs and support that cannot be provided at home. These services should not be considered as luxuries available only to those who could afford home care. Subpar standards of these services leave many individuals, rich or poor, vulnerable.

Who should carry the burden of tackling this disease? I believe that governments cannot deliver inclusive healthcare and work toward eradicating the stigma against dementia alone. It is a collective effort that we all can be a part of, as governments, private sector, non-profit organisations and societies. Investing in the number of non-profits and building the capacity, in particular, can drastically improve the lives of people living with dementia, their loved ones and carers. As too would increasing training and expertise, especially around diagnosis and coping post diagnosis. Non-profit organisations serve an important role in raising awareness of Alzheimer's disease and dementia, advocating for the rights of patients and their carers. Those types of contributions would hopefully lead to correcting the negative connotations associated with the disease, improving the way people are treated; with dignity, respect and free from prejudice.

Our strength at The King Khalid Foundation is in our ability to bring the voices of our beneficiaries forward. For the longest time, the non-profit sector in the Middle East and North Africa has focused on delivering the basic needed services on the ground, and responding to basic demands of their beneficiaries. When it comes to tackling stigma, it is essential for NGOs (Non Governmental Organisations) to spread awareness about stigmatised communities, most importantly to push forward the voices of those who are being stigmatised; not as victims but to validate the challenges that they are going through. NGOs need also provide solutions and road maps to build the awareness of and help direct policy in their developmental, health, and education, and financial plans too.

At the Foundation, we work closely with various non-profits by providing them with funding and investing in social awareness campaigns that promote social inclusion, acceptance, and celebration of the added value and benefits, those who are vulnerable provide to society and the economy once they are enabled. Through our capacity building workshops, we were fortunate to serve our local Saudi Alzheimer's Disease Association since 2011. We worked with the Association on training their team on project planning, monitoring, and measuring impact. We are proud to commend the Saudi Alzheimer Association for their advocacy efforts to normalise Alzheimer's as a legitimate disease that needs proper services in the Saudi healthcare. In 2019, the Association succeeded in making diagnosis and treatment of Alzheimer's disease available without out-of-pocket costs at the minimum mandatory health insurance coverage in Saudi Arabia, unlocking needed funding and allowing greater access for millions of people to those services. Such efforts, encompassing the consistent engagement of the public and dedicated direct advocacy with policymakers are a great example of how non-profits serve their beneficiaries directly and indirectly.

Whether it is through research, pursuing policy change, or through spreading awareness publicly, we truly believe that NGOs in the region need to spend more time and effort to bring the voices of the vulnerable forward, including the voice of people living with Alzheimer's disease. The best way to help people with Alzheimer's is not only to provide them with the needed services but to give them a voice. As NGOs, the best that we can offer them and their families is the gift of understanding and advocating, and for society to remember that the burden of disease needs to be shared publicly.

Note: *The King Khalid Foundation is an independent Saudi non-profit that works on creating prosperity in the Kingdom by mobilizing stakeholders through social investment, capacity building and advocacy. The Foundation, established in 2001, has championed the cause of expanding the non-profit sector and spreading sustainability practices in the private sector. The Foundation has a long-standing history for pioneering socioeconomic research relating to poverty, financial inclusion, and quality of life, with a special attention to put forth evidence on the characteristics of vulnerable groups in the country. For more information, kindly visit the Foundation's website: www.kkf.org.sa*

## 4.13 A view from a memory clinic in Oman

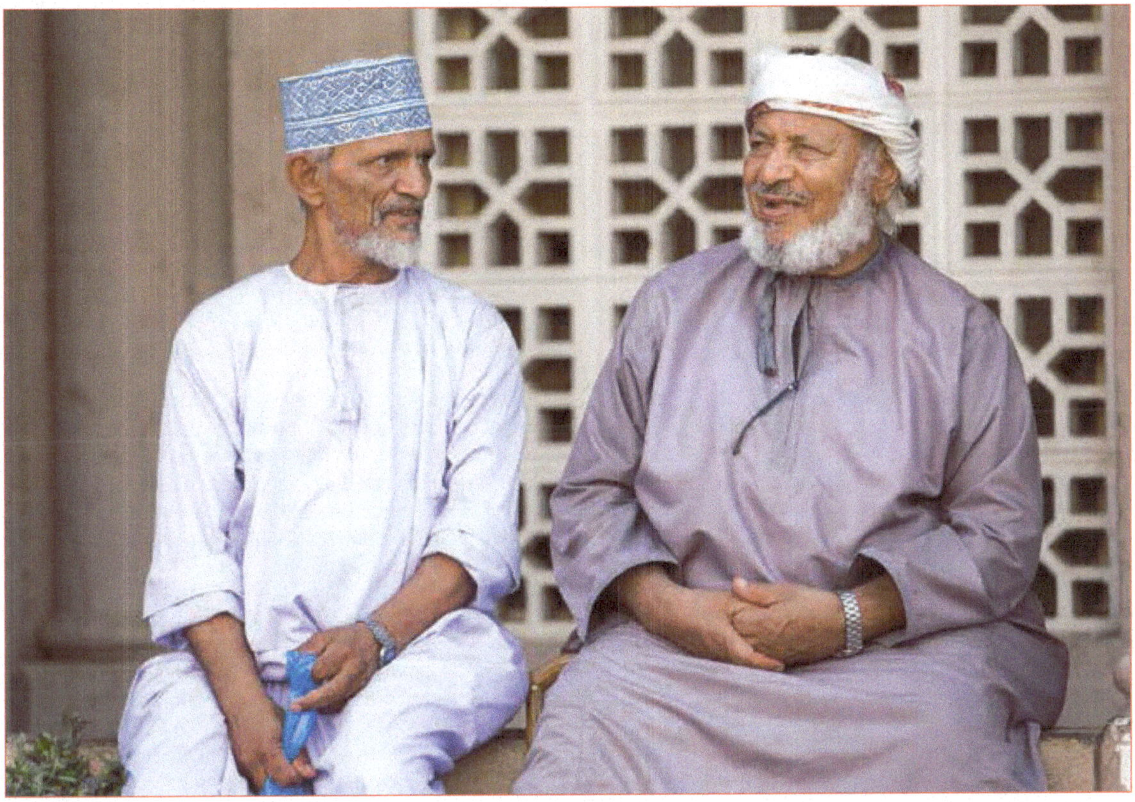

**Contributor:** Dr Hamed AL Sinawi, Senior Consultant Psychiatrist, SQUH, Chairman, Oman Alzheimer›s Society & Oman Psychiatry Society

Stigma and negative attitudes toward people with mental health problems are a global phenomenon, which is often extended to include patients, their caregivers, and also mental health professionals. In Oman, mental health services used to be provided at separate hospitals, which meant mental health workers didn't get to work with other health professions. This lack of contact with others led to them being perceived as "working with crazy people" or "acting like their patients". More recently, mental health services have been integrated with other health services. This means both patients and mental health professionals have a chance to mix with others and challenge negative stereotypes. Dementia services are relatively new in Oman with the first memory clinic being introduced in 2011. People with cognitive impairment who were admitted to medical or surgical wards often got discharged from hospital without referral to the memory service as some health workers believe that not much can be done for such patients, since there is no cure for dementia.

Unfortunately, stigma still exists and this means people are sometimes denied access to services or denied their right to make choices about their health care. At times, during the medical interview, health care professionals only talk to the caregivers without involving the person with dementia even when they are at the early stages of the disease. Some caregivers ask that the person with dementia is not told about the diagnosis, which in my opinion is also stigmatizing to the person, as it denies them the right to know about their condition.

Self-stigma is quite common in people with dementia who attend our clinic, especially those in the early stages where denial is exhibited. They may seek a second opinion abroad and refuse to accept the diagnosis. This eventually makes them endure unnecessary expenses and delays the start of treatment.

But things are slowly changing. Many people, including health care professionals, are becoming more receptive to learning about dementia and to referring patients to the memory clinic for assessment. This can be partly attributed to the dementia awareness campaign that was introduced few years back and included workshops, social media posts and lectures to non mental health workers in other department about dementia. We often come across colleagues from other hospital departments who contact us for a consultation as one of their family members is exhibiting symptoms of dementia and this personal experience makes them realize how we can support patients and their caregivers, even if there is no cure for dementia.

## 4.14 Creating an Alzheimer association; the story of the Alzheimer Indonesia Foundation

**Contributor:** DY Suharya Regional Director, Asia Pacific Alzheimer's Disease International

When my Dad informed me that my Mom (75 years old) was diagnosed with vascular dementia back in August 2009, I was shocked and confused. I was in the first year of my PhD scholarship after earning my Master of Public Health at Curtin University in Perth, Western Australia. When I had left Indonesia back in 2007, I was actually planning to move and live in Australia for good. However, my destiny seemed to bring me back home and I realised that God (and the universe) had better plans laid out for me.

Learning about my Mom's vascular dementia diagnosis in 2009 helped me reconcile almost two decades of struggling with my relationship with her. Mom had actually showed symptoms of dementia in her mid 50s. I felt real guilt.

The circumstances literally led me to a big decision, to simply 'let go' of my PhD and return to Jakarta in May 2012 and to commit to taking care of my Mom and to supporting my 80-year-old Dad. As he was the main carer, I tried my best to protect his physical and mental health in the "unknown" caring journey facing us.

The journey started when I accompanied Mom to a psychogeriatrician and was definitely not satisfied with all the answers to the questions we had. How to deal with challenging behaviour – sundowning? Refusing to eat? Agitation? Delirium? Suspicion? Hallucinations?

The doctor suggested I attend the Alzheimer's Disease International (ADI) conference in Taipei in April 2013 which led me to cross paths with the ADI "family" – at that stage, more than 80 member associations (now 100). I was inspired by members around the world who had done many things related to awareness raising, risk reduction, research, training, education, person-centered care methods, and advocacy. I learned so much from the conference and felt so lucky to have crossed paths with everyone including one of the people I admired from TADA – Secretary General Li Yu Tang. I pledged then to establish an association back home – what was to become The Alzheimer Indonesia Foundation.

On 3 August 2013, Alzheimer's Indonesia Foundation (ALZI) was officially established in Indonesia by multi-disciplinary founders, from a carer to a lawyer, a psychogeriatrician, a neurologist, a communication specialist and sports medicine doctor.

In truth, the new ALZI was actually a follow up, a transformation, from The Association of Alzheimer Indonesia which was created in 2000 and became a member of ADI in 2009. ALZI's vision was, and is, to improve quality life of people with dementia and carers and empower them with knowledge, skills and a network to support each other in the journey of caring.

I started off the new ALZI in 2013 supported by the Board of Trustees, only 5 volunteers and no funding. We were committed to conduct activities to end stigma around people with dementia and carers in Indonesia, a country with a 250 million population; where 8% of the population are over 60 and the estimated number of people with dementia is 1.2 million; with US$2 billion economic cost. We believe in our vision and mission immensely. If there's a will there is a way.

I had been inspired by Steve Jobs, who talked about why we should "connect the dots" in everyone's life, which was something that I did in my early days in kickstarting the first ever Alzheimer's awareness raising program, in September 2013. With only 500 participants, we managed to convince the Indonesian Minister of Health to support our cause.

One of my biggest goals was to influence policy makers and the Government about the importance of having a national dementia plan with sufficient budget. The Government of Indonesia subsequently launched its first ever Dementia National Plan with a modest budget in March 2016, one of the first countries in ASEAN (Association of Southeast Asian Nations) to do so.

I had a vision that nothing would be impossible if we could work together to create an inclusive society, following the principles of human rights and involving all partners – including people with living with dementia, carers, institutions, national and local government, private sector, non-profit organisations, health and care professionals and many others.

I was motivated to make things happen and to spread awareness that memory loss is not a normal part of ageing; that it's important to identify the 10 warning signs of dementia early so you can make comprehensive plans for a good quality life in the long- run. I had experienced it myself, in caring for my Mom. She was actually showing symptoms of cognitive impairment for two decades before she was diagnosed, and the entry points that affected her were hypertension, malnutrition and depression. The fact is; one person is diagnosed with dementia – but the entire family is affected and knowledge is definitely power.

My Dad is in his 90s now. He was the primary carer for my late Mom, who passed away in April 2017 - but her legacy continues. Now my Dad has been helping other husbands navigating the dementia carer path.

My sister won a traditional nationwide Poco Poco dance competition involving people in their 50s and she's now the official Poco Poco dance instructor, a dance that's designed as part of risk reduction activity around dementia - if done consistently, for example for 30 mins a day, 5 times a week, there can be 37.5% improved neuroplasticity[1].

ALZI started its movement in 2013 and 6 years on, in 2019, we have more than 50 partners, 21 chapters (18 chapters in Indonesia and 3 chapters in USA, Netherlands and Switzerland) that have committed to increasing awareness in their own communities. For the past six years our movement of "Do Not Underestimate Memory Loss", #EndStigma and "RespectYourElderly" has changed the landscape of dementia and elderly awareness in Indonesia through the production of an information materials, including the 10 warning signs, introduced carer meetings and hosted the country's first Alzheimer's walks, with over 10,000 people attending in Jakarta alone over 5 consecutive years. Twenty other cities throughout Indonesia have hosted walks, picnics, inter-generational initiatives, virtual runs and many other activities.

Through ALZI's strategy in building partnerships with all sectors, the organisation has garnered support from government departments and local and national businesses.

After three years running the organisation on a voluntary basis, the ADI Twinning Programme helped link up Alzheimer Netherlands and Alzheimer's Indonesia. In 2017 Alzheimer Netherlands and the Ministry of Health, Sports and Welfare also supported ALZI to host the first ever Asia Pacific Conference in Indonesia. A very strong partner – Atma Jaya University has been part of the journey since 2015 and as a respectable academic institution under the leadership of Dr Yuda Turana, ALZI has strengthened its programmes to deliver impact to the society involving youth and technology and innovative interventions including film, webinar, and many others.

ALZI now leads a network of dedicated volunteers who plan events, conduct advocacy, and lead carer meetings. Purple Troops in Jakarta was established to help the elderly and link them up to receive screening in the nearest clinic in Jakarta. Capacity building is indeed the key as well as conducting programs that are impactful.

Indonesia has the fourth largest population in the world at 250 million. It's made up of over 17,000 islands, and 600 cultures call these islands home. Asia, specifically Asia Pacific, has the fastest growing population of people with dementia in the world, out of 50 million people with dementia, almost half live in the region.

Often, in low- and middle- income countries health and care priorities focus on tackling and reducing the number of communicable diseases, improving access to clean water and poverty eradication. However, with the growing population of people with dementia expected to rise to 4 million by 2050, every sector of society will be impacted. How dementia is perceived in these sectors may be very different within each culture and geographic region - which is a challenging task. In the villages, outside the major cities, many families believe dementia is a normal part of aging and keep their loved one at home, isolated from society, out of shame or embarrassment.

The path forward? To continue to support and strengthen Indonesia and other members in the Asia Pacific Region to be able to maximise their resources and assets, empower and improve quality life of people with dementia and carers. For me, this is a lifetime commitment.

## References:

1 Ria, M T et al. 2019. 'The Effects Of Poco-Poco Dance On The Executive Functions Of Type 2 Diabetes Mellitus Patients With Mild Cognitive Impairment Achieved Through Improvements In Neuronal Functions And Plasticity,' *International Journal of Pharmaceutical Research,* 11(2): https://doi.org/10.31838/ijpr/2019.11.02.097 Last accessed 1 Sept 2019.

## 4.15 145 Indigenous languages and no word for dementia: use of innovation and technology to help overcome stigma

**Contributor:** Dementia Australia

In Australia today there are 145 Indigenous languages in use and within these the word dementia, cannot be found.[1] This directly results in stigma and misunderstanding associated with the condition.

Recent studies have shown Indigenous Australians are 3-5 times more likely to develop dementia and at an earlier age of onset than non-Indigenous Australians.

Generating meaningful communication pathways between dementia researchers, health service providers and Indigenous communities is critical to providing better prevention, diagnosis, treatment, and care options for Indigenous Australians living with dementia. Recent hearings at the Australian Royal Commission into Aged Care Quality and Safety highlighted the need for culturally-safe practices to be embedded into care as well as stressing the need for more research to support the development of good models of care for Indigenous Australians. Witnesses to the Commission reported a lack of respect of culture and customs in the delivery of care, including racism, lack of understanding of the Indigenous attachment to country and a lack of Indigenous carers within the aged care system.

While timely diagnosis can be problematic for anyone living with dementia, within Indigenous communities this can be heightened by a lack of culturally appropriate diagnostic tools. Poor recognition of dementia within Indigenous communities and among health care workers and service providers compounds the issue. The use of culturally appropriate validated cognitive assessment tools is critical, especially when we note that, within the 145 Indigenous languages used across Australia today the word dementia cannot be found, which in turn results in stigma and misunderstanding associated with the condition. [1]

The preferred tool is the Kimberly Indigenous Cognitive Assessment tool (KICA)[i]. This is a tool designed for Aboriginal and Torres Strait Islander people in the Kimberley region and has been modified for Aboriginal and Torres Strait Islander people in urban areas.

Innovative approaches to engaging Indigenous populations are being developed, tested and deployed in Australia programmes including Dementia Yarn Up[ii], a collaboration between Dementia Australia, the Gunditjmara community, Nathan Lovett-Murray, Winda Mara Aboriginal Corporation and Indigenous Hip Hop Projects that has resulted in the production of a hip hop music resource on dementia, wellbeing, culture and respect, going some way to reducing the stigma within Indigenous communities.

Dementia Australia's innovation and leadership in the application of virtual reality (VR), interactive video games and apps (applications) is also being adapted to assist engagement with Indigenous populations. Dementia Australia's Centre for Dementia Learning (CDL) has developed a wide range of applications in consultation with carers, people living dementia and educators. The application of VR, interactive video games, and apps continues to transform dementia care and practice for people living with dementia, families and carers across residential and community care settings. Some of the programmes have also now been introduced to Canada, Singapore and Czech Republic.

The CDL's exploration of emerging technologies such as VR and computer games has been an exciting focus for more than six years and a wide range of applications have been developed in consultation with carers, people living with dementia and educators. The drivers have been to create immersive and impactful experiences that aim to build empathy and meaningfully resonate with users to inspire positive change. The different applications are powerful tools and offer an experiential way for all who work in the industry to increase their understanding thereby improving their practice.

The impact of these technologies has been measured through ongoing and independent evaluation as well as consumer consultation that demonstrates how the use of these tools in education and information sessions is influencing change in residential and community care and improving the lives of those living with dementia.

Key products that have been developed are two apps, The Dementia-Friendly Home™ and recently, A Better Visit™, which are examples of the way technology can be accessible via everyday devices. One empowers carers to understand how they can better support a person living with dementia to maintain their independence and dignity and continue living at home, while the other has fun, engaging games to enhance communication and facilitate positive social interactions with visitors.

A third application is The Virtual Forest™, an interactive computer game which creates a beautiful, calming, natural setting, and provides people living with dementia the opportunity to reclaim a sense of control over a part of their lives by interacting with ducks, fish, a dragonfly, a butterfly and forest trees with just the wave of their hands.

(i) https://www.perkins.org.au/wacha/our-research/indigenous/kica/

(ii) https://www.dementia.org.au/resources/indigenous-hip-hop-project-yarn-up-about-dementia

For those who do not live with dementia, it can be difficult to understand what it might be like for someone experiencing changes in their brain, or to comprehend the way in which communication and the environment around them impacts on their cognitive function. The Virtual Dementia Experience™ provides an immersive, experience-based workshop which allows carers to develop a strong sense of empathy by 'virtually' being in the shoes of someone living with dementia. An evaluation by Australian-based Swinburne University found that dementia care workers who undertook the Virtual Dementia Experience training gained threefold more empathy for the person living with dementia and they were able to identify more dementia-friendly elements and care practices.

The workshop has been adapted as technology has evolved, with an updated version now available on lightweight, mobile VR googles, called EDIE (Educational Dementia Immersive Experience)™. The virtual reality experience enables participants to see, feel and hear through the eyes of a person living with dementia as he navigates his house late at night trying to find the bathroom. Participants are fully immersed and can even hear the heart beat faster as the situation becomes more and more confusing and challenging.

This portable experience has resulted in the ability to rollout EDIE workshops all over Australia, enabling aged care workers in regional and remote areas to experience the insights the technology elicits. It also offers a more economical option for providers since it minimises or removes the need for staff travel and time away from their workplaces.

An evaluation of EDIE has found it significantly improves knowledge, changes attitudes towards dementia, and stimulates greater empathy and understanding of care needs. While not all challenges are that simple to address, it shows how valuable Information Technology and applications can be for the health industry.

EDIE is also being used to break down the barriers and educate Aboriginal and Torres Strait Islander communities, with an educational programme being delivered to remote Indigenous communities in far north Queensland's Cape York region, including Wujal Wujal, Hope Vale, Lockhart River, Bamaga, Pormpuraaw, Kowanyama, Weipa. Funded by the State's Northern Queensland Primary Health Network, the programme is aimed at health, community, hospital and other staff and community members who are working with adults, older people and those living with dementia.

Dementia Australia is committed to creating unique, accessible, learning experiences for participants that touch, move and inspire them to transform their dementia practice through a change in attitudes and behaviours. A whole of society focus on educating the wider community and not just people living with dementia and their carers is key to reducing stigma, discrimination and increasing understanding of dementia in communities.

For more information on all the products and programmes above visit https://dementialearning.org.au/technology.

## References

1 Korff, J. 2019. 'Aboriginal languages' *Creative Spirits* online: https://www.creativespirits.info/aboriginalculture/language Last accessed 19 August 2019.

## 4.16 Māori, Mana and Mate Wareware: Rauawaawa Kaumātua Charitable Trust and its experience in supporting Kaumātua with Dementia

**Contributors:** Rangimahora Reddy & Pare Meha, Rauawaawa Kaumātua Charitable Trust, Dr Etuini Ma'u, Waikato District Health Board, Prof John Oetzel, University of Waikato

When asked to contribute to the World Alzheimer Report, we set out to identify the challenges of stigma, awareness raising, and diagnosis for Māori along with a unique cultural programme to address these challenges at a kaumātua (elder) serving organisation in Aotearoa (New Zealand)

With a vision of *"Hei manaaki ngā Kaumātua"* – "To enhance the quality of life and wellbeing of Kaumātua" – Rauawaawa Kaumātua Charitable Trust was established in 1997 by a group of Kaumātua (elders) concerned about loneliness and other key challenges facing Kaumātua. Based in Hamilton, New Zealand, Rauawaawa is an organisation firmly rooted in Kaupapa Māori principles (a philosophy of Māori for Māori). Central to these principles is the concept of mana (status, prestige), promoting practices that protect and uphold the dignity of Kaumātua, supporting their independence, and ensuring Kaumātua voices resonate through what we do, how we do it and when and where it is best done.

Rauawaawa is based out of Te Puna o Te Ora, a facility set up in 1941 as a residential facility for Māori moving from the rural areas into the city for work. It offers a rich history in its service to Māori and is unique in serving those that are the same age or younger. Many Kaumātua that engage with Rauawaawa today fondly recall the role the facility played in their earlier lives.

As in Maoridom, Kaumātua at Rauawaawa are revered for the mātauranga (knowledge/wisdom) gained from their lived experiences and for the central role they play in their whānau (extended family) and wider iwi (tribe). Many are also known for their experience as practitioners and custodians of tikanga (cultural customs). Kaumātua are often the first point of call in whānau crises; the cultural equivalent to the health emergency number. They are also greatly relied on by organisations to provide tikanga for events (e.g., opening a new building) and cultural training. In short, the reliance on Kaumātua has grown significantly over time.

But what happens when Kaumātua who have been the rangatira (leader) in the whānau end up needing manaaki (caring) themselves because of mate wareware (dementia)? Holding mana as a result of their rangatira role in a whānau can make it extremely challenging for both themselves and their whānau to acknowledge the symptoms, become informed, seek out a proper diagnosis, and access the support they need to enhance the quality of life and wellbeing of their Kaumātua. In a nutshell, the stigma of mate wareware may be enough for Kaumātua to resist sharing what they experience in the early stages, to disagree to having a proper assessment and to decline the opportunity to learn about the illness.

The stigma may also be enough for whānau members to try and hide what is happening with their beloved Kaumātua in an attempt to protect the mana of their Kaumātua and ensure they are not categorised or treated in a way that is not befitting of them, their whānau or their past. Other efforts to protect a kaumātua's mana may include wrapping them in "cotton wool" or surreptitiously curtailing their independence by assuming more of the decision making for them. Another challenge with this stigma is it can induce assumptions of independence no longer being possible for the Kaumātua concerned; e.g., a vehicle, bicycle or scooter maybe confiscated by whānau as they try to protect their Kaumātua and others from physical harm and yet it still may be possible for the Kaumātua to have independence.

The realities of caring for Kaumātua with mate wareware are as diverse as they are challenging, as a balance is sought between promoting independence whilst maintaining safety. Rauawaawa as a provider of culturally focussed day programmes have been tested a number of times with providing adequate care for those with mate wareware. The outcomes have not always been up to our own expectations. The realisation that, as an organisation, you are no longer able to provide the level of oversight needed for a Kaumātua can bring on a rapid and horrendous sense of panic for their safety when they go missing. The possibilities of harm that run through your mind are endless as is the hole in your stomach from worry and the ache in your heart from failing to be the safe pair of hands that Kaumātua need you to be and that Whānau rightly expect you to be.

These experiences made us realise at Rauawaawa that safely integrating Kaumātua with mate wareware into our usual programmes, whilst still maintaining their mana, would be difficult for those with a more advanced mate wareware and that a more robust programme focussed solely on kaumātua with mate wareware was needed. In 2018, Rauawaawa were supported by Alzheimer's New Zealand (NZ) to develop and implement a culturally responsive programme to promote understanding of mate wareware and the services available to support both the individual and whānau. The programme is called Hiki te Wairua (Lift the Spirit) and includes four key components:

1 A weekly group-based programme incorporating opportunities to engage and participate in activities such as te reo (Māori language), waiata (Māori

songs), poi (Māori action songs) and rakau (Māori stick games).

2 Individualized visits that incorporate opportunities to educate and share information on mate wareware with whānau and Kaumātua, as well as provide information on the services available for them to access for support.

3 The incorporation of mate wareware service providers in quarterly health expos to promote awareness, and include opportunities for providers and potential clients to develop relationships.

4 To profile mate wareware in our annual Kaumātua Olympics which hosts Kaumātua service providers and their Kaumātua from across the North Island of NZ. This programme will be launched in Alzheimer's month with Alzheimer's NZ at Rauawaawa.

Kaumātua are a cultural taonga (treasure). Symptoms that change them from what they have been in the past to who they are with mate wareware are challenging. Their significant contribution to the wellbeing of a whānau, iwi and community is a small reminder of why they deserve the best of care available to ensure *"Hei manaaki ngā Kaumātua."*

## 4.17 Federazione Alzheimer Italia – developing a model for Dementia Friendly Communities.

**Contributor:** Mario Possenti, Segretario generale, Federazione Alzheimer Italia

The Italian Dementia Friendly Community program was started in 2016 by Federazione Alzheimer Italia, the largest national non-profit organization dedicated to the promotion of medical and scientific research on the causes, care and assistance for Alzheimer's disease and dementia.

For the pilot project Abbiategrasso was chosen, a 30,000 inhabitant town in northern Italy, on the basis of a protocol developed in the United Kingdom by Alzheimer's Society. The basic idea was to evaluate the feasibility of a large-scale dissemination of these communities while always keeping in mind the peculiarities of Italian society. For this reason, the project was designed, integrating best practices from various experiences of European and non-European countries.

We used the Dementia Friends logo created by the Alzheimer's Society, however, we considered that, in Italian, the best translation for the project was "Friendly communities of people with dementia" to pay more attention to the person as the center around which the whole community revolves: listening to their voice and being guided by their indications adds meaning and great value to the whole project.

Federazione Alzheimer Italia considers every reality in creating a path towards a community that knows how to listen and support people with dementia. Through practical examples and suggestions on the main actions to be taken, the communities can then decide which activities and initiatives to use in order to make their territory welcoming for people with dementia.

From the beginning we felt the need to frame the project in the most precise way so that it was not only replicable and sustainable, but also really effective in achieving the aim of placing the person at the center and fighting the stigma of dementia. For this reason, each community starts with an active participation of people with dementia, including through an investigation of their needs.

Already in 2017 we had welcomed the review by Imogen Blood and Associates (a social research agency) in partnership with Innovations in Dementia (a UK based Community Interest Company, established to help people with dementia to keep control of their lives), which collected experiences, voices and opinions of experts, people involved and people living with dementia with the intent of providing a definition of Dementia Friendly Community and outline examples and best practices of action.

This work is part and result of Act on Dementia[1], which involves 13 States with the aim of developing consensus on the evidence of diagnosis, post diagnostic support and quality of care, and understands how these changes can be put into practice and evaluated.

When the Italian Ministry of Health asked the Abbiategrasso's community to participate in this transnational initiative, we felt it was important to give our contribution with a view to assessing whether the impact of the Dementia Friendly Community (DFC) was objectively relevant and what were the best ways to approach this project.

Federazione Alzheimer Italia, with the pilot site in Abbiategrasso, is involved together with Greece and

Bulgaria in the Work Package 7 of the Joint Action, namely the one dedicated to Dementia Friendly Communities. The aim of the pilot is to validate a series of indicators and to provide indications for the creation of a shared model.

Measuring progress during the journey to become a more welcoming Community is useful in order to demonstrate the effectiveness and impact of DFCs on the lives of people with dementia and their families. It also better clarifies the scope, responsibilities, resources and path that each initiative must have within the Community and make the long process of supporting and maintaining a DFC, traceable and repeatable.

Today in Italy there are 24 Communities: towns and portions of cities, from north to south and from east to west, which have accepted the challenge of Federazione Alzheimer Italia with conviction and commitment to launch a path on their territory where citizens have the opportunity to become a network, able to welcome and involve people with dementia. This path is made up of informative meetings, recreational, cultural and sports events aimed at the participation of citizens, never forgetting the active involvement of people with dementia at every stage of the project.

***From the beginning we felt the need to frame the project in the most precise way so that it was not only replicable and sustainable, but also really effective in achieving the aim of placing the person at the center and fighting the stigma of dementia. For this reason, each community starts with an active participation of people with dementia***

This experience is also bearing fruit at the institutional level. Together with the Ministry of Health, some representatives of the Italian regions and other dementia friendly experiences, we have written a document of recommendations for DFCs that will be approved, hopefully by the end of 2019, from all the Italian regions and will constitute the operational base for the constitution of a larger involvement. This document will allow the regions, which are public bodies, to become promoters of this initiative without, however, obscuring the fundamental role of the municipalities, associations and local communities that are the real engine of this project.

The project born from Federazione Alzheimer Italia continues to spread and grow because more and more communities have perceived the importance of initiatives like these to make dementia known but above all to fight the stigma towards people who live with dementia. However, it is necessary to monitor and evaluate these initiatives over time as it is essential to have data to be able to know, in the long term, the impact on the population and to be able to overcome those difficulties that may arise, for example, from different social contexts.

In Italy, of the 24 DFCs, 19 are located in the north and only 5 are located in southern Italy. What most characterizes the realities of the south is that the activities of the Community revolve around already consolidated experiences such as day centers or listening centers. What is lacking in the territory and in the institutions is reinforced by the presence of local associations and the richness of their initiatives.

The differences and peculiarities of the various Italian communities certainly represent a challenge for the project. For this reason it is important that local stakeholders contribute to creating a network capable of understanding the needs of people with dementia, and together with them, put in place a series of well-planned initiatives.

It should be noted that, where the networks are stronger, there is an intense collaboration between the various stakeholders, and the Community carries out more significant initiatives. However, when a real network is missing, or the fundamental contribution of an Alzheimer association, and the direct engagement of people with dementia is missing, and the initiative is left in the hands of local institutions only, the Community tends not to express its full potential.

In Italy the DFCs project is just at the beginning, however, from 2016 to date we have been able to see an increase in media coverage of the initiatives and this is undoubtedly a result that traces a path towards greater knowledge of dementia and, in perspective, towards a victory against stigma.

## References

1 European Joint Action DEM-2, 2016-2019. https://www.actondementia.eu/about Last accessed 3 September 2019.

## 4.18 Dementia in prisons; How to address the double stigma of people with dementia or memory issues in prisons and forensic institutions.

**Contributors:** Sophie N. Gaber, MSc OT, PhD Candidate at Karolinska Institutet, Sweden & Birgit Heuchemer, MSc. registered. OT at HELIX Forensic Psychiatric Clinic of Stockholm; Research Assistant at Karolinska Institutet, Sweden.

Interviews with older ex-prisoners, as well as professionals working with prison and forensic populations in the UK and Sweden, shed insight into the "double stigma" of living with dementia, or memory issues, in prisons or forensic institutions. International policies such as the United Nations' Sustainable Development Goals, strive to "leave no one behind", however, in this case study we ask whether the marginalised population of older people with dementia or memory issues, in prisons or forensic institutions, are at risk of being left behind.

### Ageing stigma: The growing population of older prisoners

Older prisoners are one of the fastest growing populations among all prisoners, in many countries (e.g. UK, US, Australia).[1] The growing population of older prisoners is attributable to several factors, including governmental policy changes. This has resulted in longer prison sentences where people age in prison, in addition to the imprisonment of older people without consideration of their specific needs.[2] The lack of consideration of the specific needs of older prisoners is compounded by insufficient research or policy on the topic.[3] Lack of information about the prevalence, incidence or experiences of older prisoners living with dementia has contributed to what prisoners have described as a "double stigma". They face not only the typical ageist assumptions that dementia is a natural part of ageing (e.g. forgetfulness, reduced ability or capacity, slowness, etc.) but also the prejudices associated with being a prisoner including views on criminals by society. One ex-prisoner described the stigma she faced, which was intensified by not only her age and memory issues but also her gender;

*"There's a stigma when you're in prison, because you're older people, especially if you're a woman, they think you should know better. There was a stigma from guards and other people. They would say 'well we can understand a young kid doing this because they don't know what they're doing or they're on drugs or something' but you're looked down upon."*

Older prisoners cost approximately two to three times more than younger prisoners.[4] Prisoners age at an escalated pace; it is estimated that the physiological age of prisoners is 10-years greater than their chronological age.[5] Consequently, the care needs of older prisoners with and without dementia tend to be higher due to the number of chronic health conditions they are living with (e.g. diabetes, high blood pressure, arthritis and mobility impairments).[3] However reports show that prison staff lack training or education about caring for older people with dementia or memory issues.[2] An older prisoner reflected that

"I think society probably doesn't expect older people to be in prison so much. And anyone that has aged in prison has been put to prison for a very long time, which must mean that their crime is something very, very serious if they've been there for many years. And the thing about being an older person in prison is that on the whole prison is a very young place. People are very busy and they run everywhere and they fight a lot. And I found it dangerous even walking down the corridors".

Due to the large amount of resources that are required to care for the complex needs of older people living with dementia in prisons, it is essential to develop knowledge about this population and consider whether prison is the appropriate place for older people with dementia convicted of a crime.

### Everyday stigma: Risk factors for dementia and cognitive decline among older prisoners

The harsh living conditions of prisons are well reported internationally, however, the potential risk that such conditions pose for dementia and their direct opposition to dementia prevention guidelines, has not been widely acknowledged.[6] Research indicates that we are able to influence between 30 to 50% of the risk factors for Alzheimer's disease, including high blood pressure (hypertension), depression, education, and limited physical inactivity.[7] Yet, this is not the case for prisoners.

- **High blood pressure:** In the case of blood pressure, prisoners described a poor diet of meals and commissary snacks rich in salts, sugars and fatty foods. Smoking is widespread with limited opportunities to visit a health professional to monitor blood pressure or one's general health and wellbeing.
- **Depression**: A high rate of depression has been reported in this population.[6] Depression has been associated with the increased sense of isolation and a lack of privacy or safety experienced by prisoners.
- **Education**: Whilst some prisons offer education programmes this is inconsistent and prisoners, as well as professionals working in prisons, described limited opportunities for cognitive stimulation.
- **Limited physical activity:** The highly-structured prison routine limited opportunities for physical activity, particularly in outdoor spaces for older

people. Additionally, the rate of alcohol and substance use, blood-borne viruses and non-communicable diseases is higher than the general population.5

The absence of cognitive stimulation or education as a risk factor for dementia or cognitive decline was highlighted by both ex-prisoners and prison staff as a key issue. One prison staff member noted that possibilities for making decisions, even minor ones such as when to make a cup of tea, are reduced.

One ex-prisoner elaborated,

*"I lost a lot of my memory. You know before I went in I used to think that I could remember numbers. I could remember my PIN code. I could remember phone numbers and things. And I found once I got in there for a while, with the strange life you live, a lot of that I couldn't remember. In fact it hasn't returned. I don't think I'm as sharp because of that experience as I was before. That's not just about old age, it's about being in a place where you're left to deteriorate, quite badly. Without the necessary stimulation that a human being needs every day."*

Another older ex-prisoner compared the stigmatising effects of the everyday living environment to the disorientating monotony of the film "Groundhog Day".

*"The film Groundhog Day - that's what it makes me think of. You wake up, you have your toast, you go back in, you have your lunch, you go back in, you have your dinner, you go back in… The only way I knew one day a week that was a point of reference for me was that on a Thursday I did my laundry."*

## Diagnostic and support stigma: Managing dementia or memory issues in prison or forensic institutions

Diagnosing dementia in prisons and forensic institutions is problematic for a variety of reasons, such as a lack of cognitive screening when a person enters prison or during their stay in prison, inadequate training of staff to identify the signs and symptoms of dementia, and a reluctance of prisoners to report memory issues or dementia due to a fear of repercussions.[4] Dementia is not a diagnosis that automatically determines whether a person convicted of a crime is sent to prison or an alternative place, such as a forensic institution. Recognising signs of a problem is based on a person's presentation of symptoms and level of functioning, which is in turn reliant on the ability of staff to identify symptoms and make the necessary actions to support the person.

Guidance for staff is inconsistent. For instance, in the United Kingdom there is no national plan for managing older prisoners.[8] One prison staff member admitted that, *"dementia is not a common part of the vocabulary"* and that the entire system is not adapted for people with dementia or cognitive impairment, with even meetings with social services being challenging. Furthermore, the staff member observed that prison services are frequently preoccupied with other mental health conditions which may even "cloak" the dementia. There is a risk for dementia to be hidden because symptoms may be dismissed as challenging behaviour. Cognitive impairment is included in many other diagnoses that are prevalent in prisons and forensic institutions (e.g. depression or psychoses) and can be attributed to the many side-effects of medications. Ageist assumptions may further cloak dementia if people do not realise that dementia affects many different people and not only the frail, very old population.[4]

A prisoner described the lack of support or activities for older people in prison;

*"There's sometimes a pastoral chaplain that could come and talk to you but it's very difficult because the medical staff are all so busy and they're only really there for serious injuries or doing things like giving out pills."*

A lack of support by fellow prisoners or opportunities for social engagement was also reported;

*"So, in there it is very difficult to find someone you can talk to and staff are constantly changing. When you talk about memory issues you are told that it is just due to the new, unfamiliar environment. You feel very isolated."*

A staff member explained the lack of support for older prisoners is due to staff members not having experience working in geriatric care and called for greater cooperation with care home or nursing home professionals, as prison may not be the most suitable place for an older person with dementia. There may also be a bias of lowered expectations for older prisoners, especially those with chronic health issues such as dementia, compared to rehabilitating young prisoners who have "their whole lives to live".

*"So, something like memory loss, would be considered I know, as something not important. Not life threatening as far as they're concerned. You'd be waiting a very long time to see anybody. It would probably be only if you requested an outside agency like Mind (a mental health charity), or something like that, if you could actually get any of them to come in. But whether you would be able to do that or not - I don't know. So, it would be very, very difficult to get help."*

One lawyer explained that, *"there is some hesitancy in addressing the issue of an ageing prison population. There is a fear that with dementia we are just uncovering the tip of the iceberg, there are serious financial, social and legal implications if we are going to address health and cognitive issues to make life fairer and better for prisoners."*

In summary, this case study is intended to be used as a launchpad for advocacy towards increased awareness and meaningful changes to support the lives of older people living with memory issues or (un)diagnosed dementia in prisons or forensic institutions internationally.

## Three recommendations for change:

1 Introduction of a mental health assessment including screening for dementia/cognitive impairment at the probation stage (prior to imprisonment).

1 An annual health and wellbeing check-up that includes a cognitive assessment for all prisoners aged 50 years and over (by mental health/dementia charities).

2 Dementia-awareness training for all professionals and volunteers working with prison populations (by dementia charities and organisations).

## References

1 Peacock, S., Hodson, A., MacRae, R., Peternelj-Taylor, C. 2018. 'Living with Dementia in Correctional Settings: A Case Report' *Journal of Forensic Nursing*. 2018; 14(3): 180-184.

2 Newcomen, N. *Dementia. Prisons and Probation Ombudsman Independent Investigations. Learning lessons bulletin* 11, 2016. online: http://www.ppo.gov.uk/app/uploads/2016/07/PPO-Learning-Lessons-Bulletins_fatal-incident-investigations_issue-11_Dementia_WEB_Final.pdf Last accessed 20 August 2019.

3 Brooke, J., Diaz-Gil, A., Jackson, D. 2018. 'The impact of dementia in the prison setting: A systematic review' *Dementia* 0(0): 1-23.

4 Cipriani, G., Danti, S., Carlesi, C., Di Fiorino, M. 2017. 'Old and dangerous: Prison and dementia' *Journal of Forensic and Legal Medicine* 51: 40-44.

5 Sindano, N. 2016. The Prison Project: Raising awareness of dementia in prisons. online: https://www.alzheimers.org.uk/blog/prison-project-raising-awareness-dementia-prisons Last accessed 20 August 2019.

6 Christodoulou, M. 2012. 'Locked up and at risk of dementia' *Lancet Neurology* 11(9): 750-751.

7 Norton, S., Matthews, FE., Barnes, DE, Yaffe, K, Brayne, C. 2014. 'Potential for primary prevention of Alzheimer's disease: an analysis of population-based data' *Lancet Neurology* 13(8): 788-794.

8 National Dementia Action Alliance. 2019. *Meeting the challenges of dementia in prisons: Roundtable discussion briefing paper* online: https://nationaldementiaaction.org.uk/wp-content/uploads/2018/09/Prisons-and-Dementia-NDAA-briefing-paper-Update.pdf Last accessed 20 August 2019.

## 4.19 Challenging stigma in mental health: What we've learnt over 10 years

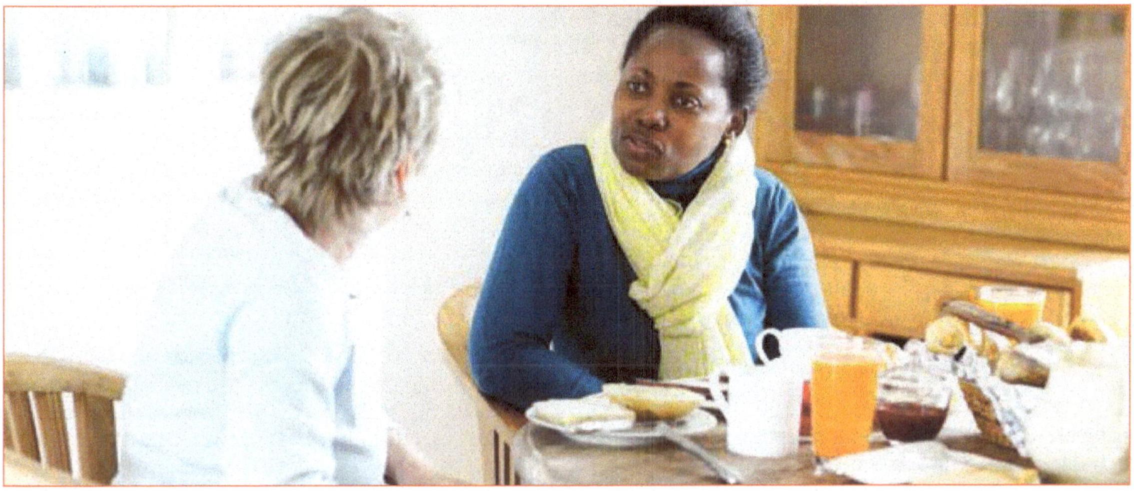

**Contributors:** Ruth Stone, Global Communications and Digital Manager, and Sue Baker, Director, Time to Change Global

This is a case study on challenging stigma in mental health as inspiration and a call for collaboration.

Ending mental health stigma is the work of a generation. I think that's the most important thing we've learnt since starting Time to Change more than 10 years ago.

Stigma is deeply ingrained, through cultural norms, families, workplace culture, the media and even the words we speak. It is present at almost every level of society, which means our work takes time, perseverance, and a broad, flexible approach.

Time to Change is one of the most evidence-based social movement campaigns in the world. We have robust, independent evaluation in place to track progress and show the difference we are making.

I am very proud to say attitudes are changing. Between 2007 and 2016, there was a 9.6% improvement in attitudes - that's around 4.1 million adults in England with better attitudes towards mental health problems. Eleven percent more people say they would be willing to live with, work with or continue a relationship with someone with mental health problems. This research carried out by the Institute of Psychiatry, Psychology and Neuroscience (IoPPN) at King's College London shows levels of discrimination have also fallen. People report experiencing 7% less discrimination from family, 15% less discrimination from friends and 10% less discrimination in dating.

We cannot be sure the precise amount of social change due to our campaign. The work of many organisations and individuals has combined to drive positive change. But we are extremely proud to have been at the forefront of social change around mental health stigma and discrimination.

More than 1,000 organisations have signed the Time to Change Employer Pledge. We've worked with more than 2,000 schools and there are over 7,000 Time to Change Champions speaking out to end stigma in their communities.

While it is important to celebrate these huge steps, there is still a long way to go.

### Going global

Mental health problems know no boundaries; neither does stigma. They affect people of all ages, all income groups, and all cultures. That's why in 2018, we launched Time to Change Global.

One in four people around the world will experience a 'mental or neurological disorder' in their lifetime. Yet nearly two-thirds of these people never seek help from a health professional.

Stigma and discrimination are a big part of this. Stereotypes, misconceptions and fear are so deep-rooted, mental health is treated as a 'poor relation' to physical heath. People with mental health problems are mistreated and misunderstood all over the world. We can be excluded by families, friends, neighbours, employers and schools.

*"I had a relapse at the prayer camp, and I was tied like a sheep. They tied my legs together, like a pig or an animal at a butcher to be carried home." (Champion, Ghana)*

Despite being a global issue, much of the evidence on how to tackle mental health stigma is concentrated to a few countries - mostly in the Global North.

The Time to Change Global programme seeks to address this balance and help build a broader evidence base for stigma reduction.

We are working with international disability and development organisation, CBM, and with local partners to pilot anti stigma campaigns in Ghana, India, Kenya, Nigeria and Uganda.

*"People say it is a waste of time to give you food – or they say you should stay outside."* Champion, India

The five pilots will look very different, depending on the needs and capacity of our local partners. Each campaign is being developed, tested and adapted with the local partner and a group of Champions. All Champions have their own experience of mental health problems.

While language, context and approach might look different, the pilots share three core elements:

- **Lived experience leadership:** People with mental health problems shape and lead all that we do.
- **Social contact**: Conversations can change lives. We know that sharing personal stories within communities is vital for ending stigma.
- **Social marketing**: Public campaigns allow us to reach more people, increase knowledge and change perceptions.

## Lived experience leadership

To effectively tackle stigma, whether you're in Accra or Accrington, we know that people with lived experience must shape, lead and deliver social change campaigns.

Those of us with personal experience of mental health problems are best placed to drive the change we want to see. It is so important that our voices are heard. It means so much to me to see Champions planning and running events and sharing their stories how they want to share them.

"When I had my crisis, I felt I was a disappo*intment to everybody that looked up to me. Now though, I can see people are still being inspired by my experience. I'm sort of giving back in my own small way."* Project Coordinator, Ghana

## Social contact

Conversations really do change lives. When those of us with experience of mental health problems start talking more openly, we can reduce stigma and discrimination in our communities. By sharing our stories and telling you how it really feels to live with a mental health problem, we can change opinions and shift attitudes.

*"We should not stay back because of our mental illness. We can all help to create awareness."* Champion, India

In the five pilot countries, Champions are planning and running social contact events to engage the public and share their stories. In Accra, Ghana, events have taken place at malls and shopping centres to reach wide sections of the public. Social contact events in Doddaballapur, near Bengaluru in India, look very different. Champions here are from rural communities. They have been sharing their stories alongside travelling actors and singers at schools and in outdoor spaces.

## Social marketing

One of the reasons our work in the UK has been so successful, is our ability to reach wide audiences through social marketing. These campaigns are effective because we take time to understand public perceptions and then we develop creative approaches which challenge and address public fears, misunderstandings and stereotypes.

Time to Change Global is replicating this approach, to help change public perceptions and behaviour in the five pilot countries. In Ghana, the work began with a set of focus groups to understand how members of the public feel about people with mental health problems.

This research has highlighted pervasive beliefs linking mental health problems to violence. One focus group member explained, *"They are not predictable. You don't know when they will strike*". Others described how people are shunned and rejected, *"mad people are not supposed to appear in public… we don't see them as humans"*.

We asked the focus groups to think about how we could challenge these negative perceptions. Building empathy was a core recommendation. As one participant explained:

"I wouldn't like to be in that situation and people rejecting me, if I see a person in that situation, I would like offer a helping hand because it might happen to me as well".

These insights will allow us to develop a campaign in Accra that is truly audience-led.

Stigma and discrimination ruin lives. We won't stop until no one has to face this injustice. No one should be made to feel alone, ashamed or worthless because of their mental health problem. Together with our local partners, we will keep fighting to remove the barriers that stop people living their lives to the full.

We want to inspire other campaigners, other organisations and anyone facing stigma in the Global South, and around the world. We want to learn from other campaigns and in turn, share our learning, our tools and our approaches.

To anyone working to end stigma – whether that's related to mental health, disability or any other issue – I want to say that we are in this together. By sharing inspiration, ideas and celebrating our successes, we can make change happen.

Find out more on our website: https://www.time-to-change.org.uk/global.

## 4.20 Case study: Advertising and dementia; the power of a cup of tea

**Contributor:** Chris Lynch, Deputy CEO & Director of Policy, Communications & Publications, ADI and Shiva Krishnamurthy, Unilever

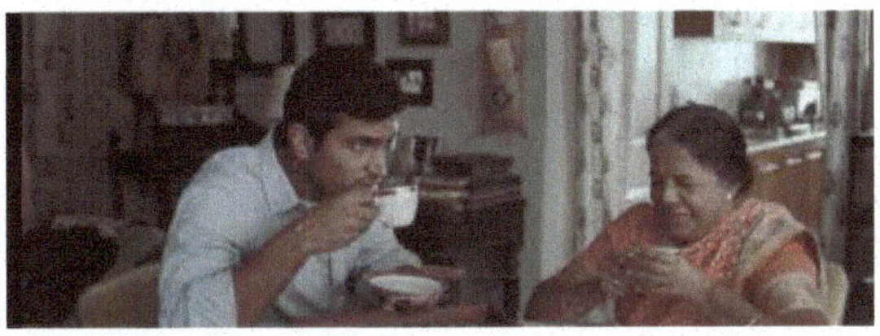

Following the launch of a TV advert in India with a strong dementia theme I interviewed Shiva Krishnamurthy, Vice President, Tea & Foods at Hindustan Unilever Ltd. about why their tea brand, Brooke Bond Red Label, decided to commission, film and distribute the advert and how they went about it.

It is really interesting, and timely, to see how the media is evolving in its depiction of dementia but also how brands are starting to engage; understanding that there is a market around dementia, for advertising their products or services, and in Brooke Bond Red Label's case, for positioning of their brand. It is a tricky area. Undoubtedly there is an economic decision by brands to engage, to sell products and services, but decisions about aligning a brand to a certain cause, challenge or disease means that a brand is making a conscious decision, perhaps based on its nature, its culture, its aspiration and the market's perception it.

The Brooke Bond Red Label advert tells the story of a lady living with dementia sharing tea with a neighbour who she mistakes for her son. It is a very well-crafted and thoughtful short film that raises lots of questions about society, dementia awareness, neighbourliness, loneliness, caring and possibly the geographically dispersed nature of families today.

Brooke Bond Red Label has an identified brand strategy to "make India more inclusive". In recent years they have explored some of the social tensions in society and produced adverts and short films in response; these have included pieces on live-in relationships, religion and eunuchs. For this advert they felt that they wanted to explore why the elderly can feel excluded and left behind, and to find an "honest" way to talk about it.

Shiva Krishnamurthy explained that they were looking for a deep story about the loneliness that can accompany old age. Dementia/Alzheimer's disease, positioned at an intersection of two big societal challenges – exclusion of the elderly and lack of awareness about mental health issues – felt like an area they wanted to tackle. The story they developed is not just about a woman who forgets; it is as much about a woman who is forgotten. A key goal of the advert is thus about bringing people together, over something as simple, but as powerful, as a cup of tea.

Brooke Bond Red Label work with the media agency Ogilvy and Mather in India and they developed this advert from the client brief. One of the writer's grandfathers had lived with Alzheimer's disease, giving the agency added insight, alongside their own research. Brooke Bond Red Label then commissioned India's top advert filmmaker, Prasoon Pandey, who showed great interest in the story. He immersed himself in research on the subject - from watching documentaries to speaking with carers. Krishnamurthy confirmed that only after thorough research and developing a deeper understanding, Prasoon took the story to the shooting floor. The aim was not to have a single moment look constructed but to convey an everyday scenario and interaction, conveyed through the natural feel of the advert.

Shiva Krishnamurthy explained that dementia, like other mental health issues, can be an awkward subject in India and in producing and airing this advert Brooke Bond Red Label has taken the subject of dementia into millions of households. It was initially screened in cinemas and then transferred to TV, guaranteeing a large audience. They feel that this advert has undoubtedly resulted in people talking about dementia, taking what was a conversation from those that are already engaged, professionals, advocates, carers, and extending the reach exponentially, by putting it on people's TV in their own homes, in a domestic setting they could relate to. "Getting a conversation started is a big job" Krishnamurthy commented.

In this report, journalist Pippa Kelly also highlights that many TV companies and film makers have developed dementia related storylines. Dementia in an advertising space, however, is still very much in its early stages and, like with Brooke Bond Red Label, often a brand statement aligned to positioning goals and societal change. Undoubtedly it raises awareness, starts a conversation and should help challenge stigma. Going forward, however, it will be interesting to see how brands, marketeers, creative agencies, etc. develop adverts around dementia. Products and services designed specifically for dementia should follow established creative routes, for example, the often emotive marketing of a drug or medical treatment, but it is the positioning of brands attracted to the market that remains to be seen. For example, Swedish furniture giant IKEA has partnered with Swedish construction company Skanska to make available 'flat-pack' dementia homes, through the BoKlok joint venture. If and how they advertise this venture will be monitored by others interested in the sector. Certainly news coverage to date has come from the design and construction press, along with some interested general press titles.

## 4.21 Young onset dementia, a personal story; time for change

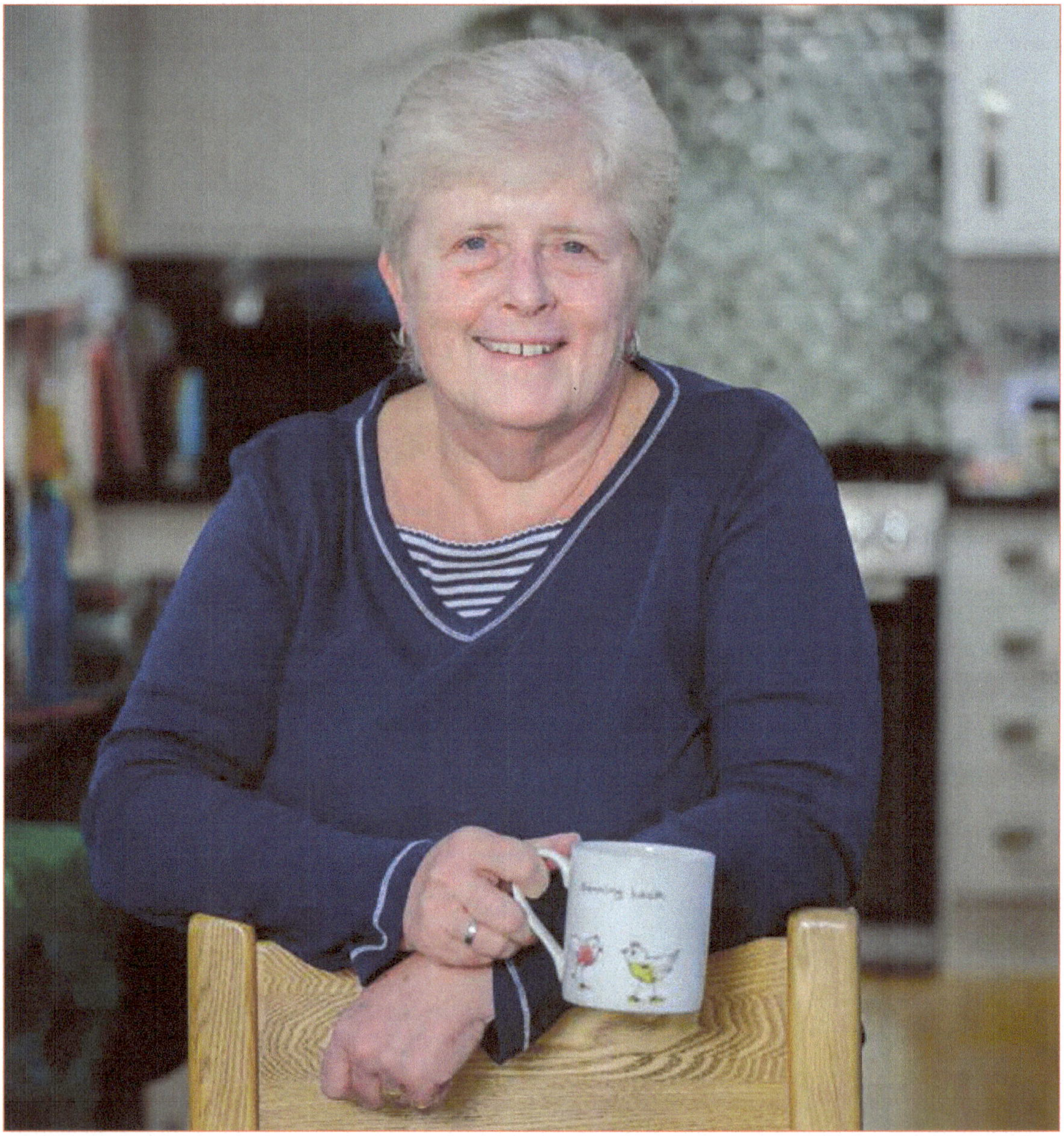

**Contributor:** Christine Maddocks

Following a stroke in 2015 I became concerned about my memory and went to see my GP (General Practitioner) who told me that she was there for my physical health and not my mental health. My GP said that, in her opinion, there was nothing wrong with my memory, even though she didn't test it, and that she would not refer me to a memory service.

This situation went on for a while until I was suddenly admitted to hospital with a suspected stroke in 2016. Despite only being 60 years old, I ended up on an elderly care unit. This led to a subsequent appointment for a memory assessment, however I was not advised that this might lead to a possible diagnosis of dementia, so I attended the appointment on my own. I was told at the end of the assessment that I had dementia. I couldn't remember anything else and just felt as though I had been given a death sentence.

I went home and cried for three months, and during this time I received no follow-up from the diagnosis appointment. I received no information about dementia and did not fully understand what it would mean for me. I became depressed and anxious and couldn't leave the house, I was referred to Mind (a mental health charity) for a therapy group, but my difficulties were very different to the other people in the group, so I didn't really find it to be helpful.

I saw some information by the Alzheimer's Society and it really made sense to me. I rang the Society and they came to see me at home and I started a 'Living Well with Dementia' group, and this felt like a life line to me.

During this time, I lost my job, and I felt that this was managed very badly. Following my stroke in 2015, I had been off work on sickness absence. During this time I had been recovering from my stroke, struggling with my memory and my mood, due to receiving my dementia diagnosis. I decided that I wanted to go back to work, but my employers said that they were not ready for me to return. They suggested a phased return, but I was not given any support, even when I struggled to remember how to log onto my computer on my first day. They were unable to find me another position and started disciplinary procedures as I was struggling to do my work, even though there was no support and no reasonable adjustment on their part. Ultimately, I had to go off sick and had to involve my union but was given ill-health retirement against my wishes. I felt that people couldn't see or understand my dementia, that I wasn't believed and that I was almost having to prove that I had the condition.

I was put in touch with an Early Onset Dementia service in the local hospital which was a specialist team, which was very good, with lots of activities tailored to younger people. I also began helping out with the Alzheimer's Society, and felt valued for contributing and being involved.

I began to struggle living alone, and I decided that I would relocate to live with my partner. I didn't feel that my family were very understanding. I felt that they were scared of dementia, because my father had the condition and had been in a very bad way towards the end of his life, and therefore they held a very negative outlook about it. I felt also that as well as my family, many of friends didn't understand the condition, and I felt that they avoided me, and stopped keeping in touch.

Since I moved to live with my partner, I have struggled to receive specialist help or advice, for example obtaining a doctor's opinion annually on whether I can continue driving. Whilst my GP is pleasant, she doesn't not seem to have much understanding about the condition and the things which help me, such as contact with other people with the condition. She has described me as a 'difficult' case, as I don't neatly fit into the 10 minutes appointment slot.

However, living with my partner has made a great difference and she is able to support me, as has doing voluntary work at a local hospice, where having a diagnosis of dementia is not held again me. I have also been very involved in working with the Alzheimer's Society, more recently becoming a Dementia Ambassador, as well as the Time for Dementia programme. I feel that lots of negative assumptions are made about the diagnosis of dementia, and therefore involvement in these activities has helped me stop feeling useless,

I decided to get involved in the programme Time for Dementia because of my own, not very good, experiences with health care professionals. I felt that it was a good opportunity to raise awareness about dementia, by telling people how it is for people living with dementia, both the positives and negatives. I thought that if I can raise awareness and help even one person to avoid what I have been through then it would be worthwhile.

My partner and I have been seeing Occupational Therapy and Physiotherapy students as part of Time for Dementia. I have been really keen that students get this exposure to dementia because it can be a hidden disability - you cannot see that people have dementia by just looking at them. I have really enjoyed doing the programme, the students are lovely. They come to our house, to our environment and this feels so much better. They are able to hear how my partner and I have been affected by dementia, and this information comes from the mouth of person with dementia, and their carer and this feels like a much better way for them to be learning. This kind of direct experience must be invaluable.

CHAPTER 5

# Programmes to reduce stigma

## 5.1 Time for Dementia; preparing the future workforce to understand and meet the challenges faced by those with dementia and their families

**Contributors:** Dr Stephanie Daley, Dr Wendy Grosvenor, Christine Maddocks, Dr Zoe Cashin, Dr Jaewon Phee, Jayme Hill, Prof Sube Banerjee

There is a need to improve how we prepare future generations of healthcare professionals to understand and support people affected by dementia to live well from diagnosis to end of life. This means enhancing the education they receive in training. Typically, healthcare education tends to focus on block clinical placements with an emphasis on crisis, or acute illness; this does not provide student learners with a true understanding of what it like to live with dementia, or other long-term conditions. This current way of learning rarely enables students to understand and challenge stigma, or to experience and create a person-centred approach to their care, or to build the compassion and understanding needed to help those affected by dementia. Seeing people with dementia only as patients and in acute settings can also build in attitudes towards and beliefs about dementia that are negative and that are not appropriately optimistic about the possibility of living well with dementia.

The ADI World Alzheimer Report 2016 advocates the development of experiential methods of teaching that involve experiences of patients; arguing that they engage staff at an emotional level to help address some of the negative perceptions about working with older people with dementia.[1] Time for Dementia is one such programme.

### What is Time for Dementia?

Time for Dementia is an innovative undergraduate educational programme, set up to address these challenges, and funded by Health Education England. It has been developed with people with dementia and the Alzheimer's Society in the United Kingdom (UK), to help create an age-friendly curriculum and lead to students building confidence in working with people with dementia that will lead to enabling improved outcomes for people with dementia when they enter clinical practice[2]. The purpose of Time for Dementia is to enhance undergraduate learning about dementia specifically, and more generally about older people's health, long-term conditions, and the role of families in care.

Along with supporting workshops and reflective assignments, students visit a person with dementia and their family in pairs for two hours every three months for two years. The programme was first established as a core component of the curricula for medical, nursing[3] and paramedic students at Brighton and Sussex Medical School (BSMS) and the University of Surrey.[4] The programme is unique in a number of ways including: the inclusion of multiple professional groups; the compulsory nature of the programme; the active involvement of people with dementia along with their carers; and the collaboration between universities, the voluntary sector (Alzheimer's Society) and local NHS trusts.

### Where are we now?

Due to the initial success of Time for Dementia as indicated by preliminary data from its integral mixed methods evaluation, in 2017, the programme was widened to include a broader range of undergraduate healthcare training programmes including Allied Health Professional (e.g. Occupational Therapy, Speech and Language Therapy, Physiotherapy and Radiography) courses at the University of Brighton, University of Greenwich, and Canterbury Christ Church University. To date the programme has involved 2,600 students and 1,200 families. This network of families is recruited and supported by staff paid for by the programme, employed by the Alzheimer's Society, which is a full partner in Time for Dementia with the universities.

### What have we found?

Emerging data from the evaluation have shown improvements in dementia knowledge and attitudes in students receiving the programme compared to those who are not. These include the development of empathy and compassion.[5] Participating in the programme as a person with dementia or as a family member was also seen as a benefit by those taking part including the understanding that they are making a positive contribution to education of the future workforce[6].

### Student accounts

Feedback from students who participated in the programme has identified four key themes: (a) Insight and understanding, (b) Challenging attitudes and stigma, (c) Relational learning, and (d) Enhanced dementia practice. Students have identified that their original perceptions of dementia had changed throughout the visits. Students felt able to see beyond negative stereotypes about dementia, and instead recognise that a person with dementia could remain intelligent, humorous, and continue to make decisions and accomplish challenges and tasks.

*"...he is still quite switched on, and he makes jokes and stuff, which is, I wasn't expecting that at all. Because you know, in, like, films and stuff, dementia is, like, so stereotyped, like, it's not really like that at all..."* Paramedic student

Students also reported that the programme has helped them to recognise that people can live well with dementia; that people can be well supported by family or services and cope well with the condition, that not everyone with dementia is isolated and struggling, and that many people with dementia still find joy in everyday life.

*"They're still enjoying life, still going out...I didn't expect that...seeing hope in their lives...I thought that they will not enjoy a good quality of life."* Nursing student

Significantly many of the students reported an increased interest in wanting to find out more about dementia, decreased apprehension and an increase in the desire to work with people with dementia in the future.

*"It's definitely made me more interested in working with people that have dementia rather than not. I think I was a little bit scared by elderly medicine and people that have dementia and cognitive deficits before this and now it's definitely changed, for sure."* Medical student

In-depth follow up of adult nursing students found that there was a broadening of views of dementia to encompass the person's life and relationships, which led to a person-centred shift in students' practice. Notably, students were able to develop an understanding of the importance of *'being'* (engaging with the person) rather than just *'doing'* (performing tasks) in practice which contributed to how they saw themselves as future nurses. Adult nursing students reported that that they could be active in their contribution to care and serve as change agents in transforming dementia care.

*"We often disable people with dementia in practice, assumption is they cannot perform their own care tasks. Visits have helped me to reframe dementia... focus on the person more and what is important to them. Staff in practice often don't know how to care for dementia, many just try and ignore it. Programmes such as this illuminate the experience of dementia... talking about it helps to reduce stigma...gives an opportunity to slowly face our misconceptions and gives the next generation of healthcare professionals a better understanding of dementia."* Adult nursing student

## Person with dementia account

*I decided to get involved in Time for Dementia because of my own not very good experiences with health care professionals. I felt that it was a good opportunity to raise awareness about dementia, by telling people how it is for people living with dementia, both the positives and negatives. I thought that if I can raise awareness and help even one person to avoid what I have been through then it would be worthwhile.*

*My partner and I have been seeing Occupational Therapy and Physiotherapy students as part of Time for Dementia. I have been really keen that students get this exposure to dementia, because it can be a hidden disability and therefore unseen, as you cannot see that people have dementia by just looking at them. I have really enjoyed doing the programme, the students are lovely. They come to our house, to our environment and this feels so much better. They are able to hear how my partner and I have been affected by dementia, and this information comes from the mouth of person with dementia and their carer and this feel a much better way for them to be learning.* Christine Maddocks.

## Newly qualified nurse and doctors accounts

*The Time for Dementia programme was extremely valuable and I continue to use my knowledge and experience gained in practice now and going forward in my career. My experience of the Time for Dementia programme has informed my practice as a junior doctor, when I meet patients with a diagnosis of dementia and their families I have a much greater insight and understanding of the potential struggles that the individual and their loved ones are going through. The treatment and management I provide patients with dementia is more individualized to their needs and their families' because I now have the insight into the journey they are on and attempt to understand what their specific needs are. I am in a position to educate and challenge misconceptions held by other members of the multidisciplinary team towards their understanding of dementia, sometimes often bleak and stereotypical perceptions of what living with dementia really means. I also feel more competent in supporting families through pre diagnosis, diagnosis and advanced care planning in dementia. Time for Dementia has also instilled in me transferable skills and understandings that ensures I treat the person behind the diagnosis in clinical practice. Remembering that people aren't their diagnosis of dementia and have other health conditions inclusive and exclusive of the disease.* Dr Zoe Cashin, junior doctor

*It is nearly four am and I have been bleeped to see a patient in the ward who has been struggling to breathe. I drag my tired body to see the patient in the dark. The patient is a 69 years old lady with a background of dementia and Huntington's disease. She is being treated for sepsis secondary to urinary tract infection. I asked her how she is and she does not say much but keeps repeating 'help'. I do a quick assessment head to toe and I am not clinically worried about her, but I can sense that she is scared. I hold her hand tightly to reassure her that she is safe here. Since I started my foundation year, I have not felt hesitant to approach patients with dementia. I try my best to be considerate and sensible. I often reflect on our patient visits of the Time for Dementia studies during the medical school and remind myself that there is always more that could be done for patients with dementia and that value of love and of family bonds never goes away and needs to be promoted and supported at all stages of the dementia journey.*

*Unfortunately, there is still stigma around dementia and we clinicians cannot help but to find ourselves focusing on presenting complaints but not the person inside. I am planning to start my GP training next year and I am grateful that I will always have something to look back into and remind myself why I am doing this.* Dr Jaewon Phee, junior doctor

*Having little experience with dementia prior to starting my degree, the Time for Dementia programme gave me an insight of how families and patients with dementia live. Working in the community I visit a lot of people who are on their own, and many of these have dementia. Previously, I visited a patient who had dementia, but unfortunately was not able to communicate verbally. Through my discussions with the patients' family, I was able to communicate with the patient through non-verbal communication. Luckily this particular patient did have family present. This isn't always the case. Time for Dementia highlighted not only how important holistic assessments are, but also how important it is that families get the support they require. I firmly believe the programme has improved my confidence and reiterated the importance of treating everyone with the dignity and respect they deserve. It has also taught me to be more patient and understanding, which I now use in my daily practice.* Jayme Hill, newly qualified nurse

## Conclusions

The definitive evaluation of the programme is not yet completed. Any impressions at this point must therefore be made with caution, however all the initial information we have suggests that Time for Dementia develops students in ways that more traditional healthcare education does not. The testimony of student participants is that it helps students to develop appropriately positive attitudes, understanding and optimism at how well people can live with dementia. The special ingredient in Time for Dementia is that it places the people with dementia and their families as the mentors and teachers of our students. They teach what is possible in dementia by sharing their experiences of life and of health care systems both positive and negative. Our students start to see the world though the experiences of their Time for Dementia families, they see what is done badly, and they resolve to act differently when they are in practice. The accounts above from the first tranche of students to transition into clinical practice following qualification give grounds for hope that this will happen.

Currently Time for Dementia is provided in the health schools in one region (Kent, Surrey and Sussex) in the UK, this is a proof of the concept. It is a complement to more traditional education and is provided at relatively low cost (administration in the universities, Alzheimer's Society support of the person with dementia and family network and travel). If the data continue to be positive, the next phase should be to roll it out in other health schools nationally and internationally. There is certainly no lack of people with dementia or family members who are willing to participate. It appears that this is one small, relatively simple thing that can be done that is likely will make modest positive changes to practice. The real challenge to healthcare in the 21st century is how to provide good quality care for older people with multimorbidity as exemplified by people with dementia.[7] Time for Dementia helps us provide a workforce willing and able to meet and beat this challenge.

## References


1 Alzheimer's Disease International. 2016. *World Alzheimer Report 2016: Improving healthcare for people living with dementia: Coverage, quality and costs now and in the future* online: https://www.alz.co.uk/research/WorldAlzheimerReport2016.pdf Last accessed 21 August 2019.

2 Banerjee, S., Farina, N., Daley, S., Grosvenor, W., Hughes, L., et al. 2017. 'How do we enhance undergraduate healthcare education in dementia? A review of the role of innovative approaches and development of the Time for Dementia programme' International *Journal of Geriatric Psychiatry* 32: 68-75.

3 Daley, S. and Grosvenor, W. 2016. Integrating dementia care into undergraduate nurse curricula London: Nursing Times Online: www.nursingtimes.net/careengland/integrating-dementia- care-into-undergraduate-nurse-curricula/7009643 Last accessed 21 August 2019.

4 Grosvenor, W., Hebditch, M., Daley, S., Vyvyan, E., Banerjee, S. 2017. 'Time for Dementia: an innovation in education' *Journal of Paramedic Practice* 9(11).

5 Bickford, B., Daley, S., Sleater, G., Hebditch, M., Banerjee, S. 2019. 'Understanding compassion for people with dementia in medical and nursing students' *BMC Education* 19:35.

6 Cashin, Z., Daley, S., Hebditch, M., Hughes, L., Banerjee, S. 2018. 'Involving people with dementia and their carers in dementia education for undergraduate healthcare professionals: a qualitative study of motivation to participate and experience' *International Psychogeriatrics* (6):869-876.

7 Banerjee, S. 2014. 'Multimorbidity—older adults need health care that can count past one' *The Lancet*. S0140-6736(14)61596-8.

## 5.2 Dementia research participation; challenging stigma

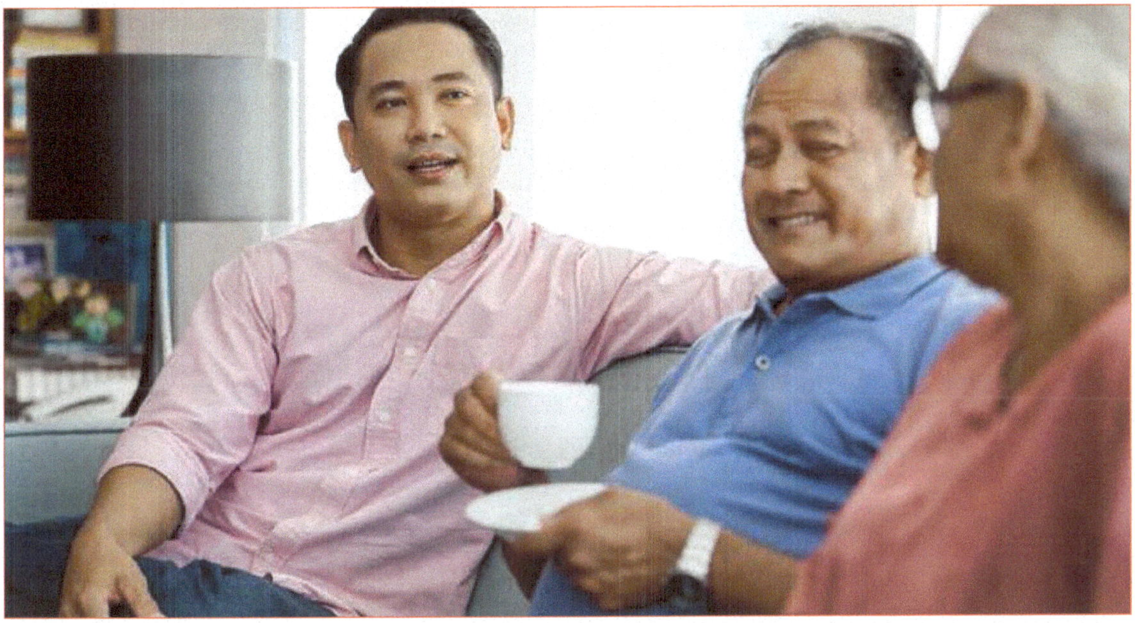

**Contributor:** Howard Gordon. Dementia Alliance International, 3 Nations Working Group

As a person living with dementia, it was important to be able to include the voice and experience of someone living with this condition in Alzheimer's Disease International's world report 2019. I am grateful for the opportunity to comment on the role of research and research participation, attitudes and stigma.

On 10th May 2019, I took part in the Alzheimer's Disease International webinar "Let's Talk Dementia Research: Maintaining hope when trials end" where we discussed the importance of researchers seeing people living with dementia as partners in research rather than participants.

People living with dementia no longer want research done for them or for others to decide what research should be undertaken.

A new Project in the UK called "Dementia Enquirers", facilitated by DEEP (Dementia Engagement and Empowerment Project) aims to put people living with dementia in the driving seat of research, showing that we can design, develop, run, report and publish research, with academics and professionals as advisors not participants.

In the last 18 months, I have taken part in over 20 research studies, one a clinical trial lasting 12 months, some as simple as a questionnaire.

On the positive side, research engages people living with dementia, giving them a purpose and whilst we understand that research may not benefit us, we do it for others, for our children, grandchildren and those that follow.

On the negative side, once research is completed, we rarely hear anymore, we may feel discarded like an old shoe or worse, we may find out that a particular study has finished early, devaluing our self-worth.

One of the greatest challenges people face following a diagnosis of dementia is stigma, which manifests itself in many ways.

The broad use of terms such as "suffering" perpetuate the misconceptions and stigma of living with a diagnosis of dementia.

Language is hugely important and changing words is important. We all suffer at times, but with increasing numbers of people being diagnosed, as young as 2 years old, it is important to differentiate the experiences of people living with dementia at different stages and abilities, while acknowledging that some, especially in the palliative stage, may feel they are suffering.

Use of the term "palliative stage" instead of "end stage", may reinforce the view that we are entitled to palliative care, not to be written off, and in a recent document there was a question asking about our "opinions" which is now going to be changed to the word "choices". A simple but powerful change.

We may still be working and driving, often we are told we have to stop at diagnosis, but may be able to continue to do so, depending on our abilities at that time.

Stigma can strip us of our personhood, belief in our own ability, to continue as we were the day before the diagnosis, leaving us with a feeling of failure, of disablement, leading us to take on the role that stigma lays out for us.

I was relieved to get the diagnosis as it put a label on what had been happening to me but the perceptions and stigma, based on working in healthcare for nearly 20 years, and on those often portrayed in media, that I carried into my neurologist's office, would have a negative, disabling effect on me during the next 12 months.

***I was relieved to get the diagnosis as it put a label on what had been happening to me but the perceptions and stigma, based on working in healthcare for nearly 20 years, and on those often portrayed in media, that I carried into my neurologist's office, would have a negative, disabling effect on me during the next 12 months.***

I was diagnosed with early onset Alzheimer's and Frontotemporal Dementia (FTD) and "Dr Google" told me my prognosis was 18 months to 20 years and told me how negative and horrendous my life would be. It didn't tell me that Christine Bryden (24 years post diagnosis), James McKillop (20 years), Kate Swaffer (12 years) et al, were still active in their communities, campaigning and changing the lives of people living with dementia. All it seemed to tell me was how bad it would be, how these diseases would strip me of who I am, leading to feelings of guilt. How I was going to put my family through such terrible torment?

With people being diagnosed at a younger age, experiences have changed, and the negative stigma and perceptions are being challenged but with the understanding that experiences change over time.

As with any chronic, terminal disease, there are differing experiences and abilities at each stage of a disease. The language and words used to describe these stages and changes need to evolve and adapt alongside with those experiences and abilities.

Often stigma informs the decision making processes of local authorities where dementia services are often one of the first to be cut, yet in 2017, according to official UK figures, dementia was the leading cause of death in the UK, which you would have thought would have led to an increase in funding for dementia services.

The United Nations has redefined dementia as a "Cognitive Disability" and since 2006 the United Nations Convention on the Rights of Persons with Disabilities (CRPD) has set out the universal rights of people living with dementia and other disabilities; rights which you cannot lose when you lose mental capacity.[1] Although these rights are part of international law, they are not yet being fully integrated and reported on at national level.

Were these fully integrated into national laws they would then go some way to challenge the stigma and often ill informed perceptions of society and professionals, removing the need for people living with dementia to fight for those rights individually, or collectively, through organisations such as ADI and Dementia Alliance International (DAI).

International law, via the CRPD, sets out the rights we have, regardless of capacity, additionally giving us the right to make mistakes, even if they have negative consequences, and in doing so it moves the power of decision making from the professional to empower people living with a disability.

In saying that, as with any chronic terminal disease, we may develop mental health problems as the disease progresses but by changing its definition, the United Nations recognises that there is not one set list of experiences of life with dementia and that we all have our own individual experiences.

In terms of research participation, I would advocate not just for more dementia research but for greater inclusion on people living with dementia in every step of the process, from design to analysis, whether a success or failure. There is a potential risk of introducing stigma by participating in research, for example if someone is identified as high risk, but my belief is that research and participation can help us tackle stigma around dementia, by introducing hope, by normalising the language and simply by helping people understand the nature of this condition.

## References

1 Mittler, P. 2018. 'Dementia is a cognitive disability' online: https://www.dementiaallianceinternational.org/dementia-as-a-cognitive-disability/ Last accessed 19 August 2019.

## 5.3 Hope through dementia research participation.

**Contributor:** Serge Gauthier MD, C.M., C.Q., MD, FRCPC, Director, AD Research Unit, McGill Center for Studies in Aging, Montreal, Canada, Member and Past Chair of ADI Medical and Scientific Advisory Panel

A 65-year-old woman came to our Research Center asking "to be tested for her risk of developing Alzheimer's disease", which had affected her mother from age 78 to 85. She was offered the opportunity to join a cohort observational study where cognitive test results are correlated with biomarkers associated with brain ageing and are measured in the brain, spinal fluid and blood, every two years. Over one thousand people have volunteered in the past three years for such a study, some of them have heard about it by word of mouth; others tell family members. This is a notable cultural shift in attitudes where people want to know more about themselves and contribute to the greater good. The motivation for many is that what is learned from their participation in observational research will help their children and grand-children in delaying age-associated cognitive decline and dementia.

*We need to find a cure but in the interim we need to encourage and facilitate research participation. Research and participation lead to hope; hope increases awareness; awareness tackles stigma.*

That being said, how do you tell a healthy 65-year-old woman that she has a significant build-up of amyloid and tau proteins in their brain? We do not yet know what the natural history is of such a finding, in terms of progression to dementia in subsequent years. There is a risk of a depressive reaction if the results of the biomarker testing are not disclosed properly. A step-by-step counselling approach akin to genetic disclosure for genetic conditions such as Huntington's disease is used.

Another concern is the proposed research classification of the National Institute of Aging that equates amyloid and tau protein build-up with some evidence of neurodegeneration (ATN positivity) to having "Alzheimer's disease", even without any cognitive symptom or measurable decline. This may lead to stigmatisation of research participants who would be labelled as having this condition even if they may never have symptoms. This is now a significant social and ethical issue that needs further discussion; discussion which must involve the research participants themselves.

The other issue is that amyloid and tau build-up alone do not explain fully the emergence of symptoms in very old persons: other proteins are at play.

Finally, neuroinflammation may be an accelerating factor whichever protein build up there is.

One hope for many research participants is that the early identification of biological risk factors towards Alzheimer's disease will accelerate the recruitment in various types of interventional studies, ranging from a ketogenic drink to a structured physical exercise program or to anti-amyloid and/or anti-tau drugs. These interventions will be done in more homogeneous groups than in the past, with better hope of therapeutic success. For instance, the lack of positive results of anti-inflammatory drugs despite the weight of evidence suggesting that they reduce significantly the risk of Alzheimer's disease, may be due to treating people without knowing if they indeed have active inflammation in their brain. New ligands for positron emission tomography are being tested in this regard in our cohort.

The other positive outcome of these observational studies is the personalisation of the risk assessment, which will eventually incorporate genetic data and biomarkers from blood tests, rather than the current multiple brain scans and lumbar puncture.

We need to find a cure but in the interim we need to encourage and facilitate research participation. Research and participation lead to hope; hope increases awareness; awareness tackles stigma.

## 5.4 Scottish working groups: advisors, advocates, influencers

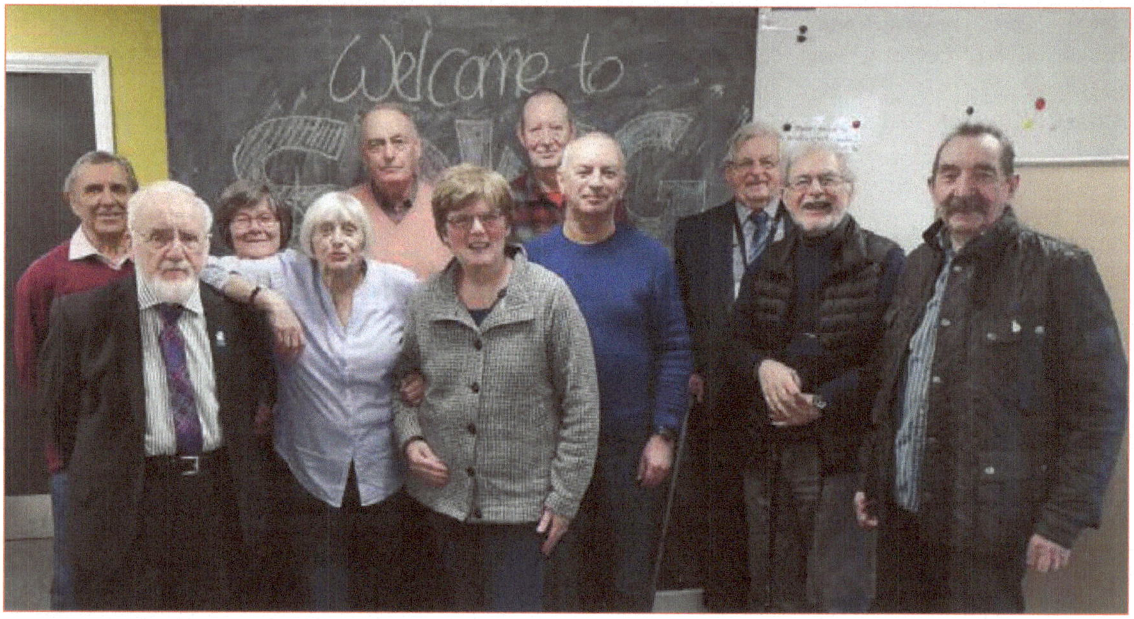


**Members of the Scottish Dementia Working Group**

**Contributor:** Jim Pearson, Director of Policy & Research, Alzheimer Scotland

For Alzheimer Scotland, the active voice of people with dementia and carers of people with dementia is central to informing everything we do. People with dementia, and carers, participate in all aspects of our work; including our governance, development of campaigning priorities, public policy reports, research priorities and our practice. Providing a platform to ensure that people with dementia and carers have meaningful opportunity to influence national and local decisions about the things that matter to them has been a key part of our work for many years. We support and fund, along with the Scottish Government, two national groups; the Scottish Dementia Working Group (SDWG) and the National Dementia Carers Action Group (NDACN). For the past several years we have worked with both groups to fund and establish local active voice networks to ensure that people with dementia and carers are able to influence the decisions of their local Health and Social Care Partnerships and elected representatives.

The SDWG is a national campaigning and awareness-raising group whose members all have a diagnosis of dementia. The group has its origin in 2001 when James McKillop, the group's founding member, began discussions with a social researcher from Edinburgh University about why there were no groups for people with dementia. They worked together to organise a conference in city of Dundee the following year for professionals and people with dementia, and it was at that conference that the idea for the SDWG took shape and a small steering group was established. Rather than set up as an independent entity the group accepted Alzheimer Scotland's invitation to join the Organisation. The group considered that Alzheimer Scotland's position as Scotland's leading dementia charity, its history campaigning for the rights of people with dementia and their families, and its ability to provide support for the group, made it the ideal partner. The group was formally established in 2002 as the independent voice of people with dementia within Alzheimer Scotland.

Over the past 17 years the SDWG has made a substantial contribution as a campaigning group working to raise awareness of dementia, challenge stigma, and crucially to shape and influence dementia policy and practice in Scotland. The group have been key partners in developing and monitoring the implementation of the commitments of Scotland three national dementia strategies and participate fully in all of dementia strategy workstreams. Members meet twice per year with Scottish Government Ministers to discuss issues that matter to them and to ask questions of the Minister relating to the gaps they experience in policy commitments and the lived experience of people with dementia in Scotland.

In addition, the members have led work in many areas to improve awareness of and educate others about dementia through the collective experience of those living with dementia. The group has been a major contributor to "Promoting Excellence" and education framework which sets out the knowledge, skills and behaviours expected of all health and social care staff who work with people with dementia. They have worked with other professionals and agencies to improve their knowledge and understanding of dementia to ensure that the services they provide are accessible to people with dementia. There are too many to list here, but these include working with transport providers across Scotland to ensure that all forms of public transport are accessible and appropriate for people with dementia. It also includes the development of "Core Principles for Research" setting out how people with dementia can be meaningfully involved in research.

***Both SDWG and NDCAN have established themselves as key partners in all aspects of dementia policy and practice within Scotland and to ensure that, alongside Alzheimer Scotland, the active collective voice of people with dementia and carers of people with dementia shape how Scotland responds to dementia now and the decades to come.***

The SDWG members participate in Alzheimer Scotland's governance as members of Alzheimer Scotland's standing committees and every chair of the group has been involved as a member of the Board of Trustees. More recently the current Chair, Archie Noone, was elected as the vice convenor of the Board of Trustees. In 2018 Archie represented Alzheimer Scotland at the Alzheimer's Disease International Council Meeting in Chicago.

Members of the SDWG speak at conferences, including national and international conferences and have participated in many ways to Alzheimer's Disease International and Alzheimer Europe Conferences over many years. The group has been recognised as world leading and has been the inspiration for national member led groups for people with dementia in countries across the world.

In 2011, Alzheimer Scotland founded the group's sister network, the NDCAN. The need for this became apparent from the work of campaigner and carer, Tommy Whitelaw, who had gathered letters from carers across Scotland sharing their experiences of caring for someone with dementia. In an event hosted by Alzheimer Scotland, Tommy delivered the letters to the then Cabinet Secretary Nicola Sturgeon (now First Minister of Scotland). The experiences shared by carers highlighted to Alzheimer Scotland the need to ensure that carers of people with dementia had a national platform to raise awareness and campaign for the things that mattered to carers. Henry Simmons, Alzheimer Scotland's Chief Executive, committed to establishing the NDCAN.

The NDCAN is a national campaigning and awareness raising group whose members all have experience of caring for someone with dementia. It is based on a core belief similar to that of SDWG, that carers should be an integral part of the planning and implementation of health and social care policy and practice, and that all professionals and organisations should acknowledge carers' experience, the issues they face as carers, and the value of their knowledge of the person they are caring for, which is valid and equal to that of health, social care and other professionals who work with people with dementia.

Though it's a decade younger than SDWG, the NDCAN has a similarly long list of achievements as a national campaigning group. It participated in the development and implementation of Scotland's National Dementia Strategies, meets regularly with Scotland's Minister for Mental Health, it trains health and social care professionals and sits on the implementation group for Scotland's Carers Act. Like SDWG, members of NDCAN speak at and participate in national and international dementia and related conferences.

### The future for SDWG and NDCAN

In the past 5 years Scotland's health and social care system has being going through the most significant change since the establishment of the welfare state in the 1940's. The development of integrated adult health and social care has meant that decisions about spending and priorities are taken locally by Integrated Health and Social Care Partnerships. For both SDWG and NDCAN this has resulted in a shift of focus to work with and support Alzheimer Scotland's local active voice networks across Scotland to influence local decision making and ensure that dementia is a priority for every Health and Social Partnership. Both groups have benefited from this local focus, seeing not only a growth in membership but a more broadly representative membership, not only geographically, but of a wider range of experiences of dementia and caring. Both have established themselves as key partners in all aspects of dementia policy and practice within Scotland; ensuring that, alongside Alzheimer Scotland, the active collective voice of people with dementia and carers of people with dementia shape how Scotland responds to dementia now and in the decades to come.

## 5.5 Dementia Advisory Group Brings Chinese Taipei to a New Era of Human Rights

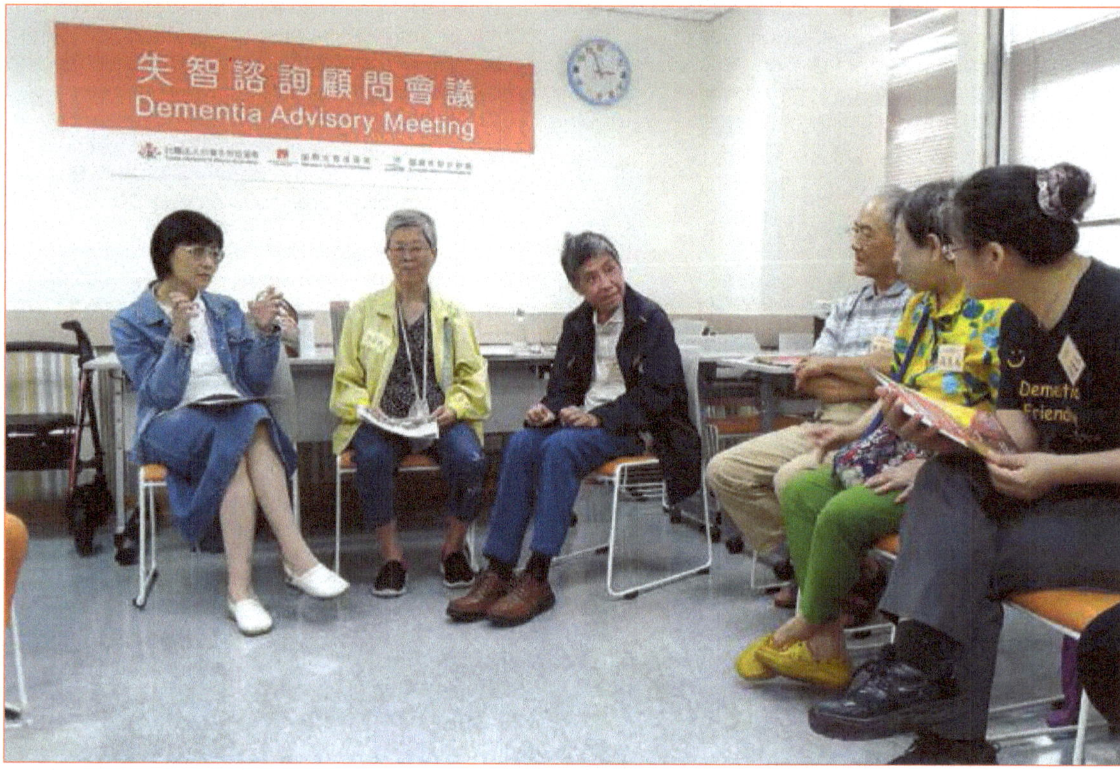


**Members of the Dementia Advisory Group**

**Contributor:** LiYu Tang Secretary General, TADA Chinese Taipei, Su-Yuan Chan, Policy Researcher, TADA Chinese Taipei

### Human rights becoming a priority in Chinese Taipei

Following the announcement of the WHO Global action plan on the public health response to dementia 2017-2025, TADA Chinese Taipei (TADA) considered the human rights of people with dementia a priority[1]. In 2017, TADA invited Glenn Rees, Chair of Alzheimer's Disease International (ADI) and Kate Swaffer, Chair and CEO of Dementia Alliance International (DAI), to advocate to the government of Chinese Taipei for human rights of people with dementia. "The Ministry of Health and Welfare referenced the Convention on the Rights of Persons with Disabilities (CRPD) when developing "Dementia Policy 2.0" and budgeted TWD 9 billion, which was equivalent to 290 million US dollars.[2]. In addition, the Control Yuan of Chinese Taipei made two investigation reports, examining all policies related to dementia, whether they were considered human rights or not. The national policy and the investigation reports provided actual situations and clear recommendations for the government departments to go onto the next step for people with dementia. Hence, human rights have become more and more important in the hearts of the people of Chinese Taipei and the government.

### Involving people with dementia in societies

TADA has involved people with dementia in many activities. In 2017, 22 persons with dementia were invited to be tour guides or to make coffee and cookies in the World Alzheimer's Month Event. In 2018, TADA expanded the activities and encouraged people with dementia to teach their unique skills to the participants. The lessons included drawing traditional Chinese paintings and making paper flowers, and about 40 people with dementia played important roles in the World Alzheimer's Month activities. It was a huge success, and more and more people with dementia got involved in various activities. These brought to the attention of the general public a new image of people with dementia and the appreciation for their contribution. It was also a great achievement for people with dementia and their families to get the confidence to join activities in the community and try to dedicate themselves into societies.

Afterwards, people with dementia started to tell the public their own stories. In 2018, Amy Su, a 70-year-old woman diagnosed with mild dementia, made the first self-advocate video in Chinese Taipei, talking about how dementia influenced her life. The video started a trend, and 3 other people living with dementia also expressed their voices through touching and inspiring videos. Amy Su also delivered a speech at the annual dementia conference.

## Chinese Taipei Dementia Advisory Group

A dementia advisory group is a good model for expressing voices, needs, and rights of people with dementia. TADA has tried hard to develop a dementia advisory group since 2017. However, it was difficult to find suitable participants in the beginning and the group did not form successfully. In 2018, with the cooperation with Integrated Dementia Care Centers (IDCC), TADA held 4 meetings to collect opinions from people with dementia. About 22 people with dementia joined the events, and 13 of them came without carers' accompanying. Most of them were able to express their feelings and thoughts; some of them even made concrete and useful suggestions for policies. The topics covered the accessibility of long-term care services, disease labelling, prevention, financial safety, the process of services application, resources to prevent people from getting lost, etc.

This year TADA formally established a self-funded dementia advisory group. Thanks to the referrals from doctors, case managers, and other resources, there are 9 participants in the advisory group, including 6 people with dementia and 3 family carers. The group meets once a month. Since April of 2019, they have focused on the topics of dementia friendly facilities, transportations, problems associated with getting lost, and financial security.

Members in the group share their experiences, thoughts, and needs at their ease. For example, when discussing driving experiences, the members sincerely shared the meaning and value of driving to them. At the same time, carers were also able to talk about their worries and the methods of convincing people with dementia to stop driving. Furthermore, people with dementia also sometimes recommended one another to stand in their carers' or passengers' shoes to consider retiring from driving. Members of the Dementia Advisory Group have established the trust between themselves.

## Keys to starting a Dementia Advisory Group

Based on the past two years of experience, TADA has found 3 keys to creating a dementia advisory group. First, participants should clearly understand their situation and be able to express their own opinions related to dementia. Not every person with dementia is ready to join the group. Second, the support of family carers, doctors, and case managers will enable the process. If doctors and case managers promote the advisory group, people with dementia and their carers will be encouraged to join the group. Last, but not least, "advisory" is a good word to use, and attitude to have, when discussing issues with people with dementia. Professionals, policymakers, and carers all need to consult people with dementia to respect their rights.

## Advocating with people with dementia in the new era of human rights

TADA would like to invite more participants through the connection with doctors and case managers. Moreover, TADA has encouraged many local city governments to invite people with dementia to participate in the policymaking process. Nowadays, people with dementia have become hosts at press conferences. People with dementia are also invited to give speeches. We truly believe that people with dementia can be empowered and advocate policies by themselves.

Not only is it important to support people living with dementia in dementia advisory groups to advocate for change and for improved support and services but through visibility and communication, with and about dementia advisory groups, it also helps to change perceptions, increase awareness and tackle stigma. TADA's dream is not only to advocate policies for people with dementia, but also to advocate with them. We believe that people with dementia will bring Chinese Taipei to a new era which promotes and ensures the human rights of people with dementia and all people.

## References


1 World Health Organization 2017. Global action plan on the public health response to dementia 2017–2025. Geneva: World Health Organization. Licence: CC BY-NC-SA 3.0. online: https://www.who.int/mental_health/neurology/dementia/action_plan_2017_2025/en/ Last accessed 19 August 2019.

2 UN General Assembly 2007. Convention on the Rights of Persons with Disabilities: resolution / adopted by the General Assembly, 24 January 2007, A/RES/61/106. online: https://www.un.org/development/desa/disabilities/convention-on-the-rights-of-persons-with-disabilities.html Last accessed 19 August 2019.

## 5.6 Forget dementia, remember the person! Breaking down stigma to move forward towards an inclusive society in Flanders (Belgium)

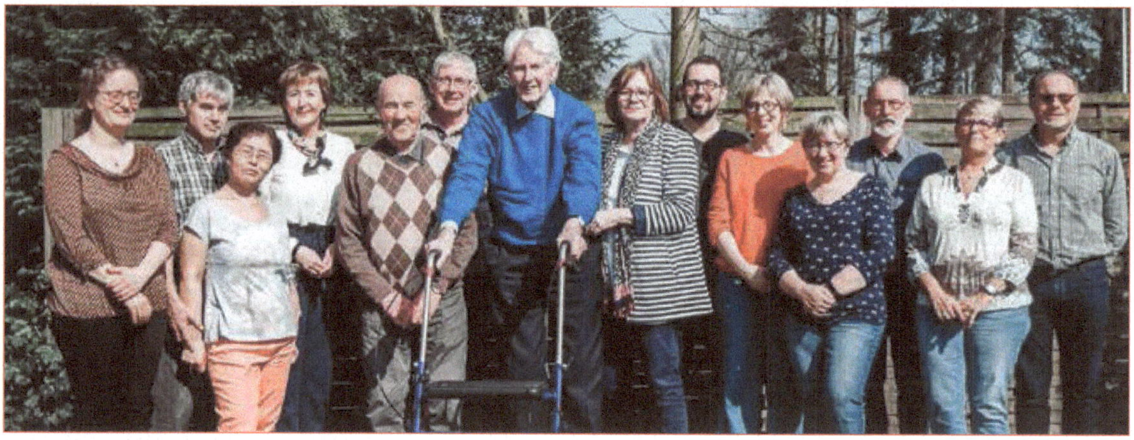

**Flemish working group of people with dementia**

**Contributor:** Olivier Constant, Flanders Centre of Expertise on Dementia

If we focus on the possibilities of people with dementia instead of their limitations, their dementia will disappear behind their talents and not the other way around; that is the starting point of the Flemish awareness raising campaign 'Vergeet dementie, onthou mens' ('Forget dementia, remember the person'). The emancipatory story of this campaign forms one of the foundations of the Dementia Strategy of Flanders (Belgium) and is written together with people with dementia and their caregivers. Their vision is the beating heart of 'Forget dementia remember the person'; respectful communication is the basis for person-centered care and an inclusive society.

*Listen to us. Give us a voice. Give us the opportunity to meet peers. Use respectful language. Include us in setting policy guidelines. Give us the opportunity to learn and experience new things.*

The best medicines for someone with an incurable condition do not come from a pillbox, we have them in our own hands; attention, empathy, a listening ear and time. People with dementia and their loved ones want to be valued, understood and included. That is exactly what we want to do in Flanders with 'Forget dementia, remember the person'. Not starting from a well-intended kind of pity for people with dementia, but from sincere compassion and a firm belief in their everlasting capacities, not only right after their diagnosis but in all stages of the condition.

As the Flanders Centre of Expertise on Dementia and official partner organization of the Flemish Authority in Belgium, we coordinate the campaign together with our partners in the field. With 'Forget dementia, remember the person' we have a clear ambition: to give more power to the people. Personal experiences are the heart and soul of this movement. Through this grassroots strategy we want to break down the walls between (in)formal care and the rest of society, bridge gaps between generations, urge more respectful communication, smash stereotypes and sustain existing dementia-friendly efforts.

### The power of visual communication

On the dynamic web platform and social media for the campaign, people can find a wide range of dementia friendly communication tools, as a starting point to break down the stigma on dementia and to give a voice to the person behind the condition. The mission statement of our campaign was translated in a short animation movie, written together with people with dementia and their caregivers. Moreover, there are series of cartoons that stress the importance of respectful language when we talk about dementia and want to invite others to stay close to people with dementia instead of avoiding them. Dementia is already difficult enough to cope with, so we pose the question, "Why don't we start to find more joy in things that people with dementia still love to do?"

Together with a professional photographer and people with young-onset dementia at a day care center in the city of Antwerp in Belgium, we also made brand new posters that explain in short poems and quotes the feelings of people with dementia and invite you to enter their world. Additionally, we designed four short graphic novel-stories about communication in the last stages of dementia, with a clear message that was written down on one of the visuals by a person with dementia, *"Learn to read the language of people with dementia. Try. Listen. Search. Feel. Find. Look. Listen to me, also when words disappear."* To distribute the campaign message, people can also order free photographs from a rich picture database that translates the baseline 'Forget dementia, remember the person' visually.

## Personal stories are the key to change

The beating heart of the campaign is the personal stories of the experts, namely people living with dementia, their carers and the people who experience dementia day-to-day. The more than 50 audiovisual testimonies that were released in Dutch during the first half of 2019 have one thing in common; the massive impact of the taboo on the challenges in the daily care and support for people with dementia, like timely diagnosis, care acceptance, advance care planning and the sustainability of their social network. This is also the reason why reducing the stigma of dementia was, and is, the foundation of the previous and current dementia strategy in Flanders. The video statements are centralised around three basic questions, which form the core of our taboo breaking initiatives of the campaign 'Forget dementia, remember the person':

- What can we learn from people with dementia?
- How can we guide them and their loved ones towards tailored care and help them to accept help?
- How can we include people with dementia and informal carers as long as possible in society?

During the second half of 2019, the personal stories will also be made available for the international audience with English translation through the YouTube channel of the Flanders Centre of Expertise on Dementia. In this way, we also want to contribute to the international movement towards advocacy and involvement of people with dementia – not only through the different communication tools described, but also through a pioneering initiative in the field: the start of the first-ever 'Working group of people with dementia' in Flanders.

## Valuing the experts by experience

The start of this working group is not a symbolic initiative, but a crucial step towards empowerment and validation of people with dementia and their caregivers. Not only to include their voice more proactively in the media, but to also include them fully in new projects, research and policy work. The Flanders Centre of Expertise on Dementia started brainstorming about the idea at the beginning of 2018, together with the other plans for the new chapter of 'Forget dementia, remember the person'. The centre joined forces with the Alzheimer's Association of Flanders to translate the ambitions for this new working group into practice.

At the moment we have six people with dementia involved, together with their family carers. It is our ambition to involve people with dementia in all stages of the condition, not only in the first phase of dementia and not only people who are younger than 65 years. Since the group held its first meeting in October 2018, we initially focused on creating an open, strong partnership between the members, as a foundation to move forward with tangible actions in 2019. After five intensive meetings we shot an introduction movie with the members of the working group as our call to action for a dementia friendly society. In May of 2019 we released the movie for the media and public in Flanders and on World Alzheimer's Day 2019 the English version of the movie will be released for the international audience.

Together with the introduction video we released the first 'Charter for a Dementia Friendly Society' written by people with dementia; another unseen initiative in our country. We want to empower people with dementia and reach out to society to respond to their needs and respect their rights. The goals were defined crystal clear by the working group: *"Listen to us. Give us a voice. Give us the opportunity to meet peers. Use respectful language. Include us in setting policy guidelines. Give us the opportunity to learn and experience new things."* These ambitions are not optional. They will form the compass for an eventual new dementia strategy in Flanders of which the realisation could start, following the elections of May 2019 and the formation of the new government later that year.

These first steps we have taken are the start of an intensive and inspiring journey that will lead to more results and an integrated vision for the coming years. We sincerely hope that the message of the 'Flemish working group of people with dementia' in Belgium gives people in other countries an extra dose of inspiration and motivation to continue building on an inclusive society that gives people with dementia and their loved ones the place they deserve; not in the margin, but at the centre of a kind and understanding society. And we also hope that our campaign baseline 'Forget dementia, remember the person' may inspire people across the globe, because in the end people with dementia should always be the reference point and quality check of a dementia friendly society. That is true inclusion and empowerment and the only way forward.

For more information on 'Forget dementia, remember the person':

- YouTube: https://www.youtube.com/channel/UCmKn3gOZLLdzneir-HIQE5g
- Website: www.onthoumens.be

## 5.7 From Seldom Heard to Seen and Heard: why communities should not be viewed as hard to reach

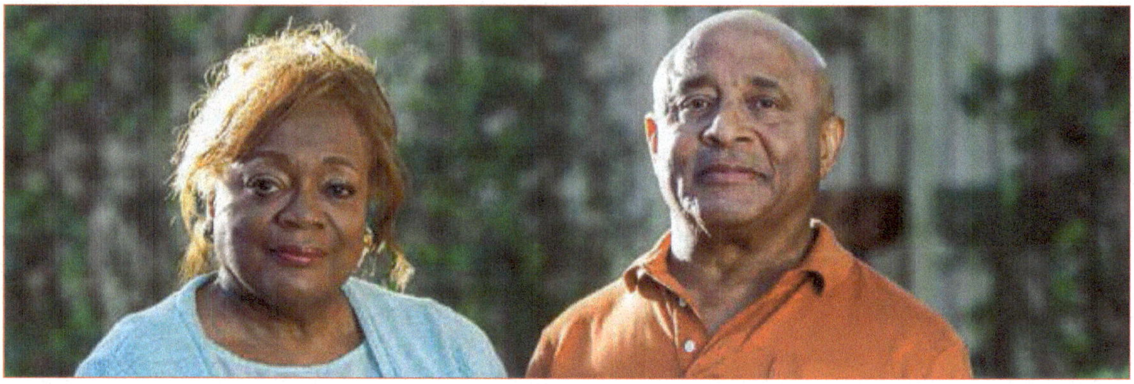

**Contributor:** Sarah Tilsed, Campaigns & Partnerships Manager, National Dementia Action Alliance

Think about the imagery that you see around dementia. Certainly, in the UK it tends to portray healthy, white, heterosexual couples, supported by a family in a comfortable environment. But as we know, dementia is not just confined to this homogenous group. People from any race or sexuality can develop dementia, as can people with no family or home. Consider people in prisons, with learning disabilities, in remote areas - no situation is the same and each has very different complexities.

It goes without saying that these groups and communities need to be researched further, to have awareness raised about them, and to be supported appropriately. Work is taking place, but as always, more can be done to ensure that the needs of people affected by dementia are being met.

The National Dementia Action Alliance (NDAA) has been working in the UK in this area since 2017 on the campaign 'From Seldom Heard to Seen and Heard'. The NDAA is a national alliance for dementia care and research organisations across England to connect, share best practice and take action on dementia. We have over 110 health and social care members, all committed to supporting people affected by dementia, with an action plan setting out what they hope to achieve.

We bring these members together through campaigns, social media, and newsletters. We run webinars, roundtables, conferences, and thematic events; and meet up with all of our members to find out what they are working on. Focussing on campaigns is a large element of our work and campaigns have included decreasing the use of antipsychotic drugs, considering the language around dementia that is used, supporting carers, and creating dementia friendly hospitals by implementing a charter that we created.

Dementia statements, created by the NDAA, are designed to represent people living with any type of dementia regardless of age, stage etc. and highlight the rights of everyone living with dementia. These rights are enshrined in the Equality Act, mental capacity legislation, health and care legislation and international human rights law, and therefore can be used as a tool to highlight the support for every person with dementia, regardless of background or community.

Dementia can be challenging enough for people who access mainstream services. For individuals with more specific needs, the challenges are even greater. Through its campaign, NDAA chose to challenge this unfair disadvantage by running three roundtables looking at learning disabilities, prisons and the LGBT+ (Lesbian, Gay, Bisexual, Transgender) community. We wanted to shine a light on these groups and look at the inequalities they face. We brought together people living with dementia, carers and people working within these groups and communities to discuss key issues. We have produced recommendations from these roundtables, which demonstrates the need for system wide change.

The campaign *'From Seldom Heard to Seen and Heard'* focusses on dementia and learning disabilities, within the LGBT+ community, and in prisons.

Prisoners over the age of 60 are the fastest growing age group in prisons and many prison staff lack the training required to spot the signs of dementia and to make the relevant referrals, meaning that prisoners' dementia can go undiagnosed. The NDAA's campaign aims to address the inequality that currently exists, where many people with dementia and carers who come from seldom heard groups face a number of additional barriers when trying to access care and support. In the first instance many are not even aware that there are services out there for them. Other times, people attend services only to find out that they are unsuitable for their needs. There are a number of reasons for this, ranging from a lack of training and awareness, insufficient funds to adapt services or in some cases, simply people's bigotry.

Many of you will have heard the term 'hard to reach' communities. When we started thinking about this campaign, this is how we referred to the different communities we wanted to support. It was then brought to our attention that people from these communities are actually not hard to reach at all. They are very much in plain sight, living where and how they have always lived. But instead they have different needs that can sometimes be overlooked. As one person put it, not so much 'hard to reach' but more 'easy to ignore'.

Through our campaign, we have tried to highlight some of the unique challenges faced by people with dementia who come from seldom heard groups. Many of these people struggle to access good quality care and support, they face a system that doesn't truly recognise their needs and cannot respond to them. It would be short-sighted not to acknowledge some of the financial strains being placed upon the health and social care sector in the UK at the moment, however this shouldn't be used as an excuse. In fact, NDAA members are demonstrating how they can, and do, provide excellent care, not just for a small group of people in England – but for all people. MacIntyre, a learning disability charity stated that "I'm extremely proud to have worked alongside NDAA for their campaign, they really have ensured that Seldom Heard Groups are 'Seen and Heard'. Thanks to the NDAA, many of their members came together, united, to pledge their support to improving outcomes for people living with dementia and their carers - many Seldom Heard Groups were represented, such as LGBT+, BAME (Black, Asian and minority ethnic), prison population as well as people living with a learning disability".

Many of the effective interventions we see do not require money, rather careful consideration, planning, and most importantly taking the time to engage with people from seldom heard groups. To engage in dialogue with them, to understand not only the challenges but what they want to receive in order to live the best possible lives.

We found there were common inequalities across the groups, such as the lack of services with joined-up working, lack of person-centred care and recognised the importance of an early diagnosis. These findings aren't surprising, and they can relate to any number of seldom heard groups. You can find the full recommendations on the NDAA website.[i] A BAME, LGBT+ person with young onset dementia said that "without my involvement with the NDAA...I would not have been able to set up the LGBT Dementia Network and show that dementia can affect anyone"

As well as holding an event on this campaign, presenting on it at an Alzheimer's Society Conference, Health Education England steering group and at Alzheimer's Disease International, it has led us to the following:

## LGBT+ communities

- held webinars on LGBT+ communities
- had an article in Diva, the largest international Lesbian magazine
- written for a London borough's LGBT+ forum
- had the CEO of Stonewall (UK LGBT+ advocacy organisation) write a blog for us
- Stonewall recommending us to speak to DHSC (Department of Health and Social Care) about the LGBT+ community and how they can adapt their internal policies
- collaborated with Alzheimer's Society, people affected by dementia from the LGBT+ community, and LGBT+ organisations to create a booklet, poster and webpage, called Bring Dementia Out
- co-presented to medical students with a person with dementia from the LGBT+ community
- an LGBT+ person with dementia forming an LGBT+ and dementia network as a result of being involved in our campaign

## BAME communities

- held webinars on BAME communities
- were consulted as a partner in a Race Equality Foundation report 'Dementia and Black, Asian and Minority Ethnic Communities'[1]

## Prisons

- sat on a national prisons steering group
- ran an event on dementia in prisons in partnership with Alzheimer's Society

## Learning Disabilities

- worked with MacIntyre (a learning, support and care charity) on an easy-read version of the Dementia Statements for people with learning disabilities
- sitting on a national learning disabilities steering group
- collaborated with The Foundation for People with a Learning Disability on its report Hidden in Plain Sight[ii]
- held webinars on learning disabilities and dementia

It is evident, through our work so far, that much more needs to be done in these areas to make sure that no one is left behind. The next immediate steps are to pull together all of this information, along with case studies, pledges and our recommendations, and this should be available within the next six months.

(i) Find out more at: https://nationaldementiaaction.org.uk/

(ii) Read the report here: https://nationaldementiaaction.org. uk/campaigns/hidden-in-plain-sight-dementia-and-learning-disability/

## References

1 Samir Jeraj, S. and Jabeer Butt, J. 2018. *Dementia and Black, Asian and Minority Ethnic Communities Report of a Health and Wellbeing Alliance project* VCSE Health & wellbeing alliance.

## 5.8 The role of technology around stigma: Marie's journey

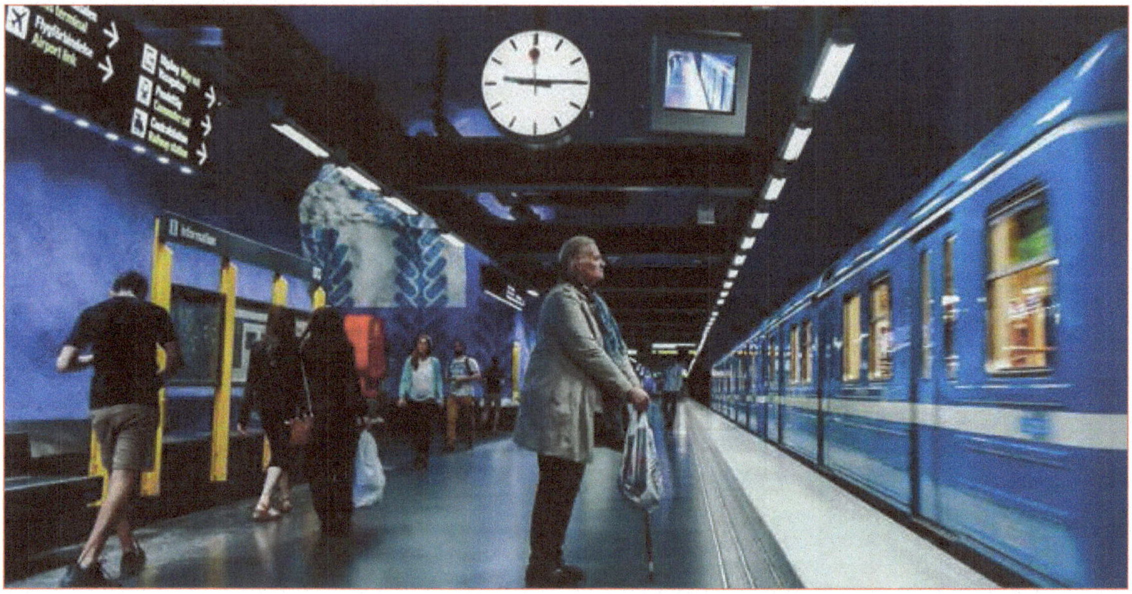

**Contributors:** Sophie N. Gaber[(i)], MSc OT, PhD Candidate at Karolinska Institutet, Sweden & Dr Anna Brorsson, MSc OT, Assistant Professor at Karolinska Institutet, Sweden.

This story is about Marie's journey; the problems she encounters whilst using Everyday Technology in places and activities in public space; the stigma these problems create; and how she manages the situations. The story is based on research about the experiences of people living with dementia in the UK and Sweden[1-5].

Marie begins the daily routine of picking up the various items she will need for going out. *Keys...check, purse... check, coat...check, phone...check, shopping list... check*! With her mental checklist ticked off, Marie steps outside her house and makes her way to the bus. Marie waits for her regular bus but there is a waiting line and the driver overshoots the stop, so Marie rushes to catch up with it. Marie breathes a sigh of relief - she has made it onto the bus. It takes a moment for Marie to steady herself and to search for her travel card in the bundle of cards wedged inside her purse. Marie can sense the people behind her are getting impatient so she asks the bus driver for help and hurriedly searches for the travel card.

Once seated, Marie sees that the electronic bus announcer is not showing the correct next stop. The bus is being diverted. Marie looks around to ask for help but notices everyone is looking down. She realises they are all looking at their phones. Marie reaches for her phone, she stares at the screen trying to recall where to find the maps. She swipes backwards and forwards through her phone but she cannot find it and so she puts the phone back in her pocket. The surroundings are not as familiar as they once were, but Marie looks out the window to try and use the local buildings as a landmark to guide herself.

Marie sees the supermarket through the bus window. She is anxious that she might miss her stop so she repeatedly presses the stop-button and makes her way as quickly as she can off the bus. Marie waits at the crossing for the green light to come up and then tries to hurry over the road as the green light flashes with a tick, tick, tick sound. Marie glances up from her shopping list and feels a little overwhelmed at the supermarket. Her senses are overloaded with so many impressions. She sees endless aisles of products, displayed in a messy and unfamiliar way. She hears many different sounds, background music, announcements, the cashier ringing, and children crying.

Marie starts to shop for the items on her shopping list. In the fruit and vegetable department, she wants to buy a couple of apples. She reaches out to collect them before realising she is touching the reflection of the apples in the mirror. Marie reaches down and collects the apples. After quite some time, Marie has located most of the items on the shopping list but she cannot find the coffee she usually buys. Eventually, she finds a shop assistant to ask for help. The shop assistant quickly mumbles the directions to the coffee then shuffles off before Marie could ask again. Marie goes up and down every aisle looking for the coffee, walking much further than she needed because the placement of the coffee is different today.

(i) The research was carried out as part of the Marie Curie Innovative Training Network (ITN) action, H2020-MSCA-ITN-2015, under grant agreement number 676265.

Marie pushes her heavy trolley to the checkout queue. This is the moment she dreads the most. Marie feels her anxiety building as she discovers it is the line for the self-service check-outs which she often experiences problems using. She glances behind at the long line and tries to follow the instructions on the self-service check-out screen. Marie manages to scan some items but one item was on sale and would not scan. Marie feels very anxious indeed. A shop assistant comes over and helps her before leaving Marie to cope alone.

By this time Marie is feeling stressed and she cannot remember the PIN number for her card. She tries two different numbers but she still cannot recall the correct number. So Marie decides to pay with cash but she cannot find which slot to put the cash in. The shop assistant comes over again and helps Marie put all her shopping back in the trolley and takes her to another till with a cashier where she can pay with cash. Marie collects her bags and takes a deep breath before she sets off on her journey back home.

## The pace of everyday technological change

In an age where technology is being adopted more and more frequently to everyday situations, often replacing a human interaction, there should be a consideration of the potential impact on people living with dementia, in the same way there could or should be for someone with a more visible disability (for example, the height of a cash machine). The speed of technological change is itself a challenge, with operators updating and adapting at a pace not previously seen. For example, self-check-in desks at airports are improving through user feedback but airports are notoriously stressful environments to begin with and introducing multiple, touch screen, scanning, printing and self-tagging requirements can be overwhelming. Some banks have been embracing dementia awareness training, especially in the UK and in Hong Kong, but as with supermarkets, the drive to reduce human costs, means not only a reduction in the number of branches, but also the introduction of more automation of tasks like transfers, cheque deposit and bill paying.

It is evident that people living with dementia can and do adapt to technology and it can be a real assistance. For example, using tablets and mobile devices enables people to keep in touch with video calling, even when distance is a challenge. Software and applications (apps) on devices are also being adapted for therapeutic use and simple touch screen and swipe technology can be a huge benefit. However, to ensure that people with dementia are engaged and benefitting from Everyday Technology advances it is vital to include them in the design and development processes. Just think how complicated choosing and watching a TV programme has become over the last few years, across multiple devices, apps and streaming services.

## Recommendations

### Dementia-friendly and usable places and services:

More service providers (e.g. retail and public transport) should consider some simple measures that could improve the experience of people with dementia when accessing their products or services, including design and layout adjustments. In addition, consider engaging people with dementia and their caregivers about what works well and not so well. Assess the implications of moving products and facilities from familiar and accessible locations and sign-posting any changes. Explain more about the vision, hearing and perception challenges and consider providing ongoing and regular dementia-friendly training to staff to enable them to recognise if a person has dementia and to provide optimal customer support, patience and consideration.

### Dementia-friendly and usable Everyday Technology:

Technology developers should engage people living with dementia and their carers in the design and testing stages, to help identify and alleviate potential issues and challenges - often simple things that are not perceived as challenges at the outset, primarily as the question is often not being asked. In retail environments, where the use of self-check-out technology is rapidly increasing, consider testing and adapting the technology from the perspective of someone with dementia. Usability testing and technology development in collaboration with people living with dementia and caregivers also conveys a thoughtful and caring approach from the business operator.

When technology is not always the answer, consider other options. In Scotland a supermarket introduced a "slow lane" for people with dementia, where check out assistants received basic awareness training and were able to assist people and simultaneously help reduce anxiety and stress. Evidently, the benefits of such a choice by the retailer also helps other people who need more time or who become anxious around technology.

## References


1 Brorsson, A., Öhman, A., Lundberg, S., & Nygård, L. 2011. 'Accessibility in public space as perceived by people with Alzheimer's disease'. *Dementia, 10*(4), 587-602.

2 Brorsson, A., Öhman, A., Cutchin, M., & Nygård, L. 2013. 'Managing critical incidents in grocery shopping by community-living people with Alzheimer's disease'. *Scandinavian Journal of Occupational Therapy*, 20(4), 292-301.

3 Brorsson, A., Öhman, A., Lundberg, S., & Nygård, L. 2016. 'Being a pedestrian with dementia: A qualitative study using photo documentation and focus groups interviews'. *Dementia, 15*(5), 1124-40.

4 Brorsson, A., Öhman, A., Lundberg, S., Cutchin, M., & Nygård, L. 2018. 'How accessible are grocery shops for people with dementia? A qualitative study using photo documentation and focus group interviews'. *Dementia,* 0(0)1-17.

5 Gaber, S., Nygård, L., Brorsson, A., Kottorp, A., and Malinowsky, C. 2019. 'Everyday Technologies and Public Space Participation among People with and without Dementia'. *Canadian Journal of Occupational Therapy.* 1-12. DOI: 10.1177/0008417419837764

## 5.9 Can design play a role in increasing awareness and challenging stigma around dementia?

**Contributor:** Prof Colm Cunningham, Director, Dementia Centre, Hammond Care, Australia

Dementia is often perceived as a hidden disability but much can be learned from the progress that has been made in response to the needs, and importantly the rights, of people living with more visible disabilities; for example, access ramps into public buildings, pavement level access for public transport, accessible height cash machines. Strategic design underpins this progress, which is equally important in public spaces, care environments and in the home. Product design, as well as built environment design, is also important and by increasing awareness of the need for design solutions for dementia, it can be argued, this goes some way to increasing overall awareness, acceptance and even helping reduce stigma, by legitimising the need for innovation in this space.

Twenty-one years ago, 'Design for Dementia' was published. It was one of the first publications to comprehensively describe the importance of design in supporting people with dementia.

It set out 8 principals that were needed to inform thinking:

- Reinforce personal identity
- Maximise independence
- Enhance self-esteem and confidence
- Compensate for disability
- Allow control of stimuli
- Be orientating and understandable
- Demonstrate care for staff
- Be welcoming to others

And the features that an environment should have:

- Be small (in scale and in numbers)
- Be domestic and familiar
- Provide good visual access
- Reduce unwanted stimulation
- Highlight important features (for residents)
- Be unobtrusively safe and secure
- Provide for planned walking (access to safe outside space)
- Provide links to the community
- Provide opportunities for privacy and social interaction
- Promote autonomy and choice

Understanding the experience of a person living with dementia is essential to providing an enabling environment and to support the person to live at home or in a care setting. To be able to 'see and sense' is critical because unfamiliar environments and situations may cause increased stress and confusion.

The majority of people with dementia live in their own home and want to be part of their communities for as long as possible. It makes good economic sense to invest in the design of cities and communities that are able to support people with dementia. Without this, premature admission to care has not only a personal but a financial cost.

When it comes to design, while familiarity is key, most people's homes and communities weren't built with dementia or ageing in mind. Companies like IKEA have only recently recognised the need for key features and adaptations in their flatpack housing options, but it's the range of positive changes that can be made to enhance the home or care environment for a person with dementia that remain a priority.

Some design changes may help support the person physically while others may assist the person in understanding their environment and overcoming specific perceptual challenges, these include:

- In the kitchen reducing clutter by clearing benches and workspaces of occasionally used items and leaving out things that are needed every day such as tea and coffee making items
- Reducing distracting noises such as both a radio and television
- Creating a special, calming space where the person has favourite and familiar items and to which they can retreat if feeling tired or overwhelmed
- Adjusting light levels is a critical issue, remembering that people with dementia and older people generally benefit from more light
- Thinking about what signs and cues would reduce confusion or uncertainty such as in the kitchen (pictures work well as the ability to read words may be lost)

### Case study

When supporting her dad David's bathroom independence, Rosemary noticed he had been having some toileting difficulties recently and often seemed quite distressed afterwards. Rosemary thought David may have been unwell, but then noticed when assisting him to the newly renovated, all white bathroom, he was unsure about locating the toilet. Later, he fumbled with the new modern tap fitting at the basin and left without washing his hands - unusual for David as he was fastidious about hygiene. When discussing this with a support person, Rosemary learned that greater contrast benefits older eyes and people with dementia, and that the shiny mixer tap would be unfamiliar to her dad. A new black toilet seat and easy to understand tap seem to have addressed most of David's difficulties and distress. Familiar handles and tap fittings often support independence especially if they clearly identify hot and cold.

In addition to changes with the ageing eye, for people with dementia, sensory changes mean that colour contrast is very important. The simple step of introducing, in some situations, contrasting colours, helps people understand the room and situation to find their way. At other times, keeping colour uniform avoids drawing attention to things that are confusing or to be avoided. For example, having contrasting bed linen so the bed is more obvious and a different colour top and bottom sheet that contrast to the floor makes finding and getting into bed easier and can be the difference between needing assistance and getting into bed independently. The recognition that the wrong flooring can slow or stop a person is now well evidenced. Pick a smooth, matte surface and ensure the same flooring is across as many rooms as possible. These surfaces are safer and easier for people with dementia. In kitchens and other wet areas, opt for a surface that is not shiny and reflective as this may look like water on the floor and a person with dementia may wisely refuse to enter! Between rooms, make the carpet bar or strip the same colour as the flooring. This can also reduce the risk of falls and prevent perceptual confusion[1]

Most design innovations and solutions around dementia have been for domestic spaces and in care settings, but is the case to translate this to public environments gathering the momentum needed and can we use disability rights to be the platform to do this? Cost is always a barrier but increasing awareness, providing advice and often introducing low-cost solutions is a route to change. It does not always have to be advocacy either, education works, for example, including design in dementia friendly community programmes; and we can decide where we spend our money, making a decision on a conference venue, a choice of hotel or restaurant and who we travel with should increasingly be based on their embracing of dementia considerate design and their investment in staff awareness.

It can be daunting for businesses such as shops, banks, cafes, theatres, transport providers, etc. to learn more about dementia and to start to look at dementia related design, but in doing so they are not only fulfilling their role from a disability rights perspective but they are also sending out a strong positive message about their nature and their brand and in doing so helping to increase awareness, which in itself can help reduce stigma.

The importance of design cannot be over-stated and much more research is required for what is needed from diagnosis through to when symptoms are advanced.

New technologies, including virtual and augmented reality, are proving to be enablers of people and designers. A key design challenge for innovators will be to span the varied and individual needs of people with dementia while creating spaces that are both aesthetically pleasing and that satisfy the functional and at times complex care requirements of the people who live there.

'Talking Sense' and 'My Home My life' are just two examples of publications on design that are 21 years later and are informed by research and the experience of people with dementia. They are free at https://www.dementiacentre.com/resources

## References

1 Judd S, Marshall M, Phippen P 1998. 'Design Dementia', Journal of Dementia Care, London: Hawker Publications.

# Conclusion & recommendations

When ADI decided to undertake a new survey on attitudes toward dementia, we had no idea that we would receive a 28-fold increase in responses from our last survey in 2012. The public has spoken – and almost 70,000 voices have told us that we still have a long way to go to 'normalise' the language, attitudes and behaviours around dementia and integrate people living with the condition fully into society in a supported way.

Almost all respondents feel they will one day develop dementia themselves, with the majority concerned by this, adding to the fear that surrounds the condition. Most of us agree that we shouldn't hide it – but with the majority of people living with dementia stating that at one time or another their opinions have not been taken seriously or they have been treated unfairly in medical, social or domestic situations, and some reporting their symptoms have even been joked about - does this encourage openness and disclosure?

In the absence of a disease-modifying treatment, we need to find ways of dealing with the condition in the 'here and now' – to ensure that people with dementia live the best quality of life they can and that those who care for them are supported. We need to tackle stigma head-on. Increased awareness leads to better understanding and empathy. Better knowledge reduces fear and changes behaviour.

A seismic shift needs to occur at all levels in society to break down the barriers of stigma; in particular in the governmental, health and care sectors, community services, and global research. Change can start with just one conversation, hence the focus of the campaign that goes with this report "Let's talk about dementia".

Now more than ever before, it's time to talk about dementia.

## Recommendations

1. Targeted public health awareness campaigns
2. Promotion of timely diagnosis and better post diagnostic support
3. Global evolution of dementia friends' programmes and dementia friendly/inclusive communities - with people living with dementia and carers at the heart of their design, implementation and evaluation
4. Increased public advocacy of people living with dementia – amplifying the voice of lived experience
5. Increase advocacy focused on carers experiences – whilst improving the understanding of first-hand experience
6. Specialised education about dementia-related stigma and person-centred care practice for healthcare practitioners
7. Call for local governments to increase the funding, range and quality of community services for people living with dementia
8. Changes to public policy relating to employment, health and insurance for both people living with dementia and their carers
9. Full adoption of a rights-based approach to dementia including full compliance with the Convention of Rights of Persons with Disabilities (CRPD)
10. Increase funded research – for both a disease-modifying drug as well as further understanding of stigma. We know from other high stigma illnesses, including cancer and HIV-AIDS, that medical treatment breakthroughs can be a catalyst to stigma reduction – and we also need to better understand the complex role stigma plays throughout society in order to tackle it and change hearts and minds.

Alzheimer's Disease International

## About ADI

Alzheimer's Disease International (ADI) is the international federation of Alzheimer associations throughout the world. Each of our 100 members is a non-profit Alzheimer association supporting people with dementia and their families. ADI's mission is to strengthen and support Alzheimer associations, to raise awareness about dementia worldwide, to make dementia a global health priority, to empower people with dementia and their care partners, and to increase investment in dementia research.

## What we do

- Support the development and activities of our member associations around the world.
- Encourage the creation of new Alzheimer associations in countries where there is no organisation.
- Bring Alzheimer organisations together to share and learn from each other.
- Raise public and political awareness of dementia.
- Stimulate research into the prevalence and impact of Alzheimer's disease and dementia around the world.
- Represent people with dementia and families on international platforms at the UN and WHO.

## Key activities

- Raising global awareness through World Alzheimer's Month™ (September every year).
- Providing Alzheimer associations with training in running a non-profit organisation through our Alzheimer University programme.
- Hosting an international conference where staff and volunteers from Alzheimer associations meet each other as well as medical and care professionals, researchers, people with dementia and their carers.
- Disseminating reliable and accurate information through our website and publications.
- Supporting the 10/66 Dementia Research Group's work on the prevalence and impact of dementia in developing countries.
- Supporting global advocacy by providing facts and figures about dementia, and monitoring as well as influencing dementia policies.

ADI is based in London and is registered as a non-profit organisation in the USA. ADI was founded in 1984, has been in official relations with the World Health Organization since 1996. ADI is partnered with Dementia Alliance International (DAI), a collaboration of individuals diagnosed with dementia providing a unified voice of strength, advocacy and support in the fight for individual autonomy for people with dementia.

You can find out more about ADI at www.alz.co.uk/adi

Alzheimer's Disease International:
The International Federation
of Alzheimer's Disease and
Related Disorders Societies, Inc.
is incorporated in Illinois, USA,
and is a 501(c)(3) not-for-profit
organization

Alzheimer's Disease International
64 Great Suffolk Street
London SE1 0BL
UK
Tel: +44 20 79810880
www.alz.co.uk

Alzheimer's Disease International
The global voice on dementia

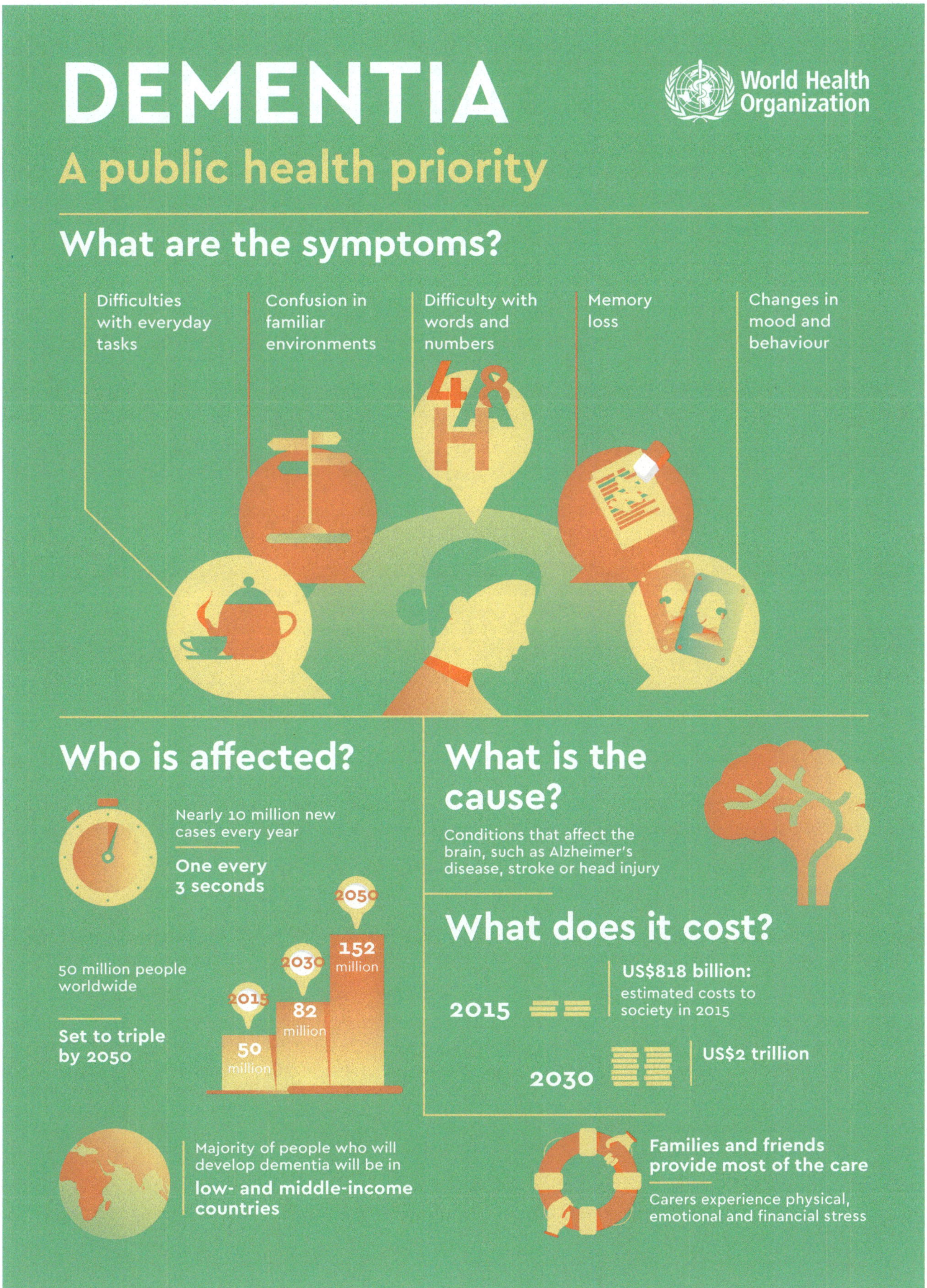
DEMENTIA
A public health priority
World Health Organization
What are the symptoms?
Difficulties with everyday tasks
Confusion in familiar environments
Difficulty with words and numbers
Memory loss
Changes in mood and behaviour
Who is affected?
Nearly 10 million new cases every year
One every 3 seconds
50 million people worldwide
Set to triple by 2050
2015
50 million
2030
82 million
2050
152 million
Majority of people who will develop dementia will be in
low- and middle-income countries
What is the cause?
Conditions that affect the brain, such as Alzheimer's disease, stroke or head injury
What does it cost?
2015
US$818 billion:
estimated costs to society in 2015
2030
US$2 trillion
Families and friends provide most of the care
Carers experience physical, emotional and financial stress

# The Global Action Plan on the Public Health Response to Dementia 2017 - 2025

## Vision

A world in which dementia is prevented and people with dementia and their carers live well and receive the care and support they need to fulfil their potential with dignity, respect, autonomy and equality.

## Goal

To improve the lives of people with dementia, their carers and families, while decreasing the impact of dementia on them as well as on communities and countries.

## The seven action areas and targets

### 1 Dementia as a public health priority

By 2025, **75%** of countries have national policies, strategies, plans or frameworks for dementia

### 2 Dementia awareness and friendliness

By 2025, **100%** of countries have a functioning public-awareness campaign on dementia

By 2025, **50%** of countries have at least one dementia-friendly initiative

### 3 Dementia risk reduction

Risk reduction targets identified in the Global action plan for prevention and control of noncommunicable diseases 2013-2020 are achieved

### 4 Dementia diagnosis, treatment & care

By 2025, **50%** of people with dementia are diagnosed, in at least 50% of countries

### 5 Support for dementia carers

By 2025, **75%** of countries provide support and training for carers and families

### 6 Information systems for dementia

By 2025, **50%** of countries routinely collect data on core dementia indicators

### 7 Dementia research and innovation

Global research output on dementia doubles between 2017 and 2025

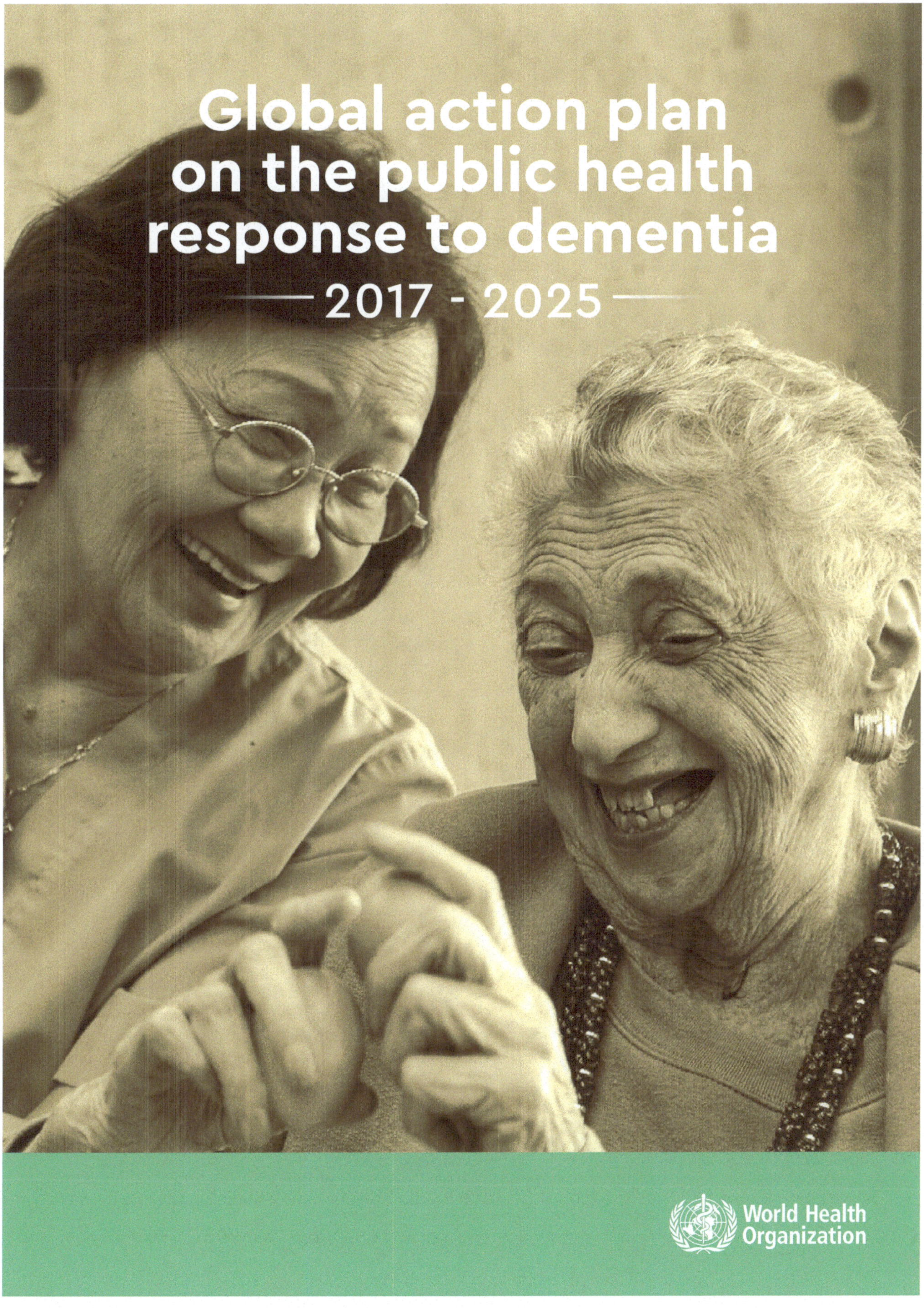
Global action plan
on the public health
response to dementia
2017 - 2025
World Health
Organization

# OVERVIEW OF THE GLOBAL SITUATION

1. Dementia is an umbrella term for several diseases that are mostly progressive, affecting memory, other cognitive abilities and behaviour, and that interfere significantly with a person's ability to maintain the activities of daily living. Alzheimer disease is the most common form of dementia and may contribute to 60–70% of cases. Other major forms include vascular dementia, dementia with Lewy bodies, and a group of diseases that contribute to frontotemporal dementia. The boundaries between different forms of dementia are indistinct and mixed forms often coexist.

2. In 2015, dementia affected 47 million people worldwide (or roughly 5% of the world's elderly population), a figure that is predicted to increase to 75 million in 2030 and 132 million by 2050. Recent reviews estimate that globally nearly 9.9 million people develop dementia each year; this figure translates into one new case every three seconds. Nearly 60% of people with dementia currently live in low- and middle-income countries and most new cases (71%) are expected to occur in those countries.[2,3]

3. Crucially, although age is the strongest known risk factor for the onset of dementia, it is not an inevitable consequence of ageing. Further, dementia does not exclusively affect older people, with young onset dementia (defined as the onset of symptoms before the age of 65 years) accounting for up to 9% of cases.[4] Some research has shown a relationship between the development of cognitive impairment and lifestyle-related risk factors that are shared with other noncommunicable diseases. These risk factors include physical inactivity, obesity, unbalanced diets, tobacco use and harmful use of alcohol as well as diabetes mellitus and mid-life hypertension. Other potentially modifiable risk factors more specific to dementia include mid-life depression, low educational attainment, social isolation and cognitive inactivity. Additionally, non-modifiable genetic risk factors exist that increase a person's risk of developing dementia.[5] There is also evidence suggesting that overall more women develop dementia than men.[3]

4. Dementia is a major cause of disability and dependency among older adults

2. WHO. The epidemiology and impact of dementia: current state and future trends. Geneva: World Health Organization; 2015, Document WHO/MSD/MER/15.3, available at http://www.who.int/mental_health/neurology/dementia/dementia_thematicbrief_epidemiology.pdf (accessed 8 March 2017).

3. Prince M, Wimo A, Guerchet M, Ali GC, Wu Yutzu, Prina M. World Alzheimer Report 2015. The global impact of dementia: an analysis of prevalence, incidence, cost and trends. London: Alzheimer's Disease International; 2015.

4. Alzheimer's Disease International and WHO. Dementia: a public health priority. Geneva: World Health Organization; 2012 (http://www.who.int/mental_health/publications/dementia_report_2012/en/, accessed 8 March 2017).

5. Loy CT, Schofield PR, Turner AM, Kwok JBJ. Genetics of dementia. Lancet. 2014;383(9919):828–40. doi:http://dx.doi.org/10.1016/S0140-6736(13)60630-3.

worldwide, having a significant impact not only on individuals but also on their carers, families, communities and societies. Dementia accounts for 11.9% of the years lived with disability due to a noncommunicable disease.[1] In light of the improved life expectancy globally, this figure is expected to increase further.

5. Dementia leads to increased costs for governments, communities, families and individuals, and to loss in productivity for economies.

   - In 2015, dementia costs[2] were estimated at US$ 818 billion, equivalent to 1.1% of global gross domestic product, ranging from 0.2% for low- and middle-income countries to 1.4% for high income countries. By 2030, it is estimated that the cost of caring for people with dementia worldwide will have risen to US$ 2 trillion, a total that could undermine social and economic development globally and overwhelm health and social services, including long term care systems specifically.[3]

   - People with dementia and their families face significant financial impact from the cost of health and social care and from reduction or loss of income. In high-income countries, the costs related to dementia are shared between informal care (45%) and social care (40%). In contrast, in low- and middle-income countries social care costs (15%) pale in comparison to informal care costs.[3] The expected disproportionate increase in dementia in low- and middle income countries will contribute further to increasing inequalities between countries and populations.

6. Currently, the gap is wide between the need for prevention, treatment and care for dementia and the actual provision of these services. Dementia is underdiagnosed worldwide, and, if a diagnosis is made, it is typically at a relatively late stage in the disease process. Long-term care pathways (from diagnosis until the end of life) for people with dementia are frequently fragmented if not entirely lacking. Lack of awareness and understanding of dementia is often to blame, resulting in stigmatization and barriers to diagnosis and care. People with dementia are frequently denied their human rights in both the community and care homes. In addition, people with dementia are not always involved in decision-making processes and their wishes and preferences for care are often not respected.

7. WHO and the World Bank estimate a need by 2030 for 40 million new health and social care jobs globally and about 18 million additional health workers, primarily in low-resource settings, in order to attain high and effective coverage with the broad range of necessary health services. In addressing dementia, expanding the health and social care workforce with appropriate skill mixes as well as available interventions and services will be essential to prevent, diagnose, treat and care for people with dementia.

1. Prince M, Albanese E, Guerchet M, Prina M. World Alzheimer Report 2014. Dementia and risk reduction: an analysis of protective and modifiable risk factors. London: Alzheimer's Disease International; 2014 (http://www.alz.co.uk/research/WorldAlzheimerReport2014.pdf, accessed 8 March 2017).
2. Direct medical and social care costs and costs of informal care.
3. Prince M, Wimo A, Guerchet M, Ali GC, Wu Yutzu, Prina M. World Alzheimer Report 2015. The global impact of dementia: an analysis of prevalence, incidence, cost and trends. London: Alzheimer's Disease International; 2015.

# VISION, GOALS AND CROSS-CUTTING PRINCIPLES

## Vision

8. The vision of the global action plan on the public health response to dementia is a world in which dementia is prevented and people with dementia and their carers live well and receive the care and support they need to fulfil their potential with dignity, respect, autonomy and equality.

## Goal

9. The goal of the global action plan is to improve the lives of people with dementia, their carers and families, while decreasing the impact of dementia on them as well as on communities and countries.

## Cross-cutting principles

10. The global action plan is grounded in the following **seven cross-cutting principles.**

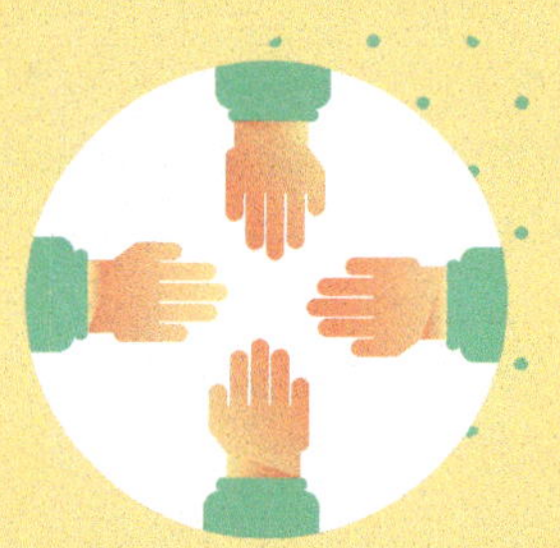

d. **Multisectoral collaboration on the public health response to dementia**

A comprehensive and coordinated response to dementia requires collaboration among all stakeholders to improve prevention, risk reduction, diagnosis, treatment and care. Achieving such collaboration requires engagement at the government level of all relevant public sectors, such as health (including alignment of existing noncommunicable disease, mental health and ageing efforts), social services, education, employment, justice, and housing, as well as partnerships with relevant civil society and private sector entities.

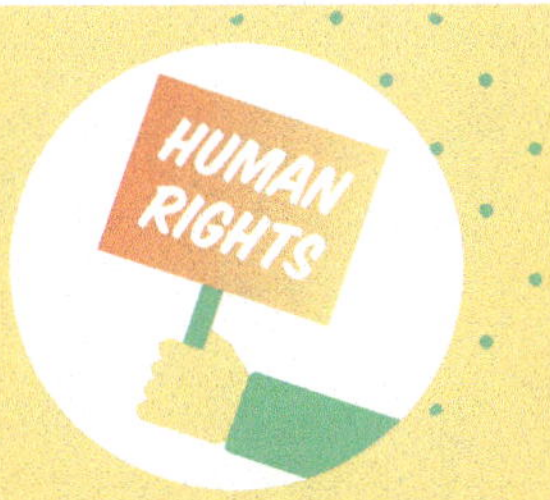


a. **Human rights of people with dementia**

Policies, plans, legislation, programmes, interventions and actions should be sensitive to the needs, expectations and human rights of people with dementia, consistent with the Convention on the Rights of Persons with Disabilities and other international and regional human rights instruments.

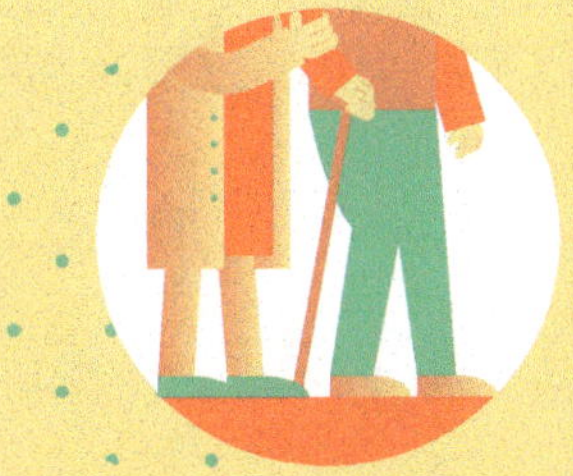

b. **Empowerment and engagement of people with dementia and their carers**

People with dementia, their carers and organizations that represent them should be empowered and involved in advocacy, policy, planning, legislation, service provision, monitoring and research of dementia.

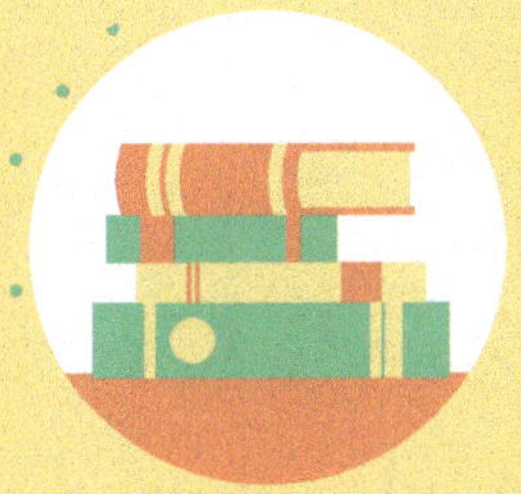

c. **Evidence-based practice for dementia risk reduction and care**

Based on scientific evidence and/or best practice, it is important to develop strategies and interventions for dementia risk reduction and care that are person-centred, cost-effective, sustainable and affordable, and take public health principles and cultural aspects into account.

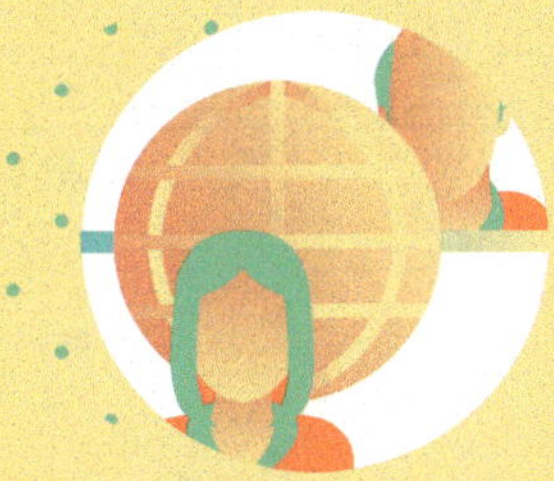

e. **Universal health and social care coverage for dementia**

Designing and implementing health programmes for universal health coverage must include financial risk protection and ensuring equitable access to a broad range of promotive, preventive, diagnostic and care services (including palliative, rehabilitative and social support) for all people with dementia and their carers.

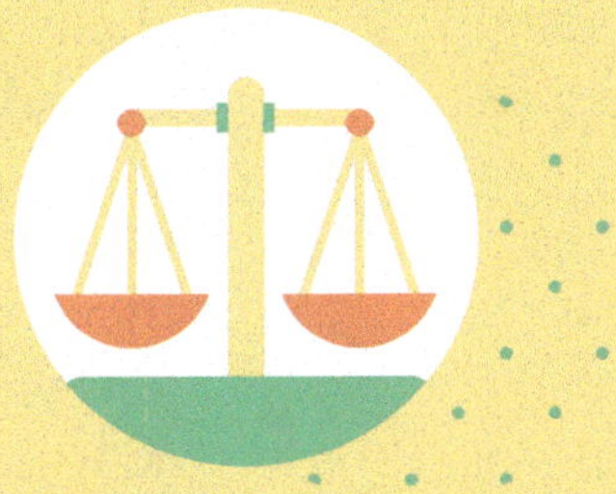

f. **Equity**

All efforts to implement public health responses to dementia must support gender equity and take a gender-sensitive perspective, keeping in mind all vulnerabilities specific to each national context, consistent with the 2030 Agenda for Sustainable Development, which recognizes that people who are vulnerable, including people with disabilities, older people and migrants, must be empowered.

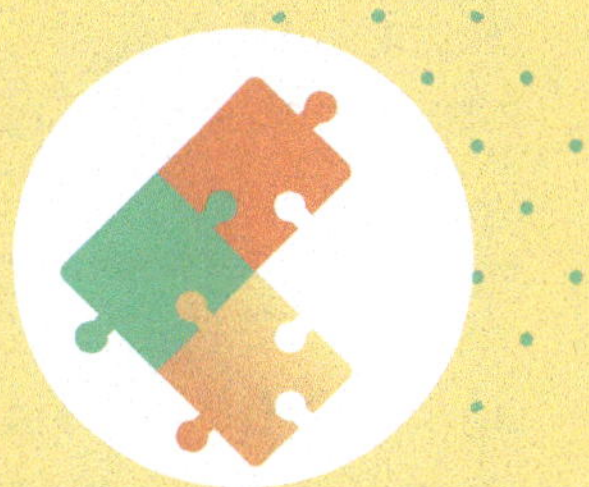

g. **Appropriate attention to dementia prevention, cure and care**

Steps to realize this focus include using existing knowledge and experience to improve prevention, risk reduction, care and support for people with dementia and their carers and generation of new knowledge towards finding disease-modifying treatments or a cure, effective risk reduction interventions and innovative models of care.

# ACTIONS AND TARGETS FOR MEMBER STATES, THE SECRETARIAT AND INTERNATIONAL, REGIONAL AND NATIONAL PARTNERS

11. Effective implementation of the global action plan on the public health response to dementia will require actions by Member States, the Secretariat and international, regional, national and subnational partners. Depending on national context, these partners include but are not limited to:

- development agencies, including international multilateral agencies (for example, OECD, United Nations development agencies and the World Bank), regional agencies (for example, regional development banks), subregional intergovernmental agencies and bilateral development aid agencies;
- academic institutions and research agencies, including the network of WHO collaborating centres for mental health, ageing, disability, human rights and social determinants of health, and other related networks;
- civil society, including people with dementia, their carers and families and associations that represent them, and other relevant organizations;
- the private sector, health insurance, and the media.

12. The roles of these four groups often overlap and can include multiple actions cutting across the areas of governance, health and social care services, promotion of understanding and prevention in dementia, and information, evidence and research. Country-based assessments of the needs and capacities of different partners will be essential to clarify the roles and actions of stakeholder groups.

13. Targets included in this global action plan are defined for achievement globally. Each Member State can be guided by these global targets when setting its own national targets, taking into account national circumstances. Each Member State will also decide how these global targets should be adapted for national planning, processes (including data collection systems), policies and strategies.

14. The global action plan recognizes that each Member State faces specific challenges in implementing these action areas and therefore suggests a range of proposed actions that each Member State will need to adapt to the national context.

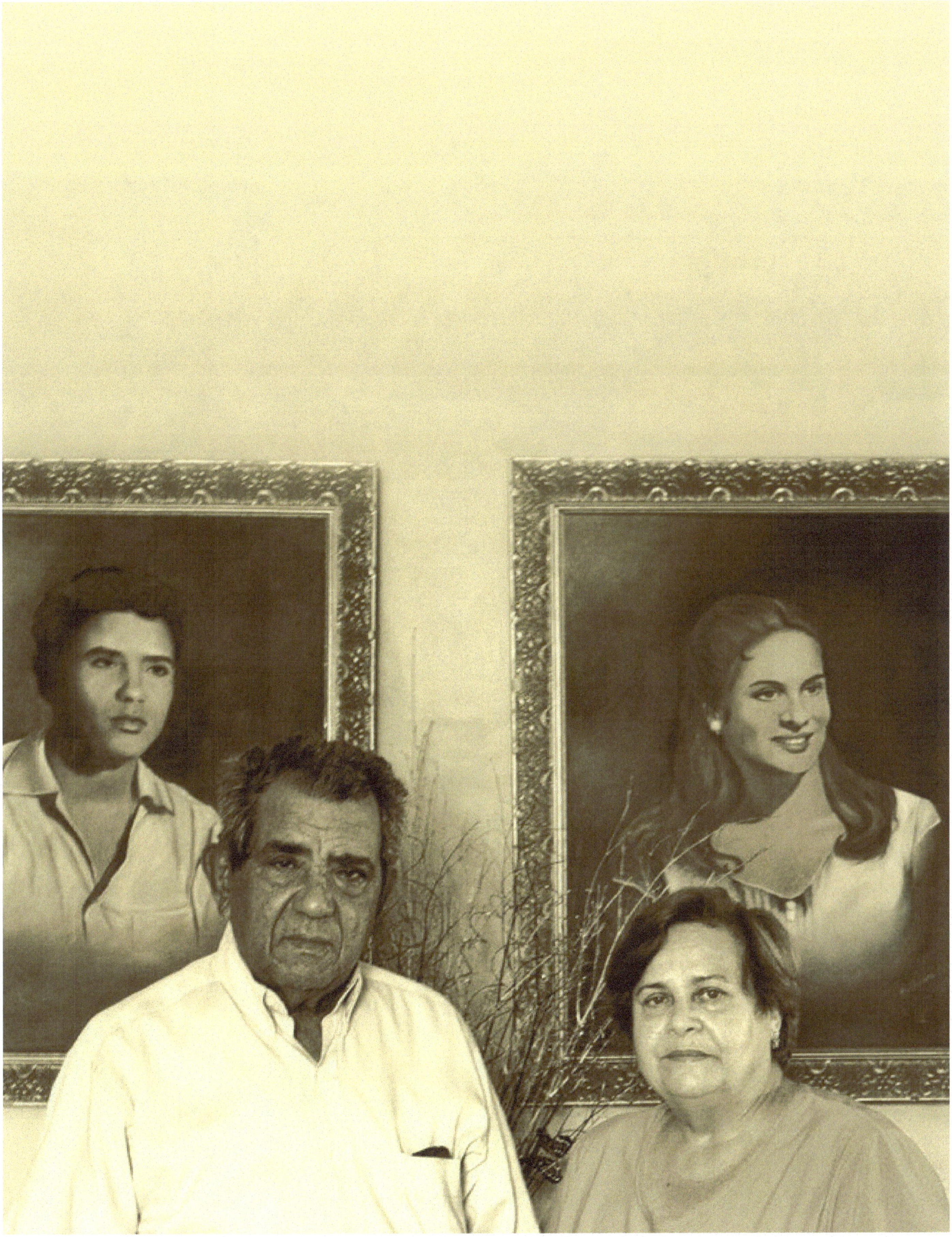

# Action areas

15. **The global action plan comprises seven action areas, which form the underlying structural framework:**

## Dementia as a public health priority

## Dementia awareness and friendliness

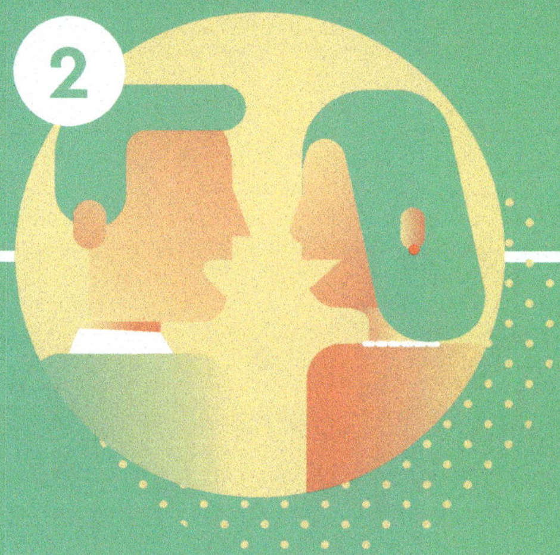


## Support for dementia carers

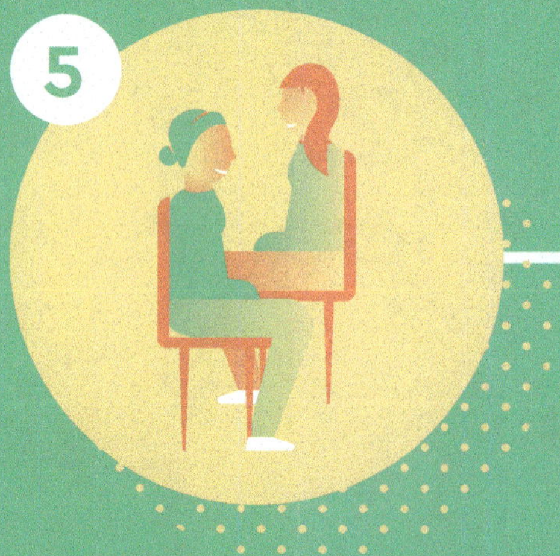


## Information systems for dementia

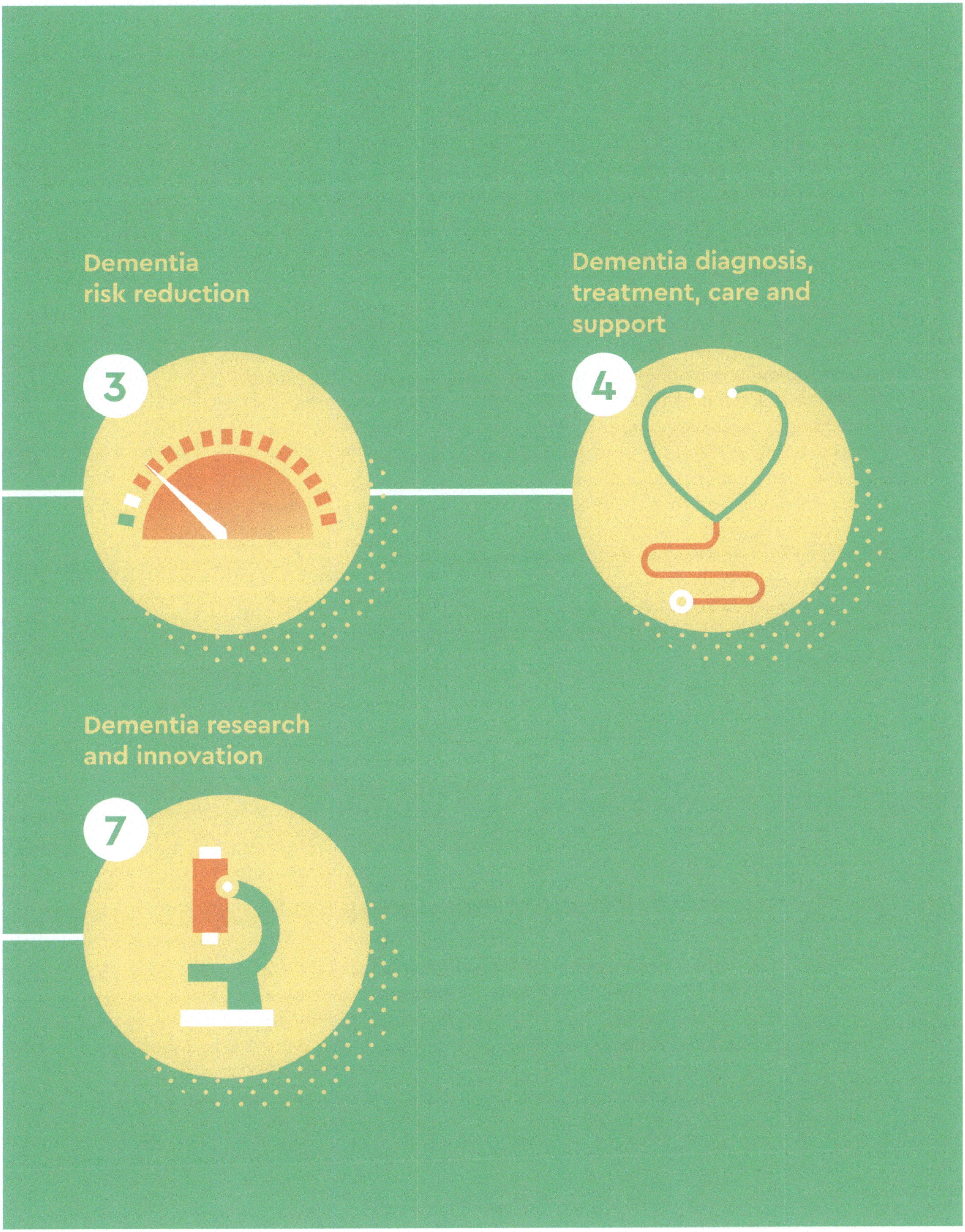
Dementia
risk reduction
3
Dementia diagnosis,
treatment, care and
support
4
Dementia research
and innovation
7

Action area 1:

# Dementia as a public health priority

16. Given the range of the population affected directly or indirectly by dementia and the complexity of this condition, dementia requires a whole-of-government, broad, multistakeholder, public health approach. Such an approach will lead to a comprehensive response from the health and social care system (both public and private) and other government sectors, and will engage people with dementia and their carers and other relevant stakeholders and partners.

17. **Rationale.** The development and coordination of policies, legislation, plans, frameworks and integrated programmes of care through a comprehensive, multisectoral approach will support the recognition, and address the complex needs, of people with dementia within the context of each country. This approach is in line with the principle of universal health coverage and the standards outlined in the Convention on the Rights of Persons with Disabilities.

18. ***Global target 1:***

***75% of countries will have developed or updated national policies, strategies, plans or frameworks for dementia, either stand-alone or integrated into other policies/plans, by 2025.***[1]

## PROPOSED ACTIONS FOR MEMBER STATES

19. Develop, strengthen and implement national and/or subnational strategies, policies, plans or frameworks that address dementia, whether as separate instruments or integrated into other planned actions for noncommunicable diseases, mental health, ageing, and disability (or equivalent). These undertakings should give consideration to equity, dignity and the human rights of people with dementia and support the needs of carers, in consultation with people with dementia and other relevant stakeholders.

1. The global target indicators and means of verification are provided in the Appendix.

20. Promote mechanisms to monitor the protection of the human rights, wishes and preferences of people with dementia and the implementation of relevant legislation, in line with the objectives of the Convention on the Rights of Persons with Disabilities and other international and regional human rights instruments. These mechanisms include safeguards for concepts such as legal capacity, self determination, supported decision-making, and power of attorney, and for protection against exploitation and abuse in institutions as well as in the community.

21. Set up a focal point, unit or functional division responsible for dementia or a coordination mechanism within the entity responsible for noncommunicable diseases, mental health or ageing within the health ministry (or equivalent body), in order to ensure sustainable funding, clear lines of responsibility for strategic planning, implementation, mechanisms for multisectoral collaboration, service evaluation, monitoring and reporting on dementia.

22. Allocate sustainable financial resources that are commensurate with the identified service need and human and other resources required to implement national dementia plans and actions, and set up mechanisms for tracking expenditures on dementia in health, social and other relevant sectors such as education and employment.

## ACTIONS FOR THE SECRETARIAT

23. Offer technical support, tools and guidance to Member States, and strengthen national capacity in:

- leadership within health ministries and other relevant sectors for the development, strengthening and implementation of evidence-based national and/or subnational strategies or plans and associated multisectoral resource planning, budgeting and tracking of expenditure on dementia;
- evaluating and implementing evidence-based options that suit Member States' needs and capacities and assessing the health impact of public policies on dementia by supporting national and international partners and establishing or strengthening national reference centres, WHO collaborating centres and knowledge-sharing networks;
- coordinating programmes on dementia with those on related noncommunicable diseases, ageing, mental health and health systems, and with service delivery and processes to ensure maximum synergy and optimal use of existing and new resources.

24. Compile and share knowledge and best practices on existing policy documents dealing with dementia, including codes of practice and mechanisms to monitor the protection of human rights and implementation of legislation,

consistent with the Convention on the Rights of Persons with Disabilities and other international and regional human rights instruments.

25. Promote and support collaboration and partnerships with countries at international, regional and national levels for multisectoral action in the response to dementia and aligning these with the principle of universal health coverage. Collaboration and partnerships should include all relevant sectors: health, justice and social services sectors, civil society, people with dementia, carers and family members, and organizations in the United Nations system, United Nations interagency groups and intergovernmental organizations.

## PROPOSED ACTIONS FOR INTERNATIONAL, REGIONAL AND NATIONAL PARTNERS

26. Create and strengthen associations and organizations of people with dementia, their families and carers, and foster their collaboration with existing disability (or other) organizations as partners in the prevention and treatment of dementia.

27. Motivate and actively engage in dialogue between associations representing people with dementia, their carers and families, health workers and government authorities in reforming health and social laws, policies, strategies, plans and programmes relevant to dementia, while paying explicit attention to the human rights of people with dementia and their carers as well as their empowerment, engagement and inclusion.

28. Support the development and application of national dementia policies, legislation, strategies and plans, and the creation of a formal role and authority for people with dementia and their carers to influence the process of designing, planning and implementing policies, laws and services related to dementia.

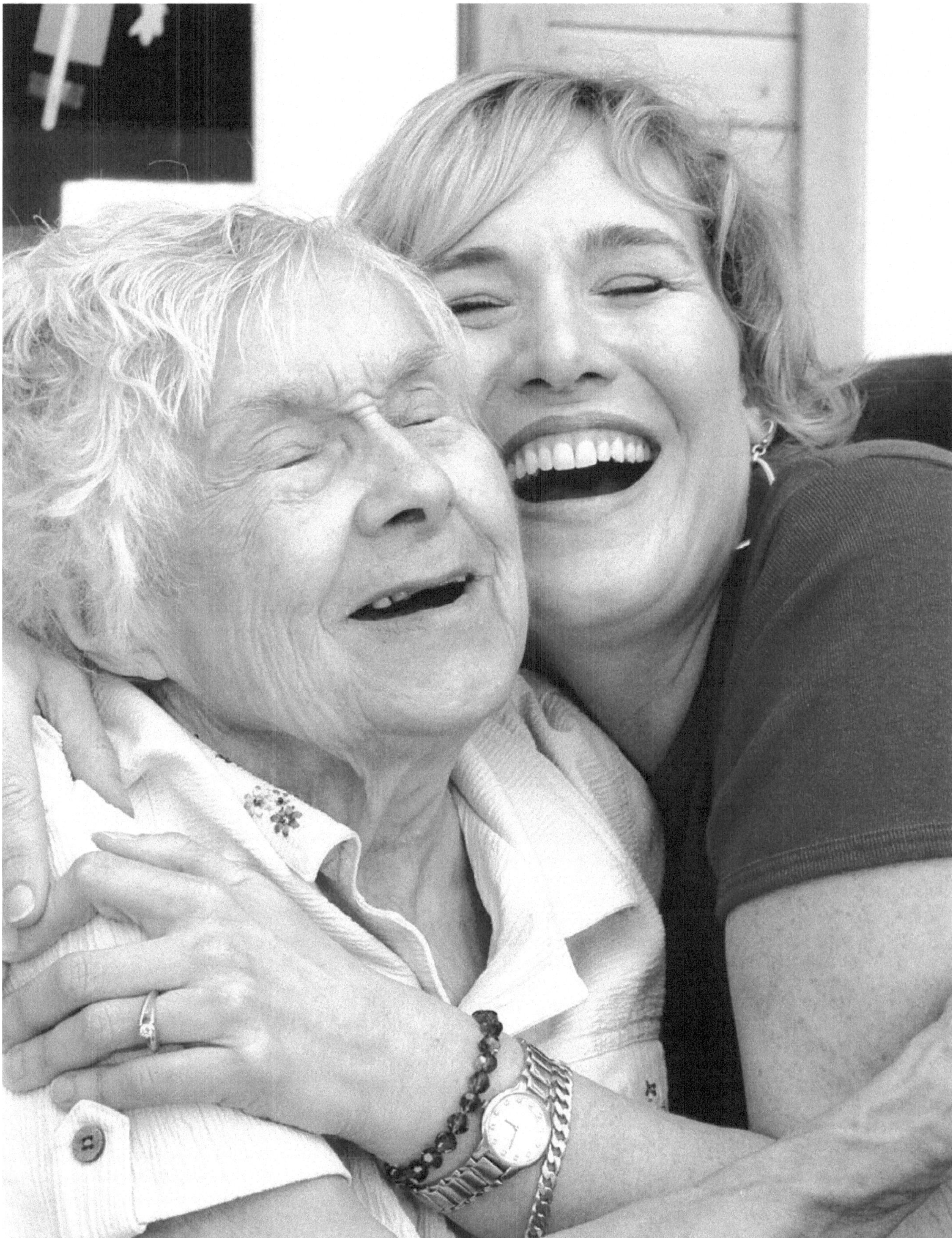

Action area 2:

# Dementia awareness and friendliness

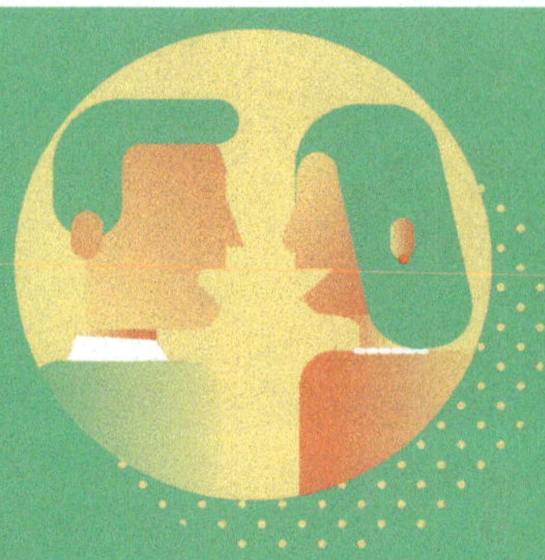

29. There is a common misconception that dementia is a natural and inevitable part of ageing rather than a disease process, resulting in barriers to diagnosis and care. The lack of understanding also causes fear of developing dementia and leads to stigmatization and discrimination. Furthermore, people with dementia are frequently denied their human rights in both the community and care homes.

30. Dementia-awareness programmes should: foster an accurate understanding of dementia and its various subtypes as clinical diseases; reduce stigmatization and discrimination associated with dementia; educate people about the human rights of people with dementia and the Convention on the Rights of Persons with Disabilities; enhance the general population's ability to recognize early symptoms and signs of dementia; and increase the public's knowledge of risk factors associated with dementia, thereby promoting healthy lifestyles and risk reduction behaviour in all.

31. A dementia-friendly society possesses an inclusive and accessible community environment that optimizes opportunities for health, participation and security for all people, in order to ensure quality of life and dignity for people with dementia, their carers and families. Shared key aspects of dementia friendly initiatives include safeguarding the human rights of people with dementia, tackling the stigmatization associated with dementia, promoting a greater involvement of people with dementia in society, and supporting families and carers of people with dementia. The concept of dementia-friendliness is tightly linked to societies also being age-friendly. Both age- and dementia-friendly initiatives should take into account the fact that a significant number of older people are living alone and are sometimes very isolated.

32. Dementia-awareness campaigns and dementia-friendly programmes that are tailored to the cultural contexts and particular needs of a community can promote enhanced health and social outcomes that reflect the wishes and preferences of people with dementia, as well as improve the quality of life for people with dementia, their carers and the broader community.

33. **Rationale.** Increasing public awareness, acceptance and understanding of dementia and making the societal environment dementia-friendly will enable people with dementia to participate in the community and maximize their autonomy through improved social participation.

34. **Global target 2.1:**

***100% of countries will have at least one functioning public awareness campaign on dementia to foster a dementia-inclusive society by 2025.[1]***

35. **Global target 2.2:**

***50% of countries will have at least one dementia-friendly initiative to foster a dementia-inclusive society by 2025.[1]***

## PROPOSED ACTIONS FOR MEMBER STATES

36. In collaboration with people with dementia, their carers and the organizations that represent them, the media and other relevant stakeholders, organize national and local public health and awareness campaigns that are community- and culture-specific. This cooperative action will improve the accuracy of the general public's knowledge about dementia, reduce stigmatization, dispel myths, promote early diagnosis, and emphasize the need for gender- and culturally-appropriate responses, recognition of human rights and respect for the autonomy of people with dementia.

37. Support changing all aspects of the social and built environments, including the provision of amenities, goods and services, in order to make them more inclusive and age- and dementia-friendly, promoting respect and acceptance in a manner that meets the needs of people with dementia and their carers and enables participation, safety and inclusion.

38. Develop programmes, adapted to the relevant context, to encourage dementia-friendly attitudes in the community and the public and private sectors that are informed by the experiences of people with dementia and their carers. Target different community and stakeholder groups, including but not limited to: school students and teachers, police, ambulance, fire brigades, transport, financial and other public service providers, education and faith-based organizations, and volunteers.

## ACTIONS FOR THE SECRETARIAT

39. Offer technical support to Member States in strengthening global, regional and national capacity:

- to engage and include people with dementia, their carers and organizations that represent them in decision-making within WHO's own processes and on issues that concern them;
- for the selection, formulation,

1. The global target indicator and means of verification are provided in the Appendix.

implementation and dissemination of best practices for awareness-raising and reduction of stigmatization and discrimination towards people with dementia.

40. Building upon the WHO Global Network of Age-friendly Cities and Communities and its dedicated website,[1] integrate and link dementia-friendly initiatives by documenting and evaluating existing dementia-friendly initiatives in order to identify evidence of what works in different contexts and disseminate this information.

41. Promote awareness and understanding of dementia, the human rights of people with dementia and the role of families and/or other carers as well as maintain and strengthen partnerships with organizations representing people with dementia and their carers.

42. Develop guidance for Member States on how to implement, monitor and evaluate dementia-friendly initiatives.

## PROPOSED ACTIONS FOR INTERNATIONAL, REGIONAL AND NATIONAL PARTNERS

43. Encourage all stakeholders to:

- raise awareness of the magnitude of the social and economic impact of dementia;
- include people with dementia, their carers and families in all aspects of developing and strengthening services that support the autonomy of people with dementia;
- protect and promote human rights of people with dementia and support their carers and their families;
- redress the inequities in vulnerable populations.

44. Ensure that people with dementia are included in activities of the wider community and foster cultural, social and civic participation by enhancing their autonomy.

45. Share in the development and implementation of all relevant programmes to raise awareness about dementia and make communities more dementia-friendly and -inclusive.

1. https://extranet.who.int/agefriendlyworld/ (accessed 8 March 2017).

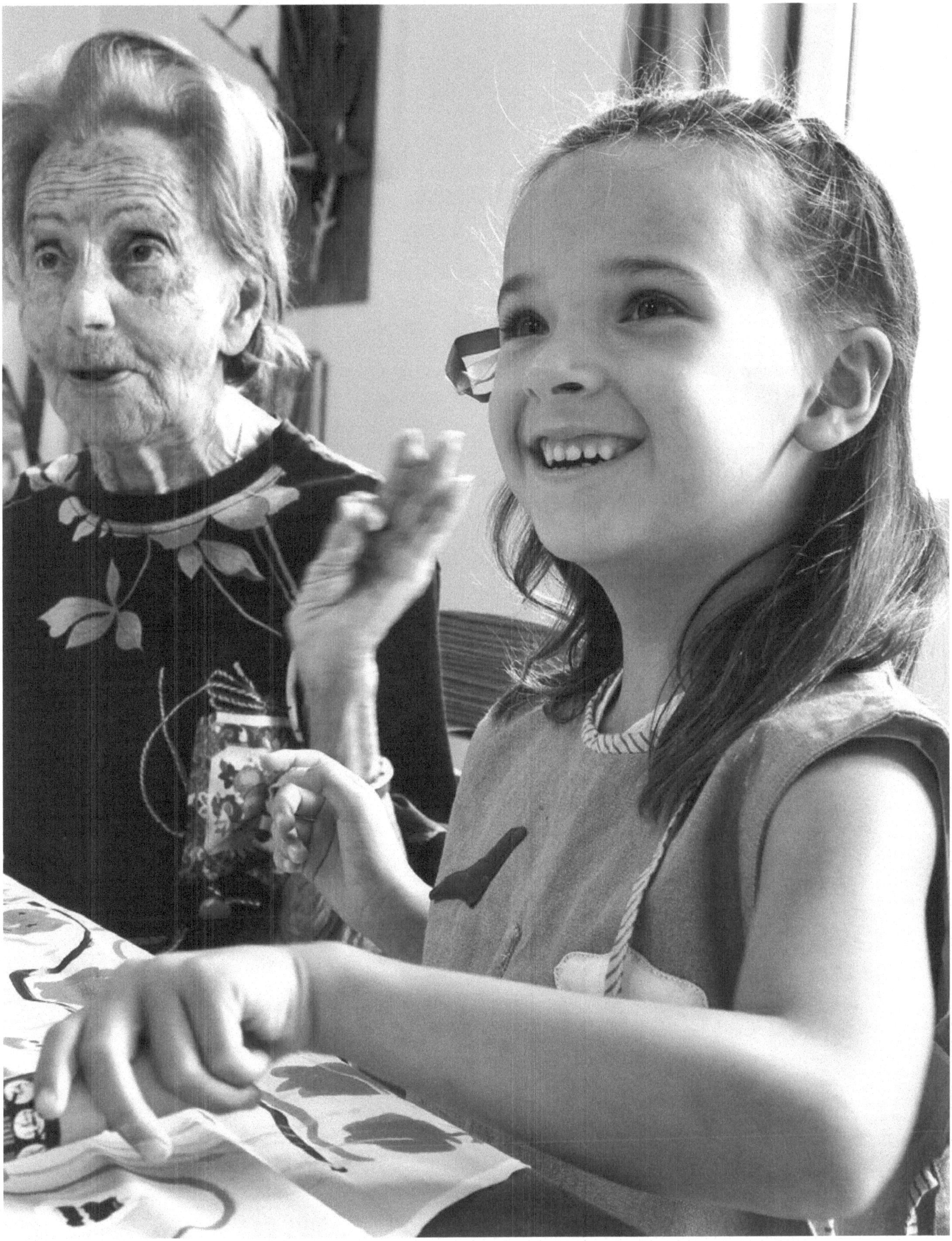

Action area 3:

# Dementia risk reduction

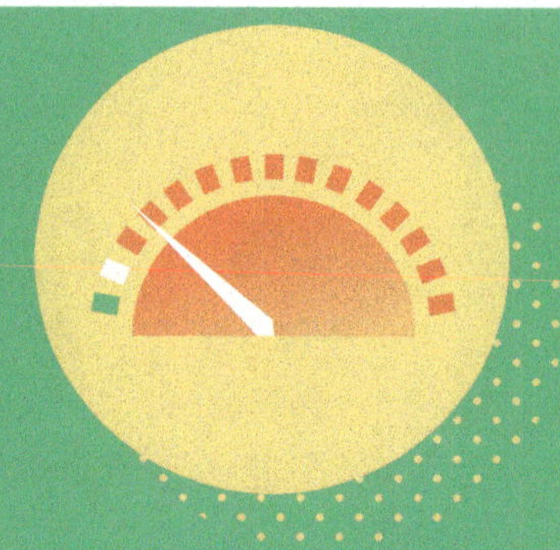

46. Growing evidence suggests an interrelationship between dementia on one side and noncommunicable disease and lifestyle-related risk factors on the other. These risk factors include physical inactivity, obesity, unbalanced diets, tobacco use, harmful use of alcohol, diabetes mellitus and mid-life hypertension. In addition, other potentially modifiable risk factors are more specific to dementia and include social isolation, low educational attainment, cognitive inactivity and mid-life depression. Reducing the level of exposure of individuals and populations to these potentially modifiable risk factors, beginning in childhood and extending throughout life, can strengthen the capacity of individuals and populations to make healthier choices and follow lifestyle patterns that foster good health.

47. There is growing consensus that the following measures are protective and can reduce the risk of cognitive decline and dementia: increasing physical activity, preventing and reducing obesity, promotion of balanced and healthy diets, cessation of tobacco use and the harmful use of alcohol, social engagement, promotion of cognitively stimulating activities and learning as well as prevention and management of diabetes, hypertension, especially in mid-life, and depression.

48. **Rationale.** By improving the capacity of health and social care professionals to provide evidence-based, multisectoral, gender and culturally-appropriate interventions to the general population, educate about and proactively manage modifiable risk factors for dementia that are shared with other noncommunicable diseases, the risk of developing dementia can be reduced or its progression delayed.

49. ***Global target 3:***

***The relevant global targets defined in the Global action plan for prevention and control of noncommunicable diseases 2013–2020 and any future revisions are achieved for risk reduction and reported.***[1]

1. See document WHA66/2013/REC/1, Annex 4, available at http://apps.who.int/gb/ebwha/pdf_files/WHA66-REC1/A66_REC1-en.pdf#page=87, accessed 20 September 2017.

## PROPOSED ACTIONS FOR MEMBER STATES

50. Link dementia with other programmes, policies and campaigns on noncommunicable disease risk reduction and health promotion across relevant sectors by promoting physical activity, healthy and balanced diets. Specific actions include weight management for obese individuals, cessation of tobacco use and the harmful use of alcohol, formal education and mentally stimulating activities as well as lifelong social engagement in line with the principle of balancing prevention and care.

51. Develop, deliver and promote evidence-based, age-, gender-, disability- and culturally sensitive interventions and training to health professionals, especially within the primary health care system, to improve knowledge and practices of such staff, and proactively manage modifiable dementia risk factors when conducting counselling about risk reduction. Routinely update these interventions as new scientific evidence becomes available.

## ACTIONS FOR THE SECRETARIAT

52. Linking to the actions specified in the global action plan for the prevention and control of noncommunicable diseases 2013–2020, offer technical support and strengthen global, regional and national capacities and capabilities to:

- raise awareness of the links between dementia and other noncommunicable diseases;
- integrate the reduction and control of modifiable dementia risk factors into national health planning processes and development agendas;
- support the formulation and implementation of evidence-based, multisectoral interventions for reducing the risk of dementia.

53. Strengthen the evidence base and share and disseminate evidence to support policy interventions for reducing potentially modifiable risk factors for dementia by providing a database of available evidence on the prevalence of those risk factors and the consequences of reducing them.

## PROPOSED ACTIONS FOR INTERNATIONAL, REGIONAL AND NATIONAL PARTNERS

54. Encourage all stakeholders to engage in activities to:

- promote and mainstream population health strategies that are age-inclusive, gender-sensitive and equity-based at national, regional and international levels in order to support a socially active lifestyle that is physically and mentally healthy for all, including people with dementia, their carers and families;
- take particular actions that have been shown to reduce the risk of dementia, particularly during mid-life;
- support national efforts for prevention and control of noncommunicable diseases in general and dementia in particular, for example, through exchange of information on evidence-based best practices and dissemination of research findings.

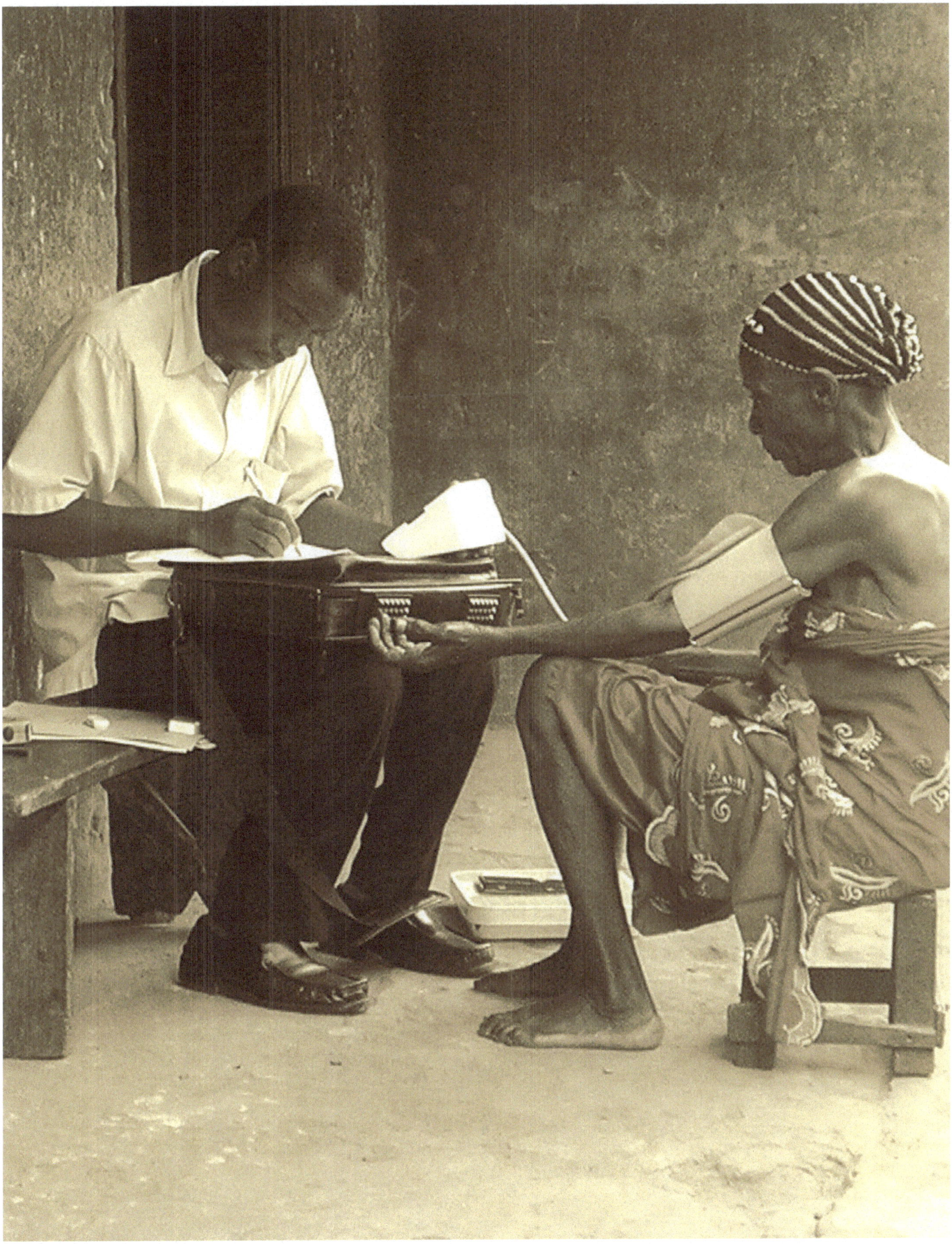

Action area 4:

# Dementia diagnosis, treatment, care and support

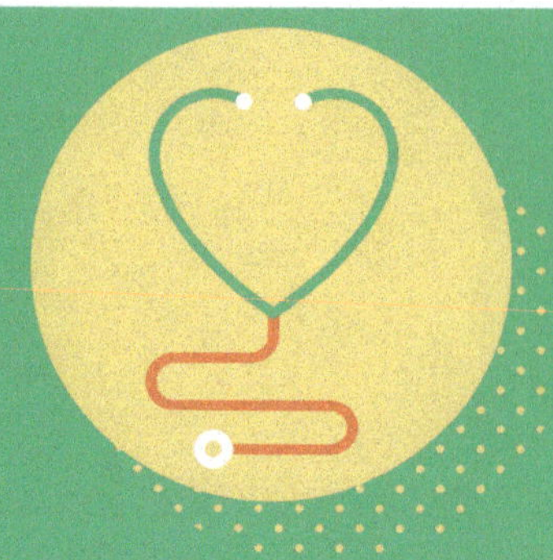

55. Dementia is associated with complex needs and high levels of dependency and morbidity in its later stages, requiring a range of health and social care, including long-term-care services. People with dementia are also less likely to be diagnosed for comorbid health conditions, which, when left untreated, can cause faster decline, and to receive the care and support they need to manage them. The services that they require include case-finding, diagnosis, treatment (including pharmacological and psychosocial), rehabilitation, palliative/end-of-life care and other support such as home help, transport, food and the provision of a structured day with meaningful activities.

56. People with dementia should be empowered to live in the community and to receive care aligned with their wishes and preferences. To ensure that people with dementia can maintain a level of functional ability consistent with their basic rights, fundamental freedoms and human dignity, they need integrated, person-centred, accessible, affordable health and social care, including long-term care. Long-term care covers all activities, whether these are provided by health, social or palliative care services or result from a dementia-friendly environment. Palliative care is a core component of the continuum of care for people living with dementia from the point of diagnosis through to the end of life and into the bereavement stages for families and carers. It provides physical, psychosocial and spiritual support for people with dementia and their carers including support with advance care planning.

57. The global action plan proposes some principles for organizing and developing health and social care, including long-term care systems for dementia. Providing sustainable care across the continuum from diagnosis to the end of life requires: timely diagnosis; the integration of dementia treatment and care into primary care; coordinated continuity of health and social care including long-term care between different providers and system levels, multidisciplinary collaboration and active cooperation between paid and unpaid carers. Planning responses to and recovery from humanitarian emergencies must ensure that individual support for

people with dementia and community psychosocial support are widely available.

58. Adequately trained and qualified workforces are required to provide these interventions. The continuity of care between different care providers, multiple sectors and system levels and active collaboration between paid and unpaid carers are crucial, from the first symptoms of dementia until the end of life. Integrated, evidence-based, person-centred care is required in all settings where people with dementia live, ranging from their homes, the community, assisted-living facilities and nursing homes to hospitals and hospices. The skills and capacity of the workforce and services are often challenged by the complex needs of people with dementia.

59. **Rationale.** The needs and preferences of people with dementia can be met and their autonomy from diagnosis to the end of life respected through integrated, culturally appropriate, person-centred, community-based health, psychosocial, long-term care and support and, where appropriate, the inputs of families and carers.

60. ***Global target 4:***

***In at least 50% of countries, as a minimum, 50% of the estimated number of people with dementia are diagnosed[1] by 2025.[2]***

## PROPOSED ACTIONS FOR MEMBER STATES

61. Develop a pathway of efficient, coordinated care for people with dementia that is embedded in the health and social care system (including long-term care), to provide integrated, person-centred care as and when it is required. The pathway should provide quality care and management that integrates multiple services, including primary health care, home care, long-term care, specialist medical care, rehabilitation and palliative services, household help, food and transport services, other social welfare services and meaningful activities, into a seamless bundle that enhances the capacity and functional ability of people with dementia.

62. Build the knowledge and skills of general and specialized staff in the health workforce to deliver evidence-based, culturally-appropriate and human rights-oriented health and social care, including long-term care services for people with dementia. (Mechanisms may include teaching the core competences of dementia diagnosis, treatment and care in undergraduate and graduate medical and paramedical training, and continuing training programmes for all health and social care professionals, in collaboration with key stakeholders such as regulatory bodies.) Earmark budgets and resources for in-service training for these

1. All people who are diagnosed should receive appropriate post-diagnostic health and social care.
2. The global target indicator and means of verification are provided in the Appendix.

professionals, or include such budgets and resources in specific programmes.

63. Improve the quality of care towards the end of life by: recognizing advanced dementia as a condition requiring palliative care; promoting awareness about advanced care planning for all people living with dementia to document their wishes for the end of their life; using validated end-of-life pathways and ensuring that people with dementia have their values and preferences respected and are cared for in their place of choice; and providing training for health care professionals and palliative care specialists.

64. Systematically shift the locus of care away from hospitals towards community-based care settings and multidisciplinary, community-based networks that integrate social and health systems and provide quality care and evidence-based interventions.

65. Enhance access to a range of person-centred, gender-sensitive, culturally-appropriate and responsive services including liaison with local nongovernmental organizations and other stakeholders in order to provide information that empowers people with dementia to make informed choices and decisions about their care. Respect their rights and preferences and foster active collaboration between the person with dementia, their families and carers and service providers from the first symptoms through to the end of life.

## ACTIONS FOR THE SECRETARIAT

66. Offer technical support to Member States for documenting and sharing best practices of evidence-based service delivery and care coordination, and provide support to Member States in developing dementia care pathways in line with the principle of universal health coverage.

67. Develop and implement guidelines, tools and training materials, such as model training curricula, covering core competencies relating to dementia for health and social care workers in the field. Provide support to Member States in the formulation of human resource strategies for dementia, including the identification of gaps, specific needs and training requirements for health and social care workers as well as graduate and undergraduate education about integrated provision of long-term care that is person-centred from diagnosis to the end of life.

68. Provide guidance on strengthening the implementation of the dementia component of the WHO Mental Health Gap Action Programme[1] to enhance capabilities of existing human resources and train more staff, and on improving the ability to provide quality care and evidence-based interventions through primary health care.

1. See http://www.who.int/mental_health/mhgap/en/ (accessed 8 March 2017).

## PROPOSED ACTIONS FOR INTERNATIONAL, REGIONAL AND NATIONAL PARTNERS

69. Support people with dementia and their families and carers, for example, by developing evidence-based, user-friendly information and training tools concerning dementia and available services to allow timely diagnosis and enhance the continued provision of long-term care, or by setting up national helplines and websites with information and advice at local levels.

70. Support the training of health and social care personnel to provide evidence-based treatment and care for people with dementia, by developing training relevant to needs, supporting teaching institutions in revising the contents of curricula so as to place greater emphasis on dementia, and ensuring that people with dementia are engaged, as appropriate, in the development and provision of education and training.

71. Promote community-based rehabilitation as an effective strategy to enable and support people with dementia in preserving their autonomy and rights and ensuring that the person with dementia remains at the centre of all discussions on diagnosis, treatment and care.

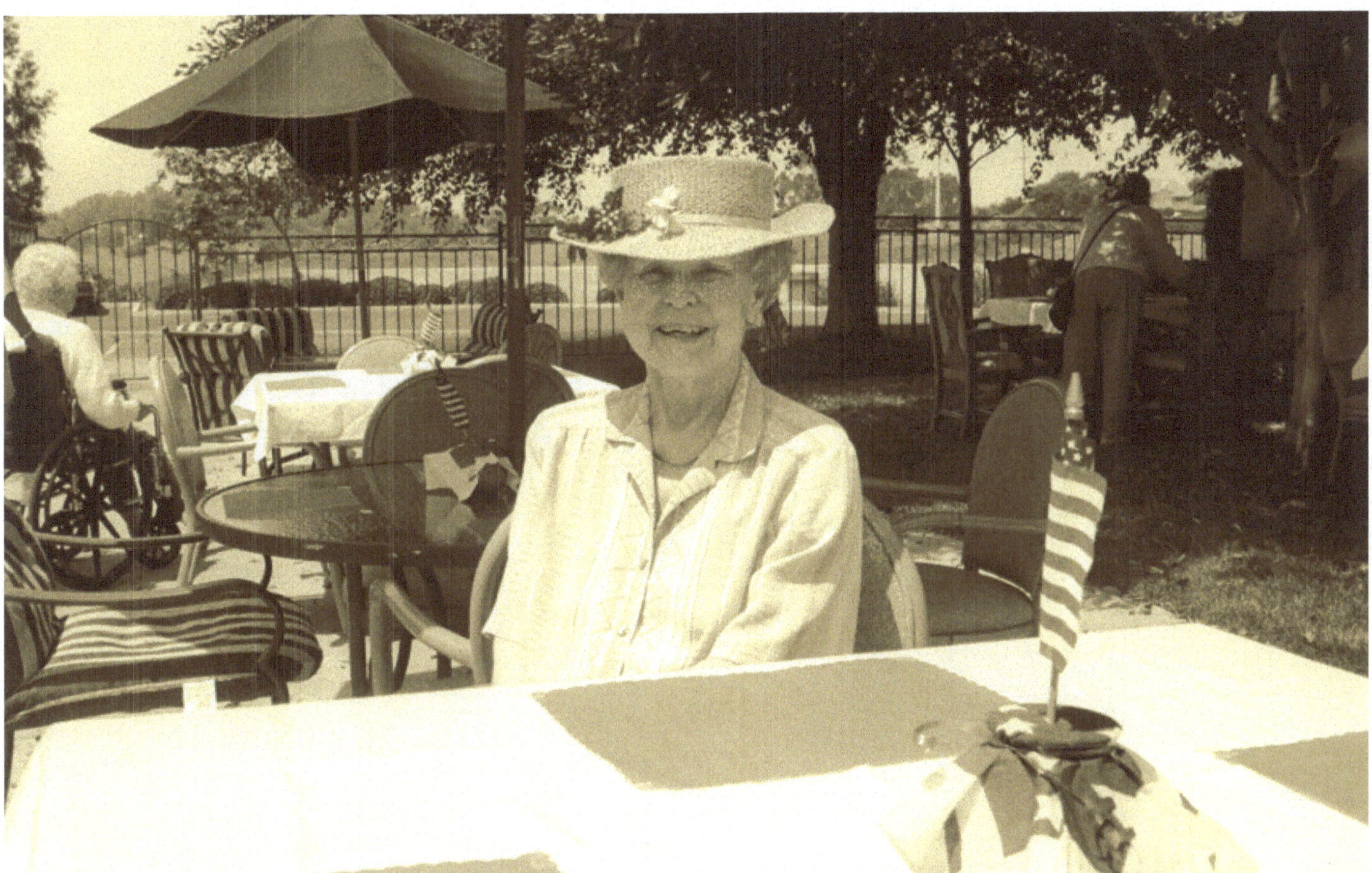

Action area 5:

# Support for dementia carers

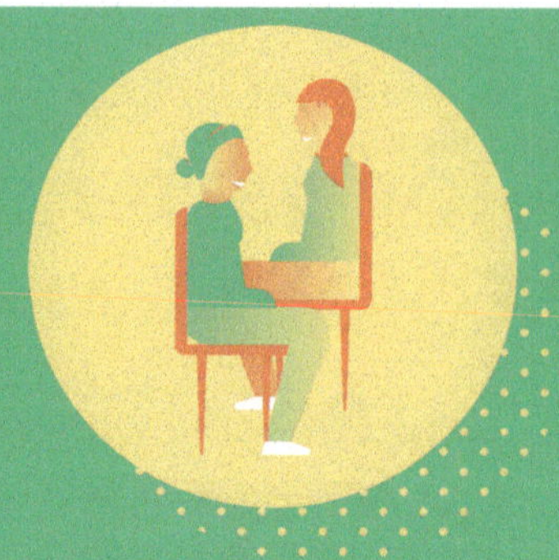

72. Carers can be defined by their relationship to the person with dementia and their care input. Many dementia carers are relatives or extended family members, but close friends, neighbours and paid lay persons or volunteers can also take on responsibilities for caring. Carers are involved in providing "hands-on" care and support for people with dementia or play a significant role in organizing the care delivered by others. Carers often know the person with dementia well, and therefore are likely to have knowledge of and information about the person with dementia that is crucial for developing effective personalized needs-based treatment and care plans. Carers should therefore be considered essential partners in the planning and provision of care in all settings according to the wishes and needs of the person with dementia.

73. It should be noted that being a carer for someone with dementia may affect the carer's physical and mental health and well-being and social relationships. Health systems must consider both the substantial need of people with dementia for help from others and its significant impact on carers and families, including economic impact. Carers should have access to support and services tailored to their needs in order effectively to respond to and manage the physical, mental and social demands of their caring role.

74. **Rationale.** The creation and implementation of means to deliver multisectoral care, support and services for carers will help to meet the needs of carers, and prevent a decline in their physical and mental health and social well-being.

75. ***Global target 5:***

***75% of countries provide support and training programmes for carers and families of people with dementia by 2025.***[1]

1. The global target indicator and means of verification are provided in the Appendix.

## PROPOSED ACTIONS FOR MEMBER STATES

76. Provide accessible and evidence-based information, training programmes, respite services and other resources tailored to the needs of carers to improve knowledge and caregiving skills, such as coping with challenging behaviour, to enable people with dementia to live in the community and to prevent stress and health problems for their carers.

77. Provide training programmes for health care and social care staff for the identification and reduction of stress and burn-out of carers.

78. Develop or strengthen protection of carers, such as social and disability benefits, policies and legislation against discrimination, for example in employment, and support them beyond their caregiving role in all settings.

79. Involve carers in the planning of care, with attention being given to the wishes and preferences of people with dementia and their families.

## ACTIONS FOR THE SECRETARIAT

80. Build evidence on and articulate the importance of carers in the lives of people with dementia, while raising awareness about the disproportionate effect on women, and offer technical support to Member States by monitoring trends in availability of carer-support services. Provide support to Member States in developing evidence-based information, training programmes and respite services for carers, using a multisectoral approach, and foster outcome measurement.

81. Facilitate access to affordable, evidence-based resources for carers to improve knowledge and skills, reduce emotional stress and improve coping, self-efficacy and health by making use of information and communication technologies such as Internet and mobile phone technologies (for instance, WHO iSupport[2]), for education, skills training and social support.

2. WHO iSupport: e-programme for caregivers of people living with dementia (http://www.who.int/mental_health/neurology/dementia/isupport/en/, accessed 8 March 2017).

## PROPOSED ACTIONS FOR INTERNATIONAL, REGIONAL AND NATIONAL PARTNERS

82. Increase awareness of the involvement, and its consequences, of carers and families in the lives of people with dementia, protecting them from discrimination, supporting their ability to continue their caregiving in a gender-sensitive manner, and empowering carers with opportunities to develop self-advocacy skills to be able to meet specific challenges in accessing health and social care, including long-term care services.

83. Assist in carrying out appropriate training programmes: for carers and families to enhance knowledge and caregiving skills across the progression of dementia; and on a person-centred approach to promote respect and well-being.

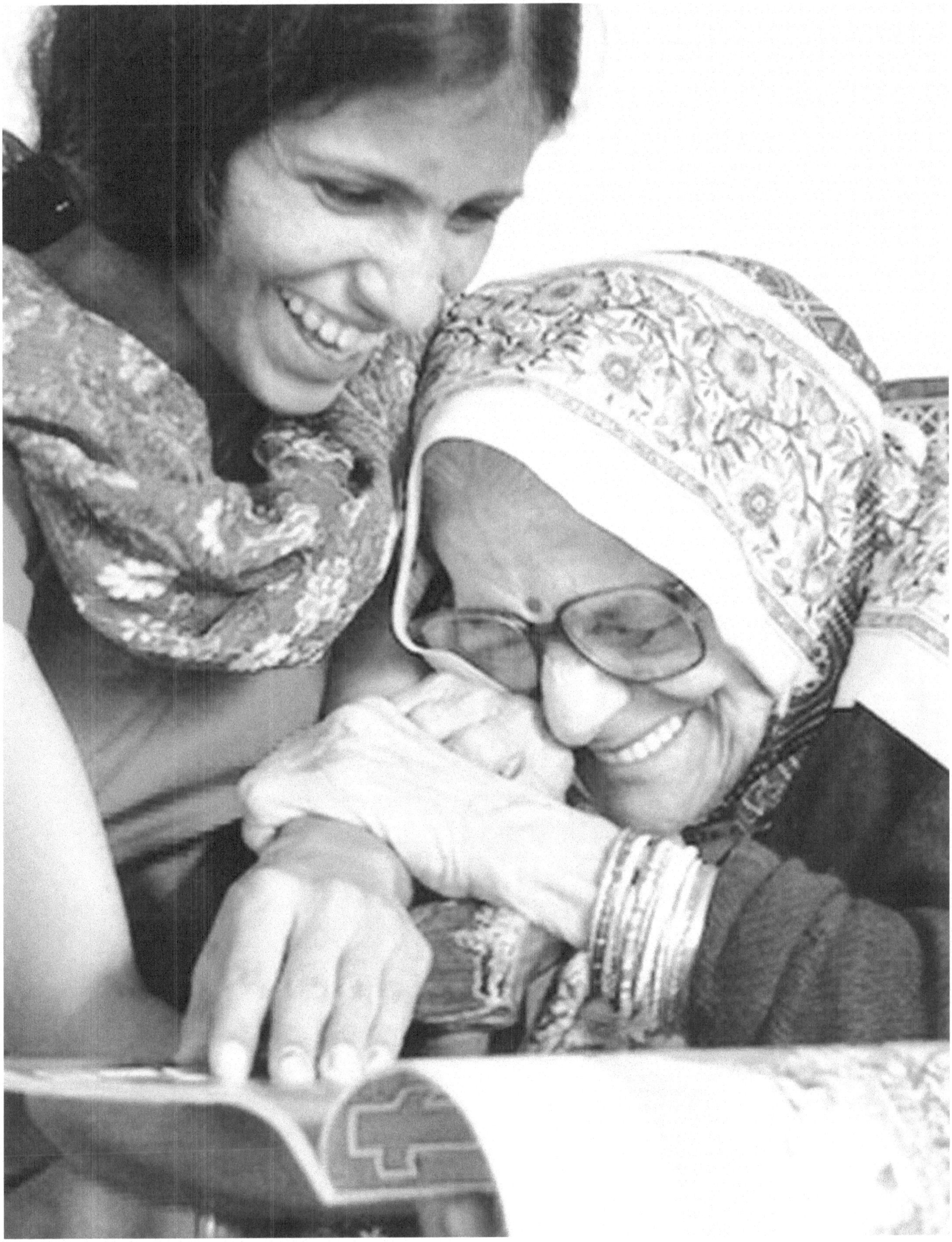

Action area 6:

# Information systems for dementia

84. Systematic, routine population-level monitoring of a core set of dementia indicators provides the data needed to guide evidence-based actions to improve services and to measure progress towards implementing national dementia policies. By building and/or strengthening information systems for dementia, the functional trajectories of people with dementia, their carers and families can be improved. However, this will require significant changes, while respecting existing regulatory frameworks, to the routine collection, recording, linkage and disaggregation for the sharing of health and administrative data of each encounter of a person with dementia with the health and social care system.

85. **Rationale.** Systematic monitoring and evaluation of the usage of health and social care systems can provide the best available evidence for policy development and service delivery, and can improve prevention and the accessibility and coordination of care for people with dementia across the continuum, from risk reduction to the end of life.

86. ***Global target 6:***

***50% of countries routinely collect a core set of dementia indicators through their national health and social information systems every two years by 2025.***[1]

## PROPOSED ACTIONS FOR MEMBER STATES

87. Develop, implement and improve, as needed, national surveillance and monitoring systems, including registers that are integrated into existing health information systems, in order to improve availability of high-quality, multisectoral data on dementia. Enable access to health and social care data and map available services and resources at national and regional levels in order to improve service delivery and coverage across the care continuum from prevention through risk reduction to the end of life.

1. The global target indicator and means of verification are provided in the Appendix.

88. Update or create supportive policy or legislation pertaining to the measurement, collection and sharing of data on health and social care for dementia and integrate this information routinely into national health information systems so as to facilitate routine reporting on dementia.

89. Collect and use the necessary data on epidemiology, care and resources relating to dementia in the country in order to implement relevant policies and plans.

## ACTIONS FOR THE SECRETARIAT

90. Offer technical support to Members States as they:

- develop and/or reform national data collection systems, including health information systems, in order to strengthen multisectoral dementia data collection;
- build national capacity and resources for systematic collection, analysis and use of dementia specific data through development of targets and indicators that account for national circumstances, yet are aligned as closely as possible with indicators and targets of the global monitoring framework.

91. Develop a core set of indicators in line with this action plan and provide guidance, training and technical assistance on capturing information and facilitating the use of these data to monitor outcomes. WHO's Global Dementia Observatory provides the mechanism to monitor systematically and facilitate the use of data from these core indicators, offering a platform for the exchange of data and knowledge in order to support evidence-based service planning, sharing of best practices and strengthening of both policies on dementia and health and social care systems.

92. Offer technical support to Member States in generating and providing information for monitoring of global, regional and national targets as required, through the Global Dementia Observatory.

## PROPOSED ACTIONS FOR INTERNATIONAL, REGIONAL AND NATIONAL PARTNERS

93. Provide support to Member States and the Secretariat in developing tools and strengthening capacity for surveillance and information systems that: capture data on core indicators on dementia; monitor usage of health and social care and support services for people with dementia, carers and families; and enable an assessment of trends over time.

94. Advocate the involvement of people with dementia and their families and carers in the creation, collection, analysis and use of data on dementia.

Action area 7:

# Dementia research and innovation

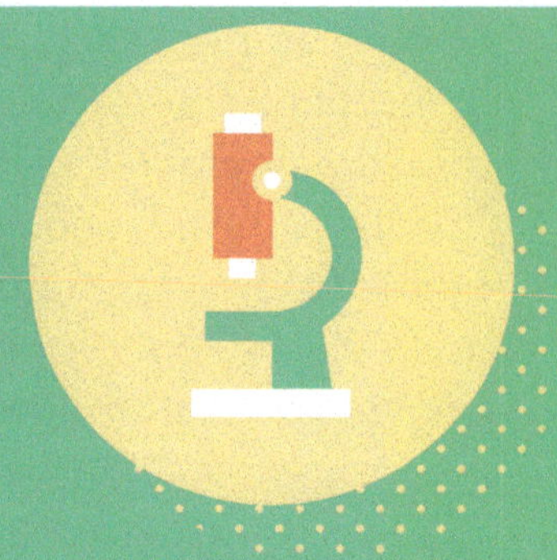

95. If the incidence of dementia is to be reduced and the lives of people with dementia are to be improved, research and innovation are crucial, as is their translation into daily practice. It is important not only that funding and appropriate infrastructures for dementia research and innovation are available but also that mechanisms are in place that assist appropriate recruitment of people with dementia, their families and carers into research studies. Research and development costs are higher for dementia than other therapeutic areas, because of lower success rates, longer development times, and low recruitment rates into trials; this disproportion discourages investment in this area. Research is needed to find a cure for dementia, but research is equally needed into prevention, risk reduction, diagnosis, treatment and care, including the disciplines of social science, public health and implementation research.

96. Collaboration among and between Member States and relevant stakeholders, with a particular focus on strengthening North-South, South-South and triangular cooperation, to implement a global dementia research agenda, will increase the likelihood of effective progress globally towards better prevention, diagnosis, treatment and care for people with dementia.

97. There is a growing interest in, and call for, the use of innovative health technologies in prevention, risk reduction, early diagnosis, treatment, care and support relating to dementia. These innovations aim to improve knowledge, skills and coping mechanisms in order to facilitate and support the daily lives of people with dementia and their carers while meeting, in particular, identified needs in an evidence-based and age-, gender- and culturally-sensitive manner.

98. **Rationale.** The successful implementation of research into dementia aligned with identified research priorities and social and technological innovations can increase the likelihood of effective progress towards better prevention, diagnosis, treatment and care for people with dementia.

99. ***Global target 7:***

***The output of global research on dementia doubles between 2017 and 2025.***[1]

1. The global target indicator and means of verification are provided in the Appendix.

## PROPOSED ACTIONS FOR MEMBER STATES

100. Develop, implement and monitor the realization of a national research agenda on prevention, diagnosis, treatment and care of people with dementia in collaboration with academic and research institutions; this work could be stand-alone or integrated into related research programmes that focus on filling gaps in evidence to support policy or practice. Strengthen research capacity for academic collaborations on national priorities for research into dementia by engaging relevant stakeholders, including people with dementia. Relevant steps may include: improving research infrastructure for dementia and related fields, enhancing competence of researchers to conduct high-quality research, and establishing centres of excellence for research into dementia.

101. Increase investment in dementia research and innovative health technologies and improve research governance as an integral component of the national response to dementia. In particular, allocate budgets to promote projects that: support collaborative national and international research; promote sharing of and open access to research data; generate knowledge on how to translate what is already known about dementia into action; and support the retention of the research workforce.

102. Foster the development of technological innovations that, in terms of design and evaluation, respond to the physical, psychological and social needs of people with dementia, their carers or people at risk of developing dementia; these innovations include but are not limited to diagnosis, disease monitoring and assessment, assistive technologies, pharmaceuticals and new models of care or forecasting/modelling techniques.

103. Following the national ethical requirements for research, promote equitable opportunities and access for people with dementia and their carers to be part of clinical and social research that concerns them.

## ACTIONS FOR THE SECRETARIAT

104. Draw up a global research agenda and work together with Member States to strengthen and build capacity in the area of dementia research by incorporating it in national and subnational policies and plans relating to dementia. Advocate increased investment in dementia research, capacities, methods and collaboration in the fields of biomedical and social sciences research, inter alia, through a network of WHO collaborating centres, countries from all WHO regions, and civil society organizations.

105. Engage relevant stakeholders, including people with dementia and their organizations, in the development and promotion of a global dementia research programme; facilitate global networks for research collaboration; and carry out multisectoral research related to the burden of disease, dementia risk reduction, treatment, care, policy and service evaluation. Promote international cooperation and intercountry exchange of research expertise, policy and practice through the systematic mapping of national investments in research and outputs of that research.

106. Support the inclusion of technological innovation in national and subnational policies and plans on dementia and offer technical support to Member States in developing and strengthening the provision of assistive and innovative technologies to maximize the functional ability of people with dementia, particularly in resource-poor settings.

## PROPOSED ACTIONS FOR INTERNATIONAL, REGIONAL AND NATIONAL PARTNERS

107. Support Member States and the Secretariat, where appropriate, by collaborating in setting priorities for dementia research, promoting increased governmental investment, mobilizing and increasing financial support, and disseminating research findings in user-friendly language to policy-makers, the public, people with dementia, their carers and families.

108. Advocate the engagement of people with dementia and their carers in applied research, clinical trials and the evaluation of new technologies that take account of the different physiology, needs and preferences of people with dementia and their carers.

109. Assist in the implementation and evaluation of innovative technologies, community-based service delivery structures and new dementia care concepts. Promote the use of information and communications technology to improve programme implementation, health outcomes, health promotion, monitoring and reporting and surveillance systems, and to disseminate, as appropriate, information on affordable, cost-effective, sustainable and high-quality interventions, best practices and lessons learned in the field of dementia.

110. Strengthen national capacity for research, development and innovation, for all aspects of dementia prevention, risk reduction, treatment and care in a sustainable and cost-effective manner, including the strengthening of institutional capacity and the creation of research fellowships and scholarships.

# 2020 Alzheimer's Disease Facts and Figures

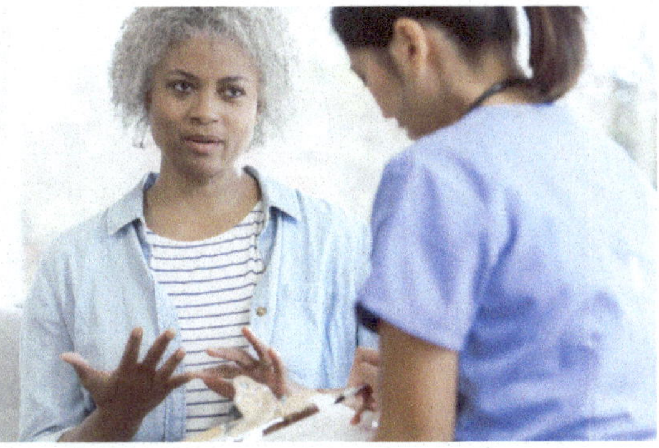

**6th** Alzheimer's disease is the leading cause of death in the United States

**50%** of primary care physicians believe the medical profession is not ready for the growing number of people with Alzheimer's or other dementias

More than **5 million** Americans are living with Alzheimer's

**1 in 3** seniors dies with Alzheimer's or another dementia

It kills more than breast cancer and prostate cancer combined

**16 million** Americans provide unpaid care for people with Alzheimer's or other dementias

These caregivers provided an estimated 18.6 billion hours valued at nearly **$244 billion**

In 2020, Alzheimer's and other dementias will cost the nation $305 billion — By 2050, these costs could rise as high as **$1.1 trillion**

Between 2000 and 2018 deaths from heart disease have decreased **7.8%**

while deaths from Alzheimer's disease have increased **146%**



alzheimer's association®

# 2020 Alzheimer's Disease Facts and Figures

**SPECIAL REPORT**

## On the Front Lines: Primary Care Physicians and Alzheimer's Care in America

alzheimer's association®

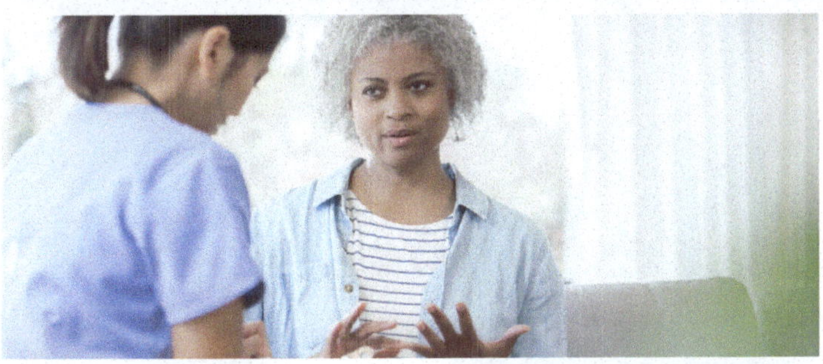

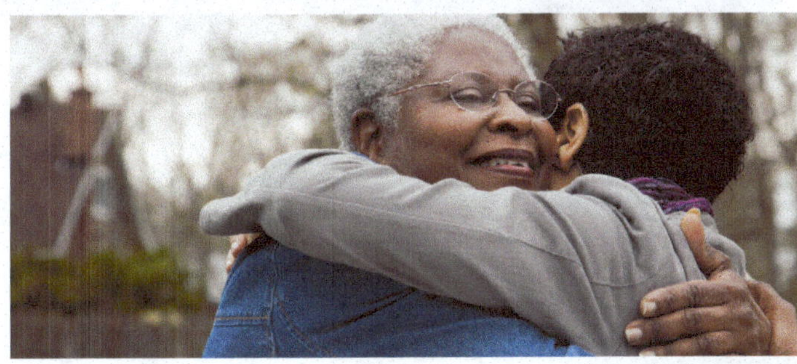

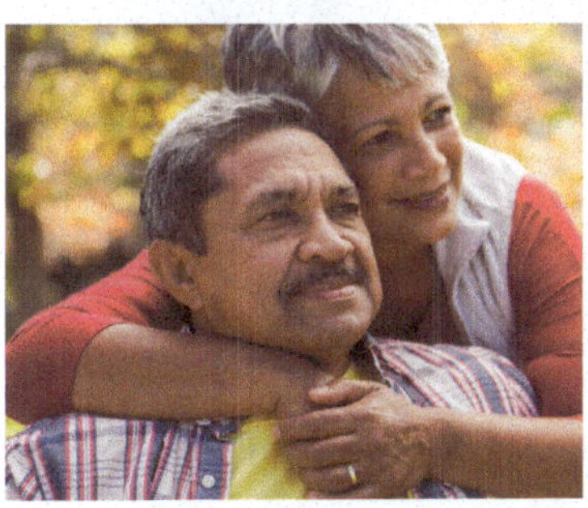

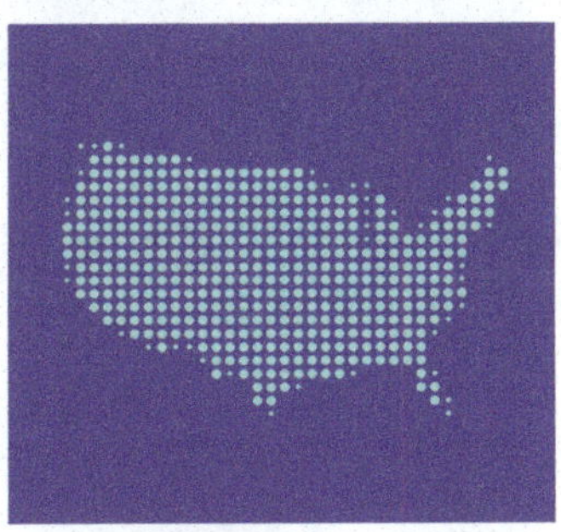

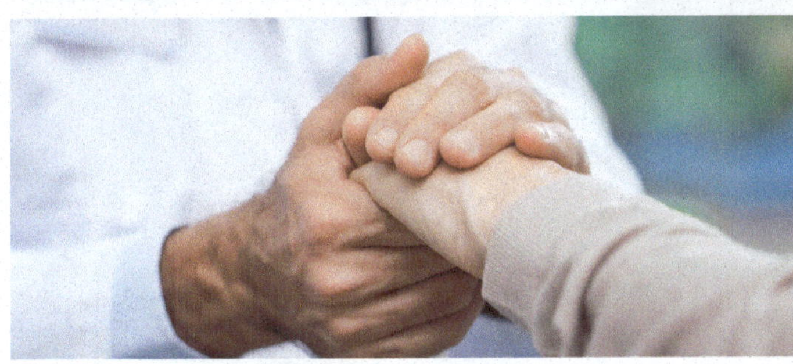

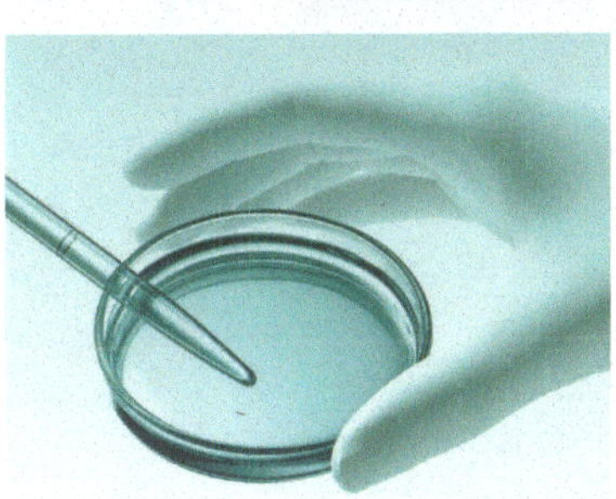

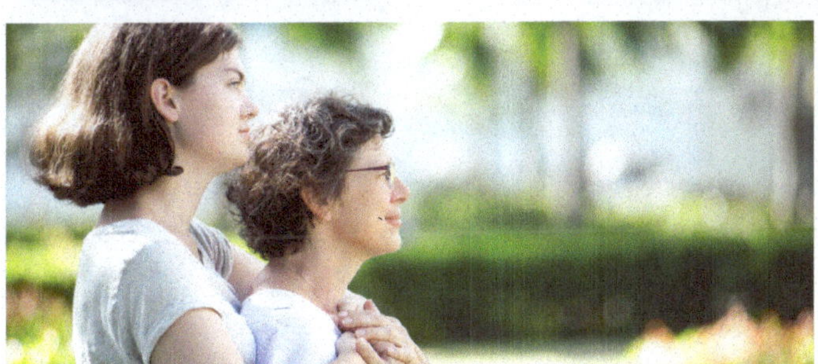

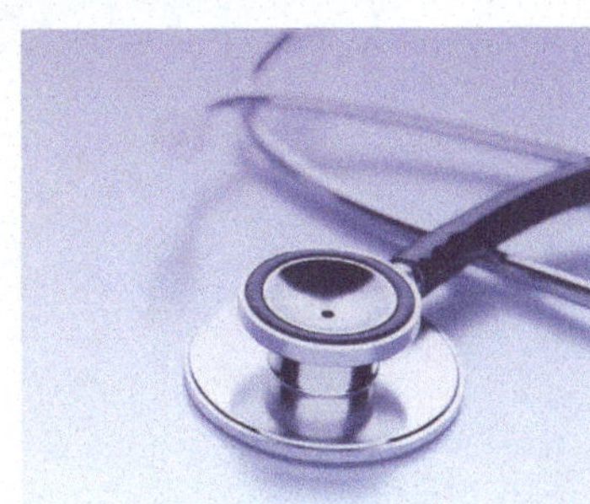

## About this report

*2020 Alzheimer's Disease Facts and Figures* is a statistical resource for U.S. data related to Alzheimer's disease, the most common cause of dementia. Background and context for interpretation of the data are contained in the Overview. Additional sections address prevalence, mortality and morbidity, caregiving and use and costs of health care and services. A Special Report examines primary care physicians' experiences, exposure, training and attitudes in providing dementia care and steps that can be taken to ensure their future readiness for a growing number of Americans living with Alzheimer's and other dementias.

Alzheimer's Association. 2020 Alzheimer's Disease Facts and Figures. Alzheimers Dement 2020;16(3):391+.

### Specific information in this year's *Alzheimer's Disease Facts and Figures* includes:

- Brain changes that occur with Alzheimer's disease (page 5).
- Risk factors for Alzheimer's dementia (page 12).
- Number of Americans with Alzheimer's dementia nationally (page 18) and for each state (page 21).
- Lifetime risk for developing Alzheimer's dementia (page 22).
- Proportion of women and men with Alzheimer's and other dementias (page 22).
- Number of deaths due to Alzheimer's disease nationally (page 27) and for each state (page 29), and death rates by age (page 30).
- Number of family caregivers, hours of care provided, and economic value of unpaid care nationally (page 33) and for each state (page 36).
- The impact of caregiving on caregivers (page 37).
- National cost of care for individuals with Alzheimer's or other dementias, including costs paid by Medicare and Medicaid and costs paid out of pocket (page 46).
- Medicare payments for people with dementia compared with people without dementia (page 47).
- Number of geriatricians needed by state in 2050 (page 65).

The Appendices detail sources and methods used to derive statistics in this report.

When possible, specific information about Alzheimer's is provided; in other cases, the reference may be a more general one of "Alzheimer's or other dementias."

# Contents

### Caregiving



### Use and Costs of Health Care, Long-Term Care and Hospice



### Special Report — On the Front Lines: Primary Care Physicians and Alzheimer's Care in America



### Appendices

# Overview

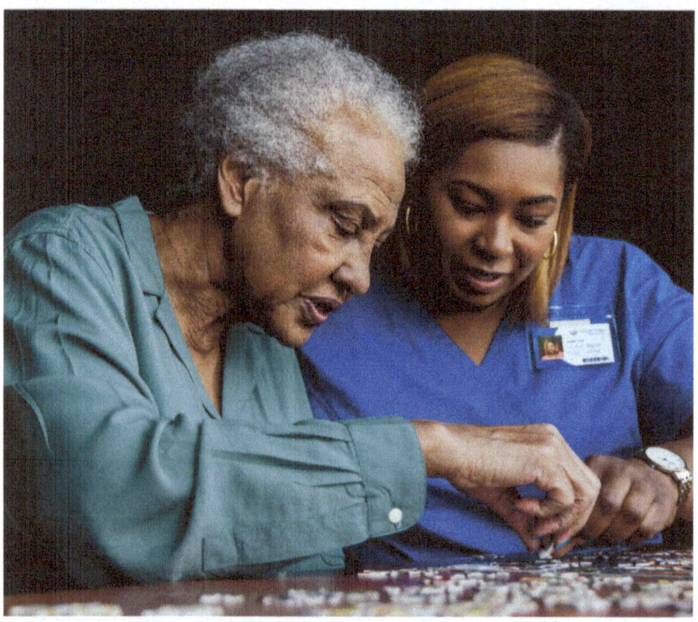

Alzheimer's disease is the most common cause of dementia, accounting for **60% to 80%** of cases.

Alzheimer's disease is a type of brain disease, just as coronary artery disease is a type of heart disease. It is also a degenerative disease, meaning that it becomes worse with time. Alzheimer's disease is thought to begin 20 years or more before symptoms arise,[1-6] with changes in the brain that are unnoticeable to the person affected. Only after years of brain changes do individuals experience noticeable symptoms such as memory loss and language problems. Symptoms occur because nerve cells (neurons) in parts of the brain involved in thinking, learning and memory (cognitive function) have been damaged or destroyed. As the disease progresses, neurons in other parts of the brain are damaged or destroyed. Eventually, nerve cells in parts of the brain that enable a person to carry out basic bodily functions, such as walking and swallowing, are affected. Individuals become bed-bound and require around-the-clock care. Alzheimer's disease is ultimately fatal.

### Alzheimer's Disease or Dementia?

Many people wonder what the difference is between Alzheimer's disease and dementia.

*Dementia* is an overall term for a particular group of symptoms. The characteristic symptoms of dementia are difficulties with memory, language, problem-solving and other thinking skills that affect a person's ability to perform everyday activities. Dementia has many causes (see Table 1, page 6). *Alzheimer's disease* is the most common cause of dementia.

## Brain Changes Associated with Alzheimer's Disease

A healthy adult brain has about 100 billion neurons, each with long, branching extensions. These extensions enable individual neurons to form connections with other neurons. At such connections, called synapses, information flows in tiny bursts of chemicals that are released by one neuron and detected by another neuron. The brain contains about 100 trillion synapses. They allow signals to travel rapidly through the brain's neuronal circuits, creating the cellular basis of memories, thoughts, sensations, emotions, movements and skills.

The accumulation of the protein fragment beta-amyloid (called beta-amyloid plaques) *outside* neurons and the accumulation of an abnormal form of the protein tau (called tau tangles) *inside* neurons are two of several brain changes associated with Alzheimer's.

Plaques and smaller accumulations of beta-amyloid called oligomers may contribute to the damage and death of neurons (neurodegeneration) by interfering with neuron-to-neuron communication at synapses. Tau tangles block the transport of nutrients and other essential molecules inside neurons. Although the complete sequence of events is unclear, beta-amyloid may begin accumulating before abnormal tau, and increasing beta-amyloid accumulation is associated with subsequent increases in tau.[7-8]

Other brain changes include inflammation and atrophy. The presence of toxic beta-amyloid and tau proteins are believed to activate immune system cells in the brain called microglia. Microglia try to clear the toxic proteins as well as widespread debris from dead and dying cells. Chronic inflammation may set in when the microglia can't keep up with all that needs to be cleared. Atrophy, or shrinkage, of the brain occurs because of cell loss. Normal brain function is further compromised in Alzheimer's disease by decreases in the brain's ability to metabolize glucose, its main fuel.

A study[5] of people with rare genetic mutations that cause Alzheimer's found that levels of beta-amyloid in the brain were significantly increased starting 22 years before symptoms were expected to develop (individuals with these genetic mutations usually develop symptoms at the same or nearly the same age as their parent with Alzheimer's). Glucose metabolism began to decrease 18 years before expected symptom onset, and brain atrophy began 13 years before expected symptom onset.

TABLE 1

Common Causes of Dementia and Associated Characteristics

| Cause | Characteristics |
|---|---|
| **Alzheimer's disease** | Alzheimer's disease is the most common cause of dementia, accounting for an estimated 60% to 80% of cases. Recent large autopsy studies show that more than half of individuals with Alzheimer's dementia have Alzheimer's disease brain changes (pathology) as well as the brain changes of one or more other causes of dementia, such as cerebrovascular disease or Lewy body disease. This is called mixed pathologies, and if recognized during life is called mixed dementia.<br><br>Difficulty remembering recent conversations, names or events is often an early clinical symptom; apathy and depression are also often early symptoms. Later symptoms include impaired communication, disorientation, confusion, poor judgment, behavioral changes and, ultimately, difficulty speaking, swallowing and walking.<br><br>The hallmark pathologies of Alzheimer's disease are the accumulation of the protein fragment beta-amyloid (plaques) *outside* neurons in the brain and twisted strands of the protein tau (tangles) *inside* neurons. These changes are accompanied by the death of neurons and damage to brain tissue. Alzheimer's is a slowly progressive brain disease that begins many years before symptoms emerge. |
| **Cerebrovascular disease** | Cerebrovascular disease refers to the process by which blood vessels in the brain are damaged and/or brain tissue is injured from not receiving enough blood, oxygen or nutrients. People with dementia whose brains show evidence of cerebrovascular disease are said to have vascular dementia. About 5% to 10% of individuals with dementia show evidence of vascular dementia alone.[9-10] However, it is more common as a mixed pathology, with most people living with dementia showing the brain changes of cerebrovascular disease and Alzheimer's disease.<br><br>Impaired judgment or impaired ability to make decisions, plan or organize may be the initial symptom, but memory may also be affected, especially when the brain changes of other causes of dementia are present. In addition to changes in cognitive function, people with vascular dementia commonly have difficulty with motor function, especially slow gait and poor balance.<br><br>Vascular dementia occurs most commonly from blood vessel blockage or damage leading to areas of dead tissue or bleeding in the brain. The location, number and size of the brain injuries determine whether dementia will result and how the individual's thinking and physical functioning will be affected. |
| **Lewy body disease** | Lewy bodies are abnormal aggregations (or clumps) of the protein alpha-synuclein in neurons. When they develop in a part of the brain called the cortex, dementia (called dementia with Lewy bodies or DLB) can result. People with DLB have some of the symptoms common in Alzheimer's, but are more likely to have initial or early symptoms of sleep disturbances, well-formed visual hallucinations and visuospatial impairment. These symptoms may occur in the absence of significant memory impairment but memory loss often occurs, especially when the brain changes of other causes of dementia are present.<br><br>About 5% of individuals with dementia show evidence of DLB alone, but most people with DLB also have Alzheimer's disease pathology. |
| **Fronto-temporal lobar degeneration (FTLD)** | FTLD includes dementias such as behavioral-variant FTLD, primary progressive aphasia, Pick's disease, corticobasal degeneration and progressive supranuclear palsy.<br><br>Typical early symptoms include marked changes in personality and behavior and/or difficulty with producing or comprehending language. Unlike Alzheimer's, memory is typically spared in the early stages of disease.<br><br>Nerve cells in the front (frontal lobe) and side regions (temporal lobes) of the brain are especially affected, and these regions become markedly atrophied (shrunken). In addition, the upper layers of the cortex typically become soft and spongy and have abnormal protein inclusions (usually tau protein or the transactive response DNA-binding protein, TDP-43).<br><br>The symptoms of FTLD may occur in those age 65 years and older, similar to Alzheimer's, but most people with FTLD develop symptoms at a younger age. About 60 percent of people with FTLD are ages 45 to 60.[11] Scientists think that FTLD is the most common cause of dementia in people younger than 60.[11] In a systematic review, FTLD accounted for about 3% of dementia cases in studies that included people 65 and older and about 10% of dementia cases in studies restricted to those younger than 65.[12] |

TABLE 1 (cont.)

Common Causes of Dementia and Associated Characteristics

| Cause | Characteristics |
|---|---|
| Parkinson's disease (PD) | Problems with movement (slowness, rigidity, tremor and changes in gait) are common symptoms of PD. Cognitive symptoms develop either just before movement symptoms or later in the disease.<br>In PD, alpha-synuclein aggregates appear in an area deep in the brain called the substantia nigra. The aggregates are thought to cause degeneration of the nerve cells that produce dopamine.[13]<br>As PD progresses, it often results in dementia secondary to the accumulation of alpha-synuclein in the cortex (similar to dementia with Lewy bodies). |
| Hippocampal sclerosis (HS) | HS is the hardening of tissue in the hippocampus of the brain. The hippocampus plays a key role in forming memories. The most pronounced symptom of HS is memory loss, and individuals may be misdiagnosed as having Alzheimer's disease.<br>HS brain changes are often accompanied by accumulations of a misfolded form of a protein called TDP-43.<br>HS is a common cause of dementia in the "oldest-old," individuals age 85 or older. |
| Mixed pathologies | When an individual shows the brain changes of more than one cause of dementia, mixed pathologies are considered the cause. When these pathologies result in dementia symptoms during life, the person is said to have mixed dementia.<br>Studies suggest that mixed dementia is more common than previously recognized, with more than 50% of people with dementia who were studied at Alzheimer's Disease Centers having pathologic evidence of more than one cause of dementia.[10] In community-based studies, the percentage of mixed dementia cases is considerably higher.[9] The likelihood of having mixed dementia increases with age and is highest in people age 85 or older.[14-15] |

It is critical to note that while the field of Alzheimer's research has made great gains over the years in understanding the brain changes associated with the disease and how the disease progresses, much of the research to date has not included sufficient numbers of blacks/African Americans, Hispanics/Latinos, Asian Americans/Pacific Islanders and Native Americans to be representative of the U.S. population. Moreover, because some studies[16-19] find blacks/African Americans and Hispanics/Latinos to be at increased risk for Alzheimer's, the underrepresentation of these populations hampers the conduct of rigorous research to understand these health disparities. Additional research involving individuals from underrepresented ethnic and racial groups is necessary to gain a comprehensive understanding of Alzheimer's disease.

## Alzheimer's Disease Continuum

The progression of Alzheimer's disease from brain changes that are unnoticeable to the person affected to brain changes that cause problems with memory and eventually physical disability is called the Alzheimer's disease continuum.

On this continuum, there are three broad phases: preclinical Alzheimer's disease, mild cognitive impairment (MCI) due to Alzheimer's disease and dementia due to Alzheimer's disease (see Figure 1).[20-23] The Alzheimer's dementia phase is further broken down into the stages of mild, moderate and severe, which reflect the degree to which symptoms interfere with one's ability to carry out everyday activities.

While we know the continuum starts with preclinical Alzheimer's and ends with severe Alzheimer's dementia, how long individuals spend in each part of the continuum varies. The length of each phase of the continuum is influenced by age, genetics, gender and other factors.[24]

### Preclinical Alzheimer's Disease

In this phase, individuals have measurable brain changes that indicate the earliest signs of Alzheimer's disease (biomarkers), but they have not yet developed symptoms such as memory loss. Examples of measurable brain changes include abnormal levels of beta-amyloid as shown on positron emission tomography (PET) scans and in analysis of cerebrospinal fluid (CSF), and decreased metabolism of glucose as shown on PET scans. When the early changes of Alzheimer's occur, the brain compensates for them, enabling individuals to continue to function normally.

FIGURE 1

Alzheimer's Disease (AD) Continuum

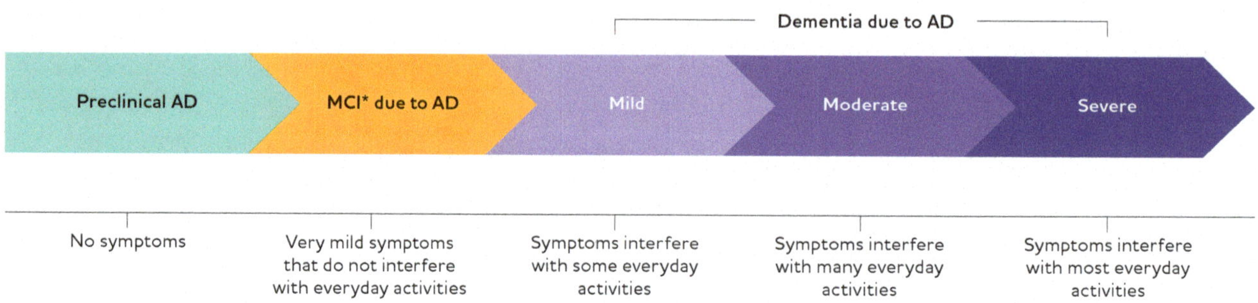


*Mild cognitive impairment

While research settings have the tools and expertise to identify some of the early brain changes of Alzheimer's, additional research is needed to fine-tune the tools' accuracy before they become available for widespread use in hospitals, doctors' offices and other clinical settings. It is important to note that not all individuals with evidence of Alzheimer's-related brain changes go on to develop symptoms of MCI or dementia due to Alzheimer's.[25-26] For example, some individuals have beta-amyloid plaques at death but did not have memory or thinking problems in life.

### MCI Due to Alzheimer's Disease

People with MCI due to Alzheimer's disease have biomarker evidence of Alzheimer's brain changes (for example, abnormal levels of beta-amyloid) plus subtle problems with memory and thinking. These cognitive problems may be noticeable to family members and friends, but not to others, and they do not interfere with individuals' ability to carry out everyday activities. The mild changes in thinking abilities occur when the brain can no longer compensate for the damage and death of nerve cells caused by Alzheimer's disease.

Among those with MCI, one analysis found that after 2 years' follow-up, 15% of individuals older than 65 had developed dementia.[27] Another study found that 32% of individuals with MCI developed Alzheimer's dementia within 5 years' follow-up.[28] A third study found that among individuals with MCI who were tracked for 5 years or longer, 38% developed dementia.[29] However, in some individuals MCI reverts to normal cognition or remains stable. In other cases, such as when a medication inadvertently causes cognitive changes, MCI is mistakenly diagnosed and cognitive changes can be reversed with medication changes. Identifying which individuals with MCI are more likely to develop Alzheimer's or other dementias is a major goal of current research.

### Dementia Due to Alzheimer's Disease

Dementia due to Alzheimer's disease is characterized by noticeable memory, thinking or behavioral symptoms that impair a person's ability to function in daily life, along with evidence of Alzheimer's-related brain changes. Individuals with Alzheimer's dementia experience multiple symptoms that change over a period of years. These symptoms reflect the degree of damage to nerve cells in different parts of the brain. The pace at which symptoms of dementia advance from mild to moderate to severe differs from person to person.

#### *Mild Alzheimer's Dementia*

In the mild stage of Alzheimer's dementia, most people are able to function independently in many areas but are likely to require assistance with some activities to maximize independence and remain safe. They may still be able to drive, work and participate in favorite activities.

#### Moderate Alzheimer's Dementia

In the moderate stage of Alzheimer's dementia, which is often the longest stage, individuals may have difficulties communicating and performing routine tasks, including activities of daily living (such as bathing and dressing); become incontinent at times; and start having personality and behavioral changes, including suspiciousness and agitation.

#### *Severe Alzheimer's Dementia*

In the severe stage of Alzheimer's dementia, individuals need help with activities of daily living and are likely to require around-the-clock care. The effects of Alzheimer's disease on individuals' physical health become especially apparent in this stage. Because of damage to areas of the brain involved in movement, individuals become bed-bound. Being bed-bound makes them vulnerable to conditions including blood clots, skin infections and sepsis, which triggers body-wide inflammation that can result in organ failure. Damage to areas of the brain that control swallowing makes it difficult to eat and drink. This can result in individuals swallowing food into the trachea (windpipe) instead of the esophagus (food pipe). Because of this, food particles may be deposited in the lungs and cause lung infection. This type of infection is called aspiration pneumonia, and it is a contributing cause of death among many individuals with Alzheimer's (see Mortality and Morbidity section, page 26).

### When Dementia-Like Symptoms Are Not Dementia

It is important to note that some individuals have dementia-like symptoms without the progressive brain changes of Alzheimer's or other degenerative brain diseases. Causes of dementia-like symptoms include depression, untreated sleep apnea, delirium, side effects of medications, Lyme disease, thyroid problems, certain vitamin deficiencies and excessive alcohol consumption. Unlike Alzheimer's and other dementias, these conditions often may be reversed with treatment. Consulting a medical professional to determine the cause of symptoms is critical to one's physical and emotional well-being.

The differences between normal age-related cognitive changes and the cognitive changes of Alzheimer's dementia can be subtle (see Table 2, page 10). People experiencing cognitive changes should seek medical help to determine if the changes are normal for one's age, reversible or a symptom of Alzheimer's or another dementia. The Medicare Annual Wellness Visit, which includes a cognitive evaluation, is an opportune time for individuals age 65 or older to discuss cognitive changes with their physician.

## Diagnosis of Dementia Due to Alzheimer's Disease

There is no single test for dementia due to Alzheimer's disease. Instead, physicians (often with the help of specialists such as neurologists, neuropsychologists, geriatricians and geriatric psychiatrists) use a variety of approaches and tools to help make a diagnosis. They include the following:

- Obtaining a medical and family history from the individual, including psychiatric history and history of cognitive and behavioral changes.
- Asking a family member to provide input about changes in thinking skills and behavior.
- Conducting problem-solving, memory and other cognitive tests, as well as physical and neurologic examinations.
- Having the individual undergo blood tests and brain imaging to rule out other potential causes of dementia symptoms, such as a tumor or certain vitamin deficiencies.
- In some circumstances, using PET imaging of the brain to find out if the individual has high levels of beta-amyloid, a hallmark of Alzheimer's; normal levels would suggest Alzheimer's is not the cause of dementia.[30]
- In some circumstances, using lumbar puncture to determine the levels of beta-amyloid and certain types of tau in CSF; normal levels would suggest Alzheimer's is not the cause of dementia.[31]

Although physicians can almost always determine if a person has dementia, it may be difficult to identify the exact cause. Alzheimer's disease is the most common cause of dementia, but there are other causes as well.[32-33] As shown in Table 1 (see page 6), different causes of dementia are associated with distinct symptom patterns and brain abnormalities. Many people with dementia have brain changes associated with more than one cause of dementia.[9,34-38] This is called mixed dementia. Some studies[9-10] report that the majority of people with the brain changes of Alzheimer's also have the brain changes of a second cause of dementia on autopsy.

As discussed in the Prevalence section (see page 17), many individuals who would meet the diagnostic criteria for Alzheimer's and other dementias are not diagnosed by a physician,[39-42] and fewer than half of Medicare beneficiaries who have a diagnosis of Alzheimer's or another dementia in their Medicare billing records report (or their caregiver reports, if the beneficiary's cognitive impairment prevented him or her from responding) being told of the diagnosis.[43-46] It is important that individuals who are living with dementia receive a diagnosis and are aware of the diagnosis. It is also important that individuals receive an *accurate* diagnosis to ensure they receive treatment or follow-up care appropriate to their specific cause of dementia.

## Treatment of Alzheimer's Dementia

### Pharmacologic Treatment

None of the pharmacologic treatments (medications) available today for Alzheimer's dementia slow or stop the damage and destruction of neurons that cause Alzheimer's symptoms and make the disease fatal. The U.S. Food and Drug Administration (FDA) has approved five drugs for the treatment of Alzheimer's — rivastigmine, galantamine, donepezil, memantine, and memantine combined with donepezil. With the exception of memantine, these drugs temporarily improve cognitive symptoms by increasing the amount of chemicals called neurotransmitters in the brain. Memantine blocks certain receptors in the brain from excess stimulation that can damage nerve cells. The effectiveness of these drugs varies from person to person and is limited in duration.

## TABLE 2

**Signs of Alzheimer's or Other Dementias Compared with Typical Age-Related Changes***

| Signs of Alzheimer's or Other Dementias | Typical Age-Related Changes |
|---|---|
| **Memory loss that disrupts daily life:** One of the most common signs of Alzheimer's is memory loss, especially forgetting recently learned information. Others include forgetting important dates or events, asking for the same information over and over, and increasingly needing to rely on memory aids (for example, reminder notes or electronic devices) or family members for things that used to be handled on one's own. | Sometimes forgetting names or appointments, but remembering them later. |
| **Challenges in planning or solving problems:** Some people experience changes in their ability to develop and follow a plan or work with numbers. They may have trouble following a familiar recipe, keeping track of monthly bills or counting change. They may have difficulty concentrating and take much longer to do things than they did before. | Making occasional errors when balancing a checkbook. |
| **Difficulty completing familiar tasks at home, at work or at leisure:** People with Alzheimer's often find it hard to complete daily tasks. Sometimes, people have trouble driving to a familiar location, managing a budget at work or remembering the rules of a favorite game. | Occasionally needing help to use the settings on a microwave or record a television show. |
| **Confusion with time or place:** People with Alzheimer's can lose track of dates, seasons and the passage of time. They may have trouble understanding something if it is not happening immediately. Sometimes they forget where they are or how they got there. | Getting confused about the day of the week but figuring it out later. |
| **Trouble understanding visual images and spatial relationships:** For some people, having vision problems is a sign of Alzheimer's. They may have difficulty reading, judging distance and determining color or contrast, which may cause problems with driving. | Vision changes related to cataracts, glaucoma or age-related macular degeneration. |
| **New problems with words in speaking or writing:** People with Alzheimer's may have trouble following or joining a conversation. They may stop in the middle of a conversation and have no idea how to continue or they may repeat themselves. They may struggle with vocabulary, have problems finding the right word or call things by the wrong name (e.g., calling a watch a "hand clock"). | Sometimes having trouble finding the right word. |
| **Misplacing things and losing the ability to retrace steps:** People with Alzheimer's may put things in unusual places, and lose things and be unable to go back over their steps to find them again. Sometimes, they accuse others of stealing. This may occur more frequently over time. | Misplacing things from time to time and retracing steps to find them. |
| **Decreased or poor judgment:** People with Alzheimer's may experience changes in judgment or decision-making. For example, they may use poor judgment when dealing with money, giving large amounts to telemarketers. They may pay less attention to grooming or keeping themselves clean. | Making a bad decision once in a while. |
| **Withdrawal from work or social activities:** People with Alzheimer's may start to remove themselves from hobbies, social activities, work projects or sports. They may have trouble keeping up with a favorite sports team or remembering how to complete a favorite hobby. They may also avoid being social because of the changes they have experienced. | Sometimes feeling weary of work, family and social obligations. |
| **Changes in mood and personality:** The mood and personalities of people with Alzheimer's can change. They can become confused, suspicious, depressed, fearful or anxious. They may be easily upset at home, at work, with friends or in places where they are out of their comfort zones. | Developing very specific ways of doing things and becoming irritable when a routine is disrupted. |

*For more information about the symptoms of Alzheimer's, visit alz.org/10signs.

No drugs are specifically approved by the FDA to treat behavioral and psychiatric symptoms that may develop in the moderate and severe stages of Alzheimer's dementia. If non-pharmacologic therapy is not successful and these symptoms have the potential to cause harm to the individual or others, physicians may prescribe medications approved for similar symptoms in people with other conditions. A type of medication called antipsychotics may be prescribed to treat hallucinations, aggression and agitation. However, research has shown that some antipsychotics are associated with an increased risk of stroke and death in individuals with dementia.[47-48] The decision to use antipsychotics must be considered with extreme caution. The FDA has ordered manufacturers to label such drugs with a "black box warning" about their risks and a reminder that they are not approved to treat dementia symptoms.

Many factors contribute to the difficulty of developing effective treatments for Alzheimer's. These factors include the slow pace of recruiting sufficient numbers of participants and sufficiently diverse participants to clinical studies, gaps in knowledge about the precise molecular changes and biological processes in the brain that cause Alzheimer's disease, and the relatively long time needed to observe whether an investigational treatment affects disease progression.

Researchers believe that future treatments to slow or stop the progression of Alzheimer's disease and preserve brain function may be most effective when administered early in the disease continuum, either at the MCI due to Alzheimer's or preclinical Alzheimer's phase. Biomarker tests will be essential to identify which individuals are in these phases of the continuum and should receive treatments when they are available. Biomarkers also will be critical for monitoring the effects of treatment. Biomarker tests are already playing an important role in drug development because they enable researchers to recruit into clinical trials only those individuals with the Alzheimer's brain changes that a drug has been designed to affect.[49] The most effective biomarker test or combination of tests may differ depending on where the individual is on the disease continuum and other factors.[50]

### Non-Pharmacologic Therapy

Non-pharmacologic therapies are those that do not involve medication. They are often used for people with Alzheimer's dementia with the goal of maintaining or improving cognitive function, overall quality of life or the ability to perform activities of daily living. They also may be used with the goal of reducing behavioral symptoms such as depression, apathy, wandering, sleep disturbances, agitation and aggression. A recent review and analysis of non-pharmacologic treatments for agitation and aggression in people with dementia concluded that non-pharmacologic interventions seemed to be more effective than pharmacologic interventions for reducing aggression and agitation.[51] Examples include computerized memory training, listening to favorite music as a way to stir recall, and using special lighting to lessen sleep disorders. As with current pharmacologic therapies, non-pharmacologic therapies do not slow or stop the damage and destruction of neurons that cause Alzheimer's symptoms and make the disease fatal.

Determining the effectiveness of non-pharmacologic therapies can be difficult because of the large number of unique therapies tested; the diversity of therapeutic aims (from improved overall quality of life to improvements in specific symptoms); the diverse dementia stages represented (from mild to moderate to severe); the diverse types of dementia that may be present among participants in a particular study given the pervasiveness of mixed dementia; and the lack of a standard method for carrying out any individual therapy. With these multiple factors to consider, it is challenging to group together and compare non-pharmacologic therapies.

Nevertheless, researchers have pooled data from multiple studies of non-pharmacologic therapies to provide insight into their potential effectiveness.

- A meta-analysis[52] found that aerobic exercise and a combination of aerobic and non-aerobic exercise had positive effects on cognitive function in people living with Alzheimer's dementia. A systematic review[53] found that exercise has a positive effect on overall cognitive function and may slow the rate of cognitive decline in people with Alzheimer's dementia.
- A systematic review[54] found that cognitive stimulation had beneficial effects on cognitive function and some aspects of well-being in people with Alzheimer's dementia. Another systematic review[55] reported that cognitive stimulation was associated with improved scores on tests of depression in people with mild-to-moderate Alzheimer's dementia. A 2019 summary[56] of systematic reviews reported that cognitive stimulation, music-based therapies and psychological treatment (for example, cognitive behavioral therapy) improved depression, anxiety and quality of life in people with dementia.
- A 2019 summary of systematic reviews[57] of cognitive training for people with mild-to-moderate dementia found cognitive training may show some benefits in overall cognition that may last for at least a few months.

## Active Management of Alzheimer's Dementia

Studies have consistently shown that active management of Alzheimer's and other dementias can improve the quality of life of affected individuals and their caregivers.[58-60] Active management includes:

- Appropriate use of available treatment options.
- Effective management of coexisting conditions.
- Providing family caregivers with effective training in managing the day-to-day life of the care recipient.
- Coordination of care among physicians, other health care professionals and lay caregivers.
- Participation in activities that are meaningful to the individual with dementia and bring purpose to his or her life.
- Having opportunities to connect with others living with dementia; support groups and supportive services are examples of such opportunities.
- Becoming educated about the disease.
- Planning for the future.

To learn more about Alzheimer's disease, as well as practical information for living with Alzheimer's and being a caregiver, visit alz.org.

## Risk Factors for Alzheimer's Dementia

The vast majority of people who develop Alzheimer's dementia are age 65 or older. This is called late-onset Alzheimer's. Experts believe that Alzheimer's, like other common chronic diseases, develops as a result of multiple factors rather than a single cause. Exceptions are cases of Alzheimer's related to uncommon genetic changes that increase risk (see page 15).

### Age, Genetics and Family History

The greatest risk factors for late-onset Alzheimer's are older age,[61-62] genetics[63-64] and having a family history of Alzheimer's.[65-68]

#### *Age*

Age is the greatest of these three risk factors. As noted in the Prevalence section (see page 17), the percentage of people with Alzheimer's dementia increases dramatically with age: 3% of people age 65-74, 17% of people age 75-84 and 32% of people age 85 or older have Alzheimer's dementia.[62] It is important to note that Alzheimer's dementia is not a normal part of aging,[69] and older age alone is not sufficient to cause Alzheimer's dementia.

#### *Genetics*

Researchers have found several genes that increase the risk of Alzheimer's. The apolipoprotein-e4 (APOE-e4) gene is the gene with the strongest impact on risk of late-onset Alzheimer's. APOE-e4 provides the blueprint for a protein that transports cholesterol in the bloodstream. Everyone inherits one of three forms (alleles) of the APOE gene — e2, e3 or e4 — from each parent, resulting in six possible APOE pairs: e2/e2, e2/e3, e2/e4, e3/e3, e3/e4 and e4/e4. Researchers have found differences in the frequency of these pairs in different racial and ethnic groups. For example, data show that a higher percentage of blacks/African Americans than European Americans have at least one copy of the e4 allele (see Table 3).[70-72]

TABLE 3

**Percentage of Blacks/African Americans and European Americans with Specified APOE Pairs**

| APOE Pair | Blacks/African Americans* | European Americans |
|---|---|---|
| e3/e3 | 45.2 | 63.4 |
| e3/e4 | 28.6 | 21.4 |
| e3/e2 | 15.1 | 10.2 |
| e2/e4 | 5.7 | 2.4 |
| e4/e4 | 4.5 | 2.4 |
| e2/e2 | 0.7 | 0.2 |

Created from data from Rajan et al.[70]

*Percentages do not total 100 due to rounding.

Having the e4 form of APOE increases one's risk of developing Alzheimer's compared with having the e3 form, but does not guarantee that an individual will develop Alzheimer's. Having the e2 form may decrease one's risk compared with having the e3 form. Those who inherit one copy of the e4 form have about three times the risk of developing Alzheimer's compared with those with two copies of the e3 form, while those who inherit two copies of the e4 form have an eight- to 12-fold risk.[73-75] In addition, those with the e4 form are more likely to have beta-amyloid accumulation[76] and Alzheimer's dementia at a younger age than those with the e2 or e3 forms of the APOE gene.[77] A meta-analysis including 20 published articles describing the frequency of the e4 form among people in the United States who had been diagnosed with Alzheimer's found that 56% had one copy of the APOE-e4 gene, and 11% had two copies of the APOE-e4 gene.[78] Another study found that among 1,770 diagnosed individuals from 26 Alzheimer's Disease Centers across the United States, 65% had at least one copy of the APOE-e4 gene.[79]

However, studies of Alzheimer's risk based on APOE status among blacks/African Americans have had inconsistent results. For example, some have found that having the e4 allele did not increase risk among blacks/ African Americans,[71-72,80] while other studies have found that it significantly increased risk.[81-82] More research is needed to better understand the genetic mechanisms involved in Alzheimer's risk among different racial and ethnic groups.

***Family History***
A family history of Alzheimer's is not necessary for an individual to develop the disease. However, individuals who have a parent or sibling (first-degree relative) with Alzheimer's dementia are more likely to develop the disease than those who do not have a first-degree relative with Alzheimer's.[65,73] Those who have more than one first-degree relative with Alzheimer's are at even higher risk.[68] A large, population-based study found that having a parent with dementia increases risk independent of known genetic risk factors such as APOE-e4.[83] When diseases run in families, heredity (genetics) and shared non-genetic factors (for example, access to healthy foods and habits related to physical activity) may play a role.

### Modifiable Risk Factors
Although age, genetics and family history cannot be changed, other risk factors can be changed or modified to reduce the risk of cognitive decline and dementia.

In 2019, the World Health Organization (WHO) published recommendations[84] to reduce risk of cognitive decline and dementia. WHO strongly recommends physical activity, quitting smoking, and managing hypertension and diabetes to reduce the risk of cognitive decline and dementia. A report[85] evaluating the state of the evidence on the effects of modifiable risk factors on cognitive decline and dementia concluded that there is sufficiently strong evidence, from a population-based perspective, that regular physical activity and management of cardiovascular risk factors (especially diabetes, obesity, smoking and hypertension) is associated with reduced risk of cognitive decline and may be associated with reduced risk of dementia. It also concluded that there is sufficiently strong evidence that a healthy diet, lifelong learning and cognitive training are associated with reduced risk of cognitive decline. A report from the National Academy of Medicine (formerly the Institute of Medicine) examined the evidence regarding modifiable risk factors for cognitive decline and reached similar conclusions.[86] More research is needed to understand the biological mechanisms by which these factors reduce risk.

It is important to note that "reducing risk" of cognitive decline and dementia is not synonymous with preventing cognitive decline and dementia. Individuals who take measures to reduce risk may still develop dementia, but may be less likely to develop it, or may develop it later in life than they would have if they had not taken steps to reduce their risk. It is also important to note that factors that increase or decrease the risk of cognitive decline and dementia may not necessarily do so by directly affecting the brain changes associated with Alzheimer's disease.[80] For example, it is possible that smoking may contribute to cerebrovascular disease, which in turn increases the risk of dementia, but it may not directly contribute to the development of the amyloid plaques and tau tangles that characterize Alzheimer's disease.

***Cardiovascular Disease Risk Factors***
Brain health is affected by the health of the heart and blood vessels. Although it makes up just 2% of body weight, the brain consumes 20% of the body's oxygen and energy supplies.[87] A healthy heart ensures that enough blood is pumped to the brain, while healthy blood vessels enable the oxygen- and nutrient-rich blood to reach the brain so it can function normally.

Many factors that increase the risk of cardiovascular disease are also associated with a higher risk of dementia.[88] These factors include smoking[89-93] and diabetes.[94-97] Some studies propose that impaired glucose processing (a precursor to diabetes) may also result in an increased risk for dementia.[98-100] The age at which some risk factors develop appears to affect dementia risk. For example, midlife obesity,[98,101-104] hypertension,[98,105-109] prehypertension (systolic blood pressure from 120 to 139 mm Hg or diastolic pressure from 80 to 89 mm Hg)[109] and high cholesterol[110-111] are associated with an increased risk of dementia. However, late-life obesity[112] and hypertension onset after age 80[113] are associated with decreased risk of dementia. More research is needed to understand why the effects of some modifiable risk factors may change with age. Regarding blood pressure, there is now evidence from a large-scale clinical trial that intensive medical treatment to reduce blood pressure may safely decrease the occurrence of MCI and dementia in older adults who have hypertension.[114]

Building on the connection between heart health and brain health, researchers have found that factors that protect the heart may also protect the brain and reduce the risk of developing Alzheimer's or other dementias. Physical activity[115-125] appears to be one of these factors. Although researchers have studied a wide variety of exercises, they do not yet know which specific types of exercises, what frequency of exercise or what duration of activity may be most effective in reducing risk. In addition to physical activity, emerging evidence suggests that consuming a heart-healthy diet may be associated with reduced dementia risk.[126-130] A heart-healthy diet emphasizes fruits, vegetables, whole grains, fish, chicken, nuts and legumes while limiting saturated fats, red meat and sugar. A systematic review[131] of the use of supplements, including (but not limited to) vitamins C, D and E, omega-3 fatty acids, and ginkgo biloba, found little to no benefit in preventing cognitive decline, MCI or Alzheimer's dementia.

Researchers have begun studying combinations of health factors and lifestyle behaviors (for example, blood pressure as a health factor and physical activity as a lifestyle behavior) to learn whether combinations of risk factors better identify Alzheimer's and dementia risk than individual risk factors. They are also studying whether intervening on multiple risk factors simultaneously is more effective at reducing risk than addressing a single risk factor. Indeed, one such study,[132] the Finnish Geriatric Intervention Study to Prevent Cognitive Impairment and Disability (FINGER), found that a multidomain lifestyle intervention was associated with beneficial effects on cognitive function in older adults at high risk for cognitive decline and dementia. The success of FINGER has led to the launch of multidomain lifestyle intervention studies in other countries, including the Alzheimer's Association U.S. Study to Protect Brain Health Through Lifestyle Intervention to Reduce Risk (U.S. POINTER).[133]

### *Education*

People with more years of formal education are at lower risk for Alzheimer's and other dementias than those with fewer years of formal education.[71,134-138] Some researchers believe that having more years of education builds "cognitive reserve." Cognitive reserve refers to the brain's ability to make flexible and efficient use of cognitive networks (networks of neuron-to-neuron connections) to enable a person to continue to carry out cognitive tasks despite brain changes[139-140] such as beta-amyloid and tau accumulation. The number of years of formal education is not the only determinant of cognitive reserve. Having a mentally stimulating job and engaging in other mentally stimulating activities may also help build cognitive reserve.[141-144]

A recent study[145] found that individuals with the APOE-e4 risk gene had a decreased risk of developing dementia if they had more years of early life education, had mentally challenging work in midlife, participated in leisure activities in late life, and/or had strong social networks in late life.

It is important to note that the underlying reason for the relationship between formal education and reduced Alzheimer's risk is unclear. It is possible that the generally higher socioeconomic status of individuals with more years of formal education is a protective factor. Having fewer years of formal education is associated with lower socioeconomic status,[146] which may:

- Increase one's likelihood of experiencing poor nutrition.
- Decrease one's ability to afford health care or medical treatments, such as treatments for cardiovascular disease risk factors that are so closely linked to brain health.
- Limit one's access to physically safe housing and employment, which could increase risk of being exposed to substances that are toxic to the nervous system such as air pollution,[147] lead[148] and pesticides.[149]

In addition, people with fewer years of education tend to have more cardiovascular risk factors for Alzheimer's, including being less physically active,[150] having a higher risk of diabetes,[151-153] and being more likely to have hypertension[154] and to smoke.[155]

### *Social and Cognitive Engagement*

Additional studies suggest that remaining socially and mentally active throughout life may support brain health and possibly reduce the risk of Alzheimer's and other dementias.[116,156-167] Remaining socially and mentally active might help build cognitive reserve, but the exact mechanism by which this may occur is unknown. It is possible that the association observed between social and cognitive engagement and reduced dementia risk reflects something else. Specifically, the presence of cognitive impairment could decrease one's interest in and ability to participate in activities involving social and cognitive skills. Therefore, the association may reflect the effect of cognitive impairment on social and cognitive engagement rather than the effect of engagement on dementia risk. More research is needed to better understand how social and cognitive engagement may affect biological processes that influence risk.

*Traumatic Brain Injury (TBI)*
TBI is the disruption of normal brain function caused by a blow or jolt to the head or penetration of the skull by a foreign object. TBI increases the risk of dementia.[168]

According to the Centers for Disease Control and Prevention (CDC), approximately 2.87 million TBI-related emergency department visits, hospitalizations and deaths occurred in 2014, the latest year for which information is available.[169] The leading causes of TBI that resulted in emergency department visits were falls, being struck by an object and motor vehicle crashes.[169]

Two ways to classify the severity of TBI are by the duration of loss of consciousness or post-traumatic amnesia[170] and by the individual's initial score on the 15-point Glasgow Coma Scale.[171]

- *Mild TBI* (also known as a concussion) is characterized by loss of consciousness or post-traumatic amnesia lasting 30 minutes or less, or an initial Glasgow score of 13-15; about 75% of TBIs are mild.[172]
- *Moderate TBI* is characterized by loss of consciousness or post-traumatic amnesia lasting more than 30 minutes but less than 24 hours, or an initial Glasgow score of 9-12.
- *Severe TBI* is characterized by loss of consciousness or post-traumatic amnesia lasting 24 hours or more, or an initial Glasgow score of 8 or less.

The risk of dementia increases with the number of TBIs sustained.[168] Even those who experience mild TBI are at increased risk of dementia compared with those who have not had a TBI. A recent study found that mild TBI is associated with a two-fold increase in the risk of dementia diagnosis.[173] Another study found that people with a history of TBI who develop Alzheimer's do so at a younger age than those without a history of TBI.[174] Whether TBI causes Alzheimer's disease, other conditions that lead to dementia, or both, is still being investigated.

Chronic traumatic encephalopathy (CTE) is a neuropathologic diagnosis (meaning it is characterized by brain changes that can only be identified at autopsy) associated with repeated blows to the head, such as those that may occur while playing contact sports. Among former amateur and professional football players, the risk of developing CTE, which is associated with dementia, increases 30% per year played.[175] Currently, there is no test to determine if someone has CTE-related brain changes during life. A review article indicates that the greatest risk factor for developing CTE-related brain changes is repetitive brain trauma — repeated, forceful blows to the head that do not, individually, result in symptoms.[176] *Like* Alzheimer's disease, CTE is characterized by tangles of an abnormal form of the protein tau in the brain. *Unlike* Alzheimer's, beta-amyloid plaques are uncommon in CTE.[177-178] How the brain changes associated with CTE are linked to cognitive or behavioral changes is unclear.

### Uncommon Genetic Changes That Increase Risk

Certain genetic mutations and the extra copy of chromosome 21 that characterizes Down syndrome are uncommon genetic factors that strongly influence Alzheimer's risk.

*Genetic Mutations*
A small percentage of Alzheimer's cases (an estimated 1% or less)[179] develop as a result of mutations to any of three specific genes. A genetic mutation is an abnormal change in the sequence of chemical pairs that make up genes. These mutations involve the gene for the amyloid precursor protein (APP) and the genes for the presenilin 1 and presenilin 2 proteins. Those inheriting an Alzheimer's mutation to these genes are virtually guaranteed to develop the disease if they live a normal life span.[180] Symptoms tend to develop before age 65, sometimes as young as age 30, while the vast majority of individuals with Alzheimer's have late-onset Alzheimer's.

*Trisomy in Down Syndrome*
In Down syndrome, an individual is born with three copies of chromosome 21 (called trisomy 21) instead of two. People with Down syndrome have an increased risk of developing Alzheimer's, and this is believed to be related to trisomy 21. Chromosome 21 includes the gene that encodes for the production of APP, which in people with Alzheimer's is cut into beta-amyloid fragments that accumulate into plaques. Having an extra copy of chromosome 21 may increase the production of beta-amyloid fragments produced in the brain.

Overall, people with Down syndrome develop Alzheimer's at an earlier age than people without Down syndrome. By age 40, most people with Down syndrome have significant levels of beta-amyloid plaques and tau tangles in their brains.[181] As with all adults, advancing age increases the likelihood that a person with Down syndrome will exhibit symptoms of Alzheimer's. According to the National Down Syndrome Society, about 30% of people with Down syndrome who are in their 50s have Alzheimer's dementia.[58] About 50% of people with Down syndrome who are in their 60s have Alzheimer's dementia.[182]

## Looking to the Future

The identification of biomarkers for Alzheimer's enables early detection of the disease and will accelerate the development of new therapies by ensuring that appropriate people are enrolled in clinical trials. With the discovery that Alzheimer's may begin 20 years or more before the onset of symptoms, a substantial window of time has been opened to intervene in the progression of the disease. In the future, more will be understood about which therapies will be most effective at which points in the Alzheimer's disease continuum.

A fuller understanding of Alzheimer's — from its causes to how to prevent it, how to manage it and how to treat it — depends on other crucial factors. Among these factors is the inclusion of participants from diverse racial and ethnic groups in all realms of Alzheimer's research. Consistent with studies of other top 10 causes of death, studies of Alzheimer's disease in underrepresented ethnic and racial groups are relatively sparse. This reflects the urgent need for current and future research to include increased numbers of blacks/African Americans, Hispanics/Latinos, Asian Americans/Pacific Islanders and Native Americans in clinical trials, observational studies and other investigations so everyone benefits from advances in Alzheimer's science.

# Prevalence

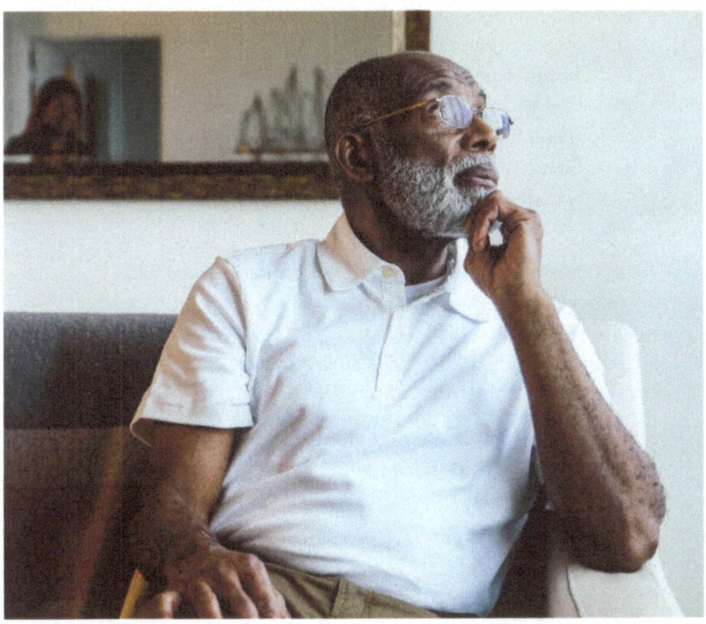

By 2050, the number of people age 65 and older with Alzheimer's dementia is projected to reach 13.8 million.

Millions of Americans have Alzheimer's or other dementias. As the size of the U.S. population age 65 and older continues to increase, the number of Americans with Alzheimer's or other dementias will grow. Both the number and proportion will escalate rapidly in coming years, as the population of Americans age 65 and older is projected to grow from 56 million in 2020 to 88 million by 2050.[183-184] The baby boom generation has already begun to reach age 65 and beyond,[185] the age range of greatest risk of Alzheimer's dementia[186]; in fact, the oldest members of the baby boom generation turn age 74 in 2020.

This section reports on the number and proportion of people with Alzheimer's dementia to describe the magnitude of the burden of Alzheimer's on the community and health care system. The prevalence of Alzheimer's dementia refers to the number and proportion of people in a population who have Alzheimer's dementia at a given point in time. Incidence refers to the number or rate of new cases per year. Estimates from selected studies on the number and proportion of people with Alzheimer's or other dementias vary depending on how each study was conducted. Data from several studies are used in this section.

FIGURE 2

Number and Ages of People 65 or Older with Alzheimer's Dementia, 2020

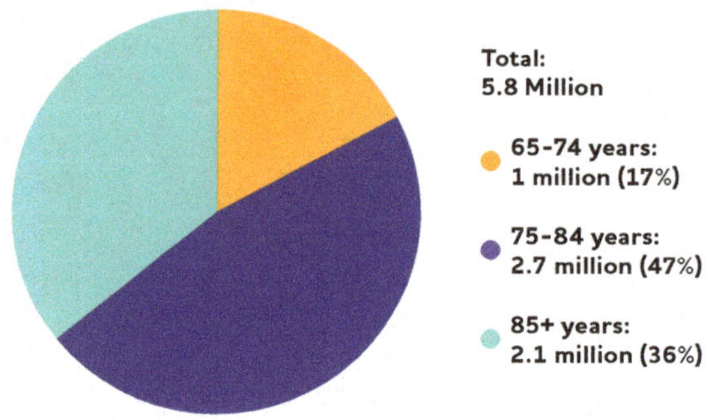


Created from data from Hebert et al.[A2,62]

## Prevalence of Alzheimer's and Other Dementias in the United States

An estimated 5.8 million Americans age 65 and older are living with Alzheimer's dementia in 2020.[A1,62] Eighty percent are age 75 or older (Figure 2).[A2,62]

Out of the total U.S. population:

- One in 10 people (10%) age 65 and older has Alzheimer's dementia.[A3,62,184]
- The percentage of people with Alzheimer's dementia increases with age: 3% of people age 65-74, 17% of people age 75-84, and 32% of people age 85 and older have Alzheimer's dementia.[62] People younger than 65 can also develop Alzheimer's dementia, but it is much less common and prevalence is uncertain.

The estimated number of people age 65 and older with Alzheimer's dementia comes from a study using the latest data from the 2010 U.S. Census and the Chicago Health and Aging Project (CHAP), a population-based study of chronic health conditions of older people.[62]

National estimates of the prevalence of all dementias are not available from CHAP, but they are available from other population-based studies including the Aging, Demographics, and Memory Study (ADAMS), a nationally representative sample of older adults.[A4,187-188] Based on estimates from ADAMS, 14% of people age 71 and older in the United States have dementia.[187]

### Prevalence Estimates

These estimates refer to people who have Alzheimer's dementia based on symptoms such as memory loss and difficulty planning or solving problems. Biomarker-based prevalence estimates could significantly affect the reported number of people with Alzheimer's disease.[189-190] The estimated 5.8 million people with Alzheimer's dementia would be lower, but the total number of people in the continuum of Alzheimer's disease (see page 7) would be higher.

Some individuals now counted as having Alzheimer's dementia may not have the biological brain changes associated with Alzheimer's disease because their diagnosis was based on clinical symptoms rather than confirmed by biomarkers. Both autopsy studies and clinical trials have found that 15% to 30% of individuals who met the criteria for Alzheimer's dementia based on symptoms did not have the required Alzheimer's-related brain changes at death.[9,69,191-193] That is, these individuals had dementia caused by something other than Alzheimer's disease.

At the same time, a biomarker-based prevalence estimate would comprise people throughout the continuum of Alzheimer's disease, including those with mild cognitive impairment (MCI) due to Alzheimer's disease and preclinical Alzheimer's disease who are not counted in current Alzheimer's prevalence estimates, which are limited to those with Alzheimer's dementia.

### Underdiagnosis of Alzheimer's and other Dementias in the Primary Care Setting

Prevalence studies such as CHAP and ADAMS are designed so that everyone in the study undergoes evaluation for dementia. But outside of research settings, a substantial portion of those who would meet the diagnostic criteria for Alzheimer's and other dementias are not diagnosed with dementia by a physician.[39-42] Furthermore, fewer than half of Medicare beneficiaries who have a diagnosis of Alzheimer's or another dementia in their Medicare billing records (or their caregiver, if the beneficiary's cognitive impairment prevented him or her from responding) report being told of the diagnosis.[43-46] Because Alzheimer's dementia is often underdiagnosed — and if it is diagnosed, people are often unaware of their diagnosis — a large portion of Americans with Alzheimer's may not know they have it. A recent survey[194] by the Alzheimer's Association found that on average, primary care physicians inform their patients 92% of the time when cognitive impairment is detected, and 64% of the physicians reported they always inform patients. Of the 36% of surveyed physicians who do not always inform their patients, 73% say it is because it is premature to do so before a full diagnostic workup, and 41% say brief cognitive assessments have high rates of false positives or false negatives.

Since 2011, the Medicare Annual Wellness Visit has included a required cognitive evaluation. The same survey by the Alzheimer's Association found that only one in three older adults were aware that these visits should include a cognitive assessment.[194] Furthermore, while 82% of older adults believe it is important to have their memory and thinking checked, only 16% report having their memory and thinking checked. Most (93%) older adults said they trust their doctor to recommend testing for memory and thinking problems; however, despite 94% of primary care physicians stating that it is important to assess all older patients for cognitive impairment, fewer than half (47%) say it is their standard protocol to do so. The primary reasons given by surveyed physicians for not assessing older patients for cognitive impairment are the patient presents with no symptoms or complaints (68%) and lack of time (58%).

### Prevalence of Subjective Cognitive Decline

The experience of worsening or more frequent confusion or memory loss (often referred to as subjective cognitive decline) is one of the earliest warning signs of Alzheimer's disease and may be a way to identify people who are at high risk of developing Alzheimer's or other dementias as well as MCI.[195-199] Subjective cognitive decline refers to self-perceived worsening of memory and other thinking abilities by an individual, separate from cognitive testing, clinical diagnosis or anyone else noticing. There is a correlation between subjective cognitive decline and worse performance on cognitive tests, as recently reported using data from the National Health and Nutrition Examination Survey, a nationally representative sample of U.S. older adults.[200] Not all of those who experience subjective cognitive decline go on to develop MCI or dementia, but many do.[201-203] One study showed those who over time consistently reported subjective cognitive decline that they found worrisome were at higher risk for developing Alzheimer's dementia.[204] The Behavioral Risk Factor Surveillance System survey, which includes questions on subjective cognitive decline, found that in the United States, 11% of Americans age 45 and older reported subjective cognitive decline, but 54% of those who reported it had not consulted a health care professional.[205] Individuals concerned about declines in memory and other cognitive abilities should consult a health care professional.

FIGURE 3

**Projected Increases Between 2020 and 2025 in Alzheimer's Dementia Prevalence by State**

6.7% - 12% | 12.1% - 17.3% | 17.4% - 22.6% | 22.7% - 27.9% | 28.0% - 33.3%

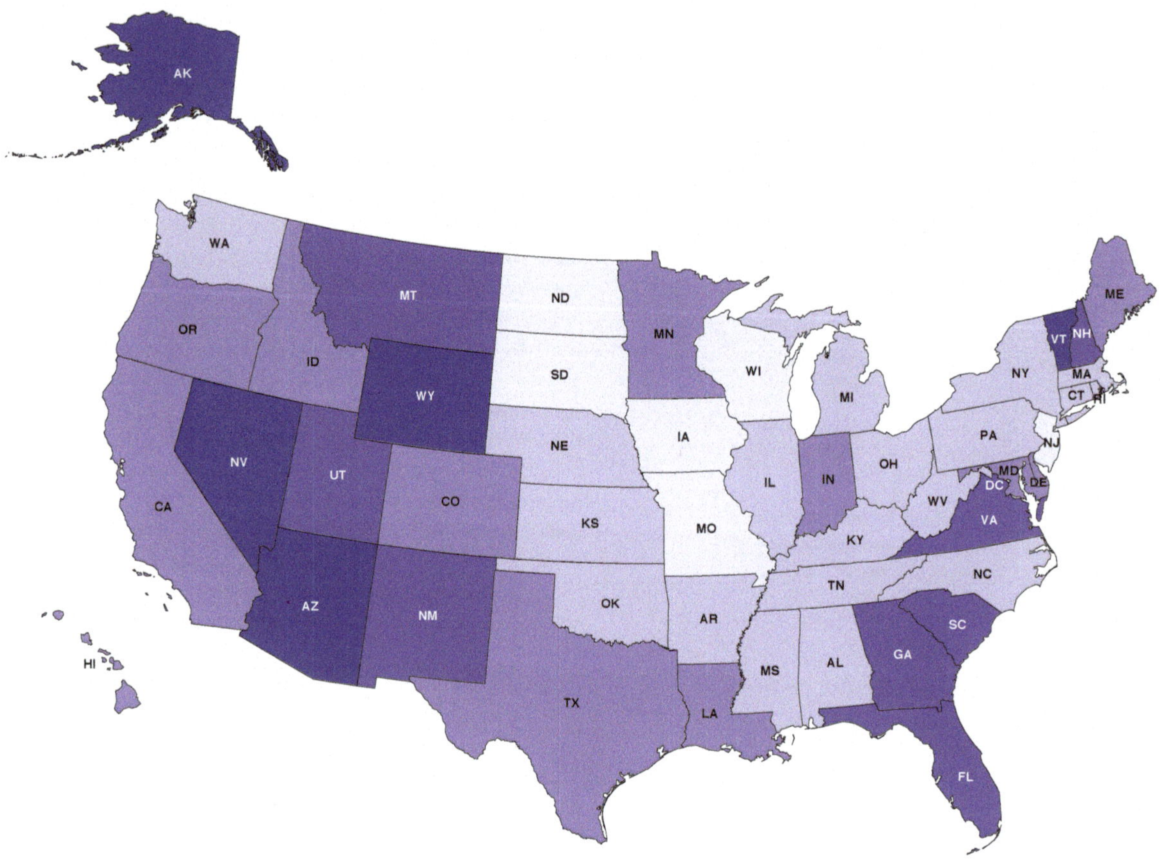


Change from 2020 to 2025 for Washington, D.C.: 1.1%

Created from data provided to the Alzheimer's Association by Weuve et al.[A5,206]

## Estimates of the Number of People with Alzheimer's Dementia by State

Table 4 (see page 21) lists the estimated number of people age 65 and older with Alzheimer's dementia by state for 2020, the projected number for 2025, and the projected percentage change in the number of people with Alzheimer's between 2020 and 2025.[A5,206]

As shown in Figure 3, between 2020 and 2025 every state across the country is expected to experience an increase of at least 6.7% in the number of people with Alzheimer's. These projected increases in the number of people with Alzheimer's are due solely to projected increases in the population age 65 and older in these states. Because risk factors for dementia such as midlife obesity and diabetes can vary dramatically by region and state, the regional patterns of future burden may be different than reported here. Based on these projections, the West and Southeast are expected to experience the largest percentage increases in people with Alzheimer's dementia between 2020 and 2025. These increases will have a marked impact on states' health care systems, as well as the Medicaid program, which covers the costs of long-term care and support for many older residents with dementia, including more than a quarter of Medicare beneficiaries with Alzheimer's or other dementias.[207]

## TABLE 4

**Projections of Total Numbers of Americans Age 65 and Older with Alzheimer's Dementia by State**

| State | Projected Number with Alzheimer's (in thousands) 2020 | 2025 | Percentage Increase 2020-2025 |
|---|---|---|---|
| District of Columbia | 8.9 | 9 | 1.1 |
| Alabama | 96 | 110 | 14.6 |
| Alaska | 8.5 | 11 | 29.4 |
| Arizona | 150 | 200 | 33.3 |
| Arkansas | 58 | 67 | 15.5 |
| California | 690 | 840 | 21.7 |
| Colorado | 76 | 92 | 21.1 |
| Connecticut | 80 | 91 | 13.8 |
| Delaware | 19 | 23 | 21.1 |
| Florida | 580 | 720 | 24.1 |
| Georgia | 150 | 190 | 26.7 |
| Hawaii | 29 | 35 | 20.7 |
| Idaho | 27 | 33 | 22.2 |
| Illinois | 230 | 260 | 13.0 |
| Indiana | 110 | 130 | 18.2 |
| Iowa | 66 | 73 | 10.6 |
| Kansas | 55 | 62 | 12.7 |
| Kentucky | 75 | 86 | 14.7 |
| Louisiana | 92 | 110 | 19.6 |
| Maine | 29 | 35 | 20.7 |
| Maryland | 110 | 130 | 18.2 |
| Massachusetts | 130 | 150 | 15.4 |
| Michigan | 190 | 220 | 15.8 |
| Minnesota | 99 | 120 | 21.2 |
| Mississippi | 57 | 65 | 14.0 |
| Missouri | 120 | 130 | 8.3 |
| Montana | 22 | 27 | 22.7 |
| Nebraska | 35 | 40 | 14.3 |
| Nevada | 49 | 64 | 30.6 |
| New Hampshire | 26 | 32 | 23.1 |
| New Jersey | 190 | 210 | 10.5 |
| New Mexico | 43 | 53 | 23.3 |
| New York | 410 | 460 | 12.2 |
| North Carolina | 180 | 210 | 16.7 |
| North Dakota | 15 | 16 | 6.7 |
| Ohio | 220 | 250 | 13.6 |
| Oklahoma | 67 | 76 | 13.4 |
| Oregon | 69 | 84 | 21.7 |
| Pennsylvania | 280 | 320 | 14.3 |
| Rhode Island | 24 | 27 | 12.5 |
| South Carolina | 95 | 120 | 26.3 |
| South Dakota | 18 | 20 | 11.1 |
| Tennessee | 120 | 140 | 16.7 |
| Texas | 400 | 490 | 22.5 |
| Utah | 34 | 42 | 23.5 |
| Vermont | 13 | 17 | 30.8 |
| Virginia | 150 | 190 | 26.7 |
| Washington | 120 | 140 | 16.7 |
| West Virginia | 39 | 44 | 12.8 |
| Wisconsin | 120 | 130 | 8.3 |
| Wyoming | 10 | 13 | 30.0 |

Created from data provided to the Alzheimer's Association by Weuve et al.[A5,206]

## Incidence of Alzheimer's Dementia

While prevalence refers to *existing* cases of a disease in a population at a given time, incidence refers to *new* cases of a disease that develop in a given period of time in a defined population — in this case, the U.S. population age 65 or older. Incidence provides a measure of risk for developing a disease. According to one study using data from the Established Populations for Epidemiologic Study of the Elderly, approximately 491,000 people age 65 or older will develop Alzheimer's dementia in the United States in 2020.[208] Other studies have arrived at incidence estimates that are much higher. For example, according to CHAP estimates, approximately 910,000 people age 65 or older developed Alzheimer's dementia in the United States in 2011, a number that would be expected to be even higher in 2020 if CHAP estimates were available for that year.[209] A study using data from the Adult Changes in Thought study, a cohort of members of Kaiser Permanente (formerly Group Health), a health care delivery system in the Northwest United States, reported similar incidence rates to the CHAP study.[210] The number of new cases of Alzheimer's increases dramatically with age: according to estimates from CHAP, in 2011 the average annual incidence in people age 65-74 was 0.4% (meaning four of every 1,000 people age 65-74 developed Alzheimer's dementia in 2011); in people age 75-84, the annual incidence was 3.2% (32 of every 1,000 people); and for age 85 and older (the "oldest-old"), the incidence was 7.6% (76 of every 1,000 people).[209] Because of the increasing number of people age 65 and older in the United States, particularly the oldest-old, the annual number of new cases of Alzheimer's and other dementias is projected to double by 2050.[208]

## Lifetime Risk of Alzheimer's Dementia

Lifetime risk is the probability that someone of a given age who does not have a particular condition will develop the condition during his or her remaining life span. Data from the Framingham Heart Study were used to estimate lifetime risks of Alzheimer's dementia by age and sex.[A6,211] As shown in Figure 4, the study found that the estimated lifetime risk for Alzheimer's dementia at age 45 was approximately one in five (20%) for women and one in 10 (10%) for men. The risks for both sexes were slightly higher at age 65.[211]

FIGURE 4

**Estimated Lifetime Risk for Alzheimer's Dementia, by Sex, at Ages 45 and 65**

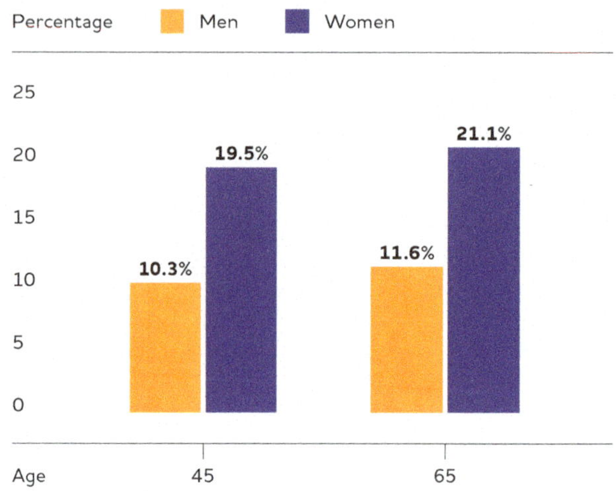


Created from data from Chene et al.[211]

## Differences Between Women and Men in the Prevalence and Risk of Alzheimer's and Other Dementias

More women than men have Alzheimer's or other dementias. Almost two-thirds of Americans with Alzheimer's are women.[A7,62] Of the 5.8 million people age 65 and older with Alzheimer's in the United States, 3.6 million are women and 2.2 million are men.[A7,62] Based on estimates from ADAMS, among people age 71 and older, 16% of women have Alzheimer's or other dementias compared with 11% of men.[187]

The prevailing reason that has been stated for the higher prevalence of Alzheimer's and other dementias in women is that women live longer than men on average, and older age is the greatest risk factor for Alzheimer's.[211-213] But when it comes to differences in the actual risk of developing Alzheimer's or other dementias for men and women of the same age, findings have been mixed. Most studies of incidence in the United States have found no significant difference between men and women in the proportion who develop Alzheimer's or other dementias at any given age.[71,210,213-215] However, some European studies have reported a higher incidence among women at older ages,[216-217] and one study from the United Kingdom reported higher incidence for men.[218] Differences in the risk of dementia between men and women may therefore depend on age and/or geographic region.[219-220]

If there is a difference in the risk of Alzheimer's or other dementias between men and women, there are a number of potential biological and social explanations.[219,221] One explanation may be differences in the distribution of or even the effect of risk factors for dementia between men and women. If women's risk for Alzheimer's or other dementias is higher, it is possible that lower educational attainment in women than in men born in the first half of the 20th century could account for some of the elevated risk, as limited formal education is a risk factor for dementia.[222] This explanation requires more research, but there is evidence that increases in educational attainment over time in the United States — which have been more substantial for women than men — have led to decreased risk for dementia.[223] Interestingly, European studies have found that the relationship of lower education with dementia outcomes may actually be stronger in women than men.[224-225] Some studies have attributed an observed difference in risk for dementia between men and women to differences in health factors. A study using Framingham Heart Study data suggested that men in the study appear to have a lower risk for dementia due to "survival bias," in which the men who survived beyond age 65 and were included in the study were the ones with a healthier cardiovascular risk profile (men have a higher rate of death from cardiovascular disease in middle age than women) and thus a lower risk for dementia.[212] More research is needed to support this interpretation.

Other research is assessing whether the risk of Alzheimer's could actually be higher for women at any given age due to genetic differences or different susceptibility to Alzheimer's pathology.[226] A number of studies have shown that the APOE-e4 genotype, the best known genetic risk factor for Alzheimer's dementia, may have a stronger association with Alzheimer's dementia[227-228] and neurodegeneration[229] in women than in men. However, a recent meta-analysis found no difference between men and women in the association between APOE genotype and Alzheimer's dementia overall, though there was an elevated risk for women with the APOE-e4 genotype at certain age ranges.[230] It is unknown why the APOE gene could convey different risk for women, but some evidence suggests that it may be due to an interaction between the APOE genotype and the sex hormone estrogen.[231-232] Finally, there is some evidence that women show more rapid cognitive decline and neurodegeneration than men despite having similar levels of beta-amyloid and tau, meaning the hallmark proteins of Alzheimer's disease may have more negative effects for women than men.[233-235]

## Racial and Ethnic Differences in the Prevalence of Alzheimer's and Other Dementias

Although there are more non-Hispanic whites living with Alzheimer's and other dementias than any other racial or ethnic group in the United States (because non-Hispanic whites are the largest racial/ethnic group in the country), older blacks/African Americans and Hispanics/Latinos are disproportionately more likely than older whites to have Alzheimer's or other dementias.[16-17,236-239] Most studies indicate that older blacks/African Americans are about twice as likely to have Alzheimer's or other dementias as older whites.[18-19,209] Some studies indicate older Hispanics/Latinos are about one and one-half times as likely to have Alzheimer's or other dementias as older whites.[A8,19,240-241] However, Hispanics/Latinos comprise a very diverse group in terms of cultural history, genetic ancestry and health profiles, and there is evidence that prevalence may differ from one specific Hispanic/Latino ethnic group to another (for example, Mexican Americans compared with Caribbean Americans).[242-243]

The higher prevalence of Alzheimer's dementia in minority racial and ethnic groups compared with whites appears to be due to a higher incidence of dementia in these groups.[244] Variations in medical conditions, health-related behaviors and socioeconomic risk factors across racial groups likely account for most of the differences in risk of Alzheimer's and other dementias.[239] Despite some evidence that the influence of genetic risk factors on Alzheimer's and other dementias may differ by race,[80,82,245] genetic factors do not appear to account for the large differences in prevalence or incidence among racial groups.[244,246] Instead, health conditions such as cardiovascular disease and diabetes, which are associated with an increased risk for Alzheimer's and other dementias, are believed to account for these differences, as they are more prevalent in black/African American and Hispanic/Latino people.[247-248] Socioeconomic characteristics, including lower levels and quality of education, higher rates of poverty, and greater exposure to adversity and discrimination, may also increase risk in black/African American and Hispanic/Latino communities (and may in turn contribute to the health conditions mentioned above).[80,247-249] Some studies suggest that differences based on race and ethnicity do not persist in rigorous analyses that account for such factors.[135,187,244]

There is evidence that missed diagnoses of Alzheimer's and other dementias are more common among older blacks/African Americans and Hispanics/Latinos than among older whites.[250-251] Based on data for Medicare beneficiaries age 65 and older, it has been estimated that Alzheimer's or another dementia had been diagnosed in 10.3% of whites, 12.2% of Hispanics/Latinos and 13.8% of blacks/African Americans.[252] Although rates of diagnosis were higher among blacks/African Americans than among whites, according to prevalence studies that detect all people who have dementia irrespective of their use of the health care system, the rates should be even higher for blacks/African Americans.

There are fewer data from population-based cohort studies regarding the national prevalence of Alzheimer's and other dementias in racial and ethnic groups other than whites, blacks/African Americans and Hispanics/Latinos. However, a study examining electronic medical records of members of a large health plan in California indicated that dementia incidence — determined by the presence of a dementia diagnosis in members' medical records — was highest in blacks/African Americans, intermediate for Latinos (the term used in the study for those who self-reported as Latino or Hispanic) and whites, and lowest for Asian Americans.[253] A follow-up study with the same cohort showed heterogeneity within Asian-American subgroups, but all subgroups studied had lower dementia incidence than whites.[254] A recent systematic review of the literature found that Japanese Americans were the only Asian-American subgroup with reliable prevalence data, and that they had the lowest prevalence of dementia compared with all other ethnic groups.[243] More studies, especially those involving population-based cohorts, are necessary to draw conclusions about the prevalence of Alzheimer's and other dementias in different racial groups and subgroups.

## Trends in the Prevalence and Incidence of Alzheimer's Dementia Over Time

A growing number of studies indicate that the prevalence[223,255-263] and incidence[218,259,263-270] of Alzheimer's and other dementias in the United States and other higher-income Western countries may have declined in the past 25 years,[218,223,258-269] though results are mixed.[61,209,271-272] These declines have been attributed to increasing levels of education and improved control of cardiovascular risk factors.[223,258,264,267,273-274] Such findings are promising and suggest that identifying and reducing risk factors for Alzheimer's and other dementias may be effective. Although these findings indicate that a person's risk of dementia at any given age may be decreasing slightly, the total number of people with Alzheimer's or other dementias in the United States and other high-income Western countries is expected to continue to increase dramatically because of the increase in the number of people at the oldest ages.

It is unclear whether these encouraging trends will continue into the future given worldwide trends showing increases in diabetes and obesity — potential risk factors for Alzheimer's dementia — which may lead to a rebound in dementia risk in coming years,[102,257,259,275-276] or if these positive trends pertain to all racial and ethnic groups.[209,255,273-274,277] Thus, while recent findings are promising, the social and economic burden of Alzheimer's and other dementias will continue to grow. Moreover, 68% of the projected increase in the global prevalence and burden of dementia by 2050 will take place in low- and middle-income countries, where there is currently no evidence that the risk of Alzheimer's and other dementias has been declining.[278]

### Looking to the Future: Aging of the Baby Boom Generation

A large segment of the American population — the baby boom generation — has reached age 65 and older, when the risk for Alzheimer's and other dementias is elevated. By 2030, the segment of the U.S. population age 65 and older will increase substantially, and the projected 74 million older Americans will make up over 20% of the total population (up from 16% in 2020).[184,279] As the number of older Americans grows rapidly, so too will the numbers of new and existing cases of Alzheimer's dementia, as shown in Figure 5.[A9,62]

- By 2025, the number of people age 65 and older with Alzheimer's dementia is projected to reach 7.1 million — almost a 22% increase from the 5.8 million age 65 and older affected in 2020.[A10,62]
- By 2050, the number of people age 65 and older with Alzheimer's dementia is projected to reach 13.8 million, barring the development of medical breakthroughs to prevent, slow or cure Alzheimer's disease.[A9,62]

FIGURE 5

**Projected Number of People Age 65 and Older (Total and by Age) in the U.S. Population with Alzheimer's Dementia, 2010 to 2050**

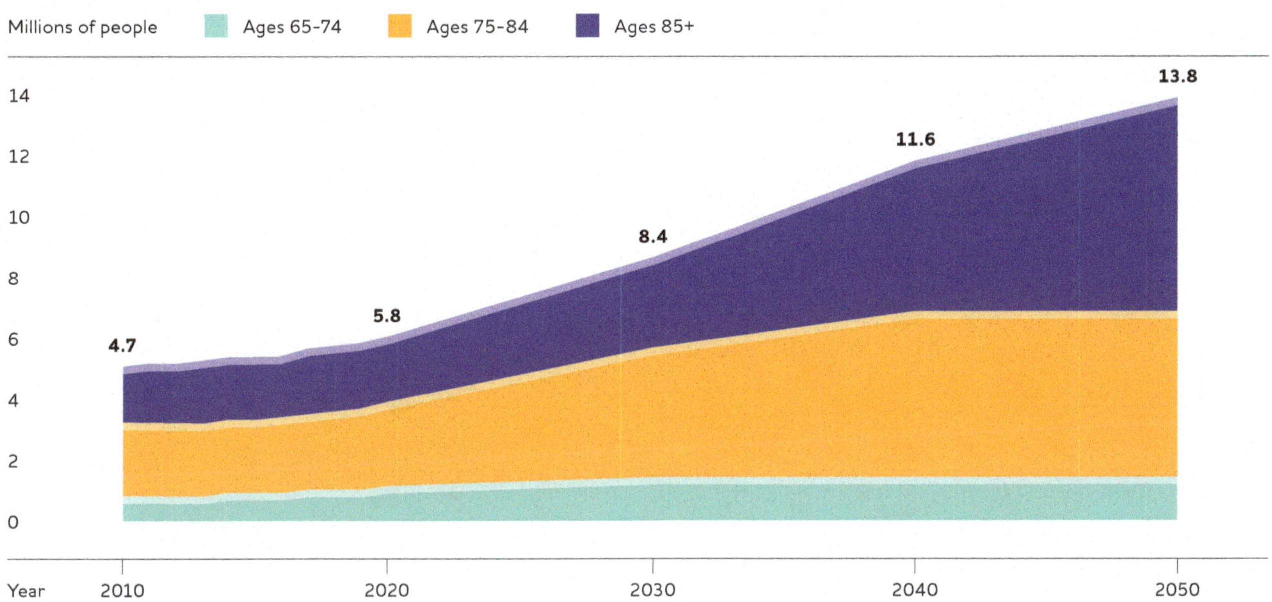


Created from data from Hebert et al.[A9,62]

### Growth of the Oldest-Old Population

The number of Americans surviving into their 80s, 90s and beyond is expected to grow dramatically due to medical advances, as well as social and environmental conditions.[279] Longer life expectancies and the aging of the large baby boom cohort will lead to an increase in the number and percentage of Americans who will be 85 and older, the oldest-old. Between now and 2050, the oldest-old are expected to comprise an increasing proportion of the U.S. population age 65 and older — from 10% in 2020 to 19% in 2050.[279] This will result in an additional 4.8 million oldest-old people — individuals at the highest risk for developing Alzheimer's dementia.[279]

- In 2020, about 2.1 million people who have Alzheimer's dementia are age 85 or older, accounting for 35% of all people with Alzheimer's dementia.[62]
- When the first wave of baby boomers reaches age 85 (in 2031), it is projected that more than 3 million people age 85 and older will have Alzheimer's dementia.[62]
- By 2050, 7 million people age 85 and older are projected to have Alzheimer's dementia, accounting for about half (51%) of all people 65 and older with Alzheimer's dementia.[62]

# Mortality and Morbidity

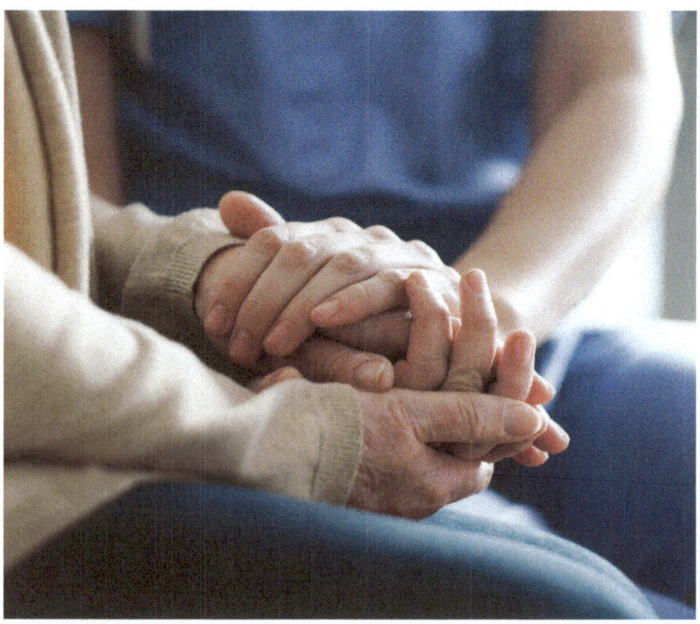

**1 in 3 seniors dies with Alzheimer's or another dementia.**

Alzheimer's disease is officially listed as the sixth-leading cause of death in the United States.[280] It is the fifth-leading cause of death for those age 65 and older.[281] However, it may cause even more deaths than official sources recognize. Alzheimer's is also a leading cause of disability and poor health (morbidity). Before a person with Alzheimer's dies, he or she lives through years of morbidity as the disease progresses.

## Deaths from Alzheimer's Disease

It is difficult to determine how many deaths are caused by Alzheimer's disease each year because of the way causes of death are recorded. According to data from the Centers for Disease Control and Prevention (CDC), 122,019 people died from Alzheimer's disease in 2018, the latest year for which data are available.[281] The CDC considers a person to have died *from* Alzheimer's if the death certificate lists Alzheimer's as the underlying cause of death, defined as "the disease or injury which initiated the train of events leading directly to death."[282]

In the United States, Alzheimer's disease is counted as a cause of death that can be ranked against other leading causes of death such as cancer and heart disease, but deaths due to other types of clinically diagnosed dementia are not ranked in this manner. The number of deaths from dementia of any type is much higher than the number of reported Alzheimer's deaths. In 2018, some form of dementia was the officially recorded underlying cause of death for 266,957 individuals (this includes the 122,019 from Alzheimer's disease).[281,283] Therefore, the number of deaths from all causes of dementia, even as listed on death certificates, is more than twice as high as the number of reported Alzheimer's deaths alone.

To add further complexity, the vast majority of death certificates listing Alzheimer's disease or dementia as an underlying cause of death are not verified by autopsy, and research has shown that about 30% of those diagnosed with Alzheimer's dementia during life do not in fact have dementia due to Alzheimer's disease, but have dementia due to another cause (see Table 1, page 6). Therefore, an underlying cause of death listed as Alzheimer's disease may not be accurate. In this section, "deaths from Alzheimer's disease" refers to what is officially reported on death certificates, with the understanding that the person filling out the report believed dementia due to Alzheimer's disease was the underlying cause of death, usually without pathologic confirmation.

Severe dementia frequently causes complications such as immobility, swallowing disorders and malnutrition that significantly increase the risk of serious acute conditions that can cause death. One such condition is pneumonia (infection of the lungs), which is the most commonly identified immediate cause of death among older adults with Alzheimer's or other dementias.[284-285] One autopsy study found that respiratory system diseases were the immediate cause of death in more than half of people with Alzheimer's dementia, followed by circulatory system disease in about a quarter.[285] Death certificates for individuals with Alzheimer's often list acute conditions such as pneumonia as the primary cause of death rather than Alzheimer's.[286-288] As a result, people with Alzheimer's dementia who die due to these acute conditions may not be counted among the number of people who die from Alzheimer's disease, even though Alzheimer's disease may well have caused the acute condition listed on the death certificate. This difficulty in using death certificates to determine the number of deaths from Alzheimer's and other dementias has been referred to as a "blurred distinction between death *with* dementia and death *from* dementia."[289]

Another way to determine the number of deaths from Alzheimer's dementia is through calculations that compare the estimated risk of death in those who have Alzheimer's dementia with the estimated risk of death in those who do not have Alzheimer's dementia. A study using data from the Rush Memory and Aging Project and the Religious Orders Study estimated that 500,000 deaths among people age 75 and older in the United States in 2010 could be attributed to Alzheimer's dementia (estimates for people age 65 to 74 were not available), meaning that those deaths would not be expected to occur in that year if those individuals did not have Alzheimer's dementia.[290]

The true number of deaths caused by Alzheimer's is somewhere between the number of deaths from Alzheimer's recorded on death certificates and the number of people who have Alzheimer's disease when they die. According to 2014 Medicare claims data, about one-third of all Medicare beneficiaries who die in a given year have been diagnosed with Alzheimer's or another dementia.[291] Based on data from the Chicago Health and Aging Project (CHAP) study, in 2020 an estimated 700,000 people age 65 and older in the United States will have Alzheimer's when they die.[292] Although some older adults who have Alzheimer's disease at the time of death die from causes that are unrelated to Alzheimer's, many of them die from Alzheimer's disease itself or from conditions in which Alzheimer's was a contributing cause, such as pneumonia.

FIGURE 6

Percentage Changes in Selected Causes of Death (All Ages) Between 2000 and 2018

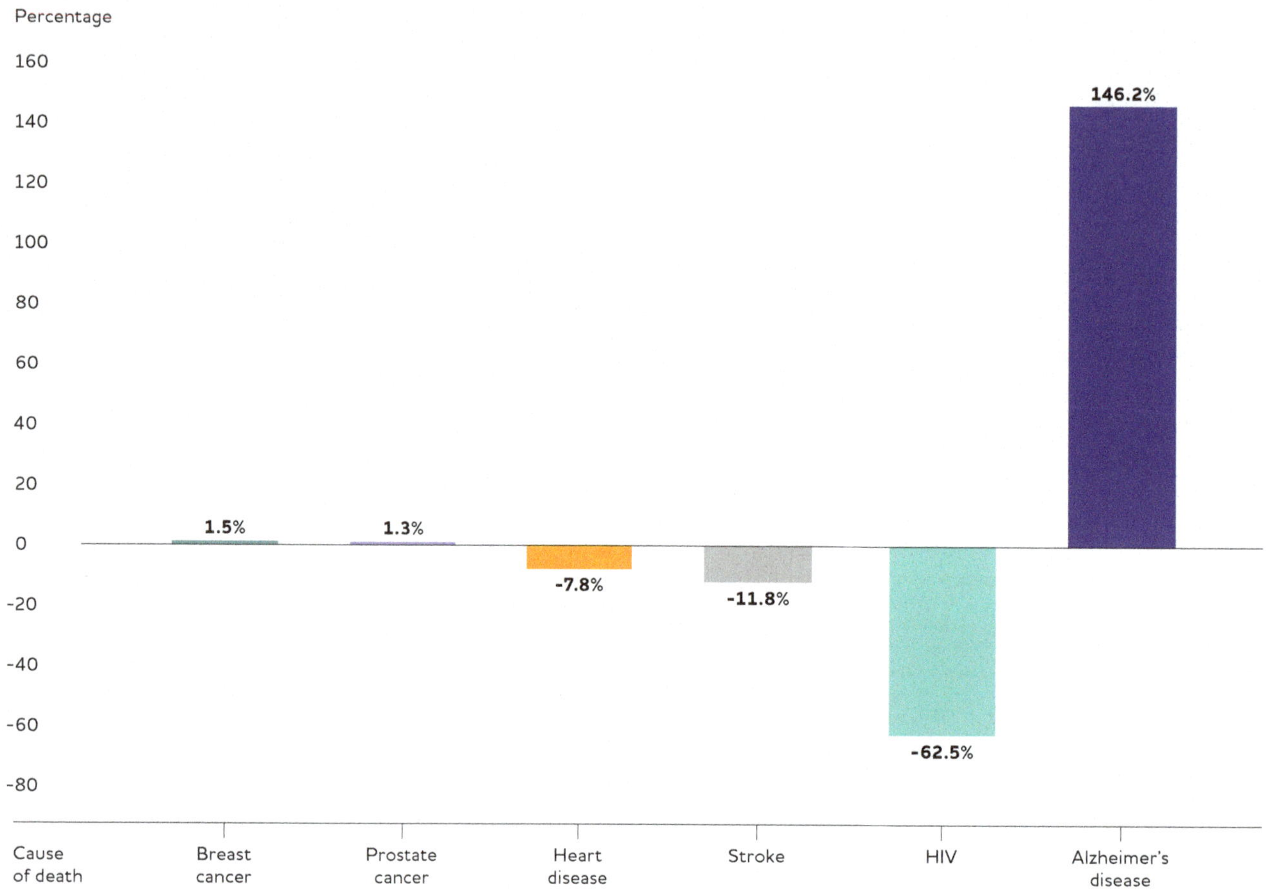


Created from data from the National Center for Health Statistics.[281,294]

Irrespective of the cause of death, among people age 70, 61% of those with Alzheimer's dementia are expected to die before age 80 compared with 30% of people without Alzheimer's dementia.[293]

## Public Health Impact of Deaths from Alzheimer's Disease

Although deaths from other major causes have *decreased* significantly or remained approximately the same, official records indicate that deaths from Alzheimer's disease have *increased* significantly. Between 2000 and 2018, the number of deaths from Alzheimer's disease as recorded on death certificates has more than doubled, increasing 146%, while the number of deaths from the number one cause of death (heart disease) decreased 7.8% (Figure 6).[281,294] The increase in the number of death certificates listing Alzheimer's as the underlying cause of death probably reflects both a real increase in the actual number of deaths from Alzheimer's due in large part to Alzheimer's becoming a more common cause of death as the population ages, as well as increased reporting of Alzheimer's deaths on death certificates over time by physicians, coroners and others who assign causes of death.[295]

## State-by-State Deaths from Alzheimer's Disease

Table 5 provides information on the number of deaths due to Alzheimer's by state in 2018, the most recent year for which state-by-state data are available. This information was obtained from death certificates and reflects the condition identified by the physician as the underlying cause of death. The table also provides annual mortality rates by state to compare the risk of death due to Alzheimer's disease across states with varying population sizes. For the United States as a whole, in 2018, the mortality rate for Alzheimer's disease was 37.3 deaths per 100,000 people.[A11,281]

TABLE 5

Number of Deaths and Annual Mortality Rate (per 100,000 People) Due to Alzheimer's Disease by State, 2018

| State | Number of Deaths | Mortality Rate |
|---|---|---|
| Alabama | 2,616 | 53.5 |
| Alaska | 131 | 17.8 |
| Arizona | 3,012 | 42.0 |
| Arkansas | 1,457 | 48.3 |
| California | 16,627 | 42.0 |
| Colorado | 1,649 | 29.0 |
| Connecticut | 986 | 27.6 |
| Delaware | 412 | 42.6 |
| District of Columbia | 105 | 14.9 |
| Florida | 6,725 | 31.6 |
| Georgia | 4,513 | 42.9 |
| Hawaii | 480 | 33.8 |
| Idaho | 666 | 38.0 |
| Illinois | 4,030 | 31.6 |
| Indiana | 2,668 | 39.9 |
| Iowa | 1,439 | 45.6 |
| Kansas | 899 | 30.9 |
| Kentucky | 1,674 | 37.5 |
| Louisiana | 2,166 | 46.5 |
| Maine | 580 | 43.3 |
| Maryland | 1,122 | 18.6 |
| Massachusetts | 1,823 | 26.4 |
| Michigan | 4,474 | 44.8 |
| Minnesota | 2,436 | 43.4 |
| Mississippi | 1,547 | 51.8 |
| Missouri | 2,641 | 43.1 |
| Montana | 310 | 29.2 |
| Nebraska | 683 | 35.4 |
| Nevada | 704 | 23.2 |
| New Hampshire | 487 | 35.9 |
| New Jersey | 2,710 | 30.4 |
| New Mexico | 583 | 27.8 |
| New York | 3,755 | 19.2 |
| North Carolina | 4,495 | 43.3 |
| North Dakota | 356 | 46.8 |
| Ohio | 5,391 | 46.1 |
| Oklahoma | 1,739 | 44.1 |
| Oregon | 1,868 | 44.6 |
| Pennsylvania | 4,064 | 31.7 |
| Rhode Island | 470 | 44.5 |
| South Carolina | 2,616 | 51.5 |
| South Dakota | 437 | 49.5 |
| Tennessee | 3,488 | 51.5 |
| Texas | 9,763 | 34.0 |
| Utah | 1,024 | 32.4 |
| Vermont | 333 | 53.2 |
| Virginia | 2,592 | 30.4 |
| Washington | 3,752 | 49.8 |
| West Virginia | 791 | 43.8 |
| Wisconsin | 2,453 | 42.2 |
| Wyoming | 277 | 47.9 |
| **U.S. Total** | **122,019** | **37.3** |

Created from data from the National Center for Health Statistics.[A11,281]

FIGURE 7

U.S. Annual Alzheimer's Death Rate (per 100,000 People) by Year

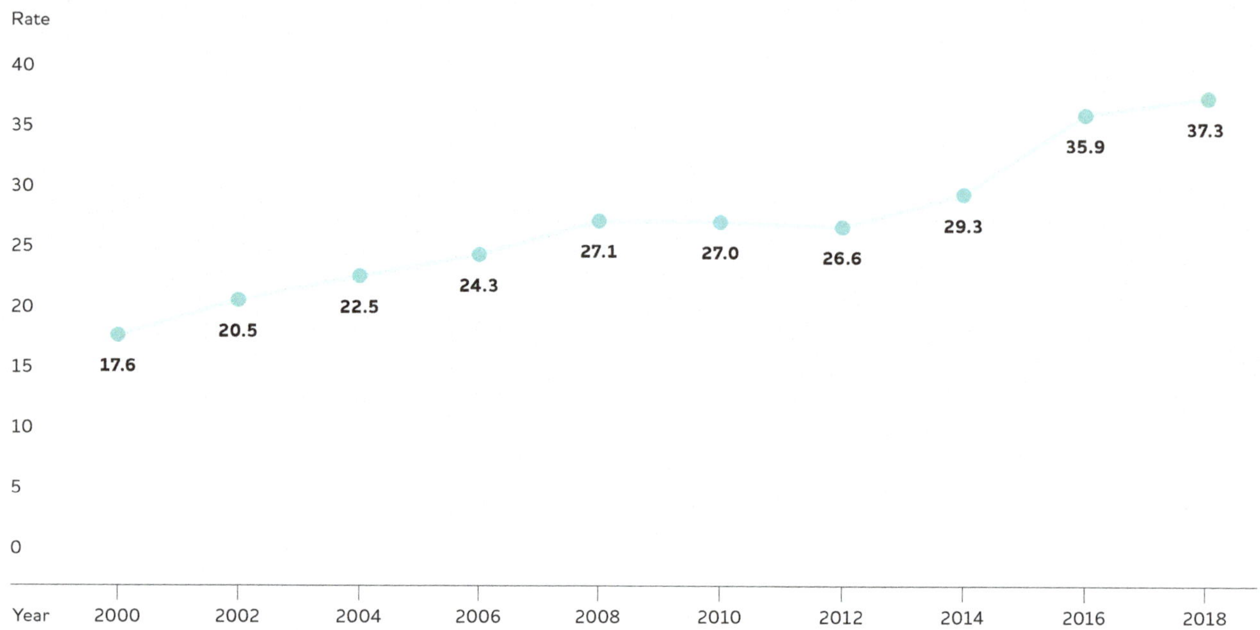


Created from data from the National Center for Health Statistics.[281]

TABLE 6

U.S. Annual Alzheimer's Death Rates (per 100,000 People) by Age and Year

| Age | 2000 | 2002 | 2004 | 2006 | 2008 | 2010 | 2012 | 2014 | 2016 | 2018 |
|---|---|---|---|---|---|---|---|---|---|---|
| 45-54 | 0.2 | 0.1 | 0.2 | 0.2 | 0.2 | 0.3 | 0.2 | 0.2 | 0.2 | 0.3 |
| 55-64 | 2.0 | 1.9 | 1.8 | 2.1 | 2.2 | 2.1 | 2.2 | 2.1 | 2.7 | 2.9 |
| 65-74 | 18.7 | 19.6 | 19.5 | 19.9 | 21.1 | 19.8 | 17.9 | 19.6 | 23.6 | 24.7 |
| 75-84 | 139.6 | 157.7 | 168.5 | 175.0 | 192.5 | 184.5 | 175.4 | 185.6 | 214.1 | 213.9 |
| 85+ | 667.7 | 790.9 | 875.3 | 923.4 | 1,002.2 | 987.1 | 936.1 | 1,006.8 | 1,216.9 | 1,225.3 |

Created from data from the National Center for Health Statistics.[281]

## Alzheimer's Death Rates

As shown in Figure 7, the rate of deaths due to Alzheimer's has risen substantially since 2000.[281] Table 6 shows that the rate of death from Alzheimer's increases dramatically with age, especially after age 65.[A11,281] The increase in the Alzheimer's death rate over time has disproportionately affected the oldest-old.[294] Between 2000 and 2018, the death rate from Alzheimer's increased 32% for people age 65 to 74, but increased 53% for people age 75 to 84 and 84% for people age 85 and older.[281] A report by the CDC determined that even after adjusting for differences in age distributions over time, the annual Alzheimer's death rate in the United States increased substantially between 1999 and 2014.[295] Therefore, the growing proportion of older adults in the country is not the only explanation for the increase in Alzheimer's death rates. Other possible reasons include fewer deaths from other common causes of death in old age such as heart disease and stroke; increased diagnosis of Alzheimer's dementia; and increased reporting of Alzheimer's as a cause of death by physicians and others who fill out death certificates.[295]

## Duration of Illness from Diagnosis to Death

Studies indicate that people age 65 and older survive an average of 4 to 8 years after a diagnosis of Alzheimer's dementia, yet some live as long as 20 years with Alzheimer's dementia.[210,296-303] This reflects the slow, insidious and uncertain progression of Alzheimer's. A person who lives from age 70 to age 80 with Alzheimer's dementia will spend an average of 40% of this time in the severe stage.[293] Much of this time will be spent in a nursing home. At age 80, approximately 75% of people with Alzheimer's dementia live in a nursing home compared with only 4% of the general population age 80.[293] In all, an estimated two-thirds of those who die of dementia do so in nursing homes, compared with 20% of people with cancer and 28% of people dying from all other conditions.[304]

## Burden of Alzheimer's Disease

The long duration of illness before death contributes significantly to the public health impact of Alzheimer's disease because much of that time is spent in a state of disability and dependence. Scientists have developed methods to measure and compare the burden of different diseases on a population in a way that takes into account not only the number of people with the condition, but also the number of years of life lost due to that disease and the number of healthy years of life lost by virtue of being in a state of disability. The primary measure of disease burden is called disability-adjusted life years (DALYs), which is the sum of the number of years of life lost due to premature mortality (YLLs) and the number of years lived with disability (YLDs), totaled across all those with the disease or injury. These measures indicate that Alzheimer's is a very burdensome disease, not only to the individuals with the disease, but also to their families and informal caregivers, and that the burden of Alzheimer's has increased more dramatically in the United States than the burden of other diseases in recent years. According to the most recent Global Burden of Disease classification system, Alzheimer's disease rose from the 12th most burdensome disease or injury in the United States in 1990 to the sixth in 2016 in terms of DALYs. In 2016, Alzheimer's disease was the fourth highest disease or injury in terms of YLLs and the 19th in terms of YLDs.[305]

Taken together, these statistics indicate that not only is Alzheimer's disease responsible for the deaths of more and more Americans, but also that the disease is contributing to more and more cases of poor health and disability in the United States.

# Caregiving

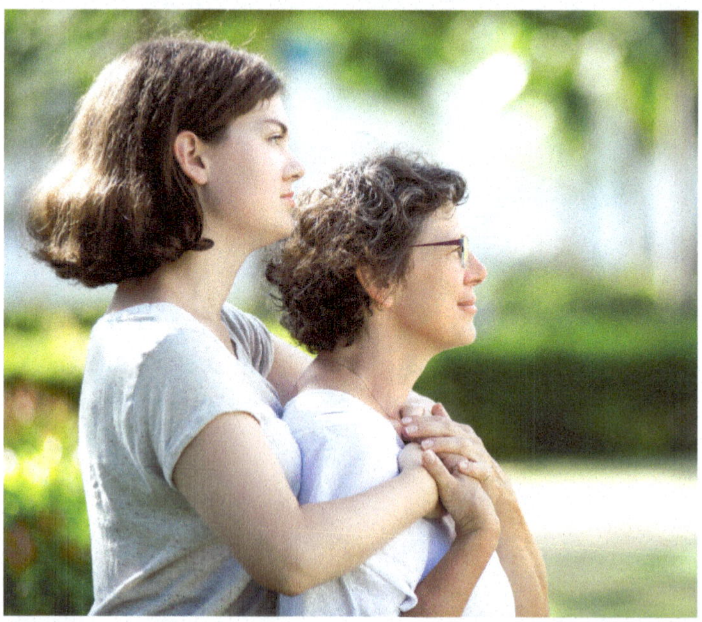

Family members and friends provided nearly **$244 billion** in unpaid care to people with Alzheimer's and other dementias in 2019.

*Caregiving* refers to attending to another person's health needs and well-being. Caregiving often includes assistance with one or more activities of daily living (ADLs), including bathing and dressing, as well as multiple instrumental activities of daily living (IADLs), such as paying bills, shopping and using transportation.[306-307] Caregivers also provide emotional support to people with Alzheimer's as well as many other forms of help (for example, communicating and coordinating care with other family members and health care providers, ensuring safety at home and elsewhere, and managing health conditions; see Table 7, page 34). In addition to providing descriptive information about caregivers of people with Alzheimer's or other dementias, this section compares caregivers of people with dementia to either caregivers of people with other medical conditions or, if that comparison is not available, to non-caregivers.

### Calculating the Number of Caregivers

It is important to note that the number of caregivers for people with Alzheimer's or other dementias is calculated using a model that incorporates, in part, data from 2009, the most recent date for which the data are available. There are indications that over the past decade, the number of family caregivers for all older Americans may have declined. The Alzheimer's Association is examining new data and recently released state-specific data on dementia caregivers and is working with experts to revise the model to take into account these recent trends. Preliminary evaluation indicates that, compared with the past, there are fewer family caregivers in total, but each individual caregiver is experiencing a greater burden by providing significantly more hours of care. If this preliminary analysis holds, future estimates of the number of Alzheimer's and dementia caregivers nationally and for each state will be lower than current estimates.

## Unpaid Caregivers

Eighty-three percent of the help provided to older adults in the United States comes from family members, friends or other unpaid caregivers.[308] Nearly half of all caregivers (48%) who provide help to older adults do so for someone with Alzheimer's or another dementia.[309] More than 16 million Americans provide unpaid care for people with Alzheimer's or other dementias.[A12]

In 2019, caregivers of people with Alzheimer's or other dementias provided an estimated 18.6 billion hours of informal (that is, unpaid) assistance, a contribution to the nation valued at $244 billion. This is approximately 47% of the net value of Walmart's total revenue in 2019 ($514.4 billion)[310] and 11 times the total revenue of McDonald's in 2018 ($21 billion).[311] The total lifetime cost of care for someone with dementia was estimated at $357,297 in 2019 dollars. Seventy percent of the lifetime cost of care is borne by family caregivers in the forms of unpaid caregiving and out-of-pocket expenses for items ranging from medications to food for the person with dementia.[312-313] Current estimates of the lifetime costs of care may underestimate the impact of a relative's dementia on family caregivers' health and workplace productivity.[314]

Three of the main reasons caregivers provide care and assistance to a person with Alzheimer's or another dementia are 1) the desire to keep a family member or friend at home (65%), 2) proximity to the person with dementia (48%) and 3) the caregiver's perceived obligation to the person with dementia (38%).[A13] Caregivers often indicate love and a sense of duty and obligation when describing what motivates them to assume care responsibilities for a relative or friend living with dementia.[315] Individuals with dementia living in the community are more likely than older adults without dementia to rely on multiple unpaid caregivers (often family members); 30% of older adults with dementia rely on three or more unpaid caregivers, whereas 23% of older adults without dementia rely on three or more unpaid caregivers.[316] Only a small percentage of older adults with dementia do not receive help from family members or other informal care providers (8%). Of these individuals, nearly half live alone, perhaps making it more difficult to ask for and receive informal care.[316] Of caregivers of spouses with dementia who are at the end of life, close to half provide care without the help of other family or friends.[317] Living alone with dementia may be a particular challenge for certain subgroups, such as lesbian, gay, bisexual and transgender (LGBT) individuals, who may

TABLE 7

**Dementia Caregiving Tasks**

| |
|---|
| Helping with instrumental activities of daily living (IADLs), such as household chores, shopping, preparing meals, providing transportation, arranging for doctor's appointments, managing finances and legal affairs, and answering the telephone. |
| Helping the person take medications correctly, either via reminders or direct administration of medications. |
| Helping the person adhere to treatment recommendations for dementia or other medical conditions. |
| Assisting with personal activities of daily living (ADLs), such as bathing, dressing, grooming and feeding and helping the person walk, transfer from bed to chair, use the toilet and manage incontinence. |
| Managing behavioral symptoms of the disease such as aggressive behavior, wandering, depressive mood, agitation, anxiety, repetitive activity and nighttime disturbances. |
| Finding and using support services such as support groups and adult day service programs. |
| Making arrangements for paid in-home, nursing home or assisted living care. |
| Hiring and supervising others who provide care. |
| Assuming additional responsibilities that are not necessarily specific tasks, such as:<br>• Providing overall management of getting through the day.<br>• Addressing family issues related to caring for a relative with Alzheimer's disease, including communication with other family members about care plans, decision-making and arrangements for respite for the main caregiver.<br>• Managing other health conditions (i.e., "comorbidities"), such as arthritis, diabetes or cancer.<br>• Providing emotional support and a sense of security. |

experience greater isolation for reasons ranging from social stigma to a diminished social network of available family or friend caregivers.[318]

### Who Are the Caregivers?

Several sources have examined the demographic background of family caregivers of people with Alzheimer's or other dementias in the United States. They have found the following[A13,319-323]:

- Approximately two-thirds of dementia caregivers are women.[A13,319-320]
- About 30% of caregivers are age 65 or older.[A13]
- Over 60% of caregivers are married, living with a partner or in a long-term relationship.[A13,320]
- Over half of caregivers are providing assistance to a parent or in-law with dementia.[323] Approximately 10% of caregivers provide help to a spouse with Alzheimer's disease or another dementia.[323-324]
- Two-thirds of caregivers are non-Hispanic white,[A13,320,323] while 10% are black/African American, 8% are Hispanic/Latino and 5% are Asian.[A13] The remaining 10% represent a variety of other racial/ethnic groups.
- Approximately 40% of dementia caregivers have a college degree or more education.[A13,320,323]
- Forty-one percent of caregivers have a household income of $50,000 or less.[A13]
- Among primary caregivers (individuals who indicate having the most responsibility for helping their relatives) of people with dementia, over half take care of their parents.[322,325-326]
- Most caregivers (66%) live with the person with dementia in the community.[316]
- Approximately one-quarter of dementia caregivers are "sandwich generation" caregivers — meaning that they care not only for an aging parent, but also for a child. [A13,323-324]

### Caregiving and Women

The responsibilities of caring for someone with dementia often fall to women. As mentioned earlier, approximately two-thirds of dementia caregivers are women.[A13,319-320,325-326] Over one-third of dementia caregivers are daughters.[308,316] It is more common for wives to provide informal care for a husband than vice versa.[327] On average, female caregivers spend more time caregiving than male caregivers.[316] According to the 2014 Alzheimer's Association Women and Alzheimer's Poll, which surveyed both men and women, of those providing care for 21 hours or more per week, 67% were women.[328] Similarly, the 2015-2017 Behavioral Risk Factor Surveillance System (BRFSS) surveys found that of all dementia caregivers who spend more than 40 hours per week providing care, 73% were women.[324] Two and a half times as many women as men

FIGURE 8

**Proportion of Caregivers of People with Alzheimer's or Other Dementias Versus Caregivers of Other Older People Who Provide Help with Specific Activities of Daily Living, United States, 2015**

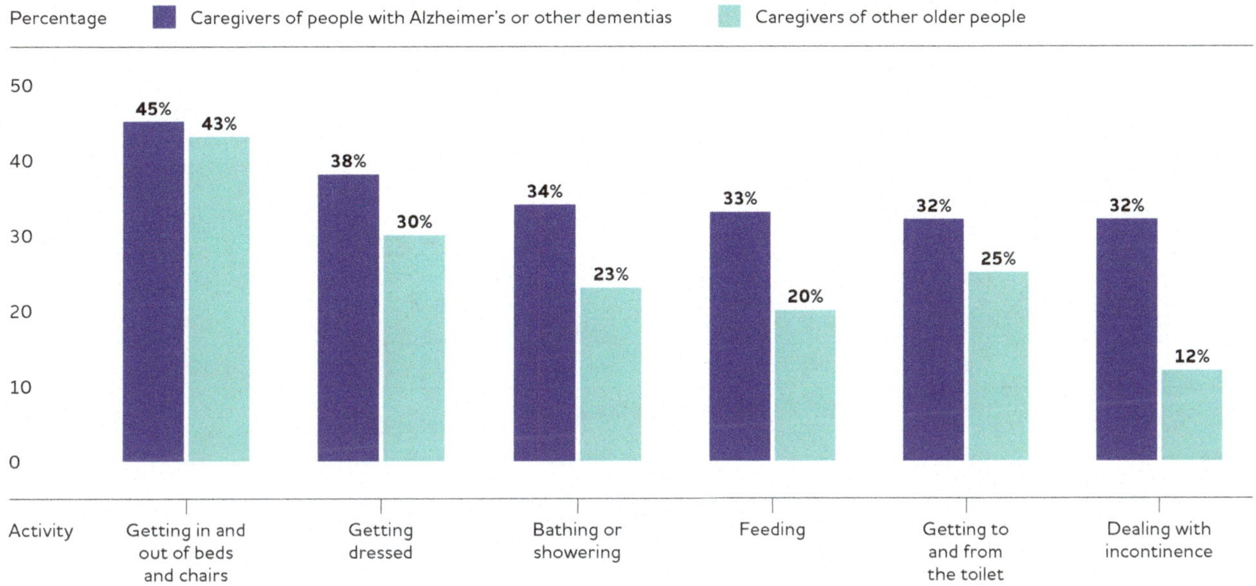


Created from data from the National Alliance for Caregiving and AARP.[323]

reported living with the person with dementia full time.[328] Of those providing care to someone with dementia for more than 5 years, 63% are women.[324] Similarly, caregivers who are women may experience slightly higher levels of burden, impaired mood, depression and impaired health than men, with evidence suggesting that these differences arise because female caregivers tend to spend more time caregiving, assume more caregiving tasks, and care for someone with more cognitive, functional and/or behavioral problems.[329-330] Of dementia caregivers who indicate a need for individual counseling or respite care, the large majority are women (individual counseling, 85%, and respite care, 84%).[324]

### Caregiving Tasks

The care provided to people with Alzheimer's or other dementias is wide-ranging and in some instances all-encompassing. Table 7 summarizes some of the most common types of dementia care provided.

Though the care provided by family members of people with Alzheimer's or other dementias is somewhat similar to the help provided by caregivers of people with other conditions, dementia caregivers tend to provide more extensive assistance. Family caregivers of people with dementia are more likely to monitor the health of the care recipient than are caregivers of people without dementia (79% versus 66%).[331] Data from the 2011 National Health and Aging Trends Study indicated that caregivers of people with dementia are more likely than caregivers of people without dementia to provide help with self-care and mobility (85% versus 71%) and health or medical care (63% versus 52%).[309,319] Figure 8 illustrates how family caregivers of people with dementia are more likely than caregivers of other older people to assist with ADLs.

In addition to assisting with ADLs, more caregivers of people with Alzheimer's or other dementias advocate for these individuals with community agencies and care providers (65%) and manage finances (68%) compared with caregivers of people without dementia (46% and 50%, respectively).[323] More caregivers of people with Alzheimer's or other dementias arrange for outside services (46%) and communicate with health care professionals (80%) compared with caregivers of people without dementia (27% and 59%, respectively).[323] One in five caregivers of people with Alzheimer's or other dementias (22%) report problems dealing with a bank or credit union when helping to manage the finances of people living with dementia, compared with 9% of caregivers of people without dementia.[323] Caring for a person with dementia also means managing symptoms that caregivers of people with other diseases may not

TABLE 8

**Number of Caregivers of People with Alzheimer's or Other Dementias, Hours of Unpaid Care and Economic Value of Unpaid Care by State, 2019***

| State | Number of Caregivers (in thousands) | Hours of Unpaid Care (in millions) | Value of Unpaid Care (in millions of dollars) |
|---|---|---|---|
| Alabama | 306 | 349 | $4,576 |
| Alaska | 33 | 38 | 495 |
| Arizona | 346 | 394 | 5,165 |
| Arkansas | 178 | 203 | 2,663 |
| California | 1,624 | 1,849 | 24,245 |
| Colorado | 256 | 292 | 3,825 |
| Connecticut | 178 | 203 | 2,655 |
| Delaware | 55 | 63 | 822 |
| District of Columbia | 29 | 33 | 433 |
| Florida | 1,152 | 1,312 | 17,206 |
| Georgia | 540 | 615 | 8,063 |
| Hawaii | 65 | 74 | 975 |
| Idaho | 87 | 99 | 1,299 |
| Illinois | 587 | 668 | 8,759 |
| Indiana | 342 | 390 | 5,112 |
| Iowa | 136 | 155 | 2,036 |
| Kansas | 152 | 173 | 2,268 |
| Kentucky | 274 | 312 | 4,089 |
| Louisiana | 231 | 264 | 3,456 |
| Maine | 70 | 79 | 1,042 |
| Maryland | 294 | 335 | 4,389 |
| Massachusetts | 340 | 387 | 5,075 |
| Michigan | 518 | 590 | 7,733 |
| Minnesota | 257 | 293 | 3,838 |
| Mississippi | 207 | 235 | 3,085 |
| Missouri | 319 | 363 | 4,755 |
| Montana | 51 | 58 | $757 |
| Nebraska | 83 | 95 | 1,240 |
| Nevada | 153 | 175 | 2,289 |
| New Hampshire | 68 | 78 | 1,016 |
| New Jersey | 448 | 510 | 6,684 |
| New Mexico | 108 | 123 | 1,617 |
| New York | 1,011 | 1,151 | 15,089 |
| North Carolina | 479 | 545 | 7,151 |
| North Dakota | 30 | 35 | 454 |
| Ohio | 604 | 688 | 9,018 |
| Oklahoma | 226 | 257 | 3,371 |
| Oregon | 188 | 214 | 2,810 |
| Pennsylvania | 677 | 771 | 10,104 |
| Rhode Island | 54 | 61 | 800 |
| South Carolina | 318 | 362 | 4,749 |
| South Dakota | 39 | 44 | 575 |
| Tennessee | 444 | 506 | 6,628 |
| Texas | 1,449 | 1,650 | 21,628 |
| Utah | 159 | 181 | 2,366 |
| Vermont | 30 | 34 | 449 |
| Virginia | 467 | 532 | 6,970 |
| Washington | 353 | 402 | 5,268 |
| West Virginia | 105 | 120 | 1,574 |
| Wisconsin | 195 | 223 | 2,918 |
| Wyoming | 28 | 31 | 413 |
| **U.S. Total** | **16,343** | **18,611** | **$243,994** |

*State totals may not add to the U.S. total due to rounding.

Created from data from the 2009 Behavioral Risk Factor Surveillance System survey, U.S. Census Bureau, Centers for Medicare & Medicaid Services, National Alliance for Caregiving, AARP and U.S. Department of Labor.[A12, A14, A15]

face, such as neuropsychiatric symptoms (for example, anxiety, apathy and lack of inhibition) and severe behavioral problems. Family caregivers of people with Alzheimer's or other dementias are more likely than family caregivers of people without dementia to help with emotional or mental health problems (41% versus 16%) and behavioral issues (15% versus 4%).[323] People with dementia tend to have larger networks of family and friends involved in their care compared with people without dementia. Family members and friends in dementia care networks tend to provide help for a larger number of tasks than do those in non-dementia care networks, where family members and friends are more likely to focus on specific care tasks.[332]

When a person with Alzheimer's or another dementia moves to an assisted living residence or a nursing home, the help provided by his or her family caregiver usually changes from the comprehensive care summarized in Table 7 (see page 34) to providing emotional support, interacting with facility staff and advocating for appropriate care. However, some family caregivers continue to help with bathing, dressing and other ADLs.[333-335]

### Duration of Caregiving

Eighty-six percent of dementia caregivers have provided care and assistance for at least the past year, according to the national 2014 Alzheimer's Association Women and Alzheimer's Poll.[A13] According to another study, well over half (57%) of family caregivers of people with Alzheimer's or other dementias in the community had provided care for 4 or more years.[316] More than six in 10 (63%) Alzheimer's caregivers expect to continue having care responsibilities for the next 5 years compared with less than half of caregivers of people without dementia (49%).[323]

### Hours of Unpaid Care and Economic Value of Caregiving

In 2019, the 16.3 million family and other unpaid caregivers of people with Alzheimer's or other dementias provided an estimated 18.6 billion hours of unpaid care. This number represents an average of 21.9 hours of care per caregiver per week, or 1,139 hours of care per caregiver per year.[A14] With this care valued at $13.11 per hour,[A15] the estimated economic value of care provided by family and other unpaid caregivers of people with dementia across the United States was nearly $244 billion in 2019. Table 8 shows the total hours of unpaid care as well as the value of care provided by family and other unpaid caregivers for the United States and each state. Unpaid caregivers of people with Alzheimer's or other dementias provided care valued at more than $4 billion in each of 22 states. Unpaid caregivers in each of the four most populous states — California, Florida, New York and Texas — provided care valued at more than $15 billion. A longitudinal study of the monetary value of family caregiving for people with dementia found that the overall value of daily family care increased 18% with each additional year of providing care, and that the value of this care further increased as the care recipient's cognitive abilities declined.[336-337] Additional research is needed to estimate the future value of family care for people with Alzheimer's disease and other dementias as the U.S. population continues to age.

Apart from its long duration, the immediate demands of caregiving are also time-intensive. Caregivers of people with dementia report providing 27 hours more care per month on average (92 hours versus 65 hours) than caregivers of people without dementia.[319] An analysis of national caregiving trends from 1999 to 2015 found that the average hours of care per week increased from 45 in 1999 to 48 in 2015 for dementia caregivers; over the same time period, weekly hours of care decreased for non-dementia caregivers from 34 to 24.[338]

### Impact of Alzheimer's Caregiving

Caring for a person with Alzheimer's or another dementia poses special challenges. For example, people in the middle to later stages of Alzheimer's experience losses in judgment, orientation, and the ability to understand and communicate effectively. Family caregivers must often help people with Alzheimer's manage these issues. The personality and behavior of a person with Alzheimer's are affected as well, and these changes are often among the most challenging for family caregivers.[339-341] Individuals with Alzheimer's also require increasing levels of supervision and personal care as the disease progresses. As symptoms worsen, the care required by family members can result in increased emotional stress and depression among caregivers; new or exacerbated health problems; and depleted income and finances due in part to disruptions in employment and paying for health care or other services for themselves and people living with dementia.[342-350]

#### *Caregiver Emotional and Social Well-Being*

The intimacy, shared experiences and memories that are often part of the relationship between a caregiver and person living with dementia may be threatened due to the memory loss, functional impairment and psychiatric/behavioral disturbances that can accompany the progression of Alzheimer's. In a national poll, however, 45% of caregivers of people with dementia indicated that providing help to someone with cognitive impairment was very rewarding.[326] Although caregivers report positive feelings about caregiving, such as family togetherness and the satisfaction of helping others,[A13,351-357] they also frequently report higher levels of stress.

*Burden and Stress*

- More dementia caregivers were classified as having a high level of burden than caregivers of people without dementia (46% versus 38%) based on the 2015 National Alliance for Caregiving/AARP survey's Burden of Care Index, which combined the number of hours of care and the number of ADL tasks performed by the caregiver into a single numerical score.[323]
- Compared with caregivers of people without dementia, twice as many caregivers of those with dementia indicate substantial emotional, financial and physical difficulties.[319]
- Fifty-nine percent of family caregivers of people with Alzheimer's or other dementias rated the emotional stress of caregiving as high or very high (Figure 9).[A13] Nearly half of dementia caregivers (49%) indicate that providing help is highly stressful compared with 35% of caregivers of people without dementia.[323]

*Depression and Mental Health*

- A meta-analysis reported that caregivers of people with dementia were significantly more likely to experience depression and anxiety than non-caregivers.[330] Approximately 30% to 40% of family caregivers of people with dementia report depression, compared with 5% to 17% of non-caregivers of similar ages.[358-362]
- The prevalence of depression is higher among dementia caregivers (30% to 40%) than other caregivers, such as those who provide help to individuals with schizophrenia (20%) or stroke (19%).[362-365]
- In a meta-analysis, the type of relationship was the strongest predictor of caregiver depression; caregivers of spouses had two and a half times higher odds of having depression than caregivers of people who were not spouses.[362]
- The prevalence of anxiety among dementia caregivers is 44%, which is higher than among caregivers of people with stroke (31%).[362-363]
- Caregivers of individuals with Alzheimer's report more subjective cognitive problems (for example, problems with memory) and experience greater declines in cognition over time than non-caregivers matched on age and other characteristics.[366-367]
- Caring for people with dementia who have four or more behavioral and psychological symptoms (for example, aggression, self-harm and wandering) represents a "tipping point" for family caregivers, as they are more likely to report clinically meaningful depression and burden (that is, negative emotional reactions to providing care).[368]

FIGURE 9

**Proportion of Caregivers of People with Alzheimer's or Other Dementias Who Report High to Very High Emotional and Physical Stress Due to Caregiving**

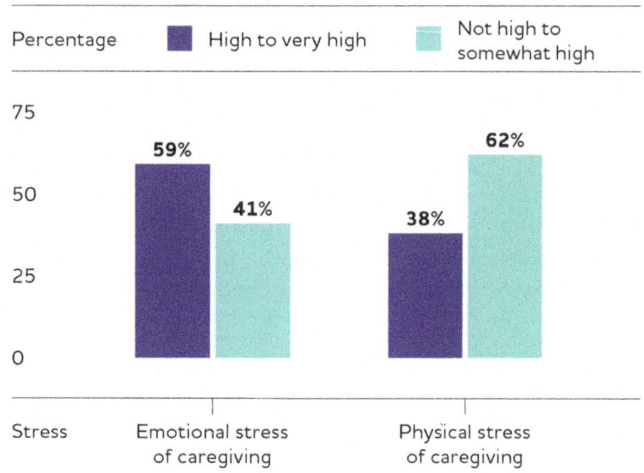


Created from data from the Alzheimer's Association.[A13]

*Strain*

- Caregivers of people with Alzheimer's or other dementias were twice as likely as caregivers of individuals without dementia (22% compared with 11%) to report that completing medical/nursing-related tasks (for example, injections, tube feedings and catheter/colostomy care) was difficult.[331]
- About half of caregivers (51%) of people with Alzheimer's or another dementia report having no experience performing medical/nursing-related tasks,[331] and they often lack the information or resources necessary to manage complex medication regimens.[369-372]
- According to the 2014 Alzheimer's Association poll of caregivers, respondents often believed they had no choice in taking on the role of caregiver.[A13]
- The poll also found that more than half of women with children under age 18 felt that caregiving for someone with dementia was more challenging than caring for children (53%).[A13]
- Many caregivers of people with Alzheimer's or other dementias provide help alone. Forty-one percent of dementia caregivers in the 2014 Alzheimer's Association poll reported that no one else provided unpaid assistance.[A13]
- A population-based sample of caregivers found that although dementia caregivers indicated greater strain than non-dementia caregivers, no substantial differences in strain between white and black/African American dementia caregivers were evident.[373]

*Stress of Care Transitions*

- Admitting a relative to a residential care facility has mixed effects on the emotional and psychological well-being of family caregivers. Some studies suggest that distress remains unchanged or even increases after a relative is admitted to a residential care facility, but other studies have found that distress declines following admission.[335,374-375]
- The demands of caregiving may intensify as people with dementia approach the end of life.[376] In the year before the death of the person living with dementia, 59% of caregivers felt they were "on duty" 24 hours a day, and many felt that caregiving during this time was extremely stressful.[377] The same study found that 72% of family caregivers experienced relief when the person with Alzheimer's or another dementia died.[377]

***Caregiver Physical Health***

For some caregivers, the demands of caregiving may cause declines in their own health. Evidence suggests that the stress of providing dementia care increases caregivers' susceptibility to disease and health complications.[378] As shown in Figure 9, 38% of Alzheimer's and other dementia caregivers indicate that the physical stress of caregiving is high to very high.[A13] Building on this, a recent analysis found that 29% of caregivers of people with Alzheimer's or other dementias report that providing care results in high physical strain compared with 17% of caregivers of people without dementia.[323] The distress associated with caring for a relative with Alzheimer's or another dementia has also been shown to negatively influence the quality of family caregivers' sleep.[379-381] Compared with those of the same age who were not caregivers, caregivers of people with dementia are estimated to lose between 2.4 hours and 3.5 hours of sleep a week.[381]

*General Health*

Seventy-four percent of caregivers of people with Alzheimer's or other dementias reported that they were "somewhat concerned" to "very concerned" about maintaining their own health since becoming a caregiver.[A13] Forty-two percent of caregivers of people with Alzheimer's or another dementia report that their health is excellent or very good, which is lower than caregivers of people without dementia (50%).[323] In addition, 35% of caregivers of people with Alzheimer's or another dementia report that their health has worsened due to care responsibilities compared with 19% of caregivers of people without dementia.[323] A 2017 poll reported that 27% of dementia caregivers delayed or did not do things they should to maintain their own health.[326] Dementia caregivers indicate lower health-related quality of life than non-caregivers and are more likely than non-caregivers or other caregivers to report that their health is fair or poor.[344,348,382-384] Data from the Health and Retirement Study showed that dementia caregivers who provided care to spouses were much more likely (41% increased odds) than other spousal caregivers of similar age to become increasingly frail during the time between becoming a caregiver and their spouse's death.[385] Other studies, however, suggest that caregiving tasks have the positive effect of keeping older caregivers more physically active than non-caregivers.[386]

Recent research has examined variations in self-rated health among dementia caregivers of diverse racial and ethnic backgrounds. Support from family and friends is associated with better self-rated health for black/African American dementia caregivers, but not for white or Mexican American caregivers. A more positive perceived relationship between the caregiver and person with dementia was associated with better self-rated health among black/African American and white caregivers.[387]

*Physiological Changes*

The chronic stress of caregiving may be associated with an increased incidence of hypertension[342,388-395] and a number of physiological changes that could increase the risk of developing chronic conditions, including high levels of stress hormones,[388] impaired immune function,[342,389] slow wound healing[390] and coronary heart disease.[391] A recent meta-analysis of studies examining the associations between family caregiving, inflammation and immune function suggests that dementia caregivers had slight reductions in immune function and modestly elevated inflammation.[396] Additional studies of physiological changes before and after the start of caregiving in diverse populations are needed to better understand the physiological effects of caregiving.

*Health Care*

Caregivers of people with dementia who are depressed, have behavioral disturbances or have low functional status are more likely to be hospitalized and have emergency department visits[397-398] than caregivers of people with dementia who do not have these symptoms. Increased depressive symptoms among caregivers over time are linked to more frequent doctor visits, increased outpatient tests and procedures, and greater use of over-the-counter and prescription medications.[398]

FIGURE 10

**Work-Related Changes Among Caregivers of People with Alzheimer's or Other Dementias Who Had Been Employed at Any Time Since They Began Caregiving**

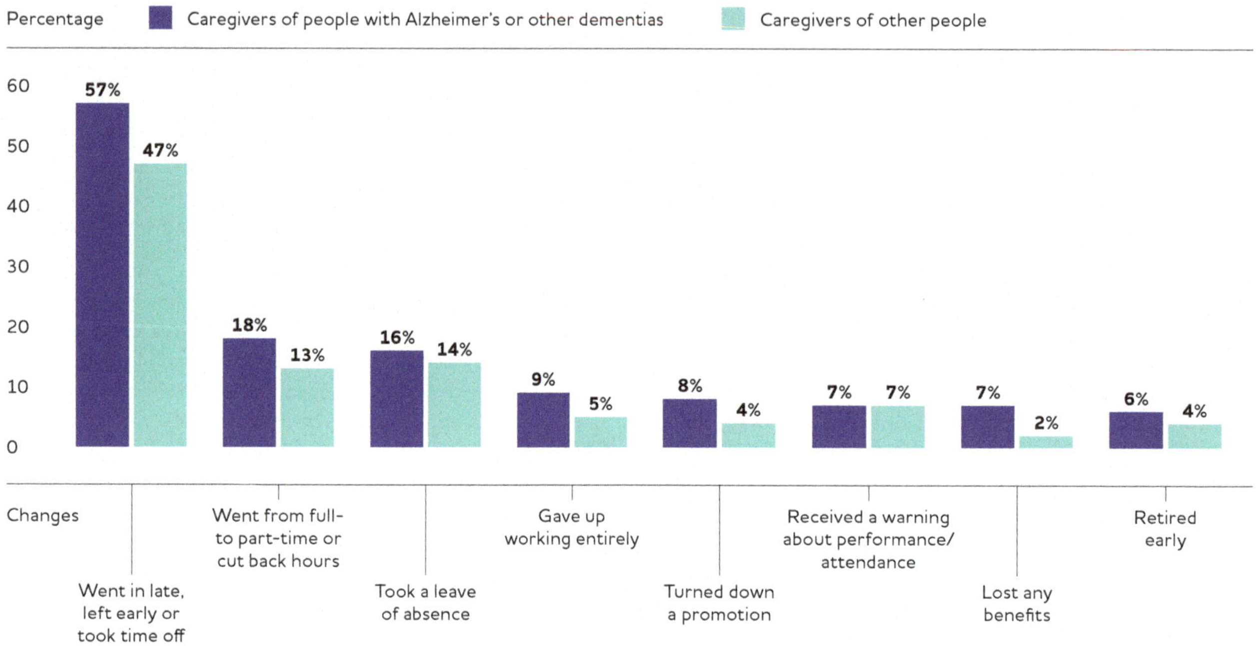


Created from data from the National Alliance for Caregiving and AARP.[323]

*Mortality*

Studies of how the health of people with dementia affects their caregivers' risk of dying have had mixed findings.[399-400] For example, caregivers of spouses who were hospitalized and had dementia were more likely to die in the following year than caregivers whose spouses were hospitalized but did not have dementia (after accounting for differences in caregiver age).[401] In addition, caregivers who perceive higher strain due to care responsibilities were at higher risk for death than caregivers who perceive little or no strain.[402] In contrast, a longitudinal study of participants in the Health and Retirement Study found that dementia caregivers were less likely to die than non-caregivers of similar age over a 12-year period. These results are consistent with a protective effect of dementia care, at least as it pertains to death.[399] The findings are also consistent with the possibility that individuals who assume dementia care roles do so in part because their initial health allows them to do so. Eighteen percent of spousal caregivers die before their partners with dementia.[403]

*Caregiver Employment and Finances*

Six in 10 caregivers of people with Alzheimer's or another dementia were employed or had been employed in the prior year while providing care.[323] These individuals worked an average of 35 hours per week while caregiving.[323] Among people who were employed in the past year while providing care to someone with Alzheimer's or another dementia, 57% reported sometimes needing to go in late or leave early compared with 47% of non-dementia caregivers. Eighteen percent of dementia caregivers reduced their work hours due to care responsibilities, compared with 13% of non-dementia caregivers. Other work-related changes among dementia and non-dementia caregivers who had been employed in the past year are summarized in Figure 10.[323]

Costs of dementia caregiving for employers may include replacement costs for employees who quit due to their caregiving responsibilities and costs of absenteeism and workday interruptions.[404] In 2010, employers lost $13 billion due to employees' elder care responsibilities.[405-406]

TABLE 9

Type and Focus of Caregiver Interventions

| Type | Focus |
|---|---|
| Case management | Provides assessment, information, planning, referral, care coordination and/or advocacy for family caregivers. |
| Psychoeducational approaches | Include structured programs that provide information about the disease, resources and services, and about how to expand skills to effectively respond to symptoms of the disease (for example, cognitive impairment, behavioral symptoms and care-related needs). Include lectures, discussions and written materials and are led by professionals with specialized training. |
| Counseling | Aims to resolve pre-existing personal problems that complicate caregiving to reduce conflicts between caregivers and care recipients and/or improve family functioning. |
| Psychotherapeutic approaches | Involve the establishment of a therapeutic relationship between the caregiver and a professional therapist (for example, cognitive-behavioral therapy for caregivers to focus on identifying and modifying beliefs related to emotional distress, developing new behaviors to deal with caregiving demands, and fostering activities that can promote caregiver well-being). |
| Respite | Provides planned, temporary relief for the caregiver through the provision of substitute care; examples include adult day services and in-home or institutional respite care for a certain number of weekly hours. |
| Support groups | Are less structured than psychoeducational or psychotherapeutic interventions. Support groups provide caregivers the opportunity to share personal feelings and concerns to overcome feelings of isolation. |
| Multicomponent approaches | Are characterized by intensive support strategies that combine multiple forms of interventions, such as education, support and respite, into a single, long-term service (often provided for 12 months or more). |

Created from data from Pinquart et al. and Gaugler et al.[346,409]

In 2019, it is estimated that dementia caregivers bore nearly twice the average out-of-pocket costs (for example, medical care, personal care and household expenses for the person with dementia and personal expenses and respite services for the caregiver) of non-dementia caregivers ($11,372 versus $6,121).[407] Data from the 2016 Alzheimer's Association Family Impact of Alzheimer's Survey indicated that among care contributors (a friend or relative who paid for dementia expenses and/or provided care for someone with dementia at least once a month in the prior year), 48% cut back on spending and 43% cut back on saving due to the out-of-pocket costs of providing help to someone with dementia.[349] Due to care responsibilities in the year prior to the survey, close to four in 10 care contributors indicated that the "food they bought just didn't last, and they didn't have money to get more," and three in 10 ate less because of care-related costs.[349]

***Effects of Caregiver Stress on People with Dementia***

Research has emerged on the effects of caregiver stress on people with dementia and their use of health care services. For example, distress on the part of family caregivers is associated with increased odds of institutionalization of the person with dementia, exacerbated behavioral and psychological challenges in the person with dementia, and increased likelihood of people with dementia being abused.[408] See the Use and Costs of Health Care, Long-Term Care, and Hospice section (page 45) for additional information.

### Interventions Designed to Assist Caregivers

For more than 30 years, strategies to support family caregivers of people with dementia have been developed and evaluated. The types and focus of these strategies (often called "interventions") are summarized in Table 9.[347,409]

In general, the goal of interventions is to improve the health and well-being of dementia caregivers by relieving the negative aspects of caregiving. Some also aim to delay nursing home admission of the person with dementia by providing caregivers with skills and resources (emotional, social, psychological and/or technological) to continue helping their relatives or friends at home. Specific approaches used in various interventions include providing education to caregivers, helping caregivers manage dementia-related symptoms, improving social support for caregivers and providing caregivers with respite from caregiving duties.

According to a publication on dementia caregiver interventions that reviewed seven meta-analyses and 17 systematic reviews of randomized controlled trials, the following characteristics distinguish interventions that are effective: family caregivers are actively involved in the intervention, in contrast to passively receiving information; the intervention is tailored and flexible to meet the changing needs of family caregivers during the course of a relative's dementia; and the intervention meets the needs not only of caregivers, but of people living with dementia as well.[410] A 2012 report examined randomized, controlled studies of caregiver interventions and identified 44 interventions that benefited individuals with dementia as well as caregivers. More such interventions are emerging each year.[411-416] A meta-analysis examining the components of dementia caregiver interventions that are most beneficial found that interventions that initially enhance caregiving competency, gradually address the care needs of the person with dementia, and offer emotional support for loss and grief when needed appeared most effective.[417]

Interventions for dementia caregivers that have demonstrated efficacy in scientific evaluations have been gradually implemented in the community, but are still not widespread or available to all family caregivers.[418-432] When interventions are implemented, they are generally successful at improving how caregiver services are delivered, and have the potential to reach a large number of families while also helping caregivers cope with their responsibilities.[433] In one example, researchers utilized an "agile implementation" process to more rapidly select, localize, evaluate and replicate a collaborative care model for dementia care. This care model has successfully operated for nearly a decade in an Indianapolis health care system.[434] Other efforts have attempted to broaden the reach and accessibility of interventions for dementia caregivers through the use of technologies (for instance, video-phone delivery and online training),[435-442] while others integrated evidence-based dementia care interventions into community-based, long-term service programs.[443] In 2019, the National Institute on Aging (NIA) awarded funding to create the NIA Imbedded Pragmatic AD/ADRD Clinical Trials (IMPACT) Collaboratory. The Collaboratory includes experts from more than 30 top research institutions and will support up to 40 pilot trials to test non-drug, care-based interventions for people living with dementia in the next five years. The goal of IMPACT is to expedite the timeline of research implementation in real-world settings to improve care for people living with dementia and their caregivers.

Because caregivers and the settings in which they provide care are diverse, more studies are required to define which interventions are most effective for specific situations and how these interventions are successful.[444-447] Improved tools and measures to personalize services for caregivers to maximize their benefits represent an emerging area of research.[448-454] More studies are also needed to adapt proven interventions or develop new intervention approaches for families from different racial, ethnic and socioeconomic backgrounds and in different geographic settings.[455-469] Additional research on interventions focused on disease stages is also needed, as well as research on specific intervention needs for LGBT caregivers.[318]

## Paid Caregivers

### Direct-Care Workers for People with Alzheimer's or Other Dementias

Direct-care workers, such as nurse aides, home health aides, and personal and home care aides, provide most of the paid long-term care to older adults living at home or in residential settings.[470-471] In nursing homes, nursing assistants make up the majority of staff who work with cognitively impaired residents.[472-474] Nursing assistants help with bathing, dressing, housekeeping, food preparation and other activities. Most nursing assistants are women, and they come from increasingly diverse ethnic, racial and geographic backgrounds.

Direct-care workers have difficult jobs, and they may not receive the training necessary to provide dementia care.[473,475-477] Turnover rates are high among direct-care workers, and recruitment and retention are persistent challenges.[476,478] Inadequate education and challenging work environments have also contributed to higher turnover rates among nursing staff across care environments.[479] Studies have shown that staff training programs to improve the quality of dementia care in nursing homes and hospitals have modest benefits.[475,480-484] The National Academies of Sciences, Engineering, and Medicine have recommended changes to federal requirements for general direct-care worker training, including an increase in training hours from 75 to 120, and instructional content that focuses more on knowledge and skills related to caring for individuals with Alzheimer's and other dementias.[476-477]

### Shortage of Geriatric Health Care Professionals

Professionals who may receive special training in caring for older adults include physicians, nurse practitioners, registered nurses, social workers, pharmacists, physician assistants and case workers.[476] It is estimated that the United States has approximately half the number of certified geriatricians that it currently needs.[485] As of 2016, there were 7,293 certified geriatricians in the United States, or one geriatrician for every 1,924 Americans age 65 or older in need of care.[486] The American Geriatrics Society estimates that, due to the increase in vulnerable older Americans who require geriatric care, an additional 23,750 geriatricians should be trained between now and 2030 to meet the needs of an aging U.S. population[487] (see the Special Report, page 63, for additional information). There were 272,000 nurse practitioners in the United States in 2019. Eleven percent of nurse practitioners had special expertise in gerontological care.[488] Less than 1% of registered nurses, physician assistants and pharmacists identify themselves as specializing in geriatrics.[476] Although 73% of social workers serve clients age 55 and older, only 4% have formal certification in geriatric social work.[476] Furthermore, the overall aging of the long-term care workforce may affect the number of paid caregivers.[479]

### Enhancing Health Care for Family Caregivers

There is a growing consensus that professionals caring for people with Alzheimer's and other dementias should acknowledge the role family caregivers play in facilitating the treatment of dementia, and that professionals should assess the well-being of family caregivers to improve overall disease management of the person with dementia.[489-493] The complex care challenges of people with dementia also require interprofessional collaboration and education.[494-497] Ongoing efforts have attempted to integrate innovative care management practices with traditional primary care for people with dementia. One example involves a skilled professional who serves as the care manager of the person with dementia. The care manager collaborates with primary care physicians and nurse practitioners to develop personalized care plans. These plans can provide support to family caregivers, help people with dementia manage care transitions (for example, a change in care provider or site of care) and ensure the person with dementia has access to appropriate community-based services. Other models include addressing the needs of family caregivers simultaneously with comprehensive disease management of people living with dementia to improve the quality of life of both.[498] Several evaluations have suggested that such approaches have considerable potential for improving outcomes for people with dementia and their family caregivers (for example, delayed nursing home admission and reduction in caregiver distress).[499-508] Current research is attempting to determine the feasibility of these models beyond the specialty settings in which they currently operate.[509-512]

In 2016, the National Academies of Sciences, Engineering, and Medicine released *Families Caring for an Aging America*, a seminal report that includes a number of recommendations to refocus national health care reform efforts from models of care that center on the patient (person-centered care) to models of care that also explicitly engage and support the patient's family (family-centered care).[404] These service models recognize the important role family members play in providing care and incorporate family caregivers during the delivery of health care to their relatives with dementia. Furthermore, these models encourage health care providers to deliver evidence-based services and support to both caregivers and people living with dementia.[404,513]

In January 2017, Medicare began reimbursing physicians, physician assistants, nurse practitioners and clinical nurse specialists for health care visits that result in a comprehensive dementia care plan. Comprehensive care planning is a core element of effective dementia care management and can result in the delivery of services that potentially enhance quality of life for people with dementia and their caregivers. In the first year the care planning benefit was available (2017), less than 1% of those with Alzheimer's disease or other dementias received a comprehensive dementia care plan. In seven states (Alaska, Montana, New Hampshire, North Dakota, Rhode Island, South Dakota and Vermont) and the District of Columbia, no fee-for-service Medicare beneficiaries received a comprehensive dementia care plan. Use of the Medicare care planning benefit did increase throughout the year, and the rate of use was 3.3 times greater in the fourth quarter of 2017 compared with the first quarter of 2017.[514] The Alzheimer's Association has developed a care planning kit (alz.org/careplanning) to help guide providers to deliver effective care planning for people with dementia and their family caregivers.

## Trends in Dementia Caregiving

There is some indication that families are now better at managing the care they provide to relatives with dementia than in the past. From 1999 to 2015, dementia caregivers were significantly less likely to report physical difficulties (from 30% in 1999 to 17% in 2015) and financial difficulties (from 22% in 1999 to 9% in 2015) related to care provision. In addition, use of respite care by dementia

FIGURE 11

Person-Centered Care Delivery

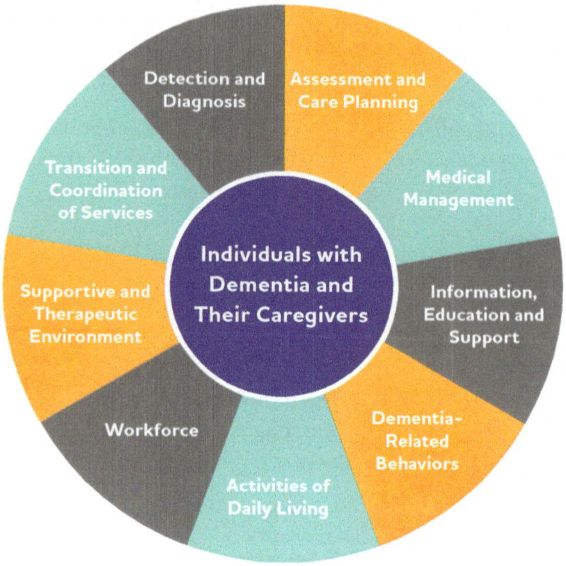


Created from data from the Alzheimer's Association.[516]

caregivers increased substantially (from 13% in 1999 to 27% in 2015).[338] However, as noted earlier, more work is needed to ensure that interventions for dementia caregivers are available and accessible to those who need them. A 2016 study of the Older Americans Act's National Family Caregiver Support Program found that over half (52%) of Area Agencies on Aging did not offer evidence-based family caregiver interventions.[515]

The Alzheimer's Association has undertaken several efforts to improve how dementia care is studied and delivered. Its recent dementia care practice recommendations[516] place individuals with dementia and their caregivers at the center of how care should be delivered (see Figure 11). Essential to this model is the need to reconsider how we measure and design care for people with dementia by moving away from an approach that focuses on loss of abilities due to dementia to an approach that emphasizes the individual's unique needs, personal experiences and strengths. This person-centered care philosophy not only values and respects the individual with dementia, but also promotes well-being and health.[517] This new framework is designed to shift how researchers and care providers think about dementia, and may point the way to a greater understanding of the resilience, adaptability, and the possibilities of maintenance or even improvement of skills and abilities when living with dementia.[518-519] A core element of this and other frameworks is to ensure that every experience and interaction is seen as an opportunity to have meaningful engagement, which in turn helps create a better quality of life for the person with dementia.

# Use and Costs of Health Care, Long-Term Care and Hospice

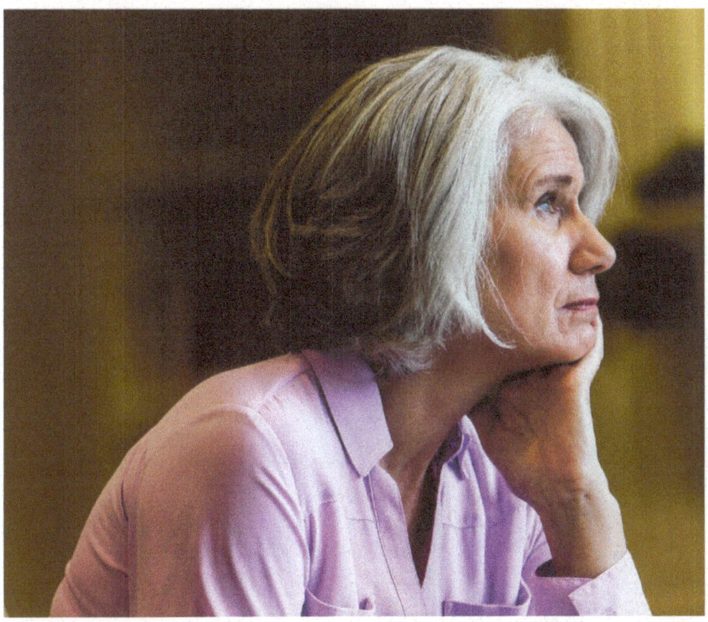

**In 2020, the total national cost of caring for people with Alzheimer's and other dementias is projected to reach $305 billion*.**

*Does not include nearly $244 billion in unpaid caregiving by family and friends.

The costs of health care and long-term care for individuals with Alzheimer's or other dementias are substantial, and dementia is one of the costliest conditions to society.[520] Total payments in 2020 (in 2020 dollars) for all individuals with Alzheimer's or other dementias are estimated at $305 billion (Figure 12), not including the value of informal caregiving that is described in the Caregiving section (see page 32). Medicare and Medicaid are expected to cover $206 billion, or 67%, of the total health care and long-term care payments for people with Alzheimer's or other dementias. Out-of-pocket spending is expected to be $66 billion, or 22% of total payments.[A16] Throughout the rest of this section, all costs are reported in 2019 dollars unless otherwise indicated.[A17]

## Total Cost of Health Care and Long-Term Care

Table 10 reports the average annual per-person payments for health care and long-term care services for Medicare beneficiaries age 65 and older with and without Alzheimer's or other dementias. Total per-person health care and long-term care payments in 2019 from all sources for Medicare beneficiaries with Alzheimer's or other dementias were over three times as great as payments for other Medicare beneficiaries in the same age group ($50,201 per person for those with dementia compared with $14,326 per person for those without dementia).[A18,207]

Twenty-seven percent of older individuals with Alzheimer's or other dementias who have Medicare also have Medicaid coverage, compared with 11% of individuals without dementia.[207] Medicaid pays for nursing home and other long-term care services for some people with very low income and low assets, and the high use of these services by people with dementia translates into high costs to Medicaid. Average annual Medicaid payments per person for Medicare beneficiaries with Alzheimer's or other dementias ($8,779) were 23 times as great as average Medicaid payments for Medicare beneficiaries without Alzheimer's or other dementias ($374) (Table 10).[207]

Despite these and other sources of financial assistance, individuals with Alzheimer's or other dementias still incur high out-of-pocket costs. These costs are for Medicare, other health insurance premiums, deductibles,

FIGURE 12

**Distribution of Aggregate Costs of Care by Payment Source for Americans Age 65 and Older with Alzheimer's or Other Dementias, 2020***

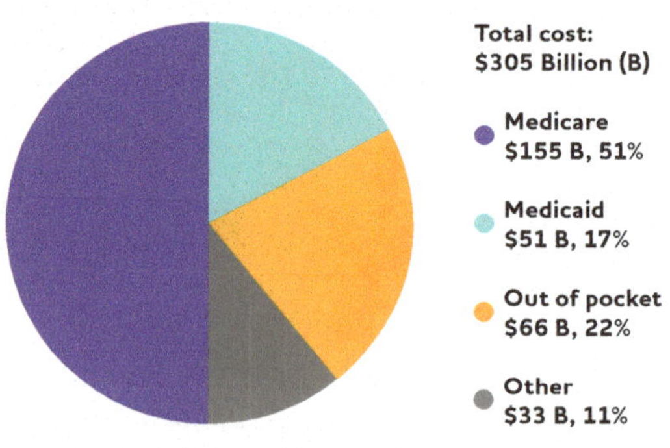


*Data are in 2020 dollars.

Percentages do not total 100 due to rounding.

Created from data from the Lewin Model.[A16] "Other" payment sources include private insurance, health maintenance organizations, other managed care organizations and uncompensated care.

TABLE 10

**Average Annual Per-Person Payments by Payment Source for Health Care and Long-Term Care Services, Medicare Beneficiaries Age 65 and Older, with and without Alzheimer's or Other Dementias, in 2019 Dollars**

| Payment Source | Beneficiaries with Alzheimer's or Other Dementias | Beneficiaries without Alzheimer's or Other Dementias |
|---|---|---|
| Medicare | $25,213 | $7,750 |
| Medicaid | 8,779 | 374 |
| Uncompensated | 390 | 392 |
| Health maintenance organization | 1,293 | 1,583 |
| Private insurance | 2,309 | 1,458 |
| Other payer | 961 | 248 |
| Out of pocket | 11,068 | 2,395 |
| **Total*** | **50,201** | **14,326** |

*Payments from sources do not equal total payments exactly due to the effects of population weighting. Payments for all beneficiaries with Alzheimer's or other dementias include payments for community-dwelling and facility-dwelling beneficiaries.

Created from unpublished data from the Medicare Current Beneficiary Survey for 2011.[207]

copayments and services not covered by Medicare, Medicaid or additional sources of support. On average, Medicare beneficiaries age 65 and older with Alzheimer's or other dementias paid $11,068 out of pocket annually for health care and long-term care services not covered by other sources (Table 10).[207]

Researchers have evaluated the additional or "incremental" health care, residential long-term care and family caregiving costs of dementia (that is, the costs specifically attributed to dementia when comparing people with and without dementia who have the same coexisting medical conditions and demographic characteristics).[312,520-522] In a recent systematic review of studies of older adults with Alzheimer's and other dementias enrolled in private Medicare managed care plans, researchers found a wide range of incremental costs attributable to Alzheimer's and other dementias.[523] One group of researchers found that the incremental health care and nursing home costs for those with dementia were $28,501 per person per year in 2010 dollars ($36,400 in 2019 dollars).[A19,520] Another group of researchers found that the incremental lifetime cost of Alzheimer's dementia was substantially higher for women than men, due to a greater lifetime risk of developing Alzheimer's dementia (see Prevalence section, page 17).[524] Additionally, because women are more likely to be widowed and living in poverty, the incremental Medicaid costs associated with Alzheimer's dementia were 70% higher for women than men. A third group of researchers found that the lifetime cost of care, including out-of-pocket costs, Medicare and Medicaid expenditures, and the value of informal caregiving, was $321,780 per person with Alzheimer's dementia in 2015 dollars ($357,297 in 2019 dollars).[312] The lifetime cost of care for individuals with Alzheimer's dementia was more than twice the amount incurred by individuals without Alzheimer's dementia, translating into an incremental lifetime cost of Alzheimer's dementia of $184,500 ($204,864 in 2019 dollars).

Several groups of researchers have examined the additional out-of-pocket costs borne by individuals with Alzheimer's or other dementias. In a recent analysis of the lifetime incremental cost of dementia, researchers found that individuals with dementia spent $38,540 (in 2014 dollars; $43,920 in 2019 dollars) more out-of-pocket between age 65 and death, due to nursing home care.[525] Another group of researchers found that community-dwelling individuals age 65 and older with Alzheimer's dementia had $1,101 (in 2012 dollars; $1,316 in 2019 dollars) higher annual out-of-pocket health care spending than individuals without Alzheimer's dementia, after controlling for differences in patient characteristics, with the largest portion of the difference being due to higher spending on home health care and prescription drugs.[526] Furthermore, individuals with Alzheimer's dementia spend 12% of their income on out-of-pocket health care services compared with 7% for individuals without Alzheimer's dementia.[527] Another research team found that the five-year incremental cost of dementia was $15,704 (in 2017 dollars; $16,389 in 2019 dollars), with the additional costs of care in the first year after diagnosis representing 46% of the five-year incremental costs.[527]

Other researchers compared end-of-life costs for individuals with and without dementia and found that the total cost in the last 5 years of life was $287,038 per person for individuals with dementia in 2010 dollars and $183,001 per person for individuals without dementia ($366,593 and $233,721, respectively, in 2019 dollars), a difference of 57%.[528] Additionally, out-of-pocket costs represented a substantially larger proportion of total wealth for those with dementia than for people without dementia (32% versus 11%).

FIGURE 13

**Reasons for Hospitalization of Individuals with Alzheimer's Dementia: Percentage of Hospitalized Individuals by Admitting Diagnosis***

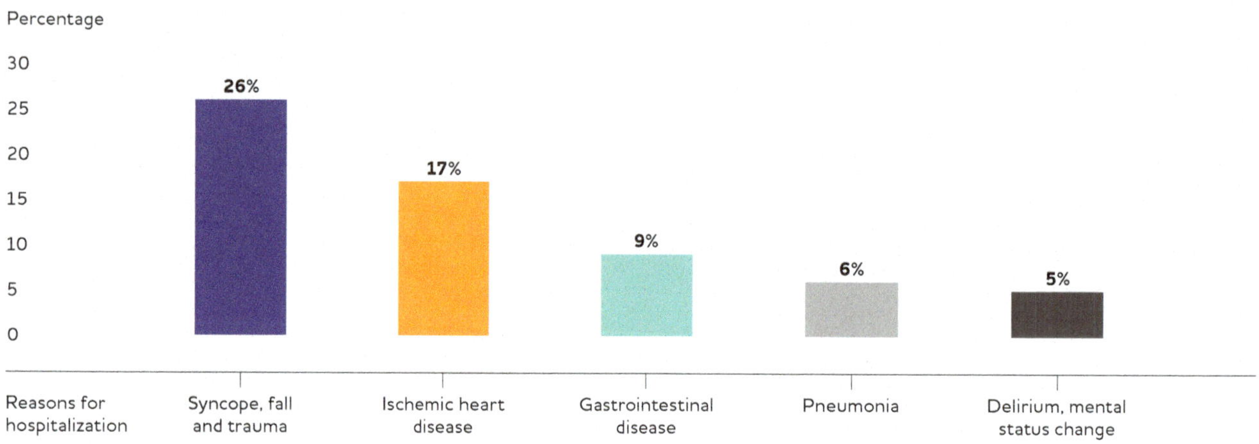


*All hospitalizations for individuals with a clinical diagnosis of probable or possible Alzheimer's were used to calculate percentages. The remaining 37% of hospitalizations were due to other reasons.

Created from data from Rudolph et al.[530]

## Use and Costs of Health Care Services

### Use of Health Care Services

People with Alzheimer's or other dementias have twice as many hospital stays per year as other older people.[291] Moreover, the use of health care services by people with other serious medical conditions is strongly affected by the presence or absence of dementia. In particular, people with coronary artery disease, diabetes, chronic kidney disease, chronic obstructive pulmonary disease (COPD), stroke or cancer who also have Alzheimer's or other dementias have higher use and costs of health care services than people with these medical conditions but no coexisting dementia.

In addition to having more hospital stays, older people with Alzheimer's or other dementias have more skilled nursing facility stays and home health care visits per year than other older people.

- Hospital. There are 538 hospital stays per 1,000 Medicare beneficiaries age 65 and older with Alzheimer's or other dementias compared with 266 hospital stays per 1,000 Medicare beneficiaries age 65 and older without these conditions.[291] A person with dementia in 2012 had, on average, 23 inpatient days — defined as days in a hospital or skilled nursing facility — compared with 5 days for the Medicare population as a whole.[529] The most common reasons for hospitalization of people with Alzheimer's dementia are syncope (fainting), fall and trauma (26%); ischemic heart disease (17%); and gastrointestinal disease (9%) (Figure 13).[530] In a study of inpatient hospitalizations of adults age 60 and older, those with Alzheimer's dementia were at 7% greater risk of dying during the hospital stay and stayed nearly a day longer than individuals without Alzheimer's dementia.[531] Among Medicare beneficiaries with Alzheimer's or other dementias, 22% of hospital stays are followed by a readmission within 30 days.[532] While not directly comparable, one study of a portion of Medicare beneficiaries found an overall readmission rate of 18%.[533] The proportion of hospital stays followed by a readmission within 30 days remained relatively constant between 2007 and 2017 (23% in 2007 versus 22% in 2017).
- Emergency department. There are 1,548 emergency department visits per 1,000 Medicare beneficiaries with Alzheimer's or other dementias per year.[532] While not directly comparable, there were 640 emergency department visits per 1,000 Medicare beneficiaries per year based on a review of utilization patterns of a subset of Medicare beneficiaries.[533] Emergency department visits for people with Alzheimer's or other dementias per 1,000 Medicare beneficiaries increased 22% between 2007 and 2017 (from 1,265 to 1,548), similar to the increases in emergency department visits for individuals with cancer, ischemic heart disease and heart failure (Figure 14, page 49).[532]

FIGURE 14

**Percentage Changes in Emergency Department Visits per 1,000 Fee-for-Service Medicare Beneficiaries for Selected Health Conditions* Between 2007 and 2017**

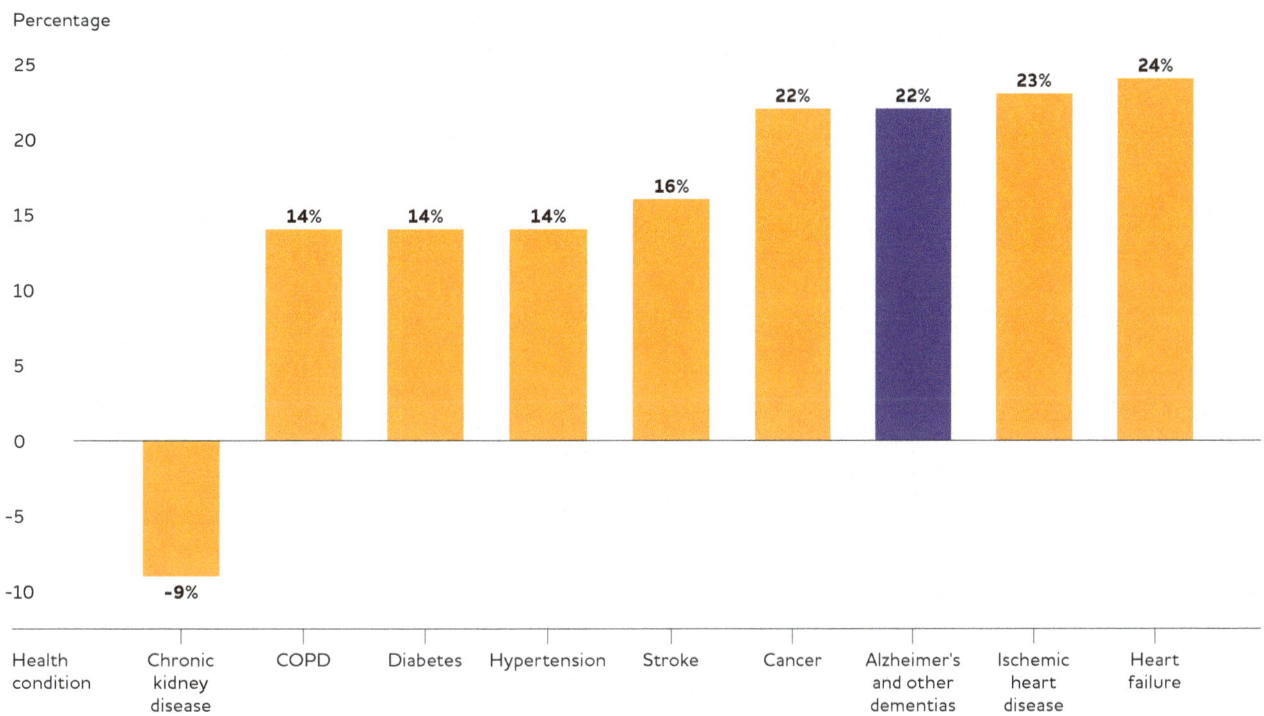


*Includes Medicare beneficiaries with a claims-based diagnosis of each chronic condition. Beneficiaries may have more than one chronic condition.

Created from data from U.S. Centers for Medicare & Medicaid Services.[532]

- Skilled nursing facility. Skilled nursing facilities provide direct medical care that is performed or supervised by registered nurses, such as giving intravenous fluids, changing dressings and administering tube feedings.[534] There are 283 skilled nursing facility stays per 1,000 beneficiaries with Alzheimer's or other dementias per year compared with 73 stays per 1,000 beneficiaries without these conditions — a rate nearly four times as great.[291]
- Home health care. Twenty-five percent of Medicare beneficiaries age 65 and older with Alzheimer's or other dementias have at least one home health visit during the year, compared with 10% of Medicare beneficiaries age 65 and older without Alzheimer's or other dementias.[291] Medicare covers home health services, such as part-time skilled nursing care, home health aide (personal hands-on) care, therapies, and medical social services in the home, but does not include homemaker or personal care services.

### Costs of Health Care Services

Average per-person payments for health care services (hospital, physician and other medical provider, nursing home, skilled nursing facility, hospice and home health care) and prescription medications were higher for Medicare beneficiaries with Alzheimer's or other dementias than for other Medicare beneficiaries in the same age group (see Table 11, page 50).[207]

### Use and Costs of Health Care Service by State

Substantial geographic variation exists in health care utilization and Medicare payments by individuals with Alzheimer's or other dementias (see Table 12, page 51), similar to the geographic variation observed for Medicare beneficiaries with other medical conditions.[535] Emergency department visits range from 1,134 per 1,000 beneficiaries in South Dakota to 1,828 per 1,000 beneficiaries in West Virginia, and the percentage of hospital stays followed by hospital readmission within

TABLE 11

**Average Annual Per-Person Payments by Type of Service for Health Care and Long-Term Care Services, Medicare Beneficiaries Age 65 and Older, with and without Alzheimer's or Other Dementias, in 2019 Dollars**

| Service | Beneficiaries with Alzheimer's or Other Dementias | Beneficiaries without Alzheimer's or Other Dementias |
|---|---|---|
| Inpatient hospital | $11,465 | $3,703 |
| Medical provider* | 5,762 | 3,589 |
| Skilled nursing facility | 7,213 | 493 |
| Nursing home | 16,523 | 800 |
| Hospice | 2,126 | 161 |
| Home health care | 2,661 | 386 |
| Prescription medications** | 3,481 | 2,986 |

*"Medical provider" includes physician, other provider and laboratory services, and medical equipment and supplies.

**Information on payments for prescription medications is only available for people who were living in the community, that is, not in a nursing home or an assisted living facility.

Created from unpublished data from the Medicare Current Beneficiary Survey for 2011.[207]

30 days ranges from 15.4% in Utah to 26.8% in the District of Columbia. Medicare spending per capita ranges from $17,572 in North Dakota to $34,875 in Nevada (in 2019 dollars).[532]

### Use and Costs of Health Care Services Across the Spectrum of Cognitive Impairment

Health care costs increase with the presence of dementia. In a population-based study of adults age 70 to 89, annual health care costs were significantly higher for individuals with dementia than for those with either mild cognitive impairment (MCI) or without cognitive impairment.[536] Annual health care costs for individuals with MCI were not significantly different, however, from costs for individuals without cognitive impairment.

Several groups of researchers have found that both health care and prescription drug spending are significantly higher in the year prior to diagnosis,[537-539] 2 years prior to diagnosis,[540] and one year after diagnosis,[527,537-538] compared with otherwise similar individuals not diagnosed with Alzheimer's or another dementia, although there are differences in the sources of increased spending. In one study, the largest differences were in inpatient and post-acute care,[538] while in another study the differences in spending were primarily due to outpatient care, home care and medical day services.[539] In a third study, the differences were due to home health care, skilled nursing care and durable medical equipment.[540] Additionally, three groups of researchers have found that spending in the year after diagnosis was higher than for individuals not diagnosed with the disease, by amounts ranging from $7,264 in 2017 dollars, based on individuals with fee-for-service Medicare coverage ($7,581 in 2019 dollars)[527] to $17,852 in additional costs in 2014 dollars, based on another group of individuals with Medicare fee-for-service coverage ($20,344 in 2019 dollars).[538] One group of researchers, however, found no difference in health care spending in the 2 years after diagnosis.[540] One possible explanation for the spike in health care costs in the year immediately prior to and after diagnosis of Alzheimer's or another dementia relates to delays in timely diagnosis. One group of researchers found that individuals with cognitive decline who sought care from a specialist (that is, a neurologist, psychiatrist or geriatrician) had a shorter time to diagnosis of Alzheimer's disease.[541] Additionally, individuals diagnosed with cognitive impairment by a specialist had lower Medicare costs in the year after receiving a diagnosis of Alzheimer's dementia than those diagnosed by a non-specialist. One research team found that health care costs were higher in each of the first four years after a dementia diagnosis, but were not significantly different in the fifth year after diagnosis.[527]

### Impact of Alzheimer's and Other Dementias on the Use and Costs of Health Care in People with Coexisting Medical Conditions

Medicare beneficiaries with Alzheimer's or other dementias are more likely than those without dementia to have other chronic conditions.[291] While 26% of Medicare beneficiaries age 65 and older with Alzheimer's or other dementias have five or more chronic conditions (including Alzheimer's or other dementias), only 4% of Medicare beneficiaries without Alzheimer's or other dementias have five or more chronic conditions.[291] Table 13 reports the percentage of people with Alzheimer's or other dementias who had certain coexisting medical conditions. In 2014, the latest year for which information is available, 38% of Medicare beneficiaries age 65 and older with dementia also had coronary artery disease, 37% had diabetes, 29% had chronic kidney disease, 28% had congestive heart failure and 25% had chronic obstructive pulmonary disease.[291]

TABLE 12

**Emergency Department (ED) Visits, Hospital Readmissions and Per Capita Medicare Payments in 2019 Dollars by Medicare Beneficiaries with Alzheimer's or Other Dementias by State, 2017**

| State | Number of ED Visits per 1,000 Beneficiaries | Percentage of Hospital Stays Followed by Readmission within 30 Days | Per Capita Medicare Payments | State | Number of ED Visits per 1,000 Beneficiaries | Percentage of Hospital Stays Followed by Readmission within 30 Days | Per Capita Medicare Payments |
|---|---|---|---|---|---|---|---|
| Alabama | 1,426.8 | 21.5 | 22,555 | Montana | 1,307.1 | 17.5 | 18,664 |
| Alaska | 1,447.9 | 19.6 | 24,801 | Nebraska | 1,166.5 | 18.1 | 21,012 |
| Arizona | 1,491.3 | 20.6 | 25,490 | Nevada | 1,712.2 | 25.4 | 34,875 |
| Arkansas | 1,563.6 | 21.8 | 22,373 | New Hampshire | 1,508.9 | 21.6 | 25,147 |
| California | 1,497.6 | 23.1 | 32,940 | New Jersey | 1,459.8 | 23.0 | 30,930 |
| Colorado | 1,437.1 | 18.3 | 23,060 | New Mexico | 1,566.1 | 20.7 | 22,711 |
| Connecticut | 1,568.0 | 22.0 | 28,461 | New York | 1,446.1 | 23.7 | 31,353 |
| Delaware | 1,600.0 | 21.8 | 28,260 | North Carolina | 1,699.3 | 21.5 | 23,226 |
| District of Columbia | 1,698.5 | 26.8 | 31,993 | North Dakota | 1,193.4 | 19.2 | 17,572 |
| Florida | 1,564.9 | 23.4 | 28,606 | Ohio | 1,633.7 | 22.6 | 26,502 |
| Georgia | 1,568.5 | 21.9 | 24,228 | Oklahoma | 1,700.7 | 21.5 | 26,351 |
| Hawaii | 1,225.2 | 17.4 | 20,009 | Oregon | 1,582.9 | 18.5 | 21,210 |
| Idaho | 1,401.8 | 17.0 | 21,051 | Pennsylvania | 1,477.7 | 22.4 | 26,839 |
| Illinois | 1,611.9 | 23.1 | 28,485 | Rhode Island | 1,614.9 | 22.8 | 26,876 |
| Indiana | 1,510.5 | 21.0 | 25,572 | South Carolina | 1,563.8 | 21.4 | 23,917 |
| Iowa | 1,344.7 | 18.5 | 18,715 | South Dakota | 1,134.0 | 19.1 | 19,070 |
| Kansas | 1,394.1 | 19.4 | 22,787 | Tennessee | 1,574.3 | 22.1 | 24,199 |
| Kentucky | 1,718.4 | 23.0 | 24,991 | Texas | 1,544.9 | 22.0 | 30,383 |
| Louisiana | 1,770.8 | 22.1 | 29,001 | Utah | 1,205.4 | 15.4 | 22,229 |
| Maine | 1,666.3 | 19.8 | 21,787 | Vermont | 1,485.6 | 19.2 | 22,588 |
| Maryland | 1,525.6 | 24.6 | 30,331 | Virginia | 1,637.2 | 22.0 | 23,846 |
| Massachusetts | 1,618.0 | 24.3 | 30,535 | Washington | 1,483.7 | 18.5 | 22,007 |
| Michigan | 1,711.5 | 24.1 | 28,325 | West Virginia | 1,827.7 | 23.6 | 24,762 |
| Minnesota | 1,447.9 | 21.0 | 22,830 | Wisconsin | 1,510.4 | 20.1 | 21,516 |
| Mississippi | 1,723.3 | 22.6 | 26,566 | Wyoming | 1,436.6 | 16.1 | 21,815 |
| Missouri | 1,515.1 | 22.4 | 23,441 | **U.S. Average** | **1,547.7** | **22.3** | **27,101*** |

*The average per capita Medicare payments differ slightly from the figure in Table 10 due to different underlying sources of data.

Created from data from the U.S. Centers for Medicare & Medicaid Services.[532]

TABLE 13

**Percentage of Medicare Beneficiaries Age 65 and Older with Alzheimer's or Other Dementias Who Have Specified Coexisting Conditions**

| Coexisting Condition | Percentage |
|---|---|
| Coronary artery disease | 38 |
| Diabetes | 37 |
| Chronic kidney disease | 29 |
| Congestive heart failure | 28 |
| Chronic obstructive pulmonary disease | 25 |
| Stroke | 22 |
| Cancer | 13 |

Created from unpublished data from the National 5% Sample Medicare Fee-for-Service Beneficiaries for 2014.[291]

Medicare beneficiaries who have Alzheimer's or other dementias and a coexisting medical condition have higher average per-person payments for most health care services than Medicare beneficiaries with the same medical condition but without dementia. Table 14 (see page 53) shows the average per-person Medicare payments for seven specific medical conditions among beneficiaries who have Alzheimer's or other dementias and beneficiaries who do not have Alzheimer's or another dementia.[291] Medicare beneficiaries with Alzheimer's or other dementias have higher average per-person payments in all categories except hospital care payments for individuals with congestive heart failure. One group of researchers found that individuals with dementia and behavioral disturbances, such as agitation, had more psychiatric comorbidities than individuals with dementia but without behavioral disturbances.[542] Additionally, larger proportions of individuals with dementia and behavioral disturbances used medications including antihypertensives, dementia treatments, antipsychotics, antidepressants, antiepileptics and hypnotics.

## Use and Costs of Long-Term Care Services

An estimated 70% of older adults with Alzheimer's or other dementias live in the community, compared with 98% of older adults without Alzheimer's or other dementias.[207] Of those with dementia who live in the community, 74% live with someone and the remaining 26% live alone.[207] As their disease progresses, people with Alzheimer's or other dementias generally receive more care from family members and other unpaid caregivers. Many people with dementia also receive paid services at home; in adult day centers, assisted living facilities or nursing homes; or in more than one of these settings at different times during the often long course of the disease. Medicaid is the only public program that covers the long nursing home stays that most people with dementia require in the late stages of their illnesses.

### Use of Long-Term Care Services by Setting

Most people with Alzheimer's or other dementias who live at home receive unpaid help from family members and friends, but some also receive paid home- and community-based services, such as personal care and adult day care. People with Alzheimer's or other dementias make up a large proportion of all elderly people who receive adult day services and nursing home care.

- Home health services. Thirty-two percent of individuals using home health services have Alzheimer's or other dementias.[543]
- Adult day services. Thirty-one percent of individuals using adult day services have Alzheimer's or other dementias.[543] Overall, 69% of adult day service programs offer specific programs for individuals with Alzheimer's or other dementias, and 14% of adult day service centers primarily serve individuals with Alzheimer's or other dementias.[544]
- Residential care facilities. Forty-two percent of residents in residential care facilities (that is, housing that includes services to assist with everyday activities, such as medication management and meals), including assisted living facilities, have Alzheimer's or other dementias.[543] Small residential care facilities (four to 25 beds) have a larger proportion of residents with Alzheimer's or other dementias than larger facilities (51% in facilities with four to 25 beds compared with 44% in facilities with 26 to 50 beds and 39% in facilities with more than 50 beds).[545] Fifty-eight percent of residential care facilities offer programs for residents with Alzheimer's or other dementias.[545]
- Nursing home care. Overall, 48% of nursing home residents have Alzheimer's or other dementias,[543] while 37% of short-stay (less than 100 days) nursing home residents have Alzheimer's or other dementias, and 59% of long stay (100 days or longer) residents have these conditions. In 2014, 61% of nursing home residents with Alzheimer's or other dementias had moderate or severe cognitive impairment.[546] Four percent of Medicare beneficiaries with Alzheimer's or other dementias reside in a nursing home,[516] and nursing home admission by age 80 is expected for 75% of people with Alzheimer's dementia compared with only 4% of the general population.[293]

## TABLE 14

**Average Annual Per-Person Payments by Type of Service and Coexisting Medical Condition for Medicare Beneficiaries Age 65 and Older, with and without Alzheimer's or Other Dementias, in 2019 Dollars***

| | Average Per-Person Medicare Payment | | | | | |
|---|---|---|---|---|---|---|
| **Medical Condition by Alzheimer's/Dementia (A/D) Status** | **Total Medicare Payments** | Hospital Care | Physician Care | Skilled Nursing Facility Care | Home Health Care | Hospice Care |
| **Coronary artery disease** | | | | | | |
| With A/D | **$28,136** | $8,644 | $2,401 | $4,832 | $2,516 | $3,087 |
| Without A/D | **17,560** | 6,226 | 1,709 | 1,553 | 1,043 | 402 |
| **Diabetes** | | | | | | |
| With A/D | **27,237** | 8,225 | 2,351 | 4,673 | 2,434 | 2,780 |
| Without A/D | **15,036** | 5,152 | 1,506 | 1,350 | 906 | 273 |
| **Congestive heart failure** | | | | | | |
| With A/D | **30,872** | 9,714 | 2,521 | 5,282 | 2,635 | 3,706 |
| Without A/D | **26,193** | 9,862 | 2,265 | 2,860 | 1,871 | 866 |
| **Chronic kidney disease** | | | | | | |
| With A/D | **30,045** | 9,308 | 2,462 | 5,141 | 2,490 | 3,302 |
| Without A/D | **21,542** | 7,694 | 1,941 | 2,075 | 1,290 | 508 |
| **Chronic obstructive pulmonary disease** | | | | | | |
| With A/D | **29,825** | 9,335 | 2,492 | 5,094 | 2,575 | 3,424 |
| Without A/D | **20,346** | 7,476 | 1,883 | 1,927 | 1,289 | 646 |
| **Stroke** | | | | | | |
| With A/D | **28,549** | 8,531 | 2,377 | 5,028 | 2,420 | 3,435 |
| Without A/D | **20,567** | 6,940 | 1,914 | 2,527 | 1,562 | 649 |
| **Cancer** | | | | | | |
| With A/D | **27,046** | 8,093 | 2,302 | 4,334 | 2,226 | 3,073 |
| Without A/D | **17,154** | 5,320 | 1,579 | 1,157 | 743 | 520 |

*This table does not include payments for all kinds of Medicare services, and as a result the average per-person payments for specific Medicare services do not sum to the total per-person Medicare payments.

Created from unpublished data from the National 5% Sample Medicare Fee-for-Service Beneficiaries for 2014.[291]

- Alzheimer's special care units and dedicated facilities. An Alzheimer's special care unit is a dedicated unit, wing or floor in a nursing home or other residential care facility that has tailored services for individuals with Alzheimer's or other dementias. Fifteen percent of nursing homes and 14% of other residential care facilities have a dementia special care unit,[543] even though 72% of Medicare beneficiaries with Alzheimer's dementia have a nursing home stay in the last 90 days of life.[547] Additionally, 9% of residential care facilities exclusively provide care to individuals with dementia, while less than 1% (0.4%) of nursing homes exclusively provide care to individuals with dementia.

*Long-Term Care Services Provided at Home and in the Community*

Nationally, state Medicaid programs are shifting long-term care services from institutional care to home- and community-based services as a means to both reduce unnecessary costs and meet the growing demand for these services by older adults. The federal and state governments share the management and funding of the program, and states differ greatly in the services covered by their Medicaid programs. In 2016, home- and community-based services represented the majority (57%) of Medicaid spending on long-term services and supports, with institutional care representing the remaining 43%.[548] Between 2013 and 2016, Medicaid spending on home- and community-based services increased 26% overall, while spending on institutional care increased only 1.5% over the same period. Additionally, total spending on home care for Medicare beneficiaries with Alzheimer's or other dementias nearly doubled between 2004 and 2011, although increases in spending may be due to a variety of factors, including more people being diagnosed with Alzheimer's dementia, more people using home care, an increase in the number of coexisting medical conditions, more intensive use of home care services and an increase in Medicaid coverage by older adults.[207,549] In two recent systematic reviews of the cost-effectiveness of home support interventions for individuals with dementia, researchers found some evidence to support occupational therapy, home-based exercise and some psychological and behavioral treatments as potentially cost-effective approaches, although the research that has evaluated both the costs and benefits of home support interventions is scant.[550-551]

*Transitions Between Care Settings*

Individuals with dementia often move between a nursing facility, hospital and home, rather than remaining solely in a nursing facility. In a longitudinal study of primary care patients with dementia, researchers found that individuals discharged from a nursing facility were nearly equally as likely to be discharged home (39%) as discharged to a hospital (44%).[552] Individuals with dementia may also transition between a nursing facility and hospital or between a nursing facility, home and hospital, creating challenges for caregivers and providers to ensure that care is coordinated across settings. Other researchers have shown that nursing home residents frequently have burdensome transitions at the end of life, including admission to an intensive care unit in the last month of life and late enrollment in hospice.[553] The number of care transitions for nursing home residents with advanced cognitive impairment varies substantially across geographic regions of the United States.[554]

### Costs of Long-Term Care Services

Long-term care services include home- and community-based services, assisted living and nursing home care. The following estimates are for all users of these services.

- Home care. The median cost for a paid non-medical home health aide is $23 per hour and $1,012 per week.[555] Home care costs increased by 3.1% annually on average over the past 5 years.
- Adult day centers. The median cost of adult day services is $75 per day.[555] The cost of adult day services has increased 2.9% annually on average over the past 5 years.
- Assisted living facilities. The median cost for care in an assisted living facility is $4,051 per month, or $48,612 per year.[555] The cost of assisted living has increased 3% annually on average over the past 5 years.
- Nursing homes. The average cost for a private room in a nursing home is $280 per day, or $102,200 per year, and the average cost of a semi-private room is $247 per day, or $90,155 per year.[555] The cost of nursing home care has increased 3.1% annually on average over the past 5 years for both private and semi-private rooms.

*Affordability of Long-Term Care Services*

Few individuals with Alzheimer's or other dementias have sufficient long-term care insurance or can afford to pay out of pocket for long-term care services for as long as the services are needed.

- Income and asset data are not available for people with Alzheimer's or other dementias specifically, but 50% of Medicare beneficiaries have incomes of $26,200 or less in 2016 dollars ($27,852 in 2019 dollars), and 25% have incomes of $15,250 or less in 2016 dollars ($16,212 in 2019 dollars).[556]

- Fifty percent of Medicare beneficiaries had total savings of $74,450 or less in 2016 dollars ($79,145 in 2019 dollars), 25% had savings of $14,550 or less in 2016 dollars ($15,468 in 2019 dollars), and 8% had no savings or were in debt. Median savings were substantially lower for black/African American and Hispanic/Latino beneficiaries than for white Medicare beneficiaries.[556]

#### *Long-Term Care Insurance*

Long-term care insurance typically covers the cost of care provided in a nursing home, assisted living facility and Alzheimer's special care facility, as well as community-based services such as adult day care and services provided in the home, including nursing care and help with personal care.[557] Results from the 2016 Alzheimer's Association Family Impact of Alzheimer's Survey revealed that 28% of adults believed Medicare covered the cost of nursing home care for people with Alzheimer's, and 37% did not know whether it covered the cost of nursing home care.[349] Although Medicare covers care in a long-term care hospital, skilled nursing care in a skilled nursing facility and hospice care, it does not cover long-term care in a nursing home.[558]

Industry reports estimate that approximately 7.2 million Americans had long-term care insurance in 2014.[559] The median income for individuals purchasing long-term care insurance was $87,500 in 2010 dollars ($102,373 in 2019 dollars), with 77% having an annual income greater than $50,000 ($58,499 in 2019 dollars) and 82% having assets greater than $75,000 ($87,748 in 2019 dollars).[559] Private health care and long-term care insurance policies funded only about 8% of total long-term care spending in 2013, representing $24.8 billion of the $310 billion total in 2013 dollars ($27.2 billion of the $340 billion in 2019 dollars).[560] The private long-term care insurance market is highly concentrated and has consolidated since 2000. In 2000, 41% of individuals with a long-term care policy were insured by one of the five largest insurers versus 56% in 2014.[559]

To address the dearth of private long-term care insurance options and high out-of-pocket cost of long-term care services, Washington became the first state in the country to pass a law that will create a public state-operated long-term care insurance program.[561] The Long-Term Services and Supports Trust Program will be funded by a payroll tax on employees of 58 cents per $100 earned that begins in 2022, and self-employed individuals will be able to opt in to the program. The program is currently structured to pay up to $36,500 in lifetime benefits, beginning in 2025.

#### *Medicaid Costs*

Medicaid covers nursing home care and long-term care services in the community for individuals who meet program requirements for level of care, income and assets. To receive coverage, beneficiaries must have low incomes. Most nursing home residents who qualify for Medicaid must spend all of their Social Security income and any other monthly income, except for a very small personal needs allowance, to pay for nursing home care. Medicaid only makes up the difference if the nursing home resident cannot pay the full cost of care or has a financially dependent spouse. Although Medicaid covers the cost of nursing home care, its coverage of many long-term care and support services, such as assisted living care, home-based skilled nursing care and help with personal care, varies by state.

Total Medicaid spending for people with Alzheimer's or other dementias is projected to be $51 billion in 2020 (in 2020 dollars).[A16] Estimated state-by-state Medicaid spending on people with Alzheimer's or other dementias in 2020 (in 2020 dollars) is included in Table 15 (see page 56). Total per-person Medicaid payments for Medicare beneficiaries age 65 and older with Alzheimer's or other dementias were 23 times as great as Medicaid payments for other Medicare beneficiaries.[207] Much of the difference in payments for beneficiaries with Alzheimer's or other dementias and other beneficiaries is due to the costs associated with long-term care (nursing homes and other residential care facilities, such as assisted living facilities) and the greater percentage of people with dementia who are eligible for Medicaid.

### Use and Costs of Care at the End of Life

Hospice care provides medical care, pain management, and emotional and spiritual support for people who are dying, including people with Alzheimer's or other dementias, either in a facility or at home. Hospice care also provides emotional and spiritual support and bereavement services for families of people who are dying. The main purpose of hospice is to allow individuals to die with dignity and without pain and other distressing symptoms that often accompany terminal illness. Medicare is the primary source of payment for hospice care, but private insurance, Medicaid and other sources also pay for hospice care. Based on data from the National Hospice Survey for 2008 to 2011, nearly all (99%) hospices cared for individuals with dementia, although only 67% of hospices cared for individuals with a primary diagnosis of dementia.[562] Fifty-two percent of individuals in for-profit hospices had either a primary or

TABLE 15

Total Medicaid Payments for Americans Age 65 and Older Living with Alzheimer's or Other Dementias by State*

| State | 2020 (in millions of dollars) | 2025 (in millions of dollars) | Percentage Increase |
|---|---|---|---|
| Alabama | $925 | $1,127 | 21.8 |
| Alaska | 76 | 110 | 44.6 |
| Arizona | 414 | 545 | 31.7 |
| Arkansas | 396 | 454 | 14.6 |
| California | 4,197 | 5,235 | 24.7 |
| Colorado | 635 | 789 | 24.1 |
| Connecticut | 1,022 | 1,187 | 16.1 |
| Delaware | 253 | 313 | 23.6 |
| District of Columbia | 126 | 135 | 6.8 |
| Florida | 2,689 | 3,453 | 28.4 |
| Georgia | 1,265 | 1,594 | 26.0 |
| Hawaii | 240 | 285 | 18.7 |
| Idaho | 149 | 196 | 31.2 |
| Illinois | 1,787 | 2,199 | 23.1 |
| Indiana | 1,054 | 1,233 | 17.1 |
| Iowa | 676 | 792 | 17.2 |
| Kansas | 473 | 543 | 14.6 |
| Kentucky | 803 | 949 | 18.2 |
| Louisiana | 765 | 934 | 22.1 |
| Maine | 212 | 274 | 29.5 |
| Maryland | 1,231 | 1,535 | 24.7 |
| Massachusetts | 1,753 | 2,031 | 15.9 |
| Michigan | 1,487 | 1,738 | 16.9 |
| Minnesota | 905 | 1,087 | 20.1 |
| Mississippi | 606 | 729 | 20.4 |
| Missouri | 973 | 1,137 | 16.8 |
| Montana | $166 | $203 | 22.2 |
| Nebraska | 372 | 411 | 10.3 |
| Nevada | 203 | 277 | 36.5 |
| New Hampshire | 254 | 335 | 31.9 |
| New Jersey | 2,186 | 2,614 | 19.6 |
| New Mexico | 227 | 279 | 22.9 |
| New York | 5,453 | 6,306 | 15.6 |
| North Carolina | 1,332 | 1,628 | 22.2 |
| North Dakota | 190 | 215 | 13.2 |
| Ohio | 2,534 | 2,940 | 16.0 |
| Oklahoma | 516 | 611 | 18.3 |
| Oregon | 253 | 317 | 25.4 |
| Pennsylvania | 3,658 | 4,029 | 10.2 |
| Rhode Island | 470 | 565 | 20.1 |
| South Carolina | 652 | 818 | 25.4 |
| South Dakota | 182 | 212 | 16.6 |
| Tennessee | 1,109 | 1,377 | 24.2 |
| Texas | 3,202 | 3,949 | 23.3 |
| Utah | 185 | 235 | 27.0 |
| Vermont | 116 | 146 | 26.4 |
| Virginia | 1,000 | 1,266 | 26.6 |
| Washington | 547 | 689 | 26.0 |
| West Virginia | 445 | 521 | 17.1 |
| Wisconsin | 777 | 924 | 18.9 |
| Wyoming | 86 | 111 | 28.8 |
| **U.S. Average** | **$51,226** | **$61,581** | **20.2** |

*All cost figures are reported in 2020 dollars. State totals may not add to the U.S. total due to rounding.

Created from data from the Lewin Model.[A16]

## TABLE 16

**Number and Percentage of Medicare Beneficiaries Admitted to Hospice with a Primary Diagnosis of Dementia by State, 2017**

| State | Number of Beneficiaries | Percentage of Beneficiaries |
|---|---|---|
| Alabama | 5,867 | 18 |
| Alaska | 95 | 14 |
| Arizona | 7,229 | 18 |
| Arkansas | 3,133 | 18 |
| California | 30,045 | 20 |
| Colorado | 3,254 | 15 |
| Connecticut | 2,380 | 15 |
| Delaware | 716 | 12 |
| District of Columbia | 263 | 18 |
| Florida | 19,897 | 15 |
| Georgia | 10,435 | 21 |
| Hawaii | 943 | 16 |
| Idaho | 1,566 | 17 |
| Illinois | 9,795 | 18 |
| Indiana | 5,922 | 17 |
| Iowa | 3,278 | 17 |
| Kansas | 2,770 | 18 |
| Kentucky | 2,895 | 15 |
| Louisiana | 4,786 | 19 |
| Maine | 1,494 | 19 |
| Maryland | 4,072 | 17 |
| Massachusetts | 7,245 | 23 |
| Michigan | 9,001 | 16 |
| Minnesota | 5,399 | 21 |
| Mississippi | 3,547 | 20 |
| Missouri | 5,991 | 17 |
| Montana | 507 | 11 |
| Nebraska | 1,648 | 18 |
| Nevada | 2,167 | 17 |
| New Hampshire | 1,007 | 17 |
| New Jersey | 8,207 | 23 |
| New Mexico | 1,523 | 15 |
| New York | 7,669 | 16 |
| North Carolina | 8,486 | 17 |
| North Dakota | 468 | 18 |
| Ohio | 12,656 | 17 |
| Oklahoma | 4,102 | 18 |
| Oregon | 3,565 | 17 |
| Pennsylvania | 12,384 | 17 |
| Rhode Island | 1,657 | 25 |
| South Carolina | 6,038 | 20 |
| South Dakota | 421 | 13 |
| Tennessee | 6,435 | 19 |
| Texas | 26,672 | 22 |
| Utah | 2,506 | 19 |
| Vermont | 543 | 17 |
| Virginia | 6,440 | 19 |
| Washington | 5,459 | 20 |
| West Virginia | 1,552 | 15 |
| Wisconsin | 5,086 | 16 |
| Wyoming | 89 | 7 |
| **U.S. Total** | **278,192** | **18** |

Created from data from the U.S. Centers for Medicare & Medicaid Services.[564]

FIGURE 15

Place of Death Due to Alzheimer's Disease, 1999 to 2017

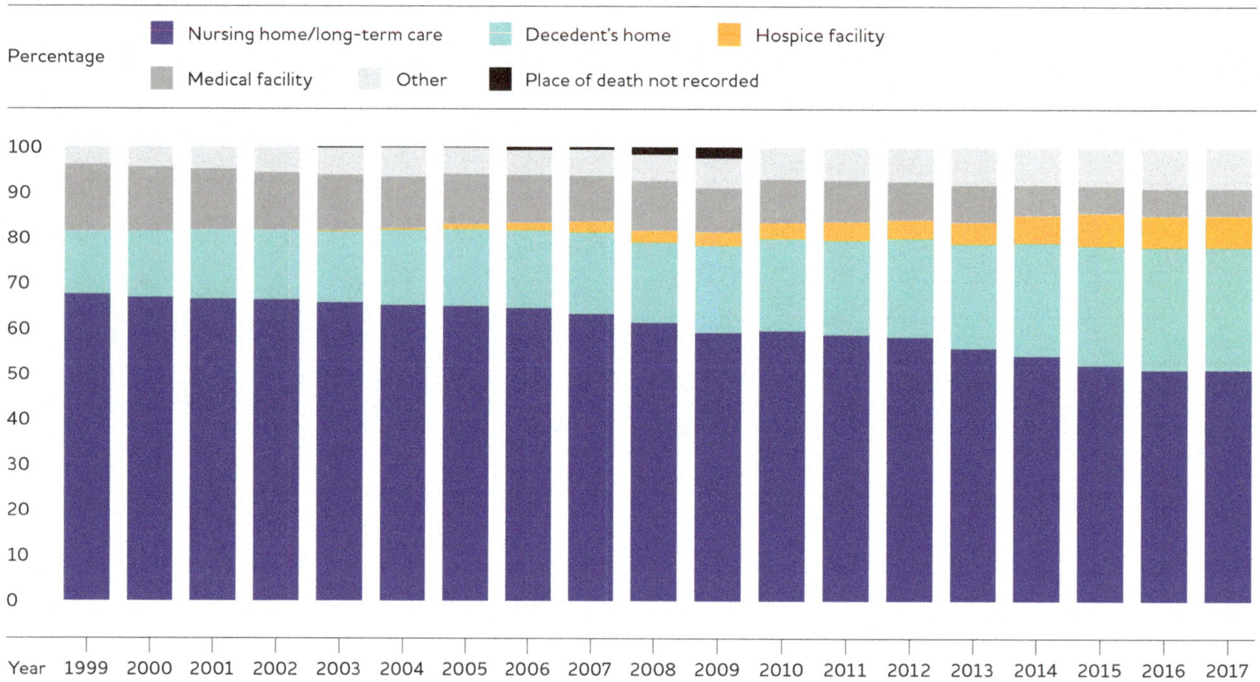


Created from data from the National Center for Health Statistics.[575]

comorbid diagnosis of dementia, while 41% of individuals in nonprofit hospices had a diagnosis of dementia. More research is needed to understand the underlying reasons for the differences in the percentage of people with dementia in for-profit versus nonprofit hospices.

Nineteen percent of Medicare beneficiaries with Alzheimer's and other dementias have at least one hospice claim annually compared with 2% of Medicare beneficiaries without Alzheimer's or other dementias.[291] Expansion of hospice care is associated with fewer individuals with dementia having more than two hospitalizations for any reason or more than one hospitalization for pneumonia, urinary tract infection, dehydration or sepsis in the last 90 days of life.[563] In 2017, there were 4,254 hospice companies in the United States that provided hospice care in the home, assisted living facilities, long-term care facilities, unskilled nursing facilities, skilled nursing facilities, inpatient hospitals, inpatient hospice facilities and other facilities.[564] Additionally, 18% of Medicare beneficiaries who received hospice care had a primary diagnosis of dementia, including Alzheimer's dementia (Table 16).[564] Dementia was the second most common primary diagnosis for Medicare beneficiaries admitted to hospice overall, with cancer being the most common primary diagnosis. Forty-five percent of hospice users in 2014 had a primary or secondary diagnosis of Alzheimer's or other dementias, suggesting that a large proportion of hospice users have Alzheimer's as a comorbid condition.[565] The average length of hospice stay for individuals with a primary diagnosis of dementia was more than 50% longer than for individuals with other primary diagnoses, based on data from the 2008 to 2011 National Hospice Survey.[562] Individuals with a primary diagnosis of dementia stayed an average of 112 days versus 74 days for individuals with other primary diagnoses.

Per-person hospice payments among all individuals with Alzheimer's dementia averaged $2,126 compared with $161 for all other Medicare beneficiaries.[207] In 2016 Medicare reimbursement for home hospice services changed from a simple daily rate for each setting to a two-tiered approach that provides higher reimbursement for days 1-60 than for subsequent days and a service intensity add-on payment for home visits by a registered nurse or social worker in the last 7 days of life. In fiscal year 2020, the routine home care rates are $194.50 per day for days 1-60 and $153.72 per day for days 61 and beyond.[566] In a simulation to evaluate whether the reimbursement

TABLE 17

**Average Annual Per-Person Payments by Type of Service and Race/Ethnicity for Medicare Beneficiaries Age 65 and Older, with Alzheimer's or Other Dementias, in 2019 Dollars**

| Race/Ethnicity | Total Medicare Payments Per Person | Hospital Care | Physician Care | Skilled Nursing Facility Care | Home Health Care | Hospice Care |
|---|---|---|---|---|---|---|
| White | $21,174 | $5,683 | $1,637 | $3,710 | $1,832 | $3,382 |
| Black/African American | 28,633 | 9,566 | 2,219 | 4,599 | 2,239 | 2,503 |
| Hispanic/Latino | 22,694 | 7,690 | 1,930 | 3,535 | 1,932 | 1,864 |
| Other | 27,548 | 8,649 | 2,171 | 3,703 | 3,969 | 2,756 |

Created from unpublished data from the National 5% Sample Medicare Fee-for-Service Beneficiaries for 2014.[291]

change will reduce costs for Medicare, a group of researchers found that the new reimbursement approach is anticipated to reduce costs for Medicare, although individuals with dementia who receive hospice care will have higher Medicare spending overall than individuals with dementia who do not receive hospice care.[567]

For Medicare beneficiaries with advanced dementia who receive skilled nursing facility care in the last 90 days of life, those who are enrolled in hospice are less likely to die in the hospital.[568] Additionally, those enrolled in hospice care are less likely to be hospitalized in the last 30 days of life[569] and more likely to receive regular treatment for pain.[570-571] Nearly half of individuals with dementia die while receiving hospice care.[547] Satisfaction with medical care is higher for families of individuals with dementia who are enrolled in hospice care than for families of individuals with dementia not enrolled in hospice care.[572]

***Feeding Tube Use at the End of Life***

Individuals with frequent transitions between health care settings are more likely to have feeding tubes at the end of life, even though feeding tube placement does not prolong life or improve outcomes.[529] The odds of having a feeding tube inserted at the end of life vary across the country and are not explained by severity of illness, restrictions on the use of artificial hydration and nutrition, ethnicity or gender. Researchers found that feeding tube use was highest for people with dementia whose care was managed by a subspecialist physician or both a subspecialist and a general practitioner. By contrast, feeding tube use was lower among people with dementia whose care was managed by a general practitioner.[573-574] With the expansion of Medicare-supported hospice care, the use of feeding tubes in the last 90 days of life has decreased for individuals with Alzheimer's or other dementias.[563] Finally, with the increased focus on the lack of evidence supporting feeding tube use for people with advanced dementia, the proportion of nursing home residents receiving a feeding tube in the 12 months prior to death decreased from nearly 12% in 2000 to less than 6% in 2014.[574]

***Place of Death for Individuals with Alzheimer's or Other Dementias***

Between 1999 and 2017, the proportion of individuals with Alzheimer's who died in a nursing home decreased from 68% to 51%, and the proportion who died in a medical facility decreased from 15% to 5%.[575] During the same period, the proportion of individuals who died at home increased from 14% to 28% (Figure 15).[575]

## Use and Costs of Health Care and Long-Term Care Services by Race/Ethnicity

Among Medicare beneficiaries with Alzheimer's or other dementias, blacks/African Americans had the highest Medicare payments per person per year, while whites had the lowest payments ($28,633 versus $21,174, respectively) (Table 17). The largest difference in payments was for hospital care, with blacks/African Americans incurring 1.7 times as much in hospital care costs as whites ($9,566 versus $5,683).[291]

In a study of Medicaid beneficiaries with a diagnosis of Alzheimer's dementia that included both Medicaid and Medicare claims data, researchers found significant differences in the costs of care by race/ethnicity.[576] These results demonstrated that blacks/African Americans had significantly higher costs of care than whites or Hispanics, primarily due to more inpatient care and more comorbidities. These differences may be

FIGURE 16

**Hospital Stays Per 1,000 Medicare Beneficiaries Age 65 and Older with Specified Coexisting Medical Conditions, with and without Alzheimer's or Other Dementias, 2014**

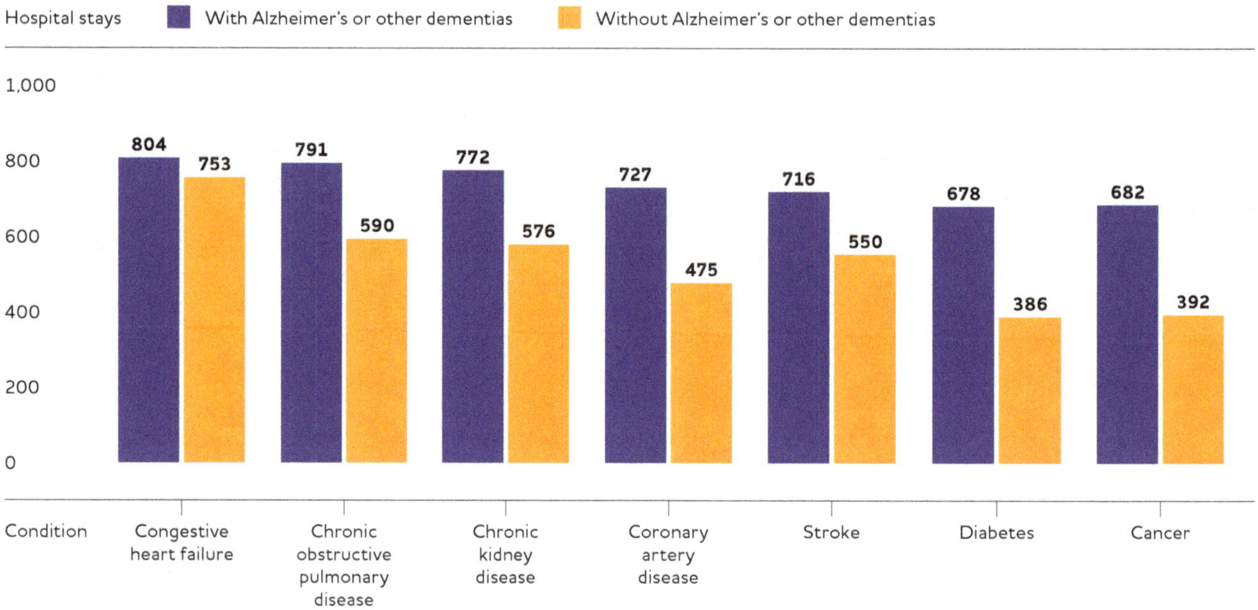


Created from unpublished data from the National 5% Sample Medicare Fee-for-Service Beneficiaries for 2014.[291]

attributable to later-stage diagnosis, which may lead to higher levels of disability while receiving care; delays in accessing timely primary care; lack of care coordination; duplication of services across providers; or inequities in access to care. However, more research is needed to understand the reasons for this health care disparity.

## Avoidable Use of Health Care and Long-Term Care Services

### Preventable Hospitalizations

Preventable hospitalizations are one common measure of health care quality. Preventable hospitalizations are hospitalizations for conditions that could have been avoided with better access to, or quality of, preventive and primary care. Unplanned hospital readmissions within 30 days are another type of hospitalization that potentially could have been avoided with appropriate post-discharge care. In 2013, 21% of hospitalizations for fee-for-service Medicare enrollees with Alzheimer's or other dementias were either for unplanned readmissions within 30 days or for an ambulatory care sensitive condition (that is, a condition that was potentially avoidable with timely and effective ambulatory care). The total cost to Medicare of these potentially preventable hospitalizations was $4.7 billion (in 2013 dollars; $5.4 billion in 2019 dollars).[577]

Of people with dementia who had at least one hospitalization, 18% were readmitted within 30 days. Of those who were readmitted within 30 days, 27% were readmitted two or more times. Ten percent of Medicare enrollees had at least one hospitalization for an ambulatory care-sensitive condition, and 14% of total hospitalizations for Medicare enrollees with Alzheimer's or other dementias were for ambulatory care sensitive conditions.

Based on Medicare administrative data from 2010 to 2015, preventable hospitalizations represented 23.5% of the total hospitalizations for individuals with Alzheimer's or other dementias.[578] Black/African American older adults had a substantially higher proportion of preventable hospitalizations (32%) compared with Hispanic/Latino and white older adults (22%).

Based on data from the Health and Retirement Study and from Medicare, after controlling for demographic, clinical and health risk factors, individuals with dementia had a 30% greater risk of having a preventable hospitalization than those without a neuropsychiatric disorder (that is, dementia, depression or cognitive impairment without dementia). Moreover, individuals with both dementia and depression had a 70% greater risk of preventable hospitalization than those without a neuropsychiatric disorder.[579] Another group of researchers found that individuals with dementia and a caregiver with depression had 73% higher rates of emergency department use over 6 months than individuals with dementia and a caregiver who did not have depression.[580]

Medicare beneficiaries who have Alzheimer's or other dementias and a serious coexisting medical condition (for example, congestive heart failure) are more likely to be hospitalized than people with the same coexisting medical condition but without dementia (Figure 16).[291] One research team found that individuals hospitalized with heart failure are more likely to be readmitted or die after hospital discharge if they also have cognitive impairment.[581] Another research team found that Medicare beneficiaries with Alzheimer's or other dementias have more potentially avoidable hospitalizations for diabetes complications and hypertension, meaning that the hospitalizations could possibly be prevented through proactive care management in the outpatient setting.[582] A third research team found that having depression, rheumatoid arthritis or osteoarthritis was associated with higher emergency department use in Medicare beneficiaries with possible or probable dementia and two more chronic conditions.[583]

Differences in health care use between individuals with and without dementia are most prominent for those residing in the community. Based on data from the Health and Retirement Study, community-residing individuals with dementia were more likely to have a potentially preventable hospitalization, an emergency department visit that was potentially avoidable, and/or an emergency department visit that resulted in a hospitalization.[584] For individuals residing in a nursing home, there were no differences in the likelihood of being hospitalized or having an emergency department visit.

### Initiatives to Reduce Avoidable Health Care and Nursing Home Use

Recent research has demonstrated that two types of programs have potential for reducing avoidable health care and nursing home use, with one type of program focusing on the caregiver and the other focusing on the care delivery team. The Caregiving section (see page 32) describes a number of caregiver support programs, and some of these also hold promise for reducing transitions to residential care for individuals with Alzheimer's or other dementias. Additionally, collaborative care models — models that include not only geriatricians, but also social workers, nurses and medical assistants, for example — can improve care coordination, thereby reducing health care costs associated with hospitalizations, emergency department visits and other outpatient visits.[502] For example, an interprofessional memory care clinic was shown to reduce per-person health care costs by $3,474 in 2012 dollars ($4,153 in 2019 dollars) over a year for individuals with memory problems compared with others with memory problems whose care was overseen by a primary care provider only.[502] More than half of the cost savings was attributed to lower inpatient hospital costs. The program was relatively low cost per person, with an average annual cost of $618 ($739 in 2019 dollars) — a nearly 6-to-1 return on investment. Another group of researchers, however, found that a dementia care program that used nurse practitioners and physicians to co-manage patients was cost neutral after taking into account the costs of the program and cost savings due to fewer long-term care nursing home admissions.[585] However, in a recent systematic review and meta-analysis of 17 randomized controlled trials from seven countries aimed at reducing avoidable acute hospital care by persons with dementia, none of the interventions reduced acute hospital use, such as emergency department visits, hospital admissions, or hospital days.[586]

A group of researchers found that individuals with dementia whose care was concentrated within a smaller number of clinicians had fewer hospitalizations and emergency department visits and lower health care spending overall compared with individuals whose care was dispersed across a larger number of clinicians.[587] More research is needed to understand whether continuity of care is a strategy for decreasing unnecessary health care use for people with Alzheimer's or other dementias.

## Projections for the Future

Total annual payments for health care, long-term care and hospice care for people with Alzheimer's or other dementias are projected to increase from $305 billion in 2020 to more than $1.1 trillion in 2050 (in 2020 dollars). This dramatic rise includes nearly four-fold increases both in government spending under Medicare and Medicaid and in out-of-pocket spending.[A16]

### Potential Impact of Changing the Trajectory of Alzheimer's Disease

While there are currently no FDA-approved pharmacologic treatments that prevent or cure Alzheimer's disease or slow its progression, several groups of researchers have estimated the cost savings of future interventions that either slow the onset of dementia or reduce the symptoms.[312,588-590] One group of researchers estimated that a treatment introduced in 2025 that delays the onset of Alzheimer's by 5 years would reduce total health care payments by 33% and out-of-pocket payments by 44% in 2050.[588] A second group of researchers estimated the cost savings of delaying the onset of Alzheimer's disease by 1 to 5 years. For individuals age 70 and older, they projected a 1-year delay would reduce total health care payments by 14% in 2050, a 3-year delay would reduce total health care payments by 27%, and a 5-year delay would reduce health care payments by 39%.[589] They also projected that a delay in onset may increase per capita health care payments through the end of life due to longer life, although the additional health care costs may be offset by lower informal care costs. A third group of researchers estimated that a treatment that slows the rate of functional decline by 10% would reduce average per-person lifetime costs by $3,880 in 2015 dollars ($4,308 in 2019 dollars), while a treatment that reduces the number of behavioral and psychological symptoms by 10% would reduce average per-person lifetime costs by $680 ($755 in 2019 dollars).[312]

The Alzheimer's Association commissioned a study of the potential cost savings of early diagnosis,[590] assuming that 88% of individuals who will develop Alzheimer's disease would be diagnosed in the MCI phase rather than the dementia phase or not at all. Approximately $7 trillion could be saved in medical and long-term care costs for individuals who were alive in 2018 and will develop Alzheimer's disease. Cost savings were due to a smaller spike in costs immediately before and after diagnosis due to 1) the diagnosis being made during the MCI phase rather than the dementia phase, which has higher costs, and 2) lower medical and long-term care costs for individuals who have diagnosed and managed MCI and dementia compared with individuals with unmanaged MCI and dementia.

A treatment that prevents, cures or slows the progression of the disease could result in substantial savings to the U.S. health care system. Without changes to the structure of the U.S. health care system, however, access to new treatments for Alzheimer's may be severely restricted by capacity constraints. For example, one group of researchers developed a model of capacity constraints that estimated that individuals would wait an average of 19 months for treatment in 2020 if a new treatment is introduced by then.[591] Under this model, approximately 2.1 million individuals with MCI due to Alzheimer's disease would develop Alzheimer's dementia between 2020 and 2040 while on waiting lists for treatment. This model assumed both that the hypothetical treatment would require infusions at infusion centers and that it would depend on people being evaluated with amyloid PET scans. While the introduction of new treatments that prevent, cure or slow the progress of Alzheimer's could have a dramatic effect on the incidence and severity of Alzheimer's, it is clear that their effectiveness could be limited by constraints on both health care system capacity and health insurance reimbursement.

# Special Report
# On the Front Lines: Primary Care Physicians and Alzheimer's Care in America

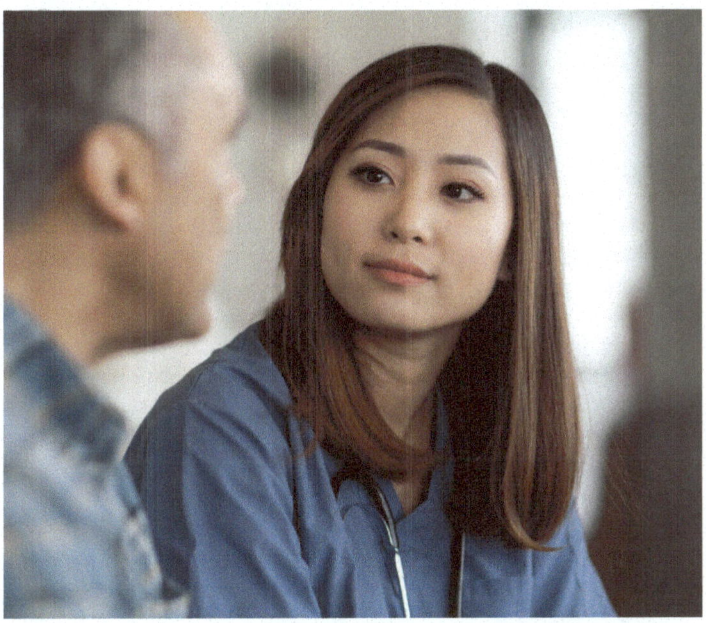

82% of primary care physicians say they are on the front lines of providing dementia care.

Alzheimer's and other dementias represent a growing crisis in America. As reported in the Prevalence section (see page 17) of this year's *Alzheimer's Disease Facts and Figures*, there are currently more than 5 million Americans living with Alzheimer's dementia, a number which is projected to increase to nearly 14 million by the year 2050. Meanwhile, there is a shortage of specialty physicians to provide care for the large and increasing number of people with Alzheimer's dementia in the United States. As a result, the responsibility for medical care rests mainly with primary care physicians. This Special Report examines the current gaps and projected future shortages in specialty care for Alzheimer's and other dementias. It also explores the challenges primary care physicians face in caring for those currently living with dementia and in meeting the future care needs of an aging U.S. population. This report concludes with recommendations to address these shortages and challenges so more Americans have access to dementia care.

## Who Diagnoses and Provides Medical Care?

Medical care for people with Alzheimer's and other dementias involves a broad array of practitioners, including physicians, nurses, neuropsychologists and allied health care professionals such as occupational and physical therapists and home health aides. In this report, we focus on primary care physicians (family medicine, internal medicine, general practice) and specialists such as geriatricians, neurologists, geriatric psychiatrists and neuropsychologists. Given the complexity of diagnosing and managing treatment for people living with dementia, there is general agreement that having a robust workforce of specialists would be ideal to optimize their care. However, the shortage of such specialists means that the major responsibility for diagnosing and treating people living with dementia lies with primary care physicians.

For example, one recent study[597] found that the vast majority of older Americans diagnosed with dementia never see a dementia care specialist and are overwhelmingly diagnosed and cared for by non-specialists. Specifically, the study found that 85% of people first diagnosed with dementia were diagnosed by a non-dementia specialist physician, usually a primary care physician. The same study found that one year after diagnosis, less than a quarter of patients had seen a dementia specialist. After five years, the percentage of patients who had seen a dementia specialist had only increased to 36%. Specialty care follow-up was particularly low for Hispanic and Asian people.

## Growing Need, Projected Shortages in Specialists

As noted in the Prevalence section, between 2020 and 2050 the size of America's older population (those 65 and over) is expected to increase dramatically. As the size of the older population grows, the number of individuals living with Alzheimer's dementia will also increase. Today approximately one in 10 people age 65 and older has Alzheimer's dementia. At the same time, however, the workforce to care for the older population is currently, and is likely to continue to be, inadequate.

According to the National Center for Health Workforce Analysis[598], there was already a shortage of geriatricians in 2013, and although a modest increase in supply was projected by 2025, it was not expected to meet demand. Trends in medical training also point to a growing shortage of geriatricians into the future. For example, geriatrics-related graduate medical education programs grew only 1.1% from the 2001-2002 academic year to the 2017-2018 academic year.[599] Similarly, a study of the current and future U.S. neurology workforce projected a 19% shortage of neurologists by 2025.[600]

We project large increases in the need for specialists to care for people living with Alzheimer's dementia in 2050. Table 18 shows state-by-state projections for the number of geriatricians needed in 2050. As a nation, we need to triple the number of geriatricians who were practicing in 2019 to have enough geriatricians to care for those 65 and older who are projected to have Alzheimer's dementia in 2050 (approximately 10% of the population age 65 and older). However, the number must increase nine times to have enough geriatricians to care for the 30% of the population age 65 and older estimated by the National Center for Health Workforce Analysis to need geriatrician care. Similar analyses also show large projected needs for neurologists, geriatric psychiatrists and neuropsychologists, specialists who provide critical expertise in dementia diagnosis and care.

These shortages will affect states differently. The gaps are small in some states. For example, New York, Hawaii and Washington, D.C., appear well-positioned to achieve the relatively modest increases they need. In contrast, 14 states need to at least quintuple the number of

## TABLE 18

### Projected Geriatrician Needs in 2050 by State

| State | Number of Geriatricians in 2019 | Number of Geriatricians Needed in 2050 to Serve 10% of Those 65 and Older | Number of Geriatricians Needed in 2050 to Serve 30% of Those 65 and Older |
|---|---|---|---|
| Alabama | 44 | 228 | 684 |
| Alaska | 6 | 31 | 92 |
| Arizona | 89 | 363 | 1,089 |
| Arkansas | 51 | 134 | 402 |
| California | 590 | 1,676 | 5,029 |
| Colorado | 89 | 289 | 867 |
| Connecticut | 99 | 166 | 497 |
| Delaware | 17 | 55 | 165 |
| District of Columbia | 37 | 28 | 83 |
| Florida | 348 | 1,365 | 4,096 |
| Georgia | 96 | 492 | 1,476 |
| Hawaii | 61 | 64 | 192 |
| Idaho | 10 | 87 | 261 |
| Illinois | 218 | 517 | 1,551 |
| Indiana | 65 | 299 | 897 |
| Iowa | 24 | 142 | 426 |
| Kansas | 23 | 121 | 364 |
| Kentucky | 34 | 207 | 622 |
| Louisiana | 31 | 198 | 595 |
| Maine | 37 | 71 | 213 |
| Maryland | 150 | 288 | 865 |
| Massachusetts | 206 | 347 | 1,042 |
| Michigan | 169 | 465 | 1,394 |
| Minnesota | 93 | 270 | 811 |
| Mississippi | 25 | 124 | 373 |
| Missouri | 103 | 283 | 849 |
| Montana | 8 | 59 | 177 |
| Nebraska | 23 | 84 | 253 |
| Nevada | 40 | 158 | 474 |
| New Hampshire | 30 | 72 | 217 |
| New Jersey | 205 | 398 | 1,193 |
| New Mexico | 29 | 93 | 279 |
| New York | 605 | 818 | 2,454 |
| North Carolina | 159 | 535 | 1,606 |
| North Dakota | 15 | 34 | 103 |
| Ohio | 163 | 537 | 1,611 |
| Oklahoma | 28 | 171 | 512 |
| Oregon | 62 | 232 | 695 |
| Pennsylvania | 278 | 601 | 1,803 |
| Rhode Island | 32 | 49 | 147 |
| South Carolina | 66 | 288 | 865 |
| South Dakota | 10 | 44 | 131 |
| Tennessee | 40 | 343 | 1,029 |
| Texas | 342 | 1,255 | 3,766 |
| Utah | 21 | 114 | 341 |
| Vermont | 5 | 32 | 95 |
| Virginia | 103 | 406 | 1,218 |
| Washington | 132 | 399 | 1,198 |
| West Virginia | 19 | 83 | 250 |
| Wisconsin | 84 | 273 | 820 |
| Wyoming | 4 | 26 | 79 |
| **U.S. Total** | 5,218 | 15,417 | 46,252 |

The 10% column shows how many geriatricians will be needed to serve *only* those age 65 and older projected to have Alzheimer's dementia in 2050, assuming the percentage of people age 65 and older with Alzheimer's dementia in that age group remains at 10%. The 30% column shows how many geriatricians will be needed to serve the 30% of people age 65 and older in 2050 who need geriatrician care, regardless of whether they have dementia, according to the National Center for Health Workforce Analysis.[598] The number of practicing geriatricians in 2019 was provided by IQVIA and includes physicians with geriatrics as either their primary or secondary specialty. Calculations for 2050 assume each geriatrician can care for up to 700 patients.[598] The underlying state-by-state estimates of the 2050 population age 65 and older were provided by Claritas Pop-Facts 2020.

practicing geriatricians by 2050 to care for those 65 and older projected to have Alzheimer's dementia, or increase the number by 15 times to care for the 30% of the population age 65 and older projected to need geriatrician care. Two states, Tennessee and Idaho, will need to increase the number of geriatricians by nine times just to meet the care needs of those projected to have Alzheimer's dementia, or by 26 times to meet the needs of all those projected to need geriatrician care.

## Primary Care Physicians

With a shortage of medical specialists to meet the current and future needs for Alzheimer's dementia care in the United States, primary care physicians (PCPs) will play an increasingly important role in caring for individuals across the disease continuum — from identifying warning signs, to providing competent diagnoses, to meeting the ongoing care and support needs for patients living with a complex, progressive and ultimately fatal disease.

While PCPs are clearly on the front lines, little is known about the extent of PCPs' preparedness to meet the growing demands for dementia care in the clinical setting. To learn more about PCPs' experiences, exposure and attitudes about their medical education and training in dementia care, the Alzheimer's Association commissioned Versta Research to conduct surveys of 1) PCPs,[A20] 2) recent medical school graduates currently completing a residency in primary care[A21] and 3) recent primary care residency graduates.[A22] All surveys were conducted December 11-26, 2019.

The Alzheimer's Association surveys revealed:

- PCPs recognize they are on the front lines of diagnosing and providing care for Alzheimer's and other dementias.
- Half of PCPs believe the medical profession is not prepared to meet the expected increase in demand.
- More than half of PCPs say there are not enough specialists to receive patient referrals.
- Medical school and residency programs in primary care offer very limited coursework and patient contact related to Alzheimer's and other dementias.
- PCPs feel a duty and are committed to staying current on the latest information about the care of patients with Alzheimer's and other dementias, particularly disease management and treatment, screening and testing, and diagnosis.
- Despite this, fewer than half of PCPs have pursued additional training in dementia care since medical school and residency, noting challenges associated with obtaining such training.
- Nearly two in five PCPs say their own experience in treating patients has been one of the most important teachers, second only to continuing medical education (CME) courses.

Overall, the results of the Alzheimer's Association surveys underscore the important role PCPs play in providing critical dementia care. Findings also highlight the need for additional dementia care training opportunities for PCPs, both during medical school and residency and in subsequent clinical practice.

### Alzheimer's Association Surveys

Physicians included in the Alzheimer's Association Primary Care Physician Dementia Training Survey[A20] were recruited via WebMD's Medscape Physician Panel, which includes 68% of all practicing primary care physicians (PCPs) in the United States. To qualify for the survey, PCPs had to have been in practice for at least two years, spend at least 50% of their time in direct patient care, and have a practice in which at least 10% of their patients were age 65 or older. A total of 1,000 PCPs, balanced by age, gender, years in practice, type of practice, specialty and region to match the total U.S. population of PCPs, were included in the survey.[A20]

A total of 202 current PCP residents in general, family or internal medicine who completed their medical school training within the last two years were recruited to participate in the Alzheimer's Association Recent Medical School Graduate Dementia Training Survey[A21] through WebMD's Medscape Healthcare Professional Panel.

PCPs who had completed their residency within the last two years were recruited to participate in the Alzheimer's Association Recent Primary Care Resident Dementia Training Survey[A22] through WebMD's Medscape Physician Panel. The sample included 200 PCPs and was matched to the full population of PCPs who are in their first two years of practice based on age, gender, specialty and region.[A22]

FIGURE 17

**Frequency of Primary Care Physicians Receiving Questions about Alzheimer's or Other Dementias from Patients Age 65 and Older**

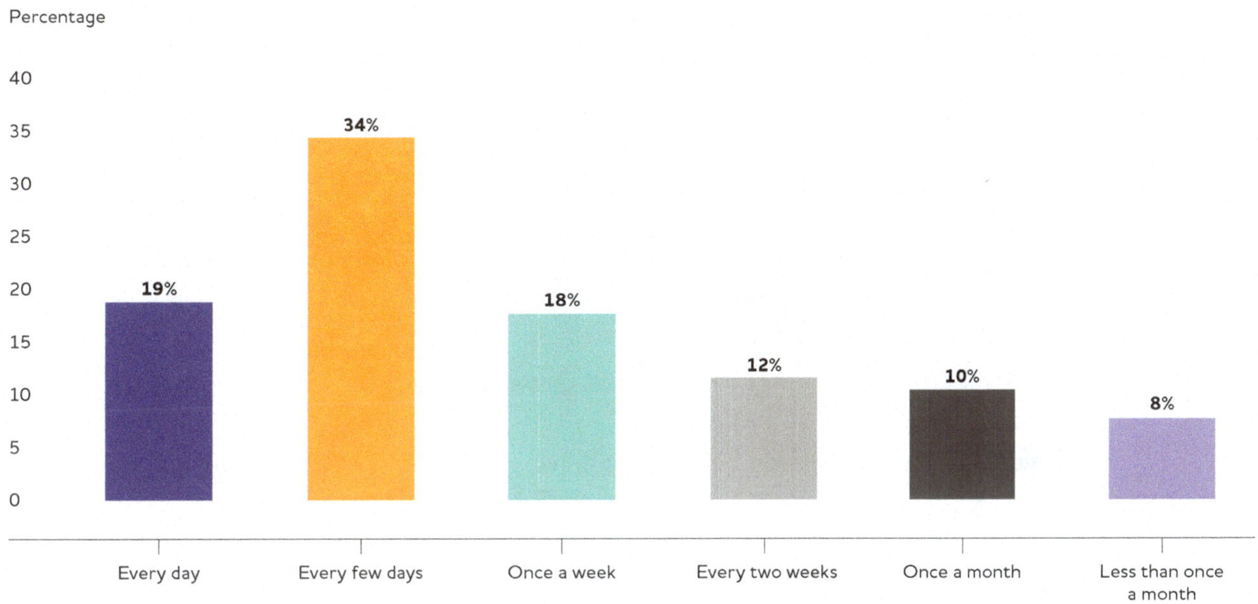


Created from data from the Alzheimer's Association Primary Care Physician Dementia Training Survey.[A20]

## Survey Results

### Patient Population

The Alzheimer's Association Primary Care Physician Dementia Care Training Survey revealed that more than four in five PCPs (82%) believe they are on the front lines of providing critical elements of dementia care for their patients. PCPs reported that, on average, 40% of their patients are age 65 and older and, of these, 13% have been diagnosed with Alzheimer's or other dementias. The survey also demonstrated that the topic of dementia is one that comes up frequently during patient visits. The majority (53%) of PCPs receive questions related to Alzheimer's or other dementias from their patients age 65 and older, or their families, every few days or more, with nearly one in five (19%) receiving these questions on a daily basis (Figure 17).

PCPs report the number of patients with Alzheimer's disease is growing. Almost nine in 10 PCPs (87%) expect the number of patients they see with dementia to increase over the next five years, and one-third (33%) expect the number of diagnosed patients to increase "a lot."

### Management of Patients

Despite knowing they are on the front lines of dementia care, a significant number of PCPs surveyed reported that they do not feel adequately prepared to care for patients with Alzheimer's and other dementias. More than one-quarter (27%) report being only sometimes or never comfortable answering patient questions about Alzheimer's or other dementias. Moreover, even though the vast majority of diagnoses are made by PCPs, nearly four in 10 PCPs (39%) report never or only sometimes being comfortable personally making a diagnosis of Alzheimer's or other dementias. In addition, half of PCPs say that the medical profession is either "not very prepared" or "not at all prepared" to care for the growing number of people living with Alzheimer's or other dementias (Figure 18, see page 68).

To care for their patients optimally, nearly one-third (32%) of PCPs make specialist referrals for their dementia patients at least once a month. However, most PCPs (55%) report that there are not enough specialists in their area to meet patient demand (Figure 19, see page 69). There was a substantial difference in PCPs' report of specialist availability depending on whether their practice was located in an urban or rural setting. While 44% of PCPs in a large city and 54% of those

FIGURE 18

Medical Profession's Preparedness to Care for People Living with Alzheimer's and Other Dementias

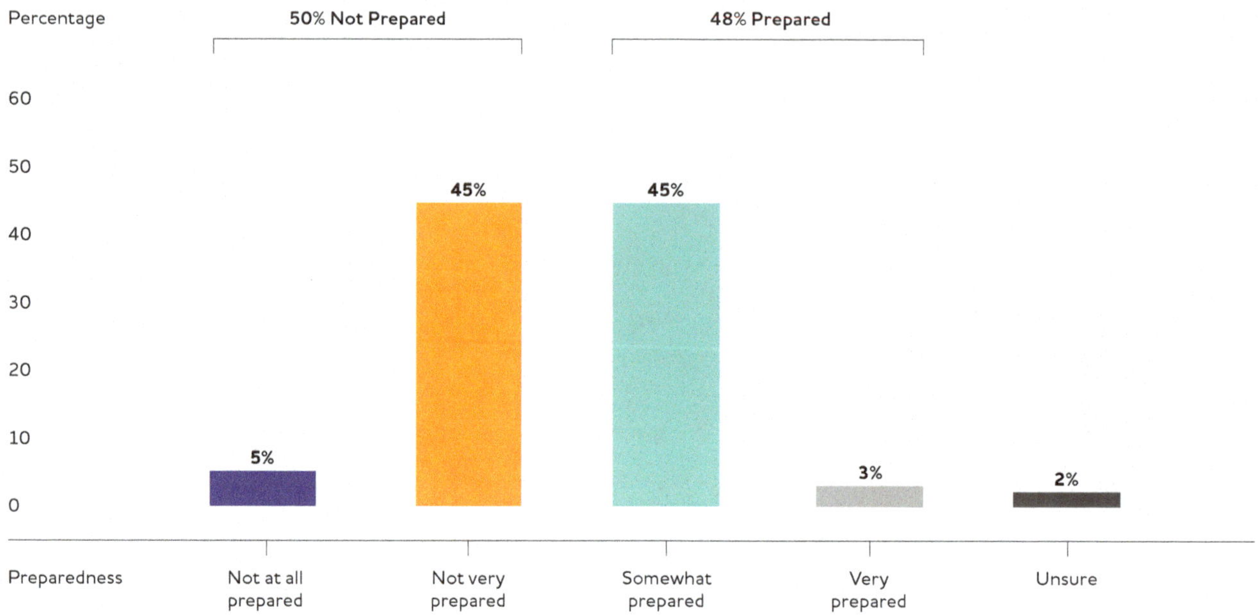


Created from data from the Alzheimer's Association Primary Care Physician Dementia Training Survey.[A20]

located in a suburb near a large city reported that there are not enough specialists in their area, 63% of PCPs in a small city or town and 71% of those in a rural area said the same.

### Medical School and Residency Training in Dementia Care

The vast majority of PCPs (91%) had at least some training in the diagnosis and care of people with Alzheimer's and other dementias in medical school, but most of those (66%) describe it as being "very little." Almost one-quarter (22%) of all PCPs had no residency training in dementia diagnosis and care. Of the 78% who did undergo training, 65% reported the amount was "very little."

Encouragingly, this trend seems to be changing. A greater proportion of recently trained PCPs report medical school and residency training in dementia care compared with PCPs with a greater number of years in practice. Ninety-eight percent of PCPs in practice for 2-9 years report at least some dementia training in medical school, compared with 81% of those with 30 or more years in practice. Similarly, 85% of PCPs in practice for 2-9 years report receiving dementia training during residency, compared with 65% of PCPs with 30 years or more of practice. However, regardless of how much training they had, most PCPs (78%) said that medical school and residency can never fully prepare a physician for dementia care.

To better understand the dementia training new PCPs undergo, the Alzheimer's Association also surveyed recent medical school and residency graduates. The survey of first- and second-year PCP residents revealed an average of 41 hours of medical school coursework that specifically focused on dementia, including Alzheimer's. However more than one in five (21%) reported having fewer than 20 hours of dementia coursework during medical school. During their clinical training in medical school, they reported seeing an average of just 20 patients with dementia.

The survey of recent residents (currently in their first or second year of practice) revealed that residents had an average of eight hours of formal curricular training focused specifically on Alzheimer's or other dementias, and one-quarter (26%) reported having fewer than two hours. On average, recent residents saw and helped 50 patients with dementia during their residency training. However, they were only involved in diagnostic workup for 10 people with dementia who were undiagnosed when initially seen. Only 18% of recent residents report feeling "very prepared" to provide dementia care in practice, compared with 82% who feel "somewhat," "not very" or "not at all" prepared.

FIGURE 19

Availability of Dementia Specialists for Patient Referral

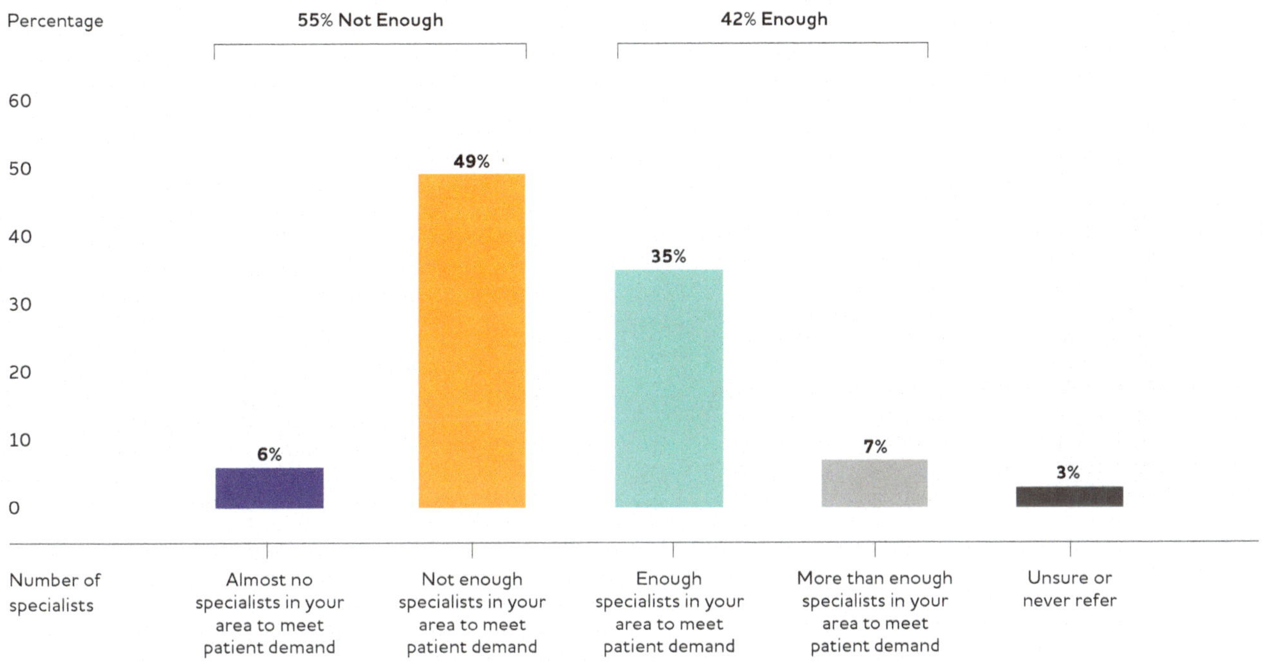


Created from data from the Alzheimer's Association Primary Care Physician Dementia Training Survey.[A20]

## Keeping Current

### Finding New Developments

The Alzheimer's Association surveys revealed that virtually all PCPs (99%) believe it is important to stay current on new developments in dementia care. Similar responses were found among recent medical school graduates (99%) and recent residents (100%). PCPs also expressed the following:

- 93% feel a duty to patients to keep up with new developments in diagnosis and care.
- 92% believe patients and caregivers expect them to know the latest thinking and best practices around dementia care.
- 92% believe dementia care is a rapidly evolving area of medicine that requires ongoing learning and training.

In addition, the surveys found that more than two-thirds of PCPs (69%) say they are always learning about the diagnosis and care of people with Alzheimer's and other dementias, and half (50%) say they put in a lot of time and effort keeping up with new developments. However, more than three in five (63%) feel they don't have enough time to keep up with all of the new developments and half (53%) say the extent to which they are keeping up with the new developments in dementia care is "only a little" or "not at all."

PCPs have enormous demands on their time and energy, across all health-related domains, so ensuring that PCPs have readily accessible, high quality training opportunities is an important challenge for the field.

The most important areas where PCPs want to stay current on Alzheimer's and other dementias include management and treatment (83%), screening and testing (69%), and diagnosis (64%). These same three areas also ranked as most important in the surveys of recent medical school graduates and recent residents. Additional areas where PCPs want to stay current include: prevention (49%), family support (49%), managing dementia alongside other conditions (46%), signs and symptoms (44%), reducing risk (41%), patient support (40%), end-of-life care (31%), palliative care and hospice (28%), coordinating care with other health care providers (24%), quality improvement measures (20%), pathophysiology (19%) and clinical trials (16%).

### Additional Training Opportunities

To keep up to date, PCPs are following new developments in dementia care mainly by scanning journals or content summaries for newly published research (77%) or scanning CME offerings for new training opportunities (66%).[A23] However, only two of five PCPs (42%) have completed

FIGURE 20

Where Primary Care Physicians Learned the Most about Dementia Diagnosis and Care

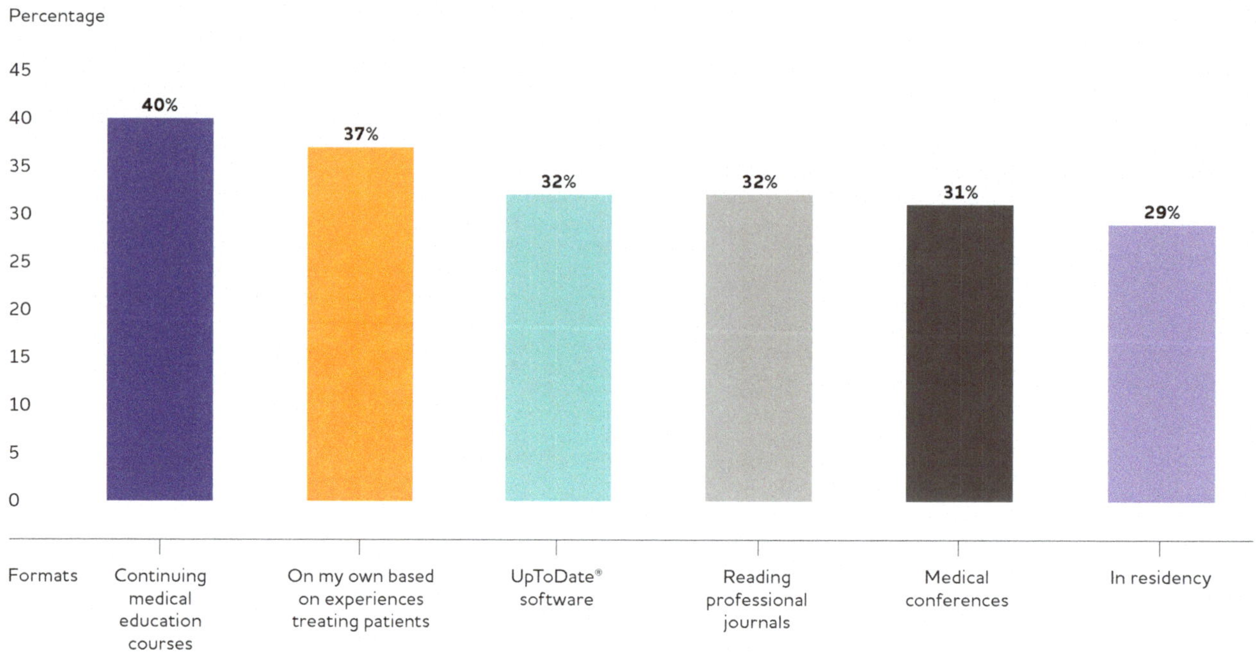


Created from data from the Alzheimer's Association Primary Care Physician Dementia Training Survey.[A20]

additional training specifically on dementia care since their residency. The most common formats for additional training are CME courses (91%), medical conferences (68%), reading professional journals (67%) and UpToDate® software that provides clinical resources to support physician practice (53%).[A24] The vast majority (89%) of PCPs feel that staying current with dementia diagnosis and care developments requires more than just fulfilling CME requirements, and when learning, the majority (55%) try to go deeper than what most CME offers.

When asked specifically about additional training opportunities, 58% of PCPs feel that the quality of existing training options is either good or excellent, though challenges in obtaining the training were noted. Nearly a third (31%) say the current options are difficult to access, and half (49%) say there are too few options for continuing education and training on dementia care. In fact, 37% reported that they learned the most about dementia care from their own experiences treating patients, second only to the 40% who reported learning the most from CME courses (Figure 20).

This finding highlights a need for better dementia training programs for PCPs. Additional sources where PCPs have learned the most about dementia diagnosis and care include UpToDate® (32%), professional journals (32%), medical conferences (31%) and in residency (29%).[A25]

The reasons provided by PCPs for pursuing additional dementia care training include general ongoing patient needs given their patient population (70%), specific patient problems or needs they are trying to solve (64%), a professional obligation to stay current (60%), or their own personal or professional interest in the topic (53%). Few PCPs have pursued additional training due to requirements for medical licensing (11%), health insurance companies or other payers (3%), or their employer (1%).

PCPs who haven't pursued additional training say it's because they don't have time (38%) and typically refer patients with Alzheimer's or other dementias to other physicians (35%). Just 19% of those who haven't pursued additional training say it's because they feel confident in how their dementia patients are being managed.[A26]

## Meeting Future Demand

This Alzheimer's Association dementia care analysis and surveys should sound an alarm regarding the future of dementia care in America. This report indicates a shortage of dementia care specialists and a PCP community committed, but not always adequately prepared, to meet the increased demands of an aging population.

One way to address shortages in the workforce is through scholarship and loan forgiveness programs offered by federal and state governments. Studies have found that loan repayment programs are correlated with increasing the number of physicians practicing in rural areas[601] and directly influence the decision of osteopathic medical graduates to become primary care physicians.[602] A large increase between 2002 and 2009 in the number of young people choosing nursing as a career followed the large increase in federal funding for nursing workforce development, which includes loan repayment and scholarships.[603] A report on the geriatric workforce by the Institute of Medicine (now known as the National Academy of Medicine) concluded that "programs that link financial support to service have been effective in increasing the numbers of health care professionals that serve in underserved areas of the country" and that such programs "serve as good models for the development of similar programs to address shortages of geriatric providers."[476]

Another approach that may increase the number of providers available to diagnose and treat those with Alzheimer's and other dementias is through educational funding. For example, federal funding of departments of family medicine at U.S. medical schools is associated with an expansion of the primary care workforce.[604] In addition, a recent demonstration project by the Centers for Medicare & Medicaid Services (CMS) found that funding for clinical education of Advanced Practice Registered Nurses (APRN) resulted in a 54% increase in APRN student enrollment, with graduations increasing 67%.[605]

In addition to policies that strengthen the specialty workforce, federal and state support is needed for programs that build capacity in primary care. One example is Project ECHO® (Extension for Community Healthcare Outcomes), a highly successful tele-mentoring program for health care providers developed by the University of New Mexico. Project ECHO has been shown to improve primary care for multiple diseases, including hepatitis C[606] and complex diabetes.[607] The Alzheimer's Association is launching a global initiative to build primary care capacity for dementia care through expanded use of this model.

Another approach to bridging the gap is to expand collaborative and coordinated care programs, which rely heavily on non-specialists. Pilot programs for individuals with dementia have reduced hospital and emergency room visits[502,608] and nursing home placement.[585] In the UCLA Alzheimer's and Dementia Care Program, dementia care management is provided by a nurse practitioner supervised by a primary care physician. After one year in the program, 58% of people living with dementia and 63% of their caregivers showed clinical benefit on validated instruments,[508] and the gross savings to Medicare on an annual basis totaled $2,404 per patient per year.[585] A similar collaborative care model in Indiana — the Healthy Aging Brain Center (HABC) — resulted in gross savings of $3,474 per patient per year.[502] While the HABC included a specialist (either a geriatrician or behavioral neurologist) as part of the care team, the bulk of the team were not physicians, and included a registered nurse, a medical assistant, a technician and a social worker. And among 780 individuals with dementia who participated in the Care Ecosystem — which uses a trained navigator, an advanced practice nurse, a social worker and a pharmacist — there were 120 fewer emergency room visits, 16 fewer ambulance use events, and 13 fewer hospitalizations than would otherwise be expected over a 12-month period.[608] Individuals in these care models still sometimes received care from specialists, but the improvement in quality care can be attributed to the well-trained, largely primary care teams.

The Alzheimer's Association also offers a variety of resources to support health systems and clinicians throughout the disease continuum, including early detection and diagnosis of Alzheimer's and other dementias, management of these conditions, and care planning and support services following a diagnosis.

For a complete listing of available Alzheimer's Association resources to support health systems and clinicians, visit alz.org/professionals/health-systems-clinicians.

## Conclusion

This Special Report underscores the urgent need to develop the medical workforce to meet current and future demands for quality diagnosis and care of people living with Alzheimer's or other dementias. Current and projected future shortages in specialist care — geriatricians, neurologists, geriatric psychiatrists and neuropsychologists — place the burden of the vast majority of patient care on PCPs. However, while PCPs recognize that they are on the front lines of this crisis and feel a duty to provide the highest quality care, they report that the medical profession is not prepared to adequately face the problem, acknowledge that there is a shortage of specialists to receive patient referrals, and note that their training opportunities are lacking or difficult to access. The severity of these needs requires solutions that develop the specialty workforce while also improving capacity in primary care.

## End Notes

A1. Estimated number (prevalence) of Americans age 65 and older with Alzheimer's dementia for 2020 (prevalence of Alzheimer's in 2020): The number 5.8 million is from published prevalence estimates based on incidence data from the Chicago Health and Aging Project (CHAP) and population estimates from the 2010 U.S. Census.[62]

A2. Percentage of total Alzheimer's dementia cases by age groups: Percentages for each age group are based on the estimated 200,000 people under 65,[62] plus the estimated numbers for people age 65 to 74 (1 million), 75 to 84 (2.7 million), and 85+ (2.1 million) based on prevalence estimates for each age group and incidence data from the CHAP study.

A3. Proportion of Americans age 65 and older with Alzheimer's dementia: The 10% of the age 65 and older population is calculated by dividing the estimated number of people age 65 and older with Alzheimer's dementia (5.8 million) by the U.S. population age 65 and older in 2020, as projected by the U.S. Census Bureau (56.4 million) = approximately 10%.[184]

A4. Differences between CHAP and ADAMS estimates for Alzheimer's dementia prevalence: ADAMS estimated the prevalence of Alzheimer's dementia to be lower than CHAP, at 2.3 million Americans age 71 and older in 2002,[187] while the CHAP estimate for 2000 was 4.5 million.[592] At a 2009 conference convened by the National Institute on Aging and the Alzheimer's Association, researchers determined that this discrepancy was mainly due to two differences in diagnostic criteria: (1) a diagnosis of dementia in ADAMS required impairments in daily functioning and (2) people determined to have vascular dementia in ADAMS were not also counted as having Alzheimer's, even if they exhibited clinical symptoms of Alzheimer's.[188] Because the more stringent threshold for dementia in ADAMS may miss people with mild Alzheimer's dementia and because clinical-pathologic studies have shown that mixed dementia due to both Alzheimer's and vascular pathology in the brain is very common,[37] the Association believes that the larger CHAP estimates may be a more relevant estimate of the burden of Alzheimer's dementia in the United States.

A5. State-by-state prevalence of Alzheimer's dementia: These state-by-state prevalence numbers are based on an analysis of incidence data from CHAP, projected to each state's population, with adjustments for state-specific age, gender, years of education, race and mortality.[206] Specific prevalence numbers for 2020 were derived from this analysis and provided to the Alzheimer's Association by a team led by Liesi Hebert, Sc.D., from Rush University Institute on Healthy Aging.

A6. Criteria for identifying people with Alzheimer's or other dementias in the Framingham Study: From 1975 to 2009, 7,901 people from the Framingham Study who had survived free of dementia to at least age 45, and 5,937 who had survived free of dementia until at least age 65 were followed for incidence of dementia.[211] Diagnosis of dementia was made according to the *Diagnostic and Statistical Manual of Mental Disorders, 4th Edition (DSM-IV)* criteria and required that the participant survive for at least 6 months after onset of symptoms. Standard diagnostic criteria (the NINCDS-ADRDA criteria from 1984) were used to diagnose Alzheimer's dementia. The definition of Alzheimer's and other dementias used in the Framingham Study was very strict; if a definition that included milder disease and disease of less than 6 months' duration were used, lifetime risks of Alzheimer's and other dementias would be higher than those estimated by this study.

A7. Number of women and men age 65 and older with Alzheimer's dementia in the United States: The estimates for the number of U.S. women (3.6 million) and men (2.2 million) age 65 and older with Alzheimer's in 2020 is from unpublished data from CHAP. For analytic methods, see Hebert et al.[62]

A8. Prevalence of Alzheimer's and other dementias in older whites, blacks/African Americans and Hispanics/Latinos: The statement that blacks/African Americans are twice as likely and Hispanics/Latinos one and one-half times as likely as whites to have Alzheimer's or other dementias is the conclusion of an expert review of a number of multiracial and multiethnic data sources, as reported in detail in the Special Report of the Alzheimer's Association's *2010 Alzheimer's Disease Facts and Figures*.

A9. Projected number of people with Alzheimer's dementia: This figure comes from the CHAP study.[62] Other projections are somewhat lower (see, for example, Brookmeyer et al.[593]) because they relied on more conservative methods for counting people who currently have Alzheimer's dementia.[A4] Nonetheless, these estimates are statistically consistent with each other, and all projections suggest substantial growth in the number of people with Alzheimer's dementia over the coming decades.

A10. Projected number of people age 65 and older with Alzheimer's dementia in 2025: The number 7.1 million is based on a linear extrapolation from the projections of prevalence of Alzheimer's for the years 2020 (5.8 million) and 2030 (8.4 million) from CHAP.[62]

A11. Annual mortality rate due to Alzheimer's disease by state: Unadjusted death rates are presented rather than age-adjusted death rates in order to provide a clearer depiction of the true burden of mortality for each state. States such as Florida with larger populations of older people will have a larger burden of mortality due to Alzheimer's — a burden that appears smaller relative to other states when the rates are adjusted for age.

A12. Number of family and other unpaid caregivers of people with Alzheimer's or other dementias: To calculate this number, the Alzheimer's Association started with data from the BRFSS survey. In 2009, the BRFSS survey asked respondents age 18 and over whether they had provided any regular care or assistance during the past month to a family member or friend who had a health problem, long-term illness or disability. To determine the number of family and other unpaid caregivers nationally and by state, we applied the proportion of caregivers nationally and for each state from the 2009 BRFSS (as provided by the CDC, Healthy Aging Program, unpublished data) to the number of people age 18 and older nationally and in each state from the U.S. Census Bureau report for July 2019. Available at: https://www.census.gov/data/tables/time-series/demo/popest/2010s-state-detail.html. Accessed on January 6, 2020. To calculate the proportion of family and other unpaid caregivers who provide care for a person with Alzheimer's or another dementia, the Alzheimer's Association used data from the results of a national telephone survey also conducted in 2009 for the National Alliance for Caregiving (NAC)/AARP.[594] The NAC/AARP survey asked respondents age 18 and over whether they were providing unpaid care for a relative or friend age 18 or older or had provided such care during the past 12 months. Respondents who answered affirmatively were then asked about the health problems of the person for whom they provided care. In response, 26% of caregivers said that: (1) Alzheimer's or another dementia was the main problem of the person for whom they provided care, or (2) the person had Alzheimer's or other mental confusion in addition to his or her main problem. The 26% figure was applied to the total number of caregivers nationally and in each state, resulting in a total of 16.343 million Alzheimer's and dementia caregivers.

A13. The 2014 Alzheimer's Association Women and Alzheimer's Poll: This poll questioned a nationally-representative sample of 3,102 American adults about their attitudes, knowledge and experiences related to Alzheimer's and dementia from Jan. 9, 2014, to Jan. 29, 2014. An additional 512 respondents who provided unpaid help to a relative or friend with Alzheimer's or a related dementia were asked questions about their care provision. Random selections of telephone numbers from landline and cell phone exchanges throughout the United States were conducted. One individual per household was selected from the landline sample, and cell phone respondents were selected if they were 18 years old or older. Interviews were administered in English and Spanish. The poll "oversampled" Hispanics/Latinos, selected from U.S. Census tracts with higher than an 8% concentration of this group. A list sample of Asian Americans was also utilized to oversample this group. A general population weight was used to adjust for number of adults in the household and telephone usage; the second stage of this weight balanced the sample to estimated U.S. population characteristics. A weight for the caregiver sample accounted for the increased likelihood of female and white respondents in the caregiver sample. Sampling weights were also created to account for the use of two supplemental list samples. The resulting interviews comprise a probability-based, nationally representative sample of U.S. adults. A caregiver was defined as an adult over age 18 who, in the past 12 months, provided unpaid care to a relative or friend age 50 or older with Alzheimer's or another dementia. Questionnaire design and interviewing were conducted by Abt SRBI of New York.

A14. Number of hours of unpaid care: To calculate this number, the Alzheimer's Association used data from a follow-up analysis of results from the 2009 NAC/AARP national telephone survey (data provided under contract by Matthew Greenwald and Associates, Nov. 11, 2009). These data show that caregivers of people with Alzheimer's or other dementias provided an average of 21.9 hours a week of care, or 1,139 hours per year. The number of family and other unpaid caregivers (16.343 million)[A12] was multiplied by the average hours of care per year, which totals 18.611 billion hours of care. This is slightly lower than the product of multiplying 1,139 by 16.343 million because of rounding.

A15. Value of unpaid caregiving: To calculate this number, the Alzheimer's Association used the method of Amo and colleagues.[595] This method uses the average of the federal minimum hourly wage ($7.25 in 2019) and the mean hourly wage of home health aides ($18.97 in July 2019).[596] The average is $13.11, which was multiplied by the number of hours of unpaid care (18.611 billion) to derive the total value of unpaid care (243.994 billion; this is slightly higher than the product of multiplying $13.11 by 18.611 billion because 18.611 billion is a rounded number for the hours of unpaid care).

A16. Lewin Model on Alzheimer's and dementia costs: These numbers come from a model created for the Alzheimer's Association by the Lewin Group. The model estimates total payments for health care, long-term care and hospice — as well as state-by-state Medicaid spending — for people with Alzheimer's and other dementias. The model was updated by the Lewin Group in January 2015 (updating previous model) and June 2015 (addition of state-by-state Medicaid estimates). Detailed information on the model, its long-term projections and its methodology are available at alz.org/trajectory. For the purposes of the data presented in this report, the following parameters of the model were changed relative to the methodology outlined at alz.org/trajectory: (1) cost data from the 2011 Medicare Current Beneficiary Survey (MCBS) were used rather than data from the 2008 MCBS; (2) prevalence among older adults was assumed to equal the prevalence levels from Hebert and colleagues[62] and included in this report (5.8 million in 2019),[A2] rather than the prevalence estimates derived by the model itself; (3) estimates of inflation and excess cost growth reflect the most recent relevant estimates from the cited sources (Centers for Medicare & Medicaid Services [CMS] actuaries and the Congressional Budget Office); and (4) the most recent (2014) state-by-state data from CMS on the number of nursing home residents and percentage with moderate and severe cognitive impairment were used in lieu of 2012 data.

A17. All cost estimates were inflated to year 2019 dollars using the Consumer Price Index (CPI): All cost estimates were inflated using the seasonally adjusted average prices for medical care services from all urban consumers. The relevant item within medical care services was used for each cost element. For example, the medical care item within the CPI was used to inflate total health care payments; the hospital services item within the CPI was used to inflate hospital payments; and the nursing home and adult day services item within the CPI was used to inflate nursing home payments.

A18. Medicare Current Beneficiary Survey Report: These data come from an analysis of findings from the 2011 Medicare Current Beneficiary Survey (MCBS). The analysis was conducted for the Alzheimer's Association by Avalere Health.[207] The MCBS, a continuous survey of a nationally representative sample of about 15,000 Medicare beneficiaries, is linked to Medicare claims. The survey is supported by the U.S. Centers for Medicare & Medicaid Services (CMS). For community-dwelling survey participants, MCBS interviews are conducted in person three times a year with the Medicare beneficiary or a proxy respondent if the beneficiary is not able to respond. For survey participants who are living in a nursing home or another residential care facility, such as an assisted living residence, retirement home or a long-term care unit in a hospital or mental health facility, MCBS interviews are conducted with a staff member designated by the facility administrator as the most appropriate to answer the questions. Data from the MCBS analysis that are included in *2020 Alzheimer's Disease Facts and Figures* pertain only to Medicare beneficiaries age 65 and older. For this MCBS analysis, people with dementia are defined as:

- Community-dwelling survey participants who answered yes to the MCBS question, "Has a doctor ever told you that you had Alzheimer's disease or dementia?" Proxy responses to this question were accepted.
- Survey participants who were living in a nursing home or other residential care facility and had a diagnosis of Alzheimer's disease or dementia in their medical record.
- Survey participants who had at least one Medicare claim with a diagnostic code for Alzheimer's or other dementias in 2008. The claim could be for any Medicare service, including hospital, skilled nursing facility, outpatient medical care, home health care, hospice or physician, or other health care provider visit. The diagnostic codes used to identify survey participants with Alzheimer's or other dementias are 331.0, 331.1, 331.11, 331.19, 331.2, 331.7, 331.82, 290.0, 290.1, 290.10, 290.11, 290.12, 290.13, 290.20, 290.21, 290.3, 290.40, 290.41, 290.42, 290.43, 291.2, 294.0, 294.1, 294.10 and 294.11.

Costs from the MCBS analysis are based on responses from 2011 and reported in 2019 dollars.

A19. Differences in estimated costs reported by Hurd and colleagues: Hurd and colleagues[520] estimated per-person costs using data from participants in ADAMS, a cohort in which all individuals underwent diagnostic assessments for dementia. *2020 Alzheimer's Disease Facts and Figures* estimated per-person costs using data from the Medicare Current Beneficiary Survey (MCBS) to be $50,201. One reason that the per-person costs estimated by Hurd and colleagues are lower than those reported in *Facts and Figures* is that ADAMS, with its diagnostic evaluations of everyone in the study, is more likely than MCBS to have identified individuals with less severe or undiagnosed Alzheimer's. By contrast, the individuals with Alzheimer's registered by MCBS are likely to be those with more severe, and therefore more costly, illness. A second reason is that the Hurd et al. estimated costs reflect an effort to isolate the incremental costs associated with Alzheimer's and other dementias (those costs attributed only to dementia), while the per-person costs in *2020 Alzheimer's Disease Facts and Figures* incorporate all costs of caring for people with the disease (regardless of whether the expenditure was related to dementia or a coexisting condition).

A20. Alzheimer's Association Primary Care Physician Dementia Training Survey: In sampling from the Medscape physician panel, data from the American Medical Association (AMA) master file of all practicing physicians in the United States were used to stratify sampling and weight final data, ensuring a representative sample based on age, gender, years in practice, type of practice, specialty and region. Of the 1,000 respondents of the survey, 18% spent less than 90% of their professional time in direct patient care, while 82% spent between 90 and 100% of their time in direct patient care. On average, 50% of their patients were age 18-64 and 40% were age 65 and older. Sixty percent of respondents were male and 39% were female. Twenty-nine percent of respondents had been in practice for 10-19 years, 28% for 20-29 years, 24% for 35 years or more, and 19% for fewer than 10 years. Eighty-three percent had office-based practices, and 14% had hospital-based practices. Fifty percent had a primary medical specialty of family medicine, 47% specialized in internal medicine, and three percent were general practitioners. Thirty-four percent of respondents practiced in the South, 25% in the West, 22% in the Midwest and 19% in the Northeast.

A21. Alzheimer's Association Recent Medical School Graduate Dementia Training Survey: Of the 202 respondents of the survey, 55% were in their first year of residency and 45% were in their second year. Ninety-seven percent of respondents were under age 40 and three percent were age 40-49. Sixty-nine percent of respondents were male and 31% were female. Sixty-eight percent had a primary medical specialty of internal medicine, 31% specialized in family medicine, and less than one percent were general practitioners. Thirty-two percent of respondents were in residency in the South, 25% in the Northeast, 23% in the Midwest and 20% in the West.

In estimating total hours of training from the survey data, 48 work weeks were assumed per year, with 5 hours of formal curriculum training each week, over the course of a three-year PCP residency.

A22. Alzheimer's Association Recent Primary Care Resident Dementia Training Survey: Data from the AMA master file were used to weight final data to ensure a sample that closely matches the full population of PCPs who are in their first two years of practice based on age, gender, specialty and region. Of the 200 respondents of the survey, 43% spent less than 90% of their professional time in direct patient care, while 57 percent spent between 90 and 100% of their time in direct patient care. Fifty-eight percent had finished residency and begun an independent practice within the last year, and 42% had done so within the last two years. Fifty-two percent of respondents were male and 48% were female. Sixty-one percent had office-based practices, and 34% had hospital-based practices. Fifty-seven percent had a primary medical specialty of family medicine, 42% specialized in internal medicine, and one percent were general practitioners. Thirty-one percent of respondents practiced in the South, 27% in the West, 25% in the Midwest and 16% in the Northeast.

To estimate total hours of training from the survey data, it was assumed that each one-week block of coursework involved 45 hours of classroom and study time.

A23. Other ways PCPs follow new developments in the diagnosis and care of Alzheimer's and other dementias: Additional responses, ranked by the percentage of participants who selected that choice, are detailed below. Participants were allowed to select more than one answer, so percentages do not add up to 100. Email or social media alerts that track new developments or offerings (31%); listening to podcasts hosted by medical professionals that focus on Alzheimer's and dementia (25%); subscribing to publications focused on disorders of the nervous system (17%); participating in online groups of physicians who discuss Alzheimer's and dementia (13%); subscribing to an online community focused on Alzheimer's and dementia (9%); other ways (12%).

A24. Other formats for additional training in dementia: Additional responses, ranked by the percentage of participants who selected that choice, are detailed below. Participants were allowed to select more than one answer, so percentages do not add up to 100. Lectures (including grand rounds, noon conferences, etc.) (38%); other online resources (such as AAN, NIH, CDC, etc.) (20%); workshops (11%); YouTube videos or other resources found on social media platforms (4%); geriatric fellowship (2%); another format (4%).

A25. Other sources where PCPs have learned the most about dementia diagnosis and care: Additional responses, ranked by the percentage of participants who selected that choice, are detailed below. Participants were allowed to select more than one answer, so percentages do not add up to 100. Own research to learn about the topic (17%); in medical school (15%); lectures (including grand rounds, noon conferences, etc.) (13%); professional discussion groups (8%); other online resources (such as AAN, NIH, CDC, etc.) (6%); workshops (5%); YouTube videos or other resources found on social media platforms (1%); another format (1%); geriatric fellowship (less than 1%).

A26. Other reasons for not pursuing additional training in dementia diagnosis and care: Additional responses, ranked by the percentage of participants who selected that choice, are detailed below. Participants were allowed to select more than one answer, so percentages do not add up to 100. Decided to focus practice on another area of medicine (17%); dementia care is less relevant than other topics (15%); do not have good access to resources for additional training (14%); do not see much Alzheimer's or other dementia among patients (7%); medical school and residency training was sufficient (5%); not much has changed in dementia care so there is no need (5%); other reasons (1%).

## References


1. Villemagne VL, Burnham S, Bourgeat P, Brown B, Ellis KA, Salvado O, et al. Amyloid β deposition, neurodegeneration, and cognitive decline in sporadic Alzheimer's disease: A prospective cohort study. Lancet Neurol 2013;12(4):357-67.
2. Reiman EM, Quiroz YT, Fleisher AS, Chen K, Velez-Pardos C, Jimenez-Del-Rio M, et al. Brain imaging and fluid biomarker analysis in young adults at genetic risk for autosomal dominant Alzheimer's disease in the presenilin 1 E280A kindred: A case-control study. Lancet Neurol 2012;11(2):1048-56.
3. Jack CR, Lowe VJ, Weigand SD, Wiste HJ, Senjem ML, Knopman DS, et al. Serial PiB and MRI in normal, mild cognitive impairment and Alzheimer's disease: Implications for sequence of pathological events in Alzheimer's disease. Brain 2009;132:1355-65.
4. Bateman RJ, Xiong C, Benzinger TL, Fagan AM, Goate A, Fox NC, et al. Clinical and biomarker changes in dominantly inherited Alzheimer's disease. N Engl J Med 2012;367(9):795-804.
5. Gordon BA, Blazey TM, Su Y, Hari-Raj A, Dincer A, Flores S, et al. Spatial patterns of neuroimaging biomarker change in individuals from families with autosomal dominant Alzheimer's disease: A longitudinal study. Lancet Neurol 2018;17(3):241-50.
6. Braak H, Thal DR, Ghebremedhin E, Del Tredici K. Stages of the pathologic process in Alzheimer disease: age categories from 1 to 100 years. J Neuropathol Exp Neurol 2011;70(11):960-9.
7. Sato C, Barthélemy NR, Mawuenyega KG, Patterson BW, Gordon BA, Jockel-Balsarotti J, et al. Tau kinetics in neurons and the human central nervous system. Neuron 2018;98(4):861-4.
8. Hanseeuw, BJ; Betensky RA, Jacobs HIL, Schultz AP, Sepulcre J, Becker JA, et al. Association of amyloid and tau with cognition in preclinical Alzheimer disease. JAMA Neurol 2019;76(8):915-24.
9. Kapasi A, DeCarli C, Schneider JA. Impact of multiple pathologies on the threshold for clinically overt dementia. Acta Neuropathol 2017;134(2):171-86.
10. Brenowitz WD, Hubbard RA, Keene CD, Hawes SE, Longstreth WT, Woltjer, et al. Mixed neuropathologies and estimated rates of clinical progression in a large autopsy sample. Alzheimers Dement. 2017;13(6):654-62.
11. National Institute on Aging. What are frontotemporal disorders? Available at: https://www.nia.nih.gov/health/what-are-frontotemporal-disorders. Accessed November 17, 2019.
12. Hogan DB, Jette N, Fiest KM, Roberts JI, Pearson D, Smith EE, et al. The prevalence and incidence of frontotemporal dementia: a systematic review. Can J Neurol Sci 2016;43(suppl):S96-109.
13. Stojkovska I, Krainc D, Mazzulli JR. Molecular mechanisms of α-synuclein and GBA1 in Parkinson's disease. Cell Tissue Res 2018;373(1):51-60.
14. De Reuck J, Maurage CA, Deramecourt V, Pasquier F, Cordonnier C, Leys D, et al. Aging and cerebrovascular lesions in pure and in mixed neurodegenerative and vascular dementia brains: A neuropathological study. Folia Neuropathol 2018;56(2):81-7.
15. James BD, Bennett DA, Boyle PA, Leurgans S, Schneider JA. Dementia from Alzheimer disease and mixed pathologies in the oldest old. JAMA 2012;307(17):1798-1800.
16. Dilworth-Anderson P, Hendrie HC, Manly JJ, Khachaturian AS, Fazio S. Diagnosis and assessment of Alzheimer's disease in diverse populations. Alzheimers Dement 2008;4(4):305-9.
17. Steenland K, Goldstein FC, Levey A, Wharton W. A meta-analysis of Alzheimer's disease incidence and prevalence comparing African-Americans and caucasians. J Alzheimers Dis 2015;50(1):71-6.
18. Potter GG, Plassman BL, Burke JR, Kabeto MU, Langa KM, Llewellyn DJ, et al. Cognitive performance and informant reports in the diagnosis of cognitive impairment and dementia in African Americans and whites. Alzheimers Dement 2009;5(6):445-53.
19. Gurland BJ, Wilder DE, Lantigua R, Stern Y, Chen J, Killeffer EH, et al. Rates of dementia in three ethnoracial groups. Int J Geriatr Psychiatry 1999;14(6):481-93.
20. Sperling RA, Aisen PS, Beckett LA, Bennett DA, Craft S, Fagan AM, et al. Toward defining the preclinical stages of Alzheimer's disease: Recommendations from the National Institute on Aging-Alzheimer's Association workgroups on diagnostic guidelines for Alzheimer's disease. Alzheimers Dement 2011;7(3):280-92.
21. Albert MS, DeKosky ST, Dickson D, Dubois B, Feldman HH, Fox N, et al. The diagnosis of mild cognitive impairment due to Alzheimer's disease: Recommendations from the National Institute on Aging-Alzheimer's Association workgroups on diagnostic guidelines for Alzheimer's disease. Alzheimers Dement 2011;7(3):270-9.
22. McKhann GM, Knopman DS, Chertkow H, Hyman BT, Jack CR, Kawas CH, et al. The diagnosis of dementia due to Alzheimer's disease: Recommendations from the National Institute on Aging-Alzheimer's Association workgroups on diagnostic guidelines for Alzheimer's disease. Alzheimers Dement 2011;7(3):263-9.
23. Jack CR, Albert MS, Knopman DS, McKhann GM, Sperling RA, Carrillo MC, et al. Introduction to the recommendations from the National Institute on Aging-Alzheimer's Association workgroups on diagnostic guidelines for Alzheimer's disease. Alzheimers Dement 2011;7(3):257-62.
24. Vermunt L, Sikkes SAM, van den Hout A, Handels R, Bos I, van der Flier WM, et al. Duration of preclinical, prodromal, and dementia stages of Alzheimer's disease in relation to age, sex, and APOE genotype. Alzheimers Dement 2019;15:888-98.
25. Bennett DA, Schneider JA, Arvanitakis Z, Kelly JF, Aggarwal NT, Shah RC, et al. Neuropathology of older persons without cognitive impairment from two community-based studies. Neurology 2006;66:1837-44.
26. Knopman DS, Parisi JE, Salviati A, Floriach-Robert M, Boeve BF, Ivnik RJ, et al. Neuropathology of cognitively normal elderly. J Neuropathol Exp Neurol 2003;62:1087-95.
27. Petersen RC, Lopez O, Armstrong MJ, Getchius TSD, Ganguli M, Gloss D, et al. Practice guideline update summary: Mild cognitive impairment. Neurology 2018;90(3):126-35.
28. Ward A, Tardiff S, Dye C, Arrighi HM. Rate of conversion from prodromal Alzheimer's disease to Alzheimer's dementia: A systematic review of the literature. Dement Geriatr Cogn Disord Extra 2013;3:320-32.
29. Mitchell AJ, Shiri-Feshki M. Rate of progression of mild cognitive impairment to dementia: Meta-analysis of 41 robust inception cohort studies. Acta Psychiatr Scand 2009;119:252-65.
30. Johnson KA, Minoshima S, Bohnen NI, Donohoe KJ, Foster NL, Herscovitch P, et al. Appropriate use criteria for amyloid PET: A report of the Amyloid Imaging Task Force, the Society of Nuclear Medicine and Molecular Imaging, and the Alzheimer's Association. Alzheimers Dement 2013;9(1):e1-e16.
31. Shaw LM, Arias J, Blennow K, Galasko D, Molinuevo JL, Salloway S, et al. Appropriate use criteria for lumbar puncture and cerebrospinal fluid testing in the diagnosis of Alzheimer's disease. Alzheimers Dement 2018;14:1505-21.
32. Wilson RS, Segawa E, Boyle, PA, Anagnos SE, Hizel LP, Bennett DA. The natural history of cognitive decline in Alzheimer's disease. Psychol Aging 2012;27(4):1008-17.
33. Barker WW, Luis CA, Kashuba A, Luis M, Harwood DG, Loewenstein D, et al. Relative frequencies of Alzheimer's disease, Lewy body, vascular and frontotemporal dementia, and hippocampal sclerosis in the State of Florida Brain Bank. Alzheimer Dis Assoc Disord 2002;16(4):203-12.
34. Viswanathan A, Rocca WA, Tzourio C. Vascular risk factors and dementia: How to move forward? Neurology 2009;72:368-74.
35. Schneider JA, Arvanitakis Z, Bang W, Bennett DA. Mixed brain pathologies account for most dementia cases in community-dwelling older persons. Neurology 2007;69:2197-204.
36. Schneider JA, Arvanitakis Z, Leurgans SE, Bennett DA. The neuropathology of probable Alzheimer disease and mild cognitive impairment. Ann Neurol 2009;66(2):200-8.

37. Jellinger KA, Attems J. Neuropathological evaluation of mixed dementia. J Neurol Sci 2007;257(1-2):80-7.
38. Jellinger KA. The enigma of mixed dementia. Alzheimers Dement 2007;3(1):40-53.
39. Boustani M, Peterson B, Hanson L, Harris R, Lohr KN. Screening for dementia in primary care: A summary of the evidence for the U.S. Preventive Services Task Force. Ann Intern Med 2003;138(11):927-37.
40. Bradford A, Kunik ME, Schultz P, Williams SP, Singh H. Missed and delayed diagnosis of dementia in primary care: Prevalence and contributing factors. Alz Dis Assoc Disord 2009;23(4):306-14.
41. Kotagal V, Langa KM, Plassman BL, Fisher GG, Giordani BJ, Wallace RB, et al. Factors associated with cognitive evaluations in the United States. Neurology 2015;84(1):64-71.
42. Taylor DH, Jr., Ostbye T, Langa KM, Weir D, Plassman BL. The accuracy of Medicare claims as an epidemiological tool: The case of dementia revisited. J Alzheimers Dis 2009;17(4):807-15.
43. Barrett AM, Orange W, Keller M, Damgaard P, Swerdlow RH. Short-term effect of dementia disclosure: How patients and families describe the diagnosis. J Am Geriatr Soc 2006;54(12):1968-70.
44. Zaleta AK, Carpenter BD, Porensky EK, Xiong C, Morris JC. Agreement on diagnosis among patients, companions, and professionals after a dementia evaluation. Alzheimer Dis Assoc Disord 2012;26(3):232-7.
45. Amjad H, Roth DL, Samus QM, Yasar S, Wolff JL. Potentially unsafe activities and living conditions of older adults with dementia. J Am Geriatr Soc 2016;64(6):1223-32.
46. Alzheimer's Association. 2015 Alzheimer's Disease Facts and Figures. Alzheimer Dement 2015;11(3):332-84.
47. Ralph SJ, Espinet AJ. Increased all-cause mortality by antipsychotic drugs: Updated review and meta-analysis in dementia and general mental health care. J Alzheimers Dis Rep 2018;2:1-26.
48. Maust DT, Kim HM, Seyfried LS, Chiang C, Kavanagh J, Schneider LS, et al. Antipsychotics, other psychotropics, and the risk of death in patients with dementia: number needed to harm. JAMA Psychiatry 2015;72:438-45.
49. McKhann GM, Albert MS, Sperling RA. Changing diagnostic concepts of Alzheimer's disease. In: Hampel H, Carrillo MC, eds. Alzheimer's disease — Modernizing concept, biological diagnosis and therapy. Basel, Switzerland: Karger; 2012: p. 115-21.
50. Bloudek LM, Spackman ED, Blankenburg M, Sullivan SD. Review and meta-analysis of biomarkers and diagnostic imaging in Alzheimer's disease. J Alzheimers Dis 2011;26:627-45.
51. Watt JA, Goodarzi Z, Veroniki AA, Nincic V, Khan PA, Ghassemi M, et al. Comparative efficacy of interventions for aggressive and agitated behaviors in dementia. Ann Internal Med October 2019.doi:10.7326/M19-0993.
52. Groot C, Hooghiemstra AM, Raijmakers PG, van Berckel BN, Scheltens P, Scherder E, et al. The effect of physical activity on cognitive function in patients with dementia: A meta-analysis of randomized control trials. Ageing Res Rev 2016;25:13-23.
53. Farina N, Rusted J, Tabet N. The effect of exercise interventions on cognitive outcome in Alzheimer's disease: A systematic review. Int Psychogeriatr 2014;26(1):9-18.
54. Aguirre E, Woods RT, Spector A, Orrell M. Cognitive stimulation for dementia: A systematic review of the evidence of effectiveness from randomised controlled trials. Ageing Res Rev 2013;12(1):253-62.
55. Fukushima RLM, do Carmo EG, do Valle Pedroso R, Micali PN, Donadelli PS, Fuzaro G, et al. Effects of cognitive stimulation on neuropsychiatric symptoms in elderly with Alzheimer's disease: A systematic review. Dement Neuropsychol 2016;10(3):178-84.
56. Bahar-Fuchs A, Martyr A, Goh AMY, Sabates J, Clare L. Cognitive training for people with mild to moderate dementia. Cochrane Database of Systematic Reviews 2019, Issue 3. Art. No.: CD013069. doi: 10.1002/14651858.CD013069.pub2.
57. Kishita N, Backhouse T, Mioshi E. Nonpharmacological interventions to improve depression, anxiety, and quality of life (QoL) in people with dementia: An overview of systematic reviews. J Geriatr Psychiatry Neurol. 2020;33(1):28-41.
58. Vickrey BG, Mittman BS, Connor KI, Pearson ML, Della Penna RD, Ganiats TG, et al. The effect of a disease management intervention on quality and outcomes of dementia care: A randomized, controlled trial. Ann Intern Med 2006;145(10):713-26.
59. Voisin T, Vellas B. Diagnosis and treatment of patients with severe Alzheimer's disease. Drugs Aging 2009;26(2):135-44.
60. Grossberg GT, Christensen DD, Griffith PA, Kerwin DR, Hunt G, Hall EJ. The art of sharing the diagnosis and management of Alzheimer's disease with patients and caregivers: Recommendations of an expert consensus panel. Prim Care Companion J Clin Psychiatry 2010;12(1):PCC.09cs00833.
61. Hebert LE, Bienias JL, Aggarwal NT, Wilson RS, Bennett DA, Shah RC, et al. Change in risk of Alzheimer disease over time. Neurology 2010;75:786-91.
62. Hebert LE, Weuve J, Scherr PA, Evans DA. Alzheimer disease in the United States (2010-2050) estimated using the 2010 Census. Neurology 2013;80(19):1778-83.
63. Saunders AM, Strittmatter WJ, Schmechel D, George-Hyslop PH, Pericak-Vance MA, Joo SH, et al. Association of apolipoprotein E allele epsilon 4 with late-onset familial and sporadic Alzheimer's disease. Neurology 1993;43:1467-72.
64. Farrer LA, Cupples LA, Haines JL, Hyman B, Kukull WA, Mayeux R, et al. Effects of age, sex, and ethnicity on the association between apolipoprotein E genotype and Alzheimer disease: A meta-analysis. JAMA 1997;278:1349-56.
65. Green RC, Cupples LA, Go R, Benke KS, Edeki T, Griffith PA, et al. Risk of dementia among white and African American relatives of patients with Alzheimer disease. JAMA 2002;287(3):329-36.
66. Fratiglioni L, Ahlbom A, Viitanen M, Winblad B. Risk factors for late-onset Alzheimer's disease: A population-based, case-control study. Ann Neurol 1993;33(3):258-66.
67. Mayeux R, Sano M, Chen J, Tatemichi T, Stern Y. Risk of dementia in first-degree relatives of patients with Alzheimer's disease and related disorders. Arch Neurol 1991;48(3):269-73.
68. Lautenschlager NT, Cupples LA, Rao VS, Auerbach SA, Becker R, Burke J, et al. Risk of dementia among relatives of Alzheimer's disease patients in the MIRAGE Study: What is in store for the oldest old? Neurology 1996;46(3):641-50.
69. Nelson PT, Head E, Schmitt FA, Davis PR, Neltner JH, Jicha GA, et al. Alzheimer's disease is not "brain aging": Neuropathological, genetic, and epidemiological human studies. Acta Neuropathol 2011;121:571-87.
70. Rajan KB, Barnes LL, Wilson RS, McAninch EA, Weuve J, Sighoko D, et al. Racial differences in the association between apolipoprotein E risk alleles and overall and total cardiovascular mortality over 18 years. JAGS 2017;65:2425-30.
71. Evans DA, Bennett DA, Wilson RS, Bienias JL, Morris MC, Scherr PA, et al. Incidence of Alzheimer disease in a biracial urban community: Relation to apolipoprotein E allele status. Arch Neurol 2003;60(2):185-9.
72. Tang M, Stern Y, Marder K, Bell K, Gurland B, Lantigua R, et al. The APOE-e4 allele and the risk of Alzheimer disease among African Americans, whites, and Hispanics. JAMA 1998;279:751-5.
73. Loy CT, Schofield PR, Turner AM, Kwok JBJ. Genetics of dementia. Lancet 2014;383:828-40.
74. Holtzman DM, Herz J, Bu G. Apolipoprotein E and apolipoprotein E receptors: Normal biology and roles in Alzheimer disease. Cold Spring Harb Perspect Med 2012;2(3):a006312.
75. Michaelson DM. APOE ε4: The most prevalent yet understudied risk factor for Alzheimer's disease. Alzheimers Dement 2014;10:861-8.
76. Jansen WJ, Ossenkoppele R, Knol KL, Tijms BM, Scheltens P, Verhey FRJ, et al. Prevalence of cerebral amyloid pathology in persons without dementia JAMA 2015;313(19):1924-38.

77. Spinney L. Alzheimer's disease: The forgetting gene. Nature 2014;510(7503):26-8.
78. Ward A, Crean S, Mercaldi CJ, Collins JM, Boyd D, Cook MN, et al. Prevalence of apolipoprotein e4 genotype and homozygotes (APOE e4/4) among patients diagnosed with Alzheimer's disease: A systematic review and meta-analysis. Neuroepidemiology 2012;38:1-17.
79. Mayeux R, Saunders AM, Shea S, Mirra S, Evans D, Roses AD, et al. Utility of the apolipoprotein E genotype in the diagnosis of Alzheimer's disease. N Engl J Med 1998;338:506-11.
80. Weuve J, Barnes LL, Mendes de Leon CF, Rajan KB, Beck T, Aggarwal NT, et al. Cognitive aging in black and white Americans: Cognition, cognitive decline, and incidence of Alzheimer disease dementia. Epidemiology 2018;29(1):151-9.
81. Hendrie HC, Murrell J, Baiyewu O, Lane KA, Purnell C, Ogunniyi A, et al. APOE ε4 and the risk for Alzheimer disease and cognitive decline in African Americans and Yoruba. Int Psychogeriatr 2014;26(6):977-85.
82. Reitz C, Jun G, Naj A, Rajbhandary R, Vardarajan BN, Wang LS, et al. Variants in the ATP-binding cassette transporter (ABCA7), apolipoprotein E epsilon 4, and the risk of late-onset Alzheimer disease in African Americans. JAMA 2013;309(14):1483-92.
83. Wolters FJ, van der Lee SJ, Koudstaal PJ, van Duijn CM, Hofman A, Ikam MK, et al. Parental family history of dementia in relation to subclinical brain disease and dementia risk. Neurology 2017;88:1642-9.
84. World Health Organization. Risk reduction of cognitive decline and dementia: WHO guidelines. https://www.who.int/mental_health/neurology/dementia/guidelines_risk_reduction/en/. Accessed September 13, 2019.
85. Baumgart M, Snyder HM, Carrillo MC, Fazio S, Kim H, Johns H. Summary of the evidence on modifiable risk factors for cognitive decline and dementia: A population-based perspective. Alzheimers Dement 2015;11(6):718-26.
86. Institute of Medicine. Cognitive Aging: Progress in Understanding and Opportunity for Action. Washington, D.C.: The National Academies Press; 2015.
87. Mergenthaler P, Lindauer U, GA Dienel, Meisel A. Sugar for the brain: The role of glucose in physiological and pathological brain function. Trends Neurosci 2013;36(10):587-97.
88. Samieri C, Perier MC, Gaye B, Proust-Lima C Helmer C, Dartigues JF, et al. Association of cardiovascular health level in older age with cognitive decline and incident dementia. JAMA 2018;320(7):657-64.
89. Anstey KJ, von Sanden C, Salim A, O'Kearney R. Smoking as a risk factor for dementia and cognitive decline: A meta-analysis of prospective studies. Am J Epidemiol 2007;166(4):367-78.
90. Rusanen M, Kivipelto M, Quesenberry CP, Zhou J, Whitmer RA. Heavy smoking in midlife and long-term risk of Alzheimer disease and vascular dementia. Arch Intern Med 2011;171(4):333-9.
91. Beydoun MA, Beydoun HA, Gamaldo AA, Teel A, Zonderman AB, Wang Y. Epidemiologic studies of modifiable factors associated with cognition and dementia: Systematic review and meta-analysis. BMC Public Health 2014;14:643.
92. Ohara T, Ninomiya T, Hata J, Ozawa M, Yoshida D, Mukai N, et al. Midlife and late-life smoking and risk of dementia in the community: The Hisayama Study. J Am Geriatr Soc 2015;63(11):2332-9.
93. Choi D, Choi S, Park SM. Effect of smoking cessation on the risk of dementia: A longitudinal study. Ann Clin Transl Neurol 2018;5(10):1192-9.
94. Wu W, Brickman AM, Luchsinger J, Ferrazzano P, Pichiule P, Yoshita M, et al. The brain in the age of old: The hippocampal formation is targeted differentially by diseases of late life. Ann Neurol 2008;64:698-706.
95. Gudala K, Bansal D, Schifano F, Bhansali A. Diabetes mellitus and risk of dementia: A meta-analysis of prospective observational studies. Diabetes Investig 2013;4(6):640-50.
96. Vagelatos NT, Eslick GD. Type 2 diabetes as a risk factor for Alzheimer's disease: The confounders, interactions, and neuropathology associated with this relationship. Epidemiol Rev 2013;35(1):152-60.
97. Reitz C, Brayne C, Mayeux R. Epidemiology of Alzheimer disease. Nat Rev Neurol 2011;7(3):137-52.
98. Rönnemaa E, Zethelius B, Lannfelt L, Kilander L. Vascular risk factors and dementia: 40-year follow-up of a population-based cohort. Dement Geriatr Cogn Disord 2011;31(6):460-6.
99. Crane PK, Walker R, Hubbard RA, Li G, Nathan DM, Zheng H, et al. Glucose levels and risk of dementia. N Engl J Med 2013;369(6):540-8.
100. Sajeev G, Weuve J, McQueen MB, Blacker D. Diabetes. The AlzRisk Database. Alzheimer Research Forum. Available at: http://www.alzrisk.org. Accessed November 17, 2019.
101. Kivimaki M, Luukkonen R, Batty GD, Ferrie JE, Pentti J, Nyberg ST, et al. Body mass index and risk of dementia: Analysis of individual-level data from 1.3 million individuals. Alzheimers Dement 2018;14:601-9.
102. Loef M, Walach H. Midlife obesity and dementia: Meta-analysis and adjusted forecast of dementia prevalence in the United States and China. Obesity (Silver Spring) 2013;21(1):E51-5.
103. Anstey KJ, Cherbuin N, Budge M, Young J. Body mass index in midlife and late-life as a risk factor for dementia: A meta-analysis of prospective studies. Obes Rev 2011;12(5):E426-37.
104. Gottesman RF, Schneider AL, Zhou Y, Coresh J, Green E, Gupta N, et al. Association between midlife vascular risk factors and estimated brain amyloid deposition. JAMA 2017;17(14):1443-50.
105. Abell JG, Kivimäki M, Dugravot A, Tabak AG, Fayosse A, Shipley M, et al. Association between systolic blood pressure and dementia in the Whitehall II cohort study: Role of age, duration, and threshold used to define hypertension. Eur Heart J 2018;39(33):3119-25.
106. Ninomiya T, Ohara T, Hirakawa Y, Yoshida D, Doi Y, Hata J, et al. Midlife and late-life blood pressure and dementia in Japanese elderly: The Hisayama Study. Hypertension 2011;58(1):22-8.
107. Debette S, Seshadri S, Beiser A, Au R, Himali JJ, Palumbo C, et al. Midlife vascular risk factor exposure accelerates structural brain aging and cognitive decline. Neurology 2011;77:461-8.
108. Livingston G, Sommerlad A, Orgeta V, Costafreda SG, Huntley H, Ames D, et al. Dementia prevention, intervention, and care. Lancet 2017;390:2673-734.
109. Gottesman RF, Albert MS, Alonso A, Coker LH, Coresh J, Davis SM, et al. Associations between midlife vascular risk factors and 25-year incident dementia in the Atherosclerosis Risk in Communities (ARIC) cohort. JAMA Neurol 2017;74(10):1246-54.
110. Solomon A, Kivipelto M, Wolozin B, Zhou, J, Whitmer, RA. Midlife serum cholesterol and increased risk of Alzheimer's and vascular dementia three decades later. Dement and Geriatr Disord 2009;28:75-80.
111. Meng XF, Yu JT, Wang HF, Tan MS, Wang C, Tan CC, et al. Midlife vascular risk factors and the risk of Alzheimer's disease: A systematic review and meta-analysis. J Alzheimers Dis 2014;42(4):1295-310.
112. Fitzpatrick A, Kuller LH, Lopez OL Diehr P, O'Meara ES, Longstreth WT, et al. Mid- and late-life obesity: Risk of dementia in the Cardiovascular Health Cognition Study. Arch Neurol 2009;66:336-42.
113. Corrada MM, Hayden KM, Paganini-Hill A, Bullain SS, DeMoss J, Aguirre C, et al. Age of onset of hypertension and risk of dementia in the oldest-old: The 90+ Study. Alzheimer Dement 2017;(13):103-10.
114. The SPRINT MIND Investigators for the SPRINT Research Group. Effect of intensive vs standard blood pressure control on probable dementia: A randomized clinical trial. JAMA 2019;321(6):553-61.
115. Ogino E, Manly JJ, Schupf N, Mayeux R, Gu Y. Current and past leisure time physical activity in relation to risk of Alzheimer's disease in older adults. Alzheimers Dement 2019;15(12):1603-11.

116. Najar J, Ostling S, Gudmundsson P, Sundh V, Johansson L, Kern S, et al. Cognitive and physical activity and dementia: A 44-year longitudinal population study of women. Neurology 2019;92(12):e1322-e1330.
117. Buchman AS, Yu L, Wilson RS, Lim A, Dawe RJ, Gaiteri C, et al. Physical activity, common brain pathologies, and cognition in community-dwelling older adults. Neurology 2019;92(8):e811-e822.
118. Harrington M, Weuve J, Jackson JW, Blacker D. Physical Activity. The AlzRisk Database. Alzheimer Research Forum. Available at: http://www.alzrisk.org. Accessed November 17, 2019.
119. Tan ZS, Spartano NL, Beiser AS, DeCarli C, Auerbach SH, Vasan RS, et al. Physical activity, brain volume, and dementia risk: The Framingham Study. J Gerontol A Biol Sci Med Sci 2017;72:789-95.
120. Willey JZ, Gardener H, Caunca MR, Moon YP, Dong C, Cheung YK, et al. Leisure-time physical activity associates with cognitive decline: The Northern Manhattan Study. Neurology 2016;86(20):1897-903.
121. Stephen R, Hongistro K, Solomon A, Lonnroos E. Physical Activity and Alzheimer's Disease: A systematic review. J Gerontol A Biol Sci Med Sci 2017;72(6):733-9.
122. Blondell SJ, Hammersley-Mather R, Veerman JL. Does physical activity prevent cognitive decline and dementia? A systematic review and meta-analysis of longitudinal studies. BMC Public Health 2014;14:510.
123. Koscak TB. Physical activity improves cognition: Possible explanations. Biogerontology 2017;18(4):477-83.
124. Guure CB, Ibrahim NA, Adam MB, Said SM. Impact of physical activity on cognitive decline, dementia, and its subtypes: Meta-analysis of prospective studies. Biomed Res Int 2017;2017:9016924.
125. Soni M, Orrell M, Bandelow S, Steptoe A, Rafnsson S, d'Orsi E, et al. Physical activity pre- and post-dementia: English Longitudinal Study of Ageing. Aging Ment Health 2017;17:1-7.
126. Barberger-Gateau P, Raffaitin C, Letenneur L, Berr C, Tzourio C, Dartigues JF, et al. Dietary patterns and risk of dementia: The Three-City Cohort Study. Neurology 2007;69(20):1921-30.
127. Hardman RJ, Kennedy G, Macpherson H, Scholey AB, Pipingas A. Adherence to a Mediterranean-style diet and effects on cognition in adults: A qualitative evaluation and systematic review of longitudinal and prospective trials. Front Nutr 2016;3:22.
128. Lourida I, Soni M, Thompson-Coon J, Purandare N, Lang IA, Ukoumunne OC, et al. Mediterranean diet, cognitive function, and dementia: A systematic review. Epidemiology 2013;24:479-89.
129. Morris MC, Tangney CC, Wang Y, Sacks FM, Barnes LL, Bennett DA, et al. MIND diet slows cognitive decline with aging. Alzheimers Dement 2015;11(9):1015-22.
130. Morris MC, Tangney CC, Wang Y, Sacks FM, Bennett DA, Aggarwal NT. MIND diet associated with reduced incidence of Alzheimer's disease. Alzheimers Dement 2015;11:1007-14.
131. Butler M, Nelson VA, Davila H, Ratner E, Fink HA Hemmy LS, et al. Over-the-counter supplement interventions to prevent cognitive decline, mild cognitive impairment, and clinical Alzheimer-type dementia. Ann Intern Med 2018;168:52-62.
132. Rosenberg A, Ngandu T, Rusanen M, Antikainen R, Bäckman L, Havulinna S, et al. Multidomain lifestyle intervention benefits a large elderly population at risk for cognitive decline and dementia regardless of baseline characteristics: The FINGER trial. Alzheimers Dement 2018;14(3):263-70.
133. Kulmala J, Ngandu T, Kivipelto M. Prevention matters: Time for global action and effective implementation. J Alzheimers Dis 2018;64(s1):S191-8.
134. Fitzpatrick AL, Kuller LH, Ives DG, Lopez OL, Jagust W, Breitner JC, et al. Incidence and prevalence of dementia in the Cardiovascular Health Study. J Am Geriatr Soc 2004;52(2):195-204.
135. Kukull WA, Higdon R, Bowen JD, McCormick WC, Teri L, Schellenberg GD, et al. Dementia and Alzheimer disease incidence: A prospective cohort study. Arch Neurol 2002;59(11):1737-46.
136. Stern Y. Cognitive reserve in ageing and Alzheimer's disease. Lancet Neurol 2012;11(11):1006-12.
137. Sando SB, Melquist S, Cannon A, Hutton M, Sletvold O, Saltvedt I, et al. Risk-reducing effect of education in Alzheimer's disease. Int J Geriatr Psychiatry 2008;23(11):1156-62.
138. Hendrie HC, Smith-Gamble V, Lane KA, Purnell C, Clark DO, Gao S. The Association of early life factors and declining incidence rates of dementia in an elderly population of African Americans. J Gerontol B Psychol Sci Soc Sci 2018;16(73, suppl 1):S82-9.
139. Stern Y. What is cognitive reserve? Theory and research application of the reserve concept. J Int Neuropsychol Soc 2002;8:448-60.
140. Stern Y, Arenaza-Urquijo EM, Bartres-Faz D, Belleville S, Cantilon M, Chetelat G, et al. Whitepaper: Defining and investigating cognitive reserve, brain reserve, and brain maintenance. Alzheimers Dement 2018;pii:S1552-5260(18)33491-5.
141. Grzywacz JG, Segel-Karpas D, Lachman ME. Workplace exposures and cognitive function during adulthood: Evidence from National Survey of Midlife Development and the O*NET. J Occup Environ Med 2016;58(6):535-41.
142. Pool LR, Weuve J, Wilson RS, Bültmann U, Evans DA, Mendes de Leon CF. Occupational cognitive requirements and late-life cognitive aging. Neurology 2016;86(15):1386-92.
143. Then FS, Luck T, Luppa M, Arelin K, Schroeter ML, Engel C, et al. Association between mental demands at work and cognitive functioning in the general population: Results of the health study of the Leipzig Research Center for Civilization Diseases. J Occup Med Toxicol 2014;9:23.
144. Fisher GG, Stachowski A, Infurna FJ, Faul JD, Grosch J, Tetrick LE. Mental work demands, retirement, and longitudinal trajectories of cognitive functioning. J Occup Health Psychol 2014;19(2):231-42.
145. Dekhtyar S, Marseglia A, Xu W, Darin-Mattsson A, Wang H, Fratiglioni L. Genetic risk of dementia mitigated by cognitive reserve: A cohort study. Ann Neurol 2019;86(1):68-78.
146. McDowell I, Xi G, Lindsay J, Tierney M. Mapping the connections between education and dementia. J Clin Exp Neuropsychol 2007;29(2):127-41.
147. Ihab M, Benson AF, Lubin TJ, Sacks JD, Richmond-Bryant J. Disparities in distribution of particulate matter emission sources by race and poverty status. Am J Public Health 2018;108:480-5.
148. Bernard SM, McGeehin MA. Prevalence of blood lead levels ≥ 5 micro g/dL among US children 1 to 5 years of age and socioeconomic and demographic factors associated with blood of lead levels of 5 to 10 micro g/dL, Third National Health and Nutrition Examination Survey, 1988-1994. Pediatrics 2003;112(6 Pt 1):1308-13.
149. Griffith M, Tajik M, Wing S. Patterns of agricultural pesticide use in relation to socioeconomic characteristics of the population in the rural U.S. South. Int J Health Serv 2007;37(2):259-77.
150. Harris CD, Watson KB, Carlson SA, Fulton JE, Dorn JM, Elam-Evans L. Adult participation in aerobic and muscle-strengthening physical activities — United States, 2011. Morb Mortal Wkly Rep 2013;62(17):326-30.
151. Menke A, Casagrande S, Geiss L, Cowie CC. Prevalence of and trends in diabetes among adults in the United States, 1988-2012. JAMA 2015;314(10):1021-9.
152. Sims M, Diez Roux AV, Boykin S, Sarpong D, Gebreab SY, Wyatt SB, et al. The socioeconomic gradient of diabetes prevalence, awareness, treatment, and control among African Americans in the Jackson Heart Study. Ann Epidemiol 2011;21(12):892-8.
153. Lee TC, Glynn RJ, Peña JM, Paynter NP, Conen D, Ridker PM, et al. Socioeconomic status and incident type 2 diabetes mellitus: Data from the Women's Health Study. PLoS One 2011;6(12):E27670.
154. Gillespie CD, Hurvitz KA. Prevalence of hypertension and controlled hypertension — United States, 2007-2010. MMWR Suppl 2013 Nov 22;62(3):144-8.

155. Centers for Disease Control and Prevention. Current Cigarette Smoking Among Adults in the United States. Available at: https://www.cdc.gov/tobacco/data_statistics/fact_sheets/adult_data/cig_smoking/index.htm. Accessed November 4, 2019.
156. Staf RT, Hogan MJ, Williams DS, Whalley LJ. Intellectual engagement and cognitive ability in later life (the "use it or lose it" conjecture): Longitudinal, prospective study. BMJ 2018;363:k4925.
157. Wang H-X, Xu W, Pei J-J. Leisure activities, cognition and dementia. BBA-Mol Basis Dis 2012;1822(3):482-91.
158. Wang H-X, Karp A, Winblad B, Fratiglioni L. Late-life engagement in social and leisure activities is associated with a decreased risk of dementia: A longitudinal study from the Kungsholmen Project. Am J Epidemiol 2002;155(12):1081-7.
159. Saczynski JS, Pfeifer LA, Masaki K, Korf ES, Laurin D, White L, et al. The effect of social engagement on incident dementia: The Honolulu-Asia Aging Study. Am J Epidemiol 2006;163(5):433-40.
160. Karp A, Paillard-Borg S, Wang H-X, Silverstein M, Winblad B, Fratiglioni L. Mental, physical and social components in leisure activities equally contribute to decrease dementia risk. Dement Geriatr Cogn Disord 2005;21(2):65-73.
161. Di Marco LY, Marzo A, Muñoz-Ruiz M, Ikram MA, Kivipelto M, Ruefenacht D, et al. Modifiable lifestyle factors in dementia: A systematic review of longitudinal observational cohort studies. J Alzheimers Dis 2014;42(1)119-35.
162. James BD, Wilson RS, Barnes LL, Bennett DA. Late-life social activity and cognitive decline in old age. J Int Neuropsychol Soc 2011;17(6):998-1005.
163. Yates LA, Ziser S, Spector A, Orrell M. Cognitive leisure activities and future risk of cognitive impairment and dementia: Systematic review and meta-analysis. Int Psychogeriatr 2016;9:1-16.
164. Ball K, Berch DB, Helmers KF, Jobe JB, Leveck MD, Marsiske M, et al. Effects of cognitive training interventions with older adults: A randomized controlled trial. JAMA 2002;288(18):2271-81.
165. Hall CB, Lipton RB, Sliwinski M, Katz MJ, Derby CA, Verghese J. Cognitive activities delay onset of memory decline in persons who develop dementia. Neurology 2009;73:356-61.
166. Sanjeev G, Weuve J, Jackson JW, VanderWeele TJ, Bennett DA, Grodstein F, et al. Late-life cognitive activity and dementia. Epidemiology 2016;27(5):732-42.
167. Wilson RS, Bennett DA, Bienias JL, Aggarwal NT, Mendes De Leon CF, Morris MC, et al. Cognitive activity and incident AD in a population-based sample of older persons. Neurology 2002;59(12):1910-4.
168. Fann JR, Ribe AR, Pedersen HS, Fenger-Grøn M, Christensen J, Benros ME, et al. Long-term risk of dementia among people with traumatic brain injury in Denmark: A population-based observational cohort study. Lancet Psychiatry 2018;5(5):424-31.
169. Centers for Disease Control and Prevention. Surveillance Report of Traumatic Brain Injury-related Emergency Department Visits, Hospitalizations, and Deaths: United States, 2014. Available at https://www.cdc.gov/traumaticbraininjury/pdf/TBI-Surveillance-Report-FINAL_508.pdf. Accessed February 10.2020.
170. Plassman BL, Havlik RJ, Steffens DC, Helms MJ, Newman TN, Drosdick D, et al. Documented head injury in early adulthood and risk of Alzheimer's disease and other dementias. Neurology 2000;55(8):1158-66.
171. Teasdale G, Jennett B. Assessment of coma and impaired consciousness: A practical scale. Lancet 1974;2(7872):81-4.
172. Centers for Disease Control and Prevention. Traumatic Brain Injury & Concussion. Potential Effects. Available at: https://www.cdc.gov/traumaticbraininjury/outcomes.html. Accessed December 5, 2019.
173. Barnes DE, Byers AL, Gardner RC Seal KH, Boscardin WJ, Yaffe K. Association of mild traumatic brain injury with and without loss of consciousness with dementia in U.S. military veterans. JAMA Neurol 2018;75(9):1055-61.
174. LoBue C, Wadsworth H, Wilmoth K, Clem M, Hart J Jr, Womack KB. Traumatic brain injury history is associated with earlier age of onset of Alzheimer disease. Clin Neuropsychol 2017;31(1):85-98.
175. Mez J, Daneshvar DH, Abdolmohammadi B, Chua AS, Alosco ML, Kiernan PT, et al. Duration of American football play and chronic traumatic encephalopathy. Ann Neurol 2019.doi:10.1002/ana.25611.
176. Asken BM, Sullan MJ, DeKosky ST, Jaffee MS, Bauer RM. Research gaps and controversies in chronic traumatic encephalopathy: A review. JAMA Neurol 2017;74(10):1255-62.
177. McKee AC, Stein TD, Kiernan PT, Alvarez VE. The neuropathology of chronic traumatic encephalopathy. Brain Pathol 2015;25(3):350-64.
178. McKee AC, Cairns NJ, Dickson DW, Folkerth RD, Keene CD, Litvan I, et al. The first NINDS/NIBIB consensus meeting to define neuropathological criteria for the diagnosis of chronic traumatic encephalopathy. ACTA Neuropathol 2016;131(1):75-86.
179. Bekris LM, Yu CE, Bird TD, Tsuang DW. Genetics of Alzheimer disease. J Geriatr Psychiatry Neurol 2010;23(4):213-27.
180. Goldman JS, Hahn SE, Bird T. Genetic counseling and testing for Alzheimer disease: Joint practice guidelines of the American College of Medical Genetics and the National Society of Genetic Counselors. Genet Med 2011;13:597-605.
181. Lott IT, Dierssen M. Cognitive deficits and associated neurological complications in individuals with Down's syndrome. Lancet Neurol 2010;9(6):623-33.
182. National Down Syndrome Society. Alzheimer's Disease and Down Syndrome. Available at: https://www.ndss.org/resources/alzheimers/. Accessed September 26, 2019.
183. He W, Goodkind D, Kowal P. U.S. Census Bureau, International Population Reports, P95/16-1, An Aging World: 2015, U.S. Government Publishing Office, Washington, D.C., 2016. Available at: http://www.census.gov/content/dam/Census/library/publications/2016/demo/p95-16-1.pdf. Accessed December 4, 2019.
184. U.S. Census Bureau. 2014 National Population Projections: Downloadable Files. Available at: https://www.census.gov/data/datasets/2014/demo/popproj/2014-popproj.html. Accessed December 4, 2019.
185. Administration on Aging, Administration for Community Living, U.S. Department of Health and Human Services. A Profile of Older Americans: 2016. Available at: https://acl.gov/sites/default/files/Aging%20and%20Disability%20in%20America/2016-Profile.pdf, Accessed February 4, 2020.
186. Guerreiro R, Bras J. The age factor in Alzheimer's disease. Genome Med 2015;7:106. doi: 10.1186/s13073-015-0232-5.
187. Plassman BL, Langa KM, Fisher GG, Heeringa SG, Weir DR, Ofstedal MB, et al. Prevalence of dementia in the United States: The Aging, Demographics, and Memory Study. Neuroepidemiology 2007;29(1-2):125-32.
188. Wilson RS, Weir DR, Leurgans SE, Evans DA, Hebert LE, Langa KM, et al. Sources of variability in estimates of the prevalence of Alzheimer's disease in the United States. Alzheimers Dement 2011;7(1):74-9.
189. Brookmeyer R, Abdalla N, Kawas CH, Corrada MM. Forecasting the prevalence of preclinical and clinical Alzheimer's disease in the United States. Alzheimers Dement 2018;14(2):121-9.
190. Jack CR Jr, Therneau TM, Weigand SD, Wiste HJ, Knopman DS, Vemuri P, et al. Prevalence of biologically vs clinically defined Alzheimer spectrum entities using the National Institute on Aging-Alzheimer's Association Research Framework. JAMA Neurol 2019;76(10):1174-83.
191. James BD, Wilson RS, Boyle PA, Trojanowski JQ, Bennett DA, Schneider JA. TDP-43 stage, mixed pathologies, and clinical Alzheimer's-type dementia. Brain 2016;139(11):2983-93.
192. Serrano-Pozo A, Qian J, Monsell SE, Blacker D, Gomez-Isla T, Betensky RA, et al. Mild to moderate Alzheimer dementia with insufficient neuropathological changes. Ann Neurol 2014;75:597-601.

193. Barnes LL, Leurgans S, Aggarwal NT, Shah RC, Arvanitakis Z, James BD, et al. Mixed pathology is more likely in black than white decedents with Alzheimer dementia. Neurology 2015;85:528-34.
194. Alzheimer's Association. 2019 Alzheimer's Disease Facts and Figures. Alzheimer Dement 2019(15):321-87.
195. Reisberg B, Gauthier S. Current evidence for subjective cognitive impairment (SCI) as the pre-mild cognitive impairment (MCI) stage of subsequently manifest Alzheimer's disease. Int Psychogeriatr 2008;20(1):1-16.
196. Jessen F, Wolfsgruber S, Wiese B, Bickel H, Mösch E, Kaduszkiewicz H, et al. AD dementia risk in late MCI, in early MCI, and in subjective memory impairment. Alzheimers Dement 2014;10(1):76-83.
197. Jessen F, Amariglio RE, van Boxtel M, Breteler M, Ceccaldi M, Chételat G, et al. A conceptual framework for research on subjective cognitive decline in preclinical Alzheimer's disease. Alzheimers Dement 2014;10(6):844-52.
198. Buckley RF, Maruff P, Ames D, Bourgeat P, Martins RN, Masters CL, et al. Subjective memory decline predicts greater rates of clinical progression in preclinical Alzheimer's disease. Alzheimers Dement 2016;12(7):796-804.
199. Gifford KA, Liu D, Lu Z, Tripodis Y, Cantwell NG, Palmisano J, et al. The source of cognitive complaints predicts diagnostic conversion differentially among nondemented older adults. Alzheimers Dement 2014;10(3):319-27.
200. Brody DJ, Kramarow EA, Taylor CA, McGuire LC. Cognitive performance in adults aged 60 and over: National Health and Nutrition Examination Survey, 2011-2014. National Health Statistics Reports; no 126. Hyattsville, MD: National Center for Health Statistics. 2019.
201. Kaup AR, Nettiksimmons J, LeBlanc ES, Yaffe K. Memory complaints and risk of cognitive impairment after nearly 2 decades among older women. Neurology 2015;85(21):1852-8.
202. Reisberg B, Shulman MB, Torossian C, Leng L, Zhu W. Outcome over seven years of healthy adults with and without subjective cognitive impairment. Alzheimers Dement 2010;6(1):11-24.
203. Fernandez-Blazquez MA, Avila-Villanueva M, Maestu F, Medina M. Specific features of subjective cognitive decline predict faster conversion to mild cognitive impairment. J Alzheimers Dis 2016;52(1):271-81.
204. Wolfsgruber S, Kleineidam L, Wagner M, Mösch E, Bickel H, Lühmann D, et al. Differential risk of incident Alzheimer's disease dementia in stable versus unstable patterns of subjective cognitive decline. J Alzheimers Dis 2016;54(3):1135-46.
205. Unpublished data from the 2015-2018 Behavioral Risk Factor Surveillance System survey, analyzed and provided to the Alzheimer's Association by the Alzheimer's Disease and Healthy Aging Program, Centers for Disease Control and Prevention.
206. Weuve J, Hebert LE, Scherr PA, Evans DA. Prevalence of Alzheimer disease in U.S. states. Epidemiology 2015;26(1):E4-6.
207. Unpublished tabulations based on data from the Medicare Current Beneficiary Survey for 2011. Prepared under contract by Avalere Health, March 2016.
208. Hebert LE, Beckett LA, Scherr PA, Evans DA. Annual incidence of Alzheimer disease in the United States projected to the years 2000 through 2050. Alzheimer Dis Assoc Disord 2001;15(4):169-73.
209. Rajan KB, Weuve J, Barnes LL, Wilson RS, Evans DA. Prevalence and incidence of clinically diagnosed Alzheimer's disease dementia from 1994 to 2012 in a population study. Alzheimers Dement 2019;15(1):1-7. doi:10.1016/j.jalz.2018.07.216 1.
210. Tom SE, Hubbard RA, Crane PK, Haneuse SJ, Bowen J, McCormick WC, et al. Characterization of dementia and Alzheimer's disease in an older population: Updated incidence and life expectancy with and without dementia. Am J Public Health 2015;105(2):408-13.
211. Chene G, Beiser A, Au R, Preis SR, Wolf PA, Dufouil C, et al. Gender and incidence of dementia in the Framingham Heart Study from mid-adult life. Alzheimers Dement 2015;11(3):310-20.
212. Seshadri S, Wolf PA, Beiser A, Au R, McNulty K, White R, et al. Lifetime risk of dementia and Alzheimer's disease. The impact of mortality on risk estimates in the Framingham Study. Neurology 1997;49(6):1498-504.
213. Hebert LE, Scherr PA, McCann JJ, Beckett LA, Evans DA. Is the risk of developing Alzheimer's disease greater for women than for men? Am J Epidemiol 2001;153(2):132-6.
214. Zahodne LB, Schofield PW, Farrell MT, Stern Y, Manly JJ. Bilingualism does not alter cognitive decline or dementia risk among Spanish-speaking immigrants. Neuropsychology 2014;28(2):238-46.
215. Kawas C, Gray S, Brookmeyer R, Fozard J, Zonderman A. Age-specific incidence rates of Alzheimer's disease: The Baltimore Longitudinal Study of Aging. Neurology 2000;54(11):2072-7.
216. Fratiglioni L, Viitanen M, von Strauss E, Tontodonati V, Herlitz A, Winblad B. Very old women at highest risk of dementia and Alzheimer's disease: Incidence data from the Kungsholmen Project, Stockholm. Neurology 1997;48:132-8.
217. Letenneur L, Gilleron V, Commenges D, Helmer C, Orgogozo JM, Dartigues JF. Are sex and educational level independent predictors of dementia and Alzheimer's disease? Incidence data from the PAQUID project. J Neurol Neurosurg Psychiatry 1999;66:177-83.
218. Matthews FE, Stephan BC, Robinson L, Jagger C, Barnes LE, Arthur A, et al. A two decade dementia incidence comparison from the Cognitive Function and Ageing Studies I and II. Nat Commun 2016;7:11398.
219. Mielke MM, Ferretti MT, Iulita MF, Hayden K, Khachaturian AS. Sex and gender in Alzheimer's disease — Does it matter? Alzheimers Dement 2018;14(9):1101-3.
220. Rocca WA. Time, Sex, gender, history, and dementia. Alzheimer Dis Assoc Disord 2017;31(1):76-9.
221. Mielke MM, Vemuri P, Rocca WA. Clinical epidemiology of Alzheimer's disease: Assessing sex and gender differences. Clin Epidemiol 2014;6:37-48.
222. Rocca WA, Mielke MM, Vemuri P, Miller VM. Sex and gender differences in the causes of dementia: A narrative review. Maturitas 2014;79(2):196-201.
223. Langa KM, Larson EB, Crimmins EM, Faul JD, Levine DA, Kabeto MU, et al. A comparison of the prevalence of dementia in the United States in 2000 and 2012. JAMA Intern Med 2017;177(1):51-8.
224. Launer LJ, Andersen K, Dewey ME, Letenneur L, Ott A, Amaducci LA, et al. Rates and risk factors for dementia and Alzheimer's disease: results from EURODEM pooled analyses. EURODEM Incidence Research Group and Work Groups. European Studies of Dementia. Neurology 1999;52(1):78-84.
225. Russ TC, Stamatakis E, Hamer M, Starr JM, Kivimaki M, Batty GD. Socioeconomic status as a risk factor for dementia death: individual participant meta-analysis of 86 508 men and women from the UK. Br J Psychiatry 2013;203(1):10-17.
226. Carter CL, Resnick EM, Mallampalli M, Kalbarczyk A. Sex and gender differences in Alzheimer's disease: Recommendations for future research. J Womens Health 2012;21(10):1018-23.
227. Altmann A, Tian L, Henderson VW, Greicius MD, Alzheimer's Disease Neuroimaging Initiative Investigators. Sex modifies the APOE-related risk of developing Alzheimer disease. Ann Neurol 2014;75(4):563-73.
228. Ungar L, Altmann A, Greicius MD. Apolipoprotein E, gender, and Alzheimer's disease: An overlooked, but potent and promising interaction. Brain Imaging Behav 2014;8(2):262-73.
229. Hohman TJ, Dumitrescu L, Barnes LL, Thambisetty M, Beecham G, Kunkle B, et al. Sex-specific association of apolipoprotein E with cerebrospinal fluid levels of tau. JAMA Neurol 2018;75(8):989-98.
230. Neu SC, Pa J, Kukull W, Beekly D, Kuzma A, Gangadharan P, et al. Apolipoprotein E genotype and sex risk factors for Alzheimer disease: A meta-analysis. JAMA Neurol 2017;74(10):1178-89.

231. Yaffe K, Haan M, Byers A, Tangen C, Kuller L. Estrogen use, APOE, and cognitive decline: Evidence of gene-environment interaction. Neurology 2000;54(10):1949-54.
232. Kang JH, Grodstein F. Postmenopausal hormone therapy, timing of initiation, APOE and cognitive decline. Neurobiol Aging 2012;33(7):1129-37.
233. Barnes LL, Wilson RS, Bienias JL, Schneider JA, Evans DA, Bennett DA. Sex differences in the clinical manifestations of Alzheimer disease pathology. Arch Gen Psychiatry 2005;62(6):685-91.
234. Koran MEI, Wagener M, Hohman TJ, Alzheimer's Neuroimaging Initiative. Sex differences in the association between AD biomarkers and cognitive decline. Brain Imaging Behav 2017;11(1):205-13.
235. Buckley RF, Mormino EC, Amariglio RE, Properzi MJ, Rabin JS, Lim YY, et al. Sex, amyloid, and APOE epsilon4 and risk of cognitive decline in preclinical Alzheimer's disease: Findings from three well-characterized cohorts. Alzheimers Dement 2018;14(9):1193-203.
236. Manly JJ, Mayeux R. Ethnic differences in dementia and Alzheimer's disease. In: Anderson N, Bulatao R, Cohen B, eds. Critical perspectives on racial and ethnic differentials in health in late life. Washington, D.C.: National Academies Press; 2004: p. 95-141.
237. Demirovic J, Prineas R, Loewenstein D, Bean J, Duara R, Sevush S, et al. Prevalence of dementia in three ethnic groups: The South Florida Program on Aging and Health. Ann Epidemiol 2003;13(6):472-78.
238. Harwood DG, Ownby RL. Ethnicity and dementia. Curr Psych Report 2000;2(1):40-5.
239. Perkins P, Annegers JF, Doody RS, Cooke N, Aday L, Vernon SW. Incidence and prevalence of dementia in a multiethnic cohort of municipal retirees. Neurology 1997;49(1):44-50.
240. Haan MN, Mungas DM, Gonzalez HM, Ortiz TA, Acharya A, Jagust WJ. Prevalence of dementia in older Latinos: The influence of type 2 diabetes mellitus, stroke and genetic factors. J Am Geriatr Soc 2003;51:169-77.
241. Samper-Ternent R, Kuo YF, Ray LA, Ottenbacher KJ, Markides KS, Al Snih S. Prevalence of health conditions and predictors of mortality in oldest old Mexican Americans and non-Hispanic whites. J Am Med Dir Assn 2012;13(3):254-9.
242. González HM, Tarraf W, Schneiderman N, Fornage M, Vásquez PM, Zeng D, et al. Prevalence and correlates of mild cognitive impairment among diverse Hispanics/Latinos: Study of Latinos-Investigation of Neurocognitive Aging results. Alzheimers Dement 2019;pii:S1552-5260(19)35376-2. doi:10.1016/j.jalz.2019.08.202. [Epub ahead of print].
243. Mehta KM, Yeo GW. Systematic review of dementia prevalence and incidence in United States race/ethnic populations. Alzheimers Dement 2017;13(1):72-83.
244. Yaffe K, Falvey C, Harris TB, Newman A, Satterfield S, Koster A, et al. Effect of socioeconomic disparities on incidence of dementia among biracial older adults: Prospective study. BMJ 2013;347:f7051.
245. Froehlich TE, Bogardus Jr. ST, Inouye SK. Dementia and race: Are there differences between African Americans and Caucasians? J Am Geriatr Soc 2001;49(4):477-84.
246. Chin AL, Negash S, Hamilton R. Diversity and disparity in dementia: The impact of ethnoracial differences in Alzheimer disease. Alzheimer Dis Assoc Disord 2011;25(3):187-95.
247. Lines LM, Sherif NA, Wiener JM. Racial and ethnic disparities among individuals with Alzheimer's disease in the United States: A literature review. Research Triangle Park, NC: RTI Press; 2014.
248. Glymour MM, Manly JJ. Lifecourse social conditions and racial and ethnic patterns of cognitive aging. Neuropsychol Rev 2008;18(3):223-54.
249. Zhang Z, Hayward MD, Yu YL. Life course pathways to racial disparities in cognitive impairment among older Americans. J Health Soc Behav 2016;57(2):184-99.
250. Clark PC, Kutner NG, Goldstein FC, Peterson-Hazen S, Garner V, Zhang R, et al. Impediments to timely diagnosis of Alzheimer's disease in African Americans. J Am Geriatr Soc 2005;53(11):2012-7.
251. Fitten LJ, Ortiz F, Ponton M. Frequency of Alzheimer's disease and other dementias in a community outreach sample of Hispanics. J Am Geriatr Soc 2001;49(10):1301-8.
252. Matthews KA, Xu W, Gaglioti AH, Holt JB, Croft JB, Mack D, et al. Racial and ethnic estimates of Alzheimer's disease and related dementias in the United States (2015-2060) in adults aged ≥ 65 years. Alzheimers Dement 2019;15(1):17-24.
253. Mayeda ER, Glymour MM, Quesenberry CP, Whitmer RA. Inequalities in dementia incidence between six racial and ethnic groups over 14 years. Alzheimers Dement 2016;12(3):216-24.
254. Mayeda ER, Glymour MM, Quesenberry CP, Jr., Whitmer RA. Heterogeneity in 14-year dementia incidence between Asian American subgroups. Alzheimer Dis Assoc Disord 2017;31(3):181-6.
255. Sheffield KM, Peek MK. Changes in the prevalence of cognitive impairment among older Americans, 1993-2004: Overall trends and differences by race/ethnicity. Am J Epidemiol 2011;174(3):274-83.
256. Hudomiet P, Hurd M, Rohwedder S. Dementia prevalence in the United States in 2000 and 2012: Estimates based on a nationally representative study. J Gerontol B Psychol Sci Soc Sci 2018;73(Suppl 1):S10-19.
257. Freedman VA, Kasper JD, Spillman BC, Plassman BL. Short-term changes in the prevalence of probable dementia: An analysis of the 2011-2015 National Health and Aging Trends Study. J Gerontol B Psychol Sci Soc Sci 2018;73(Suppl 1):S48-56.
258. Matthews FE, Arthur A, Barnes LE, Bond J, Jagger C, Robinson L, et al. A two-decade comparison of prevalence of dementia in individuals aged 65 years and older from three geographical areas of England: Results of the Cognitive Function and Ageing Study I and II. Lancet 2013;382(9902):1405-12.
259. Rocca WA, Petersen RC, Knopman DS, Hebert LE, Evans DA, Hall KS, et al. Trends in the incidence and prevalence of Alzheimer's disease, dementia, and cognitive impairment in the United States. Alzheimers Dement 2011;7(1):80-93.
260. Wiberg P, Waern M, Billstedt E, Östling S, Skoog I. Secular trends in the prevalence of dementia and depression in Swedish septuagenarians 1976-2006. Psychol Med 2013;43:2627-34.
261. Wimo A, Sjölund BM, Sköldunger A, Qiu C, Klarin I, Nordberg G, et al. Cohort effects in the prevalence and survival of people with dementia in a rural area in Northern Sweden. J Alzheimers Dis 2016;50:387-96.
262. Hall KS, Gao S, Baiyewu O, Lane KA, Gureje O, Shen J, et al. Prevalence rates for dementia and Alzheimer's disease in African Americans: 1992 versus 2000. Alzheimers Dement 2009;5(3):227-33.
263. Wu YT, Beiser AS, Breteler MMB, Fratiglioni L, Helmer C, Hendrie HC, et al. The changing prevalence and incidence of dementia over time: Current evidence. Nat Rev Neurol 2017;13(6):327-39.
264. Schrijvers EM, Verhaaren BF, Koudstaal PJ, Hofman A, Ikram MA, Breteler MM. Is dementia incidence declining? Trends in dementia incidence since 1990 in the Rotterdam Study. Neurology 2012;78(19):1456-63.
265. Qiu C, von Strauss E, Backman L, Winblad B, Fratiglioni L. Twenty-year changes in dementia occurrence suggest decreasing incidence in central Stockholm, Sweden. Neurology 2013;80(20):1888-94.
266. Satizabal CL, Beiser AS, Chouraki V, Chene G, Dufouil C, Seshadri S. Incidence of dementia over three decades in the Framingham Heart Study. N Engl J Med 2016;374:523-32.
267. Cerasuolo JO, Cipriano LE, Sposato LA, Kapral MK, Fang J, Gill SS, et al. Population-based stroke and dementia incidence trends: Age and sex variations. Alzheimers Dement 2017;13(10):1081-8.

268. Derby CA, Katz MJ, Lipton RB, Hall CB. Trends in dementia incidence in a birth cohort analysis of the Einstein Aging Study. JAMA Neurol 2017;74(11):1345-51.
269. Ahmadi-Abhari S, Guzman-Castillo M, Bandosz P, Shipley MJ, Muniz-Terrera G, Singh-Manoux A, et al. Temporal trend in dementia incidence since 2002 and projections for prevalence in England and Wales to 2040: Modelling study. BMJ 2017;358:j2856.
270. Sullivan KJ, Dodge HH, Hughes TF, Chang CH, Zhu X, Liu A, et al. Declining incident dementia rates across four population-based birth cohorts. J Gerontol A Biol Sci Med Sci 2018. doi: 10.1093/gerona/gly236. [Epub ahead of print].
271. van den Kommer TN, Deeg DJH, van der Flier WM, and Comijs HC. Time trend in persistent cognitive decline: Results from the longitudinal aging study Amsterdam. J Gerontol B Psychol Sci Soc Sci 2018;73(Suppl 1):S57-64.
272. Sekita A, Ninomiya T, Tanizaki Y, Doi Y, Hata J, Yonemoto K, et al. Trends in prevalence of Alzheimer's disease and vascular dementia in a Japanese community: The Hisayama Study. Acta Psychiatr Scand 2010;122(4):319-25.
273. Crimmins EM, Saito Y, Kim JK, Zhang Y, Sasson I, Hayward MD. Educational differences in the prevalence of dementia and life expectancy with dementia in the United States: Changes from 2000 to 2010. J Gerontol B Psychol Sci Soc Sci 2018;73(Suppl 1):S20-28.
274. Choi H, Schoeni RF, Martin LG, Langa K M. Trends in the prevalence and disparity in cognitive limitations of Americans 55-69 years old. J Gerontol B Psychol Sci Soc Sci 2018;73 (Suppl 1):S29-37.
275. Langa KM. Is the risk of Alzheimer's disease and dementia declining? Alzheimers Res Ther 2015;7(1):34.
276. Larson EB, Yaffe K, Langa KM. New insights into the dementia epidemic. N Engl J Med 2013;369(24):2275-7.
277. Weuve J, Rajan KB, Barnes LL, Wilson RS, Evans DA. Secular trends in cognitive performance in older black and white U.S. adults, 1993-2012: Findings from the Chicago Health and Aging Project. J Gerontol B Psychol Sci Soc Sci 2018;73 (Suppl 1):S73-81.
278. Prince MJ, Wimo A, Guerchet M, Ali G-C, Wu Y-T, Prina M. World Alzheimer Report 2015: The Global Impact of Dementia: An Analysis of Prevalence, Incidence, Cost and Trends; 2015.
279. U.S. Census Bureau. 2017 National Population Projections Tables. Available at: https://www.census.gov/data/tables/2017/demo/popproj/2017-summary-tables.html. Accessed December 4, 2019.
280. Xu JQ, Murphy SL, Kochanek KD, Arias E. Mortality in the United States, 2018. NCHS Data Brief; No. 355. Hyattsville, MD: National Center for Health Statistics. 2020.
281. U.S. Department of Health and Human Services, Centers for Disease Control and Prevention, National Center for Health Statistics. CDC WONDER online database: About Underlying Cause of Death, 1999-2018. Available at. https://wonder.cdc.gov/ucd-icd10.html. Accessed February 14, 2020
282. World Health Organization. International Statistical Classification of Diseases and Related Health Problems. 10th revision. 2nd edition. WHO Press: Geneva, Switzerland; 2004.
283. Kramarow EA, Tejada-Vera B. Dementia mortality in the United States, 2000-2017. National Vital Statistics Reports; vol 68 no 2. Hyattsville, MD: National Center for Health Statistics. 2019. https://www.cdc.gov/nchs/data/nvsr/nvsr68/nvsr68_02-508.pdf.
284. Burns A, Jacoby R, Luthert P, Levy R. Cause of death in Alzheimer's disease. Age Ageing 1990;19(5):341-4.
285. Brunnstrom HR, Englund EM. Cause of death in patients with dementia disorders. Eur J Neurol 2009;16(4):488-92.
286. Ives DG, Samuel P, Psaty BM, Kuller LH. Agreement between nosologist and Cardiovascular Health Study review of deaths: Implications of coding differences. J Am Geriatr Soc 2009;57(1):133-9.
287. Romero JP, Benito-Leon J, Mitchell AJ, Trincado R, Bermejo-Pareja F. Under reporting of dementia deaths on death certificates using data from a population-based study (NEDICES). J Alzheimers Dis 2014;39(4):741-8.
288. Romero JP, Benito-Leon J, Louis ED, Bermejo-Pareja F. Under reporting of dementia deaths on death certificates: A systematic review of population-based cohort studies. J Alzheimers Dis 2014;41(1):213-21.
289. Ganguli M, Rodriguez EG. Reporting of dementia on death certificates: A community study. J Am Geriatr Soc 1999;47(7):842-9.
290. James BD, Leurgans SE, Hebert LE, Scherr PA, Yaffe K, Bennett DA. Contribution of Alzheimer disease to mortality in the United States. Neurology 2014;82(12):1045-50.
291. Unpublished tabulations based on data from the National 5% Sample Medicare Fee-for-Service Beneficiaries for 2014. Prepared under contract by Avalere Health, January 2016.
292. Weuve J, Hebert LE, Scherr PA, Evans DA. Deaths in the United States among persons with Alzheimer's disease (2010-2050). Alzheimers Dement 2014;10(2):E40-6.
293. Arrighi HM, Neumann PJ, Lieberburg IM, Townsend RJ. Lethality of Alzheimer disease and its impact on nursing home placement. Alzheimer Dis Assoc Disord 2010;24(1):90-5.
294. Tejada-Vera B. Mortality from Alzheimer's disease in the United States: Data for 2000 and 2010. National Center for Health Statistics Data Brief, No. 116. National Center for Health Statistics, Hyattsville, MD; 2013.
295. Taylor C, Greenlund S, McGuire L, Lu H, Croft J. Deaths from Alzheimer's Disease — United States, 1999-2014. MMWR Morb Mortal Wkly Rep 2017;66:521-6.
296. Ganguli M, Dodge HH, Shen C, Pandav RS, DeKosky ST. Alzheimer disease and mortality: A 15-year epidemiological study. Arch Neurol 2005;62(5):779-84.
297. Waring SC, Doody RS, Pavlik VN, Massman PJ, Chan W. Survival among patients with dementia from a large multi-ethnic population. Alzheimer Dis Assoc Disord 2005;19(4):178-83.
298. Brookmeyer R, Corrada MM, Curriero FC, Kawas C. Survival following a diagnosis of Alzheimer disease. Arch Neurol 2002;59(11):1764-7.
299. Larson EB, Shadlen MF, Wang L, McCormick WC, Bowen JD, Teri L, et al. Survival after initial diagnosis of Alzheimer disease. Ann Intern Med 2004;140(7):501-9.
300. Helzner EP, Scarmeas N, Cosentino S, Tang MX, Schupf N, Stern Y. Survival in Alzheimer disease: A multiethnic, population-based study of incident cases. Neurology 2008;71(19):1489-95.
301. Xie J, Brayne C, Matthews FE. Survival times in people with dementia: Analysis from a population based cohort study with 14-year follow-up. BMJ 2008;336(7638):258-62.
302. Brodaty H, Seeher K, Gibson L. Dementia time to death: A systematic literature review on survival time and years of life lost in people with dementia. Int Psychogeriatr 2012;24(7):1034-45.
303. Todd S, Barr S, Roberts M, Passmore AP. Survival in dementia and predictors of mortality: A review. Int J Geriatr Psychiatry 2013;28(11):1109-24.
304. Mitchell SL, Teno JM, Miller SC, Mor V. A national study of the location of death for older persons with dementia. J Am Geriatr Soc 2005;53(2):299-305.
305. U.S. Burden of Disease Collaborators, Mokdad AH, Ballestros K, et al. The state of U.S. health, 1990-2016: Burden of diseases, injuries, and risk factors among U.S. states. JAMA 2018;319(14):1444-72.
306. Gaugler JE, Kane RL, Kane RA. Family care for older adults with disabilities: Toward more targeted and interpretable research. Int J Aging Hum Dev 2002;54(3):205-31.
307. Schulz R, Quittner AL. Caregiving through the life-span: Overview and future directions. Health Psychol 1998;17:107-11.
308. Friedman EM, Shih RA, Langa KM, Hurd MD. U.S. prevalence and predictors of informal caregiving for dementia. Health Aff 2015;34(10):1637-41.
309. Spillman B, Wolff J, Freedman VA, Kasper JD. Informal Caregiving for Older Americans: An Analysis of the 2011 National Health and Aging Trends Study. Available at: https://aspe.hhs.gov/pdf-report/informal-caregiving-older-americans-analysis-2011-national-health-and-aging-trends-study. Accessed December 4, 2019.

310. Walmart: 2019 Annual Report. Available at: https://s2.q4cdn.com/056532643/files/doc_financials/2019/annual/Walmart-2019-AR-Final.pdf. Accessed December 4, 2019.
311. McDonald's Corporation Report 2018. Available at: https://corporate.mcdonalds.com/content/dam/gwscorp/nfl/investor-relations-content/annual-reports/McDonalds_2018_Annual_Report.pdf. Accessed December 4, 2019.
312. Jutkowitz E, Kane RL, Gaugler JE, MacLehose RF, Dowd B, Kuntz KM. Societal and family lifetime cost of dementia: Implications for policy. J Am Geriatr Soc 2017;65(10):2169-75.
313. Official Data Foundation. CPI inflation calculator. Available at: http://www.in2013dollars.com/2017-dollars-in-2018?amount=139765. Accessed December 4, 2019.
314. Deb A, Thornton JD, Sambamoorthi U, Innes K. Direct and indirect cost of managing alzheimer's disease and related dementias in the United States. Expert Rev Pharmacoecon Outcomes Res 2017;17(2):189-202.
315. Greenwood N, Smith R. Motivations for being informal carers of people living with dementia: A systematic review of qualitative literature. BMC Geriatr 2019;19(1):169.
316. Kasper JD, Freedman VA, Spillman BC, Wolff JL. The disproportionate impact of dementia on family and unpaid caregiving to older adults. Health Aff 2015;34(10):1642-49.
317. Ornstein KA, Wolff JL, Bollens-Lund E, Rahman OK, Kelley AS. Spousal caregivers are caregiving alone in the last years of life. Health Aff (Millwood) 2019;38(6):964-72.
318. Alzheimer's Association. Issues Brief: LGBT and Dementia. Available at: https://www.alz.org/media/Documents/lgbt-dementia-issues-brief.pdf. Accessed December 4, 2019.
319. Kasper JD, Freedman VA, Spillman BC. Disability and Care Needs of Older Americans by Dementia Status: An Analysis of the 2011 National Health and Aging Trends Study. U.S. Department of Health and Human Services; 2014. Available at: http://aspe.hhs.gov/report/disability-and-care-needs-older-americans-dementia-status-analysis-2011-national-health-and-aging-trends-study. Accessed December 4, 2019.
320. Rabarison KM, Bouldin ED, Bish CL, McGuire LC, Taylor CA, Greenlund KJ. The economic value of informal caregiving for persons with dementia: Results from 38 states, the District of Columbia, and Puerto Rico, 2015 and 2016 BRFSS. Am J Public Health 2018;108(10):1370-7.
321. Langa KM, Plassman BL, Wallace RB, Herzog AR, Heeringa SG, Ofstedal MB, et al. The Aging, Demographics, and Memory Study: Study design and methods. Neuroepidemiology 2005;25(4):181-91.
322. Fisher GG, Franks MM, Plassman BL, Brown SL, Potter GG, Llewellyn D, et al. Caring for individuals with dementia and cognitive impairment, not dementia: Findings from The Aging, Demographics, and Memory Study. J Am Geriatr Soc 2011;59(3):488-94.
323. National Alliance for Caregiving in Partnership with the Alzheimer's Association. Dementia Caregiving in the U.S. Bethesda, MD. Available at: http://www.caregiving.org/wp-content/uploads/2017/02/DementiaCaregivingFINAL_WEB.pdf. Accessed December 4, 2019.
324. Unpublished data from the 2015, 2016 and 2017 Behavioral Risk Factor Surveillance System survey, analyzed by and provided to the Alzheimer's Association by the Alzheimer's Disease and Healthy Aging Program (AD+HP), Centers for Disease Control and Prevention (CDC).
325. Riffin C, Van Ness PH, Wolff JL, Fried T. Family and other unpaid caregivers and older adults with and without dementia and disability. J Am Geriatr Soc 2017;65(8):1821-8.
326. National Poll on Healthy Aging. Dementia Caregivers: Juggling, Delaying and Looking Forward. Available at: http://www.healthyagingpoll.org/sites/default/files/2017-10/NPHA_Caregivers-Report-PROOF_101817_v2.pdf. Accessed December 4, 2019.
327. National Alliance for Caregiving and AARP. Caregiving in the U.S.: Unpublished data analyzed under contract for the Alzheimer's Association; 2009.
328. Alzheimer's Association. 2014 Alzheimer's Disease Facts and Figures. Alzheimer Dement 2014;10(2):e47-e92.
329. Pinquart M, Sörensen. Gender differences in caregiver stressors, social resources, and health: An updated meta-analysis. J Gerontol B Psychol Sci Soc Sci 2006;61(1):P33-45. Available at: http://psychsocgerontology.oxfordjournals.org/content/61/1/P33.long. Accessed December 4, 2019.
330. Ma M, Dorstyn D, Ward L, Prentice S. Alzheimer's disease and caregiving: A meta-analytic review comparing the mental health of primary carers to controls. Aging Ment Health 2017;5:1-11.
331. National Alliance for Caregiving and AARP. Caregiving in the U.S. (2015). Available at: http://www.caregiving.org/wp-content/uploads/2015/05/2015_CaregivingintheUS_Final-Report-June-4_WEB.pdf. Accessed December 4, 2019.
332. Spillman BC, Freedman VA, Kasper JD, Wolff JL. Change over time in caregiving networks for older adults with and without dementia. J Gerontol B Psychol Sci Soc Sci 2019 May 18. pii: gbz065. doi: 10.1093/geronb/gbz065. [Epub ahead of print].
333. Garity J. Caring for a family member with Alzheimer's disease: Coping with caregiver burden post-nursing home placement. J Gerontol Nurs 2006;32(6):39-48.
334. Port CL, Zimmerman S, Williams CS, Dobbs D, Preisser JS, Williams SW. Families filling the gap: Comparing family involvement for assisted living and nursing home residents with dementia. Gerontologist 2005;45(Special Issue 1):87-95.
335. Schulz R, Belle SH, Czaja SJ, McGinnis KA, Stevens A, Zhang S. Long-term care placement of dementia patients and caregiver health and well-being. JAMA 2004;292(8):961-7.
336. Rattinger GB, Schwartz S, Mullins CD, Corcoran C, Zuckerman IH, Sanders C, et al. Dementia severity and the longitudinal costs of informal care in the Cache County population. Alzheimers Dement 2015;11(8):946-54.
337. Rattinger GB, Fauth EB, Behrens S, Sanders C, Schwartz S, Norton MC, et al. Closer caregiver and care-recipient relationships predict lower informal costs of dementia care: The Cache County Dementia Progression Study. Alzheimers Dement 2016;12(8):917-24.
338. Wolff JL, Mulcahy J, Huang J, Roth DL, Covinsky K, Kasper JD. Family Caregivers of Older Adults, 1999-2015: Trends in characteristics, circumstances, and role-related appraisal. Gerontologist 2018;58(6):1021-32.
339. Ornstein K, Gaugler JE. The problem with "problem behaviors": A systematic review of the association between individual patient behavioral and psychological symptoms and caregiver depression and burden within the dementia patient-caregiver dyad. Int Psychogeriatr 2012;24(10):1536-52.
340. Vaingankar JA, Chong SA, Abdin E, Picco L, Shafie S, Seow E, et al. Psychiatric morbidity and its correlates among informal caregivers of older adults. Compr Psychiatry 2016;68:178-85.
341. Feast A, Moniz-Cook E, Stoner C, Charlesworth G, Orrell M. A systematic review of the relationship between behavioral and psychological symptoms (BPSD) and caregiver well-being. Int Psychogeriatr 2016;28(11):1761-74.
342. Kiecolt-Glaser JK, Glaser R, Gravenstein S, Malarkey WB, Sheridan J. Chronic stress alters the immune response to influenza virus vaccine in older adults. Proc Natl Acad Sci 1996;93:3043-7.
343. Schulz R, Beach SR. Caregiving as a risk factor for mortality: The Caregiver Health Effects Study. JAMA 1999;282:2215-60.
344. Vitaliano PP, Zhang J, Scanlan JM. Is caregiving hazardous to one's physical health? A meta-analysis. Psychol Bull 2003;129(6):946-72.
345. Liu W, Gallagher-Thompson D. Impact of dementia caregiving: Risks, strains, and growth. In: Qualls SH, Zarit SH, eds. Aging families and caregiving. Hoboken, NJ: John Wiley & Sons, Inc.; 2009: p. 85-112.
346. Pinquart M, Sörensen S. Associations of stressors and uplifts of caregiving with caregiver burden and depressive mood: A meta-analysis. J Gerontol B Psychol Sci Soc Sci 2003;58(2):112-28.

347. Sörensen S, Duberstein P, Gill D, Pinquart M. Dementia care: Mental health effects, intervention strategies, and clinical implications. Lancet Neurol 2006;5(11):961-73.
348. Goren A, Montgomery W, Kahle-Wrobleski K, Nakamura T, Ueda K. Impact of caring for persons with Alzheimer's disease or dementia on caregivers' health outcomes: Findings from a community based survey in Japan. BMC Geriatr 2016;16:122.
349. Alzheimer's Association. 2016 Alzheimer's Disease Facts and Figures. Alzheimer Dement 2016;12(4):459-509.
350. Jones RW, Lebrec J, Kahle-Wrobleski K, Dell'Agnello G, Bruno G, Vellas B, et al. Disease progression in mild dementia due to Alzheimer disease in an 18-month observational study (GERAS): The impact on costs and caregiver outcomes. Dement Geriatr Cogn Dis Extra 2017;7(1):87-100.
351. Quinn C, Toms G. Influence of positive aspects of dementia caregiving on caregivers' well-being: A systematic review. Gerontologist 2018.doi:10.1093/geront/gny168.
352. Zarit SH. Positive aspects of caregiving: More than looking on the bright side. Aging Ment Health 2012;16(6):673-74.
353. Cheng ST, Mak EP, Lau RW, Ng NS, Lam LC. Voices of Alzheimer caregivers on positive aspects of caregiving. Gerontologist 2016;56(3):451-60.
354. Monin JK, Schulz R, Feeney BC. Compassionate love in individuals with Alzheimer's disease and their spousal caregivers: Associations with caregivers' psychological health. Gerontologist 2015;55(6):981-9.
355. Roth DL, Dilworth-Anderson P, Huang J, Gross AL, Gitlin LN. Positive aspects of family caregiving for dementia: Differential item functioning by race. J Gerontol B Psychol Sci Soc Sci 2015;70(6):813-9.
356. Lloyd J, Patterson T, Muers J. The positive aspects of caregiving in dementia: A critical review of the qualitative literature. Dementia (London) 2016;15(6):1534-61.
357. Yu DSF, Cheng ST, Wang J. Unravelling positive aspects of caregiving in dementia: An integrative review of research literature. Int J Nurs Stud 2018;79:1-26.
358. Schulz R, O'Brien AT, Bookwala J, Fleissner K. Psychiatric and physical morbidity effects of dementia caregiving: Prevalence, correlates, and causes. Gerontologist 1995;35(6):771-91.
359. Baumgarten M, Battista RN, Infante-Rivard C, Hanley JA, Becker R, Gauthier S. The psychological and physical health of family members caring for an elderly person with dementia. J Clin Epidemiol 1992;45(1):61-70.
360. Mausbach BT, Chattillion EA, Roepke SK, Patterson TL, Grant I. A comparison of psychosocial outcomes in elderly Alzheimer caregivers and noncaregivers. Am J Geriatr Psychiatry 2013;21(1):5-13.
361. Kessler RC, Chiu WT, Demler O, Merikangas KR, Walters EE. Prevalence, severity, and comorbidity of 12-month DSM-IV disorders in the National Comorbidity Survey Replication. Arch Gen Psychiatry 2005;62:617-27.
362. Sallim AB, Sayampanathan AA, Cuttilan A, Chun-Man Ho R. Prevalence of mental health disorders among caregivers of patients with Alzheimer disease. J Am Med Dir Assoc 2015;16(12):1034-41.
363. Atteih S, Mellon L, Hall P, Brewer L, Horgan F, Williams D, et al. Implications of stroke for caregiver outcomes: Findings from the ASPIRE-S Study. Int J Stroke 2015;10:918-23.
364. Thunyadee C, Sitthimongkol Y, Sangon S, Chai-Aroon T, Hegadoren KM. Predictors of depressive symptoms and physical health in caregivers of individuals with schizophrenia. J Nurs Health Sci 2015;17:412-9.
365. Collins RN, Kishita N. Prevalence of depression and burden among informal care-givers of people with dementia: A meta-analysis. Ageing and Society, 1-38. doi:10.1017/S0144686X19000527.
366. Vitaliano PP, Ustundag O, Borson S. Objective and subjective cognitive problems among caregivers and matched non-caregivers. Gerontologist 2017;57(4):637-47.
367. Dassel KB, Carr DC, Vitaliano P. Does caring for a spouse with dementia accelerate cognitive decline? Findings from the Health and Retirement Study. Gerontologist 2017;57(2):319-28.
368. Arthur PB, Gitlin LN, Kairalla JA, Mann WC. Relationship between the number of behavioral symptoms in dementia and caregiver distress: What is the tipping point? Int Psychogeriatr 2018;30(8):1099-107.
369. Gillespie R, Mullan J, Harrison L. Managing medications: The role of informal caregivers of older adults and people living with dementia: A review of the literature. J Clin Nurs 2014;23(23-24):3296-308.
370. Alsaeed D, Jamieson E, Gul MO, Smith FJ. Challenges to optimal medicines use in people living with dementia and their caregivers: A literature review. Int J Pharm 2016;512(2):396-404.
371. Polenick CA, Stanz SD, Leggett AN, Maust DT, Hodgson NA, Kales HC. Stressors and resources related to medication management: Associations with spousal caregivers' role overload. Gerontologist 2018.doi:10.1093/geront/gny130. [Epub ahead of print].
372. Aston L, Hilton A, Moutela T, Shaw R, Maidment I. Exploring the evidence base for how people with dementia and their informal carers manage their medication in the community: A mixed studies review. BMC Geriatr 2017;17(1):242.
373. Badana ANS, Marino V, Haley WE. Racial differences in caregiving: Variation by relationship type and dementia care status. J Aging Health 2019;31(6):925-46.
374. Gaugler JE, Mittelman MS, Hepburn K, Newcomer R. Clinically significant changes in burden and depression among dementia caregivers following nursing home admission. BMC Medicine 2010;8:85.
375. Mausbach BT, Chattillion EA, Ho J, Flynn LM, Tiznado D, von Känel R, et al. Why does placement of persons with Alzheimer's disease into long-term care improve caregivers' well-being? Examination of psychological mediators. Psychol Aging 2014;29(4):776-86.
376. Peacock SC. The experience of providing end-of-life care to a relative with advanced dementia: An integrative literature review. Palliat Support Care 2013;11(2):155-68.
377. Schulz R, Mendelsohn AB, Haley WE, Mahoney D, Allen RS, Zhang S, et al. End-of-life care and the effects of bereavement on family caregivers of persons with dementia. N Engl J Med 2003;349(20):1936-42.
378. Fonareva I, Oken BS. Physiological and functional consequences of caregiving for relatives with dementia. Int Psychogeriatr 2014;26(5):725-47.
379. von Känel R, Mausbach BT, Ancoli-Israel S, Mills PJ, Dimsdale JE, Patterson TL, et al. Positive affect and sleep in spousal Alzheimer caregivers: A longitudinal study. Behav Sleep Med 2014;12(5):358-72.
380. Peng H-L, Chang Y-P. Sleep disturbance in family caregivers of individuals with dementia: A review of the literature. Perspect Psychiatr C 2012;49(2):135-46.
381. Gao C, Chapagain NY, Scullin MK. Sleep Duration and Sleep Quality in caregivers of patients with dementia: A systematic review and meta-analysis. JAMA Netw Open 2019;2(8):e199891.
382. Välimäki TH, Martikainen JA, Hongisto K, Väätäinen S, Sintonen H, Koivisto AM. Impact of Alzheimer's disease on the family caregiver's long-term quality of life: Results from an ALSOVA follow-up study. Qual Life Res 2016;25(3):687-97.
383. Bremer P, Cabrera E, Leino-Kilpi H, Lethin C, Saks K, Sutcliffe C. Informal dementia care: Consequences for caregivers' health and health care use in 8 European countries. Health Policy 2015;119(11):1459-71.
384. MetLife Mature Market Institute. The MetLife Study of Alzheimer's Disease: The Caregiving Experience; August 2006. Available at: http://docplayer.net/20982840-The-metlife-study-of-alzheimer-s-disease-the-caregiving-experience.html. Accessed December 4, 2019.
385. Dassel KB, Carr DC. Does dementia caregiving accelerate frailty? Findings from the Health and Retirement Study. Gerontologist 2016;56(3):444-50.

386. Fredman L, Bertrand RM, Martire LM, Hochberg M, Harris EL. Leisure-time exercise and overall physical activity in older women caregivers and non-caregivers from the Caregiver-SOF Study. Prev Med 2006;43:226-9.
387. Rote SM, Angel JL, Moon H, Markides K. Caregiving Across Diverse Populations: New Evidence From the National Study of Caregiving and Hispanic EPESE. Innov Aging 2019;3(2):igz033.
388. von Kanel R, Dimsdale JE, Mills PJ, Ancoli-Israel S, Patterson TL, Mausbach BT, et al. Effect of Alzheimer caregiving stress and age on frailty markers interleukin-6, C-reactive protein, and D-dimer. J Gerontol A Biol Sci Med Sci 2006;61(9):963-9.
389. Kiecolt-Glaser JK, Dura JR, Speicher CE, Trask OJ, Glaser R. Spousal caregivers of dementia victims: Longitudinal changes in immunity and health. Psychosom Med 1991;53:345-62.
390. Kiecolt-Glaser JK, Marucha PT, Mercado AM, Malarkey WB, Glaser R. Slowing of wound healing by psychological stress. Lancet 1995;346(8984):1194-6.
391. Vitaliano PP, Scanlan JM, Zhang J, Savage MV, Hirsch IB, Siegler I. A path model of chronic stress, the metabolic syndrome, and coronary heart disease. Psychosom Med 2002;64:418-35.
392. Mausbach BT, Romero-Moreno R, Bos T, von Känel R, Ziegler MG, Allison MA, et al. Engagement in pleasant leisure activities and blood pressure: A 5-year longitudinal study in Alzheimer caregivers. Psychosom Med 2017;79(7):735-41.
393. Shaw WS, Patterson TL, Ziegler MG, Dimsdale JE, Semple SJ, Grant I. Accelerated risk of hypertensive blood pressure recordings among Alzheimer caregivers. J Psychosom Res 1999;46(3):215-27.
394. Mausbach BT, Roepke SK, Ziegler MG, Milic M, Von Kanel R, Dimsdale JE, et al. Association between chronic caregiving stress and impaired endothelial function in the elderly. J Am Coll Cardiol 2010;55(23):2599-606.
395. Allen AP, Curran EA, Duggan Á, Cryan JF, Chorcoráin AN, Dinan TG, et al. A systematic review of the psychobiological burden of informal caregiving for patients with dementia: Focus on cognitive and biological markers of chronic stress. Neurosci Biobehav Rev 2017;73:123-64.
396. Roth DL, Sheehan OC, Haley WE, Jenny NS, Cushman M, Walston JD. Is family caregiving associated with inflammation or compromised immunity? A meta-analysis. Gerontologist 2019;59(5):e521-e534.
397. Schubert CC, Boustani M, Callahan CM, Perkins AJ, Hui S, Hendrie HC. Acute care utilization by dementia caregivers within urban primary care practices. J Gen Intern Med 2008;23(11):1736-40.
398. Zhu CW, Scarmeas N, Ornstein K, Albert M, Brandt J, Blacker D, et al. Health-care use and cost in dementia caregivers: Longitudinal results from the Predictors Caregiver Study. Alzheimers Dement 2015;11(4):444-54.
399. Leggett AN, Sonnega AJ, Lohman MC. Till death do us part: Intersecting health and spousal dementia caregiving on caregiver mortality. J Aging Health 2019.doi: 10.1177/0898264319860975. [Epub ahead of print].
400. Roth DL, Fredman L, Haley WE. Informal caregiving and its impact on health: A reappraisal from population-based studies. Gerontologist 2015;55(2):309-19.
401. Christakis NA, Allison PD. Mortality after the hospitalization of a spouse. N Engl J Med 2006;354:719-30.
402. Perkins M, Howard VJ, Wadley VG, Crowe M, Safford MM, Haley WE, et al. Caregiving strain and all-cause mortality: Evidence from the REGARDS Study. J Gerontol B Psychol Sci Soc Sci 2013;68(4):504-12.
403. Gaugler JE, Jutkowitz E, Peterson CM, Zmora R. Caregivers dying before care recipients with dementia. Alzheimers Dement (NY) 2018;4:688-93.
404. National Academies of Sciences, Engineering, and Medicine. Families Caring for an Aging America. Washington, D.C.: The National Academies Press: 2016.
405. Albert SM, Schulz R. The MetLife Study of working caregivers and employer health care costs. New York, N.Y.: MetLife Mature Market Institute; 2010.
406. Gaugler JE, Pestka DL, Davila H, Sales R, Owen G, Baumgartner SA, et al. The complexities of family caregiving at work: A mixed-methods study. Int J Aging Hum Dev 2018;87(4):347-76.
407. AARP, Family Caregiving and Out-of-Pocket Costs: 2016 Report. Available at: https://www.aarp.org/content/dam/aarp/research/surveys_statistics/ltc/2016/family-caregiving-costs-fact-sheet.doi.10.26419%252Fres.00138.002.pdf. Accessed December 4, 2019.
408. Stall NM, Kim SJ, Hardacre KA, Shah PS, Straus SE, Bronskill SE, et al. Association of informal caregiver distress with health outcomes of community-dwelling dementia care recipients: A systematic review. J Am Geriatr So 2019;67(3):609-17.
409. Gaugler JE, Jutkowitz E, Shippee TP, Brasure M. Consistency of dementia caregiver intervention classification: An evidence-based synthesis. Int Psychogeriatr 2017;29(1):19-30.
410. Gitlin LN, Hodgson N. Caregivers as therapeutic agents in dementia care: The evidence-base for interventions supporting their role. In: Gaugler JE, Kane RL, eds. Family caregiving in the new normal. Philadelphia, Pa.: Elsevier, Inc.; 2015: p. 305-56.
411. Williams F, Moghaddam N, Ramsden S, De Boos D. Interventions for reducing levels of burden amongst informal carers of persons with dementia in the community. A systematic review and meta-analysis of randomised controlled trials. Aging Ment Health 2019;23(12):1629-42.
412. Kaddour L, Kishita N, Schaller A. A meta-analysis of low-intensity cognitive behavioral therapy-based interventions for dementia caregivers. Int Psychogeriatr 2018:1-16.
413. Nguyen H, Terry D, Phan H, Vickers J, McInerney F. Communication training and its effects on carer and care-receiver outcomes in dementia settings: A systematic review. J Clin Nurs 2019;28(7-8):1050-69.
414. Jütten LH, Mark RE, Wicherts JM, Sitskoorn MM. The effectiveness of psychosocial and behavioral interventions for informal dementia caregivers: Meta-analyses and meta-regressions. J Alzheimers Dis 2018;66(1):149-72.
415. Maslow K. Translating Innovation to Impact: Evidence-Based Interventions to Support People with Alzheimer's Disease and their Caregiver at Home and in the Community. Washington, D.C.: Administration on Aging; 2012. Available at: https://nadrc.acl.gov/sites/default/files/uploads/docs/TranslatingInnovationtoImpactAlzheimersDisease_0.pdf. Accessed December 4, 2019.
416. Rosalynn Carter Institute for Caregiving. Caregiver Intervention Database. Available at: https://www.rosalynncarter.org/research/caregiver-intervention-database/. Accessed December 4, 2019.
417. Liew TM, Lee CS. Reappraising the efficacy and acceptability of multicomponent interventions for caregiver depression in dementia: The utility of network meta-analysis. Gerontologist 2019;59(4):e380-e392.
418. Teri L, Logsdon RG, McCurry SM, Pike KC, McGough EL. Translating an evidence-based multicomponent intervention for older adults with dementia and caregivers. Gerontologist 2018;Oct 9. doi: 10.1093/geront/gny122. [Epub ahead of print].
419. Menne HL, Bass DM, Johnson JD, Primetica B, Kearney KR, Bollin S, et al. Statewide implementation of "reducing disability in Alzheimer's disease": Impact on family caregiver outcomes. J Gerontol Soc Work 2014;57(6-7):626-39.
420. Teri L, McKenzie G, Logsdon RG, McCurry SM, Bollin S, Mead J, et al. Translation of two evidence-based programs for training families to improve care of persons with dementia. Gerontologist 2012;52(4):452-9.
421. Gitlin LN, Jacobs M, Earland TV. Translation of a dementia caregiver intervention for delivery in homecare as a reimbursable Medicare service: Outcomes and lessons learned. Gerontologist 2010;50(6):847-54.
422. Burgio LD, Collins IB, Schmid B, Wharton T, McCallum D, Decoster J. Translating the REACH caregiver intervention for use by area agency on aging personnel: The REACH OUT program. Gerontologist 2009;49(1):103-16.

423. Mittelman MS, Bartels SJ. Translating research into practice: Case study of a community-based dementia caregiver intervention. Health Aff 2014;33(4):587-95.
424. Cheung KS, Lau BH, Wong PW, Leung AY, Lou VW, Chan GM, et al. Multicomponent intervention on enhancing dementia caregiver well-being and reducing behavioral problems among Hong Kong Chinese: A translational study based on REACH II. Int J Geriatr Psychiatry 2015:30(5):460-9.
425. Samia LW, Aboueissa AM, Halloran J, Hepburn K. The Maine Savvy Caregiver Project: Translating an evidence-based dementia family caregiver program within the RE-AIM Framework. J Gerontol Soc Work 2014;57(6-7):640-61.
426. Lykens K, Moayad N, Biswas S, Reyes-Ortiz C, Singh KP. Impact of a community based implementation of REACH II program for caregivers of Alzheimer's patients. PLoS One 2014;9(2):e89290.
427. Menne HL, Bass DM, Johnson JD, Kearney KR, Bollin S, Teri L. Program components and outcomes of individuals with dementia: Results from the replication of an evidence-based program. J Appl Gerontol 2017;36(5):537-52.
428. Primetica B, Menne HL, Bollin S, Teri L, Molea M. Evidence-Based Program replication: Translational activities, experiences, and challenges. J Appl Gerontol 2015;34(5):652-70.
429. Fortinsky RH, Gitlin LN, Pizzi LT, Piersol CV, Grady J, Robison JT, et al. Translation of the care of persons with dementia in their environments (COPE) intervention in a publicly-funded home care context: Rationale and research design. Contemp Clin Trials 2016;49:155-65.
430. Nichols LO, Martindale-Adams J, Burns R, Zuber J, Graney MJ. REACH VA: Moving from translation to system implementation. Gerontologist 2016;56(1):135-44.
431. McCurry SM, Logsdon RG, Pike KC, LaFazia DM, Teri L. Training Area Agencies on Aging case managers to improve physical function, mood, and behavior in persons with dementia and caregivers: Examples from the RDAD-Northwest Study. J Gerontol Soc Work 2018;61(1):45-60.
432. Czaja SJ, Lee CC, Perdomo D, Loewenstein D, Bravo M, Moxley JH, et al. Community REACH: An implementation of an evidence-based caregiver program. Gerontologist 2018;58(2):e130-7.
433. Fauth EB, Jackson MA, Walberg DK, Lee NE, Easom LR, Alston G, et al. External validity of the New York University Caregiver Intervention: Key caregiver outcomes across multiple demonstration projects. J Appl Gerontol 2019;38(9):1253-81.
434. Boustani M, Alder CA, Solid CA. Agile implementation: A blueprint for implementing evidence-based healthcare solutions. J Am Geriatr Soc 2018;66(7):1372-6.
435. Boots LM, de Vugt ME, van Knippenberg RJ, Kempen GI, Verhey FR. A systematic review of internet-based supportive interventions for caregivers of patients with dementia. Int J Geriatr Psych 2015;29(4):331-44.
436. Czaja SJ, Loewenstein D, Schulz R, Nair SN, Perdomo D. A videophone psychosocial intervention for dementia caregivers. Am J Geriatr Psychiatry 2013;21(11):1071-81.
437. Griffiths PC, Whitney MK, Kovaleva M, Hepburn K. Development and implementation of tele-savvy for dementia caregivers: A Department of Veterans Affairs Clinical Demonstration Project. Gerontologist 2016;56(1):145-54.
438. Brown EL, Ruggiano N, Li J, Clarke PJ, Kay ES, Hristidis V. Smartphone-based health technologies for dementia care: Opportunities, challenges, and current practices. J Appl Gerontol 2019;38(1):73-91.
439. Grossman MR, Zak DK, Zelinski EM. Mobile Apps for caregivers of older adults: Quantitative content analysis. JMIR mHealth and uHealth 2018;6(7):e162.
440. Gaugler JE, Zmora R, Mitchell LL, Finlay JM, Peterson CM, McCarron H, et al. Six-month effectiveness of remote activity monitoring for persons living with dementia and their family caregivers: An experimental mixed methods study. Gerontologist 2019;59(1):78-89
441. Waller A, Dilworth S, Mansfield E, Sanson-Fisher R. Computer and telephone delivered interventions to support caregivers of people with dementia: A systematic review of research output and quality. BMC Geriatr 2017;17(1):265.
442. Hopwood J, Walker N, McDonagh L, Rait G, Walters K, Iliffe S, et al. Internet-based interventions aimed at supporting family caregivers of people with dementia: Systematic review. J Med Internet Res 2018;20(6):e216.
443. Gitlin LN, Marx K, Scerpella D, Dabelko-Schoeny H, Anderson KA, Huang J, et al. Embedding caregiver support in community-based services for older adults: A multi-site randomized trial to test the Adult Day Service Plus Program (ADS Plus). Contemp Clin Trials 2019;83:97-108.
444. Gaugler JE, Potter T, Pruinelli L. Partnering with caregivers. Clin Geriatr Med 2014;30(3):493-515.
445. Gitlin LN, Marx K, Stanley IH, Hodgson N. Translating evidence-based dementia caregiving interventions into practice: State-of-the-science and next steps. Gerontologist 2015;55(2):210-26.
446. Wethington E, Burgio LD. Translational research on caregiving: Missing links in the translation process. In: Gaugler JE, Kane RL, eds. Family caregiving in the new normal. Philadelphia, Pa.: Elsevier, Inc; 2015: p. 193-210.
447. Zarit SH. Past is prologue: How to advance caregiver interventions. Aging Ment Health 2017;16:1-6.
448. Kishita N, Hammond L, Dietrich CM, Mioshi E. Which interventions work for dementia family carers?: an updated systematic review of randomized controlled trials of carer interventions. Int Psychogeriatr 2018;30(11):1679-96.
449. Zarit SH. Empirically supported treatment for family caregivers. In: Qualls SH, Zarit SH, eds. Aging families and caregiving. Hoboken, N.J.: John Wiley & Sons, Inc.; 2009: p. 131-54.
450. Zarit SH, Lee JE, Barrineau MJ, Whitlatch CJ, Femia EE. Fidelity and acceptability of an adaptive intervention for caregivers: An exploratory study. Aging Ment Health 2013;17(2):197-206.
451. Van Mierlo LD, Meiland FJ, Van Hout HP, Dröes RM. Toward an evidence-based implementation model and checklist for personalized dementia care in the community. Int Psychogeriatr 2016;28(5):801-13.
452. Gaugler JE, Reese M, Tanler R. Care to Plan: An online tool that offers tailored support to dementia caregivers. Gerontologist 2016;56(6):1161-74.
453. Jennings LA, Ramirez KD, Hays RD, Wenger NS, Reuben DB. Personalized goal attainment in dementia care: Measuring what persons with dementia and their caregivers want. J Am Geriatr Soc 2018;66(11):2120-7.
454. Whitlatch CJ, Orsulic-Jeras S. Meeting the informational, educational, and psychosocial support needs of persons living with dementia and their family caregivers. Gerontologist 2018;18;58(Suppl 1):S58-73.
455. Akarsu NE, Prince MJ, Lawrence VC, Das-Munshi J. Depression in carers of people with dementia from a minority ethnic background: Systematic review and meta-analysis of randomised controlled trials of psychosocial interventions. Int J Geriatr Psychiatry 2019;34(6):790-806.
456. Gonyea JG, López LM, Velásquez EH. The effectiveness of a culturally sensitive cognitive behavioral group intervention for Latino Alzheimer's caregivers. Gerontologist 2016;56(2):292-302.
457. Llanque SM, Enriquez M. Interventions for Hispanic caregivers of patients with dementia: A review of the literature. Am J Alzheimers Dis Other Demen 2012;27(1):23-32.
458. Kally Z, Cote SD, Gonzalez J, Villarruel M, Cherry DL, Howland S, et al. The Savvy Caregiver Program: Impact of an evidence-based intervention on the well-being of ethnically diverse caregivers. J Gerontol Soc Work 2014;57(6-7):681-93.
459. Kally Z, Cherry DL, Howland S, Villarruel M. Asian Pacific Islander dementia care network: A model of care for underserved communities. J Gerontol Soc Work 2014;57 (6-7):710-27.

460. Napoles AM, Chadiha L, Eversley R, Moreno-John G. Reviews: Developing culturally sensitive dementia caregiver interventions: Are we there yet? Am J Alzheimers Dis Other Dement 2010;25:389-406.
461. Hicken BL, Daniel C, Luptak M, Grant M, Kilian S, Rupper RW. Supporting caregivers of rural veterans electronically (SCORE). J Rural Health 2017;33(3):305-13.
462. Graham-Phillips A, Roth DL, Huang J, Dilworth-Anderson P, Gitlin LN. Racial and ethnic differences in the delivery of the resources for enhancing Alzheimer's Caregiver Health II Intervention. J Am Geriatr Soc 2016;64(8):1662-7.
463. Martindale-Adams J, Tah T, Finke B, LaCounte C, Higgins BJ, Nichols LO. Implementation of the REACH model of dementia caregiver support in American Indian and Alaska Native communities. Transl Behav Med 2017;7(3):427-34.
464. Meyer OL, Liu XL, Tancredi D, Ramirez AS, Schulz R, Hinton L. Acculturation level and caregiver outcomes from a randomized intervention trial to enhance caregivers' health: Evidence from REACH II. Aging Ment Health 2017;24:1-8.
465. Fields NL, Xu L, Richardson VE, Parekh R, Ivey D, Feinhals G. The Senior Companion Program Plus: A culturally tailored psychoeducational training program (innovative practice). Dementia (London). 2016 Jan 1:1471301216685626. doi: 10.1177/1471301216685626. [Epub ahead of print]
466. Luchsinger JA, Burgio L, Mittelman M, Dunner I, Levine JA, Hoyos C, et al. Comparative effectiveness of 2 interventions for Hispanic caregivers of persons with dementia. J Am Geriatr Soc 2018;66(9):1708-15.
467. Gilmore-Bykovskyi A, Johnson R, Walljasper L, Block L, Werner N. Underreporting of gender and race/ethnicity differences in NIH-funded dementia caregiver support interventions. Am J Alzheimers Dis Other Demen 2018;33(3):145-52.
468. Fredriksen-Goldsen KI, Jen S, Bryan AEB, Goldsen J. Cognitive impairment, Alzheimer's disease, and other dementias in the lives of lesbian, gay, bisexual and transgender (LGBT) older adults and their caregivers: Needs and competencies. J Appl Gerontol 2018;37(5):545-69.
469. U.S. Department of Health and Human Services. National Research Summit on Care, Services and Supports for Persons with Dementia and their Caregivers. Available at: https://aspe.hhs.gov/national-research-summit-care-services-and-supports-persons-dementia-and-their-caregivers. Accessed December 4, 2019.
470. Khatutsky G, Wiener J, Anderson W, Akhmerova V, Jessup EA, Squillace MR. Understanding direct care workers: A snapshot of two of America's most important jobs: Certified nursing assistants and home health aides. Washington, D.C.: U.S. Department of Health and Human Services; 2011.
471. Stone R. The Long-Term Care Workforce: From Accidental to Valued Profession. In: Wolf D, Folbre N, eds. Universal Coverage of Long-Term Care in the United States: Can We Get There from Here? New York, NY: Russell Sage Foundation; 2012: 155-78.
472. Jones AL, Dwyer LL, Bercovitz AR, Strahan GW. The National Nursing Home Survey: 2004 Overview. Vital Health Stat 13 2009;(167):1-155.
473. Kramer NA, Smith MC. Training nursing assistants to care for nursing home residents with dementia. In: Molinari V, editor. Professional psychology in long-term care. New York, N.Y.: Hatherleigh Press; 2000: p. 227-56.
474. McCabe MP, Davison TE, George K. Effectiveness of staff training programs for behavioral problems among older people with dementia. Aging Ment Health 2007;11(5):505-19.
475. Beck C, Ortigara A, Mercer S, Shue V. Enabling and empowering certified nursing assistants for quality dementia care. Int J Geriatr Psychiatry 1999;14(3):197-211.
476. Institute of Medicine. Retooling for an Aging America: Building the Health Care Workforce. Washington, D.C.: The National Academies Press 2008. Available at: http://www.nationalacademies.org/hmd/reports/2008/retooling-for-an-aging-america-building-the-health-care-workforce.aspx. Accessed December 4, 2019.
477. Warshaw GA, Bragg EJ. Preparing the health care workforce to care for adults with Alzheimer's disease and related dementias. Health Aff 2014;33(4):633-41.
478. American Health Care Association. (2011). Staffing Survey Report.
479. Stone RI. Factors affecting the future of family caregiving in the United States. In: JE Gaugler, RL Kane, eds. Family Caregiving in the New Normal. San Diego, CA: Elsevier, Inc; 2015: p. 57-77.
480. Elvish R, Burrow S, Cawley R, Harney K, Pilling M, Gregory J, et al. 'Getting to know me': The second phase roll-out of a staff training programme for supporting people with dementia in general hospitals. Dementia (London) 2016;pii:1471301216634926 [epub ahead of print].
481. Spector A, Orrell M, Goyder J. A systematic review of staff training interventions to reduce the behavioural and psychological symptoms of dementia. Ageing Res Rev 2013;12(1):354-64.
482. Bray J, Evans S, Bruce M, Carter C, Brooker D, Milosevic S, et al. Enabling hospital staff to care for people with dementia. Nurs Older People 2015;27(10):29-32.
483. Palmer JL, Lach HW, McGillick J, Murphy-White M, Carroll MB, Armstrong JL. The Dementia Friendly Hospital Initiative education program for acute care nurses and staff. J Contin Educ Nurs 2014;45(9):416-24.
484. Surr CA, Smith SJ, Crossland J, Robins J. Impact of a person-centred dementia care training programme on hospital staff attitudes, role efficacy and perceptions of caring for people with dementia: A repeated measures study. Int J Nurs Stud 2016;53:144-51.
485. Eldercare Workforce Alliance. Geriatrics Workforce Shortage: A Looming Crisis for our Families. Washington, D.C.: Eldercare Workforce Alliance; 2012.
486. The American Geriatrics Society. Current Geriatrician Shortfall. Available at: https://www.americangeriatrics.org/sites/default/files/inline-files/Current-Geriatrician-Shortfall_0.pdf. Accessed December 4, 2019.
487. The American Geriatrics Society. Projected Future Need for Geriatricians. Available at: https://www.americangeriatrics.org/sites/default/files/inline-files/Projected-Future-Need-for-Geriatricians.pdf. Accessed December 4, 2019.
488. American Association of Nurse Practitioners. NP Fact Sheet. Available at: https://www.aanp.org/all-about-nps/np-fact-sheet. Accessed December 4, 2019.
489. Hoffman D, Zucker H. A call to preventive action by health care providers and policy makers to support caregivers. Prev Chronic Dis 2016;13:E96.
490. Adelman RD, Tmanova LL, Delgado D, Dion S, Lachs MS. Caregiver burden: A clinical review. JAMA 2014;311(10):1052-60.
491. Riedel O, Klotsche J, Wittchen HU. Overlooking informal dementia caregivers' burden. Res Gerontol Nurs 2016;9(4):167-74.
492. Alzheimer's Association National Plan Care and Support Milestone Workgroup, Borson S, Boustani MA, Buckwalter KC, Burgio LD, Chodosh J, et al. Report on milestones for care and support under the U.S. National Plan to Address Alzheimer's Disease. Alzheimer's & Dementia 2016;12(3):334-69.
493. Cross AJ, Garip G, Sheffield D. The psychosocial impact of caregiving in dementia and quality of life: A systematic review and meta-synthesis of qualitative research. Psychol Health 2018;27:1-22.
494. Gaugler JE, Westra BL, Kane RL. Professional discipline and support recommendations for family caregivers of persons with dementia. Int Psychogeriatr 2016;28(6):1029-40.
495. Austrom MG, Carvell CA, Alder CA, Gao S, Boustani M, LaMantia M. Workforce development to provide person-centered care. Aging Ment Health 2016;20(8):781-92.
496. Werner P. Reflections on quality of care for persons with dementia: moving toward an integrated, comprehensive approach. Int Psychogeriatr. 2019 Mar;31(3):307-8.
497. Leggett A, Connell C, Dubin L, Dunkle R, Langa KM, Maust DT, et al. Dementia care across a tertiary care health system: What exists now and what needs to change. J Am Med Dir Assoc 2019;20(10):1307-12.e1.

498. Noel MA, Kaluzynski TS, Templeton VH. Quality dementia care. J Appl Gerontol 2017;36(2):195-212.
499. Bott NT, Sheckter CC, Yang D, Peters S, Brady B, Plowman S, et al. Systems Delivery Innovation for Alzheimer Disease. Am J Geriatr Psychiatry 2019;27(2):149-61.
500. Tan ZS, Jennings L, Reuben D. Coordinated care management for dementia in a large academic health system. Health Aff 2014;33(4):619-25.
501. Callahan CM, Sachs GA, Lamantia MA, Unroe KT, Arling G, Boustani MA. Redesigning systems of care for older adults with Alzheimer's disease. Health Aff 2014;33(4):626-32.
502. French DD, LaMantia MA, Livin LR, Herceg D, Alder CA, Boustani MA. Healthy Aging Brain Center improved care coordination and produced net savings. Health Aff 2014;33(4):613-8.
503. Borson S, Chodosh J. Developing dementia-capable health care systems: A 12-step program. Clin Geriatr Med 2014;30(3):395-420.
504. Reuben DB, Evertson LC, Wenger NS, Serrano K, Chodosh J, Ercoli L, et al. The University of California at Los Angeles Alzheimer's and Dementia Care Program for comprehensive, coordinated, patient-centered care: Preliminary data. J Am Geriatr Soc 2013;61(12):2214-8.
505. Thyrian JR, Hertel J, Wucherer D, Eichler T, Michalowsky B, Dreier-Wolfgramm A. Effectiveness and safety of dementia care management in primary care: A randomized clinical trial. JAMA Psychiatry 2017;74(10):996-1004.
506. Callahan CM. Alzheimer's Disease: Individuals, dyads, communities, and costs. J Am Geriatr Soc 2017;65(5):892-5.
507. Dreier-Wolfgramm A, Michalowsky B, Austrom MG, van der Marck MA, Iliffe S, Alder C. Dementia care management in primary care: Current collaborative care models and the case for interprofessional education. Z Gerontol Geriatr 2017;50(Suppl 2):68-77.
508. Reuben DB, Tan ZS, Romero T, Wenger NS, Keeler E, Jennings LA. Patient and caregiver benefit from a comprehensive dementia care program: 1-year results from the UCLA Alzheimer's and Dementia Care Program. J Am Geriatr Soc 2019;67:2267-73.
509. Boustani M, Alder CA, Solid CA, Reuben D. An alternative payment model to support widespread use of collaborative dementia care models. Health Aff (Millwood) 2019;38(1):54-9.
510. Clevenger CK, Cellar J, Kovaleva M, Medders L, Hepburn K. Integrated memory care clinic: Design, implementation, and initial results. J Am Geriatr Soc 2018;66(12):2401-7.
511. Odenheimer G, Borson S, Sanders AE, Swain-Eng RJ, Kyomen HH, Tierney S, et al. Quality improvement in neurology: Dementia management quality measures (executive summary). Am J Occup Ther 2013;67(6):704-10.
512. LaMantia MA, Alder CA, Callahan CM, Gao S, French DD, Austrom MG, et al. The Aging Brain Care Medical Home: Preliminary data. J Am Geriatr Soc 2015;63(6):1209-13.
513. Gaugler JE, Kane RL, eds. Family Caregiving in the New Normal. Philadelphia, Pa.: Elsevier, Inc.; 2015.
514. Alzheimer's Association. Alzheimer's Impact Movement: Use of Medicare Planning Benefit. Available at: https://alzimpact.org/media/serve/id/5d2c9620e4f5d. Accessed September 27, 2019.
515. The Lewin Group. Process Evaluation of the Older Americans Act Title IIIE-National Family Caregiver Support Program: Final Report, 2016. Available at: https://acl.gov/sites/default/files/programs/2017-02/NFCSP_Final_Report-update.pdf. Accessed December 4, 2019.
516. Alzheimer's Association. Alzheimer's Association Dementia Care Practice Recommendations. Available at: https://www.alz.org/media/Documents/alzheimers-dementia-care-practice-recommendations.pdf. Accessed November 5, 2019.
517. Camp CJ. Denial of human rights: We must change the paradigm of dementia care. Clin Gerontol 2019;42(3):221-3.
518. Gaugler JE, Bain LJ, Mitchell L, Finlay J, Fazio S, Jutkowitz E, et al. Reconsidering frameworks of Alzheimer's dementia when assessing psychosocial outcomes. Alzheimers Dement (NY) 2019;5:388-97.
519. Burton A, Ogden M, Cooper C. Planning and enabling meaningful patient and public involvement in dementia research. Curr Opin Psychiatry 2019;32(6):557-62.
520. Hurd MD, Martorell P, Delavande A, Mullen KJ, Langa KM. Monetary costs of dementia in the United States. N Engl J Med 2013;368:1326-34.
521. Yang Z, Zhang K, Lin PJ, Clevenger C, Atherly A. A longitudinal analysis of the lifetime cost of dementia. Health Serv Res 2012;47(4):1660-78.
522. Murman DL, Chen Q, Powell MC, Kuo SB, Bradley CJ, Colenda CC. The incremental direct costs associated with behavioral symptoms in AD. Neurology 2002;59:1721-9.
523. Fishman P, Coe NB, White L, Crane PK, Park S, Ingraham B, et al. Cost of dementia in Medicare Managed Care: A systematic literature review. Am J Manag Care 2019;25:e247-53.
524. Yang Z, Levey A. Gender differences: A lifetime analysis of the economic burden of Alzheimer's disease. Women Health Iss 2015;25(5):436-40.
525. Hudomiet P, Hurd MD, Rohwedder S. The relationship between lifetime out-of-pocket medical expenditures, dementia and socioeconomic status in the U.S. J Econ Ageing 2019;14:100181.
526. Dwibedi N, Findley AP, Wiener C, Shen C, Sambamoorthi U. Alzheimer disease and related disorders and out-of-pocket health care spending and burden among elderly Medicare beneficiaries. Medical Care 2018;56:240-6.
527. White L, Fishman P, Basu A, Crane PK, Larson EB, Coe NB. Medicare expenditures attributable to dementia. Health Services Res 2019;54(4):773-81.
528. Kelley AS, McGarry K, Gorges R, Skinner JS. The burden of health care costs for patients with dementia in the last 5 years of life. Ann Intern Med 2015;163:729-36.
529. Bynum JPW, Meara E, Chang C-H, Rhoads JM. Our Parents, Ourselves: Health Care for an Aging Population. A Report of the Dartmouth Atlas Project. The Dartmouth Institute for Health Policy & Clinical Practice; 2016.
530. Rudolph JL, Zanin NM, Jones RN, Marcantonio ER, Fong TG, Yang FM, et al. Hospitalization in community-dwelling persons with Alzheimer's disease: Frequency and causes. J Am Geriatr Soc 2010;58(8):1542-8.
531. Beydoun MA, Beydoun HA, Gamaldo AA, Rostant O, Dore GA, Zonderman AB, et al. Nationwide inpatient prevalence, predictors and outcomes of Alzheimer's disease among older adults in the United States, 2002-2012. J Alzheimers Dis 2015;48(2):361-75.
532. U.S. Centers for Medicare & Medicaid Services. State Level Chronic Conditions Table: Prevalence, Medicare Utilization and Spending, 2007-2017. Available at: https://www.cms.gov/Research-Statistics-Data-and-Systems/Statistics-Trends-and-Reports/Chronic-Conditions/CC_Main.html. Accessed September 13, 2019.
533. Landon BE, Keating NL, Onnela JP, Zaslavsky AM, Christakis NA, O'Malley AJ. Patient-sharing networks of physicians and health care utilization and spending among Medicare beneficiaries. JAMA Intern Med 2018;178:66-73.
534. Medicare. Glossary. Medicare: The Official U.S. Government Site for Medicare. Available at: https://www.medicare.gov/glossary/a. Accessed December 4, 2019.
535. Reschovsky JD, Hadley J, O'Malley J, Landon BE. Geographic variations in the cost of treating condition-specific episodes of care among Medicare patients. Health Services Res 2014;49(Part 1):32-51.
536. Leibson CL, Hall Lon K, Ransom JE, Roberts RO, Hass SL, Duhig AM, et al. Direct medical costs and source of cost differences across the spectrum of cognitive decline: A population-based study. Alzheimers Dement 2015;11(8):917-32.
537. Suehs BT, Davis CD, Alvir J, van Amerongen D, Patel NC, Joshi AV, et al. The clinical and economic burden of newly diagnosed Alzheimer's disease in a Medicare Advantage population. Am J Alzheimers Dis Other Dement 2013;28(4):384-92.

538. Lin P-J, Zhong Y, Fillit HM, Chen E, Neumann PJ. Medicare expenditures of individuals with Alzheimer's disease and related dementias or mild cognitive impairment before and after diagnosis. J Am Geriatr Soc 2016;64:1549-57.
539. Geldmacher DS, Kirson NY, Birnbaum HG, Eapen S, Kantor E, Cummings AK, et al. Pre-diagnosis excess acute care costs in Alzheimer's patients among a U.S. Medicaid population. Appl Health Econ Health Policy 2013;11(4):407-13.
540. Zhu CW, Cosentino S, Ornstein K, Gu Y, Scarmeas N, Andrews H, et al. Medicare utilization and expenditures around incident dementia in a multiethnic cohort. J Gerontol A Biol Sci Med Sci 2015;70(11):1448-53.
541. Kirson NY, Desai U, Ristovska L, Cummings AKG, Birnbaum HG, Ye W, et al. Assessing the economic burden of Alzheimer's disease patients first diagnosed by specialists. BMC Geriatrics 2016;16:138.
542. Aigbogun MS, Stellhorn R, Hartry A, Baker RA, Fillit H. Treatment patterns and burden of behavioral disturbances in patients with dementia in the United States: A claims database analysis. BMC Neurology 2019;19:33.
543. Harris-Kojetin L, Sengupta M, Lendon JP, Rome V, Valverde R, Caffrey C. Long-term care providers and services users in the United States, 2015-2016. Vital Health Stat 2019;3(43).
544. Rome V, Harris-Kojetin, Park-Lee E. Variation in operating characteristics of adult day services centers by center ownership: United States, 2014. NCHS Data Brief, No. 224. December 2015.
545. Caffrey C, Harris-Kojetin L, Rome V, Sengupta M. Variation in operating characteristics of residential care communities by size of community: United States, 2014. NCHS Data Brief, No. 222. November 2015.
546. U.S. Centers for Medicare & Medicaid Services. Nursing Home Data Compendium 2015 Edition. Available at: https://www.cms.gov/Medicare/Provider-Enrollment-and-Certification/CertificationandComplianc/Downloads/nursinghomedatacompendium_508-2015.pdf. Accessed December 4, 2019.
547. Teno JM, Gozalo PL, Bynum JP, Leland NE, Miller SC, Morden NE, et al. Change in end-of-life care for Medicare beneficiaries: Site of death, place of care, and health care transitions in 2000, 2005, and 2009. JAMA 2013;309(5):470-7.
548. Eiken S, Sredl K, Burwell B, Amos A. Medicaid Expenditures for Long-Term Services and Supports in FY 2016. IAP Medicaid Innovation Accelerator Program. IBM Watson. May 2018. Available at: https://www.medicaid.gov/sites/default/files/2019-12/ltssexpenditures2016.pdf. Accessed February 3, 2020.
549. Bynum J. Characteristics, Costs, and Health Service Use for Medicare Beneficiaries with a Dementia Diagnosis: Report 1: Medicare Current Beneficiary Survey. Unpublished; provided under contract with the Alzheimer's Association. Lebanon, N.H.: Dartmouth Institute for Health Policy and Clinical Care, Center for Health Policy Research, January 2009.
550. Clarkson P, Davies L, Jasper R, Loynes N, Challis D. Home Support in Dementia (HoSt-D) Programme Management Group. A systematic review of the economic evidence for home support interventions in dementia. Value in Health 2017;20:1198-209.
551. Nickel F, Barth J, Kolominsky-Rabas PL. Health economic evaluations of non-pharmacological interventions for persons with dementia and their informal caregivers: A systematic review. BMC Geriatrics 2018;18:69.
552. Callahan CM, Arling G, Tu W, Rosenman MB, Counsell SR, Stump TE, et al. Transitions in care among older adults with and without dementia. J Am Geriatr Soc 2012;60(5):813-20.
553. Gozalo P, Teno JM, Mitchell SL, Skinner J, Bynum J, Tyler D, et al. End-of-life transitions among nursing home residents with cognitive issues. N Engl J Med 2011;365(13):1212-21.
554. Teno JM, Mitchell SL, Skinner J, Kuo S, Fisher E, Intrator O, et al. Churning: The association between health care transitions and feeding tube insertion for nursing home residents with advanced cognitive impairment. J Palliat Med 2009;12(4):359-62.
555. Genworth. Genworth Cost of Care Survey 2019, Summary and Methodology. https://pro.genworth.com/riiproweb/productinfo/pdf/131168.pdf. Accessed November 3, 2019.
556. Jacobson G, Griffin S, Neuman T, Smith K. Income and Assets of Medicare Beneficiaries, 2016-2035. The Henry J. Kaiser Family Foundation Issue Brief. April 2017.
557. U.S. Department of Health and Human Services. What is Long-Term Care Insurance? Available at: http://longtermcare.gov/costs-how-to-pay/what-is-long-term-care-insurance/. Accessed December 4, 2019.
558. U.S. Centers for Medicare & Medicaid Services. Your Medicare Coverage. Long-Term Care. Available at: https://www.medicare.gov/coverage/long-term-care.html. Accessed December 4, 2019.
559. National Association of Insurance Commissioners and the Center for Insurance Policy and Research. The State of Long-Term Care Insurance: The Market, Challenges and Future Innovations. CIPR Study Series 2016-1. May 2016.
560. Reaves EL, Musumeci M. Medicaid and Long-Term Services and Supports: A Primer. Menlo Park, Calif.: Kaiser Commission on Medicaid and the Uninsured, Henry J. Kaiser Family Foundation; December 2015. Publication #8617-02.
561. House Bill 1087, 66th Legislature, 2019 Regular Session. Long-Term Services and Supports Trust Program. Available at: http://lawfilesext.leg.wa.gov/biennium/2019-20/Pdf/Bills/Session%20Laws/House/1087-S2.SL.pdf#page=1. Accessed December 4, 2019.
562. De Vleminck A, Morrison RS, Meier DE, Aldridge MD. Hospice care for patients with dementia in the United States: A longitudinal cohort study. J Am Med Dir Assoc 2018;19:633-8.
563. Gozalo P, Plotzke M, Mor V, Miller SC, Teno JM. Changes in Medicare costs with the growth of hospice care in nursing homes. N Engl J Med 2015;372:1823-31.
564. U.S. Centers for Medicare & Medicaid Services. Post-Acute Care and Hospice Provider Data 2017. Available at: https://www.cms.gov/Research-Statistics-Data-and-Systems/Statistics-Trends-and-Reports/Medicare-Provider-Charge-Data/PAC2017. Accessed December 3, 2019.
565. Harris-Kojetin L, Sengupta M, Park-Lee E, Valverde R, Caffrey C, Rome V, et al. Long-term care providers and services users in the United States: Data from the National Study of Long-Term Care Providers, 2013-2014. National Center for Health Statistics. Vital Health Stat 3 2016;(38):x-xii;1-105.
566. U.S. Centers for Medicare & Medicaid Services. Medicare Program; FY 2020 Hospice Wage Index and Payment Rate Update and Hospice Quality Reporting Requirements. Available at https://www.federalregister.gov/documents/2019/08/06/2019-16583/medicare-program-fy-2020-hospice-wage-index-and-payment-rate-update-and-hospice-quality-reporting. Accessed February 4, 2020.
567. Taylor DH, Jr., Bhavsar NA, Bull JH, Kassner CT, Olson A, Boucher NA. Will changes in Medicare payment rates alter hospice's cost-saving ability? J Palliat Med 2018;21:645-51.
568. Miller SC, Lima JC, Looze J, Mitchell SL. Dying in U.S. nursing homes with advanced dementia: How does health care use differ for residents with, versus without, end-of-life Medicare skilled nursing facility care? J Palliat Med 2012;15:43-50.
569. Miller SC, Gozalo P, Mor V. Hospice enrollment and hospitalization of dying nursing home patients. Am J Med 2001;11(1):38-44.
570. Kiely DK, Givens JL, Shaffer ML, Teno JM, Mitchell SL. Hospice use and outcomes in nursing home residents with advanced dementia. J Am Geriatr Soc 2010;58(12):2284-91.
571. Miller SC, Mor V, Wu N, Gozalo P, Lapane K. Does receipt of hospice care in nursing homes improve management of pain at the end of life? J Am Geriatr Soc 2002;50(3):507-15.

572. Shega JW, Hougham GW, Stocking CB, Cox-Hayley D, Sachs GA. Patients dying with dementia: Experience at the end of life and impact of hospice care. J Pain Symptom Manage 2008;35(5):499-507.
573. Teno JM, Meltzer DO, Mitchell SL, Fulton AT, Gozalo P, Mor V. Type of attending physician influenced feeding tube insertions for hospitalized elderly people with severe dementia. Health Aff 2014;33(4):675-82.
574. Mitchell SL, Mor V, Gozalo PL, Servadio JL, Teno JM. Tube feeding in U.S. nursing home residents with advanced dementia, 2000-2014. JAMA 2016;316(7):769-70.
575. Centers for Disease Control and Prevention, National Center for Health Statistics. Underlying Cause of Death 1999-2017 on CDC WONDER Online Database, released December, 2018. Data are from the Multiple Cause of Death Files, 1999-2017, as compiled from data provided by the 57 vital statistics jurisdictions through the Vital Statistics Cooperative Program. Available at: http://wonder.cdc.gov/ucd-icd10.html. Accessed October 14, 2019.
576. Gilligan AM, Malone DC, Warholak TL, Armstrong EP. Health disparities in cost of care in patients with Alzheimer's disease: An analysis across 4 state Medicaid populations. Am J Alzheimers Dis Other Dement 2013;28(1):84-92.
577. Lin P-J, Zhong Y, Fillit HM, Cohen JT, Neumann PJ. Hospitalizations for ambulatory care sensitive conditions and unplanned readmissions among Medicare beneficiaries with Alzheimer's disease. Alzheimers Dement 2017;13(10):1174-8.
578. Healthy People 2020. Dementias, Including Alzheimer's Disease. Available at: www.healthypeople.gov/2020/topics-objectives/topic/dementias-including-alzheimers-disease/national-snapshot. Accessed December 24, 2019.
579. Davydow DS, Zibin K, Katon WJ, Pontone GM, Chwastiak L, Langa KM, et al. Neuropsychiatric disorders and potentially preventable hospitalizations in a prospective cohort study of older Americans. J Gen Intern Med 2014;29(10):1362-71.
580. Guterman EL, Allen IE, Josephson SA, Merrilees JJ, Dulaney S, Chiong W, et al. Association between caregiver depression and emergency department use among patients with dementia. JAMA Neurol 2019;76:1166-73.
581. Patel A, Parikh R, Howell EH, Hsich E, Landers SH, Gorodeski EZ. Mini-Cog performance: Novel marker of post discharge risk among patients hospitalized for heart failure. Circ Heart Fail 2015;8(1):8-16.
582. Lin PJ, Fillit HM, Cohen JT, Neumann PJ. Potentially avoidable hospitalizations among Medicare beneficiaries with Alzheimer's disease and related disorders. Alzheimers Dement 2013;9(1):30-8.
583. MacNeil-Vroomen JL, Nagurney JM, Allore HG. Comorbid conditions and emergency department treat and release utilization in multimorbid persons with cognitive impairment. Am J Emerg Med 2020;38:127-31.
584. Feng Z, Coots LA, Kaganova Y, Wiener JM. Hospital and ED use among Medicare beneficiaries with dementia varies by setting and proximity to death. Health Aff 2014;33(4):683-90.
585. Jennings LA, Laffan AM, Schlissel AC, Colligan E, Tan Z, Wenger NS, et al. Health care utilization and cost outcomes of a comprehensive dementia care program for Medicare beneficiaries. JAMA Int Med 2019;179:161-6.
586. Godard-Sebillotte C, Le Berre M, Schuster T, Trottier M, Vedel I. Impact of health service interventions on acute hospital use in community-dwelling persons with dementia: A systematic literature review and meta-analysis. PLoS ONE 2019;14(6):e0218426.
587. Amjad H, Carmichael D, Austin AM, Chang C-H, Bynum JPW. Continuity of care and health care utilization in older adults. JAMA Intern Med 2016;176(9):1371-8.
588. Alzheimer's Association. Changing the Trajectory of Alzheimer's Disease: How a Treatment by 2025 Saves Lives and Dollars. Available at: https://www.alz.org/help-support/resources/publications/trajectory_report. Accessed December 4, 2019.
589. Zissimopoulos J, Crimmins E, St. Clair P. The value of delaying Alzheimer's disease onset. Forum Health Econ Policy. 2014;18(1):25-39.
590. Alzheimer's Association. 2018 Alzheimer's Disease Facts and Figures. Alzheimers Dement 2018;14(3):408-11.
591. Liu JL, Hlávka JP, Hillestad R, Mattke S. Assessing the preparedness of the U.S. health care system infrastructure for an Alzheimer's treatment. The RAND Corporation: Santa Monica, CA. (2017) Available at: https://www.rand.org/pubs/research_reports/RR2272.html. Accessed December 4, 2019.
592. Hebert LE, Scherr PA, Bienias JL, Bennett DA, Evans DA. Alzheimer's disease in the U.S. population: Prevalence estimates using the 2000 Census. Arch Neurol 2003;60:1119-22.
593. Brookmeyer R, Gray S, Kawas C. Projections of Alzheimer's disease in the United States and the public health impact of delaying disease onset. Am J Public Health 1998;88:1337-42.
594. National Alliance for Caregiving and AARP, Caregiving in the U.S., November 2009. Available at: https://www.caregiving.org/pdf/research/FINALRegularExSum50plus.pdf, Accessed December 22, 2019.
595. Amo PS, Levine C, Memmott MM. The economic value of informal caregiving. Health Aff 1999;18:182-8.
596. U.S. Department of Labor, Bureau of Labor Statistics. Employment, Hours, and Earnings from the Current Employment Statistics Survey. Series 10-CEU 6562160008, Home Health Care Services (NAICS code 6216), Average Hourly Earnings, July 2018. Available at: www.bls.gov/ces/data.htm. Accessed December 24, 2019.
597. Drabo EF, Barthold D, Joyce G, Ferido P, Chui HC, Zissimopoulos J. Longitudinal analysis of dementia diagnosis and specialty care among racially diverse Medicare beneficiaries. Alzheimers Dement 2019;15:1402-11.
598. U.S. Department of Health and Human Services, Health Resources and Services Administration, National Center for Health Workforce Analysis. National and Regional Projections of Supply and Demand for Geriatricians: 2013-2025. Available at: https://bhw.hrsa.gov/sites/default/files/bhw/health-workforce-analysis/research/projections/GeriatricsReport51817.pdf. Accessed February 4, 2020.
599. Petriceks AH, Olivas JC, Srivastava S. Trends in geriatrics graduate medical education programs and positions, 2001 to 2018. Gerontol Geriatr Med 2018;4:1-4.
600. Dall TM, Storm MV, Chakrabarti R, Drogan O, Keran CM, Donofri PD, et al. Supply and demand analysis of the current and future U.S. neurology workforce. Neurology 2013; 81:470-78.
601. Duffrin C, Diaz S, Cashion M, Watson R, Cummings D, Jackson N. Factors associated with placement of rural primary care physicians in North Carolina. South Med J 2014;107(11):728-33.
602. Scheckel CJ, Richards J, Newman JR, Kunz M, Fangman B, Mi L, et al. Role of debt and loan forgiveness/repayment programs in osteopathic medical graduates' plans to enter primary care. J Am Osteopath Assoc 2019;119(4):227-35.
603. Auerback DI, Buerhaus PI, Staiger DO. Registered nurse supply grows faster than projected amid surge in new entrants ages 23-26. Health Aff 2011;30(12):2286-92.
604. Meyers D, Fryer GE, Krol D, Phillips RL, Green LA, Dovey SM. Title VII funding is associated with more family physicians and more physicians serving the underserved. Am Fam Physician 2002;66(4):554.
605. Center for Medicare & Medicaid Services. Center for Medicare & Medicaid Innovation. The Graduate Nurse Education Demonstration Project: Final Evaluation Report. August 2019. Prepared by IMPAQ International, Columbia, Md. Available at https://innovation.cms.gov/Files/reports/gne-final-eval-rpt.pdf. Accessed February 7, 2020.
606. Arora S, Thornton K, Murata G, Deming P, Kalishman S, Dion D, et al. Outcomes of treatment for hepatitis C virus infection by primary care providers. NEJM. 2011; 364(23):2199-207.

607. Paul M, Saad AD, Billings J, Blecker S, Bouchonville MF, Berry C. Endo ECHO improves patient-reported measures of access to care, health care quality, self-care behaviors, and overall quality of life for patients with complex diabetes in medically underserved areas of New Mexico. J Endocr Soc April 15 2019;3(suppl 1):MON-190.
608. Possin KL, Merrilees JJ, Dulaney S, Bonasera SJ, Chiong W, Lee K, et al. Effect of collaborative dementia care via telephone and internet on quality of life, caregiver well-being, and health care use. JAMA Intern Med 2019;179(12):1658-67.

The Alzheimer's Association acknowledges the contributions of Joseph Gaugler, Ph.D., Bryan James, Ph.D., Tricia Johnson, Ph.D., Allison Marin, Ph.D., and Jennifer Weuve, M.P.H., Sc.D., in the preparation of *2020 Alzheimer's Disease Facts and Figures*.

The Alzheimer's Association leads the way to end Alzheimer's and all other dementia — by accelerating global research, driving risk reduction and early detection, and maximizing quality care and support.

Our vision is a world without Alzheimer's and all other dementia.®

Alzheimer's Association
225 N. Michigan Ave., Fl. 17
Chicago, IL 60601-7633

Alzheimer's Association
Public Policy Office
1212 New York Ave., N.W., Suite 800
Washington, DC 20005-6105

800.272.3900
alz.org®



alzheimer's association®

CDC Centers for Disease Control and Prevention

National Center for Health Statistics

# Alzheimer's Disease Mortality by State

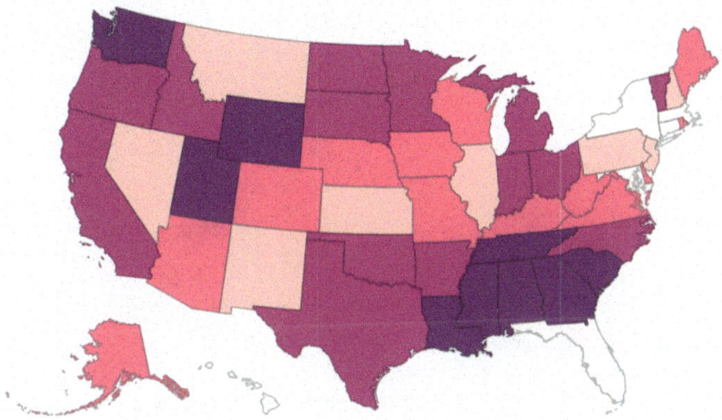

Age-Adjusted Death Rates[1]

United States: 30.5

- 13.9 — < 20.4
- 20.4 — < 26.9
- 26.9 — < 33.4
- 33.4 — < 39.9
- 39.9 — 46.5

**Filters**

Year 2018 ▼

SHARE Privacy Policy

<div data-cdc-widget="cdcMaps" dat

Data Table

| STATE | Death Rate (Click for Rankings) | Deaths (Click for Rankings) |
|---|---|---|
| New York | 13.9 | 3,755 |
| Maryland | 15.8 | 1,122 |
| Connecticut | 18.5 | 986 |
| Florida | 19.2 | 6,725 |
| Massachusetts | 19.5 | 1,823 |
| Hawaii | 20.2 | 480 |
| Pennsylvania | 20.7 | 4,064 |
| Montana | 21.7 | 310 |
| New Mexico | 22.4 | 583 |
| New Jersey | 22.7 | 2,710 |
| Kansas | 23.6 | 899 |
| Nevada | 23.6 | 704 |
| Illinois | 25.3 | 4,030 |
| New Hampshire | 26.4 | 487 |
| Virginia | 27.1 | 2,592 |
| Nebraska | 27.4 | 683 |
| Alaska | 27.5 | 131 |
| Maine | 28.4 | 580 |
| Rhode Island | 29.2 | 470 |
| Colorado | 29.6 | 1,649 |
| West Virginia | 31 | 791 |
| Iowa | 31.7 | 1,439 |
| Wisconsin | 31.7 | 2,453 |
| Kentucky | 32.5 | 1,674 |

| | | |
|---|---|---|
| Delaware | 32.7 | 412 |
| Missouri | 32.9 | 2,641 |
| Arizona | 33 | 3,012 |
| Indiana | 33.4 | 2,668 |
| Minnesota | 33.7 | 2,436 |
| North Dakota | 33.8 | 356 |
| Michigan | 34.3 | 4,474 |
| Ohio | 34.9 | 5,391 |
| Idaho | 35 | 666 |
| Oregon | 35.6 | 1,868 |
| South Dakota | 36.3 | 437 |
| California | 37.1 | 16,627 |
| Vermont | 37.7 | 333 |
| North Carolina | 37.9 | 4,495 |
| Oklahoma | 37.9 | 1,739 |
| Texas | 38.4 | 9,763 |
| Arkansas | 38.9 | 1,457 |
| Wyoming | 41.5 | 277 |
| Utah | 42.1 | 1,024 |
| Louisiana | 42.2 | 2,166 |
| South Carolina | 44.3 | 2,616 |
| Alabama | 44.9 | 2,616 |
| Tennessee | 45 | 3,488 |
| Washington | 45.2 | 3,752 |
| Mississippi | 46 | 1,547 |
| Georgia | 46.5 | 4,513 |

DOWNLOAD DATA (CSV)

[1] The number of deaths per 100,000 total population.

Source: https://wonder.cdc.gov

States are categorized from highest rate to lowest rate. Although adjusted for differences in age-distribution and population size, rankings by state do not take into account other state specific population characteristics that may affect the level of mortality. When the number of deaths is small, rankings by state may be unreliable due to instability in death rates.

Page last reviewed: April 29, 2020

# AGING

*The elderly population in the United States is growing faster than any other segment of the population, and has done so since 1900. It is estimated that this trend will continue at least through the year 2050. Although aging leads to a natural diminishment of a person's cognitive abilities, it also puts people at greater risk for dementia, with most forms of dementia-causing diseases typically affecting people 60 and older.*

Over the past decades, the number of retirement-age Americans (65+) has risen steadily and the rates are expected to increase even more in the coming decades. In 2020, 16.3 percent of the population was over 65 and by 2040 this number is expected to jump to over 20 percent. Because of the general expected increase in the population, the number of Americans over 65 is expected to jump from 54 million in 2020 to 80 million in 2040 and the number of people 85 and over to more than double from 7 to 15 million, as a result of the aging of the baby boomer generation. Predictions are that this will put a strain on the social safety net and medical resources as these elderly citizens require increased medical treatment and rely on public benefits.

Aging is not a disease, but part of the normal life cycle, and many seniors retain good health and live independently for long past the traditional age of retirement. In time, however, most will develop one or more chronic conditions; for those over 75 years of age, the most common conditions are hypertension, heart disease, hearing loss, arthritis, and cataracts. People also experience memory loss and decreased powers of cognition as they age. Although this is a normal development of aging, as people get older they also become at greater risk for mild cognitive impairment and dementia, both of which represent a range of pathologies greater than simply the normal brain deterioration that comes with aging. For example, Alzheimer's disease, the most frequent cause of dementia, becomes increasingly common the older a person gets. The disease is rare among people under 60, but people between the ages of 65 and 74 develop Alzheimer's symptoms at a rate of two new diagnoses per 1,000 people. This jumps to 11 per 1,000 for those aged 65-84, and 36 per 1,000 among those aged 85 and older.

By the year 2030, 150 million Americans are expected to have a chronic condition, and 42 million will be limited in their ability to work or live independently. Psychological and social components of well-being are also integral components of healthy aging. Approximately 15 percent of women 65 and older and 10 percent of men 65 and older have clinically relevant symptoms of depression. Additionally, older adults are at risk for social isolation. Treating this population will require many medical and nonmedical services, integrated to provide a comprehensive continuum of care.

## National Agencies & Associations

2 **AARP**
601 E Street NW
Washington, DC 20049
202-434-3525
888-687-2277
TTY: 877-434-7598
member@aarp.org
www.aarp.org

Formerly the American Association of Retired Persons. AARP is a collection of diverse individuals and ideas working as one to influence positive change and improve the lives of those 50 and over. AARP reflects a wide range of attitudes, cultures, lifestyles, and beliefs.
*Jo Ann Jenkins, CEO*

3 **ABA Commission on Law and Aging**
1050 Connecticut Avenue
Washington, DC 20003
202-662-8690
Fax: 202-662-8698
aging@americanbar.org
www.americanbar.org/aging

The Commission examines the issues that affect the elderly as victims of abuse, dispute resolution, international rights, medicare, voting, health care decision-making and other issues arising from the aging prisons populations.
*Charles P. Sabatino, JD, Director*
*Erica F. Wood, JD, Assistant Director*

4 **ACL Regional Support Center: Region I**
Administration for Community Living
John F. Kennedy Building
Boston, MA 02203
617-565-1158
Fax: 617-565-4511
www.acl.gov

Region includes CT, MA, ME, NH, RI, VT
*Jennifer Throwe, Regional Administrator*

5 **ACL Regional Support Center: Region II**
Administration for Community Living
26 Federal Plaza
New York, NY 10278
212-264-2976
Fax: 212-264-0114
www.acl.gov

Region includes NY, NJ, PR, VI
*Kathleen Otte, Regional Administrator*

6 **ACL Regional Support Center: Region III**
Administration for Community Living
801 Market Street
Philadelphia, PA 19107
267-831-2329
www.acl.gov
Region includes DC, DE, MD, PA, VA, WV
*Rhonda Schwartz, Regional Administrator*

7 **ACL Regional Support Center: Region IV**
Administration for Community Living
Atlanta Federal Center
Atlanta, GA 30303
404-562-7600
Fax: 404-562-7598
www.acl.gov

Region includes AL, FL, GA, KY, MS, NC, SC, TN
*Costas Miskis, Regional Administrator*

8 **ACL Regional Support Center: Region IX**
Administration for Community Living
90 7th Street
San Francisco, CA 94103
415-437-8780
Fax: 415-437-8782
www.acl.gov

Region includes CA, NV, AZ, HI, GU, CNMI, AS
*Percy Devine, Regional Administrator*

9 **ACL Regional Support Center: Region V**
Administration for Community Living
233 N Michigan Avenue
Chicago, IL 60601
312-938-9858
Fax: 312-886-8533
www.acl.gov

Region includes IL, IN, MI, MN, OH, WI
*Amy Wiatr-Rodriguez, Regional Administrator*

10 **ACL Regional Support Center: Region VI**
Administration for Community Living
1301 Young Street
Dallas, TX 75201
214-767-1865
Fax: 214-767-2951
www.acl.gov

Region includes AR, LA, OK, NM, TX
*Derek Lee, Regional Administrator*

11 **ACL Regional Support Center: Region VII**
Administration for Community Living
601 E 12th Street
Kansas City, MO 64106
816-702-4180
www.acl.gov
Region includes IA, KS, MO, NE
*Lacey Boven, Regional Administrator*

12 **ACL Regional Support Center: Region VIII**
Administration for Community Living
1961 Stout Street
Denver, CO 80294
303-844-2951
Fax: 303-844-2943
www.acl.gov

Region includes CO, MT, UT, WY, ND, SD
*Percy Devine, Regional Administrator*

13 **ACL Regional Support Center: Region X**
Administration for Community Living
701 Th Avenue, M/S RX-33
Seattle, WA 98104
206-615-2299
www.acl.gov
Regions include AK, ID, OR, WA
*Shelly Zylstra, Regional Administrator*

14 **ADAPT**
4513 Tyson Avenue
Philadelphia, PA 19135
215-779-1014
adapt@adapt.org
www.adapt.org

ADAPT is a national grass-roots community that organizes disability rights activists to engage in nonviolent direct action, including civil disobedience, to assure the civil and human rights of people with disabilities to live in freedom.
*Nancy Salandra, Contact*

15 **AMDA - The Society for Post-Acute and Long-Term Care Medicine**
10500 Little Patuxent Parkway
Columbia, MD 21044
410-740-9743
800-876-2632
Fax: 410-740-4572
info@paltc.org

The only medical specialty society representing the community of over 50,000 medical directors, physicians, nurse practitioners, physician assistants, and other practitioners working in the various post-acute and long-term care (PA/LTC) settings.
*Arif Nazir, MD, FACP, CMD, President*
*Karl Steinberg, MD, HMCD, Vice President*

16 **Academy for Gerontology in Higher Education**
1220 L Street NW
Washington, DC 20005
202-289-9806
membership@geron.org
www.aghe.org

Membership organization comprised of more than 130 colleges and universities that offer education and research program in the field of aging. Affiliated with the Gerontological Society of America.
*Judith L. Howe, President*
*Lisa Hollis-Sawyer, Treasurer*

17 **AgingCare**
www.agingcare.com

An online resource for aiding family caregivers. AgingCare.com covers questions on assisted living, long-term and home care, veterans benefits, Alzheimer's disease, financial aid, funeral planning, and more.

18 **Alliance for Aging Research**
1700 K Street NW
Washington, DC 20006
202-293-2856
info@agingresearch.org
www.agingresearch.org

Non-profit organization dedicated to supporting and accelerating the pace of medical discoveries to vastly improve the universal human experience of aging and health.
*Sue Peschin, President & CEO*

19 **Alliance for Retired Americans**
815 16th Street NW
Washington, DC 20006
202-637-5399
retiredamericans.org

National grassroots organization advocates for a progressive political and social agenda that improves the lives of retirees and older Americans.
*Robert Roach, Jr., President*
*Joseph Peters, Jr., Secretary & Treasurer*

20 **American Association for Geriatric Psychiatry**
6728 Old McLean Village Drive 703-556-9222
McLean, VA 22101 Fax: 703-556-8729
main@aagponline.org
www.aagponline.org
Information and resources for physician members and affiliates on improving quality of life for older persons with mental disorders. Provides news, facts, tools and expert information for adults coping with mental health issues and aging.
*Christopher Wood, Executive Director*

21 **American Association of Retired Persons**
601 E Street NW 202-434-3525
Washington, DC 20049 888-687-2277
TTY: 877-434-7598
member@aarp.org
www.aarp.org
AARP is the nation's leading organization for people age 50 and older. It serves their needs and interests through information and education, advocacy and community services provided by a network of local chapters and experienced volunteers.
*Jo Ann Jenkins, Chief Executive Officer*
*Scott Frisch, Executive Vice-President and COO*

22 **American Geriatrics Society**
40 Fulton Street 212-308-1414
New York, NY 10038 Fax: 212-832-8646
info.amger@americangeriatrics.org
www.americangeriatrics.org
The premier professional organization of healthcare providers dedicated to improving the health and well-being of older adults. With an active membership of over 6,000 health care professionals, the AGS has a long history of affecting change in the provision of healthcare in older adults. The AGS Foundation for Health in Aging (FHA) aims to build a bridge between the research and practice of geriatrics health care professionals and the public.
*Nancy E. Lundebjerg, CEO*

23 **American Public Health Association**
800 I Street NW 202-777-2742
Washington, DC 20001 Fax: 202-777-2534
TTY: 202-777-2500
www.apha.org
Public health awareness association.
*Georges C. Benjamin, Executive Director*

24 **American Society for Neurochemistry**
9037 Ron Den Lane 407-909-9064
Windermere, FL 34786 Fax: 407-876-0750
asnmanager@asneurochem.org
asneurochem.org
The Society aims to advance and promote cellular and molecular neuroscience knowledge, and to facilitate communication and the dissemination of information within the field and with related disciplines.
*Sheilah Jewart, Executive Director*
*Karen Gottlieb, Conference Coordinator*

25 **American Society on Aging**
575 Market Street 415-974-9600
San Francisco, CA 94105 800-537-9728
Fax: 415-974-0300
info@asaging.org
www.asaging.org
Health care and social service professionals, educators, researchers, administrators, businesspersons, students, and senior citizens. Works to enhance the well-being of older individuals and to foster unity among those working with and for the elderly. Offers 25 continuing education programs for professionals in aging-related fields. Publishes 'Aging Today,' a bi-monthly newspaper, and 'Generations, a quarterly journal.
*Peter Kaldes, President & CEO*
*Robert R. Lowe, COO*

26 **American Urogynecologic Society**
1100 Wayne Avenue 301-273-0570
Silver Spring, MD 20910 Fax: 301-273-0778
info@augs.org
www.augs.org
The leader in female pelvic medicine and reconstructive surgery.
*Michelle Zinnert, CEO*
*Colleen Hughes, COO*

27 **Argentum**
1650 King Street 703-894-1805
Alexandria, VA 22314 www.alfa.org
Argentum is the leading national association exclusively dedicated to supporting companies operating professionally managed, resident-centered senior living communities and the older adults and families they serve.
*James Balda, President & CEO*
*Maribeth Bersani, COO*

28 **Association for Adult Development and Aging**
5999 Stevenson Avenue www.aadaweb.org
Alexandria, VA 22304
A division of the American Counseling Association. Individuals holding a master's degree or its equivalent in adult counseling or a related field. Seeks to: improve the competence and skills of ACA and AADA members; expand professional work opportunities in adult development and aging counseling; promote the development of guidelines for professional preparation of counselors. Provides leadership and information to families, legislators, and communities.
*Amber Randolph, President*

29 **BrightFocus Foundation**
22512 Gateway Center Drive 800-437-2423
Clarksburg, MD 20871 Fax: 301-258-9454
info@brightfocus.org
www.brightfocus.org
Offers updated and trustworthy information on research, treatments, and resources. Free publications and newsletters.
*Stacy Pagos Haller, President & CEO*

30 **Brookdale Center for Healthy Aging**
2180 Third Avenue 212-396-7835
New York, NY 10035 Fax: 212-396-7852
info@brookdale.org
www.brookdale.org
Brookdale Center for Healthy Aging is one of the country's first university-based gerontology centers. The Center is dedicated to improving the lives of older adults through research, professional development, and advancements in policy and practice. Brookdale works to ensure that aging is framed not as a disease, but as another stage in the life course.
*Ruth K. Finkelstein, Executive Director*
*Jerry Antonatos, Director, Finance/Administration*

31 **Center for Benefits Access**
National Council on Aging
251 18th Street S 571-527-3900
Arlington, VA 22202 centerforbenefits@ncoa.org
www.ncoa.org/centerforbenefits
Benefits outreach and enrollment for seniors and younger adults with disabilities.
*Leslie Fried, Director*

32 **Center for Healthy Aging**
National Council on Aging
251 18th Street S 571-527-3900
Arlington, VA 22202 cha@ncoa.org
www.ncoa.org
Helping older adults live longer and healthier lives through evidence-based health promotion and disease prevention programs.
*Binod Suwal, Senior Program Manager*

33 **Center for Medicare Advocacy**
PO Box 350 860-456-7790
Willimantic, CT 06226 Fax: 860-456-2614
mshepard@medicareadvocacy.org
www.medicareadvocacy.org

Offers consultation, training, presentation, and materials on an array of topics pertaining to aging.
*Judith A. Stein, Executive Director*
*Matthew Shepard, Media Contact*

34 **Center for Positive Aging**
1440 Dutch Valley Place NE 404-872-9191
Atlanta, GA 30324 Fax: 404-872-1737
www.centerforpositiveaging.org
The Center for Positive Aging is a partnership of individuals, community organizations and congregations working together to provide health, educational and recreational opportunities for older persons and their families. Through our programs, services, and affiliations, we educate people of all ages and walks of life about living independent and creative lives.
*Ginny Helms, President & CEO*
*Jacque Thornton, SVP*

35 **Commission on Accreditation of Rehabilitation Facilities**
6951 E Southpoint Road 888-281-6531
Tucson, AZ 85756-9407 Fax: 520-318-1129
TTY: 520-495-7077
www.carf.org
CARF reviews and grants accreditation services nationally and internationally at the request of a facility or program. Standards are applied to service areas and business practices, and accreditation is ongoing in an effort to encourage service providers to continuously improve services. The CARF group also includes CARF Canada and CARF Europe.
*Brian J. Boon, PhD, President & CEO*
*Christine MacDonnell, Managing Director, Int'l Aging Services*

36 **Easter Seals**
One Concorde Gate 416-421-8377
Toronto, ON M3C 3 800-668-6252
Fax: 416-696-1035
info@easterseals.org
www.easterseals.org
Provides services to those with physical disabilities to help them achieve greater independence, accessibility, and integration.
*John M. Herhalt, Chair*

37 **Experience Works**
4401 Wilson Boulevard 703-522-7272
Arlington, VA 22203 866-397-9757
www.experienceworks.org
Helps low income seniors with multiple barriers to employment, get the training they need to find good jobs in their local community.
*Sally A. Boofer, President & CEO*
*Rosemary Schmidt, CFO*

38 **Family Caregiver Alliance/National Center on Caregiving**
101 Montgomery Street 415-434-3388
San Francisco, CA 94104 800-445-8106
www.caregiver.org
Caregiver information and assistance via phone or e-mail; fact sheets and publications describing and documenting caregiver needs and services.
*Jacquelyn Kung, PhD, Chief Executive Officer*
*Wyatt Ritchie, MBA, Managing Director*

39 **Gerontological Society of America**
1220 L Street NW 202-842-1275
Washington, DC 20005 Fax: 202-842-1150
geron@geron.org
www.geron.org
Nonprofit professional organization with more than 5,500 members in the field of aging. Provides researchers, educators, practitioners and policy makers with opportunities to understand, advance, integrate and use basic and applied research on aging populations. Also runs the National Adult Vaccination Program (www.navp.org).
*James Appleby, Chief Executive Officer*
*Karen Tracy, VP, Strategic Alliances & Communications*

40 **Goodwill Industries International, Inc.**
15810 Indianola Drive 800-466-3945
Rockville, MD 20855 contactus@goodwill.org
www.goodwill.org
A nonprofit, community-based organization whose mission is to help people achieve self-sufficiency through the dignity and power of work, serving people who are disadvantaged, disabled or elderly. The mission is accomplished through providing independent living skills, affordable housing, and training and placement in community employment. The GoodWill Network includes 160 independent, local locations across the U.S. and Canada.
*S. Dale Jenkins, Chair*
*Steven C. Preston, President & CEO*

41 **Harvey A. Friedman Center for Aging**
Washington University
St. Louis, Campus Box 8217 314-747-9212
St. Louis, MO 63110 centerforaging@wustl.edu
publichealth.wustl.edu/aging
The Center promotes research, education, policy and service initiatives that enable older adults to remain healthy, active, empowered, contributing and independent for as long as possible.
*Nancy Morrow-Howell, PhD, Director*
*Natalie Galucia, Center Manager*

42 **Heart Touch Project™**
3400 Airport Avenue 310-391-2558
Santa Monica, CA 90405 Fax: 310-391-2168
executive@hearttouch.org
www.hearttouch.org
Non-profit, educational and service organization devoted to the delivery of compassionate and healing touch to home or hospital-bound men, women, and children.
*Shawnee Isaac Smith, Co-Founder*
*Rene Russo, Co-Founder*

43 **Institute for Life Course and Aging**
246 Bloor Street W. 416-978-0377
Toronto, Ontario, M5S-1V4 Fax: 416-978-4771
aging@utoronto.ca
www.grandparentfamily.com
The Institute is a research center under the auspices of the Faculty of Social Work at the University of Toronto.
*Esme Fuller-Thomson, Director*
*Susan Murphy, Administration*

44 **International Federation on Aging**
1 Bridgepoint Drive 416-342-1655
Toronto, Ontario, M4M-2B5 Fax: 416-639-2165
jbarratt@ifa-fiv.org
www.ifa-fiv.org
The IFA seeks to inform, educate and promote policies and practice to improve the quality of life of older persons around the world.
*Greg Shaw, Director, Int'l & Corporate Relations*
*Dr. Jane Barratt, Secretary General*

45 **International Network for the Prevention of Elder Abuse**
The Somers Law Firm 518-281-2777
Nassau, NY 12123 contactus@inpea.net
www.inpea.net
Organization for the prevention of elder abuse.
*Susan B. Somers, President*
*Amanda Phelan, Secretary*

46 **Jewish Council for the Aging**
12320 Parklawn Drive 301-255-4200
Rockville, MD 20852 senior.helpline@accessjca.org
www.accessjca.org
Seeks to assist the elderly of all faiths lead independent lives. Provides transportation, job search assistance, fitness training, computer training and information and referrals. Conducts educational programs and presents an annual productive aging award. Maintains speakers' bureau.
*Norman Goldstein, President*

47 **Leadership Council of Aging Organizations**
lcao@aarp.org
www.lcao.org
Coalition of national non-profit organizations concerned with the well-being of older Americans.

48 **Leading Age**
2519 Connecticut Avenue NW 202-783-2242
Washington, DC 20008-1520 info@LeadingAge.org
www.leadingage.org

National association of more than 6,000 nonprofit nursing homes, continuing care retirement communities, independent living centers and community service providers serving more than 60,000 older Americans each year.
*Katie Smith Sloan, President & CEO*
*Nicole Fallon, Vice President, Health Policy*

49 **LeadingAge**
2519 Connecticut Avenue NW 202-783-2242
Washington, DC 20008 info@leadingage.org
www.leadingage.org
The work of LeadingAge is focused on advocacy, leadership development, and applied research and promotion of effective services, home health, hospice, community services, senior housing, continuing care communities, nursing homes, as well as technology solutions to seniors and thers with special needs.
*Lea Chambers-Johnson, Executive Team Administrator*

50 **National Adult Day Services Association**
11350 Random Hills Road 877-745-1440
Fairfax, VA 22030 info@nadsa.org
www.nadsa.org
Aims to be the leading voice of the Adult Day Services industry, representing providers, associations of providers, corporations, educators, students, and retired workers.
*Donna Hale, Executive Director*
*Lance Roberts, Associate Director, Membership*

51 **National Alliance for Caregiving**
1730 Rhode Island Avenue NW 202-918-1013
Washington, DC 20036 Fax: 202-918-1014
info@caregiving.org
www.caregiving.org
Coalition of organizations focused on improving the lives of family caregivers.
*C. Grace Whiting, President & CEO*

52 **National Asian Pacific Center on Aging**
1511 3rd Avenue 206-624-1221
Seattle, WA 98101 Fax: 206-624-1023
napca.org
Advocating for the specific needs of aging Asian Americans and Pacific Islanders.
*Joon Bang, President & CEO*
*Tina Masuda-Draughon, CFO*

53 **National Center on Elder Abuse**
Administration for Community Living
c/o USC Keck School of Medicine, De 855-500-3537
Alhambra, CA 91803 Fax: 626-457-4090
ncea-info@aoa.hhs.gov
www.ncea.acl.gov
The NCEA is an Administration on Aging Resource Center that provides up-to-date information on elder abuse, neglect and exploitation to policy makers and the public.

54 **National Clearinghouse on Abuse in Later Life**
1400 E Washington Avenue 608-255-0539
Madison, WI 53703 Fax: 608-255-3560
ncall@wcadv.org
www.ncall.us
Working to end abuse in later life.
*Bonnie Brandl, Director*

55 **National Committee to Preserve Social Security & Medicare**
111 K Street NE 202-216-0420
Washington, DC 20002 800-966-1935
Fax: 202-216-0446
webmaster@ncpssm.org
www.ncpssm.org
An advocacy and education membership organization, works to protect and enhance Federal programs vital to senior's health and economic well-being.
*Max Richtman, President & CEO*

56 **National Council for Aging Care**
1200 G Street NW 877-664-6140
Washington, DC 20005 www.aging.com
Seeks to provide older adults with information and resources on health & well-being, caregiving, money and financial planning, and lifestyle, through their Aging.com website.

57 **National Council on Aging**
251 18th Street S 571-527-3900
Arlington, VA 22202 www.ncoa.org
Emphasizes the needs for in-home and community-based health care and social services designed to help older persons remain in or return to their homes and live independently, works to educate and assist voluntary organizations to help develop such services.
*James Firman, President & CEO*

58 **National Falls Prevention Resource Center**
Center for Healthy Aging
251 18th Street S 571-527-3900
Arlington, VA 22202 www.ncoa.org
Supporting the implementation and dissemination of evidence-based falls prevention programs and strategies across the nation.

59 **National Hospice & Palliative Care Organization (NHPCO)**
1731 King Street 703-837-1500
Alexandria, VA 22314 800-646-6460
Fax: 703-837-1233
www.nhpco.org
The organization seeks to improve end-of-life care, widen access to hospice care, and improve quality of life for the dying and their loved ones.
*Edo Banach, JD, President & CEO*
*Hannah Yang Moore, MPH, Chief Advocacy Officer*

60 **National Institute of Senior Centers**
National Council on Aging
251 18th Street S 571-527-3900
Arlington, VA 22202 www.ncoa.org
Supporting the nation's senior centers.

61 **National Institute on Aging**
31 Center Drive, MSC 2292 800-222-2225
Bethesda, MD 20892 TTY: 800-222-4225
niaic@nia.nih.gov
www.nia.nih.gov
Seeks to understand the nature of aging, and to extend healthy, active years of life. Free resources are available on topics such as Alzheimer's & dementia, caregiving, cognitive heath, end of life care, and more.
*Richard J. Hodes MD, Director*
*Marie A. Bernard, MD, Deputy Director*

62 **National Institutes of Health**
9000 Rockville Pike 301-496-4000
Bethesda, MD 20892 TTY: 301-402-9612
nihinfo@od.nih.gov
www.nih.gov
The nation's medical research agency.
*Francis S. Collins, Director*

63 **National Older Worker Career Center**
3811 N Fairfax Drive 703-558-4200
Arlington, VA 22203 www.nowcc.org
National non-profit promoting experienced workers as staffing options to government agencies.
*Cito Vanegas, President & CEO*

64 **National Resource Center on Nutrition & Aging**
Meals on Wheels America
1550 Crystal Drive 703-548-5558
Arlington, VA 22202 Fax: 703-548-8024
nutritionandaging.org
Promoting better nutrition and active healthy aging.
*Ucheoma Akobundu, Director, Nutrition Strategy*
*Sharron Corle, Director, Learning & Development*

65 **National Senior Corps Association**
PO Box 360 928-523-6585
Farmington, UT 84025 sgrove@jfsmetrowest.org
www.nscatogether.org
Provides service for aging adults.
*Erin Kruse, President*
*Stephanie Grove, Membership Director*

66 **National Seniors Council**
1100 North Glebe Road 571-425-4153
Arlington, VA 22201 nationalseniorscouncil.org

The council seeks to serve the needs of the new generation of retirees, as an alternative to organizations such as the AARP.
*Carole Rhodes, National Director*

67 **Office for American Indian, Alaskan Native and Native Hawaiian Elders**
Administration for Community Living
330 C Street SW 202-401-4634
Washington, DC 20201 800-677-1116
olderindians@acl.hhs.gov
olderindians.acl.gov/about
The Office for American Indians, Alaskan Natives, and Native Hawaiians advises the Secretary, through the Assistant Secretary for Children and Families, on matters relating to Native Americans. It represents the concerns of Native Americans and serves as the focal point in the Department on the full range of developmental, social, and economic strategies that support Native American self-determination and self-sufficiency.
*Lance Robertson, Asst. Secretary for Aging*
*Mary Lazare, Principal Deputy Administrator*

68 **Quality Improvement Organizations**
qioprogram.org
Coalition of 28 organizations working to make nursing homes better places to live, work and visit.

69 **Senior Resource LLC**
questions@seniorresource.com
www.seniorresource.com
The company operates Seniorresource.com, which provides information to older adults on needed facilities and services, including through internet directories and an archive of E-zines.
*1995 pages*

70 **Society for Neuroscience**
1121 14th Street NW 202-962-4000
Washginton, DC 20005 marty@sfn.org
sfn.org
Large international organization of scientists and physicians devoted to the study of the brain and the nervous system.
*37,000 members*
*Marty Saggese, Executive Director*
*Melissa Garcia, Associate Executive Director*

71 **US Administration on Aging**
330 C Street SW 202-401-4634
Washington, DC 20201 aclinfo@acl.hhs.gov
acl.gov/about-acl/administration-aging
The Administration on Aging, an agency in the US Department of Health and Human Services, and under the Administration for Community Living, is one of the nation's largest providers of home and community-based care for older persons and their caregivers.
*Lance Robertson, Administrator & Assistant Secretary*
*Edwin Walker, Deputy Assistant Secretary*

72 **Unbound**
1 Elmwood Avenue 913-384-6500
Kansas City, KS 66103 800-875-6564
mail@unbound.org
www.unbound.org
Seeks to advance the physical, mental, spiritual, and social welfare of the economically disadvantaged, especially children and aging persons in developing countries. US sponsors provide financial support and correspond with individuals in need; volunteers help provide social services, including medical, educational, and nutritional programs.
*Scott Wasserman, President & CEO*

## State Agencies & Associations

73 **AARP Alabama**
400 South Union Street 866-542-8167
Montgomery, AL 36104 alaarp@aarp.org
states.aarp.org/region/alabama
Provides information, events, news, and resources to Alabamians over 50 years of age, and to a membership of over 430,000.
*Candi Williams, State Director*
*Lisa Billingsley, Senior Operations Administrator*

74 **AARP Alaska**
3601 C Street 866-227-7447
Anchorage, AK 99503 Fax: 907-341-2270
ak@aarp.org
states.aarp.org/region/alaska
Serves 95,000 members in Alaska, providing information, resources, news, and advocacy on matters relevant to individuals aged 50 years and older.
*Ken Helander, Advocacy Director*
*Ann Secrest, Media Contact*

75 **AARP Arizona**
7250 N 16th Street 866-389-5649
Phoenix, AZ 85020 aarpaz@aarp.org
states.aarp.org/region/arizona
The chapter seeks to enhance the quality of life for all Arizonans, with an emphasis on individuals 50 years and older.
*David Parra, Director, Community Outreach*
*Alex Suarez, Communications Contact*

76 **AARP Arkansas**
1701 Centerview Drive 866-544-5379
Little Rock, AR 72211 Fax: 501-227-7710
araarp@aarp.org
states.aarp.org/region/arkansas
Seeks to redefine and improve life for Arkansans over the age of 50.
*Charlie Wagener, State President*

77 **AARP California: Pasadena**
200 S Los Robles Avenue 866-448-3614
Pasadena, CA 91101-2422 Fax: 626-583-8500
caaarp@aarp.org
states.aarp.org/region/california
Provides news, tools, resources, and research to Californians 50 years and older.
*Nancy McPherson, State Director*
*Joy Hepp, Media Contact, Southern California*

78 **AARP California: Sacramento**
1415 L Street 866-448-3614
Sacramento, CA 95814 Fax: 916-446-2223
caaarp@aarp.org
states.aarp.org/region/california
Provides news, tools, resources, and research to Californians 50 years and older.
*Nancy McPherson, State President*
*Mark Beach, Media Contact, Northern California*

79 **AARP Colorado**
303 E 17th Avenue 866-554-5376
Denver, CO 80203-5012 Fax: 303-764-5999
coaarp@aarp.org
states.aarp.org/region/colorado
The Colorado chapter seeks to keep Coloradans 50 years and older informed, engaged, and active.
*Bob Murphy, State Director*
*Angela Cortez, Media Contact*

80 **AARP Connecticut**
21 Oak Street 866-295-7279
Hartford, CT 06106 ctaarp@aarp.org
states.aarp.org/region/connecticut
With nearly 600,000 members, the chapter provides recent news, information, and events for residents of Connecticut who are 50 years and older, as well as advocating for positive social change.
*Nora Duncan, State Director*
*Anna Doroghazi, Assoc. State Dir., Advocacy & Outreach*

81 **AARP Delaware**
222 Delaware Avenue 866-227-7441
Wilmington, DE 19801 kiapalucci@aarp.org
states.aarp.org/region/delaware
Provides news, advocacy, education, and lifestyle information for residents of Delaware who are 50 years and older.
*Lucretia Young, State Director*
*Kimberly Iapalucci, Media Contact*

82 **AARP Florida: Doral**
3750 Nw 87th Avenue 866-595-7678
Doral, FL 33178 Fax: 786-804-4544
flaarp@aarp.org
states.aarp.org/region/florida
The chapter provides information, research, and events to 2.7 million members, and Floridians 50 years and older.
*Donna L. Ginn, State President*
*Jeff Johnson, State Director*

83 **AARP Florida: St. Petersburg**
360 Central Avenue 866-595-7678
St. Petersburg, FL 33701 Fax: 727-369-5191
flaarp@aarp.org
states.aarp.org/region/florida
The chapter provides information, research, and events to 2.7 million members, and Floridians 50 years and older.
*Donna L. Ginn, State President*
*Jeff Johnson, State Director*

84 **AARP Florida: Tallahassee**
200 West College Avenue 866-595-7678
Tallahassee, FL 32301 Fax: 850-222-8968
flaarp@aarp.org
states.aarp.org/region/florida
The chapter provides information, research, and events to 2.7 million members, and Floridians 50 years and older.
*Donna L. Ginn, State President*
*Jeff Johnson, State Director*

85 **AARP Georgia**
999 Peachtree Street NE 866-295-7281
Atlanta, GA 30309 Fax: 404-815-7940
gaaarp@aarp.org
states.aarp.org/region/georgia
The chapter strives to help Georgians 50 years and older.
*Debra Tyler-Horton, State Director*
*Alisa Jackson, Media Contact*

86 **AARP Hawaii**
1132 Bishop Street 866-295-7282
Honolulu, HI 96813 Fax: 808-537-2288
hiaarp@aarp.org
states.aarp.org/region/hawaii
With 150,000 members, the chapter advocates at the state level, and provides information, resources, and volunteer opportunities.
*Jessica Wooley, Director, Advocacy*

87 **AARP Idaho**
250 S 5th Street 866-295-7284
Boise, ID 83702 Fax: 208-288-4424
aarpid@aarp.org
states.aarp.org/region/idaho
The chapter advocates for and seeks to improve the lives of residents aged 50 years and older.
*Lupe Wissel, Idaho AARP State Media Relations*
*Randy Simon, Media Contact*

88 **AARP Illinois: Chicago**
222 N LaSalle Street 866-448-3613
Chicago, IL 60601 Fax: 312-372-2204
aarpil@aarp.org
states.aarp.org/region/illinois
Advocates for and provides recent news, events, and lifestyle tips to Illinois residents aged 50 years and older.
*Bob Gallo, State Director*
*Dina Anderson, Media Contact*

89 **AARP Illinois: Springfield**
300 W Edwards Street 866-448-3613
Springfield, IL 62704 Fax: 217-522-7803
aarpil@aarp.org
states.aarp.org/region/illinois
Legislative office of the Illinois chapter.
*Bob Gallo, State Director*
*Dina Anderson, Media Contact*

90 **AARP Indiana**
One N Capitol Avenue 866-448-3618
Indianapolis, IN 46204-2025 Fax: 317-423-2211
inaarp@aarp.org
states.aarp.org/region/indiana
The chapter seeks to improve life for residents of Indiana aged 50 years and older.
*Sarah Waddle, State Director*
*Jason Tomcsi, Media Contact*

91 **AARP Iowa**
600 E Court Avenue 866-554-5378
Des Moines, IA 50309 Fax: 515-244-7767
ia@aarp.org
states.aarp.org/region/iowa
Provides news, information, and resources to Iowans aged 50 years and older.
*Brad Anderson, State Director*
*Jeremy Barewin, Media Contact*

92 **AARP Kansas**
6220 SW 29th Street 866-448-3619
Topeka, KS 66614 Fax: 785-232-1465
ksaarp@aarp.org
states.aarp.org/region/kansas
The chapter provides news, events, and more to Kansans aged 50 years and older.
*Maren Turner, Kansas AARP State Media Relations*
*Mary Tritsch, Media Contact*

93 **AARP Kentucky**
10401 Linn Station Road 866-295-7275
Louisville, KY 40223 kyaarp@aarp.org
states.aarp.org/region/kentucky
Provides news and resources for Kentuckians over the age of 50.
*Scott Wagenast, Associate State Director*

94 **AARP Louisiana: Baton Rouge**
301 Main Street 866-448-3620
Baton Rouge, LA 70825 la@aarp.org
states.aarp.org/region/louisiana
The office seeks to advocate for and provide resources to residents of Louisiana aged 50 and over.
*Denise Bottcher, State Director*
*Andrew Muhl, Director, Advocacy*

95 **AARP Louisiana: New Orleans**
3502 S Carrollton Avenue 866-448-3620
New Orleans, LA 70118 la@aarp.org
states.aarp.org/region/louisiana
AARP Louisiana's Community Resource Center.
*Denise Bottcher, State Director*
*Andrew Muhl, Director, Advocacy*

96 **AARP Maine**
53 Baxter Boulevard 866-554-5380
Portland, ME 04101 me@aarp.org
states.aarp.org/region/maine
Seeks to enhance the lives of Mainers aged 50 years and over through advocacy, information sharing, volunteer opportunities, and service. The chapter counts 230,000 members.
*Lori Parham, State Director*
*Amy Gallant, Director, Advocacy and Outreach*

97 **AARP Maryland**
200 St. Paul Place 866-542-8163
Baltimore, MD 21202 Fax: 410-837-0269
md@aarp.org
states.aarp.org/region/maryland
The chapter seeks to enhance the lives of Maryland residents aged 50 and over, as well as caregivers, through resources and a variety of social opportunities.
*Jim Campbell, State President*
*Nancy Carr, Assoc. State Director, Communications*

98 **AARP Massachusetts**
1 Beacon Street 866-448-3621
Boston, MA 02108 Fax: 617-723-4224
ma@aarp.org
states.aarp.org/region/massachusetts

Provides news, events, and resources to Massachusetts residents aged 50 and over.
*Mike Festa, State Director*
*Cindy Campbell, Director, Communications*

99 **AARP Michigan**
309 N Washington Square 866-227-7448
Lansing, MI 48933 Fax: 517-482-2794
TTY: 8
miaarp@aarp.org
states.aarp.org/region/michigan
The chapter seeks to enhance the quality of life for aging residents of Michigan through information, advocacy, and services.
*Paula D. Cunningham, State Director*

100 **AARP Minnesota**
1919 University Avenue 866-554-5381
St. Paul, MN 55104 aarpmn@aarp.org
states.aarp.org/region/minnesota
Aims to connect aging residents of Minnesota with financial and other resources to enhance quality of life.
*Will Phillips, State Director*
*Maro Jo George, Associate State Director, Advocacy*

101 **AARP Mississippi**
141 Township Avenue 866-554-5382
Ridgeland, MS 39157 Fax: 601-898-5429
msaarp@aarp.org
states.aarp.org/region/mississippi
Seeks to improve the lives of Mississippians, particularly those over 50 years of age, through events, news, resources, and advocacy.
*John McDonald, AARP Missouri State Director*
*Ronda Gooden, Media Contact*

102 **AARP Missouri**
9200 Ward Parkway 866-389-5627
Kansas City, MO 64114 Fax: 816-561-3107
aarpmo@aarp.org
states.aarp.org/region/missouri
Provides information to Missourians aged 50 and over on health, finances, and lifestyle, as well as providing advocacy.
*Craig Eichelman, State Director*
*Jamayla Long, Media Contact*

103 **AARP Montana**
30 W 14th Street 866-295-7278
Helena, MT 59601 mtaarp@aarp.org
states.aarp.org/region/montana
With 150,000 members, the chapter provides advocacy, education, information, resources, and collaborative projects for Montana residents aged 50 and over.
*Tim Summers, State Director*
*Stacia Dahl, Media Contact*

104 **AARP Nebraska: Lincoln**
301 S 13th Street 866-389-5651
Lincoln, NE 68508 Fax: 402-323-6908
neaarp@aarp.org
states.aarp.org/region/nebraska
Works on behalf of over 200,000 members and their families to provide news, services, information, resources, and advocacy for individuals 50 years and older.
*Connie Benjamin, AARP Nebraska State President*
*Devorah Lanner, Media Contact*

105 **AARP Nebraska: Omaha**
1941 S 42nd Street 402-398-9568
Omaha, NE 68105 omnebraska@aol.com
states.aarp.org/region/nebraska
AARP Nebraska's Information Center.
*Connie Benjamin, AARP Nebraska State President*
*Devorah Lanner, Media Contact*

106 **AARP Nevada**
5820 S Eastern Avenue 866-389-5652
Las Vegas, NV 89119 aarpnv@aarp.org
states.aarp.org/region/nevada
Provides news, information, and resources to 320,000 members, on matters affecting the lives of individuals aged 50 and over.
*Maria Dent, State Director*
*Scott Gulbransen, Media Contact*

107 **AARP New Hampshire**
45 South Main Street 866-542-8168
Concord, NH 03301 Fax: 603-224-6211
nh@aarp.org
states.aarp.org/region/new-hampshire
Provides information, resources, and advocacy services to 228,000 members, on matters relevant to individuals aged 50 years and older.
*Todd Fahey, State Director*
*Doug McNutt, Associate State Director, Advocacy*

108 **AARP New Jersey**
303 George Street 866-542-8165
New Brunswick, NJ 08901 Fax: 609-987-4634
aarpnJ@aarp.org
states.aarp.org/region/new-jersey
The chapter seeks to educate and advocate for New Jersey residents aged 50 and over, and their families.
*Stephanie Hunsinger, State Director*
*Jeff Abramo, Media Contact*

109 **AARP New Mexico**
535 Cerrillos Road 866-389-5636
Santa Fe, NM 87501 Fax: 505-820-2889
aarpnm@aarp.org
states.aarp.org/region/new-mexico
The chapter advocates on behalf of individuals 50 years and older, monitoring seniors' services, utility rates, transportation services, as well as providing financial planning services to members.
*Jennifer Baier, Interim State Director*
*DeAnza Valencia, Associate State Director, Advocacy*

110 **AARP New York: Albany**
1 Commerce Plaza 866-227-7442
Albany, NY 12260 nyaarp@aarp.org
states.aarp.org/region/new-york
Provides information, resources, news, and advocacy services to residents of New York who are 50 years and older.
*Beth Finkel, State President*
*Erik Kriss, Media Contact*

111 **AARP New York: New York City**
750 Third Avenue 866-227-7442
New York, NY 10017 nyaarp@aarp.org
states.aarp.org/region/new-york
Provides information, resources, news, and advocacy services to residents of New York who are 50 years and older.
*Beth Finkel, State President*
*Erik Kriss, Media Contact*

112 **AARP New York: Rochester**
435 E Henrietta Road 866-227-7442
Rochester, NY 14620 nyaarp@aarp.org
states.aarp.org/region/new-york
Provides information, resources, news, and advocacy services to residents of New York who are 50 years and older.
*Beth Finkel, State President*
*Erik Kriss, Media Contact*

113 **AARP North Carolina**
5511 Capital Center Drive 866-389-5650
Raleigh, NC 27606 ddickerson@aarp.org
states.aarp.org/region/north-carolina
Advocates for community issues such as health care, employment/income security, retirement planning, utilities, and protection from financial abuse, on behalf of a membership 1.1 million strong.
*Doug Dickerson, State Director*
*Michael Oldender, Manager, Outreach and Advocacy*

114 **AARP North Dakota**
107 W Main Avenue 866-554-5383
Bismarck, ND 58501 Fax: 701-255-2242
aarpnd@aarp.org
states.aarp.org/region/north-dakota

Provides news, information, resources, events, advocacy, and more to North Dakotans aged 50 and over.
*Josh Askvig, State Director*
*Doreen Redman, Assoc. State Dir., Community Outreach*

115 **AARP Ohio**
17 S High Street 866-389-5653
Columbus, OH 43215 Fax: 614-224-9801
ohaarp@aarp.org
states.aarp.org/region/ohio
The chapter shares information, advocates, and performs community services for 1.5 million members, 50 years and older, across the state.
*Barbara Sykes, State Director*

116 **AARP Oklahoma**
126 N Bryant Avenue 866-295-7277
Edmond, OK 73034 Fax: 405-844-7772
ok@aarp.org
states.aarp.org/region/oklahoma
Assists individuals aged 50 and over through advocacy, news, information, resources, and more.
*Sean Voskuhl, State Director*
*Chad Mullen, Associate State Director, Advocacy*

117 **AARP Oregon**
9200 SE Sunnybrook Boulevard 866-554-5360
Clackamas, OR 97015 oraarp@aarp.org
states.aarp.org/region/oregon
Strives for social change for its 500,000 members, and all individuals 50 years and over, through advocacy and community services.
*Ruby Haughton-Pitts, State Director*
*Joyce DeMonnin, Media Contact*

118 **AARP Pennsylvania: Harrisburg**
30 N 3rd Street 866-389-5654
Harrisburg, PA 17101 Fax: 717-236-4078
aarpa@aarp.org
states.aarp.org/region/pennsylvania
Seeks to enhance the quality of life for 1.8 million members across the state.
*Bill Johnston-Walsh, State Director*
*Steve Gardner, Media Contact*

119 **AARP Pennsylvania: Philadelphia**
1650 Market Street 866-389-5654
Philadelphia, PA 19103 Fax: 215-665-8529
aarpa@aarp.org
states.aarp.org/region/pennsylvania
Seeks to enhance the quality of life for 1.8 million members across the state.
*Bill Johnston-Walsh, State Director*
*Steve Gardner, Media Contact*

120 **AARP Rhode Island**
10 Orms Street 866-542-8170
Providence, RI 02904 Fax: 401-272-0596
ri@aarp.org
states.aarp.org/region/rhode-island
Provides news, information, resources, advocacy, and community services to those aged 50 and older in the state.
*Kathleen Connell, State Director*
*John Martin, Director, Communications*

121 **AARP South Carolina**
1201 Main Street 803-765-7381
Columbia, SC 29201 866-389-5655
scaarp@aarp.org
states.aarp.org/region/south-carolina
Seeks to enhance the quality of life for members and individuals aged 50 and older, through information, resources, education, advocacy, and more.
*Teresa Arnold, State Director*
*Nikki Hutchison, Associate State Director, Advocacy*

122 **AARP South Dakota**
5101 S Nevada Avenue 866-542-8172
Sioux Falls, SD 57108 sdaarp@aarp.org
states.aarp.org/region/south-dakota
Provides news, information, resources, advocacy, and community services to 110,000 members and those aged 50 and older in the state.
*Erik Gaikowski, State Director*

123 **AARP Tennessee**
150 4th Avenue N 866-295-7274
Nashville, TN 37219 tnaarp@aarp.org
states.aarp.org/region/tennessee
Strives for positive social change for 660,000 members and individuals aged 50 and over.
*Rebecca Kelly, State Director*
*Rob Naylor, Director, Communications*

124 **AARP Texas: Austin**
1905 Aldrich Street 866-227-7443
Austin, TX 78723 states.aarp.org/region/texas
The chapter offers news, information, research, and events for individuals aged 50 and over, as well as conducting advocacy on their behalf.
*Bob Jackson, State Director*
*Junita Jiminez-Soto, Associate State Director, Communications*

125 **AARP Texas: Dallas**
8140 Walnut Hill Lane 866-227-7443
Dallas, TX 75231 states.aarp.org/region/texas
The chapter offers news, information, research, and events for individuals aged 50 and over, as well as conducting advocacy on their behalf.
*Bob Jackson, State Director*
*Junita Jiminez-Soto, Associate State Director, Communications*

126 **AARP Texas: Houston**
2323 S Shepherd Drive 866-227-7443
Houston, TX 77019 states.aarp.org/region/texas
The chapter offers news, information, research, and events for individuals aged 50 and over, as well as conducting advocacy on their behalf.
*Bob Jackson, State Director*
*Junita Jiminez-Soto, Associate State Director, Communications*

127 **AARP Texas: San Antonio**
1314 Guadalupe Street 866-227-7443
San Antonio, TX 78207 states.aarp.org/region/texas
The chapter offers news, information, research, and events for individuals aged 50 and over, as well as conducting advocacy on their behalf.
*Bob Jackson, State Director*
*Junita Jiminez-Soto, Associate State Director, Communications*

128 **AARP Utah**
6975 Union Park Center 866-448-3616
Midvale, UT 84047 Fax: 801-561-2209
utaarp@aarp.org
states.aarp.org/region/utah
Serves 211,000 members in 10 regions across the state, with advocacy, communications, programming, and outreach.
*Alan Ormsby, State Director*
*Danny Harris, Director, Advocacy*

129 **AARP Vermont**
199 Main Street 866-227-7451
Burlington, VT 05401 Fax: 802-651-9805
vtaarp@aarp.org
states.aarp.org/region/vermont
Seeks to represent the concerns and interests of Vermonters aged 50 and over.
*Greg Marchildon, State Director*

130 **AARP Virginia**
707 E Main Street 866-542-8164
Richmond, VA 23219 Fax: 804-819-1923
vaaarp@aarp.org
states.aarp.org/region/virginia
Serves Virginians aged 50 and older, and their families, through advocacy, information, resources, and outreach.
*Jim Dau, State Director*

131 **AARP Washington**
18000 International Blvd. 866-227-7457
SeaTac, WA 98188 Fax: 206-517-9350
waaarp@aarp.org
states.aarp.org/region/washington
Serves 950,000 members through information, advocacy, and a variety of services.
*Doug Shadel, State Director*

132 **AARP Washington DC**
100 M Street SE 866-554-5384
Washington, DC 20003 Fax: 202-434-7946
dcaarp@aarp.org
states.aarp.org/region/washington-dc
Provides information, advocacy, and a variety of services to 87,000 members aged 50 and over.
*Louis Davis, Jr., State Director*
*Peter Rankin, Associate State Director, Advocacy*

133 **AARP West Virginia**
300 Summers Street 866-227-7458
Charleston, WV 25301 Fax: 304-344-4633
wvaarp@aarp.org
states.aarp.org/region/west-virginia
Provides information, resources, advocacy, and more to individuals aged 50 and over in West Virginia.
*Gaylene Miller, State Director*
*Tom Hunter, Associate State Director, Communications*

134 **AARP Wisconsin**
222 W Washington Avenue 866-448-3611
Madison, WI 53703 Fax: 608-251-7612
wistate@aarp.org
states.aarp.org/region/wisconsin
The chapter advocates for, and provides a variety of services to, its 840,000 members, aged 50 years and over.
*Sam Wilson, State Director*
*Jim Flaherty, Media Contact*

135 **AARP Wyoming**
2020 Carey Avenue 866-663-3290
Cheyenne, WY 82009 wyaarp@aarp.org
states.aarp.org/region/wyoming
Provides resources, information, and advocates for indviduals in Wyoming aged 50 and older, with an emphasis on health care, retirement, and utility issues.
*Sam Shumway, State Director*
*Tom Lacock, Assoc. State Dir., Advocacy & Comm.*

136 **Arizona Center on Aging**
1501 N Campbell 520-626-5800
Tucson, AZ 85724 Fax: 520-626-5801
info@aging.arizona.edu
www.aging.arizona.edu
The mission at Arizona Center of Aging (ACOA) is to promote healthy and functional lives for older adults through comprehensive programs in research, education and training, and clinical care.
*Mindy Fain, MD, Co-Director*
*Janko Nikolich-Zugish, MD, Co-Director*

137 **Goodwill Industries-Suncoast**
10596 Gandy Boulevard 727-523-1512
St. Petersburg, FL 33702 888-279-1988
TTY: 727-579-1068
www.goodwill-suncoast.org
A nonprofit, community-based organization whose mission is to help people achieve self-sufficiency through the dignity and power of work, serving people who are disadvantaged, disabled or elderly. The mission is accomplished through providing independent living skills, affordable housing, and training and placement in community employment.
*Heather Ceresoli, CPA, Chair*
*Deborah A. Passerini, President & CEO*

138 **Jewish Council for the Aging of Greater Washington**
12320 Parklawn Drive 301-255-4200
Rockville, MD 20852 senior.helpline@accessjca.org
www.accessjca.org
Seeks to assist the elderly of all faiths lead independent lives. Provides transportation, job search assistance, fitness training, computer training and information and referrals. Conducts educational programs and presents an annual productive aging award. Maintains speakers' bureau.
*Norman Goldstein, President*

139 **Legal Council for Health Justice**
17 N State Street 312-427-8990
Chicago, IL 60602 Fax: 312-427-8419
legalcouncil.org
Provides legal advice and services for persons who are HIV positive or have AIDS, as well as their families. Also serves individuals with disabilities and chronic illnesses, senior citizens, and the homeless.
*Tom Yates, Executive Director*
*Ruth Edwards, Senior Director, Program Services*

140 **Medicare Rights Center: New York**
266 W 37th Street 212-869-3850
New York, NY 10018 Fax: 212-869-3532
info@medicarerights.org
www.medicarerights.org
Seeks to ensure the rights of senior citizens and people with disabilities to quality, affordable health care. Provides counseling services to Medicare beneficiaries with health insurance problems and questions; compiles information on inquiries to detect issues and systemic problems in Medicare claims administration. Educates beneficiaries, advocates, providers, and social workers about developments in Medicare law and how to handle problems.
*Frederic Riccardi, President*

141 **Medicare Rights Center: Washington, DC**
1444 I Street NW 202-637-0961
Washington, DC 20005 Fax: 202-637-0962
info@medicarerights.org
www.medicarerights.org
A consumer service organization that works to ensure access to affordable health care for older adults and peoplw tih disabilities through counseling and advocacy, educational programs, and public policy intiatives.
*Frederic Riccardi, President*

142 **National Senior Citizens Law Center: Oakland**
1330 Broadway 510-663-1055
Oakland, CA 94612 www.justiceinaging.org
Advocates nationwide to promote the independence and well-being of low-income elderly individuals, as well as persons with disabilities, with particular emphais on women and racial and ethnic minorities. Advocates through litigation and agency representation and assistance to attotneys and paralegals in field programs.
*Kevin Prindiville, Executive Director*

143 **National Senior Citizens Law Center: Los Angeles**
3660 Wilshire Boulevard 213-639-0930
Los Angeles, CA 90010 www.justiceinaging.org
Legal services support center specializing in the legal problems of the elderly poor. Acts as advocate on behalf of elderly, poor clients in litigation and administrative affairs. Sponsors conferences and workshops on areas of the law affecting the elderly. See Legal Resources chapter for specific state resorces.
*Kevin Prindiville, Executive Director*

144 **Points of Light: Atlanta**
600 Means Street 404-979-2900
Atlanta, GA 30318 Fax: 404-979-2901
info@pointsoflight.org
www.pointsoflight.org
Mobilizing people to take action on the causes they care about.
*Natalye Paquin, President & CEO*
*Robert E. Herrera, CFO*

145 **Points of Light: Washington, DC**
1400 G Street NW 404-979-2900
Washington, DC 20005 Fax: 404-979-2901
info@pointsoflight.org
www.pointsoflight.org
Mobilizing people to take action on the causes they care about.
*Natalye Paquin, President & CEO*
*Robert E. Herrera, CFO*

146 **Virginia Center on Aging**
Virginia Commonwealth University
Box 980229 804-828-1525
Richmond, VA 23298 vcoa@vcu.edu
vcoa.chp.vcu.edu
The Virginia Center on Aging is a statewide agency created by the Virginia General Assembly, with our home at Virginia Commonwealth University. Since 1978, VCoA has worked diligently to protect and improve the quality of life of older Virginians, so that they may remain independent and contributing members in their communities. Our four program areas include: abuse in later life, dementia research, geriatrics education, and lifelong learning.
*Edward F. Ansello, PhD, Director*
*Leland Waters, PhD, Associate Director*

## Foundations & Research Centers

147 **AARP Foundation**
American Association of Retired Persons
601 E Street NW 800-775-6776
Washington, DC 20049 TTY: 877-434-7598
www.aarp.org/aarp-foundation
The foundation seeks to assist seniors living in poverty through economic opportunities and social connectedness. Legal services and grants are also offered.
*Lisa Marsh Ryerson, President*
*Emily Allen, Senior Vice President, Programs*

148 **Academy for Gerontology in Higher Education**
1220 L Street NW 202-289-9806
Washington, DC 20005 membership@geron.org
www.aghe.org
Membership organization comprised of more than 130 colleges and universities that offer education and research program in the field of aging. Affiliated with the Gerontological Society of America.
*Judith L. Howe, President*
*Lisa Hollis-Sawyer, Treasurer*

149 **Ackerman Institute for the Family**
Ackerman Institute for the Family
936 Broadway 212-879-4900
New York, NY 10010 Fax: 212-744-0206
ackerman@ackerman.org
www.ackerman.org
Provides mental health care professionals with new skills, and brings innovative perspectives to community service agencies and other health care facilities.
*John R. O'Neill, Chair*
*Lois Braverman, LCSW, President*

150 **Aging In America**
2975 Westchester Avenue 914-205-5030
Purchase, NY 10577 contact@aginginamerica.org
www.aginginamerica.org
Previously a community-based, social service agency, Aging in America is transitioning into a foundation funding technological innovations in gerontology.
*William T. Smith, PhD, President & CEO*
*Kathleen Bufano, Executive Assistant*

151 **Aging Research Institute**
LeadingAge Kansas
217 SE 8th Avenue 785-233-7443
Topeka, KS 66603 800-264-5242
Fax: 785-233-9471
Managed care and nursing facilities staff recruitment and retention.
*Kevin Reimer, Chair*
*Debra Harmon Zehr, President and CEO*

152 **Aging Research: National Institute on Aging, Public Health Service**
US Department of Health and Human Services
200 Independence Avenue, S.W. 301-496-4996
Washington, DC 20201 800-422-6237
Fax: 301-402-0010
www.hhs.gov/
To encourage biomedical, social, and behavioral research, and research training directed toward greater understanding of the aging process and the diseases, special problems, and needs of people as they age.

153 **Alliance for Aging Research**
1700 K Street NW 202-293-2856
Washington, DC 20006 info@agingresearch.org
www.agingresearch.org
Gerontologists and other medical professionals, executives and members of Congress are participants. Works to increase private and public research into aging. Supports policies concerning: productive aging; independence for older Americans; successful aging. Public and professional educational literature, newsletter web site.
*Sue Peschin, President & CEO*

154 **American Aging Association**
American Aging Association (AGE)
25373 Tyndall Falls Drive 440-793-6565
Olmsted Falls, OH 44138 Fax: 440-793-6598
americanaging@gmail.com
www.americanaging.org
Laymen and scientists primarily in the biomedical field. Dedicated to helping people live better, longer by promoting biomedical aging studies directed toward slowing down the aging process, informing the public of the progress of aging research and of practical means of achieving a long and healthy life and increasing knowledge of gerontology among physicians and other health workers.
*Mitch Harman, MD, PhD, Chair*
*LaDora Thompson, PhD, President*

155 **American Federation for Aging Research**
American Federation for Aging Research (AFAR)
55 West 39th Street 212-703-9977
New York, NY 10018 888-582-2327
Fax: 212-997-0330
www.afar.org
*William J. Lipton, JD, LLM, CPA, Chair*
*Harvey Jay Cohen, M.D., President*

156 **American Institutes for Research Center on Aging**
1000 Thomas Jefferson Street NW 202-403-5000
Washington, DC 20007 Fax: 855-459-6213
TTY: 877-334-3499
www.air.org/center/center-aging
Seeks to improve the lives of the disadvantaged through attention to aging issues, connected to existing work at AIR, and examining emerging issues.
*Marilyn Moon, Director*

157 **Archstone Foundation**
301 E Ocean Boulevard 506-590-8655
Long Beach, CA 90802 Fax: 506-495-0317
archstone@archstone.org
archstone.org
The foundation funds initiatives that meet the needs of an aging population, including stopping elder abuse, preventing falls, and compassionate end-of-life care.
*Christopher Langston, PhD, President & CEO*
*Tanisha Davis, MAG, Grants Manager*

158 **Arthur M Fishberg Research Center in Neurobiology**
Mt. Sinai Medical Center
PO Box 1065 212-659-5992
New York, NY 10029 Fax: 212-996-9785
Neurobiological systems in humans and mammals, emphasizing aging research. Specific interests include the neuroendocrinology of stress, reproduction and metabolism, the molecular biology of Alzheimer's disease, schizophrenia, and other neurological/psychiatric diseases, and growth factors and growth factor receptor gene expression in the central nervous system.

159 **Baylor College of Medicine: Roy M and Phyllis Gough Center on Aging**
Huffington Center on Aging (HCOA)
Baylor College of Medicine 713-798-5804
Houston, TX 77030 Fax: 713-798-6688
www.hcoa.org

Internal unit of Baylor College representing research into the biology of aging.
*James T. Hackett, Chair*
*Carolyn Dine King, Vice Chair and Board Secretary*

**160 Baylor University Institute for Gerontological Studies**
PO Box 97320 254-710-6400
Waco, TX 76798 Fax: 254-710-6455
www.baylor.edu/gerontology
Physical, emotional, social, and spiritual needs of older persons, including family solidarity in later life, geriatric dentistry, problems of the older offender, and life-long learning.
*Krista Barrett, Field Education Program Manager/*
*Jeanie Fitzpatrick, Assistant to the Dean*

**161 Boston University Gerontology Center**
Boston University Institute for Geriatric Social W
264 Bay State Road 617-358-2626
Boston, MA 02215 Fax: 617-358-2636
cader@bu.edu
www.bu.edu/cader/
Gerontology, including biological, psychological, social, medical, and humanistic concerns relating to aging and the elderly. Identifies socially relevant problems in the fields of gerontology and human development, socioeconomic factors impinging upon the lives and well-being of older adults, historical context in which values and attitudes toward the aging have been defined and redefined, and medical services developed to serve them.
*Scott Miyake Geron, M.S.W., Ph.D, Director*
*Bronwyn Keefe, M.S.W., M.P.H.,, Associate Director*

**162 Brain Research Institute University of California, Los Angeles**
The Brain Research Institute (BRI)
1506 Gonda (Goldschmied) Neuroscien 310-825-5061
Los Angeles, CA 90095 Fax: 310-206-5855
www.bri.ucla.edu
Brain and central nervous system, including interdisciplinary studies in developmental neurobiology, molecular neurobiology, neuroanatomy, neurobiophysics, neurochemistry, neurocytology, neuroendocrinology, neuroimaging, neuromuscular physiology, neuropathology, neuropharmacology, neurophysiology, behavior, neuroimmunology, and experimental epilepsy.
*Christopher Evans, PhD., Director*
*J. David Jentsch, PhD., Associate Director for Research*

**163 Brandeis University Institute for Health Policy**
The Heller School for Social Policy and Management
415 South Street (MS 035) 781-736-3820
Waltham, MA 02254 Fax: 781-736-3865
www.brandeis.edu/heller/ihp/ihp
Health services research and policy analysis, focusing on the design, development, implementation, and evaluation of innovative financing and delivery systems. Specific areas of research include establishing and implementing national health care expenditure limits, all-payer payment systems, an Alcohol and Drug Services Survey, changing trends of substance abuse, financing and reimbursement of drug abuse treatment programs, and long-term care.
*Lisa M. Lynch, PhD., Dean*
*Ron Etlinger, Chief Administrative Officer*

**164 Brandeis University Policy Center on Aging**
The Heller School for Social Policy and Management
415 South Street (MS 035) 781-736-3820
Waltham, MA 02254 Fax: 781-736-3865
NATWONCTR@brandeis.edu
www.brandeis.edu/heller/ihp/ihp
Retirement income adequacy and policy, long term care and health service delivery, aging and mental health, supportive service in senior housing and resource allocation for the elderly. Generates, synthesizes, and disseminates knowledge on policy alternatives affecting the economic security of the aging; analyzes the economic, legal, administrative, and political consequences and feasibility of alternative policies.
*Lisa M. Lynch, PhD., Dean*
*Ron Etlinger, Chief Administrative Officer*

**165 Brookdale Center for Healthy Aging**
2180 Third Avenue 212-396-7835
New York, NY 10035 Fax: 212-396-7852
info@brookdale.org
www.brookdale.org
Brookdale Center for Healthy Aging is one of the country's first university-based gerontology centers. The Center is dedicated to improving the lives of older adults through research, professional development, and advancements in policy and practice. Brookdale works to ensure that aging is framed not as a disease, but as another stage in the life course.
*Ruth K. Finkelstein, Executive Director*
*Jerry Antonatos, Director, Finance/Administration*

**166 Brown University Center for Gerontology and Health Care Research**
121 South Main Street 401-863-3211
Providence, RI 02912 Fax: 401-863-3489
CGCHR@brown.edu
www.chcr.brown.edu/
Fundamental and applied research relating to aging, chronic disease, and long-term care with particular emphasis on the assessment of function and health status and its application to diagnosis, prognosis and monitoring of long-term care. Offers data collection and teaching and training services.
*Christina Paxson, President*
*Elizabeth Huidekoper, Executive Vice President*

**167 Brown University Population Studies and Training Center**
Population Studies & Training Center, Brown Univer
PO Box 1836 401-863-2668
Providence, RI 02912 Fax: 401-863-3351
Population_Studies@brown.edu
www.pstc.brown.edu/
Family and household demography, health and fertility transitions in developing nations, infant mortality, child health, social and economic development, migration/immigration and population distribution, aging and health in developed societies and developing nations. Develops new methods for assessing the dynamics of population change, evaluates the causes and consequences of these changes assessment of policies to influence population change.
*Anna Aizer, Associate Professor of Economics*
*Susan M. Allen, Professor of Health Services*

**168 Case Western Reserve University Center for Biomedical Ethics**
Case Western Reserve University
10900 Euclid Avenue 216-368-2000
Cleveland, OH 44106 800-773-2633
Fax: 216-368-8713
xx245@po.cwru.edu
Bioethics, including human genetics, decisions to end life, aging, and reproductive alternatives.
*Thomas Murray PhD, Director*
*Edward M Hundert, President*

**169 Case Western Reserve University Elderly Care Research Center**
Case Western Reserve University
10900 Euclid Avenue 216-368-2000
Cleveland, OH 44106 Fax: 216-368-8713
exk@po.cwru.edu
www.cwru.edu/
Aging, health, and mental health, including public policy issues, predictors of wellness and vulnerability, environmental and social influences on well-being of the elderly, cross-national and cross-cultural comparisons, and health and mental health outcomes of stress, coping, and adaptation.
*Edward Hundert, President*

**170 Case Western Reserve University School of Medicine**
Case Western Reserve University
2103 Cornell Rd. 216-368-3611
Cleveland, OH 44106 Fax: 216-368-0494
www.case.edu/med/pathology
Immunology, immunopathology, aging, cell biology, neurobiology, Alzheimer disease, oncology, and drug delivery.
*John B Lowe MD, Chair Department of Pathology*

171 **Case Western Reserve University: University Center on Aging and Health**
Case Western Reserve University
10900 Euclid Avenue 216-368-2000
Cleveland, OH 44106 Fax: 216-368-6389
pxc127@case.edu
www.cwru.edu/
Conducts, supports, and facilitates research at the University Center on Aging and Health, including the effects of stress and strains, and elderly physical health on persons over 65 years of age. Emphasizes prevention, diagnosis, treatment, management of illness or disability, and service utilization of care giver.
*Diane Lynn Morris PhD RN, Director*
*May L Wykle PhD RN, Dean*

172 **Center for Aging Research and Education at the UW-Madison School of Nursing**
Signe Skott Cooper Hall
701 Highland Avenue 608-265-4330
Madison, WI 53705 care@son.wisc.edu
care.nursing.wisc.edu
CARE seeks to prepare healthcare professionals to work with older adults, as well as encouraging inter-professional and campus-community collaborations.
*Barbara Bowers, Founding Director*
*Barbara King, Executive Director*

173 **Center for Brain Activity Mapping**
UC San Diego
9500 Gilman Drive 858-534-2230
La Jolla, CA 92093 cbam.ucsd.edu
The Center seeks to develop new technologies for detecting neuronal activity, for reporting it out of deep brain tissue, and for processing and analyzing the resulting data, by organizing and supporting research teams and projects.
*Ralph J. Greenspan, PhD, Director*

174 **Center for Human Services**
University Research Co., LLC.
7200 Wisconsin Avenue 301-654-8338
Bethesda, MD 20814 Fax: 301-941-8427
www.urc-chs.com
Quality healthcare research
*Barbara N. Turner, President*
*Dr. David Nicholas, Director*

175 **Center for Neural Recovery and Rehabilitation Research**
Helen Hayes Hospital
51-55 Route 9W North 845-786-4000
West Haverstraw, NY 10993 888-70 -EHAB
Fax: 845-947-3097
TTY: 845-947-3187
Epilepsy, brain injury, and neuroendocrinology. Degenerative neurological disorders such as Huntington's and Alzheimer's diseases are also investigated.
*Ann C. O'Sullivan, Chair*
*Dr. Newton Shaffer, Founder*

176 **Center for the Study of Pharmacy and Therapeutics for the Elderly**
University of Maryland School of Pharmacy
20 North Pine Street 410-706-7650
Baltimore, MD 21201 877-706-2434
Fax: 410-706-4012
lamycenter@rx.umaryland.edu
www.pharmacy.umaryland.edu
Provides educational programs, researches gerontology and geriatrics. Also compiles statistics and maintains a speaker's bureau.
*Natalie D. Eddington, PhD, FAAPS,, Dean and Professor*
*William J. Cooper, Senior Associate Dean*

177 **Central Michigan University: Center for Adult Longitudinal Studies**
Central Michigan University
1200 S. Franklin St 989-774-4000
Mount Pleasant, MI 48859 Fax: 517-794-7406
Measurement of psychological and consumer behavior dimensions of the aging process for adults over the entire lifespan.
*William R. Kanine, Chair*
*George E. Ross, President*

178 **Columbia University Irving Center for Clinical Research**
Columbia University
116th Street and Broadway, 212-854-1754
New York, NY 10027 Fax: 212-305-3213
www.columbia.edu/
Multidisciplinary studies of human disease and clinical pharmacology. Areas include arrhythmia control, heart failure, atherosclerosis, nutrition, metabolism, clinical pharmacology, dermatology, endocrinology, hypertension, immunology, mineral metabolism and skeletal disease, neuromuscular disease, physiology, pulmonary disease, pulmonary physiology, reproductive research studies, andincluding dementia, stroke, and seizure disorders.
*Lee C. Bollinger, President*
*Robert Kasdin, Senior EVP*

179 **Columbia University Robert N. Butler Aging Center**
Mailman School Of Public Health
722 W 168th Street 212-305-0424
New York, NY 10032 aging.columbia.edu
Clinical research in geriatric/gerontology and long-term care, and promotes the study of aging across the university.
*Linda P. Fried, MD, MPH, Interim Co-Director*
*Kavita Sivaramakrishnan, Interim Co-Director, PhD*

180 **Coriell Institute for Medical Research**
403 Haddon Avenue 856-966-7377
Camden, NJ 08103 Fax: 856-964-0254
webmaster@coriell.org
www.coriell.org
Cell and molecular biology, microbiology, genetics, aging, cancer and cancer immunology, tumor virology, antibodies, genetic disorders, vascular disorders, infectious diseases and virus/chromosome relationships, environmental mutagenesis, and genetic probes. Studies utilization of cells grown in tissue culture for isolation and characterization of tumor cell antigens, viruses, genetic abnormalities, tumor viruses, and chromosomes.
*Joseph L Mintzer, Executive VP/COO*
*Josefina J Nash, Director Information Systems*

181 **Creighton University Center for Health Policy and Ethics**
Creighton University
2500 California Plaza 402-280-2700
Omaha, NE 68178 Fax: 402-280-5735
info@creighton.edu
www.creighton.edu/
Cross-cultural ethics, ethical issues involving the elderly and neonates, health care reform, legal ethics, medical economics, nursing ethics, pharmacy ethics, racial and ethnic health concerns, religious ethics, rural health policy, and women's issues.
*Steven Friedriche, Manager*

182 **Creighton University Center for Healthy Aging**
Creighton University
2500 California Plaza 402-280-2700
Omaha, NE 68178 Fax: 402-280-5735
info@creighton.edu
www.creighton.edu/
Focuses on human development, aging and health care for the elderly.
*Timothy R. Lannon, S.J., President*
*Colette O'Meara-McKinney, Associate Vice President*

183 **Dartmouth College Center for Evaluative Clinical Sciences**
Geisel School of Medicine
1 Rope Ferry Rd. 603-650-1200
Hanover, NH 03755 877-367-1797
Fax: 603-650-1202
Geisel.Administration@dartmouth.edu
www.dartmouth.edu/dms/cecs
Evaluative clinical science and health care delivery, including medical care epidemiology, health policy, health behavior, efficacy of medical procedures, quality of medical and surgical care, distribution of health care resources, medical interventions and consequences for patients, care at the end of life, distribution of health care resources across hospital market areas, geriatric health, and sociology of medical organizations.
*Chip Souba, MD, ScD, MBA, VP & Dean*
*Jeff Robbins, Executive Director*

184 **Duke University Center for the Study of Aging and Human Development**
Duke University
Box 3003 DUMC 919-660-7500
Durham, NC 27710 Fax: 919-668-0453
Human and animal physiology, immunology, neuroendocrinology, pharmacology, carcinogenesis, enzyme biochemistry, free radical effects, membrane and receptor function, bone metabolism and osteoporosis, central nervous system structure and function, Alzheimer's disease, dementia, cognitive processes, psychometrics, human personality and behavior, family structure and intergenerational relationships, social factors and illness.
*Harvey J Cohen MD, Director*
*Linda K. George, PhD, Associate Director*

185 **Duke University General Clinical Research Center**
Duke University
PO Box 3854 919-684-8111
Durham, NC 27708 Fax: 919-681-8829
Multidisciplinary, clinical research into the cause, progression, prevention, control, and cure of human disease. Sample projects have studied immunodeficiency diseases, Alzheimer's disease, food allergy, X-linked hypophosphatemic rickets, and cardiovascular disease.
*Harvey J Cohen MD, Director*
*Linda K. George, PhD, Associate Director*

186 **Economic and Social Research Institute**
The Economic and Social Research Institute (ESRI)
Whitaker Square 353-1 8-3200
Dublin 2, DC 20037 Fax: 353-1 8-3210
www.esri.ie/
*Frances Ruane, Director*

187 **Edmund S. Muskie School of Public Service**
University of Southern Maine
PO Box 9300 207-780-4430
Portland, ME 04104 800-800-4USM
Fax: 207-780-4417
webmaster@usm.maine.edu
usm.maine.edu/
Health, rehabilitation and special education, aging, mental health, developmental disabilities, children, youth, and families, and alcoholism. Projects include program evaluations, policy/planning analysis and research, training systems, training and curriculum materials, policy forums, and communication technologies.
*Theodora J. Kalikow, President*
*Michael R. Stevenson, PhD., Provost & VP of Academic Affairs*

188 **Ethel Percy Andrus Gerontology Center**
USC Davis School of Gerontology
3715 McClintock Avenue 213-740-5156
Los Angeles, CA 90089 Fax: 213-740-8241
ldsgero@usc.edu
http://www.usc.edu/gero
Gerontology, including interdisciplinary studies on biological, behavioral, social, and environmental aspects of aging process. Develops and evaluates curricula for training scientific and professional personnel specializing in study of aging processes and for improving associated personal, medical and social disorders, cognitive behavior, employment and retirement, state politics of aging, Alzheimer's disease, income maintenance and more.
*Pinchas Cohen, M.D., Dean*
*Jen Brewer, Administrative Assistant*

189 **Families and Work Institute**
Families and Work Institute
267 5th Avenue 212-465-2044
New York, NY 10016 Fax: 212-465-8637
www.familiesandwork.org
Child care, elder care, family and work issues, men and families, diversity, flexibility, community planning, organizational change, and public policy.
*Ellen Galinsky, President and Co-Founder*
*Anne Weisberg, Vice President - Strategy*

190 **Florida Policy Exchange Center on Aging**
Florida Policy Exchange Center on Aging (FPECA)
13301 Bruce B. Downs Blvd. 813-974-2414
Tampa, FL 33612 Fax: 813-974-5766
fpeca.cbcs.usf.edu/
Aging and aging related issues and policies, particularly effective, innovative programs for elderly in other countries. Activities include studies on crime, housing, health care, aging, service delivery issues, and other issues regarding the elderly.
*Larry Polivka, Director*
*Kathryn Hyer, Ph.D., MPP, Associate Professor and Director*

191 **Florida State University: Pepper Institute on Aging and Public Policy**
Florida State University
600 W. College Avenue 850-644-2525
Tallahassee, FL 32306 Fax: 850-644-2304
mhardy@garnet.acns.fsu.edu
Public policy issues affecting the elderly, including health care, income security, and social welfare. Research programs have included historical and comparative studies of income security programs for the elderly, the elderly in the work force, the elderly and the political system, gender and racial dimensions of poverty in old age, retirement decisions, elder abuse in Florida health care facilities, and alternatives to nursing home care.
*Melissa Hardy, Contact*

192 **Fordham University Third Age Center**
Fordham University
Rose Hill Campus 718-817-1000
Bronx, NY 10458 Fax: 718-817-4769
www.fordham.edu
Concentrates on the intellectual, emotional, economic, spiritual, and cultural opportunities that confront the elderly. Programs include studies on the interface of informal and formal support systems, long-term care and service delivery, alternative forms of housing, older persons in families, neighborhood ethnography, life styles of the suburban elderly, employment and the older worker, religion and aging.

193 **George Washington University Center for Aging, Health and Humanities**
1919 Pennsylvania Avenue NW 202-994-7901
Washington, DC 20006 Fax: 202-296-1229
aging@gwu.edu
nursing.gwu.edu
An interdisciplinary space for university faculty to collaborate on aging research, education, scholarship, and innovations.
*Melissa Batchelor-Murphy, PhD, Director*
*Elizabeth Cobbs, MD, Co-Director*

194 **Georgia Consortium on the Psychology of Aging**
Institute of Gerontology
255 E. Hancock Avenue 706-425-3222
Athens, GA 30602 Fax: 706-425-3221
gerontology@uga.edu
www.geron.uga.edu
Psychology of aging, including basic studies in cognition, and clinical diagnosis and treatment of behavioral dysfunctions most often found with the aged. The Consortium was formed to share training and research resources and to foster interaction between psychologists and other scientists.
*Toni P. Miles, Director*
*Anne P. Glass, Associate Director*

195 **Georgia State University Center for Mature Consumer Studies**
Georgia State University
P.O. Box 3965 404-880-9595
Atlanta, GA 30302 Fax: 404-651-4198
gmoschis@gsu.edu
Mature consumer marketing, with emphasis on industries of special importance to the older consumer, including financial services, health care, housing, leisure, insurance, technology, mass media, and telecommunications industries. Studies include analysis of older consumer needs, lifestyles, purchasing habits and consumption patterns. Serves as an information resource, assisting in strategy development for reaching the mature consumer market.
*Mark Becker, President*
*Jimmy George, Manager*

196 **Geriatrics Education and Research Institute**
University of North Texas Health

3500 Camp Bowie Blvd. 817-735-2600
Fort Worth, TX 76107 Fax: 817-735-2486
tfairchi@hsc.unt.edu
unthsc.edu/

Biology of aging, including fundamental chemical and molecular biological changes that may cause aging; health promotion in older adults including health programs promoting physical, psychological, and social well being; geriatric care and practice including evaluation of new clinical programs, physical/mental functions, long term care system development focusing on case management, and in-home health screen/assessment of home-bound elderly.
*Michael R Williams, DO, MD, MBA, President*
*Jennifer M Trevi□o, MBA, Vice President of Administration*

197 **Gerontological Society of America**
Gerontological Society of America
1220 L Street North West 202-842-1275
Washington, DC 20005 Fax: 202-842-1150
geron@geron.org
www.geron.org

The society was formed in 1945 to promote the scientific study of aging, to encourage exchanges among researchers and practitioners from the various disciplines related to gerontology and to foster the use of gerontological research in forming public policy. Publishes five scientific journals.
*James Appleby, Executive Director and CEO*
*Linda Krogh Harootyan, Deputy Executive Director*

198 **Harvard Brain Tissue Resource Center**
Belmont, MA 02478 800-272-4622
hbtrc@mclean.harvard.edu
www.brainbank.mclean.org

Provides tissues to the neuroscience community for studies of movement disorders, major psychoses, and dementia.
*Sabina Berretta, MD, Director*

199 **Harvard University Division of Health Policy Research and Education**
Harvard School of Public Health
Office of Admissions 617-432-1031
Boston, MA 02115 Fax: 617-432-7080
newhouse@hcp.med.harvard.edu
www.hsph.harvard.edu/

Coordinates health policy resources throughout the University, including suggestion of new research initiatives, stimulation of educational activities, coordination of research and educational efforts, promotion of multidisciplinary analysis of complex health policy issues, and dissemination of health policy findings.
*Julio Frenk, Dean*
*David Hunter, Dean for Academic Affairs*

200 **Harvey A Friedman Center for Aging Washington University**
Institute for Public Health
600 S Taylor 314-747-9192
St. Louis, MO 63110 centerforaging@wustl.edu
publichealth.wustl.edu/aging

Seeks to provide older adults with the greatest opportunity for health, security, and engagement.
*Nancy L. Morrow-Howell, PhD, Director*
*Natalie Galucia, MSW, Center Manager*

201 **Home Instead Center for Successful Aging University of Nebraska Medical Center**
730 S 38th Avenue 402-559-9600
Omaha, NE 68105 webmaster@unmc.edu
www.unmc.edu/homeinsteadcenter

Provides patient care, as well as patient education, and research into promoting independence and aging in place.
*Bradley Britigan, MD, Dean, College of Medicine*

202 **Huffington Center on Aging**
Baylor College of Medicine
1 Baylor Plaza 713-798-4951
Houston, TX 77030 Fax: 713-798-6688
www.bcm.edu/

Cell and molecular biology of aging, cardiovascular disease, and ethics in long-term care.
*Paul Klotman, M.D, President and CEO*
*Steve Sigworth, MD, VP & Chief Medical Officer*

203 **Hunter College of City University of New York: Brookdale Center on Aging**
Hunter College
695 Park Ave 212-772-4000
New York, NY 10065 Fax: 646-366-1041
www.hunter.cuny.edu

Legal support program for social workers, paralegals, attorneys and other professionals engaged in providing advocacy assistance to the elderly poor.
*Jennifer J. Raab, President*
*Vita Rabinowitz, Provost and Vice President*

204 **Indiana Family Institute**
Indiana Family Institute
140 North First Street 317-423-9178
Zionsville, IN 46077 800-269-2959
Fax: 317-423-9421
www.hoosierfamily.org

Family issues research.
*Ryan McCann, Director of Operations*
*Curt Smith, Journalist*

205 **Indiana University Bloomington Center on Aging and Aged**
Indiana University Bloomington
107 S. Indiana Ave. 812-855-4848
Bloomington, IN 47405 Fax: 812-855-6194
AskIU@iu.edu

Gerontology, including developmentally disabled, handicapped, minorities, rural-isolated, and mainstream aging populations.
*Suzanne Thorin, Manager*

206 **Indiana University School of Medicine Center for Aging Research**
545 Barnhill Drive 317-274-8438
Indianapolis, IN 46202 Fax: 317-274-1437
medicine.iu.edu

Research on aging includes brain health, decision-making, physical fitness, transitional and nursing home care, and medication.
*Mark Geraci, MD, Chair, Department of Medicine*
*Samir Gupta, MD, Vice Chair, Research*

207 **Indiana University: Purdue University at Indianapolis**
Indiana University Indianapolis
420 University Blvd. 317-274-5555
Indianapolis, IN 46202 AskIU@iu.edu

Skin diseases, including skin cancer and psoriasis and the genetic changes that occur with these conditions. Wound healing and the aging of skin are also studied.
*Daniel F Spandau, Director*
*Charles Bantz, Manager*

208 **Institute for Community Inclusion**
Institute for Community Inclusion
100 Morrissey Boulevard 617-287-4300
Boston, MA 02125 Fax: 617-287-4352
TTY: 617-287-4350
ici@umb.edu
www.communityinclusion.org

Research in health issues and the community.
*William Kiernan, Director*
*Quinn Barbour, Contact*

209 **International Center for the Disabled**
340 E 24th Street 212-585-6020
New York, NY 10010 Fax: 212-585-6002
jkirk@icdnyc.org
www.icdnyc.org

Promising techniques designed to prevent, reduce, and control disabilities arising from persistent physical disorders. Studies focus on the control of deterioration and disability associated with recurring ear infections in children, symptom magnification in those with disabling conditions, and factors associated with gainful employment. Other projects examine the parameters of post-laryngectomy speech, and nerve conduction patterns.
*Justin B. Wender, Chair*
*Dr. Richard Weber, Vice Chair*

210 **Jean Mayer USDA Human Nutrition Research Center on Aging at Tufts University**
711 Washington Street 617-556-3000
Boston, MA 02111 hnrca.tufts.edu
Makes research contributions to U.S. and international nutrition and physical activity recommendations for older adults.
*Sarah L. Booth, PhD, Director*
*Xiang-Dong Wang, MD, PhD, Associate Director*

211 **John A. Hartford Foundation**
55 E 59th Street 212-832-7788
New York, NY 10022-1713 Fax: 212-593-4913
terry.fulmer@johnahartford.org
www.johnahartford.org
The foundation is dedicated to improving care of older adults, including funding in areas such as age-friendly health systems, family caregiving, serious illness and end-of-life, and communications and special projects.
*Terry Fulmer, PhD, RN, FAAN, President*
*Rani E. Snyder, MPA, Program Director*

212 **Johns Hopkins Center on Aging and Health**
2024 E Monument Street 410-955-0491
Baltimore, MD 21205-2223 Fax: 410-614-9625
coah.jhu.edu
Sponsored by the Johns Hopkins Schools of Medicine and Public Health, COAH is an interdisciplinary group of research faculty seeking to optimize the health of older adults.
*David L. Roth, PhD, Director*
*Brian Buta, MHS, Program Manager*

213 **Johns Hopkins University Institute for Policy Studies**
Wyman Building 410-516-7174
Baltimore, MD 21218 Fax: 410-516-8233
Economic development, at risk youth, economic structural change, problems of the elderly, future of the welfare state, the role of non-profit organizations, youth employment, human resource investment, crime and delinquency, public finance, housing, regional capital flows.
*William R Brody, CEO*
*Donald Steinwachs,Ph.D., Interim Director*

214 **Johns Hopkins University: Center for Immunization Research**
Johns Hopkins University School of Hygiene
624 North Broadway 410-955-1622
Baltimore, MD 21295 Fax: 410-955-2791
Research in vaccine immunization
*Dr. Ruth Karron, Director*
*Florence C. George, Finance Manager*

215 **Kansas State University Center on Aging**
1324 Lovers Lane 785-532-5945
Manhattan, KS 66506 Fax: 785-532-5504
gerontology@k-state.edu
www.he.k-state.edu/aging
Focused on education, research, & outreach in the field of gerontology.
*Gayle Doll, Director*
*Migette Kaup, Chair, Research Committee*

216 **Kavli Foundation**
5715 Mesmer Avenue 424-353-8800
Los Angeles, CA info@kavlifoundation.org
www.kavlifoundation.org
The Foundation supports scientific research into the human brain, in the following scientific fields: Astrophysics, Nanoscience, Neuroscience and Theoretical Physics. Within Neuroscience, the study of aging and brain diseases and disorders is supported.
*Robert W. Conn, PhD, President & CEO*
*Eric Marshall, VP, Public Engagement & Prizes*

217 **Kavli Institute for Brain Science at Columbia University**
Columbia University
3227 Broadway 212-853-1016
New York, NY 10027 Fax: 212-665-9699
kavli@columbia.edu
www.kavli.columbia.edu
The Institute's primary arc of study is how signaling in neural circuits controls cognitive function and behavior, and the development of novel experimental and computational strategies for analyzing these signals.
*Eric R. Kandel, MD, Director*
*Rafael Yuste, MD, PhD, Co-Director*

218 **Kavli Institute for Brain and Mind**
UC San Diego
9500 Gilman Drive kibm@ucsd.edu
La Jolla, CA 92093-0115 kibm.ucsd.edu
The Institute supports research that furthers the understanding of the origins, evolution and mechanisms of human cognition. Of particular interest is Traumatic Brain Injury.
*Fred H. Gage, Co-Director*
*Nicholas C. Spitzer, Co-Director*

219 **Kavli Institute for Fundamental Neuroscience**
UCSF, Sandler Neurosciences Center
675 Nelson Rising Lane 415-476-2018
San Francisco, CA 94158 Fax: 415-502-7332
kavliifn@ucsf.edu
kavliifn.ucsf.edu
The Institute is the central organization for neuroscience research at UCSF and partner institutions, establishing cross-disciplinary teams of scientists and engineers devoted to advancing neuroscience in all its forms.
*Loren Frank, Co-Director*
*Roger Nicoll, Co-Director*

220 **Kavli Institute for Neuroscience at Yale University**
Yale School of Medicine
295 Congress Avenue 203-737-4461
New Haven, CT 06510 203-737-4467
pietro.decamilli@yale.edu
medicine.yale.edu/neuroscience/kavli
The institute studies nervous system development and function.
*Pietro De Camilli, MD, Director*
*Marina Picciotto, PhD, Deputy Director*

221 **Kavli Neural Systems Institute**
The Rockefeller University
1230 York Avenue 212-327-8081
New York, NY 10065 lcole@rockefeller.edu
www.rockefeller.edu/research
The Institute unites scientists at The Rockefeller University in the goal of a comprehensive look at the human brain.
*Leslie Vosshall, PhD, Director*
*Lindsey Cole, Administrator*

222 **Kavli Neuroscience Discovery Institute**
Johns Hopkins University, School of Medicine
725 N Wolfe Street 410-955-4089
Baltimore, MD 21205 Fax: 410-614-6249
KavliNDI@jhu.edu
kavlijhu.org
The Institute looks to advance neuroscience by integrating neuroscience, engineering and computational data science.
*Dwight Bergles, PhD, Director*
*Natasha Hussain, PhD, Scientific Director*

223 **Kent State University Exercise Physiology Lab**
162 Gym Annex 330-672-2930
Kent, OH 44242 Fax: 330-672-2250
eglickma@kent.edu
www.kent.edu/ehhs/exph/index.cfm
Exercise physiology, body composition, and physical fitness, including studies of protein metabolism and exercise, cardiovascular/respiratory responses during exercise in heat and cold, an neuromuscular integration/biomechanics, and psychosocial reactivity to behavioral stressors.
*Ellen L Glickman, PhD FACSM, Professor, Exercise Physiology*

224 **Landon Center on Aging University of Kansas Medical Center**
University of Kansas Medical Center
3901 Rainbow Boulevard 913-588-5000
Kansas City, KS 66160 800-766-3777
Fax: 913-588-1201
mchandler@kumc.edu
www2.kumc.edu/coa

Provides support for interdisciplinary research on the issue of age and aging.
*Matt Chandler, MBA, Program Director*
*Diane Clark, Assistant Director*

225 **Lion's Club International**
300 W 22nd Street 630-571-5466
Oak Brook, IL 60523 Fax: 630-571-8890
lions@lionsclubs.org
www.lionsclubs.org
International organization with over 1.4 million members dedicated to the largest blindness prevention program ('SightFirst').
*Barry J. Palmer, International President*
*Joseph Preston, First Vice President*

226 **Maharishi International University: Lab for Health & Aging Studies**
1000 N 4th Street 641-472-7000
Fairfield, IA 52557 www.mum.edu
*DR. Craig Pearson, Executive Vice president*

227 **Mankind Research Foundation**
1315 Apple Avenue 301-587-8686
Silver Spring, MD 20910 Fax: 301-587-8688
General health research, including conditions associated with aging.s
*Dr. Carl Schneider, President*
*Nader A Dakak MD*

228 **Massachusetts Institute of Technology General Clinical Research Center**
77 Massachusetts Ave 617-253-1000
Cambridge, MA 2139- TTY: ÿ61- 25- 934
dick@mit.edu
Normal human metabolism, physiology, and behavior, including studies on hormones (melatonin and sleep), fates of deuterated amino acids, behavioral and neuroendocrine effect of foods (carbohydrate, protein, and caffeine), effects of drugs on memory and other behaviors, and endocrine and metabolic effects on aging. Also studies human diseases such as obesity, Alzheimer's disease, brain injury, Parkinson's disease, and seasonal depression.
*Dr. Richard J Wartman, Program Director*
*Joe Graham, Manager*

229 **Mayo Clinic and Foundation-General Clinical Research Center**
St. Mary's Hospital
200 First Street SW 507-284-2511
Rochester, MN 55905 Fax: 507-538-7802
www.mayoclinic.org
Researches inpatient and outpatient sleep pattern, cardiac telemetry monitoring, endocrinology and many other medical issues.
*Jeffrey Rome, Manager*

230 **Medical University of South Carolina Center on Aging**
280 Calhoun Street 843-792-0712
Charleston, SC 29425 education.musc.edu/colleges/medicine
Engages in research, services, and education with the aim of promoting health, quality of life, and longevity for seniors.
*Heather Boger, Interim Director*

231 **Minneapolis Medical Research Foundation**
701 Park Avenue 612-875-3000
Minneapolis, MN 55415
General health research
*Paul Pentel, President*
*Carla Erickson, Director*

232 **Mount Sinai School of Medicine of City University of New York**
Department of Geriatrics & Adult Development
PO Box 1070 212-241-5561
New York, NY 10029 Fax: 212-860-9737
www.icahn.mssm.edu
Health, long-term care, and productive aging, emphasizing policy implications for future generations and institutions.
*Siu Albert, Chair*

233 **National Academy on an Aging Society**
1220 L Street NW 202-842-1275
Washington, DC 20005 Fax: 202-842-1150
geron@geron.org
www.geron.org
The policy branch of the Gerontological Society of America, the NAAS is a non-partisan institute conducting research on population aging.
*James Appleby, Chief Executive Officer*
*Judie Lieu, VP, Publishing & Professional Resources*

234 **National Institute on Aging Gerontology Research Center**
251 Bayview Boulevard 410-558-8110
Baltimore, MD 21224 longod@grc.nia.nih.gov
www.grc.nia.nih.gov/
Gerontology research, including molecular genetics, human physiology, personality, behavioral research, and Alzheimer's disease studies.
*Robin Barr, Director*

235 **National Institute on Aging: Information Center**
31 Center Drive 301-496-1752
Bethesda, MD 20892 800-222-2225
www.nia.nih.gov
Concerned with the health problems of older Americans. The Center offers free printed materials, including fact sheets about going to the hospital and about prostate problems.
*Richard J. Hodes, M.D., Director*
*Marie A. Bernard, M.D., Deputy Director*

236 **Neuropsychiatric Research Institute**
700 1st Avenue S 701-293-1335
Fargo, ND 58103 Fax: 701-293-3226
mail@nrifargo.com
Basic and clinical studies of the central nervous system. Specific applications include eating disorders, studies of Alzheimer's disease, Parkinson's disease, Huntington's disease, and schizophrenia.
*James Mitchell, President*

237 **Neuroscience Research Institute**
UC Santa Barbara
6129 Biology II 805-893-4621
Santa Barbara, CA 93106 www.nri.ucsb.edu
The Institute seeks to allow scientists from different fields to collaborate for the betterment of neurological research. Areas of interest include: Alzheimer's Disease & Related Dementias; Behavioral Neuroscience & Neuroethology; Cell Biology, Biochemistry & Biophysics of the Nervous System; Computational & Theoretical Neuroscience; Development of the Nervous System; and Stem Cells.
*Stuart Feinstein, Co-Director*
*Kenneth Kosik, Co-Director*

238 **New York State Institute for Basic Research in Developmental Disabilities**
1050 Forest Hill Road 718-494-0600
Staten Island, NY 10314 Fax: 718-494-0833
www.omr.state.ny.us/
*Dr Piotr B Kozlowski, Director*
*William T Brown MD*

239 **Nisonger Center**
Ohio State University
281 W. Lane Avenue 614-292-8365
Columbus, OH 43210 Fax: 614-292-3727
reiss.7@osu.edu
nisonger.osu.edu
Developmental disabilities, psychometric assessment, rehabilitation engineering, psychopathology, psychopharmacology, adults and aging, and family studies. Special attention given to applied research related to mental retardation and development and implementation of training programs to prepare professional personnel to work with the developmentally disabled. Provides early childhood classes for developmentally disabled preschoolers.
*Steven Reiss, Executive Director*

240 **Noll Physiological Research Center**
Pennsylvania State University
129 Noll Laboratory Building 814-865-3453
University Park, PA 16802 Fax: 814-865-4602
www.noll.psu.edu
Metabolic adaptations to stress, biology of aging, and environmental and exercise physiology. Studies the effects of aging, physical activity, nutritional status, and heat, cold, and altitude stress

on muscle metabolism and function, thermoregulation and cardiovascular control, immune function, and carbohydrate, insulin, and protein metabolism.

241 **Northwestern University: Buehler Center on Aging**
750 N Lake Shore Drive 312-503-3087
Chicago, IL 60611 Fax: 312-503-5868
Aging research
*Dr. James R Webster, Director*
*Linda Emmanuel, Executive Director*

242 **Northwestern University: General Clinical Research Center**
303 E Chicago Avenue 312-503-8649
Chicago, IL 60611 www.northwestern.edu
*Ennio C Rossi MD*

243 **Ohio State University Neuroscience Program**
333 W 10th Avenue 614-292-2379
Columbus, OH 43210 ngsp@osu.edu
www.ngsp.osu.edu
Spinal cord injury, tumor biology, neuromuscular disease, epilepsy, Parkinson Disease, multiple sclerosis, stroke, neural development, regeneration, plasticity, regeneration, molecular neurobiology, and neuroimmunology.

244 **Olive View: UCLA Education and Research Institute**
14445 Olive View Drive 818-364-3205
Sylmar, CA 91342 www.uclaoliveview.org
Researches head injury, neurology, perinatal issues, genetic counseling and other health related studies.
*Soma Wali, MD, FACP, Program Director*
*Michael Rotblatt, MD, PharmD, Sr. Associate Program Director*

245 **Oregon Research Institute**
1776 Millrace Drive 541-484-2123
Eugene, OR 97403 Fax: 541-484-1108
www.ori.org
Behavioral sciences, including studies in tobacco prevention and cessation, compliance with diabetic regimens, children's social skills, personality structure, drug abuse prevention, depression and family interaction, special education technology, adolescent depression, and community child-rearing practices. Provides behavioral research and consultation services to other public and private agencies in fields of education and mental health.
*Amy Greenwold, Manager*

246 **Orentreich Foundation for the Advancement of Science**
855 Route 301 845-265-4200
Cold Spring, NY 10516 www.orentreich.org
Dermatology, aging, endocrinology, and serum markers for human diseases.
*Norman Orentreich, President*

247 **Pennsylvania State University Center for Developmental and Health Genetics**
101 Amy Gardner House 814-865-5471
University Park, PA 16802 Fax: 814-863-4768
www.psu.edu
Role of genetics in infant, child, and adolescent behavioral development, in aging, and in common drug and health problems. Also studies molecular, nutritional and immunological genetics. Uses human and animal model research projects to study personality, cognition, functional capacity, immune system functioning, and use and effects of alcohol and tobacco.
*Gerald McCleam, Director*
*Randy Deike, Manager*

248 **Pennsylvania State University Gerontology Center**
312 Old Main 814-865-7517
University Park, PA 16802 arh1@psu.edu
Broad interdisciplinary approach to questions on aging. Major areas of research are cognition in aging, developmental methodology, family and informal supports, and animal models of aging. Specific topics include reversing cognitive decline, human services for the elderly, caregiving, urinary incontinence, and the use of pharmaceutical products.

249 **Pennsylvania State University: Noll Physiological Research Center**
129 Noll Laboratory Building 814-865-3453
University Park, PA 16802 Fax: 814-865-4602
www.noll.psu.edu
Researches metabolic adaptations to stress, the effects of physical activities, nutritional status and other related topics.

250 **Peter Lamy Center for Drug Therapy and Aging**
University of Maryland School Pharmacy
20 North Pine Street 410-706-7650
Baltimore, MD 21201 Fax: 410-706-4012
lamycenter@rx.umaryland.edu
www.pharmacy.umaryland.edu
The Lamy Center is dedicated to improving drug therapy for aging adults through innovative research, education and clinical initiatives.
*Natalie D. Eddington, PhD, FAAPS,, Dean*

251 **Population Reference Bureau**
1875 Connecticut Avenue NW 800-877-9881
Washington, DC 20009 communications@prb.org
www.prb.org
Demography, particularly national and international population trends as they relate to education, aging, employment, minority populations, health and welfare, and the environment.
*Jeffrey Jordan, President & CEO*
*Viresh Desai, CFO*

252 **Portland State University Institute on Aging**
PO Box 751 503-725-4043
Portland, OR 97207
Adult development and aging, including health and social care systems, social and economic life maintenance, political behavior, age status, economic behavior, social and psychological phenomena, and communication.
*Alba Scholz, Manager*

253 **Purdue University: Center for Research on Aging and the Life Course**
1202 W. State Street 765-494-9692
W Lafayette, IN 47907-2055 Fax: 765-494-2180
calc@purdue.edu
www.purdue.edu/aging
Social science research on aging, health and health care delivery.
*Kenneth F. Ferraro, PhD, Director*
*Paige Ebner, Assistant Director*

254 **Rehabilitation Research and Training Center on Aging With a Disability**
Rancho Los Amigos Medical Center
7601 Imperial Highway 562-401-7111
Downey, CA 90242 TTY: 562-401-8450
TDD: 562-401-
Aging research
*Jorge Orozco, PT, CEO*

255 **Research Institute of the Hebrew Home of Greater Washington**
6121 Montrose Road 301-881-0300
Rockville, MD 20852 Fax: 301-770-8309
cohen-mansfield@hebrew-home.org
Gerontology, aging, and issues concerning the elderly, focusing on nursing home residents, their families, and staff. Areas include: agitated behaviors among the elderly; stress in families caring for elderly relatives; staff stress; back injuries among staff caretakers; the preferences of nursing home residents regarding life-sustaining treatments; standardized assessment procedures of the physical and emotional states of nursing home residents.
*Warren R. Slavin, CEO/President*
*Douglas W.ÿ Sherman, Secretary*

256 **Retirement Research Foundation**
8765 W Higgins Road 773-714-8080
Chicago, IL 60631 Fax: 773-714-8089
info@rrf.org
Supports research to improve the well-being of elderly persons in the US Also provides support for model demonstration projects.
*Patrick McCarthy, President/CEO*

257 **Rockefeller University Laboratory of Neuroendocrinology**
1230 York Avenue Bruce.McEwen@rockefeller.edu
New York, NY 10065
Seeks to locate brain sites and understand the mechanisms by which hormones promote neural plasticity and thereby alter endocrine function, behavior, neurological states, and mood. Also studies the influence of gonadal and adrenal hormones on aging in the brain.

258 **Roy M and Phyllis Gough Huffington Center on Aging**
Baylor College of Medicine
One Baylor Plaza 713-798-5804
Houston, TX 77030 fincher@bcm.edu
www.hcoa.org
Internal unit of Baylor College representing research into the biology of aging.
*Hui Zheng , PhD, Director*
*Ruth Andrea Reeves, MBA, BA, AAS, Center Administrator*

259 **Rush University Neuroscience Institute**
Rush-Presbyterian-St. Luke's Medical Center
1653 W Congress Pkwy 312-942-5000
Chicago, IL 60612 www.rush.edu
Alzheimer's disease, Parkinson's disease, and stroke, including community-based studies, clinical investigations, and laboratory investigations using brain tissue and animal experimentation. Studies also focus on development of new drugs to improve symptoms of multiple sclerosis.
*Dr. Jacob H Fox, Chairperson*
*Larry J. Goodman, CEO*

260 **Rush University: Rush Institute for Healthy Aging**
1645 W Jackson Boulevard 312-421-8940
Chicago, IL 60612 Fax: 312-942-2861
devans2@rush.edu
www.rush.edu
Epidemiology of Alzheimer's disease, community-based studies of Alzheimer's disease and other common problems of older persons, physical functions among older persons, and statistical methods in aging research.
*Dennis A Evans PhD, Contact*

261 **Rutgers University Institute for Health, Health Care Policy: and Aging Research**
112 Paterson Street 848-932-8413
New Brunswick, NJ 08901 caboyer@rci.rutgers.edu
www.ihhcpar.rutgers.edu
Research divisions include and focus on the impact of stress on emotional states and health and risk behaviors and how these latter factors influence the immune system and morbidity and mortality.
*Joel C. Cantor, Sc.D., Director*

262 **Salk Institute for Biological Studies**
10010 N Torrey Pines Road 858-453-4100
La Jolla, CA 92037 www.salk.edu
Conducts groundbreaking research into cancer, aging, Alzheimer's diabetes and infectious diseases.
*Rusty Gage, PhD, President*
*Martin Hetzer, PhD, VP & Chief Science Officer*

263 **San Jose State University Gerontology Education and Training Center**
1 Washington Square 408-924-1000
San Jose, CA 95112 www.sjsu.edu/
Gerontology and the social aspects of aging, focusing on personal autonomy of elderly persons in long-term care and ethnogerontology.

264 **Sanders-Brown Center on Aging University of Kentucky**
800 S Limestone Street 859-323-6040
Lexington, KY 40536-0230 Fax: 859-323-2866
linda.vaneldik@uky.edu
www.uky.edu/coa
Investigates healthy brain aging and neurodegenerative disorders through research, education and outreach, and clinical programs.
*Linda J. Van Eldik, PhD, Director*
*Gregory A. Jicha, MD, PhD, Associate Director*

265 **Sanford Center for Aging University of Nevada, Reno**
Center for Molecular Medicine
1664 North Virginia Street 775-784-4774
Reno, NV 89557 Fax: 775-784-1814
sanford@unr.edu
med.unr.edu/aging
Aims to enhance the quality of life and well-being among older adults through education, research, and outreach.
*Peter Reed, PhD, MPH, Director*
*Heather Haslem, Director, Wellness*

266 **Sanford Consortium for Regenerative Medicine**
2880 Torrey Pines Scenic Drive 858-246-1071
La Jolla, CA 92037 www.sanfordconsortium.com
The Consortium works to achieve breakthrough discoveries in stem cell research with regards to diagnoses, treatments, and cures for degenerative diseases and injuries.
*Edward W. Holmes, MD, President & CEO*
*Jeffrey Steindorf, PhD, VP & COO*

267 **Scripps Research Institute**
10550 North Torrey Pines Road 858-784-1000
La Jolla, CA www.scripps.edu
The institute seeks to improve human wellbeing through the advancement of bioscience, including research into aging & healthspan, autoimmune diseases, cancer, infectious diseases, neurological disorders, and more.
*Peter Schultz, PhD, President & CEO*
*Eric Topol, MD, EVP, Scripps Research*

268 **SeniorNet**
5237 Summerlin Commons Boulevard 239-275-2202
Fort Myers, FL 33907 Fax: 239- 27- 250
seniornet@aol.com
www.seniornet.org
Interaction between computers and older individuals through online telecomputer system. Studies include psychological effects of the computer on the individual at the introduction, learning, and user levels.

269 **Southwest Foundation for Biomedical Research**
PO Box 760549 210-258-9400
San Antonio, TX 78245 fledford@sfbr.org
www.txbiomed.org/
Aging research
*Richard Schlosberg, Chairman*
*Lewis J. Moorman III, Vice Chairman*

270 **Stanford Center on Longevity**
Littlefield Center, Stanford University
365 Lasuen Street 650-736-8643
Stanford, CA 94305-6053 info-longevity@stanford.edu
longevity.stanford.edu
Seeks to advance scientific discoveries, advances in technology, and behavioral and social norms with the goal of enhancing century-long lives.
*Laura Carstensen, PhD, Director*
*Nancy Easterbrook, Director, External Affairs*

271 **Stein Institute for Research on Aging UC San Diego School of Medicine**
9500 Gilman Drive 858-534-6299
La Jolla, CA 92093-0012 Fax: 858-534-5475
aging@ucsd.edu
medschool.ucsd.edu/research/aging
Develops and applies recent advances in biomedical and behavioral science to issues of healthy aging, and reducing the burden of disease and disability in later life.
*Dilip V. Jeste, MD, Director*
*Deborah Kado, MD, MS, Deputy Director, Clinical Research*

272 **Syracuse University Biological Research Laboratories**
Syracuse University
114 Life Sciences Complex 315-443-3186
Syracuse, NY 13244 Fax: 314-443-2012
hrlevy@mailbox.syr.edu
Aging and aging conditions research.

273 **Syracuse University Center for Policy Research**
426 Eggers Hall 315-443-3114
Syracuse, NY 13244 Fax: 314-443-1081
ctrpol@syr.edu

Economics and demography of aging, income security policy, long-term care, gender and minority aging, and cross-national aging comparisons.
*Leonard M. Lopoo, Director*

274 **Tampa Bay Research Institute**
10900 Roosevelt Boulevard N 727-576-6675
St Petersburg, FL 33716 Fax: 727-577-9862
www.tbri.org
*Akiko Tanaka, CEO*

275 **Temple University: General Clinical Research Center**
Medical education and research Bui 215-707-4045
Philadelphia, PA 19140 Fax: 215-707-0170
www.temple.edu
*Bryant Tabb, Director*

276 **The Center on Aging and Work at Boston College**
140 Commonwealth Avenue 617-552-9195
Chestnut Hill, MA 02467 agework@bc.edu
www.bc.edu/research/agingandwork
Conducts research into quality of employment for a multi-generational workforce.
*Jacquelyn B. James, PhD, Interim Co-Director*
*Tay K. McNamara, PhD, Interim Co-Director*

277 **Thomas Jefferson University: Center for Research in Medical Education**
Jefferson Medical College
1025 Walnut Street 215-955-8907
Philadelphia, PA 19107 Fax: 215-923-6939
www.jefferson.edu
*Joseph Gonnella MD, Director*

278 **Tulane University Center For Aging**
1430 Tulane Avenue 504-988-3369
New Orleans, LA 70112 aging-studies@tulane.edu
medicine.tulane.edu
Dedicated to enhancing the quality of life of aging adults through research, education, and innovation.
*S. Michal Jazwinski, PhD, Director*

279 **Tulane University Occupational Lung Disease Center**
School of Medicine
1430 Tulane Avenue 504-988-5187
New Orleans, LA 70112 www.tulane.edu
*Dr. Hans Weill, Director*
*James V Talano MD*

280 **UCSF Memory and Aging Center**
Sandler Neurosciences Center 415-353-2057
San Francisco, CA 94143
The UCSF Memory and Aging Center provides the highest quality of care for individuals with cognitive problems, to conduct research for degenerative brain diseases, and to educate health professionals, patients, and their families. The Memory and Aging Center also publishes a biannual newsletter, as well as other publications.
*Dr. Bruce Miller, Director*

281 **USDA Human Nutrition Research Center on Aging**
711 Washington Street 617-556-3000
Boston, MA 02111 hnrca.tufts.edu
Investigates the relationship of nutrition to aging, including research programs in nutrient metabolism, nutrient requirements, nutritional epidemiology, functional systems, and drug-nutrient interactions.
*Simin Nibkin Meydani, D.V.M., Director*

282 **University at Albany: State University of New York Ringel Gerontology Institute**
State University of New York
135 West Avenue 518-442-5346
Albany, NY 12222 Fax: 518-442-3823
iog@albany.edu
Applied research on aging, primarily in the social sciences, and services for the elderly, including studies on institutional and noninstitutional care of the elderly, nursing homes, day care, foster home care, the church as service provider, retirement and preretirement, and other social aspects of aging. Collaborates in the development of community programs and their evaluation.
*Frank D Andraia, Executive Director*

283 **University of Akron Institute for Life Span Development and Gerontology**
University of Akron
340 Arts and Sciences Building 330-972-6724
Akron, OH 44325 Fax: 330-972-5174
hsterns@uakron.edu
www3.uakron.edu/ilsdg
Improving older adult cognitive functioning, aging and work, mental retardation and aging, training and retraining adult older workers, gender identity, human development, health and aging, and family and aging. Programs concentrate on aging changes in perception, perceptual style, selective attention, and learning and memory. Other studies focus on performance appraisal and selection of older adult workers.
*Harvey L Sterns, Director*

284 **University of California, San Francisco Dept of Social and Behavioral Sciences**
3333 California Street 415-476-1435
San Francisco, CA 94143 Fax: 415-476-9707
Sponsors pre- and postdoctoral research and training activities in the areas of stress and illness, cognitive factors in health behavior, mental health and aging, adult development, gerontology, Alzheimer's Disease, and AIDS.
*Morris Schambelan, MD*

285 **University of California: Center for Health & Community**
3333 California Street 415-476-7408
San Francisco, CA 94143 Fax: 415-502-1010
chc@chc.ucsf.edu
www.chc.ucsf.edu
Facilitate multidisciplinary research that will provide comprehensive understanding of problems of health, illness and health care.
*Nancy E Adler PhD, Director*
*Dina Dudum MPA, Manager*

286 **University of California: San Diego Center for Population Research**
06339500 Gilman Drive 858-534-3703
La Jolla, CA 92093 repromed@ucsd.edu
Hypothalamic control of the pituitary and gonadal function in human and animal models, focusing on issues related to neuroendicrine metabolic dysfunction in the aging population.
*Homer G Chin, Chief, Obstetrics & Gynecology*
*Steven C Plaxe, Chief, Gynecologic Oncology*

287 **University of California: San Francisco Institute for Health and Aging**
Laurel Hights Campus 3333 415-502-5200
San Francisco, CA 94143 Fax: 415-502-5208
Aging health policy issues and policy alternatives; state discretionary policies in long-term care, social services, and income maintenance; private sector involvement in supporting health and social services for the elderly; effects of intergovernmental relations and state and federal fiscal conditions on services to the elderly; coordination between state and local aging programs and health planning, financing, and regulatory programs.
*Wendy Max, Director*
*Lena Borodina, Manager*

288 **University of Chicago Brain Research Institute**
5801 South Ellis Avenue 773-702-1234
Chicago, IL 60637 infocenter@uchicago.edu
www.uchicago.edu
Alzheimer's disease, amyotrophic lateral sclerosis, myasthenia gravis, AIDS, sleep and sleep disorders, dyslexia, hyperkinesia, epilepsy and epileptoid disorders, mental retardation, mental illness, and brain and nervous system disorders such as multiple sclerosis, muscular dystrophy, cerebral palsy, encephalitis, Parkinson's disease, stroke, cerebral hemorrhage, aneurysm tumor, head injury, and intractable pain.
*Bryce Wier MD, Director*
*Sue Curtis, Manager*

289 **University of Chicago Committee on Human Development**
5736 S Woodlawn Avenue 773-702-3971
Chicago, IL 60637
Conducts research and graduate study in life course development (including child and adolescent development, adult development and aging, and philosophy of development), mental health research (including personality psychology), and cross-cultural studies (including psychological anthropology and cultural psychology). Seeks to provide education for innovative careers in research and teaching.
*Susan Cohen, Manager*

290 **University of Connecticut Center on Aging**
135 Dowling Way 860-679-8400
Farmington, CT 06030 health.uconn.edu/aging
Provides care for older adults, as well as conducting research into the aging process in order to promote health and quality of life.
*George A. Kuchel, MD, Director*

291 **University of Connecticut Health Center: Biomolecular Structure Analysis Center**
263 Farmington Avenue 860-679-2000
Farmington, CT 06030
Drug-membrane interaction, drug-receptor interaction, membrane drug design, pulmonary surfactant research, and collagen structure research as it relates to cardiology, alcoholism, Alzheimer's disease, CNS disorders, skeletal and smooth muscle disorders, and atherosclerosis.
*Dr. Leo G Herbette, Director*
*Lee Ann Maximowicz, Administrator*

292 **University of Florida Brain Institute**
JHMHC
PO Box 100015 352-273-8500
Gainesville, FL 32610 Fax: 352-846-0185
Peripheral Nerve Trauma Research Program, including biomaterials research, peripheral nerve regeneration, and mechanisms and control of pain associated with peripheral nerve trauma; Head Injury Research Program, including injury- and/or stroke-induced problems with memory, language, attention, emotion, motor skills, and epilepsy; molecular, cellular, and immunological mechanisms involved in nerve cell death and injury following stroke.
*William G Luttge PhD, Director*

293 **University of Florida Health Policy and Epidemiology**
2004 Mowry Road 352-273-5468
Gainesville, FL 32610
Policy research and evaluations of long-term care and aging, hospital cost controls, regulatory and administrative methods in the health sector, health economics and financing, maternal and child health, HIV/AIDS, community epidemiology, outcomes research.
*Dr.Thomas A. Pearson, Executice VP*

294 **University of Florida Institute on Aging**
2004 Mowry Road 352-294-5800
Gainesville, FL 32611 lcrump@ufl.edu
aging.ufl.edu
The IOA operates interdisciplinary teams in research, education and health care, dedicated to improving the health, independence, and quality of life for older adults.
*Marco Pahor, MD, Director*
*Lauren Crump, MPH, Associate Director*

295 **University of Florida: Claude D Pepper Center: Research on Oral Health & Aging**
PO Box 100405 352-273-5800
Gainesville, FL 32610 mheft@dental.ufl.edu
www.dental.ufl.edu
Health services research and basic oral-health functions of the elderly, including the development of periodontal disease, the effects of medications on saliva production, and the effects of aging on the senses.

296 **University of Florida: Institute for Gerontology**
PO Box 117335 352-392-3261
Gainesville, FL 32611 rwest@geron.ufl.edu
Faculty associates conduct interdisciplinary studies on family economic status, labor force participation and survivorship in life course perspective, alternative living environments for older people, political attitudes and policy issues in aging, preventive health self-care learning for intergenerational groups, nutritional status of elderly, memory fitness and intelligence in adulthood and old age, training needs of counselors and physicians.
*Robin Lea West, Contact*

297 **University of Georgia: Gerontology Center**
255 E. Hancock Avenue 706-425-3222
Athens, GA 30602 Fax: 706-425-3221
www.geron.uga.edu
Aging, focusing on applied gerontology, demography as it relates to the aged, mental and physical health of the oldest-old, Alzheimer's disease and other dementia in the aged, and cognitive aging, especially memory for pictures.
*Leonard W Poon PhD, Director*

298 **University of Illinois Health Systems Research**
College of Medicine
1601 Parkview Avenue 815-395-5630
Rockford, IL 61107 800-854-4461
Fax: 815-395-5602
www.rockford.uic.edu/hsr.htm
Community health, including primary care, public health, geriatrics, substance abuse, evaluation of delivery of health services, survey research, focus groups, demographic studies, health care planning, program evaluation, and feasibility studies.
*Joel B Cowen, Assistant Dean*

299 **University of Iowa Center for Health Services Research**
200 Hawkins Drive 319-384-3830
Iowa City, IA 52242 www.public-health.uiowa.edu/hmp/
Delivery, organization, and financing of health care. Studies the health practices and needs of specific populations such as individuals in rural areas. Develops multidisciplinary research teams from the University's ten colleges and facilitates interaction between researchers, policy makers, and providers to address regional health care problems.

300 **University of Kansas Laboratory of Biological Anthropology**
Department of Anthropology
622 Fraiser Hall 785-864-4172
Lawrence, KS 66045 crawford@ku.edu
Cancer etiology, twin research, aging and longevity, genetic epidemiology, anthropological genetics in Saint Vincent, Hungary, Mexico, Siberia, Belize, rural and urban US ethnic enclaves, dental anthropology, forensic medicine, and skeletal identification.
*Michael H Crawford PhD, Director*

301 **University of Kansas Neurobiology Research Laboratory**
4801 E Linwood Boulevard 816-861-4700
Kansas City, MO 64128 Fax: 816-922-3375
Development, plasticity, and diseases of the nervous system. Studies focus on synaptic formation and metabolism; roles of serine proteases and inhibitors (serpins); regulation of amyloid precursor protein processing in Alzheimer's disease; and biological markers in head injuries.
*Barry W Festoff, Director*
*Kent Hill, Executive Director*

302 **University of Kansas: Center on Aging**
Kansas University Medical Center
3901 Rainbow Boulevard 913-588-5000
Kansas City, KS 66160 Fax: 913-588-1201
www2.kumc.edu/coa
Provides support for interdisciplinary research on issues of age and aging.
*Linda J Redford, RN, PhD, Director*

303 **University of Kansas: Gerontology Center**
1000 Sunnyside Avenue 785-864-4130
Lawrence, KS 66045 Fax: 785-864-5063
www.gerontology.ku.edu
Aging and the problems of the aged, including applied and social gerontology, family caregiving, minority aging, service to the aging, cognitive aging, and housing options for elders.
*David J. Ekerdt, Director*

304 **University of Kentucky: Sanders-Brown Center on Aging**
800 S Limestone Street 859-323-6040
Lexington, KY 40536 Fax: 859-323-2866

Biology of aging, including studies on the aging nervous systems, Alzheimer's disease, stroke, immunology.
*Linda J. Van Eldik, PhD, Director*

305 **University of Maryland Division of Infectious Diseases**
10 S Pine Street 410-706-7560
Baltimore, MD 21201 800-492-5538
www.umm.edu
Infections in the elderly, including infection from urinary catheterization, epidemiology of nursing home patients, tests of antimicrobial agents, and pharmacokinetics and microbiology using animal models and clinical techniques.

306 **University of Maryland School of Public Health Center on Aging**
4200 Valley Drive 301-405-2438
College Park, MD 20742-2611 Fax: 301-405-8397
asmaa@umd.edu
sph.umd.edu
An interdisciplinary institution conducting applied and policy research, education, and public service into human aging.
*Luisa Franzini, PhD, Director*
*Jim Hagberg, PhD, Associate Director*

307 **University of Maryland: Center for the Study of Pharmacy and Therapeutics**
School of Pharmacy
20 N Pine Street 410-706-7650
Baltimore, MD 21201 Fax: 410-706-4012
Geriatrics and gerontology, focusing on drug use in the elderly and the development of artificial intelligence programs in support of optimal drug use. Also responsible for three elder care programs, the Parke-Davis Center for the Education of the Elderly, the Elder-Health Program, and the Maryland Caregiver Program.
*Natalie D Eddington, PhD, FAAPS,, Dean*

308 **University of Massachusetts at Boston: Gerontology Institute and Center**
100 Morrissey Boulevard 617-287-7300
Dorchester, MA 02125 Fax: 617-287-7080
www.geront.umb.edu
Aging Journal of Aging social policy, including health care, economics, security, long-term care, productive aging, systems delivery, older women's issues, and minority issues.
*110 pages*
*Robert P Gerary, Managing Editor*

309 **University of Miami Center for Neurological Diseases**
PO Box 16960 305-243-6732
Miami, FL 33101 800-707-5589
Fax: 305-243-1632
Neuroscience, including physiological, neurochemical, anatomical, metabolic, neuropharmacological and vascular mechanisms that account for normal brain function, and the changes in these which underlie neurological diseases such as stroke, senile dementia, epilepsy, Parkinson's syndrome, Alzheimer's disease, multiple sclerosis, amyotrophic lateral sclerosis (ALS), and other neurological dysfunctions.
*Adams David MD, Contact*
*Matilde Camjel, Manager*

310 **University of Miami Touch Research Institute**
PO Box 16820 305-585-5160
Miami, FL 33101 Fax: 305-243-6488
www.miami.edu/touch-research
Sense of touch, including the biology of touch in health and development, and the role of touch therapy in medicine and the treatment of disease. Specific research areas include the use of massage in enhancing immune function in AIDS and cancer patients, massage effects on growth in premature infants, underlying mechanism responsible for the relationship between touch and physical growth and emotional development in infants and children.
*Tiffany M Field PhD, Contact*
*Noris Reyes, Manager*

311 **University of Miami: Center on Adult Development and Aging**
1695 N.W. 9th Avenue 305-355-9080
Miami, FL 33136 Fax: 305-355-9076
Biochemistry, neuropsychiatry, and clinical treatment of Alzheimer's disease and related disorders, including brain reactive antibodies and autoimmune responses. Also studies ethnicity and aging, human factors and aging, aging and developmental disabilities, biology of aging, osteoporosis, social and behavioral patterns of older persons and families, stress and aging, nutrition and aging, and demographics of elderly population in Florida
*Chaerles B. Nemeroff, M.D., Ph.D, Director*

312 **University of Michigan Center for Human Growth and Development**
500 S. State Street 734-764-1817
Ann Arbor, MI 48109 blozoff@umich.edu
www.umich.edu/tld/chgd
Human growth and development through childhood and adolescence, including interdisciplinary studies on normal and abnormal behavioral, physical, and mental development, focusing especially on the challenges to children who grow up in adverse conditions.
*Betsy Lozoff PhD, Director*

313 **University of Michigan: Antiviral Laboratory**
4222 School of Dentistry
1500 E. Medical Center Drive 734-615-0863
Ann Arbor, MI 48109 855-855-0863
jcdrach@umich.edu
www.umich.edu
Antiviral research
*Dr. John C Drach Hd, Contact*

314 **University of Michigan: Institute of Gerontology**
300 N Ingalls Street 734-764-3493
Ann Arbor, MI 48109 Fax: 734-936-2116
www.med.umich.edu
Gerontological research studies in the behavioral, biological, clinical, and social sciences and the humanities.
*Joan A Faulkner PhD, Director*

315 **University of Minnesota: Center on Aging**
School of Public Health
PO Box 197 612-624-1185
Minneapolis, MN 55455 www.coa.umn.edu
Aging.

316 **University of Missouri Kansas City: Center for Aging Studies**
5100 Rockhill Road 816-235-1000
Kansas City, MO 64110 breytspraak@umkc.edu
Caregiving to the elderly, health care systems and costs, health promotion/disease prevention, public perceptions of Social Security, voluntarism among the elderly, the care of Chinese elderly, and rural elderly. Rural studies include program assessment and testing in areas of health promotion/disease prevention, caregiving intergenerational relationships and the elderly, transportation, and housing.
*Stephen W Lehmkuhle, Manager*

317 **University of North Carolina School of Medicine Center for Aging and Health**
5003 Old Clinic 919-966-5945
Chapel Hill, NC 27599 www.med.unc.edu/aging
Provides care for older patients, provides community resources to families and caregivers, and trains not only geriatricians, but other medical professionals in geriatric medicine.
*Jan Busby-Whitehead, Director*
*Ben Blomberg, Assistant Clinical Professor*

318 **University of North Dakota: UND Center for Rural Health**
501 North Columbia Road Stop 9037
Grand Forks, ND 58202 Fax: 701-777-6779
bgibbens@medicine.nodak.edu
http://medicine.nodak.edu/crh
Rural health care delivery, especially in the areas of health professional shortage areas, the viability of rural health facilities, aging population, Native American health care, and uncompensated care. Collaborates with other research organizations throughout the nation.
*Gary Hart, PhD, Director*

319 **University of North Texas Health Science Center at Forth Worth: Geriatrics**
3500 Camp Bowie Boulevard 817-735-2000
Fort Worth, TX 76107 tfairchi@hsc.unt.edu

Geriatric research.
*Michael R Williams, DO, MD, MBA, President*
*Jennifer M Trevi□o, MBA, VP*

320 **University of North Texas: Center for Studies in Aging**
Department of Applied Gerontology
PO Box 310919 940-565-2411
Denton, TX 76203 Fax: 940-565-4370
www.unt.edu/aging
Social gerontology, including employee job performance in nursing homes, impact of leadership on culture of nursing homes and retirement communities, the Native American elderly, development of databases and models for community services planning, geriatric programs in community health centers, mediation and aging, and the low-income minority elderly. Conducts demographic, social-psychological, and evaluation studies and surveys.
*Donald Grose, Manager*

321 **University of Northern Iowa: Center for Social and Behavioral Research**
College of Social & Behaviora 319-273-2311
Cedar Falls, IA 50614 GENE.LUTZ@UNI.EDU
Geography, history, home economics, political science, psychology, sociology, anthropology, criminology, social work, and public policy, including studies on adolescents, adult education, airline passengers, airports, educational needs assessment, elderly, environmental impact assessment, highways, human services needs assessment, outdoor recreation, radio listening habits, substance abuse, and television viewing habits.
*Robert D Koob, CEO*

322 **University of Pennsylvania Institute on Aging**
3615 Chestnut Street 215-662-2746
Philadelphia, PA 19104-2676 Fax: 215-573-8684
www.med.upenn.edu/aging
Biomedical and social science research on aging, including cellular mechanisms of aging, Alzheimer's disease, sleep disturbances, arthritis, osteoporosis, population demographics of aging, nursing home quality, organization and structure of life care communities, social security, and social support systems for the aged.
*John Q. Trojanowski, MD, PhD, Director*
*Laura Trean, Manager*

323 **University of Pennsylvania: Center for Clinical Epidemiology and Biostatistics**
School of Medicine
423 Guardian Drive 215-898-0901
Philadelphia, PA 19104 strom@cceb.upenn.edu
www.cceb.med.upenn.edu
Epidemiology of disease and risk factors of clinical importance, especially pharamacoepidemiology, molecular epidemiology, cancer, cardiovascular disease, renal disease, women's health, reproductive epidemiology, emergency medicine, injury, and aging.
*Harold I. Feldman, MD, MSCE, Director*

324 **University of Pittsburgh University Center for Social and Urban Research**
121 University Place 412-624-4141
Pittsburgh, PA 15260 Fax: 412-624-4810
Urban and regional analysis, child and family development, gerontology, intergenerational studies, and environmental policy. Conducts survey research, sampling, and data processing and analysis. Research findings are used for policy making at the international, national, regional, and local levels.

325 **University of South Dakota Social Science Research Institute**
414 E Clark Street 605-677-6240
Vermillion, SD 5706 www.usd.edu
Research includes studies on organizations, economic and social development, criminology, juvenile delinquency, child abuse, aged population, communications, social work and welfare, court administration, jury selection and community surveys for litigation, prison education, alcoholism, medical and educational problems on American Indian reservations, and follow-up on juvenile offenders. Conducts anthropological studies.
*James W. Abbott, President*

326 **University of Southern California: Inst. for Health Promotion**
Health sciences campus
Los Angeles, CA 90033
Disease prevention
*C Anderson Johnson PhD, Director*

327 **University of Tennessee: Knoxville Society for the Study of Social Problems**
906 McClung Tower 865-974-3620
Knoxville, TN 37996 Fax: 865-974-7013
tomhood@utk.edu
Community research and development; crime and juvenile delinquency; drinking and drugs; racial and ethnic minorities; conflict, social action, and change; the family; poverty, class, and inequality; psychiatric sociology; social problems theory; sociology and social welfare; youth, aging, and the life course; educational problems; environment and technology; labor studies; sexual behavior; politics and communities; law and society.
*Dr. Thomas C Hood, Executive Officer*

328 **University of Texas-Houston Health Science Center Mental Sciences Institute**
University of Texas
7000 Fannin Street 713-500-3130
Houston, TX 77030
Biochemical and behavioral aspects of psychiatric diseases, particularly physiopathology and pharmacology of alcohol and drug addiction, and affective and anxiety disorders. Performs basic and clinical studies in neuroendocrinology, metabolism, behavioral science, disorders, mental retardation, neurochemistry, psychophysiology, biochemistry, crime and delinquency, and gerontology.
*Giuseppe N. Colasurdo, M.D., President*

329 **University of Utah Human Performance Research Laboratory**
250 S 1850 E 801-581-8379
Salt Lake City, UT 84112 www.health.utah.edu
Effects of exercise and environment on muscular, cardiovascular, respiratory, nervous, and thermoregulatory systems of the human body. Programs are conducted on exercise and multiple sclerosis patients, women at risk for osteoporosis, exercise and functional abilities and health benefits.
*Kerry Jacques, Director*

330 **University of Utah: Gerontology Center**
10 South 2000 East 801-581-3414
Salt Lake City, UT 84112 nursing.utah.edu/
Health and social sciences as they relate to the aged, including long-term care, gerontology curriculum and standards, bereavement of the elderly, in-home and respite care services, the family as a support system, family caregiving, and intergenerational families.

331 **University of Vermont Larner College of Medicine Center on Aging**
89 Beaumont Avenue 802-656-0292
Burlington, VT 05405 Fax: 802-656-8380
Jeanne.Hutchins@uvm.edu
www.med.uvm.edu/centeronaging
Aims to promote well-being and a high quality of life for older adults, through university collaboration.
*William Pendlebury, MD, Director*
*Jeanne M. Hutchins, MA, Executive Director*

332 **University of Washington Northwest: Geriatric Education Center**
PO Box 357262 206-616-4276
Seattle, WA 98195 Fax: 206-616-3064
sgural@u.washington.edu
nwgec.org/
Provides education and training in geriatrics to health professionals, educators, and practitioners in Washington, Alaska, Montana, and Idaho.

333 **University of West Florida: Center on Aging**
Department of Social Work
11000 University Parkway
Pensacola, FL 32514 beechems@prodigy.net
Gerontology, including rural elderly, housing, and death. Develops and evaluates training material for aging services.
*John Cavanaugh, President*

334 **University of Wisconsin-Madison Neuropsychology Laboratory**
600 Highland Avenue 608-263-6400
Madison, WI 53792 800-323-8942
www.uwhealth.org
Clinical neuropsychology in neuropsychological correlates of epilepsy, cognitive and affective changes in aging, and differential diagnosis of dementia with a view toward cognitive and memory remediation.

335 **University of Wisconsin: Madison Institute on Aging**
1300 University Avenue 608-262-1818
Madison, WI 53706 Fax: 608-263-6211
aging@ssc.wisc.edu
www.aging.wisc.edu
Aging, including life course studies, biogerontology, social geroltology, and clinical geriatrics. Specific areas of study include, but are not limited to, Alzheimer's disease, caloric intake, coping with later life stress, demography, falls after hospital discharge, free radicals, housing and environment for older adults, muscle loss, osteoporosis, resilience in adulthood, primates, psychological well-being, swallowing disorders.
*Carol Ryff, Director*

336 **University of Wisconsin: Milwaukee Institute on Aging and Environment**
School of Architecture and Urban Planning
PO Box 413 414-229-2991
Milwaukee, WI 53201 Fax: 414-229-6976
aging@uwm.edu
www.uwm.edu/dept/iae
Interaction betweeen the aged and the environment, with emphasis on environments for people with dementia. Specific issues include innovative environmental planning, programming, and design practice for enhancement of the quality of life of older persons; behavioral and social impacts of institutional settings; constraints of zoning in the creation of innovative forms of community housing; optimal thermal and luminous conditions for seniors.
*Uriel Cohen, Director*

337 **University of Wyoming Center on Aging**
1000 E University Avenue 307-766-2829
Laramie, WY 82071 wycoa@uwyo.edu
www.uwyo.edu/wycoa
Seeks to optimize the health and well-being of older adults and caregivers in Wyoming through partnerships, research, community education, and clinical training.
*Christine McKibbin, PhD, Director*
*Catherine Phillips Carrico, PhD, Associate Director*

338 **Veterans Affairs Medical Center: Geriatric Research, Education, Center**
1601 SW Archer Road 352-374-6051
Gainesville, FL 32608 Fax: 352-371-6142
dlowenth@pharmacology.ufl.edu
Geropharmacology, including mechanisms of drug action, pharmacokinetics, therapeutic uses, drug abuse, polypharmacy and drug compliance as it applies to geriatric patients. Clinical research is conducted in the areas of exercise in the healthy, frail, and elderly, cardiovascular function, and cognitive disorders in the elderly. Basic research is conducted in pharmacologic mechanisms of temperature regulation and obesity.
*Luann Cox, Manager*

339 **Virginia Center on Aging**
Virginia Commonwealth University
Box 980229 804-828-1525
Richmond, VA 23298 vcoa@vcu.edu
vcoa.chp.vcu.edu
The Virginia Center on Aging is a statewide agency created by the Virginia General Assembly, with our home at Virginia Commonwealth University. Since 1978, VCoA has worked diligently to protect and improve the quality of life of older Virginians, so that they may remain independent and contributing members in their communities. Our four program areas include: abuse in later life, dementia research, geriatrics education, and lifelong learning.
*Edward F. Ansello, PhD, Director*
*Leland Waters, PhD, Associate Director*

340 **Virginia Commonwealth University Virginia Center on Aging**
730 East Broad Street 804-828-1525
Richmond, VA 23219 804-828-7905
vcoa@vcu.edu
vcoa.chp.vcu.edu
Interdisciplinary center for the study and research of the aged and the aging process.
*Edward F. Ansello, PhD, Director*
*Constance L. Coogle, PhD, Associate Director, Research*

341 **Wayne State University Center for Health Research**
5557 Cass Avenue 313-577-4135
Detroit, MI 48202 Fax: 313-577-5777
www.nursing.wayne.edu/
Nursing, urban health, pain reduction in hospitalized children, adolescent health, teen pregnancy, aging, chronicity, health education and promotion (e.g. smoking cessation), community health, psychosocial oncology, health behavior, self care, stress and coping, parent/child health, family health, caregivers of aged individuals, drug use, violence and abuse, sleep patterns, risk-taking with respect to teen pregnancy and STDs.

342 **Wayne State University: Institute of Gerontology**
87 E Ferry Street
Detroit, MI 48202 Fax: 313-664-2666
ioginfo@wayne.edu
www.iog.wayne.edu
Gerontology, including studies on public policy, acute and long-term health care, service delivery, aging process, family relations, and work and retirement.
*Tina Abbott, Chair*

343 **Wichita State University: Gerontology Center**
1845 Fairmount Street 316-978-3456
Wichita, KS 67260 www.webs.wichita.edu
Gerontology.
*Dr. Teresa Radebaugh, Director*

344 **Woodrow Wilson School of Public and Intl Affairs: Center for Health Car**
Princeton University
353 Nassau Street 609-258-4800
Princeton, NJ 08540 mail@chcs.org
www.chcs.org
Development and implementation of effective health and social policy for all Americans.
*Christopher Eisgruber, CEO*

345 **de Tornyay Center For Healthy Aging at University of Washington**
School of Nursing
PO Box 357260 206-616-4276
Seattle, WA 98195-7260 206-616-3064
agingctr@u.washington.edu
nursing.uw.edu
Supports gerontology research and education to promote healthy aging.
*Basia Belza, PhD, RN, FAAN, Director*
*Heather Wicklein-Sanchez, Manager*

## Support Groups & Hotlines

346 **American Association of Caregiving Youth**
1515 N Federal Hwy. 561-391-7401
Boca Raton, FL 33432 800-508-9618
info@aacy.org
www.aacy.org
Seeks to raise awareness of and provide services for youth who act as caregivers for their parents and grandparents.
*Connie Siskowski, RN, PhD, President*

347 **Caregiver Action Network**
1150 Connecticut Avenue NW 202-454-3970
Washington, DC 20036-3904 info@caregiveraction.org
caregiveraction.org
Aims to improve quality of life for Americans who care for loved ones facing chronic illnesses, disabilities, diseases, or old age.
*John Schall, Chief Executive Officer*
*Chance Browning, Senior Director, Programs*

348 **Caregiver Support Services**
PO Box 4291 866-201-6896
Omaha, NE 68104 egreen@caregiversupportservices.org
caregiversupportservices.com
Provides guidance and resources to caregivers.
*Eboni Green, President & CEO*
*Terrence Green, Vice President, Business Development*

349 **Children of Aging Parents**
PO Box 167 215-355-6611
Richboro, PA 18954 800-227-7294
Fax: 215-355-6824
info@caps4caregivers.org
www.caps4caregivers.org
A nonprofit, charitable organization that assists the nation's nearly 54 million caregivers of the elderly or chronically ill with reliable information, referrals and support, and to heighten public awareness.

350 **Hospice and Homecare**
3801 Vanesta Drive 785-537-0688
Manhattan, KS 66503 Fax: 785-537-1309
info@hcandh.org
www.homecareandhospice.org
Aims to be the premier non-profit Homecare & Hospice provider of compassionate, affordable health, wellness and support services.

351 **National Alliance for Caregiving**
4720 Montgomery Lane 301-718-8444
Bethesda, MD 20814 301-951-9067
info@caregiving.org
www.caregiving.org
Advocates on behalf of caregivers, as well as conducting research and offering support services.
*C. Grace Whiting, JD, President & CEO*
*Michael Wittke, BSW, MPA, Senior Director, Public Policy*

352 **National Health Information Center**
Office of Disease Prevention & Health Promotion
1101 Wootton Pkwy Fax: 240-453-8281
Rockville, MD 20852 odphpinfo@hhs.gov
www.health.gov/nhic
Supports public health education by maintaining a calendar of National Health Observances; helps connect consumers and health professionals to organizations that can best answer questions and provide up-to-date contact information from reliable sources; updates on a yearly basis toll-free numbers for health information, Federal health clearinghouses and info centers.
*Don Wright, MD, MPH, Director*

353 **Well Spouse Association**
63 W Main Street 732-577-8899
Freehold, NJ 07728 www.wellspouse.org
This association is a nonprofit national self-help organization serving the well spouse of the chronically ill. Members help each other develop coping and survival skills through local support groups (including bereavement), letter and telephone networks, and personal outreach and a quarterly newsletter.
*Marilyn Kamp, Executive Director*

## Magazines

354 **A Better Tomorrow**
Thomas Nelson
5301 Wisconsin Avenue NW 202-364-8000
Washington, DC 20015 Fax: 202-364-8910
www.thomasnelson.com/
Magazine focusing on issues and concerns of senior citizens.
*Bruce Barbour, Publisher*
*Dale Hanson, Editor*

355 **AARP Bulletin**
AARP
601 E Street NW 888-687-2277
Washington, DC 20049 www.aarp.org
Resources for online classes, training and more. Topics include Computers/Technology, Health/Wellbeing, Personal Finance. AARP Membership open to individuals age 50+, benefits include access to insurance services, travel discounts, advice on healthy living, financial planning, consumer protection. AARP represents members on issues like Medicare, Social Security, and consumer safety. Publications include the AARP Magazine and AARP Bulletin.

356 **AARP Magazine**
American Association of Retired Persons
601 East Street NW 202-434-3525
Washington, DC 20049 888-687-2277
TTY: 877-434-7598
member@aarp.org
www.aarp.org
Celebrity interviews. Features on health and finance. Movie reviews and more. All with an eye toward the topics and issues you care about most.
*A Barry Rand, CEO*

357 **ACE Fitness Matters**
American Council on Exercise (ACE)
4851 Paramount Drive 858-576-6500
San Diego, CA 92123 888-825-3636
Fax: 858-576-6564
support@acefitness.org
www.acefitness.org/
Consumer magazine covering health and fitness news.
*Herb Flentye, Chair*
*Scott Murdoch, PhD., RD, Vice Chair*

358 **AER Report**
Association for Education & Rehabilitation
1703 N. Beauregard Street 703-671-4500
Alexandria, VA 22311 Fax: 703-671-6391
www.aerbvi.org/
Contains organizational news, conference dates and information concerning services to visually impaired people.
*Jim Adams, President*
*Lou Tutt, Executive Director*

359 **ASN NEURO**
Sage Journals
2455 Teller Road 805-499-9774
Thousand Oaks, CA 91320 journals@sagepub.com
journals.sagepub.com/home/asn
Peer-reviewed open access journal focusing on recent advances in the cellular and molecular neurosciences. It is the official publication of the American Society for Neurochemistry.
*Douglas L. Feinstein, Editor-in-Chief*
*Sandra J. Hewitt, Deputy Editor-in-Chief*

360 **Abstracts in Social Gerontology**
National Council on Aging
1901 L Street NW 202-479-1200
Washington, DC 20036 800-677-1116
Fax: 202-479-0735
TDD: 202-479-6674
info@ncoa.org
www.ncoa.org
Detailed abstracts are provided for recent major journal articles, books, reports and other materials on many facets of aging, including adult education, demography, family relations, institutional care and work attitudes.
*Quarterly*
*James P Firman, EdD, President/CEO*

361 **Adapted Physical Activity Quarterly**
Human Kinetics
PO Box 5076 217-351-5076
Champaign, IL 61820 800-747-4457
Fax: 217-351-1549
info@hkusa.com
www.humankinetics.com
Journal on the study of physical activity for special populations.
*Brian Holding, CEO*
*Rainer Martens, Founder*

362 **Aging International**
Transaction Publishers

35 Berrue
New Brunswick, NJ 08901
732-445-1245
888-999-6778
Fax: 732-445-3138
orders@transactionpub.com
www.transactionpub.com/

Journal dedicated to the well-being of older persons worldwide. Explores productive aging, empowerment, life-long learning, health promotion, and services for the elderly, with an emphasis on sharing both common concerns and practical applications. Focuses on social and economic issues, public policies, and use of resources. Published in cooperation with the International Federation on Aging.
*Mary E. Curtis, Chair*
*Irving Louis Horowitz, Co-Founder*

363 **Aging News Alert**
CD Publications
2222 Sedwick Drive
Durham, NC 27713
301-588-6380
855-237-1396
Fax: 800-508-2592
info@cdpublications.com
www.cdpublications.com

Twice-monthly newsletter reporting on senior programs, funding opportunities and federal actions affecting the elderly.
*Michael Gerecht, President*

364 **Aging Research & Training News**
Business Publishers, Inc.
2222 Sedwick Drive
Durham, NC 27713
800-223-8720
Fax: 800-508-2592
www.bpinews.com

Compilation of studies of aging populations; reports on innovative programs with aging community; federal funding and laws.
*8 pages*
*Kimberly Gilbert, Managing Editor*
*Alexa Chew, Contributing Editor*

365 **Aging and Society**
Cambridge University Press
32 Avenue of the Americas
New York, NY 10013
212-924-3900
800-221-4512
Fax: 212-691-3239
www.cambridge.org/us/information/contact

International journal publishing on topics which further the understanding of human aging. The journal of the Centre for policy on aging and the British Socie for Gerontology.
*Ken Blakemore, Editor*
*Bill Bythwway, Editor*

366 **American Journal of Geriatric Psychiatry**
Elsevier
1600 John F Kennedy Boulevard
Philadelphia, PA 19103
www.journals.elsevier.com

Peer-reviewed articles on the rapidly developing field of geriatric psychiatry, including areas such as the diagnosis and classification of psychiatric disorders, epidemiological and biological correlates of mental health of older adults, and psychopharmacology and other somatic treatments.
*Monthly*
*Charles F. Reynolds III, MD, Editor-in-Chief*

367 **American Journal of Speech-Language Pathology**
American Speech-Language-Hearing Association (ASHA
2200 Research Boulevard
Rockville, MD 20850
301-296-5700
800-638-8255
Fax: 301-296-8580
TTY: 301-296-5650
www.asha.org/

*Elizabeth S. McCrea, PhD, CCC-SLP, President*
*Barbara K. Cone, PhD, CCC-A, Vice President for Academic Affa*

368 **American Legion Magazine**
American Legion National Headquarters
PO Box 1055
Indianapolis, IN 46206
317-630-1200
800-433-3318
Fax: 317-630-1223
www.legion.org/

General interest magazine for veterans.
*Daniel S. Wheeler, National Adjutant*
*Philip B. Onderdonk Jr., National Judge Advocate*

369 **American Rehabilitation Services Administration (RSA)**
American Rehabilitation Services Administration (R
400 Maryland Avenue, SW
Washington, DC 20202
202-205-8296
800-USA-LEAR
Fax: 202-205-9874
www2.ed.gov/about/offices/list/osers/rsa

Magazine on rehabilitation of the handicapped.
*Arne Duncan, Secretary of Education*
*Jim Shelton, Acting Deputy Secretary*

370 **Assistive Technology**
RESNA
1700 N Moore Street
Arlington, VA 22209
703-524-6686
Fax: 202-524-6630
www.resna.org

Journal focusing on assistive technology for persons with disabilities.
*Alex Mihailidis, PhD, P.Eng, President*
*Jamie Arasz Prioli, ATP, Secretary*

371 **Audecibel**
International Hearing Society
16880 Middlebelt Road
Livonia, MI 48154
734-522-7200
800-521-5247
Fax: 734-522-0200
www.ihsinfo.org/

Magazine publishing technical articles and product announcements on hearing aids and hearing.
*Amanda Ciccantelli, Administrative Assistant*
*Bernadette " Demicoli, Member Services Coordinator*

372 **Buena Vida**
Casiano Communications
1700 Fern ndez Juncos Avenue
San Juan, PR 00909
787-728-3000
800-468-8167
Fax: 787-268-1001
www.casiano.com/

Health and fitness magazine.
*Manuel A. Casiano, Chairman & CEO*
*Carlos Rom, Executive Vice President*

373 **Challenge Magazine**
Disabled Sports, USA
451 Hungerford Drive
Rockville, MD 20850
301-217-0960
Fax: 301-217-0968
dsusa@dsusa.org
www.disabledsportsusa.org/

Magazine providing information on sports for people with physical disabilities.
*Robert Meserve, President*
*Steven Goodwin, Vice President*

374 **Closing the Gap, Inc.**
P.O. Box 68
Henderson, MN 56044
507-248-3294
Fax: 507-248-3810
info@closingthegap.com
www.closingthegap.com

Online membership that includes access to the Solutions on-line magazine and archives, archived webinars and the Resource Directory, a guide to over 2,000 products for children and adults with disabilities
*Megan Turek, President*
*Marc Hagen, Vice President*

375 **Communication Outlook: Artificial Language Laboratory**
Artificial Language Laboratory
405 Computer Center
Lansing, MI 48824
517-353-0870
Fax: 517-353-4766
www.msu.edu/~artlang/CommOut.html

Magazine reporting on the newest developments in the application of technology for neurologically impaired persons.
*Dr. John B. Eulenberg, Ph.D., Director*
*Stephen R. Blosser, B.S.M.E., Technical Director*

376 **Computer-Disability News**
Easter Seals
233 South Wacker Drive
Chicago, IL 60606
312-726-6200
800-221-6827
Fax: 312-726-1494
www.easterseals.com/

Magazine highlighting news for persons with disabilities.
*Richard W. Davidson, Chairman*
*Sandra L. Bouwman, 1st Vice Chairman*

377 **Conscious Choice**
Conscious Communications
920 N Franklin Street 312-440-4373
Chicago, IL 60610 Fax: 312-751-3973
www.consciouscomms.com/
Consumer magazine covering health, nutrition and environmental issues.
*Ross Thompson, Managing Editor*
*Jim Slama, Publisher*

378 **Contemporary Gerontology**
Springer Publishing Company
11 West 42nd Street 212-431-4370
New York, NY 10036 877-687-7476
Fax: 212-941-7842
cs@springerpub.com, journals@springerpub
www.springerpub.com
Scholarly journal covering gerontology.
*James C. Costello, Vice President, Journal Publishi*
*Theodore C. Nardin, Chief Executive Officer & Publis*

379 **Dementia and Geriatric Cognitive Disorders**
S. Karger Publishers, Inc.
26 W Avon Road 860-675-7834
Unionville, CT 06085 800-828-5479
Fax: 860-675-7302
www.karger.com/DEM
Open-access journal devoted to the study of cognitive dysfunction in preclinical and clinical studies, concentrating on Alzheimer's and Parkinson's disease, Huntington's chorea and other neurodegenerative diseases.
*Victoria Chan-Pilay, Editor-in-Chief*

380 **Disability Rag's Ragged Edge Magazine**
Advocado Press
PO Box 145 502-894-9492
Louisville, KY 40201 Fax: 502-899-9562
www.advocadopress.org/
Magazine of debate on disability rights issues. ISSN# 1095-3949
*35 pages*
*Mary Johnson, Mailing Contact/Editor*

381 **Disability Rights Now**
Disability Rights Education and Defense Fund
3075 Adeline Street 510-644-2555
Berkeley, CA 94703 800-466-4232
Fax: 510-841-8645
TTY: 510-841-8645
info@dredf.org
dredf.org/
Free quarterly publication describing the activities of the Disability Rights Education and Defense Fund, available in alternative formats.
*Claudia Center, President and Chair*
*Susan Henderson, Executive Director*

382 **Disability Statistics Report**
Institute for Health & Aging
2 Koret Way, #N-319X 415-476-1435
San Francisco, CA 94143 Fax: 415-476-9707
info@nursing.ucsf.edu
nursing.ucsf.edu/iha
Magazine providing statistical data on disability in the US as collected by the Disability Statistics Program.
*David Vlahov, RN, PhD, Dean and Professor*
*Yolanda Abrea, Fiscal Analyst*

383 **Disability Studies Quarterly**
University of Hawaii at Manoa
2500 Campus Road 808-956-8111
Honolulu, HI 96822 Fax: 808-956-3162
manoa.hawaii.edu/
Scholarly journal containing articles on all aspects of disability.
*M.R.C. Greenwood, President*
*Tom Apple, Chief Executive Officer*

384 **Disabled American Veterans Magazines**
Disabled American Veterans National Headquarters
PO Box 14301 859-441-7300
Cincinnati, OH 45250 Fax: 859-441-8056
www.dav.org/
Veterans magazine on disability issues.
*Thomas K Keller, Editor*
*James Chaney, Mailing Contact*

385 **Disabled People as Second Class Citizens**
Springer Publishing Company
11 West 42nd Street 212-431-4370
New York, NY 10036 877-687-7476
Fax: 212-941-7842
cs@springerpub.com, journals@springerpub
www.springerpub.com
Disability and legal practice.
*320 pages*
*James C. Costello, Vice President, Publisher*
*Theodore C. Nardin, Chief Executive Officer*

386 **Domestic Mistreatment of the Elderly: Towards Prevention**
AARP
601 E Street NW 202-434-3525
Washington, DC 20049 888-687-2277
Fax: 202-434-3443
TTY: 877-434-7598
member@aarp.org
www.aarp.org
This comprehensive publication addresses the problem of mistreatment or neglect in the home.
*39 pages*
*Gail E. Aldrich, Board Chair*
*Robert G. Romasco, President*

387 **Duplex Planet**
Duplex Planet
PO Box 1230 518-692-7410
Saratoga Springs, NY 12866 Fax: 518-692-8208
www.duplexplanet.com/
Consumer journal covering issues of aging and popular culture.
*David Greenberger, Editor/ Founder*

388 **Eating Well Magazine**
Eating Well
6221 Shelburne Road 802-985-4500
Charlotte, VT 05482 800-344-3350
Fax: 802-425-3675
www.eatingwell.com
Food magazine with emphasis on delicious low-fat cooking and sensible nutrition.
*Thomas Witschi, President*
*Brierley Wright, Managing Editor*

389 **Educational Gerontology**
Taylor & Francis
711 3rd Avenue 212-216-7800
New York, NY 10017 800-634-7064
Fax: 212-564-7854
www.taylorandfrancis.com/
Journal publishing original research in the fields of gerontology, adult education, and the social and behavioral sciences.
*D Barry Lumsden, Editor*
*Kevin Bradley, CEO*

390 **Elderly Health Services Letter**
Health Resources Online
P.O. Box 456 800-516-4343
Allenwood, NJ 08720 Fax: 732-292-1111
info@healthresourcesonline.com
An essential tool for senior services professionals. Stays on top of the most current challenges facing senior services professionals, including financing and funding senior services, marketing, positioning senior services for managed care, getting administrative support and more.
*Robert K Jenkins, Publisher*

391 **Experimental Aging Research**
Taylor & Francis

711 3rd Avenue 212-216-7800
New York, NY 10017 800-634-7064
Fax: 212-564-7854
www.taylorandfrancis.com/

International journal devoted to the scientific study of the aging process.
*Jeffrey Elias, Editor*
*Kevin Bradley, CEO*

392 **Fitness Diet and Exercise Guide**
Family Circle
110 5th Avenue 212-463-1673
New York, NY 10011 800-627-4444
Fax: 212-463-1906
fcfeedback@familycircle.com
www.familycircle.com/

Magazine suggesting ways to eat healthier and exercise better.
*Darcy Jacobs, Executive Editor*
*Linda Fears, Vice President/Editor in Chief*

393 **Focus on Geriatric Care and Rehabilitation**
Aspen Publishers
7201 McKinney Circle 301-644-3599
Frederick, MD 21704 800-234-1660
Fax: 800-901-9075
www.aspenpublishers.com/

Monthly journal written for nurses, occupational therapists and administrators in geriatric settings.
*Bob Lemmond, President & CEO*
*Gustavo Dobles, Vice President & CCO*

394 **Generations**
American Society on Aging
575 Market Street 415-974-9600
San Francisco, CA 94105 800-537-9728
Fax: 415-974-0300
info@asaging.org
www.asaging.org

Peer-review quarterly journal featuring guest editor.
*Peter Kaldest, President & CEO*
*Robert R. Lowe, COO*

395 **Geriatrics**
ModernMedicine
7500 Old Oak Boulevard 440-891-2769
Cleveland, OH 44130 Fax: 440-891-2635

Peer-reviewed, clinical journal for physicians and laypersons relating to medical care of middle-aged and older adults.
*Don Berman, Director, Business Development*
*Terry Tetzlaff, Digital Traffic Coordinator*

396 **Gerontologist**
Gerontological Society of America
1220 L Street North West 202-842-1275
Washington, DC 20005 Fax: 202-842-1150
geron@geron.org
www.geron.org

Multidisciplinary peer-reviewed journal presenting new concepts, clinical ideas, and applied research in gerontology. Includes book and audiovisual reviews.
*James Appleby, Executive Director and CEO*
*Linda Krogh Harootyan, Deputy Executive Director*

397 **Gerontology**
S. Karger Publishers, Inc.
PO Box 529 860-675-7834
Unionville, CT 06085 800-828-5479
Fax: 860-675-7302
karger@snet.net
www.karger.com/

Medical journal.
*W Meier-Rage, Managing Editor*
*Monica Brendel, President*

398 **Get Up and Go**
Liberty Media Corporation
11551 Forest Central Drive 214-341-9429
Dallas, TX 75243 877-772-1518
Fax: 214-341-9779
www.libertymedia.com/

Magazine (tabloid) for people age 50 and over.
*John C. Malone, Chairman*
*Gregory B. Maffei, President & CEO*

399 **Impact!**
World Institute on Disability (WID)
3075 Adeline Street 510-225-6400
Berkeley, CA 94703 Fax: 510-225-0477
TTY: 510-225-0478
wid@wid.org
www.wid.org/

Magazine reporting on the activities of the World Institute on Disability.
*Paul W. Schroeder, Chair*
*Linda M. Dardarian, Vice Chair*

400 **Independent Living Provider**
Equal Opportunity Publications
1160 E Jericho Turnpike 516-421-9421
Huntington, NY 11743 Fax: 516-421-0359
info@eop.com
www.eop.com/

Business magazine for home health care.
*Tamara Flaum-Dreyfuss, President and Publisher*
*Maureen Gladstone, Account Executive*

401 **Informer**
The Simon Foundation for Continence
PO Box 815 847-864-3913
Wilmette, IL 60091 800-23S-mon
Fax: 847-864-9758
info@simonfoundation.org
www.simonfoundation.org

Magazine for persons with bladder or bowel incontinence.
*Cheryle Gartley, President and Founder*
*Elizabeth Tr LaGro, Vice President, Communications a*

402 **Innovations**
National Council on Aging
1901 L Street NW 202-479-1200
Washington, DC 20036 800-677-1116
Fax: 202-479-0735
TDD: 2024796674
info@ncoa.org
www.ncoa.org

Explores significant developments in the field of aging through opinion articles, profiles and research summaries. Features articles on social trends, articles on specific aging programs and information on NCOA's activities.
*Quarterly*
*James P Firman, EdD, President/CEO*

403 **Inside MS**
National Multiple Sclerosis Society
733 3rd Avenue 212-986-3240
New York, NY 10017 800-FIG-HTMS
Fax: 212-986-7981
editor@nmss.org
www.nationalmssociety.org/

Magazine for people with multiple sclerosis, their families, attending professionals, and interested donors. Provides information on coping, research, legislation, medical advances and disability rights advocacy.
*80 pages*
*Eli Rubenstein, Chairman of the Board*
*Cynthia Zagieboylo, President & CEO*

404 **International Journal of Aging and Human Development**
Baywood Publishing Company, Inc.
PO Box 337 631-691-1270
Amityville, NY 11701 800-638-7819
Fax: 631-691-1770
www.baywood.com/

Adult development and aging featuring original research theory, critial reviews.
*, Publisher*

405 **International Journal of Technology and Aging**
Human Sciences Press

233 Spring Street
New York, NY 10013-1522
212-620-8000
800-221-9369
Fax: 212-463-0742
www.springer.com

Designed to serve health-care professionals, researchers, academicians and industries concerned with the convergence of two recent trends, the dramatic advances in technology and the rapidly growing elderly population.

406 **International Psychogeriatrics**
Springer Publishing Company
11 West 42nd Street
New York, NY 10036
212-431-4370
877-687-7476
Fax: 212-941-7842
cs@springerpub.com, journals@springerpub
www.springerpub.com

Scholarly journal covering psychogeriatric practice, research, and education worldwide.
*James C. Costello, Vice President*
*Theodore C. Nardin, Chief Executive Officer*

407 **International Rehabilitation Review**
Rehabilitation International
125 E 21st Street
New York, NY 10010
212-420-1500
Fax: 212-505-0871
ri@riglobal.org
www.riglobal.org/

Magazine overviewing the activities programs in the disability and rehabilitation fields.
*Jan A. Monsbakken, President*
*Patrick Fougeyrollas, Vice President*

408 **JNeurosci**
Society for Neuroscience
1121 14th Street NW
Washginton, DC 20005
202-962-4000
jn@sfn.org
www.jneurosci.org

Official peer-reviewed journal of the Society for Neuroscience, publishing research on a broad range of topics of interest to those working on the nervous system.
*Marina R. Picciotto, Editor-in-Chief*
*Teresa Esch, Features Editor*

409 **Journal of AAA**
American Academy of Audiology
11480 Commerce Park Drive
Reston, VA 20191
703-790-8466
800-222-2336
Fax: 703-790-8631
www.audiology.org/

*Deborah Carlson, PhD, Chair*
*Bettie Borton, AuD, President*

410 **Journal of Aging and Ethnicity**
Springer Publishing Company
11 West 42nd Street
New York, NY 10036
212-431-4370
877-687-7476
Fax: 212-941-7842
cs@springerpub.com, journals@springerpub
www.springerpub.com

Scholarly journal for researchers and professionals in gerontology and geriatrics, emphasizing the ethnic population of North America.
*James C. Costello, Vice President*
*Theodore C. Nardin, Chief Executive Officer*

411 **Journal of Aging and Health**
Sage Publications
2455 Teller Road
Thousand Oaks, CA 91320
805-499-0721
Fax: 805-499-0871
linfo@sagepub.com
www.sagepub.in/

Journal presenting research relative to the social and behavioral factors related to aging and health.
*Kyriakos S Markides, Editor*
*C Anderson, Circulation Manager*

412 **Journal of Aging and Physical Activity**
Human Kinetics
PO Box 5076
Champaign, IL 61820
217-351-5076
800-747-4457
Fax: 217-351-1549
info@hkusa.com
www.humankinetics.com

Journal examining the relationship between physical activity and the aging process.
*Brian Holding, CEO*
*Rainer Martens, Founder*

413 **Journal of American Aging Association**
American Aging Association
52373 Tyndall Falls Drive
Olmstead Falls, OH 44138
440-793-6565
Fax: 440-793-6598
ameraging@gmail.com
www.americanaging.org

*Mitch Harman, Chairperson*
*LaDora Thompson, President*

414 **Journal of Developmental and Physical Disabilities**
Kluwer Academic Publishers
101 Philip Drive
Norwell, MA 02061
212-620-8000
Fax: 212-463-0742
vlib.ustu.ru/storon/kluwer/

Professional journal.
*Vincent B Hassett, Editor*
*V Hersen, Advertising Manager*

415 **Journal of Ethics, Law, and Aging**
Springer Publishing Company
11 West 42nd Street
New York, NY 10036
212-431-4370
877-687-7476
Fax: 212-941-7842
cs@springerpub.com, journals@springerpub
www.springerpub.com

Scholarly journal covering ethical and legal issues regarding aging for professionals who plan, administer, and provide and finance services to the elderly.
*James C. Costello, Vice President, Journal Publishing*
*Theodore C. Nardin, Chief Executive Officer & Publisher*

416 **Journal of Mental Health and Aging**
Springer Publishing Company
11 West 42nd Street
New York, NY 10036
212-431-4370
877-687-7476
Fax: 212-941-7842
www.springerpub.com

Scholarly journal covering aging population for mental health professionals.
*James C. Costello, Vice President*
*Theodore C. Nardin, Chief Executive Officer*

417 **Journal of Nuclear Medicine**
Society of Nuclear Medicine and Molecular Imaging
1850 Samuel Morse Drive
Reston, VA 20190
703-708-9000
800-513-6853
Fax: 703-708-9015
subscriptions@snm.org
jnm.snmjournals.org

Peer-reviewed journal with clinical investigations, science reports, articles benefitting continuing education, book reviews, employment opportunities, and updates on practice and research.
*Monthly*
*Johannes Czernin, MD, Editor-in-Chief*
*Susan Alexander, Associate Director, Publications*

418 **Journal of Nuclear Medicine Technology**
Society of Nuclear Medicine and Molecular Imaging
1850 Samuel Morse Drive
Reston, VA 20190
703-708-9000
800-513-6853
Fax: 703-708-9015
subscriptions@snm.org
tech.snmjournals.org

Peer-reviewed journal dedicated to nuclear medicine technology, with information on credentialing, continuing education and licensure requirements, as well as current news and updates on the field.
*Quarterly*
*Kathy S. Thomas, MHA, CNMT, PET, Editor-in-Chief*
*Susan Alexander, Associate Director, Publications*

419 **Journal of Rehabilitation**
National Rehabilitation Association
P.O. Box 150235 703-836-0850
Alexandria, VA 22315 888-258-4295
Fax: 703-836-0848
TDD: 703-836-0849
www.nationalrehab.org/
Rehabilitation journal.
*David Beach David Beach, President*
*Patricia Leahy, Interim Executive Director*

420 **Journal of Religion, Spirituality & Aging**
www.tandfonline.com
Features articles, research reports and reviews of new books and audiovisual resources on religion and aging.
*James W. Ellor, Editor*

421 **Journal of Therapeutic Horticulture**
American Horticultural Therapy Association
610 Freedom Business Center 610-992-0020
King of Prussia, PA 19406 Fax: 301-869-2397
ahta.org/
Journal containing articles on the therapeutic aspects of gardening and agriculture for persons with disabilities.
*MaryAnne Millan, HTR, President*
*Leigh Anne Starling, MS, CRC, HTR, Vice President*

422 **Journal of the Association for Persons with Severe Handicaps**
TASH
1001 Connecticut Avenue, NW 202-540-9020
Washington, DC 20036 800-482-TASH
Fax: 202-540-9019
info@tash.org
tash.org/
Special education journal presenting articles that report original research, authoritative and comprehensive reviews, and conceptual and practical position papers offering new directions for people with disabilities.
*David Westling, President*
*Jean Trainor, Vice President*

423 **Kaleidoscope: Exploring the Expirence of Disability through Literature/Fine Arts**
United Disability Services
701 S Main Street 330-762-9755
Akron, OH 44311 Fax: 330-762-0912
www.udsakron.org
Magazine featuring articles on literature and the arts. Disabilitiy related.
*64 pages*
*Karen A. Bozzelli, Chairperson*
*Bill Choler, Vice Chairperson*

424 **Macrobiotics Today**
George Ohsawa Macrobiotic Foundation
PO Box 3998 530-566-9765
Chico, CA 95927 800-232-2372
Fax: 530-566-9768
www.ohsawamacrobiotics.com/
Magazine covering macrobiotics, health, and nutrition.
*Carl Ferr,, President*
*Peter Milbury, Director*

425 **Magazines in Special Media for the Handicapped**
National Library Service for the Blind and Physic
1291 Taylor Street NW 202-707-5100
Washington, DC 20011 800-424-8567
Fax: 202-707-0712
TDD: 202-707-0744
www.loc.gov/nls
Publication includes: List of over 100 public and private organizations that publish magazines in Braille, on cassette, on disc and computer diskette, or in large print or moon type for visually impaired and physically disabled individuals. Entries include: Name of publisher, address, price. Principal content is a bibliography of periodicals, with brief description, frequency, format, and price of each.
*Karen Keninger, Director*
*Isabella Marqu,s de Castilla, Deputy Director*

426 **Massage Therapy Journal**
American Massage Therapy Association
500 Davis Street 847-864-0123
Evanston, IL 60201 877-905-0577
Fax: 847-864-5196
info@amtamassage.org
www.amtamassage.org/
Magazine focusing on professional massage therapy benefits, techniques, research, news, and practitioners.
*Winona Bontrager, President*
*Rachel Mann, Vice President*

427 **Mature Health**
New York - Haymarket
114 West 26th Street 646-638-6000
New York, NY 10001
Magazine featuring articles on health aspects of aging, as well as articles on recreation and leisure.
*Michael Heseltine, Chairman*
*Kevin Costello, Chief Group Executive*

428 **Mature Years**
United Methodist Publishing House
201 8th Avenue S 615-749-6000
Nashville, TN 37202 Fax: 615-749-6079
newscope_office@econet.org
umph.org/
Magazine promoting the physical and spiritual well-being of older adults.
*Neil Alexander, President/Publisher*
*Jeff Barnes, Executive Director*

429 **Men's Health**
Rodale Inc
400 South 10th Street 610-967-5171
Emmaus, PA 18098 800-848-4735
Fax: 610-967-7725
RodaleBooks@cdsfulfillment.com
Magazine offering health advice for men.
*Maria Rodale, CEO and Chairman*
*Scott D. Schulman, President*

430 **Mental Health Report**
Business Publishers, Inc.
2222 Sedwick Drive 301-495-5570
Durham, NC 27713 800-223-8720
Fax: 800-508-2592
custserv@bpinews.com
www.bpinews.com
Magazine reporting on legislation affecting the mentally ill and their families.
*Kimberly Gilbert, Managing Editor*
*Alexa Chew, Contributing Editor*

431 **Modern Maturity**
AARP
601 E Street NW 202-434-2277
Washington, DC 20049-0003 202-434-3525
Fax: 888-687-2277
TTY: 877-434-7598
member@aarp.org
www.aarp.org
Offers news and information of concern to those 50 and older. Features articles on current events, health, recreation, housing, family life, legislation and other issues.
*6x Year*
*Gail E. Aldrich, Board Chair*
*Robert G. Romasco, President*

432 **Molecular Imaging**
Sage Journals
2455 Teller Road 805-499-9774
Thousand Oaks, CA 91320 journals@sagepub.com
journals.sagepub.com/home/mix
Peer-reviewed open access journal focusing on molecular imaging research, including basic science, preclinical studies and human applications. Published in association with the Society of Nuclear Medicine and Molecular Imaging.
*Bimonthly*
*Henry F. VanBrocklin, PhD, Editor-in-Chief*

433 **National Easter Seal Communicator**
Easter Seals
233 South Wacker Drive 312-726-6200
Chicago, IL 60606 800-221-6827
Fax: 312-726-1494
www.easterseals.com/
Magazine for persons with any type of disability.
*Richard W. Davidson, Chairman*
*Sandra L. Bouwman, 1st Vice Chairman*

434 **New Living**
New Living Magazine
PO Box 1001 631-751-8819
Patchogue, NY 11772 800-NEW-LIVI
Fax: 631-751-8910
www.newliving.com
Features and articles about holistic health and fitness;herbal remedies, preventive medicine, nutrition, mind/body health, spirituality, fitness, recipes, book reviews and more!
*Christine Ly Harvey, Publisher and Editor-in-Chief*

435 **PN**
PVA Publications
2111 E Highland Avenue 602-224-0500
Phoenix, AZ 85016 888-888-2201
Fax: 602-224-0507
www.pn-magazine.com
Magazine spotlighting independent living for paraplegics and quadriplegics.
*Richard Hoover, Editor*
*Sherri Shea, Marketing & Circulation Director*

436 **Physical Disabilities—Education & Related Services**
Council for Exceptional Children
2900 Crystal Drive 703-620-3660
Arlington, VA 22202 888-232-7733
Fax: 703-264-1637
TTY: 866-915-5000
www.cec.sped.org/
Professional magazine covering research, instructional innovations and issues regarding education and physical disabilities.
*Robin D. Brewer, President*
*Joni L. Baldwin, Member-at-Large*

437 **Polio Network News**
Post-Polio Health International (PHI)
4207 Lindell Boulevard 314-534-0475
Saint Louis, MO 63108 Fax: 314-534-5070
info@post-polio.org
www.post-polio.org
Quarterly newsletter for polio survivors. Contains current information about the late efects of polio, encourages research and promotes networking among the post-polio community worldwide. Publish an annual Post-Polio Directory.
*12 pages*
*William G. Stothers, President/Chairperson*
*Saul J. Morse, Vice President*

438 **Post-Polio Health International**
Post-Polio Health International (PHI)
4207 Lindell Boulevard 314-534-0475
St Louis, MO 63108 Fax: 314-534-5070
info@post-polio.org
www.post-polio.org
International organization concerning advocacy and research for polio survivors and ventilator-dependent individuals. Newsletters are called Post-Polio Health and Ventilator Assisted Living.
*8 pages*
*William G Stothers, President/Chairperson*
*Saul J Morse, Vice President*

439 **Prevention**
Rodale Inc
400 South 10th Street 610-967-5171
Emmaus, PA 18098 800-848-4735
Fax: 910-967-8963
RodaleBooks@cdsfulfillment.com
rodaleinc.com/
Magazine containing articles on wellness, preventive medicine, self-care, and fitness.
*Maria Rodale, CEO and Chairman*
*Scott D. Schulman, President*

440 **Remedy**
Rx Remedies
500 Highway 51 North 601-981-0070
Ridgeland, MS 39157 800-826-1197
Fax: 800-729-0167
www.rxremediesms.com/
Consumer magazine covering health and wellness for individuals over 50 years in the US.
*Joan Montgomery, Publisher*

441 **Research on Aging**
Sage Publications
2455 Teller Road 805-499-0721
Thousand Oaks, CA 91320 Fax: 805-499-0871
info@sagepub.com
www.sagepub.in/
Social gerontology journal.
*Angela M O'Rand, Editor*
*Blaise R Simqu, CEO*

442 **SELF Magazine**
Cond, Nast
4 Times Square 212-286-2860
New York, NY 10036 800-223-0780
Fax: 212-880-8248
communications@condenast.com
www.condenast.com/
Magazine serving as a health sourcebook for contemporary women.
*Rochelle Udell, Editor-in-Chief*
*Larry Burstein, Publisher*

443 **Secure Retirement, The Newsmagazine for Mature Americans**
The National Committee to Preserve Social Security
111 K Street NE 202-216-0420
Washington, DC 20002 800-966-1935
Fax: 202-216-0446
webmaster@ncpssm.org
www.ncpssm.org
Magazine for senior citizens and others interested in politics and government and how they affect senior concerns and issues.
*Max Richtman, President & CEO*

444 **Senior Times Magazine**
Senior Times Magazine
4400 NW 36th Avenue 352-372-5468
Gainesville, FL 32601 Fax: 352-373-9178
www.seniortimesmagazine.com/
Magazine devoted to educating senior citizens on recreational, political, health and financial issues.
*Charlie Delatorre, Publisher*
*Albert Issac, Editor-in-Chief*

445 **Serenity**
Little Sisters of The Poor
601 Maiden Choice Lane 410-744-9367
Baltimore, MD 21228 Fax: 410-788-5614
serenitys@littlesistersofthepoor.org
www.littlesistersofthepoor.org/
Magazine making known the apostolate of Little Sisters of the Poor and providing a positive view of the elderly and the respect due them.
*32 pages*
*S R Marguerite, Publications Coordinator*
*Saint Jeanne Jugan, Founder*

446 **Society of Nuclear Medicine and Molecular Imaging**
1850 Samuel Morse Drive 703-708-9000
Reston, VA 20190 Fax: 703-708-9015
feedback@snmmi.org
www.snmmi.org
The mission of this nonprofit scientific and professional organization is to promote the science, technology and application of nuclear medicine and molecular imaging. Molecular imaging techniques are used to diagnose and manage the treatment of brain

disorders such as Alzheimer's and Parkinson's disease, among other conditions.
*15,000 members*
*Virginia Pappas, CEO*
*Rebecca Maxey, Director, Communications*

447 **Spirit of Change Magazine**
Spirit of Change Magazine
PO Box 405 508-278-9640
Uxbridge, MA 01569 Fax: 508-278-9641
info@spiritofchange.org
www.spiritofchange.org/
Consumer magazine covering holistic health and New Age issues.
*Carol Bedrosian, Publisher/Editor*
*Michella Bedrosian, Advertising Director*

448 **The American Wanderer**
American Volkssport Association (AVA)
1001 Pat Booker Road 210-659-2112
Universal City, TX 78148 Fax: 210-659-1212
AVAHQ@ava.org
www.ava.org
Consumer magazine covering sports and health news.
*Henry Rosales, Executive Director, AVA*

449 **Ultrasonic Imaging**
Sage Journals
2455 Teller Road 805-499-9774
Thousand Oaks, CA 91320 journals@sagepub.com
journals.sagepub.com/home/uix
The journal focuses on the rapid publication of original papers on the development and application of ultrasonic techniques, with emphasis on medical diagnosis. Also published are research notes, comments on papers appearing in the journal, book reviews, and occasional review articles.
*Ernest J. Feleppa, Editor-in-Chief*
*Roslyn Raskin, Managing Editor*

450 **VANTAGE**
Signature Group Inc.
15-598 Falconbridge Rd. 877-688-1989
Sudbury, ON P3A 5 Fax: 877-688-0808
www.signaturegroupinc.com/
Magazine for active consumers over 55 years of age.
*Paul Misniak, Publisher*
*Joanie Davies, Mailing Contact*

451 **VFW Auxiliary**
Ladies Auxiliary to the VFW
406 W 34th Street 816-561-8655
Kansas City, MO 64111 Fax: 816-931-4753
info@ladiesauxvfw.org
www.ladiesauxvfw.org/
VFW auxiliary patriotic services magazine.
*Armithea "Si Borel, National President*
*Marilyn Ebersole, Mailing Contact/Editor*

452 **Vegetarian Voice**
North American Vegetarian Society
PO Box 72 518-568-7970
Dolgeville, NY 13329 Fax: 518-568-7979
navs@telenet.net
www.navs-online.org
Consumer magazine covering vegetarianism, health, cooking, environmental and animal protection issues.
*40 pages*
*Maribeth Abrams, Managing Editor*
*Brian Graff, Executive Manager*

453 **Veggie Life**
EGW.com
4075 Papazian Way 925-671-9852
Fremont, CA 94538 Fax: 925-671-0692
www.egw.com/
Consumer magazine covering health, nutrition, and vegetarian cooking.
*68 pages*
*Shanna Masters, Editor*
*Rickie Wilson, Advertising Manager*

454 **Vim & Vigor Magazine**
McMurry
1010 E. Missouri Ave. 602-395-5850
Phoenix, AZ 85014 800-282-5850
Fax: 602-395-5853
mcmurrytmg.com/
Magazine offering articles on health, fitness, and medical research.
*Matthew Peterson, CEO*
*Fred Petrovsky, COO*

455 **WebMD Magazine**
WebMD, LLC
395 Hudson Street www.webmd.com/magazine
New York, NY 10014
*Vanessa Cognard, Publisher*
*Kristy Hammam, Editor in Chief*

456 **eNeuro**
Society for Neuroscience
1121 14th Street NW 202-312-7305
Washginton, DC 20005 eNeuro@sfn.org
www.eneuro.org
Open-access journal of the Society for Neuroscience.
*Christophe Bernard, Editor-in-Chief*
*Kelly Newton, Director, Scientific Publications*

## Web Sites

457 **60 Plus Association**
60 Plus Association
515 King Street 703-807-2070
Alexandria, VA 22314 Fax: 703-807-2073
info@60plus.org
www.60plus.org
A non-partisan seniors advocacy group with a free enterprise, less government, less taxes approach to seniors issues.
*James L. Martin, Chairman*
*Amy Noore Frederick, President*

458 **AARP**
601 E Street NW 888-687-2277
Washington, DC 20049 member@aarp.org
www.aarp.org
AARP is a nonprofit membership organization of persons 50 and older dedicated to addressing their needs and interests. AARP is dedicated to enhancing quality of life for all as we age. We lead positive social change and deliver value to members through information, advocacy and service.
*Jo Ann Jenkins, CEO*

459 **Age in place**
National Aging In Place Council
1400 16th Street NW 202-939-1770
Washington, DC 20036 Fax: 202-265-4435
jhoefer@dworbell.com
naipc.org
Web site with resources for planning for housing and care needs.
*Peter Bell, President*
*Marty Bell, Executive Director*

460 **Age of Reason**
Weird Seniors
Over 5,000 Links to sites of interest to the over 50 age group.

461 **Alliance for Aging Research**
www.agingresearch.org
Improving the health and independence of Americans as they age. Promotes medical and behavioral research into the aging process.

462 **American Association of Homes and Services for the Aging**
LeadingAge
2519 Connecticut Avenue North West 202-661-5700
Washington, DC 20008 Fax: 301-206-9789
info@LeadingAge.org
Organizations dedicated to providin high-quality health care, housing and services to the nation's elderly.
*William L. Minnix Jr., President/CEO*
*Katrinka Smith Sloan, SVP/Chief Operating Officer*

463 **American Society on Aging**
www.asaging.org
An association of diverse individuals bound together by a common goal: to support the commitment and enhance the knowledge and skills of those who seek to improve the quality of life of older adults and their families.

464 **Canadian National Seniors Council**
canada.ca/en/national-seniors-council
The council works with older Canadians, stakeholders and experts to advise the Canadian government on matters relating to the health, well-being and quality of life of seniors. The website provides links to reports and other publications featuring research on aging and senior citizens.

465 **Caresource Healthcare Communications**
CareSource
P.O. Box 8738 800-488-0134
Dayton, OH 45401 TTY: 800-750-0750
www.caresource.com/
This web site is a free information and resource pool for senior services community. It includes a community bulletin board for coming events, a database of senior and caregiver opportunities, directories of services and service providers, and extensive forms library.
*Pamela B. Morris, President & CEO*
*Bobby Jones, Chief Operating Officer*

466 **Caring.com**
www.caring.com
Online portal for family caregivers who are caring for aging loved ones.

467 **Centers for Medicare and Medicaid Services (CMS)**
Centers for Medicare and Medicaid Services
7500 Security Blvd. 410-786-3000
Baltimore, MD 21244 877-267-2323
TTY: 410-786-0727
www.cms.hhs.gov
CMS, part of the Federal Government, administers health insurance through Medicare and Medicaid. CMS regulates hospitals, nursing homes, and home health agencies.
*Jonathan Blum, Principal Deputy Administrator*
*Tim Love, Chief Operating Officer*

468 **ElderCareMatters.com**
561-406-5293
www.eldercarematters.com
National directory of elder and senior care resources.

469 **ElderConnect**
Elder Connect
107 North Main Street 864-934-5600
Anderson, SC 29621 jean@elderconnect.net
elderconnect.net/
Information of over 33,000 acute rehabilitation providers, retirement communities, and providers specializing in all levels of long-term nursing care as well as home health agencies.
*Becky Morlok, President*
*Jean Mahaffey, Ph.D., Executive Director*

470 **Eldercare Locator**
Department of Health and Human Services
800-677-1116
eldercarelocator@n4a.org
www.eldercare.gov
Eldercare Locator links those who need assistance with state and local area agencies on aging and community-based organizations that serve older adults and their caregivers.

471 **Elderhostel**
Road Scholar
11 Avenue de Lafayette 978-323-4141
Boston, MA 02111 800-454-5768
Fax: 617-426-0701
TTY: 877-426-2167
www.elderhostel.org
Elderhostel.
*Michael Zoob, Editor*
*James Moses, CEO*

472 **Fidelco Guide Dog Foundation**
Fidelco Guide Dog Foundation
103 Vision Way 860-243-5200
Bloomfield, CT 6002 Fax: 860-769-0567
www.fidelco.org
Fidelco breeds, raises, trains, and places German shepherd guide dogs with men and women who are visually impaired, primarily in the Northeast.
*Eliot D. Russman, CEO and Executive Director*

473 **Food Allergy Network**
Food Allergy Research & Education, Inc. (FARE)
7925 Jones Branch Dr. 800-929-4040
Mclean, VA 22102 Fax: 703-691-2713
www.foodallergy.org
Information to help families living with food allergies, and to increase public awareness about food allergies and anaphylaxis.
*Todd J. Slotkin, Chair*
*Janet Atwater, Vice Chair & Secretary*

474 **Friends-In-Art**
The American Council of the Blind
2220 Wilson Boulevard 202-467-5081
Arlingtonn, VA 22201 800-424-8666
Fax: 703-465-5085
info@acb.org
www.acb.org
Offers consultation to program planners in establishing accessible art and museum exhibits and presents Performing Arts Showcases.
*Kim Charlson, President*
*Jeff Thom, 1st Vice President*

475 **General Fitness**
General Fitness
425 Pleasant St 508-677-4933
Fall River, MA 2724 www.generalfitness.net/
Important reasons why senior citizens should exercise regardless of age.

476 **Generations Online**
Generations on Line
3637 Chestnut Street 215-222-6400
Philadelphia, PA 19104 www.generationsonline.com
*Tobby Dichter, CEO*
*VJ Pappas, COO*

477 **Gerontological Society of America**
Gerontological Society of America
1220 L Street North West 202-842-1275
Washington, DC 20005 Fax: 202-842-1150
geron@geron.org
www.geron.org
Provides researchers, educators, practitioners, and policy makers with opportunities to understand, advance, integrate, and use basic and applied research on aging to improve the quality of life as one ages.
*James Appleby, Executive Director and CEO*
*Linda Krogh Harootyan, Deputy Executive Director*

478 **Grand Times**
Grand Times
403 Village Drive 510-527-4337
El Cerrito, CA 94530 www.grandtimes.com
A weekly Internet magazine foe seniors. Controversial, entertaining and informative, Grand Times celebrates life's opportunities and examines life's challanges.
*Reece R. Halpern, Publisher*

479 **HMOs4seniors.com**
HealthMetrix Research
PO Box 30041 614-236-8345
Columbus, OH 43230
Dedicated to assisting seniors and caregivers with making informed choices regarding Medicare and Choice options.
*Alan Mittermaier, President*

480 **Healing Well**
HealingWell.com LLC
admin@healingwell.com
www.healingwell.com

An online health resource guide to medical news, chat, information and articles, newsgroups and message boards, books, disease-related web sites, medical directories, and more for patients, friends, and family coping with disabling diseases, disorders, or chronic illnesses.
*Peter Waite, Founder& CEO*

481 **Health Finder**
www.healthfinder.gov
Searchable, carefully developed web site offering information on over 1000 topics. Developed by the US Department of Health and Human Services, the site can be used in both English and Spanish.

482 **Healthlink USA**
www.healthlinkusa.com
Health information concerning treatment, cures, prevention, diagnosis, risk factors, research, support groups, email lists, personal stories and much more. Updated regularly.

483 **Immune Deficiency Foundation**
110 West Road
Towson, MD 21204
800-296-4433
Fax: 410-321-9165
primaryimmune.org
Offers information and referral services to immune deficient patients and their families.
*John G. Boyle, President & CEO*
*Sarah Rose, CFO*

484 **Internet Health Coalition**
iHealthCoalition.org
The mission of the Internet Healthcare Coalition is quality healthcare resources on the Internet.

485 **Living Will Form**
Easy Legal Form/Paralegal Services
33309 1st Way South
Federal Way, WA 98003
523-874-0649
kda31952@gmail.com
www.easylegalforms.net/
These are easy-to-use law documents that you individually customize for your specific needs.
*Kristen D. Alcoba, Paralegal-Owner*

486 **LongTermCare.gov**
longtermcare.acl.gov
Provides information on long-term care for patients and caregivers.

487 **Lotsa Helping Hands**
lotsahelpinghands.com
Platform for creating communities that assist in caring for loved ones, intended for caregivers, friends and family, and volunteers.

488 **Medicare**
Medicare.gov
7500 Security Boulevard
Baltimore, MD 21244
800-MED-CARE
TTY: 877-486-2048
www.medicare.gov
Official US Government website for people with Medicare.

489 **MedicineNet**
www.medicinenet.com
An online resource for consumers providing easy-to-read, authoritative medical and health information.

490 **Mediconsult**
Mediconsult Planning & Consulting Services Sdn. Bh
A13/5/5 One Ampang Business Avenue
Selangor, Ma
60 - 42-3 32
Fax: 60 - 42-3 31
info@mediconsult.com.my
www.mediconsult.com.my/
Provides links to information on disease, illness, and disorders, including such content areas as conference highlights, educational material, journal articles, research, news, and support.
*Dieter Nassler, Mediconsult Director*
*Sharif Lough Abdullah, Mediconsult Director*

491 **MedlinePlus**
U.S. National Library of Medicine
8600 Rockville Pike
Bethesda, MD 20894
custserv@nlm.nih.gov
medlineplus.gov
Produced by the National Library of Medicine - the world's largest medical library - MedlinePlus is the National Institutes of Health's Web site for patients and their families and friends.

492 **Medscape**
www.medscape.com
Medscape offers specialists, primary care physicians, and other health professionals the Web's most robust and integrated medical information and educational tools.

493 **Merck & Company**
Merck & Co.
One Merck Drive
Whitehouse Station, NJ 08889
908-423-1000
800-444-2080
www.merck.com
This site features several sections from the on-line version of the doctors' bible, the recently updated Merck Manual of Medical Information-Home Edition, the definitive guide to disease, diagnosis, prevention and treatment. Click on Publications.
*Kenneth C. Frazier, Chaairman &CEO*
*Richard R. Deluca Jr., EVP, Merck Animal Health*

494 **NIA Publishers**
National Institute on Aging
31 Center Drive, MSC 2292
Bethesda, MD 20892
800-222-2225
TTY: 800-222-4225
niaic@nia.nih.gov
Free publications online.
*Robin Barr, Director*
*Vicky Autrey, Branch Chief*

495 **NIH Senior Health**
National Institutes of Health
custserv@nlm.nih.gov
Reliable, easy to understand aging-related health information for older adults. This site was developed by the National Institute on Aging (NIA), and the National Library of Medicine (NLM) both parts of the National Institutes of Health (NIH).

496 **National Academy on Aging**
Gerontological Society of America
1220 L Street North West
Washington, DC 20005
202-842-1275
Fax: 202-842-1150
geron@geron.org
www.geron.org
Promotes the scientific study of aging.
*James Appleby, Executive Director and CEO*
*Linda Krogh Harootyan, Deputy Executive Director*

497 **National Association for Continence**
National Association for Continence (NAFC)
P.O. Box 1019
Charleston, SC 29402
843-377-0900
800-BLA-DER
Fax: 843-377-0905
memberservices@nafc.org
www.nafc.org
Committed to alleviating the social stigma associated with bladder control problems. Information to consumers and health professionals and advocating on their behalf to increase public awareness about incontinence.
*Donna Deng, MD, Chairperson*
*Nancy Hicks, Vice-Chairperson*

498 **National Association for Home Care and Hospice (NAHC)**
National Association for Home Care & Hospice
228 7th Street SE
Washington, DC 20003
202-547-7424
Fax: 202-547-3540
www.nahc.org
Providers of home health care, hospice, and homemaker-home health aide services; interested individuals and organizations. Develops and promotes high standards of patient care in home care services. Seeks to affect legislative and regulatory processes concerning home care services; gathers and disseminates home care industry data; develops public relations strategies; works to increase political visibility of home care services. Interprets home c
*Andrea Devoti, Chair*
*Lucy Andrews, Vice Chair*

499 **National Association of Professional Geriatric Care Managers (PGCM)**
3275 West Ina Road 520-881-8008
Tuscon, AZ 85741 Fax: 520-325-7925
www.caremanager.org
Information resource for those interested in the field of geriatriccare while supporting quality care and services for the elderly.
*Emily Saltz, MSW, LICSW, CMC, President*
*Amy Abrams, MPH, MSW, CMC, Director*

500 **National Association of State Units on Aging**
National Association of State Units on Aging & Dis
1201 15th Street, NW 202-898-2578
Wsahington, DC 20005 Fax: 202-898-2583
info@nasuad.org
www.nasuad.org/
Offers support, information and technical assistance to state units on aging.
*Gloria Lawlah, President*
*James Bulot, Vice President*

501 **National Council for Aging Care**
www.aging.com
Seeks to provide older adults with information and resources on health & well-being, caregiving, money and financial planning, and lifestyle, through their Aging.com website.

502 **National Council on Aging**
www.ncoa.org
The nation's first charitable organization dedicated to promoting the dignity, independence, well-being and contributions of older Americans. The council has a goal of improving the health and economic well-being of 10 million older adults by 2020. The website provides tools and resources for older adults and caregivers.

503 **National Hospice & Palliative Care Organization (NHPCO)**
www.nhpco.org
The organization seeks to improve end-of-life care, widen access to hospice care, and improve quality of life for the dying and their loved ones. NHPCO's website offers information on regulations, advocacy, quality and performance, education, and a variety of other resources.

504 **National Institute of Aging**
www.nia.nih.gov
Conducts research on aging, behavioral and social research, neuroscience and neuropsychology, geriatrics, and clinical gerontology.

505 **National Institute of Neurological Disorders and Stroke**
National Institute of Neurological Disorders &Stro
P.O. Box 5801 301-496-5751
Bethesda, MD 20824 800-352-9424
www.ninds.nih.gov
Offers a brochure on stroke. The leading supporter of research on brain and nervous system disorders, including stroke.
*Story C. Landis, Ph.D., Director*
*Caroline Lewis, Executive Officer*

506 **National Institute on Aging**
National Institute on Aging
31 Center Drive, MSC 2292 800-222-2225
Bethesda, MD 20892 TTY: 800-222-4225
niaic@nia.nih.gov
The NIA promotes healthy aging by conducting and supporting biomedical, social, and behavioral research and public education.
*Robin Barr, Director*
*Vicky Autrey, Branch Chief*

507 **National Institutes of Health**
9000 Rockville Pike 301-496-4000
Bethesda, MD 20892 TTY: 301-402-9612
nihinfo@od.nih.gov
www.nih.gov
The nation's medical research agency.
*Francis S. Collins, Director*

508 **National Meditation Center**
National Meditation Center (NMC)
936-445-0095
www.nationalmeditation.org/
A humanitarian agency with volunteer camps. We need seniors for our volunteer projects overseas and here in America.
*Master Hughes, Director*

509 **National Organization for Victim Assistance**
National Organization for Victim Assistance
510 King Street 703-535-6682
Alexandria, VA 22314 800-879-6682
Fax: 703-535-5500
www.trynova.org
NOVA's mission is to promote rights and services for victims of crime and crisis everywhere.
*Hon. Tim Jeffries, President*
*Andrew Yurick, VP for Administration*

510 **Neuronline**
Society for Neuroscience
1121 14th Street NW 202-962-4000
Washginton, DC 20005 neuronline@sfn.org
neuronline.sfn.org
Online portal for professional development and training resources for individuals in the field of neuroscience, hosted by the Society for Neuroscience.
*Amanda Kimball, Director, Digital Learning*

511 **Next Step in Care**
www.nextstepincare.org
Online platform with videos and guides for family caregivers and healthcare providers, as well as other resources.

512 **Onhealth**
MedicineNet, Inc.
www.onhealth.com
A search engine providing links to websites with information on illnesses, diseases, and disorders.

513 **Partnership for Prescription Assistance**
Partnership for Prescription Assistance (PPA)
888-4PP- NOW
www.pparx.org
Our mission is to increase awareness of patient assistance programs and boost enrollment of those who are eligible. The Partnership for Prescription Assistance offers a single point of access to more than 475 public and private patient assistance programs, including more than 150 programs offered by pharmaceutical companies.

514 **QuackWatch**
QuackWatch
Chatham Crossing, Suite 107/208 www.quackwatch.org
Chapel Hill, NC 27517
A nonprofit corporation whose purpose is to combat health-related frauds, myths, fads, fallacies, and misconduct. Its primary focus is on quackery-related information that is difficult or impossible to get elsewhere.
*Dr. Stephen Barrett, Founder*

515 **Research Center**
Online center offering information on consumer issues, demographics, independent living and other items of interest to senior citizens.

516 **Retirement Planning**
www.vanguard.com/
Helps you create a personal financial plan based on information you enter.
*F. William McNabb III, Chairman and CEO*
*John C. Bogle, Founder*

517 **Senior Housing Net**
10 Almaden Blvd. www.seniorhousing.net
San Jose, CA 95113
Comprehensive guide to retirement communities, assisted living residences, Alzheimer's facilities, and nursing homes nationwide.
*Michele Conn, VP, Corporate Development*
*Alison Schwartz, VP of Communications*

518 **Senior Job Bank**
Senior Job Bank
P.O. Box 508
Marlborough, MA 1752
888-501-0804
publisher@seniorjobbank.org
www.seniorjobbank.com

519 **Senior Law Home Page**
Senior Law Home Page
350 Fifth Avenue
New York, NY 10118
212-387-8400
goldfarb@seniorlaw.com
www.seniorlaw.com
Information about Elder Law, Medicare, Medicaid, estate planning, trusts and the rights of the elderly and disabled.
*Ira Salzman, Attorney*
*Michael Kutzin, Publisher*

520 **Senior Summer School**
Senior Summer School
P.O. Box 188
Madison, WI 53701
800-847-2466
The Education Vacation for seniors. Visit college campuses across the US and Canada from 2 to 10 weeks during the summer.

521 **Senior Times**
The Senior Times
4077 Decarie Boulevard
Montreal, QC H4A 3
514-484-5033
Fax: 514-484-8254
editor@theseniortimes.com
www.theseniortimes.com
By, for, and about exraordinary seniors.
*Barbara Moser, Publisher & Managing Editor*
*Kristine Berey, Assistant Editor*

522 **Senior Women's Travel**
20 Van Winkle Road
Hudson, NY 12534
917-880-6732
maryann@poshnosh.com
www.poshnosh.com
Senior Women's Travel brings a new dimension to senior travel and eliminates many of the annoyances of single travel. It's for 50+ women, with a large cultural appetite, who love to shop and eat.
*Mary Ann Zimmerman, President and Founder*

523 **SeniorGuidance.org**
www.seniorguidance.org
SeniorGuidance.org provides comprehensive resources on various senior living options, including: assisted living facilities, senior living communities, nursing homes, independent living communities, continuing care retirement communities (CCRC) and all other long term senior care options.

524 **Seniorresource.com**
www.seniorresource.com
Provides information to older adults on needed facilities and services, including through internet directories and an archive of E-zines.

525 **US Administration on Aging**
acl.gov/about-acl/administration-aging
An agency in the US Department of Health and Human Services, and under the Administration for Community Living, is one of the nation's largest providers of home and community-based care for older persons and their caregivers.

526 **WebMD**
WebMD, LLC
www.webmd.com
Credible information, in-depth reference material, health management tools and supportive communities.
*Kristy Hammam, SVP, Content & Programming*
*Michael Smith, Chief Medical Editor*

527 **Webhelp**
Webhelp
161, Rue de Courcelles
Paris, 75 1 44
www.webhelp.com
Provides links to information, including research, treatment, prevention, support, and more.
*Jeremy Come, Communication Director*

528 **Women's Health**
The New York Times Company
212-556-7194
800-NYT-MES
www.nytimes.com
Click on Web Specials-women's health to reach this site operated by *The New York Times*. Consult Resources for a guide to more than 100 women-related Web sites.

# ALZHEIMER'S DISEASE

*Alzheimer's disease is a degenerative neurologic disease that attacks the brain and impairs memory, thinking faculties, and behavior, leading to dementia. Sixty to seventy percent of all dementia cases are the result of Alzheimer's disease. While dementia is the umbrella term for a group of symptoms including cognitive and memory impairment, Alzheimer's is a specific condition that causes dementia.*

As of 2020, an estimated 5.8 million Americans suffer from Alzheimer's. By 2050, this number is projected to jump to 13.8 million. Alzheimer's primarily afflicts older people, with more than 95 percent of cases found in patients over 65, and it is twice as common in women as in men. The disease was first discovered by the German psychiatrist Alois Alzheimer, who witnessed the phenomenon in 1901 in a 51-year-old patient. He publicized his findings five years later when she died. By the end of the decade, numerous cases were being documented and the disease was already being known as Alzheimer's.

In spite of diligent research, the cause of Alzheimer's is unknown. There is believed to be a genetic component to the disease, with generic heritability ranging from 49% to 79% percent. There are multiple symptoms of Alzheimer's disease, the most pronounced being gradual memory loss. Other symptoms include the inability to perform routine tasks, loss of language skills, disorientation, and personality changes. The diagnosis is largely based on an interview with the patient and family members and an examination of the patient, although brain imaging tests and blood tests may add helpful information. The course of the disease is divided into four stages: pre-dementia, early, moderate, and advanced. In the final stages, the patient is completely dependent on caregivers and in many cases loses speech all together. Although the life expectancy for people with advanced-stage Alzheimer's is low, the patient typically dies of an external disease, such as pneumonia or dehydration, rather than Alzheimer's itself.

The brain's cells communicate with each other through various chemicals called neurotransmitters. In Alzheimer's disease, levels of the neurotransmitter acetylcholine are decreased. Drugs that enhance acetylcholine neurotransmission, such as donepezil, galantamine, and rivastigmine, can modestly improve memory during the early stages of Alzheimer's disease, but do not delay the overall progression of the disease. Another drug, memantine, modulates glutamate neurotransmission and can improve cognition over short periods of time, but also does not delay the progression of the disease. The antipsychotic drug, quetiapine, can control some of behavioral symptoms associated with dementia, although antipsychotics are often not recommended because they can lead to an earlier death. In 2018, 122,000 people died of Alzheimer's in the U.S. alone.

In general, non-pharmacological interventions, such as social support networks, community, and participation in hobbies are more effective treatments for Alzheimer's disease than drugs. Because Alzheimer's disease severely affects both the patient and the family, proper planning, as well as medical and social programs tailored to the individual and to family members are essential. A well-structured and safe living environment is the best way to preserve the welfare and dignity of the person with Alzheimer's disease as well as with advanced dementia.

Because of the heavy care-giving burden and the frequent need for the patient to be institutionalized in the later stages, Alzheimer's is believed to be one of the most costly diseases for society, particularly in the United States and Europe. Caregivers, who are often the patient's spouse or a close relative, often have to give up working to look after the patient, and are subject to an elevated rate of mental disorders. In 2019, caregivers for people with Alzheimer's and other dementias provided an estimated 18.6 billion hours of unpaid care, estimated in value at $244 billion.

## National Agencies & Associations

530 **Alzheimer Society of Alberta and Northwest Territories**
10430 - 61 Avenue 780-761-0030
Edmonton, Alberta, T6H-2J3 866-950-5465
Fax: 780-488-3055
reception@alzheimer.ab.ca
www.alzheimer.ca/en/ab
Provides support, education, and advocacy for all those affected by Alzheimer's disease in Alberta and the Northwest Territories, including patients, caregivers, patients' families, and the community.
*Michele Mulder, Chief Executive Officer*
*Brenda Burrell, Provincial Lead, Operations*

531 **Alzheimer Society of B.C.**
828 W 8th Avenue Street 604-681-6530
Vancouver, BC, V5C-1E2 800-667-3742
Fax: 604-669-6907
info@alzheimerbc.org
www.alzheimer.ca/en/bc
Provides support, education, and advocacy for all those affected by Alzheimer's disease in British Columbia, including patients, caregivers, patients' families, and the community.
*Maria Howard, Chief Executive Officer*
*Cathryn France, Director, Resource Development*

532 **Alzheimer Society of Canada**
20 Eglinton Avenue W 416-488-8772
Toronto, Ontario, M4R-1K8 800-618-8816
Fax: 416-322-6656
info@alzheimer.ca
www.alzheimer.ca
Identifies, develops and facilitates national priorities that enable its members to effectively alleviate the personal and social consequences of Alzheimer's disease and related disorders; promotes research and leads the search for a cure.
*Pauline Tardif, Chief Executive Officer*

533 **Alzheimer Society of Manitoba**
10 - 120 Donald Street 204-943-6622
Winnipeg, Manitoba, R3C-4G2 800-378-6699
alzmb@alzheimer.mb.ca
alzheimer.mb.ca
Provides support, education, and advocacy for all those affected by Alzheimer's disease in Manitoba, including patients, caregivers, patients' families, and the community.
*Wendy Schettler, Chief Executive Officer*
*Norma Kirkby, Program Director*

534 **Alzheimer Society of New Brunswick**
320 Maple Street 506-459-4280
Fredericton, NB, E3B-5G2 800-664-8411
Fax: 506-452-0313
info@alzheimernb.ca
alzheimer.ca/en/nb
Provides support, education, and advocacy for all those affected by Alzheimer's disease in New Brunswick, including patients, caregivers, patients' families, and the community.
*Chandra MacBean, Executive Director*

535 **Alzheimer Society of Newfoundland & Labrador**
835 Topsail Road 709-576-0608
Mount Pearl, NL, A1N-3J6 877-776-0608
Fax: 709-576-0798
info@alzheimernl.ca
alzheimer.ca/en/nl
Provides support, education, and advocacy for all those affected by Alzheimer's disease in Newfoundland and Labrador, including patients, caregivers, patients' families, and the community.
*Shirley Lucas, Chief Executive Officer*
*Jessica Flynn, Coordinator, Education Development*

536 **Alzheimer Society of Nova Scotia**
2719 Gladstone Street 902-422-7961
Halifax, Nova Scotia, B3K-4W6 800-611-6345
Fax: 902-422-7971
alzheimer@asns.ca
alzheimer.ca/en/ns
Provides support, education, and advocacy for all those affected by Alzheimer's disease in Nova Scotia, including patients, caregivers, patients' families, and the community.
*Lloyd Brown, Executive Director*
*Linda Bird, Director, Programs & Services*

537 **Alzheimer Society of Ontario**
20 Eglinton Avenue W 416-967-5900
Toronto, Ontario, M4R-1K8 800-879-4226
Fax: 416-967-3826
staff@alzon.ca
alzheimer.ca/en/on
Provides support, education, and advocacy for all those affected by Alzheimer's disease in Ontario, including patients, caregivers, patients' families, and the community.
*Cathy Barrick, Chief Executive Officer*

538 **Alzheimer Society of Prince Edward Island**
166 Fitzroy Street 902-628-2257
Charlottetown, PE, C1A-1S1 society@alzpei.ca
alzheimer.ca/en/pei
Provides support, education, and advocacy for all those affected by Alzheimer's disease in Prince Edward Island, including patients, caregivers, patients' families, and the community.
*M. Lynn Murray, QC, President*

539 **Alzheimer Society of Saskatchewan**
2550 - 12th Avenue 306-949-4141
Regina, Saskatchewan, S4P-3X1 800-263-3367
Fax: 306-949-3069
info@alzheimer.sk.ca
www.alzheimer.ca/en/sk
Provides support, education, and advocacy for all those affected by Alzheimer's disease in Saskatchewan, including patients, caregivers, patients' families, and the community.
*Joanne Bracken, Chief Executive Officer*
*Leslie Quennell, Manager, Communications & Marketing*

540 **Alzheimer's & Related Dementias Education & Referral Center**
National Institute on Aging
31 Center Drive 800-438-4380
Bethesda, MD 20892 TTY: 800-222-4225
adear@nia.nih.gov
www.nia.nih.gov/health/alzheimers
A service of the National Institute on Aging, the center distributes information on Alzheimer's disease, on current research activities and on services available to patients and family members. Offers a free list of publications available upon request.

541 **Alzheimer's Association**
225 N Michigan Avenue 800-272-3900
Chicago, IL 60601 info@alz.org
www.alz.org
Combats Alzheimer's disease and related disorders. Seeks to destroy the myth that what were once called 'senile behaviors' are a natural part of aging. Works to develop family support systems for relatives of victims of the disease.
*Harry Johns, President & CEO*
*Richard Hovland, COO*

542 **Alzheimer's Association National Office**
225 North Michigan Avenue 312-335-8700
Chicago, IL 60601 800-272-3900
Fax: 866-699-1246
TDD: 312-335-5886
info@alz.org
alz.org
Headquarters for Alzheimer's Association, an organization dedicated to helping all those with Alzheimer's disease and dementia, and their families. Funds Alzheimer's research, engages in Alzheimer's advocacy, and offers referrals, support groups, educational sessions, safety services, and publications.
*Christopher Binkley, Chair*
*Harry Johns, President and CEO*

543 **Alzheimer's Disease Education and Referral Center**
National Institute on Aging

PO Box 8250
Silver Spring, MD 20907
301-495-3311
800-438-4380
Fax: 301-495-3334
adear@nia.nih.gov
nia.nih.gov/alzheimers
The ADEAR Center provides information about Alzheimer's Disease and related disorders to health professionals, patients and their families, and the public.
*Richard J. Hodes, MD, Director*
*Patrick Shirdon, Director of Management*

544 **Alzheimer's Poetry Project**
55 Washington Street
Brooklyn, NY 11201
garyglaznerpoet@gmail.com
www.alzpoetry.com
Alzheimer's Poetry Project is dedicated to improve the quality of life of people living with Alzheimer's disease and related dementia by facilitating creative expression through poetry.
*Gary Glazner, Executive Director*

545 **American Academy of Neurology**
201 Chicago Avenue
Minneapolis, MN 55415
612-928-6000
800-879-1960
Fax: 612-454-2746
memberservices@aan.com
www.aan.com
Professional society of medical doctors specializing in brain and nervous system diseases. Maintains placement service. Sponsors research and educational programs. Compiles statistics. Publishes scientific journal, Continuum: Lifelong Learning in Neurology.
*Mary E. Post, MBA, CAE, CEO*

546 **American Board of Psychiatry and Neurology**
7 Parkway N
Deerfield, IL 60015
847-229-6500
Fax: 847-229-6600
questions@abpn.com
www.abpn.com
The mission of the ABPN is to develop and provide valid and reliable procedures for certification and maintenance of certification in psychiatry and neurology.
*Larry R. Faulkner, President & CEO*

547 **American Society for Investigative Pathology**
1801 Rockville Pike
Rockville, MD 20852
240-283-9700
Fax: 301-984-4047
www.asip.org
The Society seeks to promote experimental pathology and related disciplines through meetings, publications, and educational activities.
*William B. Coleman, PhD, Executive Officer*
*Gina LaBorde, Manager, Marketing & Communications*

548 **American Society for Neurochemistry**
9037 Ron Den Lane
Windermere, FL 34786
407-909-9064
Fax: 407-876-0750
asnmanager@asneurochem.org
asneurochem.org
The Society aims to advance and promote cellular and molecular neuroscience knowledge, and to facilitate communication and the dissemination of information within the field and with related disciplines.
*Sheilah Jewart, Executive Director*
*Karen Gottlieb, Conference Coordinator*

549 **Association for Molecular Pathology**
6120 Executive Boulvard
Rockville, MD 20852
301-634-7987
amp@amp.org
www.amp.org

550 **Brain Resources and Information Network (BRAIN)**
National Institute of Neurological Disorders & Str
PO Box 5801
Bethesda, MD 20824
301-496-5751
800-352-9424
braininfo@ninds.nih.gov
ninds.nih.gov
Federal agency focused on supporting neuroscience research and working towards reducing the burdens associated with neurological disease.
*Denise Dorsey, Chief Administrative Officer*
*Peter Soltys, Chief Information Officer*

551 **Brain Support Network**
P.O. Box 7264
Menlo Park, CA 94026
650-814-0848
Fax: 650-233-9278
www.brainsupportnetwork.org
Non-profit dedicated to facilitate brain donation for scientific study in the U.S. and Canada, to provide education on neurological conditions worldwide, and run support groups in Northern California.

552 **BrightFocus Foundation**
22512 Gateway Center Drive
Clarksburg, MD 20871
800-437-2423
Fax: 301-258-9454
info@brightfocus.org
www.brightfocus.org
Offers updated and trustworthy information on research, treatments, and resources. Free publications and newsletters.
*Stacy Pagos Haller, President & CEO*

553 **CareScout**
60 Hickory Drive
Waltham, MA 02451
800-571-1918
Fax: 800-513-8860
www.carescout.com
Care advocates help thousands of families each year find the most appropriate home health aids, assisted living facilities, and nursing homes.
*Robert N. Bua, President*

554 **Caregiver Action Network**
1150 Connecticut Avenue Northwest
Washington, DC 20036
202-454-3970
info@caregiveraction.org
caregiveraction.org
Caregiver Action Network is a nonprofit organization that acts as a support and an advocate for family caregivers of individuals with chronic conditions, diabilities, diseases, or old age. CAN provides education, peer support, and resources free of charge.
*Wes Metheny, Chair*
*John Schall, Chief Executive Officer*

555 **CaringKind**
360 Lexington Avenue
New York, NY 10017
646-744-2900
helpline@caringkindny.org
www.caringkindny.org
CaringKind provides information, tools and training to support individuals and families affected by dementia. Formerly known as the Alzheimer's Association's New York City Chapter.
*Jed A. Levine, President & CEO*
*Alex Wong, CFO*

556 **Center for Mental Health Services (CMHS)**
Substance Abuse and Mental Health Services Adminis
5600 Fishers Lane
Rockville, MD 20857
240-276-1310
877-726-4727
TTY: 800-487-4889
samhsa.gov/about-us/who-we-are/offices-c
Promotes the treatment of mental illness and emotional disorders by increasing accessibility to mental health programs; supporting outreach, treatment, rehabilitation, and support programs and networks; and encouraging the use of scientifically-based information when treating mental disorders. CMHS provides information about mental health via a toll-free number and numerous publications. Developed for users of mental health services and their families, the general public, and policy makers.
*Paolo del Vecchio, MSW, Director*
*Anne Mathews-Younes, Acting Deputy Director*

557 **Cure Alzheimer's Fund**
34 Washington Street
Wellesley Hills, MA 02481
781-237-3800
Fax: 781-658-2399
info@curealz.org
curealz.org
Dedicated to raising funds for Alzheimer research.
*Timothy W. Armour, President & CEO*

558 **Dementia & Alzheimer's Wellbeing Network**
PO Box 1934
Bonners Ferry, ID 83805
208-388-8898
info@thedawnmethod.com
www.thedawnmethod.com

The DAWN Method is a set of tools for those caring for people with dementia. Offers training to families and caregivers to meet the emotional needs and rational thought losses caused by dementia.
*Judy Cornish, Founder*

559 **Dementia Action Alliance**
732-212-9036
info@daanow.org
daanow.org
The Dementia Action Alliance USA is a non-profit national advocacy and education organization of people living with dementia, care partners, friends and dementia specialists committed to creating a stronger community through education and compassion.

560 **Dementia Alliance International**
PO Box 582 www.dementiaallianceinternational.org
Ankeny, IA 50021
A collaboration of individuals diagnosed with dementia working together to provide support and advocacy for people living with dementia. DAI promotes education and awareness through community collaboration.
*Kate Swaffer, Chair & CEO*

561 **Dementia Care Warriors**
Dallas, TX iamacarewarrior.org
A non-profit organization dedicated to providing non-medical assistance and resources to caregivers caring for those living with Alzheimer's and related dementia.

562 **Dementia Caregiver Resources Inc.**
Chicago, IL www.dcrinc.org
A non-profit assisting families and caregivers through education, support groups, and guidance.
*Karen Truman, Founder*
*Jeff Truman, Founder*

563 **Dementia Friendly America**
National Association of Area Agencies on Aging
1100 New Jersey Avenue SE 202-872-0888
Washington, DC 20003 info@dfamerica.org
www.dfamerica.org
Dementia Friendly America (DFA) is a national network of communities and organizations dedicated to supporting people living with dementia and their caregivers. DFA offers a variety of resources online and allows for communities across the country to connect and help one another.
*Sandy Markwood, Co-Chair*
*Ron Grant, Co-Chair*

564 **Dementia Redefined**
10903 Verawood Drive 941-376-2241
Riverview, FL 33579 Fax: 813-315-6906
ristow@dementiaredefined.com
dementiaredefined.com
A non-profit dedicated to providing guidance, education, and community awareness programs to people diagnosed with dementia, their families and caregivers. Offers training courses.
*Ruth Anne Ristow, Founder & Director*

565 **Dementia Society of America**
PO Box 600 800-336-3684
Doylestown, PA 18901 www.dementiasociety.org
DSA provides an information hotline and online resources to support Dementia awareness.
*Kevin Jameson, Founder, President & CEO*

566 **Dementia Spotlight Foundation**
888-695-1596
info@dementiaspotlightfoundation.org
dementiaspotlightfoundation.org
A non-profit organization dedicated to supporting people diagnosed with dementia through advocacy, the arts, and dementia education.
*Whitney DeMarlo Oeltmann, Co-Founder & CFO*
*Vincent Zangaro, Community Outreach Director*

567 **Earth Angels for Dementia**
115 Route 50 609-837-0338
Mays Landing, NJ 08330 earthangelsfordementia@gmail.com
www.earthangelsfordementia.org
A non-profit offering educational training, support groups, stress relieving activities, and other resources to assist people affected by Alzheimer's, Lewy Body and other dementias.
*Cheryl Caliri, Co-Founder*
*Hilary Van Horn, Co-Founder*

568 **Federation of Associations in Behavioral a Brain Sciences**
1001 Connecticut Avenue Northwest 202-888-3949
Washington, DC 20036 info@fabbs.org
fabbs.org
FABBS is a coalition of scientific societies focused on expanding scientific knowledge on the brain, mind, and behavior. FABBS educates the public and policymakers on the importance of brain, mind, and behavior sciences research; provides quality sources to federal agencies and the media; advocates for research-focused policy and legislation; and promotes exchange of information among scientific organizations.
*Nora Newcombe, PhD, President*
*Paula Skedsvold, JD, PhD, Executive Director*

569 **Federation of Quebec Alzheimer Societies**
5165 Sherbrooke Street W 514-369-7891
Montreal, Quebec, H4A-1T6 888-636-6473
Fax: 514-369-7900
info@alzheimerquebec.ca
alzheimer.ca/en/federationquebecoise
Provides support, education, and advocacy for all those affected by Alzheimer's disease in Quebec, including patients, caregivers, patients' families, and the community.
*Luc Pinard, President*

570 **Geoffrey Beene Alzheimer's Initiative**
Geoffrey Beene Foundation
13 E 69th Street Fax: 212-472-7711
New York, NY 10065 mara@geoffreybeenefoundation.com
geoffreybeenefoundation.com
Dedicated to raising funds for Alzheimer's research, awareness, and treatment.
*G. Thompson Hutton, CEO*
*Mara Hutton, EVP*

571 **Giving Voice Initiative**
7801 E Bush Lake Road 612-440-9660
Bloomington, MN 55439 info@givingvoicechorus.org
givingvoicechorus.org
Giving Voice Initiative inspires and equips organizations to bring together people with Alzheimer's and their caregivers to sing in choruses that foster joy, well-being, purpose and community understanding.
*Mary Lenard, Co-Founder & Executive Director*
*Marge Ostroushko, Co-Founder & Managing Director*

572 **Global Brain Health Institute**
Sandler Neurosciences Center
675 Nelson Rising Lane 415-476-3722
San Francisco, CA 94143 info@gbhi.org
www.gbhi.org
The Global Brain Health Institute (GBHI) is a collaboration between the University of California, San Francisco (UCSF) and Trinity College Dublin. GBHI is dedicated to brain health research and improving the lives of the aging population.
*Ian Robertson, Co-Director*
*Bruce Miller, Co-Director*

573 **Hilarity for Charity**
9301 Wilshire Boulevard info@wearehfc.org
Beverly Hills, CA 90210 wearehfc.org
A non-profit dedicated to raising awareness, funding research and support for people with Alzheimer's Disease and their families and caregivers.
*Bonnie Wattles, Executive Director*

574 **I'm Still Here Foundation**
10 Tower Office Park 781-674-2884
Woburn, MA 01801 www.imstillhere.org
A non-profit promoting community engagement as an initiative to support people living with dementia. The foundation places an emphasis on arts and culture, education, and public policy.
*John Zeisel, President*

575 **John Douglas French Alzheimer's Foundation**
11620 Wilshire Boulevard
Los Angeles, CA 90025-1781
323-930-6228
800-477-2243
Fax: 310-479-0516
bwelch@alz.org
www.jdfaf.org
Provides seed money for promising research including the cause cure and prevention of Alzheimer's disease. Also gives funding to scientists who might not otherwise be funded.
*Bruce L. Miller, MD, Chief Medical Officer*
*Karen Bedrosian Coyne, President*

576 **National Alzheimer's Disease Institute**
7111 Sweetgum Road
Fairview, TN 37602-9384
nationalalzdiseaseinstitute.org
Investigates and presents information on the ways in which natural or alternative medicine can slow or prevent dementia. Physician referrals are provided. The institute is overseen by the National Fund for Alternative Medicine.
*P. Anthony Chapdelaine, Jr., Executive Director*
*Mary Ann Chapdelaine, President*

577 **National Association for the Dually Diagnosed (NADD)**
132 Fair Street
Kingston, NY 12401
845-331-4336
info@thenadd.org
thenadd.org
NADD is a nonprofit organization designed to increase awareness of, and provide services for, individuals with developmental disabilities and mental illness. NADD emphasizes the importance of quality mental healthcare for people with mental health needs and offers conferences, information resources, educational programs, and training materials to professionals, parents, and organizations.
*Jeanne M. Farr, MA, Chief Executive Officer*
*Daniel Baker, PhD., President*

578 **National Association of Councils on Developmental Disabilities**
1825 K Street Northwest
Washington, DC 20006
202-506-5813
info@nacdd.org
nacdd.org/
A national membership association representing the 56 State and Territorial Councils on Developmental Disabilities. An organization with the purpose of promoting the programs and policies that its member councils advocate, as well as ensuring inclusion for Americans with developmental disabilities.
*Donna A. Meltzer, Chief Executive Officer*
*Shannon Buller, President*

579 **National Council of Certified Dementia Practitioners**
55 Main Street
Sparta, NJ 07871
973-729-6601
877-729-5191
Fax: 973-860-2244
www.nccdp.org
The NCCDP offers training programs for all health care professionals and staff. Training includes dementia education through seminars and certifications courses.
*Sandra Stimson, CEO & Founder*
*Lynn Biot-Gordon, COO & Founder*

580 **National Dementia Association**
PO Box 103
Emery, SD 57332
info@nationaldementia.org
www.nationaldementia.org
A non-profit organization dedicated to providing support to families, care givers, and persons diagnosed with some form of dementia (Alzheimer's disease, Lewy Body, Frontal Temporal Lobe disease, etc.) through education and training.

581 **National Institute on Aging**
31 Center Drive, MSC 2292
Bethesda, MD 20892
800-222-2225
TTY: 800-222-4225
niaic@nia.nih.gov
www.nia.nih.gov
Seeks to understand the nature of aging, and to extend healthy, active years of life. Free resources are available on topics such as Alzheimer's & dimentia, caregiving, cognitive heath, end of life care, and more.
*Richard J. Hodes MD, Director*
*Marie A. Bernard, MD, Deputy Director*

582 **National Mental Health Consumers' Clearinghouse**
1211 Chestnut Street
Philadelphia, PA 19107
267-507-3810
800-553-4539
Fax: 215-636-6312
info@mhselfhelp.org
mhselfhelp.org
The Clearinghouse is a peer-run national technical assistance center focused on achieving respect and equality of opportunity for those with mental illnesses. The Clearinghouse helps with the growth of the mental health consumer movement by evaluating mental health services, advocating for mental health reform, and providing consumers with news, information, publications, and consultation services.
*Joseph Rogers, Founder and Executive Director*
*Susan Rogers, Director*

583 **National Niemann-Pick Disease Foundation**
Fort Atkinson, WI 53538
920-563-0930
877-287-3672
Fax: 920-563-0931
nnpdf@nnpdf.org
nnpdf.org
The Foundations promotes research and offers support and funding for individuals with Niemann-Pick Disease and their support network.
*Lisa Chavez, Board Chair*
*Justin Hopkin, Vice Chair*

584 **Rethinking Dementia**
1551 Franklin Street SE
Grand Rapids, MI 49506
616-247-9630
contact@rethinkingdementiami.org
rethinkingdementiami.org
A non-profit organization made up of experts in senior care and aging. Rethinking Dementia is dedicated to improving the lives of people affected by dementia by promoting better access to support and services. Rethinking Dementia seeks to remove the stigma attached to dementia and memory loss, empower caregivers and provide them with better resources, and advocate for policy reform and funding.
*Lisa Misenhimer, Director*

585 **Society for Neuroscience**
1121 14th Street NW
Washginton, DC 20005
202-962-4000
marty@sfn.org
sfn.org
Large international organization of scientists and physicians devoted to the study of the brain and the nervous system.
*37,000 members*
*Marty Saggese, Executive Director*
*Melissa Garcia, Associate Executive Director*

586 **The Center for Family Support**
2811 Zulette Avenue
Bronx, NY 10461
718-518-1500
Fax: 718-518-8200
www.cfsny.org/
The Center for Family Support offers assistance to individuals with developmental and related disabilities, as well as their families, and provides support services and programs that are designed to accommodate individual needs. Offers services throughout New York City, Westchester County, Long Island, and New Jersey.
*Steven Vernikoff, Executive Director*
*Lloyd Stabiner, President*

587 **TimeSlips**
4461 N Lake Drive
Milwaukee, WI 53211
www.timeslips.org
A non-profit organization dedicated to helping people with dementia connect with their families and caregivers. TimeSlips takes a forward approach by stepping away from the expectation of memory and focuses on the present for people living with memory loss and other neurological disorders. Offers training courses and seminars, coaching, educational resources and promotes community engagement.
*Anne Basting, Founder & CEO*
*Carol Varney, Executive Director*

588 **Universal Dementia Caregivers**
24342 Ridgeview Drive
Farmington Hills, MI 48336
248-509-4357
info@universaldementia.org
www.universaldementia.org

A non-profit organization dedicated to education caregivers, families and communities supporting people diagnosed with Alzheimer's and other dementia related diseases. Services include coaching, training workshops, and family meditation.
*Paula S. Duren, Founder & CEO*

## State Agencies & Associations

589 **Alzheimer's & Dementia Resource Center**
715 Douglas Avenue 407-436-7750
Altamonte, FL 32714 Fax: 407-369-4272
info@adrccares.org
adrccares.org
A non profit organization, has been the forerunner in Central Florida bringing Alzheimer specific education and support to family caregivers as well as professional care providers.
*Kerrin Kuhn, Executive Director*

590 **Alzheimer's & Dementia Services of Memphis Inc.**
Kennedy Park Center 901-372-4585
Memphis, TN 38128 info@adsmemphis.org
www.adsmemphis.org
Dedicated to helping persons with Alzheimer's disease and related disorders live their lives with dignity and respect while providing relief to their caregivers and support for their families.
*Ruthann Shelton, Executive Director*
*Sara Todd, Programming Coordinator*

591 **Alzheimer's Aid Society of Northern California**
2641 Cottage Way 916-483-2002
Sacramento, CA 95825 800-540-3340
info@alzaid.org
Family support: provide needed support and advice for victims and their families. Counseling and emotional support are a major need. Education and information for lay and professional people. To aid and support research into the causes, treatment, prevention and cure for Alzheimer's disease. To advocate the social needs of the afflicted population, provide information to increase public awareness. Bimonthly newsletters and a multitute of direct
*Sheryl Ashby, President*
*Max Perry, Executive Officer*

592 **Alzheimer's Alliance: Texarkana Area**
104 Cypress 903-223-8021
Texarkana, TX 75503-7812 877-312-8536
Fax: 903-792-1792
*Linda Nickerson, Executive Director*
*Fran Long, Program Director*

593 **Alzheimer's Arkansas Programs and Services**
400 President Clinton Ave 501-265-0027
Little Rock, AR 72205 800-272-3900
Fax: 501-227-6303
sdavis@alz.org
www.alz.org
*Phyllis Watkins, Executive Director*
*Susie Davis, Local Contact*

594 **Alzheimer's Association San Diego/Imperial Chapter**
6632 Convoy Court 858-966-3319
San Diego, CA 92111 800-272-3900
Fax: 858-492-4406
walksandiego@alz.org
www.alz.org
The leading voluntary health organization in Alzheimer care, support and research. The mission is to eliminate Alzheimer's disease through the advancement of research; to provide and enhance care and support for all affected; to advocate for policy change; and to reduce the risk of dementia through the promotion of brain health.
*Lisa Bruner, Executive Director*
*Shelita Weinfield, Local Contact*

595 **Alzheimer's Association of Vermont and New Hampshire**
10 Ferry Street 603-226-5868
Concord, NH 03301-5004 800-272-3900
Fax: 603-225-8126
www.alz.org
*Robbie Nicol, Chair*
*Robert Dowd, First Vice Chair*

596 **Alzheimer's Association: Connecticut Chapter**
99 Trinity Street 860-956-9560
Hartford, CT 06106 800-272-3900
Fax: 860-956-9590
walkhelpct@alz.org
www.alz.org
Works with all individuals and family members affected by Alzheimer's disease and related disorders; ensures humane systems of care and support and promotes research efforts to treat and cure Alzheimer's disease.
*Christopher Rupp, Chairman*
*Daniel P Finke, Treasurer*

597 **Alzheimer's Association: Alabama**
2151 Highland Avenue S 205-379-8065
Birmingham, AL 35205 800-272-3900
info@alz.org
www.alz.org/al
*Aimee Johnson, Executive Director*

598 **Alzheimer's Association: Alaska**
225 N Michigan Avenue 312-335-8700
Chicago, IL 60601 800-272-3900
Fax: 866-699-1246
TDD: 312-335-5886
www.alz.org/alaska

599 **Alzheimer's Association: Aloha**
1130 N Nimitz Highway 808-591-2771
Honolulu, HI 96817 800-272-3900
Fax: 808-591-9071
alohainfo@alz.org
www.alz.org/hawaii
*LJ R. Duenas, Executive Director*

600 **Alzheimer's Association: Arkansas**
225 N Michigan Avenue 800-272-3900
Chicago, IL 60601 www.alz.org/arkansas

601 **Alzheimer's Association: Atlanta Chapter**
1925 Century Boulevard 404-728-6066
Atlanta, GA 30345-4021 800-272-3900
Fax: 404-636-9768
rrotunda@alz.org
www.alz.org
*Bennett Watts, Chair*
*Robyn Rotunda, Local Contact*

602 **Alzheimer's Association: Augusta Chapter**
1899 Central Avenue 706-731-9060
Augusta, GA 30904-5755 800-272-3900
Fax: 706-731-9099
kim.franklin@alz.org
www.alz.org
*Bennett Watts, Chair*
*Bruce Flechter, Treasurer*

603 **Alzheimer's Association: Big Sioux Chapter**
401 Gordon Drive 712-279-5802
Sioux City, IA 51101-3716 800-272-3900
Fax: 712-277-8076
tschroeder@alz.org
www.alz.org
*Kim McCormick, Executive Director*
*Terri Schroeder, Local Contact*

604 **Alzheimer's Association: Broward County Chapter**
201 E Sample Road 800-861-7826
Deerfield Beach, FL 33407 800-272-3900
Fax: 954-786-1538
barbara.grasch@alz.org
www.alz.org
*Barbara Grasch, Director of Program Services*
*Ellen Brown, CEO*

605 **Alzheimer's Association: California Central Chapter: Ventura County Office**
80 North Wood Road 80 - 4 - 60
Camarillo, CA 93010 800-272-3900
Fax: 805-485-4767
www.alz.org

The local chapter of the National Alzheimer's Association. The chapter stands by people with Alzheimer's disease, their families and professional caregivers through the following programs and services: a telephone help line, support groups, respite grants.
*Norma Featherston, Area Director*
*Carol Swinney, Office Manager*

606 **Alzheimer's Association: Canton Chapter**
408 Ninth St. SW 800-272-3900
Canton, OH 44707 Fax: 330-996-7757
geoachl@alz.org
www.alz.org
*Pam Schuellerman, Executive Director*
*Andy Junn, Development Director*

607 **Alzheimer's Association: Capital of Texas Chapter**
3520 Executive Center Drive 512-241-0420
Austin, TX 78731 800-272-3900
Fax: 512-241-0430
Annie.lagow@alz.org
www.alz.org
The Alzheimer Association Greater Austin Chapter is dedicated to providing leadership to enhance care and support services for individuals and their families while promoting the advancement of research eliminate Alzheimer's disease.
*Daniel Hamilton, Chair*
*Annie LaGow, Local Contact*

608 **Alzheimer's Association: Cascade/Coast Chapter**
100 Day Island Road 503-416-0209
Eugene, OR 97401 800-272-3900
Fax: 541-345-5797
kara.busick@alz.org
www.alz.org
*Judy Clarke, Vice President*
*Kara Busick, Local Contact*

609 **Alzheimer's Association: Central Indiana Chapter**
601 W. New York Street 317-575-9620
Indianapolis, IN 46202-1816 800-272-3900
Fax: 317-582-0669
IndianaWalk@alz.org
www.alz.org
*Heather Allen Hershberger, Executive Director*
*Leslie Bush, Local Contact*

610 **Alzheimer's Association: Central & Western Virginia**
355 Rio Road W 434-973-6122
Charlottesville, VA 22901 800-272-3900
alzcwva@alz.org
www.alz.org/cwva
*Marie Kolendo, Sr. Executive Director*

611 **Alzheimer's Association: Central & North Florida**
378 Centerpointe Circle 800-272-3900
Altamonte Springs, FL 32701 www.alz.org/cnfl
The Central and North Florida Chapter provides services and programs in 31 counties. Its mission is to eliminate Alzheimer's disease through the advancement of research, to provide and enhance care and support for individuals, their families and caregivers.

612 **Alzheimer's Association: Central Georgia Chapter**
277 Martin Luther King Jr Boulevard 478-746-7050
Macon, GA 31201-3498 800-272-3900
Fax: 478-746-6679
kim.franklin@alz.org
www.alz.org
*Bennett Watts, Chair*
*Bruce Flechter, Treasurer*

613 **Alzheimer's Association: Central Illinois Chapter**
606 W Glen Avenue 309-681-1100
Peoria, IL 61614-4831 800-272-3900
Fax: 309-681-1101
kgabbert@alz.org
www.alz.org
*Nikki Vulgaris, Executive Director*
*Kari Gabbert, Local Contact*

614 **Alzheimer's Association: Central Maryland Chapter**
1850 York Road 410-561-9099
Timonium, MD 21093-5122 800-272-3900
Fax: 410-561-3433
info.maryland@alz.org
www.alz.org
*Cass Naugle, Executive Director*
*Teri Bennett, Helpline Coordinator*

615 **Alzheimer's Association: Central New York Chapter**
441 W Kirkpatrick Street 315-472-4201
Syracuse, NY 13204-1361 800-272-3900
Fax: 315-472-4206
gfletcher@alz.org
www.alz.org
*Larry Malfitano, President*
*Grant Fletcher, Local Contact*

616 **Alzheimer's Association: Central Ohio Chapter**
330 Huntington Park Lane 614-442-2014
Columbus, OH 43215-2112 800-272-3900
Fax: 614-457-6634
jsega@alz.org
www.alz.org
*Kenneth Strong, Executive Director*
*Jennifer Monroe-Sega, Local Contact*

617 **Alzheimer's Association: Central Virginia Chapter**
1160 Pepsi Place 434-973-6122
Charlottesville, VA 22901 800-272-3900
Fax: 434-973-4224
alzcwva@alz.org
www.alz.org
*Sue Friedman, President and CEO*
*Brian Phelps, Chair*

618 **Alzheimer's Association: Central and Western Kansas**
1820 E Douglas Avenue 316-267-7333
Wichita, KS 67214 800-272-3900
Fax: 316-267-6369
cwkshelpline@alz.org
www.alz.org/cwkansas
Information, resources and services for patients and families. Education and Training fro family and professional caregivers. Directed Training for medical emergency and law enforcement personnel. Public awarness, Advocacy and Public Policy.
*Jenny Shipman, Program Manager*

619 **Alzheimer's Association: Clark/Champaign, Miami Valley Chapter**
1700 S. Patterson Blvd. 937-291-3332
Dayton, OH 45409-2620 800-272-3900
Fax: 937-323-9259
walkmiamivalley@alz.org
www.alz.org
*Judy Turner, Executive Director*
*Marie McLaughlin, Local Contact*

620 **Alzheimer's Association: Cleveland Area Chapter**
23215 Commerce Park Drive 216-721-8457
Beachwood, OH 44122-1013 800-272-3900
Fax: 216-831-8585
www.alz.org
*Nancy B Udelson, Executive Director*
*Robert Bazzarelli, President*

621 **Alzheimer's Association: Colorado**
455 Sherman Street 303-813-1669
Denver, CO 80203 800-272-3900
info@alz.org
www.alz.org/co
The primary provider of local information services to Alzheimer patients and families in Colorado, the leading funder of AD research and the leading voice representing those dealing with dementia on public policy issues.
*Amelia Schafer, Executive Director*

**622 Alzheimer's Association: Connecticut**
200 Executive Boulevard 860-828-2828
Southington, CT 06489 800-272-3900
Fax: 860-571-8613
info@alz.org
www.alz.org/ct

*Robin Sharp, Executive Director*

**623 Alzheimer's Association: Delaware Chapter**
240 N James Street 302-633-4420
Newport, DE 19804 800-272-3900
Fax: 302-633-4494
Wendy.Campbell@alz.org
www.alz.org

*Wendy L Campbell, President*
*Theresa Haenn, Vice President Development*

**624 Alzheimer's Association: Delaware Valley Chapter**
1 Citizens Bank Way 215-561-2919
Philadelphia, PA 19148 800-272-3900
Fax: 215-561-4663
keely.boyle@alz.org
www.alz.org

*Wendy L Campbell, President*
*Keely Boyle, Local Contact*

**625 Alzheimer's Association: Desert Southwest Chapter**
1028 E McDowell Road 602-528-0545
Phoenix, AZ 85006-2622 800-272-3900
Fax: 602-528-0546
deborah.schaus@alz.org
www.alz.org

Serving the state of Arizona and Southern Nevada offices in Phoenix, Tucson, Sun City, Prescott and Las Vegas.
*Deborah Schaus, Executive Director*
*Dawn Boeck, Development Assistant*

**626 Alzheimer's Association: Desert Southwest**
340 E Palm Lane 602-528-0545
Phoenix, AZ 85004 800-272-3900
tgspitz@alz.org
www.alz.org/dsw

Serves the state of Arizona and Southern Nevada.
*Terri Spitz, Executive Director*

**627 Alzheimer's Association: East Central Florida Chapter**
Wickham Road 407-951-7992
Melbourne, FL 32935 800-272-3900
Fax: 407-729-8044
jgiovanni@alz.org
www.alz.org

*Joan Giovanni, Local Contact*

**628 Alzheimer's Association: Eastern Tennessee Chapter**
1600 World's Fair Park Drive 865-200-6668
Knoxville, TN 37916 800-272-3900
Fax: 865-544-6249
jim.ward@alz.org
www.alz.org

*Janice Wade-Whitehea, Executive Director*
*Jim Ward, Local Contact*

**629 Alzheimer's Association: Eastern North Carolina Chapter**
1305 Navaho Dr. 919-832-3732
Raleigh, NC 27609 800-272-3900
Fax: 919-832-7989
awatkins@alznc.org
www.alz.org

Dedicated to providing program services education for patients, families and professional caregivers, advocacy and research.
*Alice Watkins, Executive Director*
*Rita Bhan, Developmental Director*

**630 Alzheimer's Association: Eastern Shore Chapter**
909 Progress Circle 410-543-1163
Salisbury, MD 21804 800-272-3900
Fax: 410-546-0184
dmagarelli@alz.org
www.alz.org

*Cass Naugle, Executive Director*
*Damian Magarelli, Local Contact*

**631 Alzheimer's Association: Eastern Tennessee**
1545 Western Avenue 800-272-3900
Knoxville, TN 37921 Fax: 865-544-6249
info@alz.org
www.alz.org/tn

**632 Alzheimer's Association: El Paso Chapter**
4687 N Mesa 915-544-1799
El Paso, TX 79912-1147 800-272-3900
Fax: 915-544-8746
susie.gorman@alz.org
www.alz.org

*Mitch Moss, Chair*
*Susie Gorman, Local Contact*

**633 Alzheimer's Association: Fargo/Moorhead Regional Center**
5225 31st Ave South 701-277-9757
Fargo, ND 58104 800-272-3900
Fax: 701-277-9785
traie.dockter@alz.org
www.alz.org

*Gretchen Dobervich, Regional Center Director*
*Traie Dockter, Local Contact*

**634 Alzheimer's Association: Florida Gulf Coast Chapter**
9365 US Highway 19 N 727-578-2558
Pinellas Park, FL 33782 800-272-3900
Fax: 727-578-2286
milnel@alzflgulf.org
www.alz.org

Provides information and services to families and professionals dealing with memory related disorders.
*Gloria JT Smith, President/CEO*
*Paul Anderson, Vice President Finance*

**635 Alzheimer's Association: Four Rivers Chapter**
401 N Wall Street 815-936-0464
Kankakee, IL 60901 800-272-3900
Fax: 815-936-9363
www.alz.org

**636 Alzheimer's Association: Georgia**
41 Perimeter Center East 404-728-1181
Atlanta, GA 30346 800-272-3900
Fax: 404-636-9768
www.alz.org/georgia

*Linda Davidson, Executive Director*

**637 Alzheimer's Association: Great Plains Chapter**
1500 S. 70th St 402-420-2540
Lincoln, NE 68506 800-272-3900
mfeit@alz.org
www.alz.org

The Alzheimer's Association of the Great Plains is dedicated to supporting those with Alzheimer's disease and their families and friends through specialized programs and services, educating families, communities, and health professionals about Alzheimer's disease.
*Karen Noel, President/CEO*
*Mark Feit, Local Contact*

**638 Alzheimer's Association: Greater Sacramento**
11th St. & N St. 916-930-9080
Sacramento, CA 95814 800-272-3900
Fax: 916-930-9085
estone@alz.org
www.alz.org

*Mary Gillon MPA, Regional Director*
*Erin Stone, Local Contact*

**639 Alzheimer's Association: Greater Beaumont Area Chapter**
8750 Phelan Blvd. 409-833-1613
Beaumont, TX 77706 800-272-3900
Fax: 713-314-1315
walk@alztex.org
www.alz.org

*Richard Elbein, Chief Executive Officer*
*Clarissa Urban, Local Contact*

640 **Alzheimer's Association: Greater Billings Area Chapter**
2100 South Shiloh Road 406-252-3053
Billings, MT 59101 800-272-3900
Fax: 406-252-2933
sshannon@alz.org
www.alz.org
*Kelly Donovan, President*
*Sharon Shannon, Local Contact*

641 **Alzheimer's Association: Greater Columbus Chapter**
5900 River Road 706-327-6838
Columbus, GA 31904-0185 800-272-3900
Fax: 706-494-0533
cvogler@alz.org
www.alz.org
*Bennett Watts, Chair*
*Christina Vogler, Local Contact*

642 **Alzheimer's Association: Greater Dallas Chapter**
4144 N Central Expressway 214-540-2413
Dallas, TX 75204-4228 800-272-3900
Fax: 214-827-2064
dhill@alz.org
www.alz.org
Provides support and assistance to persons affected by Alzheimer's disease and related dementias and their families and caregivers. Serving Collin, Cooke, Dallas, Deaton, Ellis, Fanning, Grayson, Hunt, Kaufmau, Navarro and Rockwall counties.
*John R Gilchrist Jr, Executive Director*
*Jack Broyles, Chairman*

643 **Alzheimer's Association: Greater East Ohio Chapter: Greater Youngstown Office**
3695B Boardman-Canfield Rd 330-533-3300
Canfield, OH 44406-0321 800-272-3900
Fax: 330-533-3307
geoachl@alz.org
www.alz.org
*Pam Schuellerman, Executive Director*
*Andy Junn, Development Director*

644 **Alzheimer's Association: Greater East Ohio Area**
70 W Streetsboro Street 330-650-0552
Hudson, OH 44236 800-272-3900
info@alz.org
www.alz.org/akroncantonyoungstown

645 **Alzheimer's Association: Greater Georgia Chapter**
1925 Century Boulevard 404-728-6066
Atlanta, GA 30345-4021 800-272-3900
Fax: 404-636-9768
rrotunda@alz.org
www.alz.org
*Bennett Watts, Chair*
*Robyn Rotunda, Local Contact*

646 **Alzheimer's Association: Greater Grand Junction Area Chapter**
2232 N 7th Street 970-256-1274
Grand Junction, CO 81501 800-272-3900
Fax: 970-256-0569
www.alz.org
*Linda Mitchell, President/CEO*
*Lisa Miller, Local Contact*

647 **Alzheimer's Association: Greater Idaho Chapter**
1111 S Orchard 208-384-1788
Boise, ID 83705-2878 800-272-3900
Fax: 208-385-7191
suzette.albers-tunnell@alz.org
www.alz.org
*Suzette Albers-Tunne, Executive Director*

648 **Alzheimer's Association: Greater Illinios**
207 S Prospect 309-662-8392
Bloomington, IL 61704 800-272-3900
www.alz.org/illinois
A national voluntary health agency dedicated to researching the prevention, cure and treatment of Alzheimer's disease and related disorders and to providing support and assistance to individuals with alzheimer's disease, their families and caregivers.
*L. Patrick Reedy, Chapter Executive*

649 **Alzheimer's Association: Greater Illinois Chapter: Carbondale Office**
402 E Plaza Drive 618-985-1095
Carterville, IL 62918-1429 800-272-3900
Fax: 618-457-7830
GI.Chapter@alz.org
www.alz.org
*Jill Schoenborn, Coordinator Outreach & Development*

650 **Alzheimer's Association: Greater Indiana**
50 E 91st Street 800-272-3900
Indianapolis, IN 46240 www.alz.org/indiana
*Natalie Sutton, Chapter Executive*

651 **Alzheimer's Association: Greater Iowa Chapter**
1730 28th Street 515-440-2722
W Des Moines, IA 50266 800-272-3900
Fax: 515-440-6385
Carol.Sipfle@alz.org
www.alz.org
*Carol Sipfle, Executive Director*
*Holly Bradford, Finance Director*

652 **Alzheimer's Association: Greater Maryland**
1850 York Road 800-272-3900
Timonium, MD 21093 www.alz.org/maryland

653 **Alzheimer's Association: Greater Miami Chapter**
501 Marlins Way 305-891-6228
Miami, FL 33125 800-272-3900
Fax: 305-751-5551
snewman@alz.org
www.alz.org
*Reni Rizzo, Community Education Coordinator*
*Sharon Newman, Local Contact*

654 **Alzheimer's Association: Greater Michigan Chapter: Upper Peninsula Region**
1420 Pine Street 906-228-3910
Marquette, MI 49855-4521 800-272-3900
Fax: 906-228-2455
TTY: 877-204-6924
ralmen@alz.org
www.alz.org
*Pamela Parkkila, Director*
*Ruth Almen, Local Contact*

655 **Alzheimer's Association: Greater Mid-Ohio**
1100 Liberty Avenue 412-261-5040
Pittsburgh, PA 15222 800-272-3900
Fax: 412-471-2722
mlong@alz.org
www.alz.org
Education training information support groups free newsletter telephone support services to caregivers and diagnosed individuals as well as professionals.
*Bob LeRoy, President/CEO*
*Mellisa Long, Local Contact*

656 **Alzheimer's Association: Greater Missouri**
2609 E Broadway 800-272-3900
Columbia, MO 65201 www.alz.org/greatermissouri

657 **Alzheimer's Association: Greater New Orleans Chapter**
DePaul Hospital
1040 Calhoun Street 504-648-4084
New Orleans, LA 70118-5999 800-272-3900
Fax: 504-895-0493
charrell@alz.org
www.alz.org
*Chet Harrell, Local Contact*

658 **Alzheimer's Association: Greater North Valley Chapter**
1000 Woodland Ave 530-895-9661
Chico, CA 95928-3148 800-272-3900
Fax: 530-872-7470
swatroba@alz.org
www.alz.org
*Herb Williams, President*
*Suzanne Watroba, Local Contact*

659 **Alzheimer's Association: Greater Orlando Area Chapter**
Ampitheatre at 300 Robinson St., Do 407-951-7992
Orlando, FL 32801 800-272-3900
Fax: 407-228-4201
jgiovanni@alz.org
www.alz.org
*Stu Gaines, Chair*
*Joan Giovanni, Local Contact*

660 **Alzheimer's Association: Greater Palm Beach Area Chapter**
600 N Congress Avenue 561-478-3120
Delray Beach, FL 33445 800-272-3900
Fax: 561-278-4910
www.alz.org

661 **Alzheimer's Association: Greater Richmond Chapter**
4600 Cox Road 804-967-2580
Glen Allen, VA 23060 800-272-3900
Fax: 804-967-2588
sherry.peterson@alz.org
www.alz.org
Alzheimer's Association provides support and services to those with Alzheimer's and their families services include: help line, support groups, educational programs for family and professional caregivers, monthly newsletter, lending library, and a speakers
*Sherry Peterson, CEO*
*Marry Ann Johnson, Program Director*

662 **Alzheimer's Association: Greater Wichita Falls Chapter**
901 Indiana 940-767-8800
Wichita Falls, TX 76301-3206 800-272-3900
Fax: 940-322-6259
patty.taylor@alz.org
www.alz.org
*Theresa Hocker, Executive Director*
*Patty Taylor, Local Contact*

663 **Alzheimer's Association: Greater Wisconsin Chapter**
La Crosse & Second Streets 608-784-5011
La Crosse, WI 54601 800-272-3900
Fax: 608-784-4428
bwilliams@alz.org
www.alz.org
To eliminate Alzheimer's disease through the advancement of research; to provide and enhance care and support for all affected; and to reduce the risk of dementia through the promotion of brain health.
*Brad Beckman, President*
*Brett Williams, Local Contact*

664 **Alzheimer's Association: Heart of America Chapter**
3846 W 75th Street 913-831-3888
Prairie Village, KS 66208-4126 800-272-3900
Fax: 913-831-1916
jan.horn@alz.org
www.alz.org
*Debra R Brook, Executive Director*
*Michelle Niedens, Education Director*

665 **Alzheimer's Association: Heart of Iowa Chapter**
3915 Mortensen Road 515-440-6383
Ames, IA 50014-7259 800-272-3900
Fax: 515-292-0125
cmathany@alz.org
www.alz.org
*Chantelle Mathany, Local Contact*

666 **Alzheimer's Association: Highland Rim Chapter**
201 W Lincoln Street 931-455-3345
Tullahoma, TN 37388-1004 800-272-3900
Fax: 931-455-5396
swood@alz.org
www.alz.org
*George Jensen, Chair*
*Sarah Wood, Local Contact*

667 **Alzheimer's Association: Honolulu Chapter**
1050 Ala Moana Boulevard 808-591-2771
Honolulu, HI 96814 800-272-3900
Fax: 808-591-9071
ebatalon@alz.org
www.alz.org
*Eric Batalon, Local Contact*
*Chris Shirai, Chairman*

668 **Alzheimer's Association: Houston and Southeast Texas Chapter**
400 Hamilton Street 713-314-1340
Houston, TX 77002 800-272-3900
Fax: 713-314-1315
walk@alztex.org
www.alz.org
*Richard Elbein, CEO*
*Rasheeda Daugherty, Local Contact*

669 **Alzheimer's Association: Hudson Valley**
2649 South Road 845-471-2655
Poughkeepsie, NY 12601 800-272-3900
info@alzhudsonvalley.org
www.alz.org/hudsonvalley

670 **Alzheimer's Association: Hudson Valley/ Rockland/Westchester NY Chapter**
2 Jefferson Plaza 845-471-2655
Poughkeepsie, NY 12601-4027 800-272-3900
Fax: 845-471-8960
info@alzhudsonvalley.org
www.alz.org
*Elaine Sproat, President & CEO*
*Meg Boyce, Director of Programs & Services*

671 **Alzheimer's Association: Illinois**
8430 W Bryn Mawr 847-933-2413
Chicago, IL 60631 800-272-3900
www.alz.org/illinois
To help optimize the quality of life for people with Alzheimer's Disease and their families through advocacy, education, suport and service delivery, while actively promoting research to eliminate the disease.
*L. Patrick Reedy, Chapter Executive*

672 **Alzheimer's Association: Indianhead Chapter**
Carson Park Dr 715-345-2969
Eau Claire, WI 54703-5996 800-272-3900
Fax: 715-345-2969
kdavies@alz.org
www.alz.org
*Mary B Bouche, Executive Director*
*Kathy Davies, Local Contact*

673 **Alzheimer's Association: Inland Northwest Chapter**
800 N. Howard St. 509-473-3390
Spokane, WA 99201 800-272-3900
Fax: 509-473-3389
sdruffel@alz.org
www.alz.org
*Joel Loiacono, Executive Director*
*Sandi Druffel, Local Contact*

674 **Alzheimer's Association: Iowa**
1730 28th Street 515-440-2722
West Des Moines, IA 50266 800-272-3900
Fax: 515-440-6385
iowa@alz.org
www.alz.org/iowa
*Doug Bickford, Executive Director*

675 **Alzheimer's Association: Lake Superior Chapter**
US Highway 2 East 715-392-3255
Ashland, WI 54806-1652 800-272-3900
Fax: 715-682-6561
fcarlson@alz.org
www.alz.org
*Kim Kinner, Executive Director*
*Freda Carlson, Local Contact*

676 **Alzheimer's Association: Land of Lincoln Chapter**
South Second Street & Southwind Roa 217-801-9352
Springfield, IL 62703-4833 800-272-3900
Fax: 217-726-5185
tarnold@alz.org
www.alz.org
*Jane Field, Office Manager*
*Tina Arnold, Local Contact*

677 **Alzheimer's Association: Laurel Mountains Chapter**
194 Donohoe Road 412-261-5040
Greensburg, PA 15601-1095 800-272-3900
Fax: 724-837-4567
aspreng@alz.org
www.alz.org
*Abby Spreng, Local Contact*

678 **Alzheimer's Association: Lexington/ Bluegrass Chapter**
465 E High Street 859-266-5283
Lexington, KY 40507 800-272-3900
Fax: 859-268-4764
amber.lakin@alz.org
www.alz.org
*Debbie Lacy Goodman, VP Awareness & Community Relations*
*Amber Lakin, Local Contact*

679 **Alzheimer's Association: Lincoln/Greater Nebraska Chapter**
1500 S. 70th St. 402-420-2540
Lincoln, NE 68506 800-272-3900
Fax: 402-420-2541
mfeit@alz.org
www.alz.org
*Karen Noel, President/CEO*
*Mark Feit, Local Contact*

680 **Alzheimer's Association: Long Island Chapter**
3281 Veterans Memorial Highway 631-580-5100
Ronkonkoma, NY 11779-3521 800-272-3900
Fax: 631-580-3100
Info@alzheimersli.org
www.alz.org
Voluntary health agency that provides care and consultation, information and referral, education, national safe return program and support groups to individuals with Alzheimer's, their families and/or caregivers.
*Mary Ann Malack-Ragona, Executive Director/CEO*
*Linda Cody, Director of Development*

681 **Alzheimer's Association: Los Angeles Chapter**
133 N Sunol Drive 323-930-6228
Los Angeles, CA 90063-5017 800-272-3900
Fax: 323-938-1036
bwelch@alz.org
www.alz.org
*Earl Greinetz, President*
*Brian Welch, Local Contact*

682 **Alzheimer's Association: Louisiana**
3445 N Causeway Boulevard 504-613-6505
Metairie, LA 70002 800-272-3900
www.alz.org/louisiana

683 **Alzheimer's Association: Louisville Chapter**
6100 Dutchmans Lane 502-451-4266
Louisville, KY 40205 800-272-3900
Fax: 502-456-2701
wvogel@alz.org
www.alz.org
*Teri Shirk, Chapter President & CEO*
*Whitney Vogel, Local Contact*

684 **Alzheimer's Association: Low Country Chapter**
20 Patriots Point Road 843-571-2641
Charleston, SC 29464 800-272-3900
Fax: 843-571-6020
kalmstedt@alz.org
www.alz.org
*Ashton Houghton, VP of Development & Communications*
*Kim Almstedt, Local Contact*

685 **Alzheimer's Association: Maine**
383 U.S. Route 1 207-772-0115
Scarborough, ME 04074 800-272-3900
www.alz.org/maine
*Peter Baker, Program Director*

686 **Alzheimer's Association: Maine Chapter**
383 U.S. Route 1 207-772-0115
Scarborough, ME 04074-2419 800-272-3900
Fax: 207-289-3705
laurie.trenholm@alz.org
www.alz.org
*Joy Heptner, Executive Director*
*Liz Weaver, Program Director*

687 **Alzheimer's Association: Mary's Peak Chapter**
1925 NW Circle Boulevard 541-752-1012
Corvallis, OR 97330-1312 800-272-3900
Fax: 541-757-1395
www.alz.org

688 **Alzheimer's Association: Massachusetts Chapter**
311 Arsenal Street 617-868-6718
Watertown, MA 02472 800-272-3900
Fax: 617-868-6720
www.alz.org
Nonprofit, national, voluntary health organization dedicated to Alzheimer research and care. Provides 24 hour help line, support groups, a wanderers prevention program early stage patient programs, family educators, professional training, and advocacy.
*James Wessle MBA, President & CEO*
*Betsy Fitzgerald-Cam, Vice President Communications*

689 **Alzheimer's Association: Massachusetts - New Hampshire**
309 Waverley Oaks Road 617-868-6718
Watertown, MA 02452 800-272-3900
Fax: 617-868-6720
info@alz.org
www.alz.org/manh

690 **Alzheimer's Association: Memphis Area Office**
500 North Pine Lake Drive 901-565-0011
Memphis, TN 38134 800-272-3900
Fax: 901-565-9550
sgraham@alz.org
www.alz.org
*George Jensen, Chair*
*Susan Graham, Local Contact*

691 **Alzheimer's Association: Miami Valley**
31 W Whipp Road 937-291-3332
Dayton, OH 45459 800-272-3900
www.alz.org/dayton
*Eric VanVlymen, Executive Director*

692 **Alzheimer's Association: Michigan Great Lakes Chapter: West Shore Region**
1740 Village Drive 734-475-7043
Muskegon, MI 49442-5546 800-272-3900
Fax: 231-780-1494
mglcwalk@alz.org
www.alz.org
Providing caregiver support groups a help line informational materials community education and a quarterly newsletter.
*Barb Betts, Program Coordinator*
*Stephanie Barnhill, Local Contact*

693 **Alzheimer's Association: Mid South**
478 Craighead 800-272-3900
Nashville, TN 37204 www.alz.org/altn
*Dawne Bunn, Executive Director*

694 **Alzheimer's Association: Mid-Michigan Chapter**
4604 N Saginaw Road 989-839-9910
Midland, MI 48640 800-272-3900
Fax: 989-839-5910
TTY: 877-204-6924
boneill@alz.org
www.alz.org
*Dawn Spicer, Director*
*Betty O'Neill, Local Contact*

695 **Alzheimer's Association: Mid-Missouri Chapter**
2400 Bluff Creek Drive 573-443-8665
Columbia, MO 65201 800-272-3900
Fax: 573-499-9701
cbaker@alz.org
www.alz.org

*Linda Newkirk, Executive Director*
*Chris Baker, Local Contact*

696 **Alzheimer's Association: Mid-State South Carolina Chapter**
3223 Sunset Blvd 803-791-3430
W Columbia, SC 29169-7044 800-272-3900
Fax: 803-791-8388
www.alz.org

*Adelle Stanley, Program Director*
*Lynee Moore, Director of Development*

697 **Alzheimer's Association: Mid-Willamette Chapter**
PO Box 12768 503-371-7728
Salem, OR 97309-0768 800-272-3900
Fax: 503-571-9842
midwillamatte@alz.org
www.alz.org

698 **Alzheimer's Association: Middle Tennessee Chapter**
4205 Hillsboro Pike 615-292-4938
Nashville, TN 37215-2859 800-272-3900
Fax: 615-386-9768
ajackson1@alz.org
www.alz.org

*George Jensen, Chair*
*Andrew Jackson, Local Contact*

699 **Alzheimer's Association: Midstate Wisconsin Chapter**
1800 S Central Ave 715-845-7440
Marshfield, WI 54449 800-272-3900
Fax: 715-387-5727
aswatek@alz.org
www.alz.org

700 **Alzheimer's Association: Minnesota/Dakotas**
1 Twins Way 952-830-0512
Minneapolis, MN 55403 800-272-3900
Fax: 952-830-0513
mnnd-walk@alz.org
www.alz.org

*Mary Birchard, Executive Director*
*Libby Wilhelmy, Local Contact*

701 **Alzheimer's Association: Mississippi Chapter**
1900 Dunbarton Drive 601-987-0020
Jackson, MS 39216 800-272-3900
Fax: 601-987-9020
rruello@alz.org
www.alz.org

*Barb Dobrosky, Program Director*
*Rachel Ruello, Local Contact*

702 **Alzheimer's Association: Montana**
3010 11th Avenue N 406-252-3053
Billings, MT 59101 800-272-3900
www.alz.org/montana

703 **Alzheimer's Association: Monterey County Chapter**
5 Custom House Plaza 831-647-9890
Monterey, CA 93940-5337 800-272-3900
Fax: 831-655-9241
janderson@alz.org
www.alz.org

*Herb Williams, President*
*Joy Anderson, Local Contact*

704 **Alzheimer's Association: N Central West Virginia Chapter**
1299 Pineview Drive 304-599-1159
Morgantown, WV 26505-4543 800-272-3900
Fax: 304-291-2577
wvinfo@alz.org
www.alz.org

*Jane Marks, Executive Director*
*Jane Siers, Development Director*

705 **Alzheimer's Association: National Capital Area Chapter**
3701 Pender Drive 703-359-4440
Fairfax, VA 22030 800-272-3900
Fax: 703-359-4441
Danielle.Otsuka@alz.org
www.alz.org

Provides support and services to those diagnosed with Alzheimer's disease and related disorders and their families. Services include information on the disease, care options, caregiving techniques and research, support groups, education and training, and advocacy.
*Matthew B Aaron, Chair*
*Danielle Otsuka, Director of Development*

706 **Alzheimer's Association: Nebraska**
11711 Arbor Street 800-272-3900
Omaha, NE 68144 sstephens@alz.org
www.alz.org/nebraska

Serves persons with Alzheimer's disease and their families in 80 counties across Nebraska and the entire state of Wyoming. The mission is to enhance the quality of life for all persons affected by Alzheimer's disease and related disorders through comprehensive educational programs, compassionate services, access to resources and support for research.
*Sharon Stephens, Executive Director*

707 **Alzheimer's Association: New Mexico Chapter**
9500 Montgomery Boulevard NE 505-266-4473
Albuquerque, NM 87111 800-272-3900
Fax: 505-266-0108
nlawrie@alz.org
www.alz.org

*Agnes Vallejos, Executive Director*
*Nika Lawrie, Local Contact*

708 **Alzheimer's Association: New York City Chapter**
360 Lexington Avenue 646-744-2900
New York, NY 10017 800-272-3900
Fax: 212-490-6037
helpline@alznyc.org
www.alz.org/nyc

*Lou-Ellen Barkan, President/CEO*
*Jed A. Levine, Executive Vice President*

709 **Alzheimer's Association: North Alabama Chapter**
4747 Bob Wallace Avenue SW 256-880-1575
Huntsville, AL 35805-4872 800-272-3900
Fax: 256-880-8596
cwhite2@alz.org
www.alz.org

*Al Wiggins, Chair*
*Courtney White, Local Contact*

710 **Alzheimer's Association: North Bay Chapter**
4340 Redwood Highway 415-472-4340
San Rafael, CA 94903 800-272-3900
Fax: 415-472-4350
info@alznorcal.org
www.alz.org

Provides a continuum of services for Alzheimer's families, education and referral in Marin, Sonoma and Napa counties. To provide leadership and to eliminate Alzheimer's disease through the advancement of research while enhancing care and support services.
*Herb Williams, President*
*Eduardo Salaz, Vice President*

711 **Alzheimer's Association: North Central Wisconsin Chapter**
1205 Lincoln St 715-362-7779
Rhinelander, WI 54501 800-272-3900
Fax: 715-362-1879
jstpierre@alz.org
www.alz.org

*Kim Kinner, Executive Director*
*Julie St. Pierre, Local Contact*

712 **Alzheimer's Association: Northeast Florida**
4237 Salisbury Rd
Jacksonville, FL 32216
904-281-9077
800-272-3900
Fax: 866-281-9078
mdrinks@alz.org
www.alz.org
*Michelle Drinks, Local Contact*

713 **Alzheimer's Association: Northeast Texas Chapter**
211 Winchester
Tyler, TX 75701-8732
903-509-8323
800-272-3900
Fax: 903-509-8373
www.alz.org
*Jana Humphrey, Executive Director*
*Sherlon Spurling, Client Services Coordinator*

714 **Alzheimer's Association: Northeastern New York Chapter**
4 Pine West Plaza
Albany, NY 12205-2083
518-867-4999
800-272-3900
Fax: 518-867-4997
infoneny@alz.org
www.alz.org
Regional affiliate of national association. Works to educate and support families, while raising funds in support of research.
*Paul A Wajda, Chair*
*Warren E Garling, Vice Chair*

715 **Alzheimer's Association: Northern Arizona**
225 Grove Avenue
Prescott, AZ 86301-2911
928-771-9257
800-272-3900
Fax: 520-771-9297
pwinkels@alz.org
www.alz.org
*Don Connell, Regional Director*
*Patty Winkels, Local Contact*

716 **Alzheimer's Association: Northern Central Florida Chapter**
1001 NW 34th St
Gainesville, FL 32605
904-281-9077
800-272-3900
Fax: 352-372-2038
mdrinks@alz.org
www.alz.org
*Michelle Drinks, Local Contact*
*Tish Sheesley, CEO*

717 **Alzheimer's Association: Northern Idaho Chapter**
2003 Kootenai Health Way
Coeur D Alene, ID 83814
208-666-2996
800-272-3900
Fax: 509-473-3389
pchristo@alz.org
www.alz.org
*PJ Christo, Outreach Coordinator*
*Joel Loiacono, Executive Director*

718 **Alzheimer's Association: Northern Indiana Chapter**
922 E Colfax Avenue
S Bend, IN 46617-3112
57 - 2 - 41
800-272-3900
Fax: 57 - 2 - 42
www.alz.org

719 **Alzheimer's Association: Northern Nevada**
225 Grove Avenue
Prescott, AZ 86301
928-771-9257
800-272-3900
Fax: 520-771-9297
pwinkels@alz.org
www.alz.org
*Meg Fenzi, Regional Director*
*Patty Winkels, Local Contact*

720 **Alzheimer's Association: Northwest Florida Chapter**
119 Hollywood Boulevard
Ft. Walton Beach, FL 32548
850-302-0581
800-272-3900
Fax: 850-302-0583
www.alz.org

721 **Alzheimer's Association: Northwest Ohio Chapter**
75 N. Main St.
Mansfield, OH 44902-7906
419-537-1999
800-272-3900
Fax: 419-522-5318
nvargas@alz.org
www.alz.org
Voluntary health organization committed to finding a cure for Alzheimer's and helping those affected by the disease.
*Michael Malone, President*
*Nick Vargas, Local Contact*

722 **Alzheimer's Association: Oklahoma**
6601 Broadway
Oklahoma City, OK 73116
405-319-0780
800-272-3900
oksocial@alz.org
www.alz.org/oklahoma

723 **Alzheimer's Association: Oklahoma Chapter**
2448 E. 81st Street
Tulsa, OK 74137-7804
918-392-5012
800-272-3900
Fax: 918-481-7745
TTY: 800-493-1411
shauptman@alz.org
www.alz.org
Dedicated to serving Alzheimer's patients, their families, and caregivers through education, outreach, programs, support services and public advocacy.
*Judi A Ver Hoef, President/CEO*
*Sarah Hauptam, Local Contact*

724 **Alzheimer's Association: Omaha/Eastern Nebraska Chapter**
3220 Farnam St
Omaha, NE 68131-2167
402-502-4301
800-272-3900
Fax: 402-502-7001
cenoviso@alz.org
www.alz.org
*Duane Gross, President and CEO*
*Cathy Enoviso, Local Contact*

725 **Alzheimer's Association: Orange County Chapter**
17771 Cowan
Irvine, CA 92614
949-955-9000
800-272-3900
Fax: 949-757-3700
helpoc@alz.org
www.alz.org
Dedicated to providing services, education and advocacy for individuals, families and the community affected by Alzheimer's disease and related memory disorders. Services include: 24/7 help line, support groups, family orientation program and care managers.
*Norma Castellano, Program Specialist*
*Bobbie Babbage, Family Services Coordinator*

726 **Alzheimer's Association: Oregon**
1650 NW Naito Parkway
Portland, OR 97209
800-272-3900
www.alz.org/oregon
Alzheimer's information and resources.

727 **Alzheimer's Association: Piedmont-Valley Area Chapter**
1160 Pepsi Place
Charlottesville, VA 22901
434-973-6122
800-272-3900
Fax: 434-973-4224
mhanson@alz.org
www.alz.org
*Sue Friedman, President and CEO*
*Mary Pat Hanson, Local Contact*

728 **Alzheimer's Association: Putnam County Chapter**
Robin Hill Corporate Park
15 Mount Ebo Road S
Brewster, NY 10509-2164
845-278-0343
800-272-3900
info@alzhudsonvalley.org
www.alz.org
*Stuart Greif, Program Development Specialist*

729 **Alzheimer's Association: Rhode Island Chapter**
245 Waterman Avenue
Providence, RI 02906
401-421-0008
800-272-3900
Fax: 401-941-8988
Donna.McGowan@alz.org
www.alz.org
*Elizabeth Morancy, Executive Director*
*Marge Angilly, Program Director*

730 **Alzheimer's Association: Rio Grande Valley Region**
222 E Van Buren 956-440-0636
Harlingen, TX 78550 800-272-3900
Fax: 956-440-9290
www.alz.org

A nonprofit organization designed to educate and support individuals with Alzheimer's, their families and caregivers.

731 **Alzheimer's Association: Riverside/San Bernardino Counties Chapter**
5900 Wilshire Boulevard 323-930-6228
Los Angeles, CA 90036 800-272-3900
Fax: 323-938-1036
bwelch@alz.org
www.alz.org

Help line, support groups, information and education for caregivers and community.
*400 Members*
*Earl Greinetz, President*
*Brian Welch, Local Contact*

732 **Alzheimer's Association: Roanoke Salem Chapter**
3959 Electric Rd 540-345-7600
Roanoke, VA 24018 800-272-3900
Fax: 540-345-7900
mhanson@alz.org
www.alz.org

*Sue Friedman, President and CEO*
*Mary Pat Hanson, Local Contact*

733 **Alzheimer's Association: Rochester Chapter**
85 Adams Street 585-760-5472
Rochester, NY 14608 800-272-3900
Fax: 585-760-5401
rochesterwalk@alz.org
www.alz.org

*Chris Lacey, Local Contact*
*Judy Lemoncelli, Local Contact*

734 **Alzheimer's Association: Rocky Mountain Chapter**
455 Sherman Street 303-813-1669
Denver, CO 80203 800-272-3900
Fax: 303-813-1670
jlorentz@alz.org
www.alz.org

*Linda Mitchell, President/CEO*
*Jill Lorentz, Local Contact*

735 **Alzheimer's Association: STAR Chapter, Midland Region**
4400 N Big Spring 432-570-9191
Midland, TX 79705 800-272-3900
Fax: 432-683-2345
derdwurm@alz.org
www.alz.org

*Mitch Moss, Chair*
*Debbie Erdwurm, Local Contact*

736 **Alzheimer's Association: San Antonio & South Texas**
10223 McAllister Freeway 210-822-6449
San Antonio, TX 78216 800-272-3900
www.alz.org/sanantonio

737 **Alzheimer's Association: San Francisco Bay Area Chapter**
1060 La Avenida 650-962-8111
Mountain View, CA 94043 800-272-3900
Fax: 650-962-9644
info@alznorcal.org
www.alz.org

*Herb Williams, President*
*Eduardo Salaz, Vice President*

738 **Alzheimer's Association: Santa Barbara Central Coast Chapter**
3400 Calle Real 805-892-4259
Santa Barbara, CA 93105-8820 800-272-3900
Fax: 805-892-4250
gbolton@alz.org
www.alz.org

The Alzheimer's Association California Central Coast Chapter serves families caring for people with Alzheimer's disease and related dementia throughout San Luis Obispo, Santa Barbara and Ventura Counties, offering a variety of educational and supportive programs.
*Rhonda Spiegel, Executive Director*
*Genny Bolton, Local Contact*

739 **Alzheimer's Association: Santa Cruz County Chapter**
1777-A Capitola Road 831-464-9982
Santa Cruz, CA 95062 800-272-3900
Fax: 831-464-8930
info@alznorcal.org
www.alz.org

*Herb Williams, President*
*Eduardo Salaz, Vice President*

740 **Alzheimer's Association: South Carolina**
4124 Clemson Boulevard 864-224-3045
Anderson, SC 29621 800-272-3900
Fax: 864-225-1387
info@alz.org
www.alz.org/sc

*Cindy Alewine, President & CEO*

741 **Alzheimer's Association: South Central Connecticut Chapter**
2911 Dixwell Avenue 203-230-1777
Hamden, CT 06518 800-272-3900
Fax: 203-230-1712
www.alz.org

*Patricia Clark, Executive Director*

742 **Alzheimer's Association: South Dakota**
4304 S Technology Drive 605-339-4543
Sioux Falls, SD 57106 800-272-3900
www.alz.org/sd

743 **Alzheimer's Association: South Jersey Chapter**
3 Eves Drive 856-797-1212
Marlton, NJ 08053 800-272-3900
Fax: 609-784-8486
Wendy.Campbell@alz.org
www.alz.org

*Wendy L Campbell, President & CEO*
*Theresa Haenn, Vice President Development*

744 **Alzheimer's Association: South West Virginia Chapter**
601 Morris St. 304-343-2717
Charleston, WV 25301 800-272-3900
Fax: 304-343-2723
kford@alz.org
www.alz.org

*Jane Marks, Executive Director*
*Kaarmin Ford, Local Contact*

745 **Alzheimer's Association: Southeast Alabama Chapter**
PO Box 609 334-677-6799
Dothan, AL 36302 800-272-3900
Fax: 334-671-3715
www.alz.org

*Kay Jones, Executive Director*

746 **Alzheimer's Association: Southeastern Virginia Chapter**
6350 Center Drive 757-459-2405
Norfolk, VA 23502 800-272-3900
Fax: 757-461-7902
InfoSEVA@alz.org
www.alz.org

Provides support to people with Alzheimer's disease or related dementia and their families; educates professionals and the public about Alzheimer's disease and related dementia; supports research into causes, improved diagnosis, therapies and cures.
*Gino V Colombara, Executive Director*
*Patricia Far Lacey, Director of Education & Family Services*

747 **Alzheimer's Association: Southern Arizona**
5132 East Pima Street 520-322-6601
Tucson, AZ 85712 800-272-3900
Fax: 520-322-6739
kraach@alz.org
www.alz.org

*Tormay Newman, Director*
*Kelly Raach, Local Contact*

748 **Alzheimer's Association: Southern Arizona Region**
3003 S Country Club Road 520-322-6601
Tucson, AZ 85713 800-272-3900
Fax: 520-322-6739
kraach@alz.org
www.alz.org
*Heriberto Contreras, Regional Director*
*Kelly Raach, Local Contact*

749 **Alzheimer's Association: Southern Nevada Chapter**
5190 S Valley View Boulevard 702-248-2770
Las Vegas, NV 89118-6062 800-272-3900
Fax: 702-248-2771
achavez@alz.org
www.alz.org
*Luis Carrillo, Regional Director*
*Albert Chavez, Local Contact*

750 **Alzheimer's Association: Southern Tier Chapter**
401 Hayes Avenue 607-785-7852
Endicott, NY 13760-5421 800-272-3900
Fax: 607-785-4004
alzcny@alzcny.org
www.alz.org
*L Jane Hudreck, Regional Director*

751 **Alzheimer's Association: Southside Virginia Chapter**
120 S Hill Avenue 434-447-3963
S Hill, VA 23970-0310 800-272-3900
Fax: 434-447-9024
gino.colombara@alz.org
www.alz.org
*Gino V Colombara, Executive Director*
*June Rainey, Education & Family Services Coordinator*

752 **Alzheimer's Association: Southwest Alabama Chapter**
PO Box 9272 334-660-5661
Mobile, AL 36691 800-272-3900
Fax: 334-660-5667
www.alz.org
*Bunnie Sutton, Executive Director*

753 **Alzheimer's Association: St. Louis Chapter**
700 Clark Avenue 314-801-0465
Saint Louis, MO 63102-3214 800-272-3900
Fax: 314-432-3824
stlwalksupport@alz.org
www.alz.org
*Joan D'Ambrose, President*
*Alyssa Vorhies, Local Contact*

754 **Alzheimer's Association: Sunflower Chapter**
347 S Laura 316-267-7333
Wichita, KS 67211-4109 800-272-3900
Fax: 316-267-6369
lbelton@alz.org
www.alz.org
*Marsha Hills, Executive Director*
*Lanette Belton, Local Contact*

755 **Alzheimer's Association: Tampa Bay Chapter**
601 N Old Coachman Rd 727-259-2317
Clearwater, FL 33765 800-272-3900
Fax: 941-380-5701
farinasr@alzflgulf.org
www.alz.org
*Gloria JT Smith, President/CEO*
*Rachel Farinas, Local Contact*

756 **Alzheimer's Association: Tarrant County Chapter**
101 Summit Avenue 817-336-4949
Fort Worth, TX 76102 800-272-3900
Fax: 817-336-4966
lyn.downing@alz.org
www.alz.org
Offers support to those afflicted with Alzheimer's disease and their families through education, support groups, case management, telephone help line and referral to services (i.e. long term care, adult daycare, medical assistance, legal assistance etc.).
*Theresa Hocker, Executive Director*
*Lyn Downing, Local Contact*

757 **Alzheimer's Association: Upstate South Carolina Chapter**
3027 MLK Jr. Blvd 864-224-3045
Anderson, SC 29625-5528 800-272-3900
Fax: 864-225-1387
kwilliams@alz.org
www.alz.org
*Cindy Alewine, President/CEO*
*Kimberly Williams, Local Contact*

758 **Alzheimer's Association: Utah**
12894 S Pony Express Road 801-265-1944
Draper, UT 84020 800-272-3900
www.alz.org/utah

759 **Alzheimer's Association: Utah Chapter**
296 E. Murray Park Ave 801-265-1944
Salt Lake City, UT 84107 800-272-3900
Fax: 801-269-1226
Emartini@alz.org
www.alz.org
*Nick Sussman, Program Director*
*Elaine Martini, Local Contact*

760 **Alzheimer's Association: Vermont**
300 Cornerstone Drive 802-316-3839
Williston, VT 05495 800-272-3900
www.alz.org/vermont
The Alzheimer's Association is the only voluntary health organization dedicated to research aimed at the prevention, care, and treatment of Alzheimer's disease and related disorders, while providing support and assistance to those affected with the disease and their families.
*Grace Gilbert-Davis, Executive Director*

761 **Alzheimer's Association: Volusia/Flagler Branch**
111 N Frederick Avenue 407-951-7992
Daytona Beach, FL 32114-5126 800-272-3900
Fax: 386-238-8293
jgiovanni@alz.org
www.alz.org
*Joan Giovanni, Local Contact*

762 **Alzheimer's Association: West Central Florida Chapter**
PO Box 2070 813-848-8888
New Port Richey, FL 34656-2070 800-272-3900
Fax: 813-849-6124
www.alz.org

763 **Alzheimer's Association: West Hawaii Chapter**
PO Box 390247 808-591-2771
Kailua Kona, HI 96739-0247 800-272-3900
Fax: 808-322-0008
ebatalon@alz.org
www.alz.org
*Eric Batalon, Local Contact*

764 **Alzheimer's Association: West Texas**
4400 N Big Spring C-32 432-570-9191
Midland, TX 79705 800-272-3900
www.alz.org/westtexas

765 **Alzheimer's Association: West Virginia**
1601 Second Avenue 304-343-2717
Charleston, WV 25387 800-272-3900
info@alz.org
www.alz.org/wv

766 **Alzheimer's Association: Western Arkansas Chapter**
121 Riverfront Drive 479-426-5541
Fort Smith, AR 72901-3454 800-272-3900
Fax: 479-782-3185
sdavis@alz.org
www.alz.org
*Rebecca Freeman, Executive Director*
*Susie Davis, Local Contact*

767 **Alzheimer's Association: Western & Central Washington Chapter**
100 W. Harrison St 206-529-3898
Seattle, WA 98119 800-272-3900
Fax: 206-363-5700
walk@alzwa.org
www.alz.org
*Nancy Dapper, Executive Director*
*Justine Stevens, Local Contact*

768 **Alzheimer's Association: Western Maryland Chapter**
101 Clarke Pl. 301-696-0315
Frederick, MD 21701 800-272-3900
Fax: 301-696-9061
kweddle@alz.org
www.alz.org
To eliminate Alzheimer's disease through the advancement of research and to enhance care and support for individuals their families and caregivers.
*Cathy Hanson, Program Coordinator*
*Kristen Weddle, Local Contact*

769 **Alzheimer's Association: Western New York Chapter**
2805 Wehrle Drive 716-626-0600
Williamsville, NY 14421 800-272-3900
Fax: 717-626-2255
Donna.McKenzie@alz.org`
www.alz.org
*David Cascio, President*
*Linda Sabo, Executive Director*

770 **Alzheimer's Association: Western Regional Office: Massachusetts Chapter**
264 Cottage Street 413-787-1113
Springfield, MA 01104 800-272-3900
Fax: 413-787-1109
www.alz.org
Nonprofit organization serving family and professional caregivers in seven counties in southwest Michigan. Provides information on Alzheimer's and other diseases, educational programs, resource libraries. Train-the-trainer agency referral, autopsy liaison, and other services.
*Marcia McKen Med, Manager*
*Annie Clattenburg, Coordinator Administrative Services*

771 **Alzheimer's Association: Wyoming**
2232 Dell Range Boulevard 307-316-2892
Cheyenne, WY 82009 800-272-3900
www.alz.org/wyoming

772 **Alzheimer's Disease Resource Agency of Alaska**
1750 Abbott Road 907-561-3313
Anchorage, AK 99507 800-272-3900
Fax: 907-561-3315
dnobre@alzalaska.org
www.alz.org
*Jackie Brunton, President*
*Debbie Newsham, Vice President*

773 **Alzheimer's Foundation of Staten Island**
789 Post Avenue 718-667-7110
Staten Island, NY 10310-6427 877-574-7068
Fax: 718-667-8431
Not-for-profit health and human services organization, serving people with Alzheimer's disease and related dementias.
*Leilani Joven Pelletie, Executive Director*
*David Cascio, President*

774 **Alzheimer's Foundation of the South: Mississippi Division**
PO Box 2394 228-867-6251
Gulfport, MS 39503 800-272-3900
Fax: 228-864-8843
alzms@cs.com
www.alz.org
*Rosemary Hudgins, Executive Director*

775 **Alzheimer's Services of the Capital Area**
3772 N Boulevard 225-334-7494
Baton Rouge, LA 70806 800-548-1211
Fax: 225-387-3664
info@alzbr.org
www.alzbr.org
The mission of Alzheimer's Services of the Capital Area is to provide education and support services to memory impaired individuals as well as caregivers and professionals; and to enhance community awareness of Alzheimer's disease and related disorders.
*Barbara Auten, Executive Director*

776 **Alzheimer's Wyoming**
900 Werner Court 307-265-7960
Casper, WY 82602 Fax: 307-265-7960
Alzheimer's Affiliation of Wyoming is an independent organization that makes presentations about Alzheimer's Disease; assists Alzheimer support groups; provides funds for respite care; maintains a lending library; refers patients and their families to services.
*Mary Hein, Executive Director*

777 **American Homes for the Aging: Midwest Regional Office**
911 N Elm Street 630-323-6755
Hinsdale, IL 60521-3641 800-272-3900
Fax: 630-325-0749
www.alz.org
Regional office of the AHA, a national professional association of nonprofit nursing homes, retirement communities and homes for the aging.

778 **American Homes for the Aging: Western**
5010 Aspen Drive 303-795-5465
Littleton, CO 80123 Fax: 303-794-0487
Part of the national association representing retirement communities, nursing homes and community services for the elderly.

779 **Dementia Alliance of North Carolina**
9131 Anson Way 919-832-3732
Raleigh, NC 27615 800-228-8738
info@dementianc.org
dementianc.org
A non-profit dedicated to improving the lives of North Carolinians impacted by dementia, engaging and empowering them through support, education and research.
*Heather Hooper, Executive Director*
*Dee Dee Harris, Family Services Director*

780 **Dementia Education Inc.**
PO Box 434 614-519-2843
Inverness, FL 34450 dementiaeducationinc@gmail.com
dementiaedu.org
A local non-profit dedicated to identifying and funding projects, publications, and events that promote education and raise awareness about dementia and memory loss disorders. The organization offers community engagement across Citrus County, Florida.
*Ed Youngblood, President*
*Susan Fogarty, Vice President*

781 **Dementia Family Pathways**
1038 Jenks Avenue 850-215-7078
Panama City, FL 32401 info@dementiafamilypathways.org
www.dementiafamilypathways.com
A non-profit organization dedicated to raising funds and promoting initiatives to serve the people diagnosed with dementia and Parkinson's Disease. Dementia Family Pathways strives to continue activities that have been established and to create new resources for those in need.

782 **Dementia Friendly Community Coalition Marinette County**
715-732-3850
dfcwi.com
A non-profit organization based in Marinette County, Wisconsin dedicated to creating a dementia-friendly community that is safe, respectful, and welcoming for people living with dementia through awareness, education, and community engagement. Works in partnership with other local non-profits.

783 **Greater Iowa Chapter Alzheimer's Association Quadcity Office**
736 Federal Street 563-324-1022
Davenport, IA 52803-5750 800-272-3900
Fax: 563-324-6267
Jerry.Schroeder@alz.org
www.alz.org
*Jerry Schroeder, Program Specialist*
*Julie Seier, Community Relations Coordinator*

784 **Long Island Alzheimer's & Dementia Center**
1025 Old Country Road 516-767-6856
Westbury, NY 11590 Fax: 516-767-6864
tcohen@lidementia.org
www.lidementia.org
Dedicated to improving the quality of life for individuals living with Alzheimer's disease and related memory disorders, and their caregivers. Mission is centered around community engagement and support.
*Tori Cohen, Executive Director*
*Frank Abrignani, Director, Finance & Operations*

785 **Maine Alzheimer's Care Center**
154 Dresden Avenue 207-626-1770
Gardiner, ME 04345

786 **New York Memory Center**
199 14th Street 718-499-7701
Brooklyn, NY 11215 jbrown@nymemorycenter.org
www.nymemorycenter.org
A community-based agency providing services to adults with cognitive, physical, and emotional limitations. The NY Memory Center's mission is to improve the quality of life for those diagnosed with memory loss.
*Josephine Brown, Executive Director*
*Susan Ramos, Operations Manager*

787 **San Diego Dementia Consortium**
PO Box 230725 858-412-7337
Encinitas, CA 92024 Fax: 858-630-5484
webmaster@sddementiaconsortium.org
www.sddementiaconsortium.org
A non-profit dedicated to raising awareness of dementia and cognitive health. The SDDC offers meetings and events in support of people affected by dementia and cognitive diseases.
*Rachel Hagopian, Outreach Director*

788 **The Tender: New Jersey**
4501 Church Road 856-234-5999
Mt. Laurel, NJ 08054 Fax: 856-234-9074
tenderADC@gmail.com
www.thetender.org
Caring for frail seniors and people with Alzheimer's in Burlington County, NJ since 1977.
*Barbara Fetty, Executive Director*

789 **Wyoming Dementia Care**
2546 E 2nd Street 307-232-3385
Casper, WY 82609 www.wyomingdementiacare.com
A non-profit organization dedicated to providing support services to families and caregivers of those with Alzheimer's disease and other dementia-related illnesses.
*Dani Mandelstam-Guerttman, Executive Director*

## Libraries & Resource Centers

790 **Green-Field Library-Alzheimer's Association**
225 N. Michigan Avenue 847-324-0356
Chicago, IL 60601-7633 800-272-3900
Fax: 866-699-1238
TTY: 312-335-5886
TDD: 312-335-8700
greenfield@alz.org
www.alz.org
Located at the national Alzheimer's Association in Chicago this library offers a sizable collection of videos on a variety of subjects that may interest the Alzheimer's patient family members and caregivers.
*Richard Hovland, COO*

## Foundations & Research Centers

791 **Aging and Alzheimer's Disease Center Oregon Health Sciences University**
Oregon Health Sciences University
3181 SW Sam Jackson Park Road 503-494-8311
Portland, OR 97239-3098 Fax: 503-494-6695
kaye@ohsu.edu
www.ohsu.edu/research/alzheimers
Researches causes and consequences of Alzheimer's disease and ways of clinical services. Publishes a newsletter twice a year.
*Jeffrey Kaye, Director*
*Joan Benedict, Administrative Coordinator*

792 **Alzheimer's Disease Center Emory University/VA Medical Center**
201 Dowman Drive 404-727-6069
Atlanta, GA 30322 Fax: 404-286-55
emoryadrc@emory.edu
www.med.emory.edu/ADRC
Researchers work to translate advances into improved care and diagnosis for Alzheimer's patients.
*Allan Levey, Director*
*Stuart Zola, Co-Director*

793 **Alzheimer's Disease Center Kentucky University**
Sanders-Brown Center on Aging
1030 South Broadway 859-257-1412
Lexington, KY 40504-0230 Fax: 859-323-2866
rdavi3@email.uky.edu
/www.mc.uky.edu/coa
Researchers work to translate advances into improved care and diagnosis for Alzheimer's patients.
*Linda J. Van Eldik, Ph.D., Director*
*Vince J Kellen, Chief Information Officer*

794 **Alzheimer's Disease Center Mayo Clinic Mayo Medical School**
Mayo Medical School
200 First Street SW 507-284-2511
Rochester, MN 55905 Fax: 507-538-0161
TDD: 507-2849786
mayoADC@mayo.edu
www.mayoclinic.com
Researchers work to translate advances into improved care and diagnosis for Alzheimer's patients.
*John H Noseworhty MD, President*
*William C Rupp MD, Vice President, CEO*

795 **Alzheimer's Disease Center Pennsylvania University School of Medicine**
Ralston House
3615 Chestnut Street 215-662-7810
Philadelphia, PA 19104 Fax: 215-662-7812
jason.karlawish@uphs.upenn.edu
www.pennadc.org
Researchers work to translate advances into improved care and diagnosis for Alzheimer's patients.
*John Q Trojanowski, Director*

796 **Alzheimer's Disease Center: Boston University**
Boston University School of Medicine
72 E Concord Street 617-638-5426
Boston, MA 02118 888-458-2823
Fax: 617-414-1197
buad@bu.edu
www.bu.edu/alzresearch
Researchers work to translate advances into improved care and diagnosis for Alzheimer's patients.
*Neil W Kowall, Director*
*Richard Fine, Associate Director*

797 **Alzheimer's Disease Center: Johns Hopkins University School of Medicine**
Johns Hopkins University Department of Pathology
720 Rutland Avenue 410-502-5164
Baltimore, MD 21205 Fax: 410-955-9777
edelman1@jhmi.edu
www.alzresearch.org

Researchers work to translate advances into improved care and diagnosis for Alzheimer's patients.
*Marilyn Albert, Director*
*Philip Wong, Associate Director*

798 **Alzheimer's Disease Center: University of Alabama at Birmingham**
1720 7th Avenue S 205-934-3847
Birmingham, AL 35294-0017 Fax: 205-975-7365
adbrain@uab.edu
Researchers work to translate advances into improved care and diagnosis for Alzheimer's patients.
*Daniel C Marson, Director*
*J Michael Wyss, Associate Director*

799 **Alzheimer's Disease Center: Washington University**
1660 S Columbian Way 206-764-2069
Seattle, WA 98108-1597 800-317-5382
Fax: 206-768-5456
wamble@u.washington.edu
www.depts.washington.edu/adrcweb
Researchers work to translate advances into improved care and diagnosis for Alzheimer's patients.
*Sydney Lewis, Education and Outreach Coordinator*
*Nancy Brown, Lead Psychometrist and Autopsy Coordinat*

800 **Alzheimer's Disease Research Center Washington University School of Medicine**
Washington University School of Medicine
4488 Forest Park Avenue 314-286-2683
St Louis, MO 63108 Fax: 314-286-2763
morrisj@abraxas.wustl.edu
www.adrc.wustl.edu
Researchers work to translate advances into improved care diagnosis and treatment for Alzheimer's patients.
*John Morris, Director*
*Virginia D Buckles, Executive Director*

801 **Alzheimer's Disease Research Center Duke University**
Bryan ADRC
2200 W Main Street Suite A200 919-668-0820
Durham, NC 27705 866-444-2372
kwe@duke.edu
adrc.mc.duke.edu
Researchers work to translate advances into improved care and diagnosis for Alzheimer's patients.
*Kathleen A Welsh-Bohmer, Director*
*James Robert Burke, Associate Director*

802 **Alzheimer's Drug Discovery Foundation**
57 W 57th Street 212-901-8000
New York, NY 10019 info@alzdiscovery.org
www.alzdiscovery.org
Funds the most promising Alzheimer's drug research worldwide.
*Howard Fillit, Executive Director*

803 **Alzheimer's Foundation of America**
322 Eighth Avenue 646-638-1542
New York, NY 10001 866-232-8484
Fax: 646-638-1546
info@alzfdn.org
www.alzfdn.org
To provide support, services and education to individuals, families and caregivers affected by Alzheimer's disease and related dementias nationwide.
*Charles J. Fuschillo Jr., President & CEO*

804 **Alzheimer's Research Foundation**
3152 Little Road 813-920-2922
Trinity, FL 34655
A non-profit dedicated to funding research for Alzheimer's Disease and other dementias. The foundation focuses on prevention, caregiver support, drug treatments, and education.

805 **American Brain Foundation**
201 Chicago Avenue 866-770-7570
Minneapolis, MN 55415 www.americanbrainfoundation.org
A national foundation for the brain dedicated to the relentless pursuit of early diagnoses, improved treatments, and the discovery of cures for brain diseases and disorders.
*Jane Ransom, Executive Director*
*Kim Howard, Operations & Executive Manager*

806 **Arizona Alzheimer's Consortium**
4745 N 7th Street 602-839-6525
Phoenix, AZ 85014 david.jerman@bannerhealth.com
azalz.org
A leader in statewide collaboration in Alzheimer's Disease research.

807 **Banner Alzheimer's Institute**
Stead Family Memory Center 602-839-6900
Phoenix, AZ 85006 www.banneralz.org
*Eric M. Reiman, Executive Director*
*Pierre N. Tariot, Director*

808 **Baylor College of Medicine Center for Allergy & Immunological Disorders**
1 Baylor Plaza 713-798-4951
Houston, TX 77030 www.bcm.edu
*Paul Klotman, President & CEO*

809 **Beacham Center for Geriatric Medicine**
John Hopkins Bayview Medical Campus
5505 Hopkins Bayview Circle 410-550-0925
Baltimore, MD 21224 www.hopkinsmedicine.org
Nonprofit organization focusing on gerontology research including Alzheimer's disease studies.
*Samuel C. Durso, Director*

810 **Boston University Alzheimer's Disease Center**
Boston University School of Medicine
72 E Concord Street 857-364-2140
Boston, MA 02118 888-458-2823
Fax: 617-358-6544
mpober@bu.edu
www.bu.edu/alzresearch
One of 29 Alzheimer's Disease Centers funded by the National Institutes of Health.
*Beverly Young, Administrator*
*Maria Ober, Asst. Dean for Communications*

811 **Center for Brain Activity Mapping**
UC San Diego
9500 Gilman Drive 858-534-2230
La Jolla, CA 92093 cbam.ucsd.edu
The Center seeks to develop new technologies for detecting neuronal activity, for reporting it out of deep brain tissue, and for processing and analyzing the resulting data, by organizing and supporting research teams and projects.
*Ralph J. Greenspan, PhD, Director*

812 **Cognitive Neurology and Alzheimer's Disease Center**
CNADC
320 E Superior Street 312-908-9339
Chicago, IL 60611 Fax: 312-908-8789
CNADC-Admin@northwestern.edu
www.brain.northwestern.edu
Researchers work to translate advances into improved care and diagnosis for Alzheimer's patients.
*Megan Atchu, MA, Research Administrator*
*Kevin Connolly, Business Administrator*

813 **Columbia University Alzheimer's Disease Research Center**
Department of Pathology & Cell Biology
630 W 168th Street Fax: 212-342-3013
New York, NY 10032 pathology@columbia.edu
pathology.columbia.edu
Alzheimer's disease and elderly care. Serves as a resource for tissue, cells, and DNA from Alzheimer's disease and control patients. Areas of research include epidemiology, cell biology, molecular biology, and care-giving.
*Joann Li, CFO*

814 **Cornell University: Winifred Masterson Burke Medical Research-Dementia**
1300 York Avenue 212-746-5454
New York, NY 10065 Fax: 212-821-0576
publicaffairs@med.cornell.edu
www.med.cornell.edu
Clinical and basic studies in metabolic aspects of the nervous system especially Alzheimer's disease.
*David J Skorton MD, President*
*Thomas H Blair lll, Senior Director Administrator*

815 **Duke University Center for the Study of Aging and Human Development**
Duke University
Box 3003 919-660-7500
Durham, NC 27710 Fax: 919-668-0453
webmaster@geri.duke.edu
Basic and clinical research into geriatrics and gerontology focusing on a number of chronic diseases in the elderly including osteoporosis cancer heart disease infectious diseases Alzheimer's disease and other disorders leading to dysmobility.
*Harvey Jay Cohen MD, Director*
*Linda K George, Associate Director*

816 **Duke University Clinical Research Institute**
Headquarters
2400 Pratt Street 919-668-8700
Durham, NC 27705 www.dcri.duke.edu
Multidisciplinary clinical research into the cause and prevention of human diseases such as Alzheimer's.
*Robert A Harrington, Director*
*Elizabeth Be Reed, Chief Operating Officer*

817 **Duke University General Clinical Research Center**
Durham, NC 27710 919-668-1755
medicine.duke.edu/research
Multidisciplinary, clinical research into the cause and prevention of human diseases such as Alzheimer's.
*Heather E. Whitson, Division Director*
*Laurie Snyder, Medical Director*

818 **Fisher Center for Research on Alzheimer's Disease**
Rockefeller University
FDR Station 212-915-1328
New York, NY 10150 800-259-4636
Fax: 212-915-1319
info@alzinfo.org
www.alzinfo.org
An organization that provides millions of dollars for novel Alzheimer's research primarily conducted by the late Nobel Laureate Dr. Paul Greengard and his team of over 45 internationally renowned scientists at the Fisher Center lab at The Rockefeller University, plus other leading research institutes around the world. The center's mission is to understand the causes of Alzheimer's disease, improve the care of those with it, and find a cure.
*Lucretia Holden, Executive Director*

819 **Georgetown University: International Center for Interdiciplinary Studies**
3800 Reservoir Road NW 202-687-8227
Washington, DC 20007 bellantj@georgetown.edu
www.georgetown.edu
Studies of immunology and allergic disorders.
*Joseph A. Bellanti, Director*

820 **Goizueta Alzheimer's Disease Research Center**
Emory Brain Health Center
12 Executive Park Drive NE 404-778-3444
Atlanta, GA 30329 www.alzheimers.emory.edu
One of 27 active centers in the nation supported by the National Institutes of Health. The center hopes to bring scientists together to facilitate their research and help learn more about Alzheimer's and related diseases.
*Allan Levey, Director*

821 **I'm Still Here Foundation**
10 Tower Office Park 781-674-2884
Woburn, MA 01801 www.imstillhere.org
A non-profit promoting community engagement as an initiative to support people living with dementia. The foundation places an emphasis on arts and culture, education, and public policy.
*John Zeisel, President*

822 **Indiana University Center for Aging Research**
The Center for Aging Research
1050 Wishard Blvd 317-630-6083
Indianapolis, IN 46202-2872 Fax: 317-423-5695
www.medicine.iupui.edu/iucar/?
Researchers work to translate advances into improved care and diagnosis for Alzheimer's patients.
*Christopher Callahan, Director*
*Douglas K Miller, Associate Director*

823 **Indiana University-Purdue University at Indianapolis: Center for Alzheimer's**
420 University Boulevard 317-274-5555
Indianapolis, IN 46202 www.iupui.edu
Alzeheimer's Disease and related neuropsychiatric disorders characterized by memory loss and mood disorders in the elderly.

824 **Indiana University: Human Genetics Center of Medical & Molecular Genetics**
School of Medicine
340 West 10th Street 317-274-8157
Indianapolis, IN 46202-3082 kcornett@iupui.edu
www.medicine.iu.edu
Comprised of a core group of scientists with primary appointments in the Department and a group of molecular biologists from other departments who hold joint appointments in Medical and Molecular Genetics.
*D Craig Brater MD, Dean*
*John F. Fitzgerald, MD, MBA, Executive Associate Dean*

825 **Institute for Basic Research in Developmental Disabilities**
1050 Forest Hill Road 718-494-0600
Staten Island, NY 10314-0001 866- 94- 973
TTY: 866- 933-488
ibr@opwdd.ny.gov
www.opwdd.ny.gov/institute-for-basic-res
*James F Moran, Acting Commissioner*

826 **John Douglas French Alzheimer's Foundation**
11620 Wilshire Boulevard 323-930-6228
Los Angeles, CA 90025-1781 800-477-2243
Fax: 310-479-0516
bwelch@alz.org
www.jdfaf.org
Provides seed money for promising research including the cause cure and prevention of Alzheimer's disease. Also gives funding to scientists who might not otherwise be funded.
*Bruce L. Miller, MD, Chief Medical Officer*
*Karen Bedrosian Coyne, President*

827 **Johns Hopkins University: Alzheimer's Disease Research Center**
1620 McElderry Street 410-502-9272
Baltimore, MD 21205 brodzon@jhu.edu
www.alzresearch.org
Alzheimer's disease, including basic and applied studies of symptoms and psychiatric problems.
*Marilyn Albert, Director*

828 **Kavli Foundation**
5715 Mesmer Avenue 424-353-8800
Los Angeles, CA info@kavlifoundation.org
www.kavlifoundation.org
The Foundation supports scientific research into the human brain, in the following scientific fields: Astrophysics, Nanoscience, Neuroscience and Theoretical Physics. Within Neuroscience, the study of aging and brain diseases and disorders is supported.
*Robert W. Conn, PhD, President & CEO*
*Eric Marshall, VP, Public Engagement & Prizes*

829 **Kavli Institute for Brain Science at Columbia University**
Columbia University
3227 Broadway 212-853-1016
New York, NY 10027 Fax: 212-665-9699
kavli@columbia.edu
www.kavli.columbia.edu

The Institute's primary are of study is how signaling in neural circuits controls cognitive function and behavior, and the development of novel experimental and computational strategies for analyzing these signals.
*Eric R. Kandel, MD, Director*
*Rafael Yuste, MD, PhD, Co-Director*

830 **Kavli Institute for Brain and Mind**
UC San Diego
9500 Gilman Drive kibm@ucsd.edu
La Jolla, CA 92093-0115 kibm.ucsd.edu
The Institute supports research that furthers the understanding of the origins, evolution and mechanisms of human cognition. Of particular interest is Traumatic Brain Injury.
*Fred H. Gage, Co-Director*
*Nicholas C. Spitzer, Co-Director*

831 **Kavli Institute for Fundamental Neuroscience**
UCSF, Sandler Neurosciences Center
675 Nelson Rising Lane 415-476-2018
San Francisco, CA 94158 Fax: 415-502-7332
kavliifn@ucsf.edu
kavliifn.ucsf.edu
The Institute is the central organization for neuroscience research at UCSF and partner institutions, establishing cross-disciplinary teams of scientists and engineers devoted to advancing neuroscience in all its forms.
*Loren Frank, Co-Director*
*Roger Nicoll, Co-Director*

832 **Kavli Institute for Neuroscience at Yale University**
Yale School of Medicine
295 Congress Avenue 203-737-4461
New Haven, CT 06510 203-737-4467
pietro.decamilli@yale.edu
medicine.yale.edu/neuroscience/kavli
The institute studies nervous system development and function.
*Pietro De Camilli, MD, Director*
*Marina Picciotto, PhD, Deputy Director*

833 **Kavli Neural Systems Institute**
The Rockefeller University
1230 York Avenue 212-327-8081
New York, NY 10065 lcole@rockefeller.edu
www.rockefeller.edu/research
The Institute unites scientists at The Rockefeller University in the goal of a comprehensive look at the human brain.
*Leslie Vosshall, PhD, Director*
*Lindsey Cole, Administrator*

834 **Kavli Neuroscience Discovery Institute**
Johns Hopkins University, School of Medicine
725 N Wolfe Street 410-955-4089
Baltimore, MD 21205 Fax: 410-614-6249
KavliNDI@jhu.edu
kavlijhu.org
The Institute looks to advance neuroscience by integrating neuroscience, engineering and computational data science.
*Dwight Bergles, PhD, Director*
*Natasha Hussain, PhD, Scientific Director*

835 **Knight Alzheimer's Disease Research Center**
4488 Forest Park 314-286-2683
St. Louis, MO 63108 knightadrc.wustl.edu

836 **Long Island Alzheimers Foundation**
5 Channel Drive 516-767-6856
Port Washington, NY 11050 Fax: 516-767-6856
info@liaf.org
www.liaf.org
Researchers work to translate advances into improved care and diagnosis for Alzheimer's patients.
*Fred Jenny, Executive Director*
*Anna Maria Warmuz, Executive Assistant*

837 **Massachusetts Alzheimer's Disease Research Center**
Massachusetts General Hospital
Building, Suite 2011 617-726-3987
Charlestown, MA 02129 Fax: 617-724-1480
www.madrc.org
Coordinates research on Alzheimer's disease, including memory loss, dementia, neuropathology, neuropsychology, neurochemistry, and investigational drug studies. Projects focus on biochemical studies on the abnormal proteins that accumulate in the brains of Alzheimer's patients, possible genetic markers or familial traits, anatomical and neurotransmitter abnormalities, and clinical studies of behavior and neuropharmacology.
*Bradley T. Hyman, Director*

838 **Massachusetts Alzheimers Disease Research Center**
Massachusetts ADRC
16th Street 617-726-3987
Charlestown, MA 02129 Fax: 617-724-1480
www.madrc.org
Multi-institutional consortium of Harvard affiliated facilities encompasses five Core units: an Administrative Core a Clinical Core a Database Management and Statistics Core a Neuropathology Core and an Education and Information Transfer Core. The ADRC also supports four specific research projects funded for 3-5 years and annually designates three or four pilot research projects that are funded for 1 year.
*John H Growdon, Clinic Director*
*Bradley T Hyman, Center Director*

839 **Mayo Clinic Alzheimer's Disease Research Center**
Mayo Clinic
200 First Street SW 507-284-1324
Rochester, MN 55905 Fax: 507-538-0878
potaracke.ryan@mayo.edu
www.mayo.edu/research
The Alzheimer's Disease Research Center at Mayo Clinic promotes research and education about healthy brain aging, mild cognitive impairment, Alzheimer's disease, Lewy body dementia, frontotemporal dementia and other related dementia disorders.
*Ronald C. Petersen, Director*

840 **Medical College of Georgia Alzheimers Research Center**
1120 15th Street 706-721-0211
Augusta, GA 30912 Fax: 706-721-7063
Clinical and basic research of Alzheimer's disease.
*Jerry Buccaf MD, Director*
*J Warren Beach, Member*

841 **Michigan Alzheimer's Disease Research Center**
University of Michigan
2101 Commonwealth Blvd., 734-936-4000
Ann Arbor, MI 48105-0316 www.med.umich.edu/alzheimers
Researchers work to translate advances into improved care and diagnosis for Alzheimer's patients.
*Sid Gilman MD, Director*
*Bruno Giordani Ph.D., Core Director*

842 **Mount Sinai School of Medicine of CUNY Alzheimer's Disease**
University of New York
1 Gustave L. Levy Place 212-241-8329
New York, NY 10029 Fax: 212-996-0987
adrc@mssm.edu
icahn.mssm.edu/research/adrc
Etiology, diagnosis, and treatment of Alzheimer's disease and related dementias. Clinical studies include trials of new drugs and biological markers and longitudinal follow-up studies. An active autopsy network obtains brain material from Alzheimer patients.
*Mary Sano, Director*

843 **Mount Sinai School of Medicine: Alzheimers Disease Research Center**
Alzheimer's Disease Research Center
One Gustave L Levy Place 212-241-6696
New York, NY 10029-6574 Fax: 212-369-2344
mary.sano@mssm.edu
www.mssm.edu
Focuses on Alzheimer's disease research.
*Mary Sano, Director*
*Samuel Gandy, Associate Director*

844 **NHI Clinical Center**
9000 Rockville Pike 301-496-2563
Bethesda, MD 20892 Fax: 301-402-9033
ccpressgroup@cc.nih.gov
www.cc.nih.gov

Established as the research hospital of the National Institutes of Health. Designed so that patient care facilities are close to research laboratories so new findings of basic and clinical scientists can be quickly applied to the treatment of patients. Upon referral by physicians or self-referral, qualifying patients are admitted to NIH clinical studies.
*Dr. James K. Gilman, CEO*

845 **Nathan Kline Institute for Psychiatric Research: Center for Alzheimer's Disease**
140 Old Orangeburg Road 845-398-5500
Orangeburg, NY 10962 Fax: 914-398-5510
David.AlcantaraG@nki.rfmh.org
www.rfmh.org
Molecular neuroscience and aging, including molecular neurobiology of proteases, signal transduction, neurodegenerative disease, protein/peptide analytical techniques, molecular genetics, vesicle biology, transgenic modeling.
*Donald C. Goff M.D., Director*
*Antonio Convit M.D., Deputy Director*

846 **National Alzheimer's Coordinating Center**
4311 11th Avenue NE 206-543-8637
Seattle, WA 98105 Fax: 206-616-5927
naccmail@uw.edu
www.alz.washington.edu
Coordinating data collection and fostering collaborative research among Alzheimer's Disease centers.
*Walter A. Kukull, Director/Principal Investigator*

847 **National Cell Repository for Alzheimer's Disease**
800-526-2839
alzstudy@iu.edu
ncrad.iu.edu
Providing biological samples and data to researchers to help them find genetic factors in Alzheimer's Disease and dementia.
*Tatiana Foroud, Principal Investigator*

848 **Neuroscience Research Institute**
UC Santa Barbara
6129 Biology II 805-893-4621
Santa Barbara, CA 93106 www.nri.ucsb.edu
The Institute seeks to allow scientists from different fields to collaborate for the betterment of neurological research. Areas of interest include: Alzheimer's Disease & Related Dementias; Behavioral Neuroscience & Neuroethology; Cell Biology, Biochemistry & Biophysics of the Nervous System; Computational & Theoretical Neuroscience; Development of the Nervous System; and Stem Cells.
*Stuart Feinstein, Co-Director*
*Kenneth Kosik, Co-Director*

849 **Neurosciences Institute of the Neurosciences Research Program**
The Neurosciences Institute
10640 John Jay Hopkins Drive 858-626-2000
San Diego, CA 92121 Fax: 858-626-2099
info@nsi.edu
www.nsi.edu
Nonprofit organization focusing on Alzheimer's and related disorders.
*Gerald M Edelman, President*

850 **Ohio State University Neuroscience Program**
1835 Neil Avenue 614-292-8185
Columbus, OH 43210 Fax: 614-921-44
ASC-psychmainoffice@osu.edu
psychology.osu.edu
Specializes in brain disorders such as Alzheimer's disease.
*Richard Petty, Chair*
*Scott Burch, Behavioral Neurosciences Area Assistant*

851 **Oregon Health & Science University: Brain Institute**
3181 SW Sam Jackson Park Road 503-494-7198
Portland, OR 97239 zitzelbe@ohsu.edu
ohsu.edu/brain-institute
The OHSU Brain Institute funds several research centres dedicated to neurological disorders, including Alzheimer's and Dementia.
*Jeffrey Kaye, Director*
*Tracy Zitzelberger, Administrator*

852 **Rush Alzheimer's Disease Center**
Rush University
1653 W Congress Parkway 888-352-7874
Chicago, IL 60612 www.rush.edu
Alzheimer's disease, including causes, treatment, and cure. Conducts clinical trials of new drug treatments and analyzes potential risk factors in the development of Alzheimer's disease.

853 **Salk Institute for Biological Studies**
10010 N Torrey Pines Road 858-453-4100
La Jolla, CA 92037 www.salk.edu
Conducts groundbreaking research into cancer, aging, Alzheimer's diabetes and infectious diseases.
*Rusty Gage, PhD, President*
*Martin Hetzer, PhD, VP & Chief Science Officer*

854 **Sanford Consortium for Regenerative Medicine**
2880 Torrey Pines Scenic Drive 858-246-1071
La Jolla, CA 92037 www.sanfordconsortium.com
The Consortium works to achieve breakthrough discoveries in stem cell research with regards to diagnoses, treatments, and cures for degenerative diseases and injuries.
*Edward W. Holmes, MD, President & CEO*
*Jeffrey Steindorf, PhD, VP & COO*

855 **Scripps Research Institute**
10550 North Torrey Pines Road 858-784-1000
La Jolla, CA www.scripps.edu
The institute seeks to improve human wellbeing through the advancement of bioscience, including research into aging & healthspan, autoimmune diseases, cancer, infectious diseases, neurological disorders, and more.
*Peter Schultz, PhD, President & CEO*
*Eric Topol, MD, EVP, Scripps Research*

856 **Sun Health Research Institute: Alzheimer's Center**
14719 W Grand Avenue 623-471-9550
Surprise, AZ 85374 info@sunhealth.org
www.sunhealth.org
Alzheimer's disease, Parkinson's disease, rheumatoid arthritis, and other age-related diseases. Research focuses on molecular genetics molecular/cell biology, protein chemistry, and immunology of degenerative disorders affecting the elderly.
*Joseph E. La Rue, CEO*

857 **Taub Institute for Research on Alzheimer 's Disease and the Aging Brain**
Columbia University
630 W 168th Street 212-305-1818
New York, NY 10032 Fax: 212-342-2849
taubinstitute@columbia.edu
columbianeuroresearch.org/taub
Dedicated to epidemiological and cell biological research to study Alzheimer's Disease and other dementia related disorders. The Institute collaborates with several departments at Columbia University, including Neurology, Pathology, Psychiatry, Radiology, and the Huntington's Disease Center.
*Richard Mayeux, Director*
*Michael Shelanski, Director*

858 **The Alzheimer's Disease & Memory Disorders Center**
ADMDC
One Baylor Plaza 713-798-5971
Houston, TX 77030 Fax: 713-798-7434
neurons@bcm.edu
www.bcm.edu/neurology/admdc
Researchers work to translate advances into improved care and diagnosis for Alzheimer's Disease and other memory disorders.
*Eli M Mizrahi, Chair, Department of Neurology*
*Keith Davis, Department Administrator*

859 **The Sam and Rose Stein Institute for Research on the Aging**
University of California San Diego
9500 Gilman Drive 858-534-6299
La Jolla, CA 92093-0664 Fax: 858-534-5475
steininstitute@ucsd.edu
Research on aging and Alzheimer's disease.
*Debra Kaine, Director*
*Maureen Halp MS, Executive Director*

860 **UC Irvine Alzheimer's Disease Research Center**
UCI MIND
2642 Biological Sciences III 949-824-3253
Irvine, CA 92697 Fax: 949-824-0885
research@mind.uci.edu
www.mind.uci.edu
Internationally recognized research into age-related disorders of the brain.
*Carl W. Cotman, Founding Director*

861 **UT Southwestern Medical Center Alzheimer 's Disease Center**
UT Southwestern Medical Center 214-648-3111
Dallas, TX 75390 www.utsouthwestern.edu
Funded by the National Institute on Aging, the Alzheimer's Disease Center (ADC) is an interdisciplinary research team focused on the nature of Alzheimer's disease.
*Marc Diamond, Director*

862 **University Alzheimer Center University of Alabama at Birmingham**
University of Alabama at Birmingham
1530 3rd Avenue S 205-934-4011
Birmingham, AL 35294-1150 800-333-6543
Fax: 205-975-7365
TTY: 205-934-4642
adbrain@uab.edu
Researchers work to translate advances into improved care and diagnosis for Alzheimer's patients.
*Dr. Carol Garrison, President*
*Kristen N Burdick, Director of Executive Affairs*

863 **University Alzheimer Center UHC: Case Western Reserve University**
12200 Fairhill Road 216-844-6400
Cleveland, OH 44120 Fax: 216-844-6446
Kathy.Shaw@Case.Edu
www.ohioalzcenter.org
Researchers work to translate advances into improved care and diagnosis for Alzheimer's patients.
*Alan Lerner, Co-Director*
*Kathleen A Smyth, Administrator*

864 **University of Chicago Dept of Neurology University of Chicago Hospital**
University of Chicago Hospital
5841 S Maryland Avenue 773-702-6390
Chicago, IL 60637-1470 Fax: 773-702-9076
cgomez@neurology.bsd.uchicago.edu
neurology.uchicago.edu
Covers Translational Neuroscience Research and research programs in neuroimmunology neuromuscular disease and neurovirology provided the initial foundation and brought national recognition.
*Kenneth Goodell, Senior Executive Administrator*
*Judith Maratea, Administrative Assistant*

865 **University of Chicago: Brain Research Institute**
Department of Neurology
5841 S Maryland Avenue 773-702-6222
Chicago, IL 60637 neurology.uchicago.edu
Studies brain disorders including Alzheimer's disease.

866 **University of Illinois Health Services Research**
University of Illinois College of Medicine
1601 Parkview Avenue 815-395-0600
Rockford, IL 61107 Fax: 815-395-5887
prrockford@uic.edu
A unit of the University of Illinois College of Medicine at Rockford serves faculty students health care providers human services agencies and other community organizations throughout Illinois with demographic health social and economic data. The skills data and resources available to faculty and students at the college are also available to individuals and organizations needing assistance.
*Joann Glacken, Research Support Services*

867 **University of Iowa: Alzheimer's Disease Research Center**
College of Medicine
451 Newton Road 319-335-6707
Iowa City, IA 52242 www.medicine.uiowa.edu
Alzheimer's disease and related conditions. Departments with participating specialists include anatomy, radiology, pathology, ophthalmology, psychology.

868 **University of Kentucky: Alzheimer's Disease Research Center**
Sanders-Brown Center on Aging
800 S Limestone Street 859-323-6040
Lexington, KY 40536 Fax: 859-323-2866
www.uky.edu/coa/adc
Alzheimer's disease, focusing on the cause, treatment, and eventual cure.
*Linda J. Van Eldik, Director*

869 **University of Maryland: Division of Infectious Diseases**
UM Baltimore Department of Medicine
655 West Baltimore Street 410-706-7410
Baltimore, MD 21201 Fax: 410-706-0235
rredfield@ihv.umaryland.edu
www.medschool.umaryland.edu
Focuses research on elderly studies including drug use treatments and infectious diseases of the aged.
*E. Albert Reece, Vice President*
*Richard Pierson III MD, Senior Associate Dean*

870 **University of Miami: Center for Neurological Diseases**
1501 NW 9th Avenue 305-547-6946
Miami, FL 33136 uhealthsystem.com
Focuses on aged disorders such as Alzheimer's research.

871 **University of Miami: Center on Aging**
Center on Aging
1695 NW 9th Avenue 305-355-9080
Miami, FL 33136 Fax: 305-355-9076
ajaret@med.miami.edu
Focuses on aged disorders such as Alzheimer's research.
*Sara J Czaja, Co-Director*
*Charles B. Nemeroff, M.D., Ph.D, Director*

872 **University of Michigan: Alzheimer's Disease Research Center**
Department of Neurology
2101 Commonwealth Boulevard 734-936-8803
Ann Arbor, MI 48105 UM-Ask-MADC@med.umich.edu
alzheimers.med.umich.edu
Alzheimer's disease and other neurodegenerative diseases associated with dementia, including Parkinson's disease, multiple system atrophy, progressive supranuclear palsy, and olivopontocerebellar atrophy. Studies involve positron emission tomography (PET) scanning of patients with neurological disorders, neuropathological studies of patients with neurodegenerative illnesses, animal models, and a statewide public opinion survey.
*Arijit K. Bhaumik, Research Administrator*

873 **University of Texas Southwestern Medical Center at Dallas: Alzheimer's Disease**
Department of Psychiatry
5323 Harry Hines Boulevard 214-648-3111
Dallas, TX 75235 Fax: 214-648-2450
www.utsouthwestern.edu
Alzheimer's diseaese and aging in the brain, focusing on loss of cognitive functions and test measurements including IQ, problem solving, abstract thinking, spatial and dexterity skills, attention and concentration, language function, and memory.
*Marc Diamond, Director*

874 **University of Washington: Alzheimer's Disease Research Center**
Harborview Medical Center 206-744-0588
Seattle, WA 98104 855-744-0588
www.depts.washington.edu/adrcweb
Basic mechanisms underlying the development of adult dementing disorders, with particular attention to heritable susceptibility factors underlying Alzheimer's disease.
*Thomas J. Grabowski, Director*

875 **Wisconsin Alzheimer's Disease Research Center**
600 Highland Avenue 608-263-2582
Madison, WI 53792 adrc@medicine.wisc.edu
www.adrc.wisc.edu
Investigators conduct basic, clinical and behavioral research.
*Sanjay Asthana, Director*

876 **Yeshiva University: Resnick Gerontology Center**
Albert Einstein College of Medicine
Jack and Pearl Resnick Campus 718-920-6722
Bronx, NY 10467 866-633-8255
Fax: 718-655-9672
ljacobs@aecom.yu.edu
www.aecom.yu.edu
Alzheimer's disease and other dementia studies.
*Allen M Spiegel MD, Dean*
*Amy R Ehrlich, Geriatrics Fellowship Program Director*

## Support Groups & Hotlines

877 **Alzheimer's Association Autopsy Assistance Network**
Alzheimer s Association
Western/Central Washington Chapter 206-363-5500
Seattle, WA 98125 800-848-7097
Fax: 206-363-5700
rowena.rye@alz.org
http://alzwa.org/resources6.htm
The primary purposes of the Autopsy Assistance Network are: to provide families with information regarding autopsy; to assist in obtaining a confirmed diagnosis; provide tissue for Alzheimer's disease research; and establish diagnosis for purpose of clinical and epidemiological studies.
*Nancy Dapper, Executive Director*
*Rowena Rye, Community Resources*

878 **Alzheimer's Support Group**
Columbus Health Rehabilitation Center
2100 Midway Street 812-372-8447
Columbus, IN 47201 Fax: 812-375-5117
www.columbushrc.com/
The skilled Nursing Center includes a separate unit dedicated to the care of residents with Alzheimer's disease and other forms of dementia. The Alzheimer's program is designed to celebrate the spirit of their residents, striving to offer a comfortable and compassionate environment that emphasizes positive life experiences and active involvement in a daily routine.
*Mike Spencer, Executive Director*

879 **National Health Information Center**
Office of Disease Prevention & Health Promotion
1101 Wootton Pkwy Fax: 240-453-8281
Rockville, MD 20852 odphpinfo@hhs.gov
www.health.gov/nhic
Supports public health education by maintaining a calendar of National Health Observances; helps connect consumers and health professionals to organizations that can best answer questions and provide up-to-date contact information from reliable sources; updates on a yearly basis toll-free numbers for health information, Federal health clearinghouses and info centers.
*Don Wright, MD, MPH, Director*

## Magazines

880 **ADRC Pathways**
University of Pittsburgh
UPMC Montefiore, 4th Floor, Suite 4 412-692-2700
Pittsburgh, PA 15213 Fax: 412-692-2710
www.adrc.pitt.edu
A bi-annual newsletter covering recent news on Dementia and Alzheimer's Disease research.
*Oscar Lopez, Director*

881 **ASN NEURO**
Sage Journals
2455 Teller Road 805-499-9774
Thousand Oaks, CA 91320 journals@sagepub.com
journals.sagepub.com/home/asn
Peer-reviewed open access journal focusing on recent advances in the cellular and molecular neurosciences. It is the official publication of the American Society for Neurochemistry.
*Douglas L. Feinstein, Editor-in-Chief*
*Sandra J. Hewitt, Deputy Editor-in-Chief*

882 **Alzheimer Disease and Associated Disorders: An International Journal**
Raven Press
1185 Ave of the Americas 212-930-9500
New York, NY 10036-2601 800-777-2295
journals.lww.com
A leading international forum for reports of new research findings and new approaches to diagnosis and treatments. Contributions are offered from all scientific and medical fields.
*Quarterly*
*ISBN: 0-89303H- -*
*Charles DeCarli, MD, Editor-in-Chief*

883 **American Journal of Geriatric Psychiatry**
Elsevier
1600 John F Kennedy Boulevard www.journals.elsevier.com
Philadelphia, PA 19103
Peer-reviewed articles on the rapidly developing field of geriatric psychiatry, including areas such as the diagnosis and classification of psychiatric disorders, epidemiological and biological correlates of mental health of older adults, and psychopharmacology and other somatic treatments.
*Monthly*
*Charles F. Reynolds III, MD, Editor-in-Chief*

884 **American Journal of Pathology**
Elsevier
1600 John F Kennedy Boulevard 301-634-7959
Philadelphia, PA 19103 Fax: 301-634-7961
ajp@asip.org
ajp.amjpathol.org
Official journal of the American Society for Investigative Pathology, publishing original research reports, reviews, and commentaries related to the molecular and cellular basis of disease.
*Martha Furie, Editor-in-Chief*

885 **BMC Neuroscience**
Springer Nature
One New York Plaza 800-777-4643
New York, NY 10004-1562 info@biomedcentral.com
bmcneurosci.biomedcentral.com
A peer-reviewed, open-access journal devoted to all aspects of the nervous system (including molecular, cellular, developmental and animal model studies), as well as cognitive and behavioral research, and computational modeling.
*Darren Byrne, Editor*
*Ana Donnelly, Manuscript Editor*

886 **Brain & Life**
American Academy of Neurology
201 Chicago Avenue 612-928-6000
Minneapolis, MN 55415 800-879-1960
Fax: 612-454-2748
BrainandLife@wolterskluwer.com
www.brainandlife.org
Official magazine of the American Academy of Neurology, aimed at parents and home-caregivers interested in neurology in everyday life.
*Orly Avitzur, MD, MBA, FAAN, Editor-in-Chief*
*Mary Bolster, Managing Editor*

887 **Brain: A Journal of Neurology**
Oxford University Press
2001 Evans Road 919-677-0977
Cary, NC 27513 800-852-7323
Fax: 919-677-1714
brain@ucl.ac.uk
academic.oup.com/brain
Focus is clinical neurology and translational neuroscience.
*Dimitri M. Kullmann, Editor*
*Joanne Bell, Managing Editor*

888 **Continuum: Lifelong Learning in Neurology**
American Academy of Neurology
201 Chicago Avenue 612-928-6000
Minneapolis, MN 55415 800-879-1960
continuumcme@aan.com
journals.lww.com/continuum

Official journal of the American Academy of Neurology, aiding professionals in patient care and continuing education.
*Bimonthly*
*Steven L. Lewis, MD, FAAN*
*Andrea J. Weiss, MA, Executive Editor*

889 **Dementia and Geriatric Cognitive Disorders**
S. Karger Publishers, Inc.
26 W Avon Road 860-675-7834
Unionville, CT 06085 800-828-5479
Fax: 860-675-7302
www.karger.com/DEM
Open-access journal devoted to the study of cognitive dysfunction in preclinical and clinical studies, concentrating on Alzheimer's and Parkinson's disease, Huntington's chorea and other neurodegenerative diseases.
*Victoria Chan-Pilay, Editor-in-Chief*

890 **Dimensions**
UW Alzheimer's Disease Research Center
Box 359791 206-744-0588
Seattle, WA 98104 855-744-0588
uwadrc@uw.edu
www.uwadrc.org
Dimensions is a bi-annual magazine focused on all facets of dementia and the lives of people diagnosed with dementia.
*Thomas Grabowski, Director*

891 **JNeurosci**
Society for Neuroscience
1121 14th Street NW 202-962-4000
Washginton, DC 20005 jn@sfn.org
www.jneurosci.org
Official peer-reviewed journal of the Society for Neuroscience, publishing research on a broad range of topics of interest to those working on the nervous system.
*Marina R. Picciotto, Editor-in-Chief*
*Teresa Esch, Features Editor*

892 **Journal of Alzheimer's Disease**
IOS Press
6751 Tepper Drive 703-830-6300
Clifton, VA 20124 Fax: 703-830-2300
editorial@j-alz.com
www.j-alz.com
Research into the etiology, pathogenesis, epidemiology, genetics, behavior, treatment and psychology of Alzheimer's disease.
*George Perry, PhD, Editor-in-Chief*
*Beth Kumar, Managing Editor*

893 **Journal of Molecular Diagnostics**
Elsevier
1600 John F Kennedy Boulevard 301-634-7959
Philadelphia, PA 19103 Fax: 301-634-7961
jmd@asip.org
jmd.amjpathol.org
Official journal of the American Society for Investigative Pathology and the Association for Molecular Pathology, focusing on molecular discoveries in medicine translating into the clinical diagnostic setting, as well as the description and application of technological advances in the field of molecular diagnostic medicine.
*Monthly*
*Barbara Zehnbauer, PhD, Editor-in-Chief*

894 **Journal of NeuroEngineering and Rehabilitation**
Springer Nature
One New York Plaza 800-777-4643
New York, NY 10004-1562 info@biomedcentral.com
jneuroengrehab.biomedcentral.com
An open-access journal devoted to integrated research from the fields of neuroscience, biomedical engineering, and physical medicine and rehabilitation.
*David J. Reinkensmeyer, Editor-in-Chief*

895 **Journal of Neurodevelopmental Disorders**
Springer Nature
One New York Plaza 800-777-4643
New York, NY 10004-1562 info@biomedcentral.com
jneurodevdisorders.biomedcentral.com
An open-access journal devoted to integrating research from neurobiology, genetics, cognitive neuroscience, psychiatry and psychology.
*Joseph Piven, Editor-in-Chief*

896 **Journal of Neuroinflammation**
Springer Nature
One New York Plaza 800-777-4643
New York, NY 10004-1562 info@biomedcentral.com
jneuroinflammation.biomedcentral.com
A peer-reviewed, open-access journal focusing on the interactions of the immune system with the nervous system as a means of expanding understanding of chronic neurological diseases.
*Monica J. Carson, Editor-in-Chief*
*Sue T. Griffin, Editor-in-Chief*

897 **Journal of Nuclear Medicine**
Society of Nuclear Medicine and Molecular Imaging
1850 Samuel Morse Drive 703-708-9000
Reston, VA 20190 800-513-6853
Fax: 703-708-9015
subscriptions@snm.org
jnm.snmjournals.org
Peer-reviewed journal with clinical investigations, science reports, articles benefitting continuing education, book reviews, employment opportunities, and updates on practice and research.
*Monthly*
*Johannes Czernin, MD, Editor-in-Chief*
*Susan Alexander, Associate Director, Publications*

898 **Journal of Nuclear Medicine Technology**
Society of Nuclear Medicine and Molecular Imaging
1850 Samuel Morse Drive 703-708-9000
Reston, VA 20190 800-513-6853
Fax: 703-708-9015
subscriptions@snm.org
tech.snmjournals.org
Peer-reviewed journal dedicated to nuclear medicine technology, with information on credentialing, continuing education and licensure requirements, as well as current news and updates on the field.
*Quarterly*
*Kathy S. Thomas, MHA, CNMT, PET, Editor-in-Chief*
*Susan Alexander, Associate Director, Publications*

899 **Journal of the Neurological Sciences**
Elsevier
LSU Health Sciences Center JNS_England@lsuhsc.edu
New Orleans, LA 70112 www.jns-journal.com
Original articles in neurology and neuroscience from around the world.
*Monthly*
*John D. England, Editor-in-Chief*

900 **Mature Health**
Haymarket Group, Ltd.
45 W 34th Street 212-239-0855
New York, NY 10001-3073
Magazine featuring articles on health aspects of aging, as well as articles on recreation and leisure.

901 **Molecular Imaging**
Sage Journals
2455 Teller Road 805-499-9774
Thousand Oaks, CA 91320 journals@sagepub.com
journals.sagepub.com/home/mix
Peer-reviewed open access journal focusing on molecular imaging research, including basic science, preclinical studies and human applications. Published in association with the Society of Nuclear Medicine and Molecular Imaging.
*Bimonthly*
*Henry F. VanBrocklin, PhD, Editor-in-Chief*

902 **Molecular Neurodegeneration**
Springer Nature
One New York Plaza 800-777-4643
New York, NY 10004-1562 info@biomedcentral.com
www.biomedcentral.com

A peer-reviewed, open-access journal devoted to all aspects of neurodegeneration research at the molecular and cellular levels.
*Guojun Bu, Editor-in-Chief*
*Huaxi Xu, Editor-in-Chief*

903 **Neurocase: The Neural Basis of Cognition**
Taylor & Francis Group
530 Walnut Street www.tandfonline.com/toc/nncs20/current
Philadelphia, PA 19106
Rapid response journal featuring case and group studies in neuropsychology, neuropsychiatry and behavioral neurology, with a focus on the neural basis of cognition.
*Bruce L. Miller, Editor*
*Hans J. Markowitsch, Editor*

904 **Neurology**
American Academy of Neurology
201 Chicago Avenue 612-928-6000
Minneapolis, MN 55415 800-879-1960
Fax: 612-454-2748
journal@neurology.org
n.neurology.org
Official journal of the American Academy of Neurology, peer-reviewed, highlighting clinical neurology research.
*Jose G. Merino, MD, MPhil, FAAN, Editor-in-Chief*
*Patricia K. Baskin, MS, Executive Editor*

905 **Neurology Clinical Practice**
American Academy of Neurology
201 Chicago Avenue 612-928-6000
Minneapolis, MN 55415 800-879-1960
Fax: 612-454-2748
journal@neurology.org
cp.neurology.org
Official peer-reviewed journal of the American Academy of Neurology for practicing neurologists.
*John R. Corboy, MD, FAAN, Editor*
*Patricia K. Baskin, MS, Executive Editor*

906 **Neurology: Genetics**
American Academy of Neurology
201 Chicago Avenue 612-928-6000
Minneapolis, MN 55415 800-879-1960
Fax: 612-454-2748
journal@neurology.org
ng.neurology.org
Official journal of the American Academy of Neurology, publishing online open-access peer-reviewed reports in the field of neurogenetics.
*Stefan M. Pulst, MD, FAAN, Editor*
*Patricia K. Baskin, MS, Executive Editor*

907 **Neurology: Neuroimmunology & Neuroinflammation**
American Academy of Neurology
201 Chicago Avenue 612-928-6000
Minneapolis, MN 55415 800-879-1960
Fax: 612-454-2748
journal@neurology.org
nn.neurology.org
Official journal of the American Academy of Neurology, publishing online open-access peer-reviewed reports of original research and in-depth reviews of topics in neuroimmunology & neuroinflammation.
*Josep O. Dalmau, MD, PhD, Editor*
*Patricia K. Baskin, MS, Executive Editor*

908 **Research & Practice**
Alzheimer's Association
225 North Michigan Avenue 312-335-8700
Chicago, IL 60601-1696 800-272-3900
Fax: 866-699-1246
TDD: 312-335-5886
info@alz.org
www.alz.org
Provides practical information for healthcare professionals on the current status of prominent areas of Alzheimer research.
*Quarterly*
*ISBN: 2-909342-84-0*

909 **Society of Nuclear Medicine and Molecular Imaging**
1850 Samuel Morse Drive 703-708-9000
Reston, VA 20190 Fax: 703-708-9015
feedback@snmmi.org
www.snmmi.org
The mission of this nonprofit scientific and professional organization is to promote the science, technology and application of nuclear medicine and molecular imaging. Molecular imaging techniques are used to diagnose and manage the treatment of brain disorders such as Alzheimer's and Parkinson's disease, among other conditions.
*15,000 members*
*Virginia Pappas, CEO*
*Rebecca Maxey, Director, Communications*

910 **Translational Neurodegeneration**
Springer Nature
One New York Plaza 800-777-4643
New York, NY 10004-1562 info@biomedcentral.com
www.biomedcentral.com
A peer-reviewed, open-access journal covering research, therapeutics and education for all areas of neurodegenerative diseases.
*Shengdi Chen, Editor-in-Chief*

911 **Ultrasonic Imaging**
Sage Journals
2455 Teller Road 805-499-9774
Thousand Oaks, CA 91320 journals@sagepub.com
journals.sagepub.com/home/uix
The journal focuses on the rapid publication of original papers on the development and application of ultrasonic techniques, with emphasis on medical diagnosis. Also published are research notes, comments on papers appearing in the journal, book reviews, and occasional review articles.
*Ernest J. Feleppa, Editor-in-Chief*
*Roslyn Raskin, Managing Editor*

912 **eNeuro**
Society for Neuroscience
1121 14th Street NW 202-312-7305
Washginton, DC 20005 eNeuro@sfn.org
www.eneuro.org
Open-access journal of the Society for Neuroscience.
*Christophe Bernard, Editor-in-Chief*
*Kelly Newton, Director, Scientific Publications*

## Web Sites

913 **Alzheimer Research Forum**
1 Main Street contact@alzforum.org
Cambridge, MA 02142 www.alzforum.org
Dedicated to understanding Alzheimer's disease and related disorders.
*Stacie Weninger, President*

914 **Alzheimer Support**
www.alzheimersupport.com
Serves Alzheimer's sufferers and their loved ones by reporting the latest news in research and treatment, making hard-to-find, recommended nutritional supplements available at manufacturer-direct low prices, and, most importantly, donating profits from each purchase to fund Alzheimer's medical research.

915 **Alzheimer's Association**
www.alz.org
The leading, global voluntary health organization in Alzheimer care and support, and the largest private, nonprofit funder of Alzheimer research.

916 **Alzheimer's Association Hotline**
www.alz.org/help-support
A 24-hour telephone information line offering information on Alzheimer's and local chapters across the country to Alzheimer's patients, families and caregivers.

917 **Alzheimer's Disease Center**
UW Alzheimer's Disease Research Center

PO Box 359791
Seattle, WA 98104
206-744-0588
800-744-0588
uwadrc@uw.edu
depts.washington.edu/mbwc/adrc
Researchers work to translate advances into improved care and diagnosis for Alzheimer's patients.

918 **Alzheimer's Disease International**
57A Great Suffolk Street
London, UK SE1 0
info@alz.co.uk
www.alz.co.uk
Aims to help establish and strengthen Alzheimer associations throughout the world, and to raise global awareness about Alzheimer's disease and all other causes of dementia.
*Paola Barbarino, CEO*
*Michael Lefevre, General Manager*

919 **Alzheimer's Foundation of America**
322 Eighth Avenue
New York, NY 10001
646-638-1542
866-232-8484
Fax: 646-638-1546
info@alzfdn.org
www.alzfdn.org
To provide support, services abd education to individuals, families and caregivers affected by Alzheimer's disease and related dementias nationwide.
*Charles J. Fuschillo Jr., President & CEO*

920 **Alzheimer's Speaks**
lori@alzheimersspeaks.com
alzheimersspeaks.wordpress.com
A blog that provides insight, guidance, and support for people living with Alzheimer's, their families and caregivers.
*Lory La Bey, Author*

921 **Alzheimers.gov**
800-438-4380
adear@nia.nih.gov
alzheimers.gov
Alheizers.gov is an official U.S. government website managed by the National Institute on Aging, National Institutes of Health, U.S. Department of Health & Human Services providing the public access to information related to Alzheimer's Disease.

922 **Alzheimers.net**
866-567-4049
content@alzheimers.net
www.alzheimers.net
An online community dedicated to advocacy, education, and supporting those impacted by Alzheimer's disease and other forms of dementia. Offers a variety of resources. Publishes an educational blog.

923 **American Academy of Neurology**
201 Chicago Avenue
Minneapolis, MN 55415
612-928-6000
800-879-1960
Fax: 612-454-2746
memberservices@aan.com
www.aan.com
Professional society of medical doctors specializing in brain and nervous system diseases. Maintains placement service. Sponsors research and educational programs. Compiles statistics. Publishes scientific journal, Continuum: Lifelong Learning in Neurology.
*Mary E. Post, MBA, CAE, CEO*

924 **American Board of Psychiatry and Neurology**
7 Parkway N
Deerfield, IL 60015
847-229-6500
Fax: 847-299-6600
questions@abpn.com
www.abpn.com
Physicians with specialized training in psychiatry, neurology, child neurology, child adolescent psychiatry, clinical neurophysiology, and geriatric psychiatry. Determines eligibility requirements, administers examinations, and certifies physicians.
*Larry R. Faulkner, President & CEO*

925 **Brain Health**
National Institute on Aging
brainhealth.nia.nih.gov
The Brain Health campaign is an online resource dedicated to promoting healthy living. Offers tips and activities to keep your brain engaged, as well as educational resources. The campaign was created by Administration for Community Living, a division of the US Department of Health and Human Services.

926 **BrainFacts.org**
Society for Neuroscience
1121 14th Street NW
Washington, DC 20005
brainfactsinfo@sfn.org
brainfacts.org
Online public information portal founded by the Kavli Foundation, the Gatsby Charitable Foundation and the Society for Neuroscience, with topics on brain function and anatomy, diseases and disorders, and more.
*Richard Wingate, DPhil, Editor-in-Chief*
*Charles Yokoyama, PhD, Associate Editor*

927 **BrainTest**
35 E Gay Street
Columbus, OH 43215
braintest.com
BrainTest is a medical software company that provides scientifically validated cognitive screening instruments on a wide range of tablets and mobile devices. BrainTest works in partnership with the Ohio State University to hold the exclusive digital rights to the Self-Administered Gerocognitive Examination (SAGE Test), an assessment tool to detect early dementia.
*Michael Kader, President & Legal Counsel*
*Frederick Ghahramani, Founder*

928 **BrightFocus Foundation**
25512 Gateway Center Drive
Clarksburg, MD 20871
800-437-2423
Fax: 301-258-9454
info@brightfocus.org
www.brightfocus.org
Funds research programs for heart disease, glaucoma, and Alzheimer's disease. Provides financial assistance through Alzheimer's Family Relief Program. Formerly known as American Health Assistance Foundation.
*Stacy Pagos Haller, President & CEO*

929 **Dementia Care Central**
www.dementiacarecentral.com
An online resource for caregivers. In addition to providing information on dementia as a diseas, the website offers advice on providing care, hiring care, and paying for care. Also provides self-administered online tests for Alzheimer's Disease, mild cognitive impairment and aging-related mental decline.

930 **Healing Well**
www.healingwell.com
A social network and support community for patients, caregivers, and families coping with the daily struggles of diseases, disorders and chronic illness.

931 **Health Finder**
www.healthfinder.gov
A government website where individuals can find information and tools to help you and those you care about stay healthy.

932 **Healthlink USA**
www.healthlinkusa.com
Health information concerning treatment, cures, prevention, diagnosis, risk factors, research, support groups, email lists, personal stories and much more. Updated regularly.

933 **HelpGuide**
1250 6th Street
Santa Monica, CA 90401
www.helpguide.org
An online resource guide to mental health and wellness. HelpGuide has a section dedicated to Alzheimer's and Dementia within its Aging catagory. HelpGuide publishes articles focused on how to recognize the signs and symptoms, coping, and advice on how to move forward following diagnosis.
*Robert Segal, Executive Director*
*Melinda Smith, Editor in Chief*

934 **MEDLINEplus Health Information**
www.nlm.nih.gov/medlineplus
MedlinePlus is the National Institutes of Health's Web site for patients and their families and friends.

935 **MedicineNet**
www.medicinenet.com

An online resource for consumers providing easy-to-read, authoritative medical and health information.

936 **Medscape**

www.medscape.com

Medscape offers specialists, primary care physicians, and other health professionals the Web's most robust and integrated medical information and educational tools.

937 **National Alzheimer's and Dementia Resource Center**

Administration for Community Living

erin.long@acl.hhs.gov
nadrc.acl.gov

Funded by the Administration for Community Living (ACL), the National Alzheimer's and Dementia Resource Center (NADRC) provides expert technical assistance to AoA'ACL and its grantees, as well as making program information and resources available to individuals and organizations outside the AlzheimerBs grantee community.

938 **Neurology Channel**

www.healthcommunities.com

Find clearly explained, medically accurate information regarding conditions, including an overview, symptoms, causes, diagnostic procedures and treatment options. On this site it is possible to ask questions and get information from a neurologist and connect to people who have similar health interests.

939 **Neuronline**

Society for Neuroscience
1121 14th Street NW 202-962-4000
Washginton, DC 20005 neuronline@sfn.org
neuronline.sfn.org

Online portal for professional development and training resources for individuals in the field of neuroscience, hosted by the Society for Neuroscience.
*Amanda Kimball, Director, Digital Learning*

940 **Steps for Caregivers: Caring for Persons with Alzheimer's Disease**

www.alz.org/help-support/caregiving

Provides guidance and support for caregivers of those with Alzheimer's.

941 **WebMD**

www.webmd.com

Provides credible information, supportive communities, and in-depth reference material about health subjects. A source for original and timely health information as well as material from well known content providers.

942 **www.aan.com**

American Academy of Neurology
Provides information for both professionals and the public on neurology subjects, covering Alzheimer's and Parkinson's diseases to stroke and migraine, includes comprehensive fact sheets.

943 **www.agelessdesign.com**

Ageless Design
Information on age related diseases such as Alzheimer's disease.

944 **www.ahaf.org/alzdis/about/adabout.htm**

American Health Assistance Foundation
Alzheimer's resource for patients and caregivers.

945 **www.alz.co.uk**

Alzheimer's Disease International
Umbrella organization of associations that support people with dementia.

946 **www.alzforum.org**

Alzheimer Research Forum
Information in layman's terms, plus many references and resources listed.

947 **www.alzheimersupport.Com**

AlzheimerSupport.com
Information and products for people dealing with Alzheimer's Disease.

948 **www.biostat.wustl.edu**

Washington University - Saint Louis
Page on Alzheimer's information, from basic care to friends and family networking experiences for support.

949 **www.cyberpsych.org**

CyberPsych
Hosts the American Psychoanalyists Foundation, American Association of Suicideology, Society for the Exploration of Psychotherapy Intergration, and Anxiety Disorders Association of America. Also subcategories of the anxiety disorders, as well as general information, including panic disorder, phobias, obsessive compulsive disorder (OCD), social phobia, generalized anxiety disorder, post traumatic stress disorder, and phobias of childhood. Book reviews and links to web pages sharing the topics.

950 **www.mayohealth.org/mayo/common/htm/**

MayoClinic.com
Information for dealing with Alzheimer's Disease.

951 **www.mentalhealth.com**

Internet Mental Health
On-line information and a virtual encyclopedia related to mental disorders, possible causes and treatments. News, articles, on-line diagnostic programs and related links. Designed to improve understanding, diagnosis and treatment of mental illness throughout the world. Awarded the Top Site Award and the NetPsych Cutting Edge Site Award.

952 **www.mindstreet.com/training.html**

Cognitive Therapy: A Multimedia Learning Program
The basics of cognitive therapy are presented.

953 **www.nia.nih.gov/Alzheimers**

Alzheimer's Disease Education and Referral

Fax: 301-495-3334

A division of the National Institute on Aging of the National Institute of Health. Solid information and a list of federally funded centers for evaluation, referral, treatment.

954 **www.planetpsych.com**

Planetpsych.com
Learn about disorders, their treatments and other topics in psychology. Articles are listed under the related topic areas. Ask a therapist a question for free, or view the directory of professionals in your area. If you are a therapist sign up for the directory. Current features, self-help, interactive, and newsletter archives.

955 **www.psych.org/clin_res/pg_dementia.cfm**

American Psychiatric Association
Practice guidelines for the treatment of patients with Alzheimer's.

956 **www.psychcentral.com**

Psych Central
Personalized one-stop index for psychology, support, and mental health issues, resources, and people on the Internet.

957 **www.rcpsych.ac.uk/info/help/memory**

Royal College of Psychiatrists
Memory and Dementia

958 **www.store.samhsa.gov**

Substance Abuse and Mental Health Services Adminis
Resources on mental disorders as well as treatment and recovery.

959 **www.zarcrom.com/users/alzheimers**

Alzheimer's Outreach
Detailed and practical information.

# ARGYROPHILIC GRAIN DISEASE

*Argyrophilic Grain Disease is a newly-discovered form of late-onset dementia — meaning that it is first diagnosed when patients are 70 years and older. It is believed to account, according to some studies, for between 4 and 13 percent of dementia cases, typically afflicting patients who are well into their senior years. AGD is marked by a reduction of short term memory, behavioral disturbances, disorientation, and reading and writing disorders.*

AGD was first described by German anatomist Heiko Braak and his team in 1987. Clinically similar to Alzheimer's Disease, AGD is distinguished by the presence of silver-staining (argyrophilic) grains or coiled bodies located within the cytoplasm of the brain's neurons. To date, no study has been able to definitively demonstrate any clinical symptom associated with the disease. In most cases, dementia and other symptoms are found, although some 30 percent of cases are diagnosed in subjects with no cognitive impairment. Compared with Alzheimer's Disease, cognitive impairment that does occur with AGD is believed to be milder, and AGD patients maintain verbalization and articulation skills two years longer than Alzheimer's patients. Diagnosis of AGD is based exclusively on postmortem findings, made after microscopic examination of the brain tissue.

Very little is known about Argyrophilic Grain Disease. With no clinical knowledge available as to the origins of the grains or the specific causes of the disease, and no way to properly diagnosis the disease before death, AGD remains very much a subject for further study.

## National Agencies & Associations

961 **American Academy of Neurology**
201 Chicago Avenue 612-928-6000
Minneapolis, MN 55415 800-879-1960
Fax: 612-454-2746
memberservices@aan.com
www.aan.com
Professional society of medical doctors specializing in brain and nervous system diseases. Maintains placement service. Sponsors research and educational programs. Compiles statistics. Publishes scientific journal, Continuum: Lifelong Learning in Neurology.
*Mary E. Post, MBA, CAE, CEO*

962 **American Society for Investigative Pathology**
1801 Rockville Pike 240-283-9700
Rockville, MD 20852 Fax: 301-984-4047
www.asip.org
The Society seeks to promote experimental pathology and related disciplines through meetings, publications, and educational activities.
*William B. Coleman, PhD, Executive Officer*
*Gina LaBorde, Manager, Marketing & Communications*

963 **American Society for Neurochemistry**
9037 Ron Den Lane 407-909-9064
Windermere, FL 34786 Fax: 407-876-0750
asnmanager@asneurochem.org
asneurochem.org
The Society aims to advance and promote cellular and molecular neuroscience knowledge, and to facilitate communication and the dissemination of information within the field and with related disciplines.
*Sheilah Jewart, Executive Director*
*Karen Gottlieb, Conference Coordinator*

## Foundations & Research Centers

964 **Neuroscience Research Institute**
UC Santa Barbara
6129 Biology II 805-893-4621
Santa Barbara, CA 93106 www.nri.ucsb.edu
The Institute seeks to allow scientists from different fields to collaborate for the betterment of neurological research. Areas of interest include: Alzheimer's Disease & Related Dementias; Behavioral Neuroscience & Neuroethology; Cell Biology, Biochemistry & Biophysics of the Nervous System; Computational & Theoretical Neuroscience; Development of the Nervous System; and Stem Cells.
*Stuart Feinstein, Co-Director*
*Kenneth Kosik, Co-Director*

965 **Sanford Consortium for Regenerative Medicine**
2880 Torrey Pines Scenic Drive 858-246-1071
La Jolla, CA 92037 www.sanfordconsortium.com
The Consortium works to achieve breakthrough discoveries in stem cell research with regards to diagnoses, treatments, and cures for degenerative diseases and injuries.
*Edward W. Holmes, MD, President & CEO*
*Jeffrey Steindorf, PhD, VP & COO*

## Magazines

966 **ASN NEURO**
Sage Journals
2455 Teller Road 805-499-9774
Thousand Oaks, CA 91320 journals@sagepub.com
journals.sagepub.com/home/asn
Peer-reviewed open access journal focusing on recent advances in the cellular and molecular neurosciences. It is the official publication of the American Society for Neurochemistry.
*Douglas L. Feinstein, Editor-in-Chief*
*Sandra J. Hewitt, Deputy Editor-in-Chief*

967 **American Journal of Geriatric Psychiatry**
Elsevier
1600 John F Kennedy Boulevard www.journals.elsevier.com
Philadelphia, PA 19103
Peer-reviewed articles on the rapidly developing field of geriatric psychiatry, including areas such as the diagnosis and classification of psychiatric disorders, epidemiological and biological correlates of mental health of older adults, and psychopharmacology and other somatic treatments.
*Monthly*
*Charles F. Reynolds III, MD, Editor-in-Chief*

968 **American Journal of Pathology**
Elsevier
1600 John F Kennedy Boulevard 301-634-7959
Philadelphia, PA 19103 Fax: 301-634-7961
ajp@asip.org
ajp.amjpathol.org
Official journal of the American Society for Investigative Pathology, publishing original research reports, reviews, and commentaries related to the molecular and cellular basis of disease.
*Martha Furie, Editor-in-Chief*

969 **BMC Neuroscience**
Springer Nature
One New York Plaza 800-777-4643
New York, NY 10004-1562 info@biomedcentral.com
bmcneurosci.biomedcentral.com
A peer-reviewed, open-access journal devoted to all aspects of the nervous system (including molecular, cellular, developmental and animal model studies), as well as cognitive and behavioral research, and computational modeling.
*Darren Byrne, Editor*
*Ana Donnelly, Manuscript Editor*

970 **Brain & Life**
American Academy of Neurology
201 Chicago Avenue 612-928-6000
Minneapolis, MN 55415 800-879-1960
Fax: 612-454-2748
BrainandLife@wolterskluwer.com
www.brainandlife.org
Official magazine of the American Academy of Neurology, aimed at parents and home-caregivers interested in neurology in everyday life.
*Orly Avitzur, MD, MBA, FAAN, Editor-in-Chief*
*Mary Bolster, Managing Editor*

971 **Brain: A Journal of Neurology**
Oxford University Press
2001 Evans Road 919-677-0977
Cary, NC 27513 800-852-7323
Fax: 919-677-1714
brain@ucl.ac.uk
academic.oup.com/brain
Focus is clinical neurology and translational neuroscience.
*Dimitri M. Kullmann, Editor*
*Joanne Bell, Managing Editor*

972 **Continuum: Lifelong Learning in Neurology**
American Academy of Neurology
201 Chicago Avenue 612-928-6000
Minneapolis, MN 55415 800-879-1960
continuumcme@aan.com
journals.lww.com/continuum
Official journal of the American Academy of Neurology, aiding professionals in patient care and continuing education.
*Bimonthly*
*Steven L. Lewis, MD, FAAN*
*Andrea J. Weiss, MA, Executive Editor*

973 **Dementia and Geriatric Cognitive Disorders**
S. Karger Publishers, Inc.
26 W Avon Road 860-675-7834
Unionville, CT 06085 800-828-5479
Fax: 860-675-7302
www.karger.com/DEM
Open-access journal devoted to the study of cognitive dysfunction in preclinical and clinical studies, concentrating on Alzheimer's and Parkinson's disease, Huntington's chorea and other neurodegenerative diseases.
*Victoria Chan-Pilay, Editor-in-Chief*

974 **Journal of Alzheimer's Disease**
IOS Press
6751 Tepper Drive 703-830-6300
Clifton, VA 20124 Fax: 703-830-2300
editorial@j-alz.com
www.j-alz.com
Research into the etiology, pathogenesis, epidemiology, genetics, behavior, treatment and psychology of Alzheimer's disease.
*George Perry, PhD, Editor-in-Chief*
*Beth Kumar, Managing Editor*

975 **Journal of Molecular Diagnostics**
Elsevier
1600 John F Kennedy Boulevard 301-634-7959
Philadelphia, PA 19103 Fax: 301-634-7961
jmd@asip.org
jmd.amjpathol.org
Official journal of the American Society for Investigative Pathology and the Association for Molecular Pathology, focusing on molecular discoveries in medicine translating into the clinical diagnostic setting, as well as the description and application of technological advances in the field of molecular diagnostic medicine.
*Monthly*
*Barbara Zehnbauer, PhD, Editor-in-Chief*

976 **Journal of Neuroinflammation**
Springer Nature
One New York Plaza 800-777-4643
New York, NY 10004-1562 info@biomedcentral.com
jneuroinflammation.biomedcentral.com
A peer-reviewed, open-access journal focusing on the interactions of the immune system with the nervous system as a means of expanding understanding of chronic neurological diseases.
*Monica J. Carson, Editor-in-Chief*
*Sue T. Griffin, Editor-in-Chief*

977 **Journal of Nuclear Medicine**
Society of Nuclear Medicine and Molecular Imaging
1850 Samuel Morse Drive 703-708-9000
Reston, VA 20190 800-513-6853
Fax: 703-708-9015
subscriptions@snm.org
jnm.snmjournals.org
Peer-reviewed journal with clinical investigations, science reports, articles benefitting continuing education, book reviews, employment opportunities, and updates on practice and research.
*Monthly*
*Johannes Czernin, MD, Editor-in-Chief*
*Susan Alexander, Associate Director, Publications*

978 **Journal of Nuclear Medicine Technology**
Society of Nuclear Medicine and Molecular Imaging
1850 Samuel Morse Drive 703-708-9000
Reston, VA 20190 800-513-6853
Fax: 703-708-9015
subscriptions@snm.org
tech.snmjournals.org
Peer-reviewed journal dedicated to nuclear medicine technology, with information on credentialing, continuing education and licensure requirements, as well as current news and updates on the field.
*Quarterly*
*Kathy S. Thomas, MHA, CNMT, PET, Editor-in-Chief*
*Susan Alexander, Associate Director, Publications*

979 **Journal of the Neurological Sciences**
Elsevier
LSU Health Sciences Center JNS_England@lsuhsc.edu
New Orleans, LA 70112 www.jns-journal.com
Original articles in neurology and neuroscience from around the world.
*Monthly*
*John D. England, Editor-in-Chief*

980 **Molecular Imaging**
Sage Journals
2455 Teller Road 805-499-9774
Thousand Oaks, CA 91320 journals@sagepub.com
journals.sagepub.com/home/mix
Peer-reviewed open access journal focusing on molecular imaging research, including basic science, preclinical studies and human applications. Published in association with the Society of Nuclear Medicine and Molecular Imaging.
*Bimonthly*
*Henry F. VanBrocklin, PhD, Editor-in-Chief*

981 **Molecular Neurodegeneration**
Springer Nature
One New York Plaza 800-777-4643
New York, NY 10004-1562 info@biomedcentral.com
www.biomedcentral.com
A peer-reviewed, open-access journal devoted to all aspects of neurodegeneration research at the molecular and cellular levels.
*Guojun Bu, Editor-in-Chief*
*Huaxi Xu, Editor-in-Chief*

982 **Neurocase: The Neural Basis of Cognition**
Taylor & Francis Group
530 Walnut Street www.tandfonline.com/toc/nncs20/current
Philadelphia, PA 19106
Rapid response journal featuring case and group studies in neuropsychology, neuropsychiatry and behavioral neurology, with a focus on the neural basis of cognition.
*Bruce L. Miller, Editor*
*Hans J. Markowitsch, Editor*

983 **Neurology**
American Academy of Neurology
201 Chicago Avenue 612-928-6000
Minneapolis, MN 55415 800-879-1960
Fax: 612-454-2748
journal@neurology.org
n.neurology.org
Official journal of the American Academy of Neurology, peer-reviewed, highlighting clinical neurology research.
*Jose G. Merino, MD, MPhil, FAAN, Editor-in-Chief*
*Patricia K. Baskin, MS, Executive Editor*

984 **Neurology Clinical Practice**
American Academy of Neurology
201 Chicago Avenue 612-928-6000
Minneapolis, MN 55415 800-879-1960
Fax: 612-454-2748
journal@neurology.org
cp.neurology.org
Official peer-reviewed journal of the American Academy of Neurology for practicing neurologists.
*John R. Corboy, MD, FAAN, Editor*
*Patricia K. Baskin, MS, Executive Editor*

985 **Neurology: Genetics**
American Academy of Neurology
201 Chicago Avenue 612-928-6000
Minneapolis, MN 55415 800-879-1960
Fax: 612-454-2748
journal@neurology.org
ng.neurology.org
Official journal of the American Academy of Neurology, publishing online open-access peer-reviewed reports in the field of neurogenetics.
*Stefan M. Pulst, MD, FAAN, Editor*
*Patricia K. Baskin, MS, Executive Editor*

986 **Neurology: Neuroimmunology & Neuroinflammation**
American Academy of Neurology
201 Chicago Avenue 612-928-6000
Minneapolis, MN 55415 800-879-1960
Fax: 612-454-2748
journal@neurology.org
nn.neurology.org
Official journal of the American Academy of Neurology, publishing online open-access peer-reviewed reports of original research and in-depth reviews of topics in neuroimmunology & neuroinflammation.
*Josep O. Dalmau, MD, PhD, Editor*
*Patricia K. Baskin, MS, Executive Editor*

987 **Society of Nuclear Medicine and Molecular Imaging**
1850 Samuel Morse Drive 703-708-9000
Reston, VA 20190 Fax: 703-708-9015
feedback@snmmi.org
www.snmmi.org

The mission of this nonprofit scientific and professional organization is to promote the science, technology and application of nuclear medicine and molecular imaging. Molecular imaging techniques are used to diagnose and manage the treatment of brain disorders such as Alzheimer's and Parkinson's disease, among other conditions.
*15,000 members*
*Virginia Pappas, CEO*
*Rebecca Maxey, Director, Communications*

988 **Translational Neurodegeneration**
Springer Nature
One New York Plaza 800-777-4643
New York, NY 10004-1562 info@biomedcentral.com
www.biomedcentral.com

A peer-reviewed, open-access journal covering research, therapeutics and education for all areas of neurodegenerative diseases.
*Shengdi Chen, Editor-in-Chief*

989 **Ultrasonic Imaging**
Sage Journals
2455 Teller Road 805-499-9774
Thousand Oaks, CA 91320 journals@sagepub.com
journals.sagepub.com/home/uix

The journal focuses on the rapid publication of original papers on the development and application of ultrasonic techniques, with emphasis on medical diagnosis. Also published are research notes, comments on papers appearing in the journal, book reviews, and occasional review articles.
*Ernest J. Feleppa, Editor-in-Chief*
*Roslyn Raskin, Managing Editor*

# BRAIN TUMORS

*Although not among the leading causes of dementia, brain tumors often lead to cognitive dysfunction which can sometimes match the official definition for dementia. Dementia brought on by brain tumors has some features in common with other forms of dementia while exhibiting some distinctive characteristics of its own. Common features of brain tumor-induced dementia include poor concentration, paraphasia, disorientation, social withdrawal, and intellectual decline. There is typically no marked memory loss, which is a common symptom of dementia. The onset of dementia among brain tumor patients is generally quick and is often associated with other symptoms such as headaches and incontinence.*

Brain tumors are either primary (originate in the brain) or metastatic (travel from other cancer sites). About 80,000 people in the United States are diagnosed with primary brain tumors each year; approximately 70 percent of those are benign (noncancerous). Cancerous brain tumors originating in the brain make up roughly 2 percent of all cancers, but they constitute 20 percent of all childhood cancers. They may occur at any age but are most common in early adult and middle life. Metastatic brain tumors (those that spread from other cancers) occur in 20-40 percent of all cancers.

There are more than 120 different types of brain tumors, each with a distinctive appearance under the microscope and a characteristic pattern of onset, progression, genetic abnormalities, location and response to treatment. Depending on the exact site and rate of growth of the tumor, symptoms may include change in personality, moodiness, impaired vision and hearing, headaches, nausea, vomiting, seizures, lethargy, and a varying degree of weakness. The most common group of primary brain tumors are gliomas, which arise from glial cells, which are the support cells in the central nervous system. Neuronal tumors, or tumors that arise from neurons (those cells that conduct nerve impulses within the nervous system) are far less common than gliomas and tend to occur in younger adults and cause seizures. About 5-10 percent of brain tumors result from genetic factors that are inherited. In most cases, the cause of an individual's brain tumor is not known.

The treatment of brain tumors, as in many other cancers, consists of a combination of surgical removal, chemotherapy and radiation therapy. The types of chemotherapeutic agents available to treat brain tumors is limited, since most anti-cancer agents do not penetrate the blood-brain barrier. This limitation can be circumvented by injecting agents directly into the brain. Steroids reduce swelling, and anti-seizure medications are commonly given. If the disease or its treatment has caused damage to the brain's functioning, the patient may also need physical therapy, speech therapy, or general supportive care. The prognosis depends on the patient's age and on the location, extent and precise type of the tumor.

## National Agencies & Associations

991 **American Academy of Neurology**
201 Chicago Avenue
Minneapolis, MN 55415
612-928-6000
800-879-1960
Fax: 612-454-2746
memberservices@aan.com
www.aan.com
Professional society of medical doctors specializing in brain and nervous system diseases. Maintains placement service. Sponsors research and educational programs. Compiles statistics. Publishes scientific journal, Continuum: Lifelong Learning in Neurology.
*Mary E. Post, MBA, CAE, CEO*

992 **American Brain Tumor Association**
8550 W Bryn Mawr Avenue
Chicago, IL 60631
773-577-8750
800-886-2282
Fax: 773-577-8738
info@abta.org
www.abta.org
Services includes over 40 publications which address brain tumors, their treatment and coping with the disease. Materials address brain tumors in all age groups. Provides free social service consultations and a mentorship program for new brain tumor support groups.
*Ralph DeVitto, President & CEO*
*Nicole Willmarth, PhD, Chief Mission Officer*

993 **American Society for Neurochemistry**
9037 Ron Den Lane
Windermere, FL 34786
407-909-9064
Fax: 407-876-0750
asnmanager@asneurochem.org
asneurochem.org
The Society aims to advance and promote cellular and molecular neuroscience knowledge, and to facilitate communication and the dissemination of information within the field and with related disciplines.
*Sheilah Jewart, Executive Director*
*Karen Gottlieb, Conference Coordinator*

994 **National Brain Tumor Society**
55 Chapel Street
Newton, MA 02458
617-924-9997
Fax: 617-924-9998
development@braintumor.org
www.braintumor.org
Exists to find a cure for brain tumors and strives to improve the quality of life of brain tumor patients and their families. Disseminates educational information and provides access to psycho-social support and raises funds.
*David F. Arons, JD, Chief Executive Officer*
*Kirk Tanner, PhD, Chief Scientific Officer*

995 **National Institute of Neurological Disorders and Stroke**
NIH Neurological Institute
Bethesda, MD 20824
301-496-5751
800-352-9424
www.ninds.nih.gov
Seeks to reduce the burden of neurological disease affecting individuals from all walks of life.
*Walter J. Koroshetz, MD, Director*
*Amy B. Adams, Director, Office of Scientific Liaison*

996 **Society for Neuroscience**
1121 14th Street NW
Washginton, DC 20005
202-962-4000
marty@sfn.org
sfn.org
Large international organization of scientists and physicians devoted to the study of the brain and the nervous system.
*37,000 members*
*Marty Saggese, Executive Director*
*Melissa Garcia, Associate Executive Director*

## Foundations & Research Centers

997 **Brain Research Center**
Children s Hospital National Medical Center
111 Michigan Avenue NW
Washington, DC 20010
202-476-3000
800-884-5433
Fax: 202-884-5226
tbear@cnmc.org
www.dcchildrens.com
*Edwin K Zechman Jr, President*
*Mark L Batshaw, Chief Medical Officer*

998 **Brain Research Foundation**
111 W Washington Street
Chicago, IL 60602
312-759-5150
Fax: 312-759-5151
info@theBRF.org
www.thebrf.org
Supports cutting-edge neuroscience research that will lead to novel treatments and prevention of neurological disease and disorders in children and adults. Deliver this commitment through seed grants, which provide early stage fundinf for innovative research projects, as well as educational programs for researchers and the general public.
*Nathan Hansom, President*
*Terre A Constantine PhD, Executive Director*

999 **Brain Tissue Resource Center McLean Hospital**
McLean Hospital
115 Mill Street
Belmont, MA 02478
617-855-2000
800-272-4622
Fax: 617-855-3199
mcleaninfo@mclean.harvard.edu
A centralized resource for the collection and distribution of human brain specimens for brain research.
*Francine M Benes, Director*
*Edward D Bird, Director Emeritus*

1000 **Brain Tumor Foundation of Canada**
205 Horton Street E
London, Ontario, N6B-1K7
519-642-7755
800-265-5106
www.braintumour.ca
Seeks to find the cause of, and a cure for, brain tumors while also assisting affected individuals.
*Susan Marshall, Chief Executive Officer*
*Suzanne Fratschko Elliott, Manager, Fundraising & Engagement*

1001 **Central Brain Tumor Registry of the US**
244 E Ogden avenue
Hinsdale, IL 60521
630-655-4786
Fax: 630-655-1756
cbtrus@aol.com
www.cbtrus.org
Nonprofit resource for gathering and distributing current statistics on all primary brain tumors for the entire US. Includes data on benign borderline and malignant primary brain tumors.
*Carol Kruchko, President /Administrator*
*Jeri Dolan, Executive Administrator*

1002 **Kavli Foundation**
5715 Mesmer Avenue
Los Angeles, CA
424-353-8800
info@kavlifoundation.org
www.kavlifoundation.org
The Foundation supports scientific research into the human brain, in the following scientific fields: Astrophysics, Nanoscience, Neuroscience and Theoretical Physics. Within Neuroscience, the study of aging and brain diseases and disorders is supported.
*Robert W. Conn, PhD, President & CEO*
*Eric Marshall, VP, Public Engagement & Prizes*

1003 **Kavli Institute for Fundamental Neuroscience**
UCSF, Sandler Neurosciences Center
675 Nelson Rising Lane
San Francisco, CA 94158
415-476-2018
Fax: 415-502-7332
kavliifn@ucsf.edu
kavliifn.ucsf.edu
The Institute is the central organization for neuroscience research at UCSF and partner institutions, establishing cross-disciplinary teams of scientists and engineers devoted to advancing neuroscience in all its forms.
*Loren Frank, Co-Director*
*Roger Nicoll, Co-Director*

1004 **Kavli Neural Systems Institute**
The Rockefeller University

1230 York Avenue 212-327-8081
New York, NY 10065 lcole@rockefeller.edu
www.rockefeller.edu/research

The Institute unites scientists at The Rockefeller University in the goal of a comprehensive look at the human brain.
*Leslie Vosshall, PhD, Director*
*Lindsey Cole, Administrator*

1005 **Kavli Neuroscience Discovery Institute**
Johns Hopkins University, School of Medicine
725 N Wolfe Street 410-955-4089
Baltimore, MD 21205 Fax: 410-614-6249
KavliNDI@jhu.edu
kavlijhu.org

The Institute looks to advance neuroscience by integrating neuroscience, engineering and computational data science.
*Dwight Bergles, PhD, Director*
*Natasha Hussain, PhD, Scientific Director*

1006 **Salk Institute for Biological Studies**
10010 N Torrey Pines Road 858-453-4100
La Jolla, CA 92037 www.salk.edu
Conducts groundbreaking research into cancer, aging, Alzheimer's diabetes and infectious diseases.
*Rusty Gage, PhD, President*
*Martin Hetzer, PhD, VP & Chief Science Officer*

1007 **Scripps Research Institute**
10550 North Torrey Pines Road 858-784-1000
La Jolla, CA www.scripps.edu
The institute seeks to improve human wellbeing through the advancement of bioscience, including research into aging & healthspan, autoimmune diseases, cancer, infectious diseases, neurological disorders, and more.
*Peter Schultz, PhD, President & CEO*
*Eric Topol, MD, EVP, Scripps Research*

1008 **University of California, San Francisco Brain Tumor Research Center**
Department of Neurological Surgery
505 Parnassus Avenue 415-353-7500
San Francisco, CA 94143-0112 Fax: 415-353-2889
garritye@neurosurg.ucsf.edu
Continuously funded by grants from the National Institutes of Health Since 1072, the Brain Tumor Research Center at UCSF is internationally recognized as a major research and treatment center for adults and children with tumors of the brain and spinal cord. This center emphasizes translational research into the biology and behavior of brain tumors - research in which scientists and health care clinicians work in partnership to translate laboratory findings of new or improved forms of therapy.
*Charles B Wilson, Director*
*Michael Gillis, Administrative Director*

## Support Groups & Hotlines

1009 **All Ages Support Group**
Brain Tumor Foundation for Children
6065 Roswell Road NE 404-252-4107
Atlanta, GA 30328-4015 Fax: 404-252-4108
info@braintumorkids.org
www.braintumorkids.org/
Patient Support Group Activities includes bowling, fishing, craft parties, picnics, sporting events, holiday parties, etc. These activities, social events and more are provided for children of all ages and their families.
*Mary Campbell, Executive Director*
*R Hal Meeks Jr, President*

1010 **American Brain Tumor Association**
8550 W Bryn Mawr Avenue 800-886-2282
Chicago, IL 60631 info@abta.org
www.abta.org
CareLine offered for newly diagnosed patients with brain tumors.
*Ralph DeVitto, President & CEO*
*Nicole Willmarth, PhD, Chief Mission Officer*

1011 **Angels in the Sun Brain Tumor Support Group**
Wellness Community
3900 Clark Road 941-921-5539
Sarasota, FL 34233 www.braintumorfoundation.org
*John Kleinbaum, Program Director*

1012 **Arizona Brain Tumor Support Group**
Barrow Neurological Ins of St. Joe's Hospital
350 W Thomas Road 623-205-6446
Phoenix, AZ 85013 www.braintumorfoundation.org
*Lanette Veres, Director*

1013 **Bereavement Group for Children**
The Center for Attitudinal Healing
33 Buchanan Drive 415-331-6161
Sausalito, CA 94965 www.braintumor.org
*Jimmy Pete, Contact*

1014 **Brain Cancer Support Group**
St John's Hospital
Main Hospital 417-820-3157
Springfield, MO 65804 laura.flowers@mercy.net
*Laura Flowers, Contact*

1015 **Brain Cancer Support Group: Port Orchard**
2186 Yukon Harbor Rd SE 360-536-5042
Port Orchard, WA 98366 ideas56@msn.com
*Victoria Tierney MA RC, Contact*

1016 **Brain Cancer Support Group: Seattle**
Northwest Hospital
Professional Building 206-297-2500
Seattle, WA 98133

1017 **Brain Injury/Brain Tumor Support Group**
Frisbie Memorial Hospital
11 Whitehall Rd
Rochester, NH 03867
*Wendy Mitchell LMSW, Contact*

1018 **Brain Tumor Community Group**
Lancaster General Health Campus
Wellness Conference Room 800-860-9949
Lancaster, PA 17601
*Christine Burfete RN, Contact*

1019 **Brain Tumor Education & Support Group**
Legacy Good Samaritan Hospital Cancer Center
1130 NW 22nd Ave 503-413-7921
Portland, OR 97210
*Wendy Talbot MSW LCSW, Contact*
*Selma Annala RT CLC, Contact*

1020 **Brain Tumor Networking Club**
Gilda's Club Metro Detroit
3517 Rochester Road 248-577-0800
Royal Oak, MI 48073 Fax: 248-577-0898
*Kristen Bernat, Contact*

1021 **Brain Tumor Networking Group**
10628 Falls Road 410-832-2719
Lutherville, MD 21022 www.loyolamedicine.org
*Ronald Petrocelli, Chairÿ*
*Michael Cathey, Vice Chair*

1022 **Brain Tumor Patient and Caregiver Support Group**
Dana Farber Cancer Institute
Boston, MA 02115 617-632-3634
*Nancy Tharler LICSW, Contact*

1023 **Brain Tumor Resource and Vital Encouragement**
Childrens Hospital
1056 19th Avenue 303-861-8888
Denver, CO
Pediatric focus. Education and support. Retreats for parents of brain tumor patients.
*Jim Shmerling, DHA, FACHE, President & CEO*

1024 **Brain Tumor Society**
National Brain Tumor Society

22 Battery Street 415-834-9970
San Francisco, CA 94111-5520 800-770-8287
Fax: 415-834-9980
info@braintumor.org
www.braintumor.org
*N Paul TonThat, Executive Director*

**1025 Brain Tumor Support Group**
Miami Children's Hospital Foundation
3000 SW 62nd Avenue 305-662-8386
Miami, FL 33155 maria.penate@mch.com
*Maria Penate RN, Facilitator*
*Raquel Pasaron, Facilitator*

**1026 Brain Tumor Support Group for Patients and Families**
Albany Medical Center
Office of NY Oncology/Hematology 845-338-4820
Albany, NY 12208-3412 eehauser@gmail.com
www.braintumor.org/patients-family-frien
*Emilie Hauser, Contact*

**1027 Brain Tumor Support Group for Patients & Families**
University of Michigan Medical Center
1500 E Medical Center Drive 734-936-9071
Ann Arbor, MI 48109-0316
*Christina Crandall, Contact*
*Kathy Wilson, Contact*

**1028 Brain Tumor Support Group of Maine**
Maine Medical Center
22 Bramhall Street 207-871-4527
Portland, ME 04102
Meets on the second Tuesday of each month from 7:00 to 9:00 p.m.
*Nancy Fortier LCSW, Contact*

**1029 Brain Tumor Support Group: Ann Arbor**
St Joseph Mercy Hospital, Cancer Care Center
5301 E Huron River Drive 734-712-3658
Ann Arbor, MI 48106 www.sjmh.com
*Paula Nedela RN, Contact*

**1030 Brain Tumor Support Group: Charleston**
Hollings Cancer Center
86 Jonathon Lucas Street 843-792-8257
Charleston, SC 29445 lizzic@musc.edu
www.braintumor.org
*Christa Lizzi RN, Contact*

**1031 Brain Tumor Support Group: Cincinnati**
Wellness Community
4918 Cooper Road 513-791-4060
Cincinnati, OH 45242 Fax: 513-791-8239

**1032 Brain Tumor Support Group: Duarte**
City of Hope National Medical Center
55 Chapel Street 617-924-9997
Newton, MA 02458 Fax: 617-924-9998
www.braintumor.org
Help you learn more about brain tumors including symptoms, treatment options, and considerations for caregivers.
*Heather Ducksworth, Contact*

**1033 Brain Tumor Support Group: El Paso**
Rio Grande Cancer Foundation
10460 Vista Del Sol Drive 915-562-7660
El Paso, TX 79925
*Jutta Ramirez, Contact*
*Robert Lefferts, Contact*

**1034 Brain Tumor Support Group: Florence**
Florence Neurosurgery and Spine
1204 E Cheves Street 843-206-1910
Florence, SC 29506 info@florenceneurosurgery.com
www.braintumor.org

**1035 Brain Tumor Support Group: Fresno**
Cancer Center at St. Agnes
7130 N Millbrook Avenue 559-450-5528
Fresno, CA 93720 karen.kennedy@samc.com
www.braintumor.org
*Karen Kennedy, Contact*

**1036 Brain Tumor Support Group: Fullerton**
St. Jude Medical Plaza
2151 N Harbor Blvd 714-446-7182
Fullerton, CA 92835 kathy.pearson@stjoe.org
www.braintumor.org
*Kathy Pearson RN, Contact*

**1037 Brain Tumor Support Group: John Sierzant Lutheran Hospital, Gunderson Clinic**
1836 S Avenue 608-791-9862
LaCrosse, WI
*Esther Lindeman RN*

**1038 Brain Tumor Support Group: Johnstown**
John P Murtha Neuroscience and Pain Institute
1450 Scalp Avenue 814-534-3797
Johnstown, PA 15904 dlehew@conemaugh.org
www.braintumor.org
*N. Paul TonThat, Chief Executive Officer*
*Michele Rhee, Director of Program Initiatives*

**1039 Brain Tumor Support Group: Kansas City**
St Luke's Hospital of Kansas City
4321 Washington Suite 4000 816-932-6015
Kansas City, MO 64111
*Michelle Martin, Contact*

**1040 Brain Tumor Support Group: Lahey**
Lahey Clinic Medical Center
41 Mall Road 617-726-1061
Burlington, MA 01805 www.lahey.org
*Michele Lucas MSW LICSW, Contact*

**1041 Brain Tumor Support Group: Long Island**
230 Main St. Emma Clark Library 516-747-8749
Setauket, NY
*Billie Wilczek*

**1042 Brain Tumor Support Group: Maryland**
NIH Clinical Research Center
9000 Rockville Pike 301-496-6380
Bethesda, MD 20892 garrenn@mail.nih.gov
www.braintumor.org
*Nancy Garren, Contact*

**1043 Brain Tumor Support Group: New Jersey**
90 Bergen Street 973-972-1164
Newark, NJ 07103
*LaDawn McClamb, Contact*

**1044 Brain Tumor Support Group: Newport Beach**
Hoag Hospital
Advanced Technology Pavilion 949-764-6036
Newport Beach, CA 92663 lberberet@hoaghospital.org
www.braintumor.org
*Lori Berberet RN, Contact*

**1045 Brain Tumor Support Group: Orange**
UC Irvine-Chao Family Comprehensive Cancer Center
101 The City Drive 714-456-8609
Orange, CA 92868 bakerd@uci.edu
www.braintumor.org
*N. Paul TonThat, Chief Executive Officer*
*Michele Rhee, Director of Program Initiatives*

**1046 Brain Tumor Support Group: Philadelphia**
University of PA Hospital-Neurological Institute
3400 Spruce Street 215-615-5240
Philadelphia, PA 19104
*Alisha Amendt MSN CRNP, Contact*
*Arbena Merolli MSW, Contact*

**1047 Brain Tumor Support Group: Pittsburgh**
Cancer Caring Center
4117 Liberty Avenue 412-622-1212
Pittsburgh, PA 15224

**1048 Brain Tumor Support Group: Providence**
Brown University Campus

BioMedical Center 401-789-0126
Providence, RI 02912
*Judy Allenson, Contact*
*Betty Bentley, Contact*

1049 **Brain Tumor Support Group: Raleigh Area**
Raleigh Community Hospital
3400 Wake Forest Road 919-846-0923
Raleigh, NC 27609-7373 www.raleighcommunity.com
Lectures, educational materials, and newsletter. Home and hospital visitation.
*Louise Clark, Director*

1050 **Brain Tumor Support Group: Redding**
American Cancer Society
3290 Bechelli Lane 530-222-1058
Redding, CA 96002 www.braintumor.org

1051 **Brain Tumor Support Group: Richmond**
St Mary's Hospital
Education Center 877-284-3905
Richmond, VA 23226 curebt@hotmail.com
www.abta.org
*Ronald Petrocelli, M.D., Chair*
*Michael Cathey, Vice Chair*

1052 **Brain Tumor Support Group: Sacramento**
UC Davis Ambulatory Care Center
4860 Y Street 916-734-5613
Sacramento, CA 95817 kksmith@ucdavis.edu
www.braintumor.org
*Karen Smith RN, Contact*
*Carolyn Guadagnolo LCSW, Contact*

1053 **Brain Tumor Support Group: San Diego**
Kaiser's Pt Loma Medical Facility
3250 Fordham 619-515-9908
San Diego, CA 92117 www.braintumor.org
*Connie Campbell, Contact*

1054 **Brain Tumor Support Group: San Francisco**
UCSF
521 Parnassus Avenue 415-990-4461
San Francisco, CA 94143 mlovely@braintumor.org
www.braintumor.org
*Sharon Lamb RN, Contact*
*Mary Lovely RN, Contact*

1055 **Brain Tumor Support Group: Santa Barbara**
Cancer Center of Santa Barbara
300 W Pueblo Street 805-563-5852
Santa Barbara, CA 93105 www.braintumor.org
*Rosario Campuzano, Contact*

1056 **Brain Tumor Support Group: Southern West Virginia**
First Presbyterian Church
16 Broad Street 304-744-0393
Charleston, WV 25301-2487
*Jeri McDonald*

1057 **Brain Tumor Support Group: Stanford**
Stanford Cancer Center
875 Blake Wilbur Drive 415-990-4461
Stanford, CA 94305 mlovely@braintumor.org
www.braintumor.org
*Joanie Taylor RN, Contact*
*Sharon Lamb RN, Contact*

1058 **Brain Tumor Support Group: Toms River**
Community Medical Center
99 Highway 37 W 732-557-8270
Toms River, NJ 08755
*Sherry Laniado LCSW, Contact*

1059 **Brain Tumor Support Group: West Bloomfield**
Henry Ford Hospital
6777 W Maple 313-916-1796
West Bloomfield, MI 48322
*Sandy Remer RN, Contact*

1060 **Brain Tumor Support Group: Westlake Village**
The Wellness Community
530 Hampshire Road 805-379-4777
Westlake Village, CA 91361 www.braintumor.org
*Rebecca Dekker MFT, Contact*

1061 **Brain Tumor Support Group: Worcester**
UMass Memorial Medical Center-University Campus
55 Lake Avenue N 508-334-7595
Worcester, MA 01655 Fax: 800-697-2593
ellen.sharenow@umassmemorial.org
www.braintumor.org
*Ellen Sharenow PhD, Contact*

1062 **Brain Tumor Support and Networking Group**
Wellness Community of Greater St. Louis
1058 Old Des Peres Road 314-238-2000
Saint Louis, MO 63131 www.wellnesscommunitystl.org/
*Mitchell L Baris, Chair of the Board*
*Mary Jane Pieroni, CPA, Treasurer*

1063 **Brain Tumor/Pituitary Patient Support Group**
John Wayne Cancer Institute
2200 Santa Monica Blvd 949-515-9595
Santa Monica, CA 90404 pituitarybuddy@hotmail.com
www.braintumor.org
*Sharmyn McGraw, Contact*

1064 **Brainiacs**
Perryville Library 410-459-8157
Perryville, MD 21903
*Liz Carrino, Contact*

1065 **Cancer Patient/Caregiver Support Group**
Wellness Community
1820 W Lincoln Street 406-582-1600
Bozeman, MT 59715 twcmontana@qwest.net
*Becky Robideaux, Contact*

1066 **Cancer Support Group**
Sanford Cancer Cetner Oncology Clinic
1020 W 18th Street 605-328-8000
Sioux Falls, SD 57104 www.lls.org/aboutlls/chapters/mn/patient
*Sue Halbritter RN NP, Contact*

1067 **Cancer Support Group: Knoxville**
Wellness Community of East Tennessee
2230 Sutherland Avenue 865-546-4661
Knoxville, TN 37919 Fax: 865-522-0938
www.cancersupportet.org
*Christi Branscom, President*
*Beth Lee, Secretary*

1068 **Cancer Support Group: Nashville**
Gilda's Club Nashville
1707 Division Street 615-329-1124
Nashville, TN 37203

1069 **Cancer Wellness House**
59 S 1100 E 801-236-2294
Salt Lake City, UT 84102
*Karen Elliott*

1070 **Central New Jersey Brain Tumor Support Group**
St. Luke's Roman Catholic Church
300 Clinton Avenue 732-321-7000
North Plainfield, NJ 07063
*Patty Anthony RN, Contact*
*Virginia Shrodo, Contact*

1071 **Central Oregon Brain Tumor Support Group**
900 SW 23rd Place 541-350-7243
Redmond, OR 97756 rgklug@crestviewcable.com
*Rubyanne Klug, Contact*

1072 **Central Texas Brain Tumor Support Group**
Brain and Spine Center at Brackenridge Hospital
274 Madison Avenue 512-636-1578
New York, NY 10016 866-228-4673
info@cbtf.org
www.cbtf.org

Contains practical information to sort out the complexities of medical procedures, interruptions in school and social life, and uncertainty about the future.
*Thomas Lewman, Contact*

1073 **Colorado Brain Tumor Support Group**
Swedish Medical Center 303-806-7420
Englewood, CO 80113 lgibson@thecni.org
www.braintumorfoundation.org
*Lorre Gibson, Contact*

1074 **Connecticut Brain Tumor Support Group**
20 York Street 203-785-7528
New Haven, CT 06510 Fax: 203-688-2395
www.braintumorfoundation.org
*Angela Thomas LCSW, Contact*

1075 **Emory Brain Tumor Support Group**
Emory Clinic
Department of Neurosurgery 404-778-3091
Atlanta, GA 30322
Meets the first Thursday of each month with the purpose of providing an opportunity for information-sharing and suport for brain tumor patients, as well as their family, friends and caregivers.
*Maxine Brown, Contact*

1076 **Florida Brain Tumor Association**
PO Box 770182 954-755-4307
Coral Springs, FL 33077-0182 sshetsky@fbta.info
www.fbta.info
Provides hope, support and education to brain tumor survivors, their families and friends; conquers brain tumors by funding research into their causes and cures; and enriches the quality of life of those touched by brain tumors
*Sheryl Shetsky, President*
*Gary L Kornfeld, VP*

1077 **Florida Brain Tumor Support Group**
Healthpark Medical Ctr, Meeting Rm 239-433-4396
Ft Meyers, FL 33919 www.braintumorfoundation.org
*Dona Ross, Contact*

1078 **Florida Brain Tumor Support Group: Deerfield Beach**
North Broward Medical Center 954-755-4307
Deerfield Beach, FL 33441 www.fbta.info
*Sheryl Shetsky, President*
*Gary L Kornfeld, VP*

1079 **Glendale Adventist Medical Center Brain Tumor Support Group**
Cancer Services
381 Merrill Avenue 818-409-3530
Glendale, CA 91026 www.braintumor.org
*Connie Munoz LCSW, Contact*

1080 **Gray Matters Support: Kansas City**
24050 W 57th Street graymatters2007@yahoo.com
Shawnee, KS 66226
*Debbie Stephenson, Contact*

1081 **Heads Up!**
Northridge Hospital Medical Center
18300 Roscoe Blvd 818-885-8500
Northridge, CA 91325 www.braintumor.org
*Wanda Martin, Contact*
*Robert Salazar, Additional Contact*

1082 **Headstrong Brain Tumor Support Group**
Victory in the Valley
3755 E Douglas 316-682-7400
Wichita, KS 67218 info@victoryinthevalley.com
www.victoryinthevalley.org
*Cary Cozby, Golf Pro & CEO*
*Tim Farrell, President, RST Ventures, Inc*

1083 **Hearts and Minds**
Piedmont Hospital
1968 Peachtree Road NW 404-373-5202
Atlanta, GA Fax: 404-605-5000
www.piedmonthospital.org
*H.M McFarling, M.D, Chairman*
*Leslie A. Donahue, President & CEO*

1084 **Hollywood Area Brain Tumor Support Group**
Memorial Regional Hospital 954-265-4725
Hollywood, FL 33021 csurloff@mhs.net
www.floridabraintumor.com
*Sheryl Shetsky, Founder & President*
*Gary L. Kornfeld, Vice President*

1085 **Houston Area Brain Tumor Network**
MD Anderson Cancer Center Brain & Spine Center
1515 Holcombe Blvd 713-794-1777
Houston, TX 77030 spanju@mdanderson.org
*Mark Anderson, Contact*
*Suki Panju, Contact*

1086 **Iowa Brain Tumor Support Group**
University of Iowa Hospitals
Iowa City, IA 52242 319-356-2557
*Lori Roetlin, Contact*
*Sue May, Additional Contact*

1087 **Johns Hopkins Brain Tumor Education Group**
Weinberg Building 410-502-2789
Baltimore, MD 21231
*Liz Carrino, Contact*

1088 **LODAT: Brain Tumor Support Group**
Children's Hospital of Wisconsin
Room 888 414-962-8984
Milwaukee, WI www.braintumor.org
Living One Day At a Time is a parent support group for families of chidren with cancer. Monthly newsletter, informational meetings, social activities for families, and bereavement support.
*Frances Swigart*

1089 **Long Island Brain Tumor Support Group**
Old Bethpage Public Library
999 Old Country Road 516-996-3705
Plainview, NY 11803
*Bob Crescenzo, Contact*

1090 **Memphis Regional Brain Tumor Survivors Group**
Methodist University Hospital
1265 Union Ave 904-757-0806
Memphis, TN 38104
*Cherry Welborn, Contact*

1091 **Meningioma/Benign Brain Tumor Support Group**
Michael Quinlan Brain Tumor Foundation
4012 Dupont Circle 502-896-1701
Louisville, KY 40207
*Kathy Quinlan-Thompson, Contact*

1092 **Mount Sinai Medical Center Brain Tumor Support Group**
Ruttenberg Care Center-Guggenheim Pavilion
1190 Fifth Ave 212-717-3527
New York, NY 10029
*Kathleen Maloney-Lutz RN, Contact*

1093 **National Health Information Center**
Office of Disease Prevention & Health Promotion
1101 Wootton Pkwy Fax: 240-453-8281
Rockville, MD 20852 odphpinfo@hhs.gov
www.health.gov/nhic
Supports public health education by maintaining a calendar of National Health Observances; helps connect consumers and health professionals to organizations that can best answer questions and provide up-to-date contact information from reliable sources; updates on a yearly basis toll-free numbers for health information, Federal health clearinghouses and info centers.
*Don Wright, MD, MPH, Director*

1094 **Neuro-Oncology Information and Support Group**
Sister Mary Pia Regional Cancer Center
1800 N California Street 209-467-6550
Stockton, CA 95204-6019 www.stjosephscares.org
For patients and family members living with primary and metastatic brain tumors as well as spinal cord tumors. Free child care and refreshments are provided.
*Jim Linderman*

1095 **Neurological Center of Iowa**
Iowa Clinic
5950 University Avenue 515-875-9100
Des Moines, IA 50266-1418 Fax: 515-241-6090
www.iowaclinic.com/
Networks people in similar situations.
*Mark A. Reece, Chairman of the Board*
*Steven A. Keller, Chair Patient Care Committee*

1096 **Neurological Support Group of St. Luke's Hospital**
101 Page Street 508-997-1515
New Bedford, MA 02740-3464
*Diane Robinson RN*

1097 **Neuroscience Institute Brain Tumor Hotline**
Hospital of the Good Samaritan
637 Lucas Avenue 800-762-1692
Los Angeles, CA 90017-1912 info@goodsam.org
www.goodsam.org
*Diana Selover, LCSW*

1098 **New York Brain Tumor Support Group**
525 E 68th Street 212-746-3986
New York, NY 10021 wem9011@nyp.org
www.braintumor.org
*Wendy Mitchell LMSW, Contact*

1099 **Parent Education/Support Group**
Dana Farber Cancer Institute
44 Binney Street 617-632-3301
Boston, MA 2115 800-525-5068
www.dfci.harvard.edu
For parents of children with brain tumors. Please call for schedule.
*Beverly Lavalley Run, Facilitator*
*Edward Benz Jr, President*

1100 **Patient Services**
22 Battery Street 415-834-9970
San Francisco, CA 94111-5520 800-934-2873
Fax: 415-834-9980
info@braintumor.org
www.braintumor.org
Quickly access brain tumor information and resources.
*12 pages*
*George Gellert, Chief Medical Officer*
*N. Paul TonThat, Executive Director*

1101 **People Living Through Cancer Support Groups**
3411 Candelaria NE 505-242-3263
Albuquerque, NM 87107 888-441-4439
Fax: 505-242-6756
info@pltc.org
www.pltc.org
A not for profit organization that connects and supports cancer survivors and caregivers by transforming shared individual experiences into enduring hope.
*Beth Brown, Executive Director*
*Mary Ellen Kurucz, Program Director*

1102 **Preston Robert Tisch Brain Tumor Center at Duke**
Cornucopia Cancer Support Center
5517 Durham Chapel Hill Blvd 919-668-6178
Durham, NC 27707 stephanie.english@duke.edu
www.cancer.duke.edu
*Stephanie English MSW LCSW, Contact*

1103 **Primary Brain Cancer Support Group**
Women's Cancer Center at Lutheran Hospital
7950 W Jefferson Boulevard 260-435-7959
Fort Wayne, IN 46804
*Linda Jordan RN, Contact*

1104 **Quad Cities Brain Tumor Support Group**
Genesis Medical Center
1401 W Central Park 563-421-1907
Davenport, IA 52804
*Deb Ide, Contact*

1105 **Rhode Island Brain & Spine Tumor Foundation**
Bethany Home
229 Medway Street 401-272-4177
Providence, RI 02906 ribstf@gmail.com
*Colin Shaw, Contact*

1106 **SBTF Brain Tumor Support Group**
PO Box 422471 404-843-3700
Atlanta, GA 30342 info@sbtf.org
www.sbtf.org
To improve the quality of life for brain tumor patients and their families.
*Costas Hadjipanayis, President*
*Jennifer Kee Giliberto, Vice President*

1107 **Sarasota Area Brain Tumor Support Group**
Institute of Advanced Medicine
5880 Rand Avenue www.fbta.info
Sarasota, FL
*Sheryl R Shetsky, President*
*Gary L Kornfeld, VP*

1108 **South Texas Brain Tumor Foundation Support Group**
San Antonio Employees Federal Credit Union
6000 NW Loop 410 210-670-9323
San Antonio, TX 78201
*Susie Soriano, Contact*

1109 **Southern Arizona Brain Tumor Support Group**
Arizona Cancer Cetner
1515 N Campbell Avenue 520-694-4605
Tucson, AZ www.braintumorfoundation.org
*Marsha Drozdoff, Contact*

1110 **Southwest Ohio Brain Tumor Support Group**
Kettering Medical Center
3535 Southern Boulevard 937-298-3399
Kettering, OH 45429-1221
*Ronald Petrocelli, M.D., Chair*
*Michael Cathey, Vice Chair*

1111 **Support Group for Caregivers of Brain Tumor Patients**
UCLA Medical Center
200 UCLA Medical Plaza 310-206-6731
Los Angeles, CA 90095 cabe@mednet.ucla.edu
*Cheryl Abe LCSW, Clinical Social Worker*
*Pamela Hoff LCSW, Clinical Social Worker*

1112 **Valley Brain Tumor Support Group**
Rehab2Health
Shenandoah Memorial Hospital 540-984-4921
Woodstock, VA 22664 vbtsg@shentel.net
*Valorie Hockman, Contact*

1113 **Virginia Mason Brain Tumor Support Group**
1201 Terry Avenue 206-223-7552
Seattle, WA 98111
*Michelle Handler RN, Contact*

1114 **Vital Options International**
4419 Coldwater Canyon Avenue 818-508-5657
Studio City, CA 91604-1479 Fax: 818-788-5260
info@vitaloptions.org
www.vitaloptions.org
A not-for-profit cancer communications, support, and advocacy organization with a mission, to facilitate a global cancer dialogue.
*Selma R Schimmel, CEO/Founder*
*Juliana Lee, Production Manager*

1115 **Washington DC Metropolitan Area Brain Tumor Support Group**
George Washington Ambulatory Center
I & 22nd Street 301-371-8660
Middletown, MD 21769
*Lionel Chaiken, Contact*
*Jeff Schanz, Contact*

1116 **Washington DC Metropolitan Area Support Group**
George Washington University
2150 Pennsylvania Aveneu NW 202-994-4035
Washington, DC 20037-3201
*Margaret Fiore, RN*

1117 **Wellness Community Cancer Support Groups**
San Francisco/East Bay

3276 Mc Nutt Avenue 925-933-0107
Walnut Creek, CA 94597 emaslan@yahoo.com
www.braintumor.org
*Erika Maslan MFCC, Contact*

1118 **Wellness Community: Kentucky**
1717 Dixie Highway 859-331-5568
Fort Wright, KY 41011 www.cancersupportcincinnati.org
*Rick Bryan, Executive Director*
*Gail Lauleÿ, Office Manager*

1119 **Wellness Community: South Bay Cities**
109 W Torrance Blvd www.braintumor.org
Redondo Beach, CA 90277
*Tom May, Contact*

1120 **Wellness Community: West Los Angeles**
2716 Ocean Park Blvd www.braintumor.org
Santa Monica, CA 90405

1121 **Wenatchee Valley Brain Tumor Support Group**
Wellness Place
1610 Fifth Street 509-679-9574
Wenatchee, WA 98801
*Jeff Hastings, Contact*
*Mary Lowe, Contact*

1122 **West Palm Beach Area Brain Tumor Support Group**
Good Samaritan Medical Center 561-655-5511
West Palm Beach, FL 33401
*Sheryl R Shetsky, President*
*Gary L Kornfeld, VP*

1123 **Delware Valley Brain Tumor Support Group at Jefferson**
Jefferson Health System
Bluemle Life Sciences Building 215-955-4429
Philadelphia, PA 19107
*Ann Marie DiBona RN, Contact*
*Janis Haaf RN, Contact*

## Magazines

1124 **ASN NEURO**
Sage Journals
2455 Teller Road 805-499-9774
Thousand Oaks, CA 91320 journals@sagepub.com
journals.sagepub.com/home/asn
Peer-reviewed open access journal focusing on recent advances in the cellular and molecular neurosciences. It is the official publication of the American Society for Neurochemistry.
*Douglas L. Feinstein, Editor-in-Chief*
*Sandra J. Hewitt, Deputy Editor-in-Chief*

1125 **BMC Neuroscience**
Springer Nature
One New York Plaza 800-777-4643
New York, NY 10004-1562 info@biomedcentral.com
bmcneurosci.biomedcentral.com
A peer-reviewed, open-access journal devoted to all aspects of the nervous system (including molecular, cellular, developmental and animal model studies), as well as cognitive and behavioral research, and computational modeling.
*Darren Byrne, Editor*
*Ana Donnelly, Manuscript Editor*

1126 **Brain & Life**
American Academy of Neurology
201 Chicago Avenue 612-928-6000
Minneapolis, MN 55415 800-879-1960
Fax: 612-454-2748
BrainandLife@wolterskluwer.com
www.brainandlife.org
Official magazine of the American Academy of Neurology, aimed at parents and home-caregivers interested in neurology in everyday life.
*Orly Avitzur, MD, MBA, FAAN, Editor-in-Chief*
*Mary Bolster, Managing Editor*

1127 **Brain: A Journal of Neurology**
Oxford University Press
2001 Evans Road 919-677-0977
Cary, NC 27513 800-852-7323
Fax: 919-677-1714
brain@ucl.ac.uk
academic.oup.com/brain
Focus is clinical neurology and translational neuroscience.
*Dimitri M. Kullmann, Editor*
*Joanne Bell, Managing Editor*

1128 **Continuum: Lifelong Learning in Neurology**
American Academy of Neurology
201 Chicago Avenue 612-928-6000
Minneapolis, MN 55415 800-879-1960
continuumcme@aan.com
journals.lww.com/continuum
Official journal of the American Academy of Neurology, aiding professionals in patient care and continuing education.
*Bimonthly*
*Steven L. Lewis, MD, FAAN*
*Andrea J. Weiss, MA, Executive Editor*

1129 **JNeurosci**
Society for Neuroscience
1121 14th Street NW 202-962-4000
Washginton, DC 20005 jn@sfn.org
www.jneurosci.org
Official peer-reviewed journal of the Society for Neuroscience, publishing research on a broad range of topics of interest to those working on the nervous system.
*Marina R. Picciotto, Editor-in-Chief*
*Teresa Esch, Features Editor*

1130 **Journal of NeuroEngineering and Rehabilitation**
Springer Nature
One New York Plaza 800-777-4643
New York, NY 10004-1562 info@biomedcentral.com
jneuroengrehab.biomedcentral.com
An open-access journal devoted to integrated research from the fields of neuroscience, biomedical engineering, and physical medicine and rehabilitation.
*David J. Reinkensmeyer, Editor-in-Chief*

1131 **Journal of Neurodevelopmental Disorders**
Springer Nature
One New York Plaza 800-777-4643
New York, NY 10004-1562 info@biomedcentral.com
jneurodevdisorders.biomedcentral.com
An open-access journal devoted to integrating research from neurobiology, genetics, cognitive neuroscience, psychiatry and psychology.
*Joseph Piven, Editor-in-Chief*

1132 **Journal of Neuroinflammation**
Springer Nature
One New York Plaza 800-777-4643
New York, NY 10004-1562 info@biomedcentral.com
jneuroinflammation.biomedcentral.com
A peer-reviewed, open-access journal focusing on the interactions of the immune system with the nervous system as a means of expanding understanding of chronic neurological diseases.
*Monica J. Carson, Editor-in-Chief*
*Sue T. Griffin, Editor-in-Chief*

1133 **Journal of Nuclear Medicine**
Society of Nuclear Medicine and Molecular Imaging
1850 Samuel Morse Drive 703-708-9000
Reston, VA 20190 800-513-6853
Fax: 703-708-9015
subscriptions@snm.org
jnm.snmjournals.org
Peer-reviewed journal with clinical investigations, science reports, articles benefitting continuing education, book reviews, employment opportunities, and updates on practice and research.
*Monthly*
*Johannes Czernin, MD, Editor-in-Chief*
*Susan Alexander, Associate Director, Publications*

1134 **Journal of Nuclear Medicine Technology**
Society of Nuclear Medicine and Molecular Imaging

1850 Samuel Morse Drive 703-708-9000
Reston, VA 20190 800-513-6853
Fax: 703-708-9015
subscriptions@snm.org
tech.snmjournals.org

Peer-reviewed journal dedicated to nuclear medicine technology, with information on credentialing, continuing education and licensure requirements, as well as current news and updates on the field.

*Quarterly*
*Kathy S. Thomas, MHA, CNMT, PET, Editor-in-Chief*
*Susan Alexander, Associate Director, Publications*

1135 **Journal of the Neurological Sciences**
Elsevier
LSU Health Sciences Center JNS_England@lsuhsc.edu
New Orleans, LA 70112 www.jns-journal.com

Original articles in neurology and neuroscience from around the world.

*Monthly*
*John D. England, Editor-in-Chief*

1136 **Molecular Imaging**
Sage Journals
2455 Teller Road 805-499-9774
Thousand Oaks, CA 91320 journals@sagepub.com
journals.sagepub.com/home/mix

Peer-reviewed open access journal focusing on molecular imaging research, including basic science, preclinical studies and human applications. Published in association with the Society of Nuclear Medicine and Molecular Imaging.

*Bimonthly*
*Henry F. VanBrocklin, PhD, Editor-in-Chief*

1137 **Molecular Neurodegeneration**
Springer Nature
One New York Plaza 800-777-4643
New York, NY 10004-1562 info@biomedcentral.com
www.biomedcentral.com

A peer-reviewed, open-access journal devoted to all aspects of neurodegeneration research at the molecular and cellular levels.

*Guojun Bu, Editor-in-Chief*
*Huaxi Xu, Editor-in-Chief*

1138 **Neurology**
American Academy of Neurology
201 Chicago Avenue 612-928-6000
Minneapolis, MN 55415 800-879-1960
Fax: 612-454-2748
journal@neurology.org
n.neurology.org

Official journal of the American Academy of Neurology, peer-reviewed, highlighting clinical neurology research.

*Jose G. Merino, MD, MPhil, FAAN, Editor-in-Chief*
*Patricia K. Baskin, MS, Executive Editor*

1139 **Neurology Clinical Practice**
American Academy of Neurology
201 Chicago Avenue 612-928-6000
Minneapolis, MN 55415 800-879-1960
Fax: 612-454-2748
journal@neurology.org
cp.neurology.org

Official peer-reviewed journal of the American Academy of Neurology for practicing neurologists.

*John R. Corboy, MD, FAAN, Editor*
*Patricia K. Baskin, MS, Executive Editor*

1140 **Neurology: Genetics**
American Academy of Neurology
201 Chicago Avenue 612-928-6000
Minneapolis, MN 55415 800-879-1960
Fax: 612-454-2748
journal@neurology.org
ng.neurology.org

Official journal of the American Academy of Neurology, publishing online open-access peer-reviewed reports in the field of neurogenetics.

*Stefan M. Pulst, MD, FAAN, Editor*
*Patricia K. Baskin, MS, Executive Editor*

1141 **Neurology: Neuroimmunology & Neuroinflammation**
American Academy of Neurology
201 Chicago Avenue 612-928-6000
Minneapolis, MN 55415 800-879-1960
Fax: 612-454-2748
journal@neurology.org
nn.neurology.org

Official journal of the American Academy of Neurology, publishing online open-access peer-reviewed reports of original research and in-depth reviews of topics in neuroimmunology & neuroinflammation.

*Josep O. Dalmau, MD, PhD, Editor*
*Patricia K. Baskin, MS, Executive Editor*

1142 **Society of Nuclear Medicine and Molecular Imaging**
1850 Samuel Morse Drive 703-708-9000
Reston, VA 20190 Fax: 703-708-9015
feedback@snmmi.org
www.snmmi.org

The mission of this nonprofit scientific and professional organization is to promote the science, technology and application of nuclear medicine and molecular imaging. Molecular imaging techniques are used to diagnose and manage the treatment of brain disorders such as Alzheimer's and Parkinson's disease, among other conditions.

*15,000 members*
*Virginia Pappas, CEO*
*Rebecca Maxey, Director, Communications*

1143 **Translational Neurodegeneration**
Springer Nature
One New York Plaza 800-777-4643
New York, NY 10004-1562 info@biomedcentral.com
www.biomedcentral.com

A peer-reviewed, open-access journal covering research, therapeutics and education for all areas of neurodegenerative diseases.

*Shengdi Chen, Editor-in-Chief*

1144 **Ultrasonic Imaging**
Sage Journals
2455 Teller Road 805-499-9774
Thousand Oaks, CA 91320 journals@sagepub.com
journals.sagepub.com/home/uix

The journal focuses on the rapid publication of original papers on the development and application of ultrasonic techniques, with emphasis on medical diagnosis. Also published are research notes, comments on papers appearing in the journal, book reviews, and occasional review articles.

*Ernest J. Feleppa, Editor-in-Chief*
*Roslyn Raskin, Managing Editor*

1145 **eNeuro**
Society for Neuroscience
1121 14th Street NW 202-312-7305
Washginton, DC 20005 eNeuro@sfn.org
www.eneuro.org

Open-access journal of the Society for Neuroscience.

*Christophe Bernard, Editor-in-Chief*
*Kelly Newton, Director, Scientific Publications*

## Web Sites

1146 **American Brain Tumor Association**
www.abta.org

Provide free social service consultations; a mentorship program for new brain tumor support group leaders; a nationwide database of established support groups; the Connections pen-pal program; networking with organizations that provide services to patients and families; a resource listing of physicians offering investgative treatments.

1147 **Brain Tumor Society**
braintumor.org

Disseminates educational information and provides access to psycho-social support and raises funds to advance carefully selected scientific research projects, improve clinical care and find a cure.

1148 **BrainFacts.org**
Society for Neuroscience

1121 14th Street NW brainfactsinfo@sfn.org
Washington, DC 20005 brainfacts.org
Online public information portal founded by the Kavli Foundation, the Gatsby Charitable Foundation and the Society for Neuroscience, with topics on brain function and anatomy, diseases and disorders, and more.
*Richard Wingate, DPhil, Editor-in-Chief*
*Charles Yokoyama, PhD, Associate Editor*

1149 **Healing Well**
www.healingwell.com
An online health resource guide to medical news, chat, information and articles, newsgroups and message boards, books, disease-related web sites, medical directories, and more for patients, friends, and family coping with disabling diseases, disorders, or chronic illnesses.

1150 **Health Finder**
www.healthfinder.gov
Searchable, carefully developed web site offering information on over 1000 topics. Developed by the US Department of Health and Human Services, the site can be used in both English and Spanish.

1151 **Healthlink USA**
www.healthlinkusa.com
Health information concerning treatment, cures, prevention, diagnosis, risk factors, research, support groups, email lists, personal stories and much more. Updated regularly.

1152 **MedicineNet**
www.medicinenet.com
An online resource for consumers providing easy-to-read, authoritative medical and health information.

1153 **Medscape**
www.medscape.com
Medscape offers specialists, primary care physicians, and other health professionals the Web's most robust and integrated medical information and educational tools.

1154 **National Brain Tumor Foundation**
braintumor.org
Disseminates educational information and provides access to psycho-social support and raises funds to advance carefully selected scientific research projects, improve clinical care and find a cure.

1155 **Neuronline**
Society for Neuroscience
1121 14th Street NW 202-962-4000
Washginton, DC 20005 neuronline@sfn.org
neuronline.sfn.org
Online portal for professional development and training resources for individuals in the field of neuroscience, hosted by the Society for Neuroscience.
*Amanda Kimball, Director, Digital Learning*

1156 **WebMD**
www.webmd.com
Provides credible information, supportive communities, and in-depth reference material about health subjects. A source for original and timely health information as well as material from well known content providers.

# CHRONIC DRUG OR ALCOHOL MISUSE

*Chronic drug and alcohol abuse has been linked to changes in mental state and cognitive function and is believed, in some cases, to lead to dementia in later life. These cognitive functional changes are usually found in heavy users of both drugs and alcohol. In some cases, the dementia brought on by these substances can be reversed if the patient stops using the drug; in other cases, the damage may be permanent.*

Chronic substance abuse is a broad term that refers to any illegal, dangerous, or destructive use of a substance. This use may be legal (binge drinking by an adult) or illegal (smoking crystal methamphetamine). Abused substances include alcohol, nicotine, marijuana, heroin, prescription painkillers and tranquilizers, stimulants such as amphetamines and cocaine, and hallucinogens such as LSD. The abuse may be a danger to the user, family members, business associates, close friends or even total strangers. Substance dependence refers to a state of strong compulsion to use the substance, in many cases accompanied by physical withdrawal symptoms if the substance is not regularly available. In addition, the chronic use and abuse of alcohol and other drugs has been linked to changes in mental state and cognitive function and is believed, in some cases, to lead to dementia in later life.

The cause of substance abuse is very complex, and involves the relationship between the individual's behavioral choices, genetic background, and past and present social environment. Some substance abusers also have a psychiatric disorder such as depression or schizophrenia, making treatment especially challenging.

The consequences of substance abuse are serious, and include job loss, arrest, family breakup, automobile and other accidents, birth defects (fetal alcohol syndrome), direct toxic effects (cirrhosis of the liver or lung cancer), and infections (HIV or hepatitis B). Substance abuse, unless it occurs in persons who are extremely isolated from other individuals, greatly affects family members and loved ones, who often deny the reality of the abuse, and may help, or enable, the abuser to cover up the problem.

Although mild or moderate alcohol consumption does not usually have a negative impact on cognitive function, heavy, long-term consumption is known to have such an impact and is believed to cause—or at least to put the patient at greater risk for—dementia. Other drugs, such as bendzodiazpenes, when used chronically, have been shown to reduce cognitive function as well, and may also lead to dementia. Although evidence of drug-induced dementia remains far from definitive, the continued abuse of drugs and alcohol is known to have a negative effect on cognition. In some cases, the cognitive damage can be reversed by stopping the drug use, though the longer the drug use, the more unlikely reversal becomes.

There is no quick and universally effective treatment for substance abuse. Options range from inexpensive peer-based organizations such as Alcoholics Anonymous to expensive long-term inpatient programs. Some programs are defined by sex, race, age, or religious affiliation. Treatment is much more likely to succeed if it is freely chosen by the individual rather than mandated by a court. Dropout during treatment and relapse after initial success are common, but many people do achieve life-long cures with abstinence from further substance abuse. Family members should look for education and support through groups like Al-Anon, which bring them together with people facing similar situations.

## National Agencies & Associations

1158 **AAA Foundation for Traffic Safety**
607 14th Street NW
Washington, DC 20005
202-638-5944
Fax: 202-638-5943
info@aaafoundation.org
www.aaafoundation.org

A non-profit foundation conducting research with the goal of preventing traffic deaths. Raises awareness on road safety measures and driver education.

*C. Y. David Yang, Executive Director*
*Tara Kelley-Baker, Group Leader*

1159 **AMERSA**
135 Lyndon Road
Cranston, RI 02905
401-230-2165
Fax: 877-418-8769
doreen@amersa.org
amersa.org

AMERSA, founded in 1976, is a nonprofit organization of healthcare professionals dedicated to improving education and clinical care in the management of problems related to substance abuse.

*Sharon Levy, MD. MPH, President*
*Doreen MacLane-Baeder, Executive Director*

1160 **Adult Children of Alcoholics World Service Organization, Inc.**
PO Box 811
Lakewood, CA 90714
310-534-1815
adultchildren.org

Adult Children of Alcoholics is a 12 Step, 12 Tradition program for adult women and men who grew up in alcoholic or otherwise dysfunctional homes, and for adults who have experienced abuse or neglect in the past. The program involves ACA members meeting with each other in a mutually respectful, safe environment and sharing their experiences, as well as applying the program's 12 Steps for recovery to their own lives.

1161 **African American Family Services**
310 Groveland Avenue S
Minneapolis, MN 55403
612-813-5034
Fax: 651-925-0044
www.aafs.net

African American Family Services works with individuals, families and communities affected by addiction and mental illness. Provides culturally-specific mental health services.

*Freddie Davis-English, Chairman of the Board*
*Thomas Adams, PhD (ABD), MSW, Chief Executive Officer*

1162 **Al-Anon Family Group Headquarters**
1600 Corporate Landing Parkway
Virginia Beach, VA 23454-5617
757-563-1600
888-425-2666
Fax: 757-563-1656
wso@al-anon.org
al-anon.org

A fellowship of relatives and friends of alcoholics whose lives have been affected by someone else's drinking and a self-help recovery program based on the 12 steps of Alcoholics Anonymous. The single purpose of this organization is to help families and friends of alcoholics, whether the alcoholic is still drinking or not.

1163 **Alabama Division of Mental Illness and Substance Abuse Community Programs**
The Alabama Department of Mental Health
100 N Union Street
Montgomery, AL 36130
334-242-3454
800-367-0955
Fax: 334-242-0725
alabama.dmh@mh.alabama.gov
www.mh.alabama.gov

Promoting the health and well-being of Alabamians with mental illnesses, developmental disabilities and substance use disorders.

*Kim Boswell, Chief of Staff*

1164 **Alcohol Justice**
24 Belvedere Street
San Rafael, CA 94901
415-456-5692
alcoholjustice.org

Promote evidence-based public health policies and organize campaigns with diverse communities and youth against the alcohol industry's harmful practices.

*Karen Kuhn, Administrative Director*
*Bruce Lee Livingston, Executive Director*

1165 **Alcohol Research Group: Public Health Institute**
Alcohol Research Group
6001 Shellmound Street
Emeryville, CA 94608
510-898-5800
info@arg.org
www.arg.org

ARG's mission is to improve public health through deepening our understanding of alcohol and other drug use and investigating innovative approaches to reduce its consequences for individuals, families, and communities.

*Dominique Lampert, Executive Director*
*Thomas K Greenfield, Scientific Director*

1166 **Alcohol-Drug Treatment Referral**
Recovery Now
800-281-4731
charlick@spencerrecovery.com

National Help and Referral Network, a nonprofit organization available 24 hours a day to assist people troubled by drug or alcohol abuse. Here to provide information on addiction treatment and support services and to help save lives and mend broken dreams.

1167 **Alcoholics Anonymous (AA): Worldwide**
475 Riverside Drive at West 120th S
New York, NY 10115
212-870-3400
aa.org

A fellowship of men and women around the world who share experiences, strength, and hope with each other with the goal of solving their drinking problem and helping others to recover from alcoholism.

*Bill Wilson, Co-Founder*
*Dr. Bob Smith, Co-Founder*

1168 **American Academy of Addiction Psychiatry (AAAP)**
400 Massasoit Avenue
East Providence, RI 02914
401-524-3076
Fax: 401-272-0922
aaap.org

An organization of healthcare professionals dedicated to helping those with mental health disorders. Promotes the use of evidence-based research in the assessment and treatment of substance abuse and mental disorders, as well as in public policy and clinical practice. Provides education to healthcare professionals and the public on patient care, recovery, and the safe treatment of those suffering from substance abuse disorders.

*Shelly F. Greenfield, MD, MPH, President*
*Larissa Mooney, MD, Vice President*

1169 **American Chronic Pain Association**
PO Box 850
Rocklin, CA 95677
800-533-3231
ACPA@theacpa.org
www.theacpa.org

The ACPA facilitates peer support and education for individuals with chronic pain in its many forms, in order to increase quality of life. Also raises awareness among the healthcare community, and with policy makers.

*Penney Cowan, Founder & CEO*
*Daniel Galia, Director, Global Support*

1170 **American Council on Addiction & Alcohol Problems**
2376 Lakeside Drive
Birmingham, AL 35244
205-989-8177
ccorley@alcap.com
sapacap.com

The American Council on Addiction and Alcohol Problems is a non-profit organization whereby state organizations, national religious bodies, and other concerned groups unite to solve the issues caused by addiction.

*Rob Chambers, President*
*Joe Godfrey, President-Elect*

1171 **American Council on Addiction and Alcohol Problems**
2376 Lakeside Drive
Birmingham, AL 35244
205-989-8177
sapacap.com

Provides the forum and the mechanism through which concerned people can find common ground on alcohol and other drug problems and address these issues with a united voice. Members of the organization include 36 state temperance organizations, 22 national Christian denominations and other fraternal organizations which support the ACAP's philosophy of abstinence.

*Ed Wolkin, President*
*William E. Day, Executive Director*

1172 **American Council on Alcoholism**
1000 East Indian School Road 800-527-5344
Phoenix, AZ 85014
ACA is a nonprofit organization committed to educating the public about alcoholism and the effects of alcohol abuse, and the necessity of having readily accessible, affordable, and effective alcoholism treatment.
*Lloyd R. Vacovsky, Executive Director*

1173 **American Public Human Services Association**
1133 19th Street Northwest 202-682-0100
Washington, DC 20036 Fax: 202-289-6555
memberservice@aphsa.org
aphsa.org
APHSA is a nonprofit organization dedicated to improving health and human services by supporting state and local agencies, and working with partners and policymakers to drive effective policies.
*Tracy Wareing Evans, President/CEO*
*Nicole York, Human Resources Director*

1174 **American Society of Addiction Medicine**
11400 Rockville Pike 301-656-3920
Rockville, MD 20852 Fax: 301-656-3815
email@asam.org
asam.org
ASAM's mission is to support the practice of Addiction Medicine and to improve the quality of care and treatment for people struggling with addiction.
*Kelly J. Clark, MD, MBA, DFAPA, President*
*Penny S. Mills, MBA, Executive VP and CEO*

1175 **Association of Halfway House Alcoholism Programs of North America (AHHAP)**
2360 Corporate Circle 650-618-9889
Henderson, NV 89074 888-843-8169
TTY: 650-618-1414
contact.omics@omicsonline.org
www.omicsonline.org
Open-access publisher running over 700 scientific journals in the medical, clinical, pharmaceutical, and engineering technology fields. Current literature and research on addictions can be accessed, as well as connections to halfway houses across North America.
*Olivia Howard, President*
*David Logan, Vice President*

1176 **Betty Ford Center**
Eisenhower Medical Center
39000 Bob Hope Drive 866-831-5700
Rancho Mirage, CA 92270 www.hazeldenbettyford.org
Provides effective drug and alcohol dependency treatment services.
*Jim Steinhagen, Vice President Administrator*
*Steve Eickelberg, Medical Director*

1177 **Center for Mental Health Services (CMHS)**
Substance Abuse and Mental Health Services Adminis
5600 Fishers Lane 240-276-1310
Rockville, MD 20857 877-726-4727
TTY: 800-487-4727
samhsa.gov/about-us/who-we-are/offices-c
Promotes the treatment of mental illness and emotional disorders by increasing accessibility to mental health programs; supporting outreach, treatment, rehabilitation, and support programs and networks; and encouraging the use of scientifically-based information when treating mental disorders. CMHS provides information about mental health via a toll-free number and numerous publications. Developed for users of mental health services and their families, the general public, and policy makers.
*Paolo del Vecchio, MSW, Director*
*Anne Mathews-Younes, Acting Deputy Director*

1178 **Center for Substance Abuse Prevention**
1 Choke Cherry Road 240-276-2420
Rockville, MD 20857 www.samhsa.gov
This organization's goal is to connect people and resources with innovative ideas, strategies and programs designed to encourage creative and effective efforts aimed at reducing and eliminating alcohol, tobacco and other drug problems in our society.
*Frances M. Harding, Director*

1179 **Center for Substance Abuse Research**
4321 Hartwick Road 301-405-9770
College Park, MD 20740 Fax: 301-403-8342
cesar@umd.edu
www.cesar.umd.edu
*Eric Wish, Director*

1180 **Center of Alcohol Studies**
Smithers Hall 848-445-2190
Piscataway, NJ 08854 Fax: 732-445-3500
alcoholstudies.rutgers.edu
Studies the causes and effective treatment of alcoholism. Also operates a controlled drug-delivery research center.
*Marsha Bates, Acting Director*

1181 **Centre for Addiction and Mental Health**
1001 Queen Street West 416-535-8501
Toronto, ON M6J 1H4, 800-463-2338
info@camh.ca
camh.ca
The Centre for Addiction and Mental Health is a mental health and addiction teaching hospital and research centre based in Canada. CAMH seeks to support people affected by mental health and addiction issues through research, education, policy development, clinical care, and the promotion of health.
*David Wilson, Board Chair*
*Dr Catherine Zahn, President and CEO*

1182 **Cocaine Anonymous**
C.A. World Services Office
21720 S Wilmington Avenue 310-559-5833
Long Beach, CA 90810 Fax: 310-559-2554
cawso@ca.org
www.ca.org
Fellowship of men and women who share their experience, strength and hope with each other that they may solve their common problem and help others recover from their addiction.

1183 **Cocaine Anonymous World Services**
21720 S Wilmington Avenue 310-559-5833
Long Beach, CA 90810-1641 Fax: 310-559-2554
cawso@ca.org
www.ca.org
Members are recovering from addiction, and offer support and maintain their sobriety by working together.

1184 **Community Anti-Drug Coalition of America**
625 Slaters Lane 800-542-2322
Alexandria, VA 22314 Fax: 703-706-0565
cadca.org
Community Anti-Drug Coalition of America is a national organization representing the interests of over 5,000 anti-drug coalitions across the United States. CADCA participates in public policy advocacy and provides community coalitions with marketing programs, technical assistance and training, and special events with the purpose of making communities safe and drug-free.
*Arthur T. Dean, Chairman and CEO*
*Jerilyn Simpson-Jordon, Vice Chairman*

1185 **Cornerstone Treatment Facilities Network**
159-05 Union Turnpike 800-233-9999
Fresh Meadows, NY 11366 info@cornerstoneny.com
www.cornerstoneny.com
Offers a complete integrated program for alcohol assessment, alcohol and drug rehabilitation, continuing care, community education and comprehensive family recovery.

1186 **Dentists Concerned for Dentists**
651-275-0313
800-632-7643
dcdmn.com
Dentists Concerned for Dentists (DCD) is a group of recovering alcoholic and chemically dependent dentists concerned about other dentists who are having problems with alcohol and/or other mood-altering drugs.

1187 **Do It Now Foundation**
Do It Now Foundation
P.O. Box 27921
Tempe, AZ 85285
480-736-0599
info@doitnow.org
www.doitnow.org

An information clearinghouse for service providers that publishes well-written pamphlets, booklets, and materials on chemical dependency amd recovery.
*James Parker, Executive Director*

1188 **Drug Abuse Resistance Education of America : D.A.R.E.**
PO Box 512090
Los Angeles, CA 90051-0090
310-215-0575
800-223-3273
Fax: 310-215-0180
www.dare.com

Provides information, resources, tips, warning signs and other information for parents and kids to help keep children off drugs.
*Michele M. Leonhart, Chair*
*Robert J. Strang, Vice Chair*

1189 **Drug-Free Workplace Helpline**
Substance Abuse & Mental Health Services Admin.
5600 Fishers Lane
Rockville, MD 20857
800-967-5752
www.samhsa.gov

A helpline for businesses to obtain information on a wide range of drug abuse related problems, issues and services.

1190 **Facing Addiction with NCADD**
217 Broadway
New York, NY 10007
212-269-7797
800-622-2255
Fax: 212-269-7510
national@ncadd.org
www.ncadd.org

Facing Addiction with the National Council on Alcoholism and Drug Dependence (NCADD) have merged to form into a national leading organization dedicated to fighting the addiction epidemic, providing awareness, support, and resources.
*James L. Abernathy, Chairman & CEO*
*Michael Ballue, CADC II, BSBA, Director*

1191 **Families Anonymous**
701 Lee Street
Des Plaines, IL 60016
847-294-5877
800-736-9805
Fax: 847-294-5837
www.familiesanonymous.org

Addresses the needs of families who are concerned about a relative with a drug problem and with related behavioral problems. Offers informational packets, meetings and support networks for these families.

1192 **Families Anonymous, Inc. Recovery Fellowship**
701 Lee Street
Des Plaines, IL 60016
800-736-9805
847-294-5877
Fax: 847-294-5837
info@familiesanonymous.org
www.familiesanonymous.org

Addresses the needs of families who are concerned about a relative with a drug problem and with related behavioral problems. Offers informational packets, meetings and support networks for these families.

1193 **Goodwill's Community Employment Services**
Goodwill Industries-Suncoast, Inc.
10596 Gandy Blvd.
St. Petersburg, FL 33702
727-523-1512
888-279-1988
TDD: 727-579-1068
goodwill-suncoast.org

Program providing job coaching and community job placements for people with disabilities.
*Heather Ceresoli, CPA, Chair*
*Deborah A. Passerini, President*

1194 **Grief Recovery After a Substance Passing (GRASP)**
40569 Calle Balderas
Indio, CA 92203
302-492-7717
administrator@grasphelp.org
grasphelp.org

GRASP provides information resources, offers support, and organizes meetings and events for families or individuals who have experienced the death of a loved one as a result of substance abuse or addiction.
*Denise Cullen, Executive Director*

1195 **Hazelden Betty Ford Foundation**
P.O. Box 11 CO9
Center City, MN 55012-0011
866-286-3140
www.hazeldenbettyford.org

A nonprofit organization dedicated to providing quality rehabilitation, education and professional services for chemical dependency and related addictive behaviors. Services offered include assessment and rehabilitation, family services, community prevention and professional education, counselor and clergy training and educational materials.
*Dawne Calrson, VP, Human Resources*
*James A Blaha, VP, CFO, CAO*

1196 **Indian Health Service**
5600 Fishers Lane
Rockville, MD 20857
301-443-3593
www.ihs.gov

The Indian Health Service an agency within the Department of Health Services, is responsible for providing federal health services to American indians and Alaska natives.
*Michael Weahkee, Acting Director*
*Chris Buchanan, Deputy Director*

1197 **International Lawyers in Alcoholics Anonymous**
5371 Sherbrooke Street
Vancouver, BC V5W 3
604-644-9254
foot3@telus.net
www.ilaa.org

International Lawyers in Alcoholics Anonymous is a group of recovered lawyers and judges carrying the message of recovery within our profession. Our purpose is to act as a bridge between reluctant (in denial) lawyers/judges and Alcoholics Anonymous.
*Barry Kerfoot, Chairman*
*David Crawford, Trustee*

1198 **Lawyers Concerned for Lawyers**
2550 University Avenue W
Saint Paul, MN 55114
651-646-5590
866-525-6466
help@mnlcl.org
www.mnlcl.org

A non-profit organization of recovering lawyers, judges, law students, and concerned others. Educates and arranges interventions and offers lawyer-only AA meetings.
*Howard Bolter, Chair*
*Warren Maas, Treasurer*

1199 **Marijuana Anonymous World Services**
340 S Lemon Avenue
Walnut, CA 91789-2706
800-766-6779
office@marijuana-anonymous.org
www.marijuana-anonymous.org

Non-profit fellowship of individuals with marijuana addiction, seeking sobriety and support.

1200 **Mental Health America**
500 Montgomery Street
Alexandria, VA 22314
703-684-7722
800-969-6642
Fax: 703-684-5968
mentalhealthamerica.net

Mental Health America is a community-based nonprofit organization committed to enabling the mental wellness of all Americans. MHA advocates for greater access to quality health services and seeks to educate individuals on identifying symptoms, as well as intervention and prevention.
*Reginald Williams, Chair of the Board*
*Paul Gionfriddo, President and CEO*

1201 **MindWise Innovations**
270 Bridge Street
Dedham, MA 02026
781-239-0071
Fax: 781-320-9136
info@mindwise.org
www.mindwise.org

Formerly known as Screening For Mental Health, MindWise Innovations provides resources to schools, workplaces, and communities to address mental health issues, substance abuse, and suicide.
*Bryan Kohl, Senior Vice President*
*Marjie McDaniel, Vice President*

1202 **NAADAC, The Association for Addiction Professionals**
44 Canal Center Plaza 703-741-7686
Alexandria, VA 22314 800-548-0497
Fax: 703-741-7698
naadac@naadac.org
naadac.org

The Association for Addiction Professionals is an organization representing the professional interests of over 85,000 healthcare professionals. Members consist of addiction counselors, healthcare professionals, and educators who specialize in addiction, including the areas of education, treatment, prevention, and recovery support. Dedicated to promoting and enabling healthier individuals, families, and communities.
*Gerard J. Schmidt, MA, MAC, LPC, President*
*Diane Sevening, EdD, LAC, President Elect*

1203 **NAATP:National Association of Addiction Treatment**
1120 Lincoln Street 888-574-1008
Denver, CO 80203 info@naatp.org
naatp.org

NAATP ensures the availability and accessibility of high quality addiction treatment across the country through leadership, advocacy, training, and other member support services.
*Marvin Ventrell, JD, Executive Director*
*Katie Strand, CMP, Director of Operations*

1204 **Narcotics Anonymous World Services**
P.O. Box 9999 818-773-9999
Van Nuys, CA 91409 Fax: 818-700-0700
fsmail@na.org
www.na.org

Narcotics Anonymous is a global, community-based organization with a multilingual and multicultural membership. NA was founded in 1953, and members hold nearly 67,000 meetings weekly in 139 countries today.

1205 **National Alliance on Mental Illness**
3803 North Fairfax Drive 703-524-7600
Arlington, VA 22203 800-950-6264
info@nami.org
nami.org

NAMI is an organization dedicated to raising awareness on mental health and providing support and education for Americans affected by mental illness. NAMI advocates for access to services and treatment and fosters an environment of awareness and understanding for those concerned with mental health.
*Steve Pitman, JD, President*
*Lacey Berumen, PhD, MNM, First Vice President*

1206 **National Association for Alcoholism and Drug Abuse Counselors**
1001 N Fairfax Street 703-741-7686
Alexandria, VA 22314 800-548-0497
Fax: 703-741-7698
naadac@naadac.org
www.naadac.org

This organization is comprised of addiction focused professionals who enhance the health and recovery of individuals, families and communities. NAADAC's mission is to lead, unify and empower addiction focused professionals to achieve excellence through education, advocacy, knowledge, standards of practice, ethics, professional development and research.
*Cynthia Moreno Tuohy, Executive Director*
*HeidiAnne Werner, Director of Operations & Finance*

1207 **National Association of Addiction Treatment Providers**
PO Box 6693 888-574-1008
Denver, CO 80206 www.naatp.org
*Marvin Ventrell, Executive Director*
*Katie Strand, Director of Operations*

1208 **National Association of Alcoholism and Drug Abuse Counselors (NAADAC)**
44 Canal Center Plaza 703-741-7686
Alexandria, VA 22314 Fax: 703-741-7698
naadac@naadac.org
www.naadac.org

Largest membership organization serving addiction counselors, educators and other addiction-focused health care professionals who specialize in addiction prevention, treatment and education.
*Cynthia Moreno Tuohy, BSW, SAP, Executive Director*
*Jessica Gleason, JD, Deputy Director*

1209 **National Association of State Alcohol/Drug Abuse Directors**
1919 Pennsylvania Avenue NW 202-293-0090
Washington, DC 20006 Fax: 202-293-1250
dcoffice@nasadad.org
nasadad.org

The National Association of State Alcohol and Drug Abuse Directors is a private, not-for-profit organization focused on the promotion of educational and scientific materials on alcohol, drug abuse, and related fields. NASADAD seeks to support and further the development of effective alcohol and other drug abuse treatment programs in the United States.
*Cassandra Price, President*
*Robert Morrison, Executive Director*

1210 **National Association on Drug Abuse Problems**
355 Lexington Avenue 212-986-1170
New York, NY 10017 info@nadap.org
www.nadap.org

Private non-profit corporation providing skills, evaluation, job training and job placement to recovering drug addicts in the metropolitan New York area.
*John A. Darin, President & CEO*
*Tyler H. Beebe, Treasurer*

1211 **National Clearinghouse for Alcohol and Drug Information**
Substance Abuse & Mental Health Administration
PO Box 2345 301-468-2600
Rockville, MD 20847 800-729-6686
Fax: 301-468-6433
TDD: 800-487-4889

A resource for alcohol and other drug information. It carries a wide variety of publications dealing with alcohol and other drug abuse.

1212 **National Coalition for the Homeless**
2201 P Street Northwest 202-462-4822
Washington, DC 20037 info@nationalhomeless.org
nationalhomeless.org

The National Coalition for the Homeless is an organization serving to protect the needs of those experiencing homelessness, while striving to prevent and end homelessness. NCH promotes effective treatment, services, and programs for those struggling with homelessness as well as substance abuse problems.
*Bob Erlenbusch, President*
*Megan Hastings, Interim Director*

1213 **National Council for Behavioral Health**
1400 K Street Northwest 202-684-7457
Washington, DC 20005 communications@thenationalcouncil.org
thenationalcouncil.org

The National Council for Behavioral Health serves to unify America's behavioral health organizations. The council is dedicated to ensuring that quality mental health and addictions care is readily accessible to all Americans.
*Jeff Richardson, Chair*
*Linda Rosenberg, President and CEO*

1214 **National Council on Alcoholism and Drug Dependence**
217 Broadway 212-269-7797
New York, NY 10007 Fax: 212-269-7510
national@ncadd.org
www.ncadd.org

Provides education, information, help and hope in the fight against addictions. Founded in 1944, NCADD, with its nationwide network of affiliates, advocates prevention, intervention and treatment, is committed to ridding the disease of its stigma and its sufferers of their denial and shame.
*Andrew N. Pucher, President & CEO*

1215 **National Families in Action (NFIA)**
PO Box 133136 404-248-9676
Atlanta, GA 30333-3136 nfia@nationalfamilies.org
www.nationalfamilies.org

Non-profit organization that obtained the nation's first state laws banning the sale of drug paraphernalia. Leads a national effort to

help parents replicate Georgia's laws in other states to prevent the marketing of drugs and drug use to children.
*Sue Rusche, President*
*Carol S. Reeder, Treasurer*

1216 **National Institute on Alcohol Abuse and Alcoholism**
National Institute on Health
9000 Rockville Pike 301-443-3860
Rockville, MD 20892 niaaaweb-r@exchange.nih.gov
niaaa.nih.gov
NIAAA seeks to reduce alcohol-related problems by conducting scientific research in a range of areas, including neuroscience, treatment, prevention, and epidemiology; working with other research institutes, federal programs, and organizations focused on the issues surrounding alcohol abuse; and disseminating information to healthcare providers, researchers, policymakers, and the public.
*Dr. George F. Koob, PhD, Director*
*Patricia Powell, Deputy Director*

1217 **National Institute on Drug Abuse**
6001 Executive Boulevard 301-443-1124
Rockville, MD 20852 www.drugabuse.gov
NIDA's mission is to lead the nation in bringing the power of science to bear drug abuse and addiction. The Institute operate's a toll-free hotline at the above number, with drug information and a nationwide alcohol and drug abuse treatmanet referral line.
*Nora D. Volkow, Director*

1218 **National Mental Health Consumers' Self-Help Clearinghouse**
1211 Chestnut Street 267-507-3810
Philadelphia, PA 19107 800-553-4539
Fax: 215-636-6312
info@mhselfhelp.org
mhselfhelp.org
The Clearinghouse is a peer-run national technical assistance center focused on achieving respect and equality of opportunity for those with mental illnesses. The Clearinghouse helps with the growth of the mental health consumer movement by evaluating mental health services, advocating for mental health reform, and providing consumers with news, information, publications, and consultation services.
*Joseph Rogers, Founder and Executive Director*
*Susan Rogers, Director*

1219 **Office of Women's Services Substance Abuse & Mental Health Services**
5600 Fishers Lane 877-726-4727
Rockville, MD 20857-0001 www.samhsa.gov
Provides leadership and guidance in creating and maintaining an agency-wide focus for addressing the substance abuse and mental health needs of women.

1220 **Office on Smoking and Health: Centers for Disease Control & Prevention**
1600 Clifton Road 800-232-4636
Atlanta, GA 30329-4027 TTY: 888-232-6348
tobaccoinfo@cdc.gov
www.cdc.gov/tobacco
Offers reference services to researchers through the Technical Information Center. Publishes and distributes a number of titles in the field of smoking and health.

1221 **Partnership for a Drug-Free America**
352 Park Avenue S 212-922-1560
New York, NY 10010 855-378-4373
Fax: 212-922-1570
www.drugfree.org
Committed to helping families whose son or daughter is struggling with substance use by empowering families with information, support and guidance to get the help their loved one needs and deserves.
*Fred Muench, PhD, President & CEO*
*Andrea Castiello, Development Manager*

1222 **Phoenix House**
888-671-9392
www.phoenixhouse.org
Phoenix House is committed to serving those persons, families, and communities whose lives are threatened, disrupted, or otherwise burdened by addiction and related behavioral concerns.

1223 **Pride Institute**
14400 Martin Drive 952-353-5929
Eden Prairie, MN 55344 800-547-7433
Fax: 952-934-8764
www.pride-institute.com
An inpatient treatment center run by and for gay men and lesbians with addiction problems. The program lasts one month and has a Twelve-Step orientation.
*Rick Pliszka, Chief Executive Officer*
*J Heinz, Admissions Counselor*

1224 **Remove Intoxicated Drivers (RID-USA)**
PO Box 520 877-823-9235
Schenectady, NY 12301 888-283-5144
ridusa@verizon.net
rid-usa.org
Volunteers working to deter impaired driving, to help its victims obtain justice, restitution and peace of mind while navigating the criminal justice systems, and to curb the alcohol abuse which leads to drunk driving.
*Doris Aiken, Founder & President*
*Bill Aiken, Vice President & Manager*

1225 **SAMHSA Prevention of Substance Abuse and Mental Illness**
Substance Abuse & Mental Health Services Admin.
5600 Fishers Lane 877-726-4727
Rockville, MD 20857 www.samhsa.gov
Promotes, monitors, evaluates and coordinates programs for the prevention and treatment of alcoholism and alcohol abuse.
*Frances M Harding, Director*
*Gregory Goldstein, Deputy Director*

1226 **Section for Psychiatric and Substance Abuse Services**
155 North Wacker Drive 312-422-3000
Chicago, IL 60606 800-424-4301
www.aha.org
A membership section that represents over 1,660 behavioral health providers and professionals who are members of the American Hospital Association (AHA). The Section applies AHA policy, advocacy, and service efforts to advance understandings of behavioral health care and to emphasize its importance.
*Mary Lou Mastro, FACHE, Chair*
*John A. Miller, PhD, Chair-Elect*

1227 **Society for Neuroscience**
1121 14th Street NW 202-962-4000
Washginton, DC 20005 marty@sfn.org
sfn.org
Large international organization of scientists and physicians devoted to the study of the brain and the nervous system.
*37,000 members*
*Marty Saggese, Executive Director*
*Melissa Garcia, Associate Executive Director*

1228 **State University of New York at Buffalo Toxicology Research Center**
3435 Main Street 716-829-2125
Buffalo, NY 14214 Fax: 716-829-2806
www.smbs.buffalo.edu/CENTERS/trc/
Toxicology-related research and services, including the development of tests to evaluate toxins, chemicals and drugs.
*Paul J Kostyniak PhD, Director*
*James R. Olson, PhD, Associate Director*

1229 **Substance Abuse & Mental Health Services Administration**
5600 Fishers Lane 877-726-4727
Rockville, MD 20857 www.samhsa.gov
Mission is to reduce the impact of substance abuse and mental illness on American communities.
*Michael E Etzinger, Executive Officer*
*Frances M Harding, Director*

1230 **Substance Abuse and Mental Health Services Administration (SAMHSA)**
5600 Fishers Lane
Rockville, MD 20857
877-726-4727
Fax: 240-221-4292
TTY: 800-487-4889
findtreatment.samhsa.gov
www.samhsa.gov
Part of the U.S. Department of Health and Human Services, SAMHSA promotes, monitors, evaluates and coordinates programs for the prevention and treatment of alcoholism and alcohol abuse.
*Thomas Clarke, PhD, Director*
*Elinore F. McCance-Katz, MD, PhD, Assistant Secretary*

1231 **Susbstance Use Disorder Program, Policy and Fiscal Division**
Department of Health Care Services
1501 Capitol Avenue, MS 4000
Sacramento, CA 95899
877-685-8333
www.dhcs.ca.gov
Directs prevention and treatment programs that address substance use disorders (SUD). Its core functions include developing and implementing SUD prevention strategies, reviewing and approving county SUD treatment program contracts, and granting applications submitted for state and federal funds for SUD services.
*Jennifer Kent, Director*

1232 **Tennessee Prescription Drug Overdose Program**
Tennessee Department of Health
710 James Robertson Parkway
Nashville, TN 37243
615-741-5735
800-889-9789
Fax: 615-532-5369
tn.health@tn.gov
www.tn.gov/health
This program is designed to combat the prescription drug overdose epidemic through education, research and communication.
*Melissa L McPheeters, PhD, Dir., Informatics & Analytics*

1233 **The Council on Alcohol and Drugs**
270 Peachtree Street NW
Atlanta, GA 30303
404-223-2480
cwade@livedrugfree.org
www.livedrugfree.org
The Council on Alcohol and Drugs is a substance abuse prevention and education agency that develops programs and resource material based on research on drug use and its impact on community.
*Chuck Wade, Executive Director & CEO*
*Scott E Yost, Director of Operations*

1234 **WFS' New Life Program**
Women For Sobriety
P.O. Box 618
Quakertown, PA 18951
215-536-8026
Fax: 215-538-9026
contact@womenforsobriety.org
www.womenforsobriety.org
A self-help program for women that can be used independent from AA or with AA. Groups are in many states in the United States.
*Karen Hamm, President*
*Rebecca Fenner, Director*

1235 **Women for Sobriety**
P.O. Box 618
Quakertown, PA 18951
215-536-8026
Fax: 215-538-9026
contact@womenforsobriety.org
www.womenforsobriety.org
A national organization with local units that address the specific needs of women with alcohol-related problems.
*Karen Hamm, President*
*Rebecca Fenner, Director*

1236 **Workplace Program**
Substance Abuse & Mental Health Services Admin.
5600 Fishers Lane
Rockville, MD 20857
877-726-4727
www.samhsa.gov
This program sets standards for drug testing in workplace settings.
*Ron Flegel, Director*

## State Agencies & Associations

1237 **Alcohol and Drug Abuse Bureau: Department of Human Resources**
4126 Technology Way
Carson City, NV 89706
775-684-5943
Fax: 775-684-5964
MHDS@MHDS.NV.GOV
*Maria Canfield, Chief*

1238 **Alcohol and Drug Abuse Division Department of Human Services**
Department of Human Services
4055 S Lowell Boulevard
Denver, CO 80236-3120
303-866-7480
Fax: 303-866-7481
jaqueline.enriques@state.co.us
*Janet Wood, Director*
*Mary McCann, Acting Manager*

1239 **Alcohol and Drug Abuse Program Department Of Children And Families**
Department Of Children And Families
1317 Winewood Boulevard
Tallahassee, FL 32399-6570
850-487-2920
Fax: 850-414-7474
www.dcf.state.fl.us/mentalhealth/sa
The Substance Abuse and Mental Health (SAMH) Program, within the Florida Department of Children and Families, is the single state authority on substance abuse and mental health as designated by the federal Substance Abuse and Mental Health Services Administration (SAMHSA). The Department's SAMH Program oversees a statewide system of care for the prevention, treatment, and recovery of children and adults with serious mental illnesses and/or substance abuse disorders.
*Cynthea Panzarino, Director*

1240 **Alcohol and Drug Abuse Programs of Vermont Department Of Health**
Department Of Health
108 Cherry Street
Burlington, VT 05402-1531
802-651-1550
Fax: 802-651-1573
www.healthvermont.gov

1241 **Alcohol and Drug Abuse Section**
Division of Mental Health & Mental Retardation
2001 Mail Service Center
Raleigh, NC 27699-3007
919-733-7011
800-662-7030
Fax: 919-508-0951
www.dhhs.state.nc.us
*Leza Wainwright, Director*
*Michael S Lancaster, Director*

1242 **Alcohol and Drug Abuse Services**
915 Harrison Street
Topeka, KS 66612
785-296-3959
800-586-3690
Fax: 785-296-7275
TTY: 785-296-1491
dxmd@srskansas.org
www.srskansas.org
*Don Jordan, Secretary*
*Laura Howard, Deputy Secretary/CFO*

1243 **Alcohol and Drug Services Addictive Diseases Program**
Addictive Diseases Program
Two Peachtree Street NW
Atlanta, GA 30303-3171
404-657-2331
Fax: 404-657-2160
www.mhddad.dhr.georgia.gov
DBHDD contracts with providers in all 6 regions to provide outpatient and residential substance abuse treatment to men and women who are struggling with the disease of addiction
*Frank Berry, Commissioner*

1244 **Alcoholism and Drug Abuse: Office of Community Behavioral Health**
Department of Health Services
150 N 18th Avenue
Phoenix, AZ 85007-3228
602-364-4558
Fax: 602-364-4570
cancerlr@azdhs.gov
www.azdhs.gov
The Arizona Department of Health Services promotes and protects the health of Arizona's children and adults. Its mission is to set the

standard for personal and community health through direct care, science, public policy, and leadership.
*January Contreras, Acting Director*

**1245 Arizona Substance Abuse Task Force**
Arizona Governor's Office of Youth, Faith & Family
1700 W Washington Street 602-542-4043
Phoenix, AZ 85007 azsubstanceabusepartnership@gmail.com
substanceabuse.az.gov
The Arizona Substance Abuse Task Force is a coalition of leading substance abuse experts, providers and community members focused on addressing and reversing the growing epidemic of drug abuse and addiction in Arizona communities by finding the best treatments and reducing barriers to care.
*Debbie Moak, Director*

**1246 Arkansa Substance Abuse Prevention, Education and Early Intervention**
Arkansas Department of Human Services
305 South Palm Street 501-686-9164
Little Rock, AR 72205 Fax: 501-686-9182
TDD: 501-686-9176
jay.hill@dhs.arkansas.gov
humanservices.arkansas.gov
The Division of Behavioral Health Services is responsible for ensuring the provision of public behavioral health services, including mental health and substance abuse prevention, treatment, and recovery services throughout the State of Arkansas. The Division supports, certifies, licenses, and funds behavioral health providers throughout the state. In addition, the Division of Behavioral Health Service operates two behavioral health institutions:
*Jay Hill, Director*
*Kirk Lane, State Drug Director*

**1247 Bureau on Alcohol Abuse and Recovery Ohio Department of Health**
Ohio Department of Health
30 East Broad Street 614-466-3445
Columbus, OH 43215-2550 Fax: 614-752-8645
info@ada.ohio.gov
www.odadas.state.oh.us
The mission of the Ohio Department of Mental Health and Addiction Services (OhioMHAS) is to provide statewide leadership of a high-quality mental health and addiction prevention, treatment and recovery system that is effective and valued by all Ohioans.
*Tracy J. Plouck, Director*
*Orman Hall, Director of the Governor's Cabinet Opiat*

**1248 Bureau on Drug Abuse: Ohio Department of Health**
Ohio Department of Health
30 East Broad Street 614-466-3445
Columbus, OH 43215 Fax: 614-752-8645
info@ada.ohio.gov
The mission of the Ohio Department of Mental Health and Addiction Services (OhioMHAS) is to provide statewide leadership of a high-quality mental health and addiction prevention, treatment and recovery system that is effective and valued by all Ohioans.
*Tracy J. Plouck, Director*
*Orman Hall, Director of the Governor's Cabinet Opiat*

**1249 California Friday Night Live Partnership**
Department of Health Care Services
6200 S Mooney Boulevard 559-733-6496
Visalia, CA 93278 Fax: 559-737-4231
www.fridaynightlive.org
These groups, located in California, are all run by students with a faculty adviser. They arrange local alcohol and drug free events, from dances and movies to visiting hospitalized children. Students not only have fun but they learn to have fun sober.
*Jim Kooler, Administrator*
*Lynne Goodwin, Program Director*

**1250 California Women's Commission on Alcohol and Drug Dependencies**
14622 Victory Boulevard 818-376-0470
Van Nuys, CA 91411
Dedicated to improving the quality and increasing the quantity of services to women with alcohol-related problems.

**1251 Chemical Dependency Program Division Department of Human Services**
Department of Human Services
Saint Paul, MN 55164-3899 651-431-2460
800-627-3529
Fax: 651-582-1865
dhs.info@state.mn.us
mn.gov/dhs/about-dhs/
The Minnesota Department of Human Services, working with many others, helps people meet their basic needs so they can live in dignity and achieve their highest potential.

**1252 Connecticut Alcohol and Drug Abuse Commission**
410 Capitol Avenue 860-418-7000
Hartford, CT 06134 800-446-7348
Fax: 860-418-6780
TTY: 860-418-6707
The mission of the Department of Mental Health and Addiction Services is to improve the quality of life of the people of Connecticut by providing an integrated network of comprehensive, effective and efficient mental health and addiction services that foster self-sufficiency, dignity and respect.
*Patricia Rehmer, Commissioner*

**1253 Connecticut Department of Mental Health and Addiction Services**
State of Connecticut
410 Capitol Avenue 860-418-7000
Hartford, CT 06134 800-446-7348
TTY: 860-418-6707
miriam.delphin-rittmon@ct.gov
www.ct.gov/dmhas
The Connecticut Department of Mental Health and Addiction Services is a health care agency whose mission is to promote the overall health and wellness of persons with behavioral health needs through an integrated network of holistic, comprehensive, effective, and efficient services and supports that foster dignity, respect, and self-sufficiency.
*Miriam E Delphin-Rittmon, PhD, Commissioner*
*Nancy Navarretta, Deputy Commissioner*

**1254 Delaware Division of Alcoholism, Drug Abuse and Mental Health**
Alcohol And Drug Services
1901 North DuPont Highway 302-255-9399
New Castle, DE 19720 Fax: 302-255-4427
DHSSInfor@state.de.us
Our mission is to promote health and recovery by ensuring that Delawareans have access to quality prevention and treatment for mental health, substance use, and gambling conditions.
*Renata J. Henry, Director*

**1255 Dentists Concerned for Dentists**
450 N Syndicate 651-641-0730
Saint Paul, MN 55104 www.medhelp.org/amshc/amshc53.htm
A nonprofit organization for chemically dependent Minnesota dentists and concerned others.

**1256 Department of Alcohol and Drug Programs**
1700 K Street 916-445-0834
Sacramento, CA 95811-4037 800-879-2772
Fax: 916-323-1270
www.colorado.gov/CDHS
*Kathryn P Jett, Director*

**1257 Department of Alcoholism and Substance Abuse**
Department Of Human Services
100 W Randolph Street 312-814-3840
Chicago, IL 60601 800-843-6154
Fax: 312-814-2419
TTY: 800-447-6404
www.dhs.state.il.us
*Theodora Binion-Tayl, Director*

**1258 Department of Health and Welfare Department Of Health And Welfare**
Department Of Health And Welfare

1720 Westgate Drive
Boise, ID 83704-0036
208-334-6747
800-926-2588
Fax: 208-334-6738
rossil@dhw.idaho.gov
www.healthandwelfare.idaho.gov

*Landis Rossi, Regional Director*
*Richard Armstrong, Director*

1259 **Department of Institutions, Alcohol and Drug Abuse Division**
Helena, MT 59620-2905
406-444-3964
Fax: 406-444-9389

1260 **Department of Mental Health and Mental Retardation, Alcohol & Drug Service**
Bureau Of Alcohol And Drug Abuse Services
601 Mainstream Drive
Nashville, TN 37243-4401
615-532-6500
800-560-5767
Fax: 615-532-2419
www.state.tn.us

*Michael A. Rabin, Director and Meida Contact*
*Lorene Lambert, Publications & Web Management*

1261 **Department of Public Health: Division of Substance Abuse and Health**
Lucas State Office Building
321 E 12th Street
Des Moines, IA 50319-0075
515-281-7689
866-227-9878
Fax: 515-281-4535
www.idph.state.ia.us

The Iowa Department of Public Health (IDPH) partners with local public health, policymakers, health care providers, business and many others to fulfill our mission of promoting and protecting the health of Iowans.
*Kathy Stone, Director*

1262 **Department of Public Instruction: Division of Alcoholism and Drug Abuse**
Division Of Behavioral Health
Lincoln, NE 68509-8925
402-471-7818
800-648-4444
Fax: 402-479-5162
www.hhs.state.ne.us

*Scot Adams, Director*
*GibsonBlaine Shaffer, CEO*

1263 **Department of Social Services: Division of Substance Abuse**
Department Of Human Services
195 North 1950 West
Salt Lake City, UT 84116
801-538-3939
Fax: 801-538-9892
jemarrott@utah.gov

The Utah Division of Substance Abuse and Mental Health is the State agency responsible for ensuring that prevention and treatment services for substance abuse and mental health are available statewide. If you, a friend, or family member is struggling with a mental health problem or a problem with alcohol, tobacco, or other drugs there is help available. Hope and recovery are possible.
*Paula Bell, Chairperson*
*Darryl Wagner, Vice Chairman*

1264 **Division of Addiction Services Department of Mental Health**
Department of Mental Health
402 W Washington Street
Indianapolis, IN 46204-3614
317-232-7800
800-662-4357
Fax: 317-233-3472
www.in.gov/fssa

*Gina Eckart, Director*
*Alma Burrus, Operations Manager*

1265 **Division of Alcohol & Drug Abuse: Mississippi**
Department of Mental Health
1101 Robert E Lee Building
Jackson, MS 39201
601-359-1288
877-210-8513
Fax: 601-359-6295
TTY: 601-359-6230
www.dmh.state.ms.us

Supporting a better tomorrow by making a difference in the lives of Mississippians with mental illness, substance abuse problems and intellectual/developmental disabilities one person at a time.
*Rose Roberts, Chair*
*Jim Herzog, Vice Chair*

1266 **Division of Alcohol & Drug Abuse: South Department of Mental Health**
1101 Robert E Lee Building
Jackson, MS 39201
601-359-1288
877-210-8513
Fax: 601-359-6295
TTY: 601-359-6230
www.dmh.state.ms.us

Supporting a better tomorrow by making a difference in the lives of Mississippians with mental illness, substance abuse problems and intellectual/developmental disabilities one person at a time.
*Rose Roberts, Chair*
*Jim Herzog, Vice Chair*

1267 **Division of Alcoholism & Drug Abuse: Department of Human Services**
Department Of Human Services
1237 W Divide Avenue
Bismarck, ND 58501
701-328-8920
800-755-2719
Fax: 701-328-8969
www.nd.gov/dhs/services/mentalhealth/

The Mental Health and Substance Abuse Services Division provides leadership for the planning, development, and oversight of a system of care for children, adults, and families with severe emotional disorders, mental illness, and/or substance abuse issues.

1268 **Division of Mental Illness and Substance Abuse Community Programs**
Department of Mental Health
Montgomery, AL 36130-1410
334-242-3454
800-367-0955
Fax: 334-242-0725
Alabama.DMH@mh.alabama.gov
www.mh.alabama.gov

*Kent Hunt, Associate Commissioner Substance Abuse*
*Susan P Chambers, Associate Commissioner Mental Illness*

1269 **Division of Narcotic and Drug Abuse Control**
120 S Stockton Street
Trenton, NJ 08625-0362
609-292-5760
800-238-2333
Fax: 609-292-3816
www.state.nj.us/humanservices

*Jeffers, Director*

1270 **Division of Substance Abuse**
250 Washington Street
Boston, MA 02108-4619
617-624-5111
800-327-5050
Fax: 617-624-5185
TTY: 888-448-8321
bsas.questions@state.ma.us
www.mass.gov/eohhs/gov/departments/dph/p

*Michael Botticelli, Director*

1271 **Division of Substance Abuse Services**
Substance Abuse Services
1450 Western Avenue
Albany, NY 12203-3526
518-473-3460
877-846-7369
Fax: 518-457-5474
communications@oasas.ny.gov
www.oasas.ny.gov

*Karen M Carpenter-Palumbo, Commissioner*
*Kathleen Caggiano-Si, Executive Deputy Commissioner*

1272 **Division of Substance Abuse: Department of Mental Health**
Department For MH/MR Services
100 Fair Oaks Lane
Frankfort, KY 40621
502-564-2880
Fax: 502-564-7152
TTY: 502-564-5777

1273 **Drug and Alcohol Programs Department Of Health**
Department Of Health
02 Kline Plaza
Harrisburg, PA 17104-0090
717-783-8200
877-724-3258
Fax: 717-787-6285
rkauffman@state.pa.us
www.ddap.pa.gov

*Gary Tennis, Secretary*
*Kim Bowman, Deputy Secretary*

1274 **Florida Substance Abuse and Mental Health Program (SAMH)**
Florida Health

4052 Bald Cypress Way 850-245-4444
Tallahassee, FL 32399 800-662-4357
health@flhealth.gov
www.floridahealth.gov

Provides free and confidential information in English and Spanish for individuals and family members facing substance abuse and mental health issues. 24 hours a day, 7 days a week.
*Mike Carroll, Secretary*
*David Fairbanks, Deputy Secretary*

1275 **Fresh Start Alcohol and Drug Recovery Group**
Cambridge Health Alliance
454 Broadway 617-591-6051
Revere, MA 02151 www.challiance.org

Fresh Start is an AA-affiliated, 12-step anonymous alcohol and drug recovery peer support group. It's free and open to everyone at any stage of their recovery. Meetings every Thursday evening from 6:30 - 7:30 p.m. on the 1st floor at CHA Revere Care Center.

1276 **Georgia Alcohol & Substance Abuse Prevention Project (ASAPP)**
Department of Behavioral Health
Two Peachtree Street, NW 404-657-2252
Atlanta, GA 30303 dbhdd.georgia.gov

Georgia's Alcohol & Substance Abuse Prevention Project uses the Strategic Prevention Framework (SPF) and a public health approach to tackle Georgia's leading substances of abuse and misuse issues.
*Kimberly Ryan, Chair*
*David Glass, Vice Chair*

1277 **Hawaii Alcohol and Drug Abuse Division**
Department of Health
601 Kamokila Boulevard 808-692-7506
Kapolei, HI 96707 health.hawaii.gov/substance-abuse

The Alcohol and Drug Abuse Division (ADAD) is the primary and often sole source of public funds for substance abuse treatment. ADAD's treatment efforts are designed to promote a statewide culturally appropriate, comprehensive system of services to meet the treatment and recovery needs of individuals and families.
*Virginia Pressler, MD, Director*
*Keith Y Yamamoto, Deputy Director*

1278 **Health Planning and Development**
825 N Capitol Street NE 202-727-8473
Washington, DC 20002 Fax: 202-727-8411
doh@dc.gov
doh.dc.gov/service/doh-substance-abuse

1279 **Illinois Church Action on Alcohol Problems**
1132 W Jefferson Street 217-546-6871
Springfields, IL 62702 Fax: 217-546-2814
www.ilcaaap.org

An interdenominational Christian agency representing church groups in Illinois. Works to prevent alcohol and other drug-related problems through education legislative action and public awareness.

1280 **Illinois Department of Alcoholism and Substance Abuse**
Illinois Department of Human Services
401 South Clinton Street 800-843-6154
Chicago, IL 60607 TTY: 866-324-5553
www.dhs.state.il.us

The mission of the Division of Alcoholism and Substance Abuse is to provide a system of care along the continuum of prevention, intervention, treatment and recovery support where individuals with SUD, those in recovery and those at risk are valued and treated with dignity and where stigma, accompanying attitudes, discrimination, and other barriers to recovery are eliminated.
*James T Dimas, Secretary*

1281 **Iowa Bureau of Substance Abuse**
Iowa Department of Public Health
Lucas State Office Building 515-281-7689
Des Moines, IA 50319 855-581-8111
idph.iowa.gov/substance-abuse

The Bureau of Substance Abuse is part of the Division of Behavioral Health, in the Iowa Department of Public Health. The Bureau focuses on and provides oversight for all aspects related to substance abuse prevention and treatment services in Iowa, in addition to injury prevention programs. The bureau actively works to address Prevention and Treatment needs by providing focus for training efforts, identifying and securing available grant funding,
*DeAnn Decker, Bureau Chief*

1282 **Maine Association of Substance Abuse Programs**
295 Water Street 207-621-8118
Augusta, ME 04330 Fax: 207-621-8362
mshaughnessy@masap.org
thealliancemaine.org

Statewide membership association for community behavioral health organizations that provide multi-level services, programming and coordinated leadership to ensure that Mainers have full access to the continuum of recovery-oriented systems of care for mental illness and substance use disorder - from prevention through treatment and into peer recovery support.
*Malory Shaughnessy, Executive Director*
*Steven Cotreau, Manager*

1283 **Maryland State Alcohol and Drug Abuse Administration**
55 Wade Avenue 410-402-8600
Catonsville, MD 21228 Fax: 410-402-8601
adaainfo@dhmh.state.md.us
www.maryland-adaa.org

The Alcohol and Drug Abuse Administration is committed to providing access to a quality and effective substance abuse prevention, intervention and treatment service system for the citizens of Maryland.
*Kathleen Rebbert-Fra, Acting Director*
*Steve Bocian, Acting Deputy Director*

1284 **Minnesota Recovery Connection**
822 S Third Street 612-584-4158
Minneapolis, MN 55415 Fax: 612-886-3940
nfo@minnesotarecovery.org
minnesotarecovery.org

A recovery community organization serving the seven county metro area of Minnesota and supporting recovery communities in both St. Cloud and Duluth. The Minnesota Recovery Connection's mission is to strengthen the recovery community through peer-to-peer support, public education, and advocacy.
*Julia Alexander, Co-Executive Director*
*Kris Kelly, Co-Executive Director*

1285 **Mississippi Division of Alcohol and Drug Abuse**
Department of Mental Health
239 N Lamar Street 601-359-1288
Jackson, MS 39201 877-210-8513
Fax: 601-359-6295
TDD: 601-359-6230
www.dmh.ms.gov

The Bureau of Alcohol and Drug Services has the responsibility of administering fiscal resources (state and federal) to the public system of prevention, treatment, and recovery supports for persons with substance use disorders. The overall goal of the state's substance use disorder service system is to provide quality care within a continuum of accessible community-based services including: prevention, outpatient, withdrawal management, intensi

1286 **Missouri Division of Alcohol and Drug Abuse**
Department of Mental Health
1706 E Elm Street 573-751-4942
Jefferson City, MO 65102 800-575-7480
Fax: 573-751-8224
TTY: 573-526-1201
dmhmail@dmh.mo.gov
dmh.mo.gov/ada/

*Keith Schafer, Director*
*Heidi DiBiaso, Administrative Assistant*

1287 **Montana Division of Addictive & Mental Disorders**
Department of Public Health and Human Services
100 N Park, Suite 300 406-444-3964
Helena, MT 59620 Fax: 406-444-4435
hhsamdemail@mt.gov
dphhs.mt.gov/amdd

To implement and improve an appropriate statewide system of prevention, treatment, care and rehabilitation for Montanans with mental disorders or addictions to drugs or alcohol. Provides sub-

stance abuse and adult mental health services by contracting with behavioral health providers throughout Montana.
*Zoe Barnard, Administrator*
*Bobbi Perkins, Bureau Chief*

1288 **Nebraska Division of Alcoholism and Drug Abuse**
Nebraska Department of Health & Human Services
301 Centennial Mall S 402-471-7818
Lincoln, NE 68509 Fax: 402-471-7859
dhhs.ne.gov
Provides information on substance abuse prevention and treatment in the state of Nebraska.
*Courtney N Phillips, Chief Executive Officer*
*Tom Williams, MD, Chief Medical Officer*

1289 **Nevada State Board of Examiners For Alcohol, Drug and Gambling Counselors**
4600 Kietzke Lane 775-689-0563
Reno, NV 89502 Fax: 775-689-0564
agawronski@adgc.nv.gov
alcohol.nv.gov
Mission is to reduce the impact of substance abuse in Nevada.
*Agata Gawronski, Executive Director*
*Darlene Dufault, President*

1290 **New Jersey Division of Mental Health & Addiction Services**
201 S Shore Road 609-645-5932
Northfield, NJ 08225 widitz_robert@aclink.org
www.nj.gov/health
Provides information and support for prevention and treatment services for alcohol, tobacco and other drugs in New Jersey.
*Robert Widitz, Director*

1291 **New Mexico Behavioral Health Services**
New Mexico Human Services Department
P.O. Box 2348 505-476-9266
Santa Fe, NM 87504 Fax: 505-476-9277
www.hsd.state.nm.us/bhsd
To address need, services, planning, monitoring and continuous quality systemically across the state.
*Wayne Lindstrom, Director*

1292 **New York State Office of Alcoholism and Substance Abuse Services**
1450 Western Avenue 518-473-3460
Albany, NY 12203 www.oasas.ny.gov
To improve the lives of all New Yorkers by leading a comprehensive premier system of addiction services for prevention, treatment, and recovery.
*Arlene Gonzalez-Sanchez, Commissioner*

1293 **North Carolina Division of Mental Health , Developmental Disabilities and Abuse S**
Department of Human Resources
2001 Mail Service Center 919-733-7011
Raleigh, NC 27699 contactdmh@dhhs.nc.gov
www.ncdhhs.gov
Providing quality support to achieve self-determination for individuals with intellectual and or developmental disabilities and quality services to promote treatment and recovery for individuals with mental illness and substance use disorders.

1294 **North Dakota Mental Health & Substance Abuse**
1237 W Divide Avenue 701-328-8920
Bismarck, ND 58501 800-755-2719
Fax: 701-328-8969
dhsbhd@nd.gov
www.nd.gov
Provides information on substance abuse prevention and treatment in the state of North Dakota.

1295 **Office of Alcohol and Drug Abuse Prevention**
305 South Palm Street 501-686-9866
Little Rock, AR 72205 877-726-4727
Fax: 501-686-9035
SAMHSA's mission is to reduce the impact of substance abuse and mental illness on America's communities.

1296 **Office of Alcohol and Drug Abuse Programs**
500 Summer Street NE 503-945-5763
Salem, OR 97301-1118 Fax: 503-378-8467
TTY: 800-375-2863

1297 **Office of Alcohol and Other Drug Abuse**
1 W Wilson Street 608-266-1865
Madison, WI 53703-7851 Fax: 608-266-1533
TTY: 608-267-7371
dhswebmaster@wisconsin.gov
*John Easterday, Administrator*
*Susan Gadacz, Contact*

1298 **Office of Alcohol and Substance Abuse Department of Health and Social Services**
Department of Health and Social Services
350 Main Street 907-465-3030
Juneau, AK 99811 800-465-4828
Fax: 907-465-3068
Stacy.Toner@Alaska.gov
dhss.alaska.gov/Pages/default.aspx
*William J. Streuss, Commissioner*
*Tara Horton, Special Assistant*

1299 **Office of Human Services: Division of Alcohol and Drug Abuse**
628 N 4th Street 225-342-9500
Baton Rouge, LA 70802-2790 855-229-6848
Fax: 225-342-3875
TTY: 225-342-5568
dhhwebinfo@la.gov
www.dhh.louisiana.gov

1300 **Office of Substance Abuse Services Department of Public Health**
Department of Public Health
320 S Walnut Street 517-373-4700
Lansing, MI 48913 888-736-0253
Fax: 517-335-2121
TTY: 517-373-3573
www.michigan.gov/mdch
*Yvonne Blackmond, Director*

1301 **Oklahoma Department of Mental Health and Substance Abuse Services**
Substance Abuse Program
1200 NE 13th Street 405-522-3908
Oklahoma City, OK 73117-3277 800-522-9054
Fax: 405-522-3650
TTY: 405-522-3851
jglover@odmhsas.org
www.odmhsas.org
*J. Andy Sullivan, Chairperson*
*Larry McCauley, Vice Chair*

1302 **Oregon Alcohol and Drug Policy Commission**
Department of Human Services
500 Summer Street NE 503-378-5796
Salem, OR 97301 www.oregon.gov/adpc
The Alcohol and Drug Policy Commission is an independent state government agency that was created by the Oregon Legislature to improve the effectiveness and efficiency of state and local alcohol and drug abuse prevention and treatment services.
*Rem Nivens, Executive Director*

1303 **Parkside Medical Services Corporation**
205 W Touhy Avenue 847-698-9866
Park Ridge, IL 60068-4256 800-727-5723
This establishment offers treatment and hope for the alcoholic/substance abuser. A resource center that provides information books and resources pertaining to substance abuse and offers treatment facilities in various states across the country.

1304 **Pennsylvania Drug and Alcohol Programs**
P.O. Box 60769 717-526-1010
Harrisburg, PA 17106 Fax: 717-526-1020
www.pacdaa.org
The Pennsylvania Association of County Drug and Alcohol Administrators (PACDAA) is a professional association that represents the Single County Authorities (SCAs) across the commonwealth who receive state and federal dollars through contracts with the Department of Drug and Alcohol Programs (DDAP), to plan, coordinate, programmatically and fiscally man-

age and implement the delivery of drug and alcohol prevention, intervention, and treatment servi
*Cheryl Andrews, Chair*
*April Brown, Vice Chair*

1305 **SMART Recovery**
Cambridge Health Alliance
195 Canal Street 508-878-2291
Malden, MA 02148 www.challiance.org
SMART Recovery is a science-based program and addresses all kinds of addictive behaviors using a four point cognitive approach: building and maintaining motivation, coping with urges, managing thoughts, feelings and behaviors and living a balanced life. Meetings are held every Friday afternoon from noon to 1 p.m. at the CHA Malden Care Center.
*Gail Cardelle, Contact*

1306 **South Carolina Commission on Alcohol and Drug Abuse**
Department Of Alcohol And Drug Abuse Services
2414 Bull Street 803-896-5555
Columbia, SC 29201-9498 Fax: 803-896-5557
The department's mission is to ensure the provision of quality services to prevent or reduce the negative consequences of substance use and addictions.
*Bob Toomey, Director*
*Kaitlin Blanco-Silva, Project Manager*

1307 **South Carolina Department of Alcohol & Other Drug Abuse Services**
1801 Main Street 803-896-5555
Columbia, SC 29201 Fax: 803-896-5557
mtaylor@daodas.sc.gov
www.daodas.sc.gov
The mission of DAODAS is to ensure the availability and quality of substance use services, improving the health status, safety, and quality of life of individuals, families, and communities across South Carolina.
*Sara Goldsby, Interim Director*
*Mitchell Taylor, Administrative Coordinator*

1308 **Substance Abuse Bureau**
1190 Saint Francis Drive 505-827-2601
Santa Fe, NM 87502 800-362-2013
Fax: 505-827-0097

1309 **Substance Abuse Services Office of Virginia**
Department of Mental Health & Mental Retardation
1220 Bank Street 804-786-3921
Richmond, VA 23218-1797 800-451-5544
Fax: 804-371-6638
TTY: 804-371-8977
Available to citizens statewide, Virginia's public mental health, intellectual disability and substance abuse services system is comprised of 16 state-operated facilities and 40 locally-run community services boards (CSBs) The CSBs and facilities serve children and adults who have-or who are at risk of-mental illness, serious emotional disturbance, intellectual disabilities, or substance abuse disorders.
*Jim Stewart, Commissioner*
*Olivia Garland, Deputy Commissioner*

1310 **Texas Commission on Alcohol and Drug Abuse Department Of State Health**
Department Of State Health
Austin, TX 78714 512-206-5000
866-378-8440
Fax: 512-458-7477
TTY: 800-735-2989
TDD: 800-735-2989
web.master@dshs.state.tx.us
www.dshs.state.tx.us/mhsa/
Mission is to improve health and well-being in Texas.
*David L. Lakey, Commissioner*

1311 **Texas of Mental Health & Substance Abuse Division**
Texas Department of State Health Services
P.O. Box 149347 512-776-7111
Austin, TX 78714 866-378-8440
customer.service@dshs.texas.gov
dshs.texas.gov
To improve health and well-being in Texas by providing leadership and services that promote hope, build resilience, and foster recovery.
*John William Hellerstedt, Commissioner*

1312 **The Center for Family Support**
2811 Zulette Avenue 718-518-1500
Bronx, NY 10461 Fax: 718-518-8200
www.cfsny.org/
The Center for Family Support offers assistance to individuals with developmental and related disabilities, as well as their families, and provides support services and programs that are designed to accommodate individual needs. Offers services throughout New York City, Westchester County, Long Island, and New Jersey.
*Steven Vernikoff, Executive Director*
*Lloyd Stabiner, President*

1313 **Utah Department of Human Services: Substance Abuse and Mental Health**
195 North 1950 West 801-538-3939
Salt Lake City, UT 84116 Fax: 801-538-9892
dsamh@utah.gov
dsamh.utah.gov
Oversees publicly funded prevention and treatment services through locally designed programs throughout Utah.
*Doug Thomas, Director*
*Lana Stohl, Deputy Director*

1314 **Vermont Office of Alcohol & Drug Abuse Programs: Agency of Human Services**
Vermont Department of Health
108 Cherry Street 802-651-1550
Burlington, VT 05402 AHS.VDHADAP@vermont.gov
healthvermont.gov
Provides resources to those suffering from substance abuse across Vermont.
*Mark Levine, MD, Commissioner*
*Tracy Dolan, Deputy Health Commissioner*

1315 **Virginia Division of Substance Abuse Services**
Department of Mental Health and Mental Retardation
1220 Bank Street 804-786-3921
Richmond, VA 23219 Fax: 804-371-6638
TDD: 804-371-8977
www.dbhds.virginia.gov
In collaboration with its state and community partners, DBHDS plans, develops, directs, funds and monitors the delivery of comprehensive substance abuse services throughout the Commonwealth of Virginia.
*Mellie Randall, Administrator*

1316 **Washington Department of Social and Health Services, Alcohol and Drug Prog.**
Department Of Social And Health Services
Olympia, WA 98504-5330 877-301-4557
800-737-0617
Fax: 360-438-8078
TTY: 877-301-4557
starkkd@dshs.wa.gov
www1.dshs.wa.gov

1317 **Washington Division of Alcoholism & Substance Abuse**
Washington Department of Social & Mental Health
877-501-2233
www.dshs.wa.gov
Provide a basic overview of alcohol/substance abuse system and guidelines to assist in determining if a client is in need of alcohol or substance abuse treatment.
*Robin Arnold-Williams, Secretary*
*Tracy Guerin, Chief Of Staff*

1318 **West Virginia Division of Alcohol & Drug Abuse**
Department Of Health And Human Resources
350 Capitol Street 304-356-4811
Charleston, WV 25304-3702 Fax: 304-558-1008
www.dhhr.wv.gov
The Division on Alcoholism and Drug Abuse, an operating division of the Bureau for Behavioral Health and Health Facilities (BBHHF) within the West Virginia Division of Health and Human Services is charged in code with being the Single State Authority

(SSA) primarily responsible for prevention, control, treatment, rehabilitation, educational research and planning for substance abuse related services
*Craig A. Richards, Deputy Commissioner*

1319 **West Virginia Division of Alcohol and Drug Abuse**
WV Bureau for Behavioral Health
350 Capitol Street 304-356-4811
Charleston, WV 25301 Fax: 304-558-1008
www.dhhr.wv.gov/bhhf
Responsible for prevention, control, treatment, rehabilitation, educational research and planning for substance abuse related services.
*Nancy Sullivan, Commissioner*

1320 **Wisconsin Bureau of Substance Abuse Services**
Wisconsin Department of Health Services
1 West Wilson Street 608-266-9485
Madison, WI 53703 TTY: 800-947-3529
scott.stokes@wi.gov
www.dhs.wisconsin.gov/substabuse
Privodes resources and treatment services for persons suffering of substance abuse problems.
*Scott Stokes, Contact*

1321 **Wyoming Behavioral Health Division**
Wyoming Department of Health
6101 Yellowstone Road 307-777-6494
Cheyenne, WY 82002 800-535-4006
Fax: 307-777-5849
health.wyo.gov/behavioralhealth
Oversees programs and grants for communities to provide outpatient and regional mental health and substance use treatment services and supports, including Court Supervised Treatment programs, that are accessible, affordable and provided in the least restrictive and most appropriate environment.
*Chris Newman, Administrator*

## Libraries & Resource Centers

1322 **Do it Now Foundation**
PO Box 27658 480-736-0599
Tempe, AZ 85285-7658 Fax: 480-736-0599
An information clearinghouse for service providers that publishes well-written pamphlets booklets and materials on chemical dependency and recovery.

1323 **Families in Action National Drug Abuse Center**
National Drug Abuse Center
PO Box 3553 252-237-1242
Wilson, NC 27895 Fax: 252-237-6544
phil@familiesinaction.org
www.familiesinaction.org
Publish prevention materials and serves as an information clearinghouse for families with a member suffering from a drug or alcohol addiction.
*Phillip A Mooring, Executive Director*
*Anna Godwin, Coordinator*

1324 **Hazeldon Foundation: Library and Information Resources**
Hazelden
15251 Pleasant Valley Road 651-213-4200
Center City, MN 55012 800-257-7810
Fax: 651-213-4793
info@hazelden.org
www.hazelden.org
Since its 1949 founding in a rural Minnesota lakeside farmhouse, Hazelden has grown into one of the world's largest, most respected, and best-known private alcohol and drug rehabilitation centers in the world. Thousands of people from all 50 states and 42 foreign countries have turned to Hazelden to find expertise, quality care, and leading authorities on addiction and recovery issues. Our mission today remains the same.
*Mark Mishek, President & CEO*
*James A. Blaha, Vice President*

1325 **Maine State Office of Substance Abuse: Information and Resource Center**
Substance Abuse
41 Anthony Ave.ÿ 207-287-2595
Augusta, ME 04333 Fax: 207-287-4334
TTY: 800-606-0215
osa.ircosa@maine.gov
www.maine.gov
The Maine Office of Substance Abuse is the single state administrative authority responsible for the planning, development, implementation, regulation, and evaluation of substance abuse services. The Office provides leadership in substance abuse prevention, intervention, and treatment. Its goal is to enhance the health and safety of Maine citizens through the reduction of the overall impact of substance use, abuse, and dependency.
*Guy Cousins, Director*
*Geoff Miller, Associate Director*

1326 **National Clearinghouse for Alcohol and Drug Information**
Rockville, MD 20847-2345 240-221-4019
800-729-6686
Fax: 240-221-4292
TDD: 800-487-4889
A resource for alcohol and other drug information. It carries a wide variety of publications dealing with alcohol and other drug abuse.
*John Noble, Director*

1327 **National Treatment Consortium for Alcohol and Other Drugs**
PO Box 1294 202-434-4780
Washington, DC 20013 www.ntc-usa.org

1328 **National Volunteer Training Center for Substance Abuse Prevention**
CSAP Division of Communications Programs
5600 Fishers Lane 301-443-9936
Rockville, MD 20857
Volunteers are always on hand to provide answers, information, referrals and resources pertaining to alcohol, drugs and substance abuse.

1329 **RADAR Network National Clearinghouse**
National Clearinghouse for Alcohol & Drug Info
PO Box 2345 301-468-2600
Rockville, MD 20847-2345 800-729-6686
Fax: 240-221-4292
TTY: 800-487-4889
TDD: 800-487-4889
Consists of state clearinghouses specialized information centers of national organizations and the Department of Education Regional Training Centers. Each RADAR member can offer the public a variety of information services.
*John Noble, Director*

1330 **Resource Institute for Drug Education**
160 Vanderbilt Court 800-279-6361
Bowling Green, KY 42103 Fax: 270-746-9598
info@pridesurveys.com
www.pridesurveys.com
Offers national information and educational materials pertaining to alcohol and drug dependency.
*Thomas J Gleaton, EdD, President*
*Janie Pitcock, President*

## Foundations & Research Centers

1331 **Alcohol Disease Foundation**
33 Eglantine Avenue 609-737-0088
Pennington, NJ 08534-2308
Founded in 1988 to promote research on testing systems that could diagnose the metabolic aspects of alcoholism. Seeks to educate the public on the validity of the disease concept of alcoholism.

1332 **Alcohol Research Group Public Health Institute**
Public Health Institute
6475 Christie Avenue 510-597-3440
Emeryville, CA 94608-1324 Fax: 510-985-6459
info@arg.org
www.arg.org
The Alcohol Research Group (ARG) of the Public Health Institute was established in 1959 to conduct and disseminate high-quality research in epidemiology of alcohol consumption and problems in-

cluding alcohol use disorders, alcohol-related health services research, and analyses of alcohol policy and its impacts.
*Dominique La MPH, Executive Director*
*Thomas K. Greenfield, Scientific Director*

1333 **American Academy of Addiction Psychiatry**
American Academy of Addictionÿ
400 Massasoit Ave 401-524-3076
East Providence, RI 02914 Fax: 401-272-0922
info@aaap.org
www.aaap.org
Psychiatrists and other health care and mental health professionals treating people with addictions. Promotes excellence in the treatment of addictions; seeks to insure availability of addiction treatment programs; encourages improvement in the training of health and mental health care providers treating people with addictions.
*Kathrynÿ Cates-Wessel, Executive Director*
*Isabelÿ Vieira, Director of Education*

1334 **Boston University Laboratory of Neuropsychology**
Dept of Behavioral Neuroscience
80 E Concord Street M9 617-638-4803
Boston, MA 02118 Fax: 617-638-4806
www.bu.edu
Offers research and studies into the effects of Alcoholism pertaining to aphasia apraxia dementia memory disorders and various other neurological malfunctions.
*Marlene Osca Berman PhD, Director*

1335 **Center for Alcohol & Addiction Studies**
Brown University
PO Box G-B 401-863-1000
Providence, RI 02912-0001 Fax: 401-444-1850
denise_bayles@brown.edu
brown.edu
The Center for Alcohol and Addiction Studies, through its affiliation with the Brown Medical School, occupies a unique position within the University. The Center brings together more that 90 faculty and professional staff members, from 11 University departments and eight affiliated hospitals, to promote the identification, prevention, and effective treatment of alcohol and other substance abuse.
*Christina Paxson, President*
*Mark S.ÿ Schlissel, Provost*

1336 **Center for Applied Prevention Research**
Community Prevention Initiative
708 College Ave. 877-568-4227
Santa Rosa, CA 95404 Fax: 707-568-3810
www.ca-cpi.org
Prevention of alcohol and drug abuse is the main focus of the research studies.
*Jo%ol L. Phillips, Executive Director*
*Kerrilyn Scott-Nakai, CPI and SIG Project Director*

1337 **Cornerstone Medical Arts Center Hospital**
Medical Arts Center Hospital
159-05 Union Turnpike 718-906-6700
Fresh Meadows, NY 11366-2802 800-233-9999
Fax: 718-906-6840
admin@cornerstoneny.com
www.cornerstoneny.com
Offers a complete integrated program for alcohol assessment alcohol and drug rehabilitation continuing care community education and comprehensive family recovery.
*Norine Hurtado, Senior Vice President of Human Resources*

1338 **Do it Now Foundation**
PO Box 27658 480-736-0599
Tempe, AZ 85285-7658 Fax: 480-736-0599
An information clearinghouse for service providers that publishes well-written pamphlets booklets and materials on chemical dependency and recovery.

1339 **Dorothea Dix Hospital Clinical Research Unit**
809 Ruggles Drive 919-733-5227
Raleigh, NC 27603 866-349-5627
Fax: 919-733-5351
www.med.unc.edu
Researches the biological risk factors of alcoholism using young adults without the disease but with history of familial alcoholism.
*Terry Spell, Director*
*William L Roper, CEO*

1340 **Ernest Gallo Clinic and Research Center**
San Francisco General Hospital
5858 Horton Street 510-985-3100
Emeryville, CA 94608 Fax: 510-985-3101
Alcoholism studies with a special emphasis on genetics.
*John A. De Luca, Chairman of the Board*
*William R. Sawyers, Chief Administrative Officer*

1341 **Families in Action National Drug Abuse Center**
National Drug Abuse Center
PO Box 3553 252-237-1242
Wilson, NC 27895 Fax: 252-237-6544
phil@familiesinaction.org
www.familiesinaction.org
Publish prevention materials and serves as an information clearinghouse for families with a member suffering from a drug or alcohol addiction.
*Phillip A Mooring, Executive Director*
*Anna Godwin, Coordinator*

1342 **Friends Medical Science Research Center**
1229 West Mount Royal Avenue 410-752-4218
Baltimore, MD 21217 Fax: 310-477-9601
www.wellness.com
Studies narcotic addictions.
*John Valenty, President*
*Rob Greenstein, President*

1343 **Hahnemann University Laboratory of Human Pharmacology**
Department of Pharmacology
Broad and Vine 215-762-7000
Philadelphia, PA 19102 Fax: 215-762-8109
www.hahnemannhospital.com
Hahnemann University hospital is committed to providing quality patient care in an academic setting.
*Benjamin Cal MD, Director*

1344 **Hamot Medical Center: Research Department**
UPMC Hamot
200 Lothrop St. 412-647-8762
Pittsburgh, PA 15213 800-533-8762
Fax: 814-877-7590
www.upmc.com
Drug evaluations and medical products.
*Desmond J. McDonald, Chairman*
*V. James Fiorenzo, President*

1345 **Harvard Cocaine Recovery Project**
1493 Cambridge Street 617-498-1000
Cambridge, MA 02139-1099 Fax: 617-642-58
Six-year study of relapse and recovery in cocaine addicts.
*William McAu MD, Principal Investigator*

1346 **Hazeldon Foundation: Library and Information Resources**
Hazelden
15251 Pleasant Valley Road 651-213-4200
Center City, MN 55012 800-257-7810
Fax: 651-213-4793
info@hazelden.org
www.hazelden.org
Since its 1949 founding in a rural Minnesota lakeside farmhouse, Hazelden has grown into one of the world's largest, most respected, and best-known private alcohol and drug rehabilitation centers in the world. Thousands of people from all 50 states and 42 foreign countries have turned to Hazelden to find expertise, quality care, and leading authorities on addiction and recovery issues. Our mission today remains the same as our early founders ha
*Mark Mishek, President & CEO*
*James A. Blaha, Vice President*

1347 **Interdisciplinary Program in Cell and Molecular Pharmacology**
Medical University of South Carolina
173 Ashley Avenue BSB 358 843-792-8975
Charleston, SC 29425 Fax: 843-792-0481

Research into pharmacology and toxicology.
*Kenneth D Tew, Ph.D., D.Sc., Professor and Chairman*
*Michelle Shorter, Administrative Coordinator*

1348 **Johns Hopkins Behavioral Pharmacology Research Unit**
School of Medicine
4940 Eastern Avenue 410-550-0616
Baltimore, MD 21224 Fax: 410-550-0030
www.hopkinsmedicine.org
*Paul B. Rothman, Chief Executive Officer*
*Ronald R. Peterson, Executive Vice President*

1349 **Johns Hopkins University: Behavioral Pharmacology Research Unit**
John Hopkins Bay View Campus
5510 Nathan Shock Drive 410-955-5000
Baltimore, MD 21224-2735 Fax: 410-550-0030
bigelow@jhmi.edu
www.hopkinsmedicine.org
An internationally recognized center of excellence in research on psychoactive drugs. As the name implies BPRU's orientation is behavioral and pharmacological emphasizing a behavioral analysis of drug action.
*George E Bigelow PhD, Scientific Director*
*Eric C Strain MD, Medical Director*

1350 **Kettering-Scott Magnetic Resonance Laboratory**
Wright State University, School of Medicine
PO Box 927 937-775-2934
Dayton, OH 45435-0927 www.med.wright.edu
No information found on the website.
*Marjorie Bowman, MD and Dean*
*Betty Kangas, Assistant to the dean*

1351 **Maine State Office of Substance Abuse: Information and Resource Center**
Substance Abuse
41 Anthony Ave.ÿ 207-287-2595
Augusta, ME 04333 Fax: 207-287-4334
TTY: 800-606-0215
osa.ircosa@maine.gov
www.maine.gov
The Maine Office of Substance Abuse is the single state administrative authority responsible for the planning, development, implementation, regulation, and evaluation of substance abuse services. The Office provides leadership in substance abuse prevention, intervention, and treatment. Its goal is to enhance the health and safety of Maine citizens through the reduction of the overall impact of substance use, abuse, and dependency.
*Guy Cousins, Director*
*Geoff Miller, Associate Director*

1352 **Marin Institute**
24 Belvedere Street 415-456-5692
San Rafael, CA 94901-4817 Fax: 415-456-0491
www.marinInstitute.org
The mission of this Institute is to reduce the toll of alcohol and other drug problems on Marin County and society in general. The Institute fulfills this mission by developing implementing evaluating and disseminating innovative approaches to prevention locally nationally and internationally.
*Bruce Lee Livingston MPP, Executive Director*
*Michele Simo JD MPH, Research & Policy Director*

1353 **Narcotic and Drug Research**
Informa Healthcare
11 Beach Street 212-966-8700
New York, NY 10013-2429 Fax: 212-334-8058
informahealthcare.com
Nonprofit organization that is devoted to drug abuse education, treatment and prevention.
*Douglas S Lipton PhD, Director*
*Arthur Liu, CEO*

1354 **National Center on Addiction and Substance Abuse**
Columbia University
633 3rd Avenue 212-841-5200
New York, NY 10017-6706 800-622-4357
Fax: 212-956-8020
www.casacolumbia.org
The only nation-wide organization that brings together under one roof all the professional disciplines needed to study and combat abuse of all substances-alcohol nicotine as well as illegal prescription and performance enhancing drugs-in all sectors of society.
*Lee C. Bollinger, President*
*Ursula M. Burns, Chairman and CEO*

1355 **National Clearinghouse for Alcohol and Drug Information Library (NCADI)**
Substance Abuse & Mental Health Services Offices
1 Choke Cherry Road 301-468-2600
Rockville, MD 20857 877-726-4727
Fax: 301-468-2600
TTY: 800-487-4889
TDD: 800-487-4889
webmaster@samhsa.hhs.gov
beta.samhsa.gov
National Clearinghouse for Alcohol and Drug Information (NCADI) is the Nation's one-stop resource for information about substance abuse prevention and addiction treatment. We staff both English- and Spanish-speaking information specialists who are skilled at recommending appropriate publications, posters, and videocassettes; conducting customized searches; providing grant and funding information; and referring people to appropriate organizations.
*Pamela S. Hyde, Administrator*
*Kana Enomoto, Principal Deputy Administrator*

1356 **National Development and Research Institutes: Library/Resource Center**
National Development and Research Institute
71 West 23rd Street 212-845-4400
New York, NY 10010 Fax: 212-438-0894
*Natalieÿ Becker, PhD, President*
*Erik M. Bagin, Vice President*

1357 **National Institute on Drug Abuse Addiction Research Center Library (NIDA)**
National Institute on Drug Abuse
6001 Executive Boulevard 301-443-1124
Bethesda, MD 20892 Fax: 410-550-1438
mpfeiffe@intra.nida.nih.gov
www.drugabuse.gov
NIDA's mission is to lead the Nation in bringing the power of science to bear on drug abuse and addiction. Recent scientific advances have revolutionized our understanding of drug abuse and addiction. The majority of these advances, which have dramatic implications for how to best prevent and treat addiction, have been supported by the National Institute on Drug Abuse (NIDA).
*Nora Volkow, Director*
*Wilson Compton, Deputy Director*

1358 **National Prevention Resource Center CSAP Division of Communications Programs**
CSAP Division of Communications Programs
5600 Fishers Lane 301-443-9936
Rockville, MD 20857-0001
Supports an array of prevention program evaluation approaches including individual grantee evaluations program evaluations and a National Evaluation Project. Also offers a National Data Base to provide information on programs for prevention of substance abuse.

1359 **National Treatment Consortium for Alcohol and Other Drugs**
PO Box 1294 202-434-4780
Washington, DC 20013 www.ntc-usa.org

1360 **National Volunteer Training Center for Substance Abuse Prevention**
CSAP Division of Communications Programs
5600 Fishers Lane 301-443-9936
Rockville, MD 20857
Volunteers are always on hand to provide answers, information, referrals and resources pertaining to alcohol, drugs and substance abuse.

1361 **National Volunteer Training Center for Sub CSAP Division of Communications Programs**
5600 Fishers Lane 301-443-9936
Rockville, MD 20857

Volunteers are always on hand to provide answers information referrals and resources pertaining to alcohol drugs and substance abuse.

1362 **Office of Applied Studies**
Substance Abuse & Mental Health Services Offices
1 Choke Cherry Road
Rockville, MD 20857
301-468-2600
877-726-4727
Fax: 301-468-2600
TTY: 800-487-4889
TDD: 800-487-4889
webmaster@samhsa.hhs.gov
beta.samhsa.gov
Provides the leadership needed for collecting data on mental illness and substance abuse, including incidence and prevalence studies.
*Pamela S. Hyde, Administrator*
*Kana Enomoto, Principal Deputy Administrator*

1363 **Ohio State University Clinical Pharmacology Division**
College of Medicine
370 Western 9th Avenue
Columbus, OH 43210-1239
614-292-2220
800-252-3636
Fax: 614-292-4293
Substance abuse and alcohol related research.
*Robert Bornstein PHD, Dean of Academic Affairs*
*Glen Apsloss, Director*

1364 **Ohio State University: Division of Clinical Trials**
The Ohio State University
281 W. Lane Ave.
Columbus, OH 43210
614-292-8600
800-854-4461
Fax: 614-292-7232
Clinical studies and clinical pharmacology research.
*Wolfgang Sadee, Professor/Chairman*
*Melinda Church, Vice President*

1365 **Research Institute on Alcoholism**
1021 Main Street
Buffalo, NY 14203
716-887-2566
Fax: 716-887-2252
webmaster@ria.buffalo.edu
Research center within the University at Buffalo, part of the State University of New York.
*Kenneth E. Leonard, Director*
*Kimberly S. Walitzer, Deputy Director*

1366 **Research Society on Alcoholism**
7801 North Lamar Boulevard
Austin, TX 78752
512-454-0022
Fax: 512-454-0812
rsastaff@sbcglobal.net
rsoa.org
The Research Society on Alcoholism, founded in 1976, serves as a forum for scientists and researchers focused on the fields of alcoholism and alcohol-related problems. The Society promotes research with the purpose of advancing treatment of alcoholism and finding potential cures.
*Cristine Czachowski, PhD, President*
*Mary Larimer, PhD, Vice President*

1367 **Rockefeller University Laboratory of Biology**
1230 York Avenue
New York, NY 10065
212-327-8000
Fax: 212-327-7974
www.rockefeller.edu
*Marc Tessier Lavigne, President*

1368 **Rutgers University Center of Alcohol Studies**
Busch Campus
607 Allison Road
Piscataway, NJ 08854
732-445-2190
Fax: 732-445-3500
alclib@rci.rutgers.edu
alcoholstudies.rutgers.edu
Causes and treatment of alcoholism.
*Robert Pandi PhD, Director*

1369 **Rutgers University: Controlled Drug- Delivery Research Center**
College of Pharmacy
PO Box 789
Piscataway, NJ 08855-0789
732-932-3834
Fax: 732-932-5767
*Yie W Chien, Director*

1370 **Ruth E Golding Clinical Pharmacokinetics Laboratory**
College of Pharmacy
1703 E Mabel
Tucson, AZ 85721-1427
520-626-1938
www.pharmacy.arizona.edu
Conducts studies of drugs in humans and animals.
*Michael Maye MD, Head*

1371 **Salk Institute for Biological Studies**
10010 N Torrey Pines Road
La Jolla, CA 92037
858-453-4100
www.salk.edu
Conducts groundbreaking research into cancer, aging, Alzheimer's diabetes and infectious diseases.
*Rusty Gage, PhD, President*
*Martin Hetzer, PhD, VP & Chief Science Officer*

1372 **Southern California Research Institute**
Journal Studies on Alcohol and Drugs
11912 W Washington Boulevard
Los Angeles, CA 90066
213-427-3200
Fax: 310-398-6651
www.jsad.com
Effects of alcohol and drugs on behavior studies.
*Dr. M Burns, Director*
*Dirk Stoehr, Manager*

1373 **Stanford Center for Research in Disease Prevention**
Stanford University School of Medicine
211 Quarry Road
Palo Alto, CA 94304
650-723-6028
Fax: 650-725-6906
Prevention and control of alcohol and drug abuse related disorders.
*Philip A. Pizzo, Former Dean*
*John W Farquhar MD, Director*

1374 **State University of New York at Buffalo Toxicology Research Center**
3435 Main Street
Buffalo, NY 14214
716-831-2125
Fax: 716-829-2806
www.smbs.buffalo.edu
Toxicology-related research and services including the development of tests to evaluate toxins chemicals and drugs.
*Michale E. Cain, Director*
*Dr James R Olson, Assistant Director*

1375 **Substance Abuse and Mental Health Services Administration**
Substance Abuse & Mental Health Services Offices
1 Choke Cherry Road
Rockville, MD 20857
301-468-2600
877-726-4727
Fax: 301-468-2600
TTY: 800-487-4889
TDD: 800-487-4889
webmaster@samhsa.hhs.gov
The goal of this organization is to reduce incidence and prevalence of mental disorders and substance abuse and improve treatment outcomes for persons suffering from addictive and mental health problems and disorders.
*Pamela S. Hyde, Administrator*
*Kana Enomoto, Principal Deputy Administrator*

1376 **UAMS Psychiatric Research Institute**
4224 Shuffield Drive
Little Rock, AR 72205
501-526-8100
Fax: 501-660-7542
kramerteresal@uams.edu
www.psychiatry.uams.edu
Combining research, education and clinical services into one facility, PRI offers inpatiend and outpatient services, with 40 psychiatric beds, therapy options, and specialized treatment for specific disorders, including: addictive eating, anxiety, deppressive and post-traumatic stress disorders. Research focuses on evidence-based care takes into consideration the education of future medical personnel while relying on research scientists to provide innovative forms of treatment.

1377 **University of Alabama: Center for Alcohol and Addiction Studies**
3211 Providence Drive
Anchorage, AK 99508
907-786-1805
Fax: 907-786-4866
Basic, applied and evaluative research into alcohol and substance abuse.
*Dennis Fisher, Director*

1378 **University of California: Los Angeles Alcohol Research Center**
405 Hilgard Ave 310-825-4321
Los Angeles, CA 90095-8353 Fax: 310-206-7309
www.ucla.edu
Causes of alcoholism including genetics.
*Dr Ernest Noble, Director*

1379 **University of Delaware: Center for Drug and Alcohol Studies**
University of Delaware ÿ
77 E Main Street 302-831-2792
Newark, DE 19716 Fax: 302-831-3307
butzin@udel.edu
www.udel.edu/butzin/cdas.html
Substance abuse research
*Patrick T. Harker, President*
*Domenico Grasso, Provost*

1380 **University of Michigan Alcohol Research Center**
University of Michigan Health System
1500 E. Medical Center Drive 734-615-0863
Ann Arbor, MI 48109 855-855-0863
Fax: 734-615-6085
zuckerra@umich.edu
www.med.umich.edu
Alcohol abuse among the elderly, including the relationship of alcohol and aging on the central nervous system. Also does general research pertaining to the effects of alcholoism and drug abuse.
*Ora Hirsch Pescovitz, Executive Vice President*
*Douglas L. Strong, Chief Executive Officer*

1381 **University of Michigan: Alcohol Research Center**
400 E Eisenhower Parkway 734-764-1817
Ann Arbor, MI 48108-3318 Fax: 734-998-7994
www.umich.edu
Alcohol abuse studies among the elderly including the relationship between alcohol and aged disorders.
*Robert A Zucker PhD, Contact*

1382 **University of Michigan: Psychiatric Center**
4250 Plymouth road 734-936-5900
Ann Arbor, MI 48109-0001 Fax: 734-936-9761
www.umich.edu
Psychiatric disease research pertaining to the effects of alcoholism and drug abuse.
*Gregory W Dalack, MD*

1383 **University of Minnesota: Program on Alcohol/Drug Control**
Stadium Gate 27 612-624-6861
Minneapolis, MN 55455
Alcohol tobacco and drug research.
*Dr James Schaefer, Director*

1384 **University of Missouri: Kansas City Drug Information Service**
University of Missouri
2411 Holmes Street 816-235-1000
Kansas City, MO 64110-2640 webmaster@umkc.edu
www.umkc.edu
Literature research and evaluation of clinical drug problems and questions.
*Patrick J Bryant PharmD, Director*
*Antoine D Richardson PharmD, Assistant Director*

1385 **University of Tennessee Drug Information Center**
UT Health Science Center
920 Madison Ave. 901-448-8423
Memphis, TN 38163-1 Fax: 901-524-4545
TDD: 901-448-7382
www.uthsc.edu
*Dr. Peter A Chyka, Director*
*Cheryl R. Scheid, Vice Chancellor*

1386 **University of Texas Health Science Center Neurophysiology Research Center**
Speech & Hearing Institute
7000 Fannin 713-500-4472
Houston, TX 77030-3405 Fax: 713-792-4513
Conducts clinical and animal studies aimed at combating alcohol drug and tobacco dependence.
*Giuseppe N Colasurdo, Director*

1387 **University of Texas at Austin: Drug Synamics Institute**
1 University Station 512-475-9746
Austin, TX 78712 Fax: 512-471-2746
www.utexas.edu
Pharmaceutical and drug research.
*Janet C Walkow PhD, Director*
*Carla Van Den Berg PhD, Associate Professor*

1388 **University of Utah: Center for Human Toxicology**
30 South 2000 East 801-581-6731
Salt Lake City, UT 84112-1210 Fax: 801-581-3716
dwilkins@alanine.pharm.utah.edu
www.pharmacy.utah.edu
Clinical forensic and toxicology research.
*Chris M . Ireland PHd, Dean*
*Dennis Crouch, Director*

1389 **University of Washington: Alcohol & Drug Abuse Institute Library**
University of Washington
1107 Northeast 45th Street, Suite 1 206-543-0937
Seattle, WA 98105 Fax: 206-543-5473
library@adai.uw.edu
lib.adai.washington.edu/
The ADAI Library collection represents the spectrum of research and scientific literature on alcohol and other drug use from all relevant disciplines, including medicine, nursing, social work, criminal justice, sociology and psychology.
*Nancy Sutherland, Director*
*Meg Brunner, Librarian*

1390 **University of Wisconsin Milwaukee Medicinal Chemistry Group**
University of Wisconsin
PO Box 413 414-229-1122
Milwaukee, WI 53201-413 www4.uwm.edu
Research on drugs including studies of valium receptors.
*Michael R. Lovell, Chancellor*

1391 **University of Wisconsin: Milwaukee Medicinal Chemistry Group**
Medical College of Wisconsin
8701 Watertown Plank Road 414-955-8296
Milwaukee, WI 53226 www.mcw.edu
Research on drugs, including studies of valium receptors.
*John R. Raymond, President and CEO*
*Dr. Kerschne , Dean and Executive Vice Presiden*

1392 **Marin Institute**
24 Belvedere Street 415-456-5692
San Rafael, CA 94901-4817 Fax: 415-456-0491
www.marinInstitute.org
The mission of this Institute is to reduce the toll of alcohol and other drug problems on Marin County and society in general. The Institute fulfills this mission by developing implementing evaluating and disseminating innovative approaches to prevention locally, nationally and internationally.
*Bruce Lee Livingston MPP, Executive Director*
*Michele Simo JD MPH, Research & Policy Director*

## Support Groups & Hotlines

1393 **Adult Children of Alcoholics**
PO Box 3216 562-595-7831
Torrance, CA 90510 info@adultchildren.org
adultchildren.org
An anonymous Twelve Step, Twelve Tradition program of women and men who grew up in an alcoholic or otherwise dysfunctional homes.

1394 **Alcohol Drug Treatment Referral**
1316 South Coast Highway 800-454-8966
Laguna Beach, CA 92651-3118 Fax: 949-281-1933
National Help and Referral Network, a nonprofit organization available 24 hours a day to assist people troubled by drug or alcohol abuse. Here to provide information on addiction treatment and support services and to help save lives and mend broken dreams.
*Mike Cohan, Director*

1395 **Alcoholics Anonymous (AA): World Services**
475 Riverside Drive at West 120th S 212-870-3400
New York, NY 10115 aa.org
For men and women who share the common problems of alcoholism.

1396 **Alcoholics Anonymous World Services**
PO Box 459 212-870-3400
New York, NY 10163-4059 Fax: 212-870-3003
www.aa.org
Alcoholics Anonymous is a fellowship of men and women who share their experience, strength and hope with each other that they may solve their common problem and help others to recover from alcoholism. The only requirement for membership is a desire to stop drinking. There are no dues or fees for AA membership; they are self-supporting through their own contributions.
*Greg M, General Manager*

1397 **Chemically Dependent Anonymous**
PO Box 423 888-232-4673
Severna Park, MD 21146 www.cdaweb.org
A 12-step fellowship for anyone seeking freedom from drug and alcohol addiction. The basis of the program is abstinence from all mood-changing and mind-altering chemicals, including street-type drugs, alcohol and unnecessary medication.

1398 **Cocaine Anonymous**
21720 S. Wilmington Ave 310-559-5833
Long Beach, CA 90810 Fax: 310-559-2554
cawso@ca.org
ca.org
Fellowship of men and women who share their experience, stength and hope with each other in hope that they may solve their common problem and help others recover from their addiction.

1399 **Drug Free Workplace Hotline**
Division of Workplace Programs
Samhsa Diagonal CSAP 1 Choke Cherry 240-276-2612
Rockville, MD 20857 877-726-4727
Fax: 240-276-1210
TDD: 800-457-4889
webmaster@samhsa.hhs.gov
A hotline for businesses to obtain information on a wide range of drug abuse related problems, issues and services.
*Robert Stephenson II, Director*

1400 **Infoline**
United Way of Connecticut
1344 Silas Deane Highway 860-571-7500
Rocky Hill, CT 06067 800-203-1234
Fax: 860-571-7525
TTY: 800-671-0737
ctunitedway.org
Infoline is a free, confidential, help-by-telephone service for information, referral, and crisis intervention. Trained professionals help callers find information, discover options or deal with a crisis by locating hundreds of services in their area on many different issues, from substance abuse to elder needs to suicide to volunteering in your community. Infoline is certified by the American Association of Suicidology. Operates 24 hours a day, everyday. Multilingual caseworkers are available.
*Richard Porth, CEO*

1401 **International Lawyers in Alcoholics Anonymous**
39 Smith Neck Road 860-529-7474
Old Lyme, CT 6371 www.ilaa.org
Provides 40 independent local groups.
*Scoot Huyghebaert, Chairman*

1402 **Join Together Online**
352 Park Avenue South 212-922-1560
New York, NY 10010 855-378-4373
Fax: 212-922-1570
www.drugfree.org/join-together
Join Together is a collaboration of the Boston University School of Public Health and The Partnership at Drugfree.org, dedicated to advancing effective drug and alcohol policy, prevention and treatment.
*Patricia F Russo, Chairman*
*Stephen J Pasierb, President,CEO*

1403 **Marijuana Anonymous**
PO Box 7807 800-766-6779
Torrance, CA 90504 office@marijuana-anonymous.org
marijuana-anonymous.org
A fellowship of men and women who share experience, strength and hope with each other to solve common problem and help others to recover from marijuana addiction.

1404 **Nar-Anon Family Groups**
22527 Crenshaw Blvd 310-534-8188
Torrance, CA 90505 800-477-6291
Fax: 310-534-8688
nar-anon.org
Twelve-step program for families and friends of addicts.
*Cathy Khaledi, Executive Director*

1405 **Narcotics Anonymous**
PO Box 9999 818-773-9999
Van Nuys, CA 91409 Fax: 818-700-0700
na.org
For narcotic addicts: Peer support for recovered addicts.

1406 **National Health Information Center**
Office of Disease Prevention & Health Promotion
1101 Wootton Pkwy Fax: 240-453-8281
Rockville, MD 20852 odphpinfo@hhs.gov
www.health.gov/nhic
Supports public health education by maintaining a calendar of National Health Observances; helps connect consumers and health professionals to organizations that can best answer questions and provide up-to-date contact information from reliable sources; updates on a yearly basis toll-free numbers for health information, Federal health clearinghouses and info centers.
*Don Wright, MD, MPH, Director*

1407 **Pathways to Promise**
5400 Arsenal Street Fax: 314-516-8405
Saint Louis, MO 63139 info@pathways2promise.org
pathways2promise.org
An interfaith cooperative of many faith groups, providing assistance and a resource center which offers liturgical and educational materials, program models, caring ministry with people experiencing a mental illness and their families.

1408 **Rational Recovery**
PO Box 800 530-621-2667
Lotus, CA 95651 rational.org
Exclusive, worldwide source of counseling, guidance and direct instruction on self-recovery from addiction to alcohol and other drugs through planned, permanent abstinence.
*Jack Trimpey, President*

1409 **SMART-Self Management and Recovery Training**
7304 Mentor Avenue 440-951-5357
Mentor, OH 44060 866-951-5357
Fax: 440-951-5358
info@smartrecovery.org
smartrecovery.org
The leading self-empowering addiction recovery support group. Participants learn tools for addiction recovery based on the latest scientific research and participate in a world-wide community which includes free, self-empowering, science-based mutual help groups.
*Shari Allwood, Executive Director*

1410 **WFS' New Life Program**
Women for Sobriety
PO Box 618 215-536-8026
Quakertown, PA 18951-0618 Fax: 215-538-9026
newlife@nni.com
www.womenforsobriety.org
A self-help program for women that can be used independent from AA or with AA. Groups are in many states in the United States. Donations suggested.
*Rebecca M Fenner, Director*

## Magazines

1411 **ACAP Recap**
American Council on Alcohol Problems
2376 Lakeside Drive 205-989-8177
Birmingham, AL 35244-2603 Fax: 314-739-0848
sapacap.com
Offers information on organization activities and events, updates on resources and publications and legislative information for affiliate executives.
*Monthly*
*Mark Creech, President*
*Ed Wolkin, President-Elect*

1412 **American Issue**
American Council on Alcohol Problems
2376 Lakeside Drive 205-989-8177
Birmingham, AL 35244-2603 Fax: 314-739-0848
Offered to contributors of the organization.
*Monthly*
*Mark Creech, President*
*Ed Wolkin, President-Elect*

1413 **Drug Abuse Update**
2296 Henderson Mill Road 770-934-6364
Atlanta, GA 30345-2739
A journal of news and information for persons interested in drug prevention.
*Quarterly*

1414 **Forum Magazine**
Al-Anon Alateen Family Group Headquarters
1600 Corp Landing Pkwy 757-563-1600
Virginia Beach, VA 23454-970 888-425-2666
Fax: 757-563-1655
www.al-anon.alateen.org
Contains many personal stories of inspiration, some of which are maade available each month on the Internet by authorization of Al-Anon Family Group Headquarters, Inc.
*Ric Buchanan, Executive Director*

1415 **JNeurosci**
Society for Neuroscience
1121 14th Street NW 202-962-4000
Washginton, DC 20005 jn@sfn.org
www.jneurosci.org
Official peer-reviewed journal of the Society for Neuroscience, publishing research on a broad range of topics of interest to those working on the nervous system.
*Marina R. Picciotto, Editor-in-Chief*
*Teresa Esch, Features Editor*

1416 **Journal of Neurodevelopmental Disorders**
Springer Nature
One New York Plaza 800-777-4643
New York, NY 10004-1562 info@biomedcentral.com
jneurodevdisorders.biomedcentral.com
An open-access journal devoted to integrating research from neurobiology, genetics, cognitive neuroscience, psychiatry and psychology.
*Joseph Piven, Editor-in-Chief*

1417 **Journal of Neuroinflammation**
Springer Nature
One New York Plaza 800-777-4643
New York, NY 10004-1562 info@biomedcentral.com
jneuroinflammation.biomedcentral.com
A peer-reviewed, open-access journal focusing on the interactions of the immune system with the nervous system as a means of expanding understanding of chronic neurological diseases.
*Monica J. Carson, Editor-in-Chief*
*Sue T. Griffin, Editor-in-Chief*

1418 **Lead Line**
Grapevine
PO Box 1980 212-870-3400
New York, NY 10163-1980 Fax: 212-870-3301
AA members all over the world communicate with each other through the pages of this magazine. It contains: insight into how AAs stay sober; readers' views; old-timers corner, beginners meeting, youth enjoying sobriety, and spotlight on service.
*Monthly*

1419 **eNeuro**
Society for Neuroscience
1121 14th Street NW 202-312-7305
Washginton, DC 20005 eNeuro@sfn.org
www.eneuro.org
Open-access journal of the Society for Neuroscience.
*Christophe Bernard, Editor-in-Chief*
*Kelly Newton, Director, Scientific Publications*

## Web Sites

1420 **Indian Health Service**
www.ihs.gov
Charged with providing a comprehensive program of alcoholism and substance abuse prevention and treatment for Native Americans and Alaskan natives.

1421 **Lawyers Concerned for Lawyers**
www.mnlcl.org/
Lawyers Concerned for Lawyers provides free, confidential peer and professional assistance to Minnesota lawyers, judges, law students, and their immediate family members on any issue that causes stress or distress.

1422 **MedicineNet**
www.medicinenet.com
An online resource for consumers providing easy-to-read, authoritative medical and health information.

1423 **Medscape**
www.medscape.com
Medscape offers specialists, primary care physicians, and other health professionals the Web's most robust and integrated medical information and educational tools.

1424 **National Clearinghouse for Alcohol and Drug Information**

1425 **Neuronline**
Society for Neuroscience
- - 0
neuronline@sfn.org
neuronline.sfn.org
Online portal for professional development and training resources for individuals in the field of neuroscience, hosted by the Society for Neuroscience.
*Amanda Kimball, Director, Digital Learning*

1426 **Peter Lamy Center for Drug Therapy and Aging**
University of Maryland School of Pharmacy
20 North Pine Street Baltimore 410-706-7650
Maryland, MD 21201 Fax: 410-706-4012
www.pharmacy.umaryland.edu
The Lamy Center is dedicated to improving drug therapy for aging adults through innovative research, education and clinical initiatives.
*Natalie D. Eddington, Dean and Professor*
*William J. Cooper, Senior Associate Dean for Admini*

1427 **Safe Homes**
This national organization encourages parents to sign a contract stipulating that when parties are held in one another's homes they will adhere to a strict no-alcohol/no-drug-use rule.

1428 **Substance Abuse and Mental Health Services Administration**
www.samhsa.gov
The goal of this organization is to reduce incidence and prevalence of mental disorders and substance abuse and improve treatment outcomes for persons suffering from addictive and mental health problems and disorders.

1429 **WebMD**
www.webmd.com
Provides credible information, supportive communities, and in-depth reference material about health subjects. A source for original and timely health information as well as material from well known content providers.

1430 **www.aa.org**
AA-Alcoholics Anonymous
Group sharing their experience, strength and hope with each other to recover from alcoholism.

1431 **www.addictionresourceguide.com**
Addiction Resource Guide
A comprehensive directory of addiction treatment facilities online.

1432 **www.adultchildren.org**
Adult Children of Alcoholics World Services Organi
12 step and 12 tradition program for adults raised in an environment including alcohol or other dysfunctions.

1433 **www.alcoholism.about.com**
The Alcoholism Home Page
Information about addictive drug use, behaviors, and alcoholism.

1434 **www.cfsny.org**
Center for Family Support (CFS)
Devoted to providing support and assistance to individuals with developmental and related disabilities, and to the family members who care for them.

1435 **www.doitnow.org**
The Do It Now Foundation
Copies of brochures on drugs, alcohol, smoking, drugs and kids, and street drugs.

1436 **www.drugabuse.gov**
National Institute on Drug Abuse
Many publications useful for patients. Research Reports, summaries about chemicals and treatments.

1437 **www.drugabuse.gov/drugpages**
Commonly Abused Drugs: Street Names for Drugs of A
Current names, periods of detection, medical uses.

1438 **www.drugfree.org/join-together**
Join Together
Alcohol and substance abuse information, legislative alerts, new and updates.

1439 **www.higheredcenter.org**
National Clearinghouse for Alcohol & Drug Informat
One-stop resource for information about abuse prevention and addiction treatment.

1440 **www.jacsweb.org**
Jewish Alcoholics Chemically Dependent Persons
Ten articles dealing with denial and ignorance.

1441 **www.lifering.org**
LifeRing
Offers nonreligious approach with links to groups.

1442 **www.mentalhealth.com**
Internet Mental Health
On-line information and a virtual encyclopedia related to mental disorders, possible causes and treatments. News, articles, on-line diagnostic programs and related links. Designed to improve understanding, diagnosis and treatment of mental illness throughout the world. Awarded the Top Site Award and the NetPsych Cutting Edge Site Award.

1443 **www.mhselfhelp.org**
National Mental Health Consumers Self-Help Clearin
Encourages the development and growth of consumer self-help groups.

1444 **www.naadac.org**
The Association for Addiction Professionals
NAADAC is the premier global organization of addiction focused professionals who enhance the health and recovery of individuals, families and communities. NAADAC's mission is to lead, unify and empower addiction focused professionals to achieve excellence through education, advocacy, knowledge, standards of practice, ethics, professional development and research.

1445 **www.niaaa.nih.gov**
National Institute on Alcohol Abuse & Alcoholism
Supports research nationwide on alcohol abuse and alcoholism.

1446 **www.psychcentral.com**
Psych Central
Personalized one-stop index for psychology, support, and mental health issues, resources, and people on the Internet.

1447 **www.samhsa.gov**
Substance Abuse and Mental Health Services Adminis
Provides links to government resources related to substance abuse and mental health.

1448 **www.sapacap.com**
American Council on Alcohol Problems
Referrals to DWI classes and treatment centers.

1449 **www.smartrecovery.org**
Self Help for Substance Abuse & Addiction
Four-Point program includes maintaining motivation, coping with urges, managing feelings and behavior, balancing momentary/enduring satisfactions.

1450 **www.soulselfhelp.on.ca/coda.html**
Souls Self Help Central
Discusses self-help, mental health, issues of co-dependency.

1451 **www.store.samhsa.gov**
SAMHSA's National Mental Health Info Center
Information about resources, technical assistance, research, training, networks, and other federal clearing houses, and fact sheets and materials.

1452 **www.thenationalcouncil.org**
National Council for Commuity Behavioral Healthcar
A network for sharing information and provding assistance among those working in the healthcare management field.

1453 **www.well.com**
Web of Addictions
Links to fact sheets from trustworthy sources.

# CREUTZFELDT-JAKOB DISEASE

*Affecting about one million people in the United States every year, Creutzfeldt-Jakob disease is a deadly degenerative brain disorder. With a typical onset age of between 60 and 65, the disease initially manifests as memory loss, a set of behavioral changes, and a number of visual disturbances. Before long, these symptoms degenerate into dementia, involuntary movements, and blindness. Involuntary movements occur in roughly 90 percent of patients. Additional symptoms include anxiety, depression, paranoia, speech impairment, and ataxia. About 70 percent of patients die within a year of diagnosis and no patient has lived longer than two and a half years after diagnosis.*

Cretuzfeldt-Jakob disease is caused by prions, proteins that occur in the neurons of the central nervous system. In CJD, the prions become misfolded. This affects the signaling process, damages the neurons, and leads to the progressive death of brain cells. By the late stages of the disease, the brain takes on a spongiform appearance. Although the vast majority of cases appear spontaneously, 7.5 percent of cases are inherited. In addition, CJD can be transmitted by contaminated harvested human brain products, grafts, and human growth hormone, although such transmissions are relatively rare. Diagnosis of CJD is difficult and is usually made by observation supported with one or more of the following tests: electroencephalography, cerebral spinal fluid analysis, and magnetic resource imaging (MRI).

First described by German neurologist Hans Gerhard Creutzfeldt in 1920, CJD is a disease without a cure and which is, in every case, fatal. Individual symptoms such as twitching, anxiety, and depression can be treated with benzodiazepines and antidepressants. Otherwise, treatment is limited to palliative care. Although the disease is quite rare, with a worldwide rate of one case per million, it is believed that some percentage of cases that have been diagnosed as Alzheimer's were actually instances of CJD instead.

## National Agencies & Associations

1455 **American Academy of Neurology**
201 Chicago Avenue
Minneapolis, MN 55415
612-928-6000
800-879-1960
Fax: 612-454-2746
memberservices@aan.com
www.aan.com
Professional society of medical doctors specializing in brain and nervous system diseases. Maintains placement service. Sponsors research and educational programs. Compiles statistics. Publishes scientific journal, Continuum: Lifelong Learning in Neurology.
*Mary E. Post, MBA, CAE, CEO*

1456 **American Society for Investigative Pathology**
1801 Rockville Pike
Rockville, MD 20852
240-283-9700
Fax: 301-984-4047
www.asip.org
The Society seeks to promote experimental pathology and related disciplines through meetings, publications, and educational activities.
*William B. Coleman, PhD, Executive Officer*
*Gina LaBorde, Manager, Marketing & Communications*

1457 **American Society for Neurochemistry**
9037 Ron Den Lane
Windermere, FL 34786
407-909-9064
Fax: 407-876-0750
asnmanager@asneurochem.org
asneurochem.org
The Society aims to advance and promote cellular and molecular neuroscience knowledge, and to facilitate communication and the dissemination of information within the field and with related disciplines.
*Sheilah Jewart, Executive Director*
*Karen Gottlieb, Conference Coordinator*

1458 **CJD International Support Alliance**
cjdisa.com
A group of non-profit organizations from around the world dedicated to prion disease victims, their families, and those at risk for the disease. Activities include educational initiatives, information dissemination, resource allocation, program design and implementation and advocacy.
*Suzanne Solvyns, Co-Chair*
*Deana Simpson, Co-Chair*

1459 **Canadian CJD Association**
905-536-8996
terrichaston@cogeco.ca
www.canadiancjdassociation.com
The Association seeks to connect individuals and families dealing with Creutzfeldt-Jakob Disease, with families who have gone through it before, as well as healthcare professionals.
*Terri Chaston, Co-Founder*
*Michelle Santos, Co-Founder*

1460 **Prion Alliance**
Cambridge, MA
www.prionalliance.org
Non-profit devoted to scientific research and towards a treatment or cure for human prion disease.
*Sonia Vallabh, President*

## Foundations & Research Centers

1461 **Creutzfeldt-Jakob Disease Foundation**
3634 W. Market St.
Akron, OH 44333
800-659-1991
Fax: 234-466-7077
help@cjdfoundation.org
cjdfoundation.org
The Foundation seeks to support families affected by Prion Disease, raise awareness, and support medical education and research through support services, education and information, political advocacy, conference and workshops, scientific collaboration, and research grants.
*Debbie Yobs, President*
*Lori Nusbaum, Program Director*

1462 **Kavli Foundation**
5715 Mesmer Avenue
Los Angeles, CA
424-353-8800
info@kavlifoundation.org
www.kavlifoundation.org
The Foundation supports scientific research into the human brain, in the following scientific fields: Astrophysics, Nanoscience, Neuroscience and Theoretical Physics. Within Neuroscience, the study of aging and brain diseases and disorders is supported.
*Robert W. Conn, PhD, President & CEO*
*Eric Marshall, VP, Public Engagement & Prizes*

1463 **Neuroscience Research Institute**
UC Santa Barbara
6129 Biology II
Santa Barbara, CA 93106
805-893-4621
www.nri.ucsb.edu
The Institute seeks to allow scientists from different fields to collaborate for the betterment of neurological research. Areas of interest include: Alzheimer's Disease & Related Dementias; Behavioral Neuroscience & Neuroethology; Cell Biology, Biochemistry & Biophysics of the Nervous System; Computational & Theoretical Neuroscience; Development of the Nervous System; and Stem Cells.
*Stuart Feinstein, Co-Director*
*Kenneth Kosik, Co-Director*

1464 **Sanford Consortium for Regenerative Medicine**
2880 Torrey Pines Scenic Drive
La Jolla, CA 92037
858-246-1071
www.sanfordconsortium.com
The Consortium works to achieve breakthrough discoveries in stem cell research with regards to diagnoses, treatments, and cures for degenerative diseases and injuries.
*Edward W. Holmes, MD, President & CEO*
*Jeffrey Steindorf, PhD, VP & COO*

## Support Groups & Hotlines

1465 **Creutzfeldt-Jakob Disease Foundation**
3634 W. Market St.
Akron, OH 44333
800-659-1991
Fax: 234-466-7077
help@cjdfoundation.org
cjdfoundation.org
The Foundation seeks to support families affected by Prion Disease, raise awareness, and support medical education and research. Support services include a 7-day HelpLine, referrals, support groups and teleconference speaker series.
*Debbie Yobs, President*
*Lori Nusbaum, Program Director*

## Magazines

1466 **ASN NEURO**
Sage Journals
2455 Teller Road
Thousand Oaks, CA 91320
805-499-9774
journals@sagepub.com
journals.sagepub.com/home/asn
Peer-reviewed open access journal focusing on recent advances in the cellular and molecular neurosciences. It is the official publication of the American Society for Neurochemistry.
*Douglas L. Feinstein, Editor-in-Chief*
*Sandra J. Hewitt, Deputy Editor-in-Chief*

1467 **American Journal of Pathology**
Elsevier
1600 John F Kennedy Boulevard
Philadelphia, PA 19103
301-634-7959
Fax: 301-634-7961
ajp@asip.org
ajp.amjpathol.org
Official journal of the American Society for Investigative Pathology, publishing original research reports, reviews, and commentaries related to the molecular and cellular basis of disease.
*Martha Furie, Editor-in-Chief*

1468 **BMC Neuroscience**
Springer Nature
One New York Plaza
New York, NY 10004-1562
800-777-4643
info@biomedcentral.com
bmcneurosci.biomedcentral.com

A peer-reviewed, open-access journal devoted to all aspects of the nervous system (including molecular, cellular, developmental and animal model studies), as well as cognitive and behavioral research, and computational modeling.
*Darren Byrne, Editor*
*Ana Donnelly, Manuscript Editor*

1469 **Brain & Life**
American Academy of Neurology
201 Chicago Avenue 612-928-6000
Minneapolis, MN 55415 800-879-1960
Fax: 612-454-2748
BrainandLife@wolterskluwer.com
www.brainandlife.org
Official magazine of the American Academy of Neurology, aimed at parents and home-caregivers interested in neurology in everyday life.
*Orly Avitzur, MD, MBA, FAAN, Editor-in-Chief*
*Mary Bolster, Managing Editor*

1470 **Brain: A Journal of Neurology**
Oxford University Press
2001 Evans Road 919-677-0977
Cary, NC 27513 800-852-7323
Fax: 919-677-1714
brain@ucl.ac.uk
academic.oup.com/brain
Focus is clinical neurology and translational neuroscience.
*Dimitri M. Kullmann, Editor*
*Joanne Bell, Managing Editor*

1471 **Continuum: Lifelong Learning in Neurology**
American Academy of Neurology
201 Chicago Avenue 612-928-6000
Minneapolis, MN 55415 800-879-1960
continuumcme@aan.com
journals.lww.com/continuum
Official journal of the American Academy of Neurology, aiding professionals in patient care and continuing education.
*Bimonthly*
*Steven L. Lewis, MD, FAAN*
*Andrea J. Weiss, MA, Executive Editor*

1472 **Dementia and Geriatric Cognitive Disorders**
S. Karger Publishers, Inc.
26 W Avon Road 860-675-7834
Unionville, CT 06085 800-828-5479
Fax: 860-675-7302
www.karger.com/DEM
Open-access journal devoted to the study of cognitive dysfunction in preclinical and clinical studies, concentrating on Alzheimer's and Parkinson's disease, Huntington's chorea and other neurodegenerative diseases.
*Victoria Chan-Pilay, Editor-in-Chief*

1473 **Journal of Alzheimer's Disease**
IOS Press
6751 Tepper Drive 703-830-6300
Clifton, VA 20124 Fax: 703-830-2300
editorial@j-alz.com
www.j-alz.com
Research into the etiology, pathogenesis, epidemiology, genetics, behavior, treatment and psychology of Alzheimer's disease.
*George Perry, PhD, Editor-in-Chief*
*Beth Kumar, Managing Editor*

1474 **Journal of Molecular Diagnostics**
Elsevier
1600 John F Kennedy Boulevard 301-634-7959
Philadelphia, PA 19103 Fax: 301-634-7961
jmd@asip.org
jmd.amjpathol.org
Official journal of the American Society for Investigative Pathology and the Association for Molecular Pathology, focusing on molecular discoveries in medicine translating into the clinical diagnostic setting, as well as the description and application of technological advances in the field of molecular diagnostic medicine.
*Monthly*
*Barbara Zehnbauer, PhD, Editor-in-Chief*

1475 **Journal of Neuroinflammation**
Springer Nature
One New York Plaza 800-777-4643
New York, NY 10004-1562 info@biomedcentral.com
jneuroinflammation.biomedcentral.com
A peer-reviewed, open-access journal focusing on the interactions of the immune system with the nervous system as a means of expanding understanding of chronic neurological diseases.
*Monica J. Carson, Editor-in-Chief*
*Sue T. Griffin, Editor-in-Chief*

1476 **Journal of Nuclear Medicine**
Society of Nuclear Medicine and Molecular Imaging
1850 Samuel Morse Drive 703-708-9000
Reston, VA 20190 800-513-6853
Fax: 703-708-9015
subscriptions@snm.org
jnm.snmjournals.org
Peer-reviewed journal with clinical investigations, science reports, articles benefitting continuing education, book reviews, employment opportunities, and updates on practice and research.
*Monthly*
*Johannes Czernin, MD, Editor-in-Chief*
*Susan Alexander, Associate Director, Publications*

1477 **Journal of Nuclear Medicine Technology**
Society of Nuclear Medicine and Molecular Imaging
1850 Samuel Morse Drive 703-708-9000
Reston, VA 20190 800-513-6853
Fax: 703-708-9015
subscriptions@snm.org
tech.snmjournals.org
Peer-reviewed journal dedicated to nuclear medicine technology, with information on credentialing, continuing education and licensure requirements, as well as current news and updates on the field.
*Quarterly*
*Kathy S. Thomas, MHA, CNMT, PET, Editor-in-Chief*
*Susan Alexander, Associate Director, Publications*

1478 **Journal of the Neurological Sciences**
Elsevier
LSU Health Sciences Center JNS_England@lsuhsc.edu
New Orleans, LA 70112 www.jns-journal.com
Original articles in neurology and neuroscience from around the world.
*Monthly*
*John D. England, Editor-in-Chief*

1479 **Molecular Imaging**
Sage Journals
2455 Teller Road 805-499-9774
Thousand Oaks, CA 91320 journals@sagepub.com
journals.sagepub.com/home/mix
Peer-reviewed open access journal focusing on molecular imaging research, including basic science, preclinical studies and human applications. Published in association with the Society of Nuclear Medicine and Molecular Imaging.
*Bimonthly*
*Henry F. VanBrocklin, PhD, Editor-in-Chief*

1480 **Molecular Neurodegeneration**
Springer Nature
One New York Plaza 800-777-4643
New York, NY 10004-1562 info@biomedcentral.com
www.biomedcentral.com
A peer-reviewed, open-access journal devoted to all aspects of neurodegeneration research at the molecular and cellular levels.
*Guojun Bu, Editor-in-Chief*
*Huaxi Xu, Editor-in-Chief*

1481 **Neurocase: The Neural Basis of Cognition**
Taylor & Francis Group
530 Walnut Street www.tandfonline.com/toc/nncs20/current
Philadelphia, PA 19106
Rapid response journal featuring case and group studies in neuropsychology, neuropsychiatry and behavioral neurology, with a focus on the neural basis of cognition.
*Bruce L. Miller, Editor*
*Hans J. Markowitsch, Editor*

1482 **Neurology**
American Academy of Neurology
201 Chicago Avenue 612-928-6000
Minneapolis, MN 55415 800-879-1960
Fax: 612-454-2748
journal@neurology.org
n.neurology.org
Official journal of the American Academy of Neurology, peer-reviewed, highlighting clinical neurology research.
*Jose G. Merino, MD, MPhil, FAAN, Editor-in-Chief*
*Patricia K. Baskin, MS, Executive Editor*

1483 **Neurology Clinical Practice**
American Academy of Neurology
201 Chicago Avenue 612-928-6000
Minneapolis, MN 55415 800-879-1960
Fax: 612-454-2748
journal@neurology.org
cp.neurology.org
Official peer-reviewed journal of the American Academy of Neurology for practicing neurologists.
*John R. Corboy, MD, FAAN, Editor*
*Patricia K. Baskin, MS, Executive Editor*

1484 **Neurology: Genetics**
American Academy of Neurology
201 Chicago Avenue 612-928-6000
Minneapolis, MN 55415 800-879-1960
Fax: 612-454-2748
journal@neurology.org
ng.neurology.org
Official journal of the American Academy of Neurology, publishing online open-access peer-reviewed reports in the field of neurogenetics.
*Stefan M. Pulst, MD, FAAN, Editor*
*Patricia K. Baskin, MS, Executive Editor*

1485 **Neurology: Neuroimmunology & Neuroinflammation**
American Academy of Neurology
201 Chicago Avenue 612-928-6000
Minneapolis, MN 55415 800-879-1960
Fax: 612-454-2748
journal@neurology.org
nn.neurology.org
Official journal of the American Academy of Neurology, publishing online open-access peer-reviewed reports of original research and in-depth reviews of topics in neuroimmunology & neuroinflammation.
*Josep O. Dalmau, MD, PhD, Editor*
*Patricia K. Baskin, MS, Executive Editor*

1486 **Society of Nuclear Medicine and Molecular Imaging**
1850 Samuel Morse Drive 703-708-9000
Reston, VA 20190 Fax: 703-708-9015
feedback@snmmi.org
www.snmmi.org
The mission of this nonprofit scientific and professional organization is to promote the science, technology and application of nuclear medicine and molecular imaging. Molecular imaging techniques are used to diagnose and manage the treatment of brain disorders such as Alzheimer's and Parkinson's disease, among other conditions.
*15,000 members*
*Virginia Pappas, CEO*
*Rebecca Maxey, Director, Communications*

1487 **Translational Neurodegeneration**
Springer Nature
One New York Plaza 800-777-4643
New York, NY 10004-1562 info@biomedcentral.com
www.biomedcentral.com
A peer-reviewed, open-access journal covering research, therapeutics and education for all areas of neurodegenerative diseases.
*Shengdi Chen, Editor-in-Chief*

1488 **Ultrasonic Imaging**
Sage Journals
2455 Teller Road 805-499-9774
Thousand Oaks, CA 91320 journals@sagepub.com
journals.sagepub.com/home/uix
The journal focuses on the rapid publication of original papers on the development and application of ultrasonic techniques, with emphasis on medical diagnosis. Also published are research notes, comments on papers appearing in the journal, book reviews, and occasional review articles.
*Ernest J. Feleppa, Editor-in-Chief*
*Roslyn Raskin, Managing Editor*

## Web Sites

1489 **BrainFacts.org**
Society for Neuroscience
1121 14th Street NW brainfactsinfo@sfn.org
Washington, DC 20005 brainfacts.org
Online public information portal founded by the Kavli Foundation, the Gatsby Charitable Foundation and the Society for Neuroscience, with topics on brain function and anatomy, diseases and disorders, and more.
*Richard Wingate, DPhil, Editor-in-Chief*
*Charles Yokoyama, PhD, Associate Editor*

1490 **Prion Registry**
prionregistry.org
An online portal for individuals affected by or at risk for prion disease, who want to be involved in research into the disease.

# DELIRIUM

*Delirium is a mental state in which the patient suddenly becomes confused or disoriented or experiences difficulty with memory or concentration. Delirium and dementia are similar conditions and, in many cases, can occur together, with dementia sometimes serving as a cause of delirium. The main difference, though, between delirium and dementia is that delirium comes on suddenly and the symptoms may get better or worse. With dementia, the onset is gradual and the symptoms usually remain stable over the course of a number of years. In addition, delirium may produce hallucinations, while dementia generally does not.*

There are three major types of delirium: hypoactive, where the patient is sleepy or depressed; hyperactive, where the patient is restless and agitated; and mixed, where the patient vacillates between the other two types. There are numerous conditions that can trigger delirium, including dementia, alcohol or drug withdrawal or intoxication, dehydration, metabolic disorders, medicinal side effects, sleep deprivation, poisoning, and infections. In addition to confusion, disorientation, and cognitive problems, some symptoms of delirium include disrupted sleep patterns, emotional changes, incontinence, and hallucinations and delusions.

Delirium is usually diagnosed by a combination of techniques including taking a medical history, performing physical and neurological exams, and doing lab tests. Once delirium is diagnosed and the cause is determined, the attention is turned toward treating the cause rather than the symptoms. While treating the underlying cause, it is important that the patient remain in a controlled environment, one that is quiet and well-lit and one where they are around family members. In some cases, medications such as antipsychotics and benzodiazepines may be used, although their effectiveness is clinically inconclusive. For delirium brought on by alcohol withdrawal, benzodiazepines are usually recommended. Among older patients, delirium tends to result in poor long-term health even if the condition is resolved.

## National Agencies & Associations

1492 **American Academy of Neurology**
201 Chicago Avenue
Minneapolis, MN 55415
612-928-6000
800-879-1960
Fax: 612-454-2746
memberservices@aan.com
www.aan.com
Professional society of medical doctors specializing in brain and nervous system diseases. Maintains placement service. Sponsors research and educational programs. Compiles statistics. Publishes scientific journal, Continuum: Lifelong Learning in Neurology.
*Mary E. Post, MBA, CAE, CEO*

## Magazines

1493 **BMC Neuroscience**
Springer Nature
One New York Plaza
New York, NY 10004-1562
800-777-4643
info@biomedcentral.com
bmcneurosci.biomedcentral.com
A peer-reviewed, open-access journal devoted to all aspects of the nervous system (including molecular, cellular, developmental and animal model studies), as well as cognitive and behavioral research, and computational modeling.
*Darren Byrne, Editor*
*Ana Donnelly, Manuscript Editor*

1494 **Brain & Life**
American Academy of Neurology
201 Chicago Avenue
Minneapolis, MN 55415
612-928-6000
800-879-1960
Fax: 612-454-2748
BrainandLife@wolterskluwer.com
www.brainandlife.org
Official magazine of the American Academy of Neurology, aimed at parents and home-caregivers interested in neurology in everyday life.
*Orly Avitzur, MD, MBA, FAAN, Editor-in-Chief*
*Mary Bolster, Managing Editor*

1495 **Brain: A Journal of Neurology**
Oxford University Press
2001 Evans Road
Cary, NC 27513
919-677-0977
800-852-7323
Fax: 919-677-1714
brain@ucl.ac.uk
academic.oup.com/brain
Focus is clinical neurology and translational neuroscience.
*Dimitri M. Kullmann, Editor*
*Joanne Bell, Managing Editor*

1496 **Continuum: Lifelong Learning in Neurology**
American Academy of Neurology
201 Chicago Avenue
Minneapolis, MN 55415
612-928-6000
800-879-1960
continuumcme@aan.com
journals.lww.com/continuum
Official journal of the American Academy of Neurology, aiding professionals in patient care and continuing education.
*Bimonthly*
*Steven L. Lewis, MD, FAAN*
*Andrea J. Weiss, MA, Executive Editor*

1497 **Journal of Neuroinflammation**
Springer Nature
One New York Plaza
New York, NY 10004-1562
800-777-4643
info@biomedcentral.com
jneuroinflammation.biomedcentral.com
A peer-reviewed, open-access journal focusing on the interactions of the immune system with the nervous system as a means of expanding understanding of chronic neurological diseases.
*Monica J. Carson, Editor-in-Chief*
*Sue T. Griffin, Editor-in-Chief*

1498 **Journal of the Neurological Sciences**
Elsevier
LSU Health Sciences Center
New Orleans, LA 70112
JNS_England@lsuhsc.edu
www.jns-journal.com
Original articles in neurology and neuroscience from around the world.
*Monthly*
*John D. England, Editor-in-Chief*

1499 **Molecular Neurodegeneration**
Springer Nature
One New York Plaza
New York, NY 10004-1562
800-777-4643
info@biomedcentral.com
www.biomedcentral.com
A peer-reviewed, open-access journal devoted to all aspects of neurodegeneration research at the molecular and cellular levels.
*Guojun Bu, Editor-in-Chief*
*Huaxi Xu, Editor-in-Chief*

1500 **Neurocase: The Neural Basis of Cognition**
Taylor & Francis Group
530 Walnut Street
Philadelphia, PA 19106
www.tandfonline.com/toc/nncs20/current
Rapid response journal featuring case and group studies in neuropsychology, neuropsychiatry and behavioral neurology, with a focus on the neural basis of cognition.
*Bruce L. Miller, Editor*
*Hans J. Markowitsch, Editor*

1501 **Neurology**
American Academy of Neurology
201 Chicago Avenue
Minneapolis, MN 55415
612-928-6000
800-879-1960
Fax: 612-454-2748
journal@neurology.org
n.neurology.org
Official journal of the American Academy of Neurology, peer-reviewed, highlighting clinical neurology research.
*Jose G. Merino, MD, MPhil, FAAN, Editor-in-Chief*
*Patricia K. Baskin, MS, Executive Editor*

1502 **Neurology Clinical Practice**
American Academy of Neurology
201 Chicago Avenue
Minneapolis, MN 55415
612-928-6000
800-879-1960
Fax: 612-454-2748
journal@neurology.org
cp.neurology.org
Official peer-reviewed journal of the American Academy of Neurology for practicing neurologists.
*John R. Corboy, MD, FAAN, Editor*
*Patricia K. Baskin, MS, Executive Editor*

1503 **Neurology: Genetics**
American Academy of Neurology
201 Chicago Avenue
Minneapolis, MN 55415
612-928-6000
800-879-1960
Fax: 612-454-2748
journal@neurology.org
ng.neurology.org
Official journal of the American Academy of Neurology, publishing online open-access peer-reviewed reports in the field of neurogenetics.
*Stefan M. Pulst, MD, FAAN, Editor*
*Patricia K. Baskin, MS, Executive Editor*

1504 **Neurology: Neuroimmunology & Neuroinflammation**
American Academy of Neurology
201 Chicago Avenue
Minneapolis, MN 55415
612-928-6000
800-879-1960
Fax: 612-454-2748
journal@neurology.org
nn.neurology.org
Official journal of the American Academy of Neurology, publishing online open-access peer-reviewed reports of original research and in-depth reviews of topics in neuroimmunology & neuroinflammation.
*Josep O. Dalmau, MD, PhD, Editor*
*Patricia K. Baskin, MS, Executive Editor*

1505 **Translational Neurodegeneration**
Springer Nature

One New York Plaza 800-777-4643
New York, NY 10004-1562 info@biomedcentral.com
www.biomedcentral.com

A peer-reviewed, open-access journal covering research, therapeutics and education for all areas of neurodegenerative diseases.
*Shengdi Chen, Editor-in-Chief*

## Web Sites

1506 **BrainFacts.org**
Society for Neuroscience
1121 14th Street NW brainfactsinfo@sfn.org
Washington, DC 20005 brainfacts.org
Online public information portal founded by the Kavli Foundation, the Gatsby Charitable Foundation and the Society for Neuroscience, with topics on brain function and anatomy, diseases and disorders, and more.
*Richard Wingate, DPhil, Editor-in-Chief*
*Charles Yokoyama, PhD, Associate Editor*

# DEMENTIA WITH LEWY BODIES

*Considered by many medical experts to be the third most common cause of dementia (after Alzheimer's and vascular dementia), Lewy body dementia is a form of progressive dementia that leads to disturbances in thinking, movement, behavior, and mood. Caused by abnormal deposits of protein in the brain, called Lewy bodies, LBD is believed to account for between 5 and 10 percent of all dementia cases, although most people with the disease also exhibit pathologies consistent with Alzheimer's.*

Lewy body dementia is a progressive disease with a relatively slow onset. It typically affects those who are 50 years or older, and is slightly more common in men than women. The average time between diagnosis and death is 5 to 8 years, although some patients can live as long as 20 years after diagnosis. The early symptoms are often mild and are, in many cases, similar to those of Alzheimer's. Nonetheless, people suffering from Lewy body dementia are more likely to experience sleep disturbances, visual hallucinations, and visuospatial impairment (difficulty distinguishing spatial relationships of objects). These early symptoms may occur without significant memory loss, although memory loss almost always occurs eventually.

Lewy bodies were first discovered in 1912 by a German neurologist named Friedrich Lewy. These bodies are made from a protein known as alpha-synuclein, which is an important element in the regular functioning of neurons, particularly in the communication of brain cells with each other. In Lewy body dementia, the alpha-synuclein forms into clumps inside the neurons, causing them to lose effectiveness and eventually die. Lewy bodies most commonly affect the cerebral cortex, the limbic cortex, the hippocampus, the midbrain and basal ganglia, and the brain stem.

Diagnosis of Lewy body dementia, as with other forms of dementia, is difficult. This difficulty is compounded by the similarities between Lewy body dementia and Parkinson's disease. Indeed, many experts believe the two diseases to be different expressions of the same underlying causes. In addition, medical practitioners often have a hard time differentiating Lewy body dementia from Alzheimer's. LBD cannot be slowed or stopped by medical intervention, but treatment of the symptoms is often undertaken, generally using cholinesterase inhibitors, antipsychotic drugs, and antidepressants.

## National Agencies & Associations

1508 **American Academy of Neurology**
201 Chicago Avenue
Minneapolis, MN 55415
612-928-6000
800-879-1960
Fax: 612-454-2746
memberservices@aan.com
www.aan.com
Professional society of medical doctors specializing in brain and nervous system diseases. Maintains placement service. Sponsors research and educational programs. Compiles statistics. Publishes scientific journal, Continuum: Lifelong Learning in Neurology.
*Mary E. Post, MBA, CAE, CEO*

1509 **American Society for Investigative Pathology**
1801 Rockville Pike
Rockville, MD 20852
240-283-9700
Fax: 301-984-4047
www.asip.org
The Society seeks to promote experimental pathology and related disciplines through meetings, publications, and educational activities.
*William B. Coleman, PhD, Executive Officer*
*Gina LaBorde, Manager, Marketing & Communications*

1510 **American Society for Neurochemistry**
9037 Ron Den Lane
Windermere, FL 34786
407-909-9064
Fax: 407-876-0750
asnmanager@asneurochem.org
asneurochem.org
The Society aims to advance and promote cellular and molecular neuroscience knowledge, and to facilitate communication and the dissemination of information within the field and with related disciplines.
*Sheilah Jewart, Executive Director*
*Karen Gottlieb, Conference Coordinator*

1511 **Brain Support Network**
P.O. Box 7264
Menlo Park, CA 94026
650-814-0848
Fax: 650-233-9278
www.brainsupportnetwork.org
Non-profit dedicated to facilitate brain donation for scientific study in the U.S. and Canada, to provide education on neurological conditions worldwide, and run support groups in Northern California.

1512 **Lewy Body Dementia Association**
912 Killian Hill Road SW
Lilburn, GA 30047
404-935-6444
800-539-9767
Fax: 480-422-5434
www.lbda.org
A non-profit dedicated to raising awareness of the Lewy Body dementials (known as LBD). The association aims to better the quality of life of people with LBD and offers support to their families and caregivers.
*Christina M. Christie, President*
*Angela Taylor, Director of Programs*

1513 **Lewy Body Dementia Resource Center**
750 W Broadway
Long Beach, NY 11561
516-218-2026
norma@lbdny.org
lewybodyresourcecenter.org
A non-profit organization focused on providing resources and assistance to those diagnosed with Lewy Body Dementia and their caregivers.
*Norma Loeb, Founder & Executive Director*
*Suzanne Pargament, Director, Social Services*

1514 **Society for Neuroscience**
1121 14th Street NW
Washginton, DC 20005
202-962-4000
marty@sfn.org
sfn.org
Large international organization of scientists and physicians devoted to the study of the brain and the nervous system.
*37,000 members*
*Marty Saggese, Executive Director*
*Melissa Garcia, Associate Executive Director*

## Libraries & Resource Centers

1515 **Lewy Body Dementia Resource Center**
750 W Broadway
Long Beach, NY 11561
516-218-2026
norma@lbdny.org
lewybodyresourcecenter.org
A non-profit organization focused on providing resources and assistance to those diagnosed with Lewy Body Dementia and their caregivers.
*Norma Loeb, Founder & Executive Director*
*Suzanne Pargament, Director, Social Services*

## Foundations & Research Centers

1516 **Center for Brain Activity Mapping**
UC San Diego
9500 Gilman Drive
La Jolla, CA 92093
858-534-2230
cbam.ucsd.edu
The Center seeks to develop new technologies for detecting neuronal activity, for reporting it out of deep brain tissue, and for processing and analyzing the resulting data, by organizing and supporting research teams and projects.
*Ralph J. Greenspan, PhD, Director*

1517 **Kavli Foundation**
5715 Mesmer Avenue
Los Angeles, CA
424-353-8800
info@kavlifoundation.org
www.kavlifoundation.org
The Foundation supports scientific research into the human brain, in the following scientific fields: Astrophysics, Nanoscience, Neuroscience and Theoretical Physics. Within Neuroscience, the study of aging and brain diseases and disorders is supported.
*Robert W. Conn, PhD, President & CEO*
*Eric Marshall, VP, Public Engagement & Prizes*

1518 **Kavli Institute for Brain Science at Columbia University**
Columbia University
3227 Broadway
New York, NY 10027
212-853-1016
Fax: 212-665-9699
kavli@columbia.edu
www.kavli.columbia.edu
The Institute's primary are of study is how signaling in neural circuits controls cognitive function and behavior, and the development of novel experimental and computational strategies for analyzing these signals.
*Eric R. Kandel, MD, Director*
*Rafael Yuste, MD, PhD, Co-Director*

1519 **Neuroscience Research Institute**
UC Santa Barbara
6129 Biology II
Santa Barbara, CA 93106
805-893-4621
www.nri.ucsb.edu
The Institute seeks to allow scientists from different fields to collaborate for the betterment of neurological research. Areas of interest include: Alzheimer's Disease & Related Dementias; Behavioral Neuroscience & Neuroethology; Cell Biology, Biochemistry & Biophysics of the Nervous System; Computational & Theoretical Neuroscience; Development of the Nervous System; and Stem Cells.
*Stuart Feinstein, Co-Director*
*Kenneth Kosik, Co-Director*

1520 **Salk Institute for Biological Studies**
10010 N Torrey Pines Road
La Jolla, CA 92037
858-453-4100
www.salk.edu
Conducts groundbreaking research into cancer, aging, Alzheimer's diabetes and infectious diseases.
*Rusty Gage, PhD, President*
*Martin Hetzer, PhD, VP & Chief Science Officer*

1521 **Sanford Consortium for Regenerative Medicine**
2880 Torrey Pines Scenic Drive
La Jolla, CA 92037
858-246-1071
www.sanfordconsortium.com
The Consortium works to achieve breakthrough discoveries in stem cell research with regards to diagnoses, treatments, and cures for degenerative diseases and injuries.
*Edward W. Holmes, MD, President & CEO*
*Jeffrey Steindorf, PhD, VP & COO*

1522 **Scripps Research Institute**
10550 North Torrey Pines Road 858-784-1000
La Jolla, CA www.scripps.edu
The institute seeks to improve human wellbeing through the advancement of bioscience, including research into aging & healthspan, autoimmune diseases, cancer, infectious diseases, neurological disorders, and more.
*Peter Schultz, PhD, President & CEO*
*Eric Topol, MD, EVP, Scripps Research*

## Magazines

1523 **ASN NEURO**
Sage Journals
2455 Teller Road 805-499-9774
Thousand Oaks, CA 91320 journals@sagepub.com
journals.sagepub.com/home/asn
Peer-reviewed open access journal focusing on recent advances in the cellular and molecular neurosciences. It is the official publication of the American Society for Neurochemistry.
*Douglas L. Feinstein, Editor-in-Chief*
*Sandra J. Hewitt, Deputy Editor-in-Chief*

1524 **American Journal of Pathology**
Elsevier
1600 John F Kennedy Boulevard 301-634-7959
Philadelphia, PA 19103 Fax: 301-634-7961
ajp@asip.org
ajp.amjpathol.org
Official journal of the American Society for Investigative Pathology, publishing original research reports, reviews, and commentaries related to the molecular and cellular basis of disease.
*Martha Furie, Editor-in-Chief*

1525 **BMC Neuroscience**
Springer Nature
One New York Plaza 800-777-4643
New York, NY 10004-1562 info@biomedcentral.com
bmcneurosci.biomedcentral.com
A peer-reviewed, open-access journal devoted to all aspects of the nervous system (including molecular, cellular, developmental and animal model studies), as well as cognitive and behavioral research, and computational modeling.
*Darren Byrne, Editor*
*Ana Donnelly, Manuscript Editor*

1526 **Brain & Life**
American Academy of Neurology
201 Chicago Avenue 612-928-6000
Minneapolis, MN 55415 800-879-1960
Fax: 612-454-2748
BrainandLife@wolterskluwer.com
www.brainandlife.org
Official magazine of the American Academy of Neurology, aimed at parents and home-caregivers interested in neurology in everyday life.
*Orly Avitzur, MD, MBA, FAAN, Editor-in-Chief*
*Mary Bolster, Managing Editor*

1527 **Brain: A Journal of Neurology**
Oxford University Press
2001 Evans Road 919-677-0977
Cary, NC 27513 800-852-7323
Fax: 919-677-1714
brain@ucl.ac.uk
academic.oup.com/brain
Focus is clinical neurology and translational neuroscience.
*Dimitri M. Kullmann, Editor*
*Joanne Bell, Managing Editor*

1528 **Continuum: Lifelong Learning in Neurology**
American Academy of Neurology
201 Chicago Avenue 612-928-6000
Minneapolis, MN 55415 800-879-1960
continuumcme@aan.com
journals.lww.com/continuum
Official journal of the American Academy of Neurology, aiding professionals in patient care and continuing education.
*Bimonthly*
*Steven L. Lewis, MD, FAAN*
*Andrea J. Weiss, MA, Executive Editor*

1529 **Dementia and Geriatric Cognitive Disorders**
S. Karger Publishers, Inc.
26 W Avon Road 860-675-7834
Unionville, CT 06085 800-828-5479
Fax: 860-675-7302
www.karger.com/DEM
Open-access journal devoted to the study of cognitive dysfunction in preclinical and clinical studies, concentrating on Alzheimer's and Parkinson's disease, Huntington's chorea and other neurodegenerative diseases.
*Victoria Chan-Pilay, Editor-in-Chief*

1530 **JNeurosci**
Society for Neuroscience
1121 14th Street NW 202-962-4000
Washginton, DC 20005 jn@sfn.org
www.jneurosci.org
Official peer-reviewed journal of the Society for Neuroscience, publishing research on a broad range of topics of interest to those working on the nervous system.
*Marina R. Picciotto, Editor-in-Chief*
*Teresa Esch, Features Editor*

1531 **Journal of Alzheimer's Disease**
IOS Press
6751 Tepper Drive 703-830-6300
Clifton, VA 20124 Fax: 703-830-2300
editorial@j-alz.com
www.j-alz.com
Research into the etiology, pathogenesis, epidemiology, genetics, behavior, treatment and psychology of Alzheimer's disease.
*George Perry, PhD, Editor-in-Chief*
*Beth Kumar, Managing Editor*

1532 **Journal of Molecular Diagnostics**
Elsevier
1600 John F Kennedy Boulevard 301-634-7959
Philadelphia, PA 19103 Fax: 301-634-7961
jmd@asip.org
jmd.amjpathol.org
Official journal of the American Society for Investigative Pathology and the Association for Molecular Pathology, focusing on molecular discoveries in medicine translating into the clinical diagnostic setting, as well as the description and application of technological advances in the field of molecular diagnostic medicine.
*Monthly*
*Barbara Zehnbauer, PhD, Editor-in-Chief*

1533 **Journal of NeuroEngineering and Rehabilitation**
Springer Nature
One New York Plaza 800-777-4643
New York, NY 10004-1562 info@biomedcentral.com
jneuroengrehab.biomedcentral.com
An open-access journal devoted to integrated research from the fields of neuroscience, biomedical engineering, and physical medicine and rehabilitation.
*David J. Reinkensmeyer, Editor-in-Chief*

1534 **Journal of Neurodevelopmental Disorders**
Springer Nature
One New York Plaza 800-777-4643
New York, NY 10004-1562 info@biomedcentral.com
jneurodevdisorders.biomedcentral.com
An open-access journal devoted to integrating research from neurobiology, genetics, cognitive neuroscience, psychiatry and psychology.
*Joseph Piven, Editor-in-Chief*

1535 **Journal of Neuroinflammation**
Springer Nature
One New York Plaza 800-777-4643
New York, NY 10004-1562 info@biomedcentral.com
jneuroinflammation.biomedcentral.com

A peer-reviewed, open-access journal focusing on the interactions of the immune system with the nervous system as a means of expanding understanding of chronic neurological diseases.
*Monica J. Carson, Editor-in-Chief*
*Sue T. Griffin, Editor-in-Chief*

1536 **Journal of Nuclear Medicine**
Society of Nuclear Medicine and Molecular Imaging
1850 Samuel Morse Drive 703-708-9000
Reston, VA 20190 800-513-6853
Fax: 703-708-9015
subscriptions@snm.org
jnm.snmjournals.org
Peer-reviewed journal with clinical investigations, science reports, articles benefitting continuing education, book reviews, employment opportunities, and updates on practice and research.
*Monthly*
*Johannes Czernin, MD, Editor-in-Chief*
*Susan Alexander, Associate Director, Publications*

1537 **Journal of Nuclear Medicine Technology**
Society of Nuclear Medicine and Molecular Imaging
1850 Samuel Morse Drive 703-708-9000
Reston, VA 20190 800-513-6853
Fax: 703-708-9015
subscriptions@snm.org
tech.snmjournals.org
Peer-reviewed journal dedicated to nuclear medicine technology, with information on credentialing, continuing education and licensure requirements, as well as current news and updates on the field.
*Quarterly*
*Kathy S. Thomas, MHA, CNMT, PET, Editor-in-Chief*
*Susan Alexander, Associate Director, Publications*

1538 **Journal of the Neurological Sciences**
Elsevier
LSU Health Sciences Center JNS_England@lsuhsc.edu
New Orleans, LA 70112 www.jns-journal.com
Original articles in neurology and neuroscience from around the world.
*Monthly*
*John D. England, Editor-in-Chief*

1539 **Molecular Imaging**
Sage Journals
2455 Teller Road 805-499-9774
Thousand Oaks, CA 91320 journals@sagepub.com
journals.sagepub.com/home/mix
Peer-reviewed open access journal focusing on molecular imaging research, including basic science, preclinical studies and human applications. Published in association with the Society of Nuclear Medicine and Molecular Imaging.
*Bimonthly*
*Henry F. VanBrocklin, PhD, Editor-in-Chief*

1540 **Molecular Neurodegeneration**
Springer Nature
One New York Plaza 800-777-4643
New York, NY 10004-1562 info@biomedcentral.com
www.biomedcentral.com
A peer-reviewed, open-access journal devoted to all aspects of neurodegeneration research at the molecular and cellular levels.
*Guojun Bu, Editor-in-Chief*
*Huaxi Xu, Editor-in-Chief*

1541 **Neurocase: The Neural Basis of Cognition**
Taylor & Francis Group
530 Walnut Street www.tandfonline.com/toc/nncs20/current
Philadelphia, PA 19106
Rapid response journal featuring case and group studies in neuropsychology, neuropsychiatry and behavioral neurology, with a focus on the neural basis of cognition.
*Bruce L. Miller, Editor*
*Hans J. Markowitsch, Editor*

1542 **Neurology**
American Academy of Neurology
201 Chicago Avenue 612-928-6000
Minneapolis, MN 55415 800-879-1960
Fax: 612-454-2748
journal@neurology.org
n.neurology.org
Official journal of the American Academy of Neurology, peer-reviewed, highlighting clinical neurology research.
*Jose G. Merino, MD, MPhil, FAAN, Editor-in-Chief*
*Patricia K. Baskin, MS, Executive Editor*

1543 **Neurology Clinical Practice**
American Academy of Neurology
201 Chicago Avenue 612-928-6000
Minneapolis, MN 55415 800-879-1960
Fax: 612-454-2748
journal@neurology.org
cp.neurology.org
Official peer-reviewed journal of the American Academy of Neurology for practicing neurologists.
*John R. Corboy, MD, FAAN, Editor*
*Patricia K. Baskin, MS, Executive Editor*

1544 **Neurology: Genetics**
American Academy of Neurology
201 Chicago Avenue 612-928-6000
Minneapolis, MN 55415 800-879-1960
Fax: 612-454-2748
journal@neurology.org
ng.neurology.org
Official journal of the American Academy of Neurology, publishing online open-access peer-reviewed reports in the field of neurogenetics.
*Stefan M. Pulst, MD, FAAN, Editor*
*Patricia K. Baskin, MS, Executive Editor*

1545 **Neurology: Neuroimmunology & Neuroinflammation**
American Academy of Neurology
201 Chicago Avenue 612-928-6000
Minneapolis, MN 55415 800-879-1960
Fax: 612-454-2748
journal@neurology.org
nn.neurology.org
Official journal of the American Academy of Neurology, publishing online open-access peer-reviewed reports of original research and in-depth reviews of topics in neuroimmunology & neuroinflammation.
*Josep O. Dalmau, MD, PhD, Editor*
*Patricia K. Baskin, MS, Executive Editor*

1546 **Society of Nuclear Medicine and Molecular Imaging**
1850 Samuel Morse Drive 703-708-9000
Reston, VA 20190 Fax: 703-708-9015
feedback@snmmi.org
www.snmmi.org
The mission of this nonprofit scientific and professional organization is to promote the science, technology and application of nuclear medicine and molecular imaging. Molecular imaging techniques are used to diagnose and manage the treatment of brain disorders such as Alzheimer's and Parkinson's disease, among other conditions.
*15,000 members*
*Virginia Pappas, CEO*
*Rebecca Maxey, Director, Communications*

1547 **Translational Neurodegeneration**
Springer Nature
One New York Plaza 800-777-4643
New York, NY 10004-1562 info@biomedcentral.com
www.biomedcentral.com
A peer-reviewed, open-access journal covering research, therapeutics and education for all areas of neurodegenerative diseases.
*Shengdi Chen, Editor-in-Chief*

1548 **Ultrasonic Imaging**
Sage Journals
2455 Teller Road 805-499-9774
Thousand Oaks, CA 91320 journals@sagepub.com
journals.sagepub.com/home/uix
The journal focuses on the rapid publication of original papers on the development and application of ultrasonic techniques, with

emphasis on medical diagnosis. Also published are research notes, comments on papers appearing in the journal, book reviews, and occasional review articles.
*Ernest J. Feleppa, Editor-in-Chief*
*Roslyn Raskin, Managing Editor*

1549 **eNeuro**
Society for Neuroscience
1121 14th Street NW 202-312-7305
Washginton, DC 20005 eNeuro@sfn.org
www.eneuro.org
Open-access journal of the Society for Neuroscience.
*Christophe Bernard, Editor-in-Chief*
*Kelly Newton, Director, Scientific Publications*

## Web Sites

1550 **BrainFacts.org**
Society for Neuroscience
1121 14th Street NW brainfactsinfo@sfn.org
Washington, DC 20005 brainfacts.org
Online public information portal founded by the Kavli Foundation, the Gatsby Charitable Foundation and the Society for Neuroscience, with topics on brain function and anatomy, diseases and disorders, and more.
*Richard Wingate, DPhil, Editor-in-Chief*
*Charles Yokoyama, PhD, Associate Editor*

1551 **Neuronline**
Society for Neuroscience
1121 14th Street NW 202-962-4000
Washginton, DC 20005 neuronline@sfn.org
neuronline.sfn.org
Online portal for professional development and training resources for individuals in the field of neuroscience, hosted by the Society for Neuroscience.
*Amanda Kimball, Director, Digital Learning*

# EMOTIONAL ISSUES

*The emotional issues tied to dementia can be divided into two categories: those that affect the patient and those that affect the patient's caregivers and loved ones. People suffering from dementia often exhibit a wide range of emotions, including negative feelings such as anger, anxiety, depression, fear, and loneliness. For caregivers and loved ones, the difficulty of seeing a family member or friend deteriorate can often have strong psychological effects, leading to feelings of depression and despair.*

As dementia patients lose neurons in parts of their brain, this leads to inevitable changes in behavior and often triggers uncontrollable emotions. Patients can often be moody or angry and often switch between behaviors very quickly so that one minute a patient is calm and the next, they are hurling angry insults. Although dementia affects different patients differently, common behaviors include suspiciousness, irritability, agitation, and depression. Some patients become completely apathetic and passive, losing interest in things they used to enjoy. Often, patients exhibit frustration because they can no longer do or remember the things they once could. They also may lose confidence in themselves and their abilities. Anywhere from 30 to 90 percent of dementia patients suffer from behavioral disorders.

For caregivers, who in the majority of cases are family members or other loved ones, the emotional burden can be immense. Care-giving is an all-encompassing pursuit. As the patient's mind, and inevitably, health begins to deteriorate caregivers often feel overwhelmed and defeated. Almost all caregivers experience sadness, anxiety, or loneliness at some point. Many experience clinical depression or an intense feeling of burnout.

There are many strategies that caregivers and loved ones can take to help them cope with the immense emotional burden of dementia. Reaching out to other family members or friends can help enormously, as can joining one of the many support groups that exist for caregivers. In addition, practicing meditation or yoga, exercising regularly, or talking with a therapist can aid caregivers in maintaining their mental and physical health. For those who can afford it, in-home help and day programs can relieve some of the burden. In many cases, antidepressants can be of great use is easing feelings of depression and anxiety.

## National Agencies & Associations

**1553 Action Autonomie**
3958 Rue Dandurand
Montreal, Quebec, H1X-1P7
514-525-5060
Fax: 514-525-5580
lecollectif@actionautonomie.qc.ca
www.actionautonomie.qc.ca
Community organization for individuals with mental illness who unite their efforts collectively in order to defend their rights. Action Autonomie educates others on their rights while navigating the mental health care system.

**1554 American Association on Intellectual and Developmental Disabilities**
8403 Colesville Road
Silver Spring, MD 20910
202-387-1968
Fax: 202-387-2193
mnygren@aaidd.org
www.aamr.org
Promotes progressive policies, scientific research, effective practices and universal human rights for people with intellectual and developmental disabilities.
*Margaret A. Nygren, EdD, Executive Director & CEO*

**1555 American Psychiatric Association**
800 Maine Avenue SW
Washington, DC 20024
202-559-3900
apa@psych.org
www.psychiatry.org
A medical specialty society representing a growing membership of psychiatrists. Offers information for psychiatrists, medical students, patients and families.

**1556 American Psychological Association**
750 First Street NE
Washington, DC 20002-4242
202-336-5500
800-374-2721
TTY: 202-336-6123
www.apa.org
Advancing the creation, communication and application of psychological knowledge to benefit society and improve people's lives.
*Rosie Phillips Davis, PhD, President*
*Jean A. Carter, PhD, Treasurer*

**1557 Canadian Federation of Mental Health Nurses**
7270 Woodbine Avenue
Markham, Ontario, L3R-4B9
www.cfmhn.ca
A national voice for psychiatric and mental health nurses in Canada, providing resources relevant to the field.
*Florence Budden, President*
*Sherette Currie, Director of Membership*

**1558 Canadian Mental Health Association (CMHA)**
250 Dundas Street W
Toronto, Ontario, M5T-2Z5
416-646-5557
info@cmha.ca
www.cmha.ca
Promotes the mental health of all and supports the recovery of people experiencing mental illness.

**1559 Community Access, Inc.**
17 Battery Place
New York, NY 10004
212-780-1400
www.communityaccess.org
A non-profit agency providing housing and advocacy for people with disabilities.
*Stephen H. Chase, President*
*Dan Wurtzel, Vice President*

**1560 Goodwill Industries International, Inc.**
15810 Indianola Drive
Rockville, MD 20855
800-466-3945
contactus@goodwill.org
www.goodwill.org
A nonprofit, community-based organization whose mission is to help people achieve self-sufficiency through the dignity and power of work, serving people who are disadvantaged, disabled or elderly. The mission is accomplished through providing independent living skills, affordable housing, and training and placement in community employment. The GoodWill Network includes 160 independent, local locations across the U.S. and Canada.
*S. Dale Jenkins, Chair*
*Steven C. Preston, President & CEO*

**1561 Mental Health America**
500 Montgomery Street
Alexandria, VA 22314
703-684-7722
800-969-6642
Fax: 703-684-5968
www.mentalhealthamerica.net
Formerly known as the National Mental Health Association, Mental Health America is committed to helping all people live mentally healthier lives by promoting awareness of mental health.
*340+ Members*
*Tom Starling, EdD, Chair*
*Jennifer L. Bright, MPA, Secretary & Treasurer*

**1562 National Alliance for Hispanic Health**
1501 16th Street NW
Washington, DC 20036-1401
866-783-2645
www.healthyamericas.org
Members are Spanish-speaking mental health professionals and patients and those interested in services and decision-making that consider culture and community.
*Augustine Chris Baca, MPA, Chairperson*
*Jane L. Delgado, PhD, MS, President & CEO*

**1563 National Alliance on Mental Illness (NAMI)**
3803 N Fairfax Drive
Arlington, VA 22203
703-524-7600
800-950-6264
info@nami.org
www.nami.org
Committed to building better lives for the millions of Americans affected by mental illness by raising awareness and offering community support.
*Adrienne Kennedy, MA, President*
*Lacey Berumen, PhD, LAC, MNM, First Vice President*

**1564 National Association of State Mental Health Program Directors**
66 Canal Center Plaza
Alexandria, VA 22314
703-739-9333
Fax: 703-548-9517
www.nasmhpd.org
Offers referrals to state mental health programs, services and physicians for persons with mental illness.
*Brian Hepburn, MD, Executive Director*
*Aaron J. Walker, MPA, Senior Policy Associate*

**1565 National Council for Behavioral Health**
1400 K Street NW
Washington, DC 20005
202-684-7457
communications@thenationalcouncil.org
www.thenationalcouncil.org
Represents community mental health centers working on Capitol Hill to ensure funding for community mental health services. Offers technical support and guidance and serves as a liaison with state organizations and other mental health related organizations.
*Linda Rosenberg, MSW, President & CEO*
*Jeannie Campbell, Executive Vice President & COO*

**1566 National Institute of Mental Health**
6001 Executive Boulevard
Rockville, MD 20852-9663
866-615-6464
Fax: 301-443-4279
TTY: 866-415-8051
nimhinfo@nih.gov
www.nimh.nih.gov
The National Institute of Mental Health works to transform the understanding and treatment of mental illnesses through basic and clinical research, paving the way for prevention, recovery, and cure.
*Joshua A. Gordon, MD, PhD, Director*

**1567 Option Institute**
2080 South Undermountain Road
Sheffield, MA 01257
413-229-2100
800-714-2779
Fax: 413-229-8931
participantsupport@option.org
www.option.org
Self-defeating beliefs, along with attitudes and judgments, can lead to a host of physical and psychological challenges. The Option Institute offers programs designed to help people gain new perspectives on the attitudes and judgments that may be affecting their lives.
*Barry Kaufman, Co-Founder*
*Samahria Lyte Kaufman, Co-Founder*

1568 **The Coalition of Behavioral Health**
123 William Street 212-742-1600
New York, NY 10038 Fax: 212-742-2080
jalvarez@coalitionny.org
www.coalitionny.org

An advocacy organization of New York's mental health community representing over 100 non-profit community health agencies that serve clients in the five boroughs of New York City.
*Amanda Saake, Director*
*Marlo Pasion, Associate Director*

1569 **World Federation for Mental Health**
PO Box 807 Fax: 703-490-6926
Occoquan, VA 22125 info@wfmh.com
www.wfmh.com

International organization dedicated to improving the care and treatment of individuals with mental disorders, and raising public awareness and understanding of mental health.
*Alberto Trimboli, President*
*Janet Paleo, Treasurer*

## State Agencies & Associations

1570 **All Access Mental Health**
Information
819 Alexander Road 609-452-2088
Princeton, NJ 08540 Fax: 609-452-0627
info@aamh.org
www.aamh.org

This organization was founded to create a permanent community support system for mentally ill and developmentally disabled adults and their families living in the Greater Mercer County area of New Jersey.
*Cynthia Murphy, President*
*Lauren Murphy, Vice-President*

1571 **Alliance for the Mentally Ill in Delaware (AMID)**
2400 W 4th Street 302-427-0787
Wilmington, DE 19805-3306 888-427-2643
Fax: 302-427-2075
namide@namide.org
www.namide.org

*Mary Berger, President*
*John P Smoots, Treasurer*

1572 **Community Mental Health Foundation**
610 Industrial Avenue 201-986-5070
Paramus, NJ 07652 Fax: 201-265-3543
*Perrin, President*
*Sylvia Axelrod, Executive Director*

1573 **DC Threshold Alliance for the Mentally Ill**
422 8th Street SE 202-546-0646
Washington, DC 20003-2832 Fax: 202-546-6817
www.nami.org/MSTemplate.cfm?MicrositeID=
*Lois Fitzgerald, President*
*Mary J DiPietro, Secretary*

1574 **Families Together in New York State**
737 Madison Avenue 518-432-0333
Albany, NY 12209 888-326-8644
Fax: 518-434-6478
info@ftnys.org
www.ftnys.org

*Vicky McCarthy, President*
*Paige Pierce, Executive Director*

1575 **Families United For CMH, Inc.**
PO Box 151 860-537-6125
New London, CT 06320 Fax: 860-537-6130
www.familiesunited.org

*Morgan Correll, President*
*Sheila King, Executive Director*

1576 **Family Action Network**
PO Box 322 765-643-4357
Winnetka, IN 60093-2206 info@familyactionnetwork.net
www.familyactionnetwork.net

*Susan Rooney, Co-Chair*
*Lonnie Stonitsch, Co-Chair*

1577 **Family Advocacy and Support Association**
PO Box 74884 202-234-2325
Washington, DC 20056 Fax: 202-576-7154
*Lynne M Gladysz, Chair*
*R Lee Waits, President*

1578 **Family Support Network**
1002 10th Street W 406-256-7783
Billings, MT 59102 877-376-4850
Fax: 406-256-9879
www.mtfamilysupport.org

*Barbara Milhelish, President*
*Matt Kuntz, Executive Director*

1579 **Florida Alliance for the Mentally Ill**
1030 E. Lafayette Street 850-671-4445
Tallahassee, FL 32301-2646 877-626-4352
Fax: 850-671-5272
Info@namiflorida.org
www.namiflorida.org

*James Sleeper, President*
*Judith Evans, Executive Director*

1580 **Georgia Alliance for the Mentally Ill**
3050 Presidential Drive 770-234-0855
Atlanta, GA 30340-3916 800-728-1052
Fax: 770-234-0237
namigeorgia@namiga.org
www.namiga.org

*Bill Kissel, President*
*Eric Spencer, Executive Director*

1581 **Goodwill Industries-Suncoast**
10596 Gandy Boulevard 727-523-1512
St. Petersburg, FL 33702 888-279-1988
TTY: 727-579-1068
www.goodwill-suncoast.org

A nonprofit, community-based organization whose mission is to help people achieve self-sufficiency through the dignity and power of work, serving people who are disadvantaged, disabled or elderly. The mission is accomplished through providing independent living skills, affordable housing, and training and placement in community employment.
*Heather Ceresoli, CPA, Chair*
*Deborah A. Passerini, President & CEO*

1582 **Idaho Alliance for the Mentally Ill**
4097 Bottle Bay Road 208-242-7430
Sagle, ID 83860-0068 800-572-9940
Fax: 208-673-6685
namiidaho@yahoo.com
www.nami.org/MSTemplate.cfm?MicrositeID=
*Douglas McKnight, President*
*Tom Hanson, Vice President*

1583 **Illinois Alliance for the Mentally Ill**
218 W Lawrence Avenue 217-522-1403
Springfield, IL 62704-2612 800-346-4572
Fax: 217-522-3598
namiil@sbcglobal.net
il.nami.org

*Hugh Brady, President*
*Brian Allen, Vice President*

1584 **Illinois Federation of Families**
PO Box 413 847-265-0500
McHenry, IL 60051 800-871-8400
Fax: 847-265-0501
www.iffcmh.net

*Cynthia Hamilton*

1585 **JIMHO Affiliated Centers (Justice in Mental Health Organization)**
520 Cherry Street
Lansing, MI 48933
517-371-2221
800-831-8035
Fax: 517-371-5770
brwellwood@aol.com
www.jimho.org
JIMHO advocates for the rights and dignity that all people suffering from mental or emotional illness deserve.
*Huebl, President*
*Sharon Solomon, Executive Director*

1586 **Kentucky Alliance for the Mentally Ill**
808 Monticello Street
Somerset, KY 42501-1277
606-451-6935
800-257-5081
Fax: 606-677-4052
namiky@nami.org
www.nami.org/MSTemplate.cfm?micrositeID=
*Wendy Morris, Chair*
*Bertha Diaz-Story, 1st Vice Chair*

1587 **Louisiana Alliance for the Mentally Ill**
5534 Galeria Drive
Baton Rouge, LA 70816-2398
225-291-6262
800-437-0303
Fax: 225-926-8773
info@namilouisiana.org
www.namilouisiana.org
*Stephanie Boyd, President*
*Mitch Bergeron, Vice President*

1588 **MO-SPAN**
440 Rue Saint Francois
Florissant, MO 63031
314-972-0600
Fax: 314-972-0606
www.mo-span.org
*Donna Dittrich, Executive Director*
*Tina VarVera, Administrative Assistant*

1589 **Maine Alliance for the Mentally Ill**
1 Bangor Street
Augusta, ME 04330-4701
207-622-5767
800-464-5767
Fax: 207-621-8430
info@namimaine.org
www.namimaine.org
*Valerie Gamache, President*
*Cathy Kidman, Interim Executive Director*

1590 **Massachusetts Alliance for the Mentally Ill**
400 W Cummings Park
Woburn, MA 01801-6528
781-938-4048
800-370-9085
Fax: 781-938-4069
helpline@namimass.org
www.namimass.org
*Lynda Cutrell, President*
*Laurie Martinelli, Executive Director*

1591 **Mental Health Association of Delaware**
100 W 10th Street
Wilmington, DE 19801
302-654-6833
800-287-6423
Fax: 302-654-6838
jlafferty@mhainde.org
www.mhainde.org
*Janet M Brown, President*
*James Lafferty, Executive Director*

1592 **Michigan Alliance for the Mentally Ill**
921 N Washington Avenue
Lansing, MI 48906-5137
517-485-4049
800-331-4264
Fax: 517-485-2333
namimichigan@acd.net
mi.nami.org
*Hubert Lloyd, President*
*Sue Abderholden, Executive Director*

1593 **Minnesota Alliance for the Mentally Ill**
800 Transfer Road
Saint Paul, MN 55114-1146
651-645-2948
888-NAM-IHEL
Fax: 651-645-7379
namihelps@namimn.org
www.namihelps.org
*Barb Lindberg, President*
*Sue Abderholden, Executive Director*

1594 **Mississippi Alliance for the Mentally Ill**
411 Briarwood Drive
Jackson, MS 39206-3058
601-899-9058
800-357-0388
Fax: 601-956-6380
stateoffice@namims.org
www.namims.org/
*Debbie Waller, President*
*Hank Rainer, Vice President*

1595 **Mississippi Families as Allies**
5166 Keele Street
Jackson, MS 39206
601-355-0915
800-833-9671
Fax: 601-355-0919
info@msfaacmh.org
www.msfaacmh.org
*Joy Hogge, PhD, Executive Director*
*Cynthia Moore-Hardy, MS, Director of Respite Services*

1596 **Missouri Coalition Alliance for the Mentally Ill**
230 W Dunklin Street
Jefferson City, MO 65101-3260
573-634-7727
800-374-2138
Fax: 573-761-5636
Keele@aol.com
*Keele, Executive Director*
*Karren Jones, President*

1597 **Montana Alliance for the Mentally Ill Mihelish's Residence**
Mihelish's Residence
616 Helena Avenue
Helena, MT 59601-6946
406-443-7871
888-280-6264
Fax: 406-862-6352
info@namimt.org
www.namimt.org
*Matt Kuntz, Executive Director*
*Carole Denton, President*

1598 **NAMI Arkansas**
1012 Autumn Road
Little Rock, AR 72211-2222
501-661-1548
800-844-0381
Fax: 501-312-7540
nami-ar@namiarkansas.org
www.nami.org
Grassroots organization that focuses on improving mental health services. The mission is three prong: Support, Education, and Advocacy. Support Group meetings are held at 11 locations across the state.
*Rick Scott, First Vice President*
*Karen H Henry, President*

1599 **NAMI California**
1851 Heritage Lane
Sacramento, CA 95815-3218
916-567-0163
Fax: 916-567-1757
nami.california@namicalifornia.org
www.namicalifornia.org
*Dorothy Hendrickson, President*
*Jessica Cruz, Executive Director*

1600 **NAMI Indiana**
PO Box 22697
Indianapolis, IN 46222-0697
317-925-9399
800-677-6442
Fax: 317-925-9398
info@namiindiana.org
www.namiindiana.org/
Grass roots advocacy support and educational group for families affected by severe and persistent mental illnesses.
*Joshua G Sprunger, Executive Director*
*Joanne Abbott, Program Director*

1601 **NAMI Iowa: National Alliance on Mental Illness**
5911 Meredith Drive
Des Moines, IA 50322-1903
515-254-0417
800-417-0417
Fax: 515-254-1103
www.namiiowa.com
*Dawn Adams*

1602 **NAMI Kansas: Kansas' Voice on Mental Illness**
610 SW 10th Ave 785-233-0755
Topeka, KS 66612-0675 800-539-2660
Fax: 785-233-4804
info@namikansas.org
www.nami.org/MSTemplate.cfm?Site=NAMI_Ka
*John Brennan, President*
*Mr Richard D Cagan, Executive Director*

1603 **NAMI South Dakota**
PO Box 88808 605-271-1871
Sioux Falls, SD 57109-1204 800-551-2531
Fax: 605-271-1871
namisd@midconetwork.com
*Shelly Jablonski, President*
*Sita Diehl, Executive Director*

1604 **NAMI Washington (National Alliance for the Mentally Ill of Washington)**
7500 Greenwood Avenue North 206-783-4288
Seattle, WA 98103-5580 800-782-9264
office@namiwa.org
www.namiwa.org/
Advocacy, support and education for the mentally ill, their families and friends.
*Gordon Bopp, President*
*Jim Bloss, Vice President*

1605 **NAMI West Virginia**
PO Box 2706 304-342-0497
Charleston, WV 25330-2706 800-598-5653
Fax: 304-342-0499
namiwv@aol.com
Educational advocacy and support for families consumers and friends of people with mental illnesses.
*Randal Rutkowski, Co-President*
*Terence Schnapp, Interim Executive Director*

1606 **NAMI of Missouri**
1001 SW Boulevard 573-634-7727
Jefferson City, MO 65109-2501 800-374-2138
Fax: 573-761-5636
namimosjf@yahoo.com
www.nami.org/MSTemplate.cfm?MicrositeID=
A nonprofit education adudcacy, referal and support organization serving people with mental illness and their families.
*12 pages newsletter*
*Cinda Holloway, President and Chairman*
*Cindi Keele, Executive Director*

1607 **NAMI-Oregon**
4701 SE 24th Avenue 503-230-8009
Portland, OR 97202-1552 800-343-6264
Fax: 503-230-2751
namioregon@namior.org
www.nami.org/MSTemplate.cfm?Site=NAMI_Or
Providing support education and advocacy for people with biological mental illness and their families. The in-state 800 phone number is Oregon's NAMI-Line. Callers to this line are provided with information about mental illnesses and referrals to support and treatment services.
*Chris Bouneff, Executive Director*
*Michelle Madison, Events Manager/Outreach Coordinator*

1608 **NAMI-SC: National Alliance on Mental Illness: South Carolina**
PO BOX 1267 803-733-9592
Columbia, SC 29202-1267 800-788-5131
Fax: 803-733-9593
namisc@namisc.org
www.namisc.org
Advocacy, Education and Support
*Joan Herbert, MS, President*
*Bill Lindsey, Executive Director*

1609 **NAMI: The Local Affiliate of the National Alliance for the Mentally Ill**
770 Kapiolani Boulevard 808-591-1297
Honolulu, HI 96813-2025 Fax: 808-591-2058
info@namihawaii.org
namihawaii.org
Members include consumers families health professionals and interested persons/organizations. Programs include advocacy support and education and are free and open to the public. Office has lending library of books and videos. Newsletter is published.
*6 pages Quarterly*
*Carol Kozlovich, President*
*Kathleen Hasegawa, Executive Director*

1610 **National Alliance for the Mentally Ill of Colorado**
2280 S Albion Street 303-321-3104
Denver, CO 80222-3334 888-566-6264
Fax: 303-321-0912
admin@namicolorado.org
www.namicolorado.org
The National Alliance for the Mentally Ill Of Colorado is a statewide, grassroots, nonprofit organization whose mission is; To give strength and hope to individuals with mental illness and their families.
*Greg C Coleman, President*
*Scott Glaser, Executive Director*

1611 **National Alliance for the Mentally Ill of Connecticut**
576 Farmington Avenue 860-882-0236
Hartford, CT 06105 800-215-3021
Fax: 860-882-0240
membership@namict.org
www.namict.org
*Kate Mattias, Executive Director*

1612 **National Alliance for the Mentally Ill: Maryland**
10630 Little Patuxent Parkway 410-884-8691
Columbia, MD 21044-4486 877-878-2371
Fax: 410-884-8695
amimd@aol.com
md.nami.org
*Chris Griffin, President*
*Kate Farinholt, Executive Director*

1613 **National Alliance on Mental Illness of Alabama: NAMI Alabama**
1401 I-85 Parkway 334-396-4797
Montgomery, AL 36106-1902 800-626-4199
Fax: 334-396-4794
wlaird@namialabama.org
www.namialabama.org
*Will O'Rear, President*
*Sue Guffey, 1st Vice President*

1614 **Nevada Alliance for the Mentally Ill**
2251 N Rampart Boulevard 702-310-5764
Las Vegas, NV 89128 Fax: 775-329-1618
*Joe Abate*

1615 **New Jersey Alliance for the Mentally Ill**
1562 Route 130 732-940-0991
N Brunswick, NJ 08902-3004 Fax: 732-940-0355
info@naminj.org
www.naminj.org
*Mark Perrin, MD, President*
*Sylvia Axelrod, Executive Director*

1616 **New Mexico Alliance for the Mentally Ill**
8015 Mountain Rd NE 505-260-0154
Albuquerque, NM 87110-3086 Fax: 505-260-0342
naminm@aol.com
www.nami.org/MSTemplate.cfm?MicrositeID=
*Patricia D Romero, President*

1617 **New York Alliance for the Mentally Ill**
99 Pine Street 518-462-2000
Albany, NY 12207 800-950-3228
Fax: 518-462-3811
info@naminys.org
www.naminys.org
*Thomas Easterly, President*
*Paul A Capofari, 1st Vice President*

1618 **North Dakota Alliance for the Mentally Ill**
PO Box 3215 701-770-8063
Minot, ND 58702-6016 Fax: 701-725-4334
l.lund8@hotmail.com
www.namind.org/
*Linda Lund, President*

1619 **Ohio Alliance for the Mentally Ill**
1225 Dublin Road 614-224-2700
Columbus, OH 43215 800-686-2646
Fax: 614-224-5400
TTY: 866-924-1478
namiohio@namiohio.org
www.namiohio.org
*Bob Spada, President*
*Terry Russell, Executive Director*

1620 **Oklahoma Alliance for the Mentally Ill**
4200 Perimeter Drive 405-230-1900
Oklahoma City, OK 73112-6200 800-583-1264
Fax: 405-230-1903
namiok@coxinet.net
www.namioklahoma.org/
*Paula Walker, President*
*Traci Cook, Executive Director*

1621 **Oregon Family Support Network**
1300 Broadway Street 503-363-8068
Salem, OR 97301 800-323-8521
Fax: 503-390-3161
www.ofsn.org
*David De Fiebre, Board President*
*Sandy Bumpus, Executive Director*

1622 **Pennsylvania Alliance for the Mentally Ill**
2149 N 2nd Street 717-238-1514
Harrisburg, PA 17011-1005 800-223-0500
Fax: 717-238-4390
TTY: 800-890-6093
nami-pa@nami-pa.org
www.nami-pa.org/
*Suzanne Vogel-Scibilia, M.D, President*
*James W Jordan, Jr, Executive Director*

1623 **Tennessee Alliance for the Mentally Ill**
1101 Kermit Drive 615-361-6608
Nashville, TN 37217-2126 800-467-3589
Fax: 615-361-6698
rpbaxter@comcast.net
www.namitn.org
*Dick Baxter, President*
*Jeff Fladen, Executive Director*

1624 **Texas Alliance for the Mentally Ill**
Foundtain Park Plaza III 512-693-2000
Austin, TX 78704 800-633-3760
Fax: 512-693-8000
kjeschke@namitexas.org
www.namitexas.org
*Andrea Hazlitt, Board President*
*Ed Dickey, Vice President*

1625 **Utah Alliance for the Mentally Ill**
1600 West 2200 South 801-323-9900
West Valley City, UT 84119-1701 877-230-6264
Fax: 801-323-9799
rebecca@namiut.org
www.namiut.org
*Zara Juillerat, President*
*Rebecca Glathar, Executive Director*

1626 **Vermont Alliance for the Mentally Ill**
162 S Main Street 802-244-1396
Waterbury, VT 05676-1519 800-639-6480
Fax: 802-244-1405
info@namivt.org
www.nami.org/MSTemplate.cfm?Site=NAMI_Ve
*Karen Kelley, Chair*
*Wendy Beinner, President/CEO*

1627 **Virginia Alliance for the Mentally Ill**
PO Box 8260 804-285-8264
Richmond, VA 23226-1903 888-486-8264
Fax: 804-285-8464
namiva@verizon.net
www.namivirginia.org/
*Robert Cluck, President*
*Mira Signer, Executive Director*

1628 **Wisconsin Alliance for the Mentally Ill**
4233 W Beltline Highway 608-268-6000
Madison, WI 53711-3814 800-236-2988
Fax: 608-268-6004
nami@namiwisconsin.org
www.namiwisconsin.org
*Jim Connors, President*
*Julianne Carbin, Executive Director*

1629 **Wisconsin Family Ties**
16 N Carroll Street 608-267-6888
Madison, WI 53703 800-422-7145
Fax: 608-267-6801
info@wifamilyties.org
www.wifamilyties.org
*Hugh Johnson, President*
*Deion Hagemeister, Vice-President*

1630 **Wyoming Alliance for the Mentally Ill**
133 W 6th Street 307-265-2573
Casper, WY 82601-3124 888-882-4968
Fax: 307-234-0440
www.namiwyoming.org/
*Marty Coe, President*
*Tammy Noel, Executive Director*

## Libraries & Resource Centers

1631 **Alta Bates Summit Medical Center**
2001 Dwight Way 510-204-4444
Berkeley, CA 94704-2608 www.altabatessummit.org/
Alta Bates Summit Medical Center has made community healthcare a priority. We are proud of our many areas of clinical excellence including cardiovascular, behavioral health, women and infants, orthopedics, rehabilitation, and oncology care.
*Carolyn McGee, Medical Librarian*

1632 **Central Louisiana State Hospital Medical and Professional Library**
242 West Shamrock Street 318-484-6363
Pineville, LA 71360 Fax: 318-484-6284
bentonmcgee@hotmail.com
The Consortium was established to increase and better utilize the health information resources of Central Louisiana. Information offered on psychiatry, psychology and mental health.
*Carol Rogers, Director*

1633 **National Mental Health Consumer's Self-Help Clearinghouse**
1211 Chestnut Street 267-507-3810
Philadelphia, PA 19107 800-553-4539
Fax: 215-636-6312
info@mhselfhelp.org
www.mhselfhelp.org
The National Mental Health Consumers' Self-Help Clearinghouse, the nation's first national consumer technical assistance center, has played a major role in the development of the mental health consumer movement. The consumer movement strives for dignity, respect, and opportunity for those with mental illnesses.
*Joseph Rogers, Executive Director*
*Susan Rogers, Director*

## Foundations & Research Centers

1634 **Anxiety Disorders Center University of Wisconsin**
University of Wisconsin
Department of Psychiatry 608-263-6100
Madison, WI 53719-0001

Provides evaluation and treatment for individuals suffering from anxiety disorders as well as training and education for clinicians.
*Andy Alexander, PhD, Professor*
*Ruth Benca, MD, PhD, Professor*

**1635 Central Louisiana State Hospital Medical and Professional Library**
242 West Shamrock Street 318-484-6363
Pineville, LA 71360 Fax: 318-484-6284
bentonmcgee@hotmail.com
The Consortium was established to increase and better utilize the health information resources of Central Louisiana. Information offered on psychiatry, psychology and mental health.
*Carol Rogers, Director*

**1636 Institute of Psychiatry and Human Behavior: University of Maryland**
655 West Baltimore Street 410-706-7410
Baltimore, MD 21201-1542 Fax: 410-706-0235
alehman@psych.umaryland.edu
www.medschool.umaryland.edu
Studies in psychiatric disorders.
*Anthony Lehm MD, Director*
*Craig Vantyke, Chief Executive Officer*

**1637 Jane & Terry Semel Institute for Neuroscience & Human Behavior**
Neuropsychiatric Institute
760 Westwood Plaza 310-825-2631
Los Angeles, CA 90095 800-825-9989
www.semel.ucla.edu
Studies behavior disorders and psychosocial adaptation and the future.
*Peter Whybrow, Director*
*Fawzy Fawzy, Associate Director*

**1638 Langley Porter Psychiatric Institute University of California**
University of California
401 Parnassus Avenue 415-476-7365
San Francisco, CA 94143-9911 www.universityofcalifornia.edu
Conducts clinical studies of psychiatric disorders.
*Samuel Barno Faucher, Director*

**1639 Medical College of Pennsylvania: Eastern Psychiatric Institute**
3200 Henry Avenue 215-842-6990
Philadelphia, PA 19129-1137
Offers research into all aspects of mental illness.
*Michael Spohn, Director*

**1640 Menninger Clinic: Department of Research**
12301 S. Main Street 713-275-5140
Houston, TX 77035-0829 800-351-9058
Fax: 785-350-5392
www.menningerclinic.com/
Focuses research on mental illness and mental health issues.
*B. Christoph Frueh, PhD, Director of Clinical Research*
*Chris Fowler, PhD, Associate Director of Clinical Research*

**1641 Mental Illness Research and Education Institute**
Eastern State Hospital
PO Box 800 509-299-3121
Medical Lake, WA 99022-800 Fax: 509-997-15
Governmental organization focusing on mental illness research.
*Harold David, Director*

**1642 NIH Clinical Center**
National Institute of Health
9000 Rockville Pike 301-496-4000
Bethesda, MD 20892 800-411-1222
Fax: 301-402-2984
TTY: 866-411-1010
prpl@mail.cc.nih.gov
www.cc.nih.gov
Established in 1953 as the research hospital of the National Institutes of Health. Designed so that patient care facilities are close to research laboratories so new findings of basic and clinical scientists can be quickly applied to the treatment of patients. Upon referral by physicians patients are admitted to NIH clinical studies.
*John I Gallin, MD, Clinical Center Director*
*David Henderson, MD, Deputy Director for Clinical Care*

**1643 State University of New York at Stony Brook: Mental Health Research**
450 Clarkson Avenue 718-270-1270
Brooklyn, NY 11203-2056 www.stonybrook.edu
*Benjamin S Hsiao, Phd, Vice President for Research*

**1644 University of Michigan: Mental Health Research Institute**
205 Washtenaw Place 734-763-1817
Ann Arbor, MI 48109 UMresearch@umich.edu
www.umich.edu
Focuses on the diagnosis treatment and prevention of mental illnesses and disorders.
*Dr Bernard Schulz, Chair of Psychiatry*

**1645 University of Minnesota Department of Psychiatry**
420 Delaware Street SE 612-624-2430
Minneapolis, MN 55455-374 Fax: 612-265-91
www.umn.edu
Behavior and mental illness research.
*S Charles PhD, Director*

**1646 University of Missouri: Columbia Missouri Institute of Mental Health**
5247 Fyler Avenue 573-634-8787
Saint Louis, MO 63139-1300 Fax: 314-644-8834
Mental health policy and ethics studies.
*Danny Weddin MD, Director*

**1647 University of Pittsburgh: Western Psychiatric Institute & Clinic**
3811 Ohara Street 412-246-6356
Pittsburgh, PA 15213-2593 Fax: 412-246-6350
reitzpm@msx.upmc.edu
www.pitt.edu
Advancement of basic and clinical knowledge in mental health and psychiatric care.
*Thomas Detre Camarata, Acting Director*

**1648 Vanderbilt Kennedy Center**
Vanderbilt University
110 Magnolia Center 615-322-8240
Nashville, TN 37203-5701 Fax: 615-228-36
kc@vanderbilt.edu
Mental health research.
*Donna G Eskind, Chair*
*Cathy S Brown, Past Chair*

**1649 Veterans Medical Center: Mental Health Clinical Research Center**
3801 Miranda Avenue 650-858-3941
Palo Alto, CA 94304-1207 www.va.gov
*Jerome Gallin, Director*
*David Henderson, Deputy Director for Clinical Care*

**1650 Yeshiva University: Soundview-Throgs Neck Community Mental Health Center**
2527 Glebe Avenue 718-904-4400
Bronx, NY 10461-3109 Fax: 718-931-7307
Mental health mental illness and recovery from mental illness research.
*Dr Itamar , Director*

## Support Groups & Hotlines

**1651 Emotional Health Anonymous**
PO Box 4245 651-647-9712
St Paul, MN 55104-0245 Fax: 651-647-1593
www.emotionsanonymous.org
A twelve-step organization, similar to Alcoholics Anonymous. Compsed of people who come together in weekly meetings for the purpose of working toward recovery from emotional difficulties.
*Karen Mead, Executive Director*

1652 **Federation of Families of South Carolina**
810 Dutch Square Boulevard 803-772-5210
Columbia, SC 29210-2344 866-779-0402
Fax: 803-772-5212
FedFamSC@yahoo.com
www.fedfamsc.org/
*Kathleen Scharer, President*
*Roxann McKinnon, Vice President*

1653 **Florida Institute for Family Involvement ( FIFI)**
3927 Spring Creek Highway 305-293-7626
Crawfordville, FL 32327 877-926-3514
Fax: 863-582-9358
HewFLMOM@aol.com
Florida Institute for Family Involvement (FIFI), an affiliate of Federation of Families for Children's Mental Health (FFCMH), enhances, facilitates, and supports family and consumer involvement in the development of responsive, family centered, and community based systems of care. FIFI works in collaboration with state, federal, and private programs to develop a resource and training information center to enable individuals to advocate for appropriate services and make wise service choices.
*Connie Hawke, Co-Director*
*Tara Bremer, Co-Director*

1654 **Hawaii Families As Allies (HFAA)**
99-209 Moanalua Road 808-487-8785
Aiea, HI 96701 866-361-8825
Fax: 808-487-0514
hfaa@hfaa.net
www.hfaa.net/
Hawaii Families as Allies (HFAA) is a statewide parent-controlled family network organization that provides support, services and information for families of children and adolescents with emotional and/or behavioral challenges. HFAA is the Hawaii state chapter of the Federation of Families for Children's Mental Health, a national organization that advocates for service system change so that families are valued and treated as true partners.
*Linda Machado, Executive Director*
*Charlene Daraban, Family Resource Specialist*

1655 **KALEIDOSCOPE**
1340 S. Damen Avenue 773-278-7200
Chicago, IL 60608 Fax: 773-278-5663
TTY: 773-292-4086
info@kaleidoscope4kids.org
www.kaleidoscope4kids.org
*William J Binder, Chair*
*Ivy Walker, Vice Chairman-Secretary*

1656 **Kentucky IMPACT**
275 E Main Street 502-564-7610
Frankfort, KY 40621
*Sandra Welles, Executive Director*

1657 **Laradon Services for Children and Adults with Developmental Disabilities**
5100 Lincoln Street 303-296-2400
Denver, CO 80216 866-381-2163
Fax: 303-296-4012
TDD: 7209746821
www.laradon.org/
Laradon specializes in services to children and adults with developmental disabilities, operating 15 programs that are designed to help each individual develop to his or her fullest potential and maximize self-sufficiency.
*John Galvin, Chairman*
*Frank Lucero, PhD, Executive Director*

1658 **MOSPAN Northwest Region**
440 Rue Street Fran‡ois 314-972-0600
Jefferson City, MO 63031 Fax: 314-720-06
*Donna Taycher, Executive Director*

1659 **MOSPAN Southwest Region**
210 W Vine Street 660-679-5767
Butler, MO 64730
*Eldonna Dittrich, Executive Director*
*Tina Vervara, Administrative Assistant*

1660 **Mental Health Association in Dutchess County**
253 Mansion Street 845-473-2500
Poughkeepsie, NY 12601 Fax: 845-473-4870
www.mhadc.com/
The Mental Health Association in Dutchess County promotes mental well-being and advances the recovery from mental illness, provides rehabilitation programs and support services for adults with a history of mental illness and their families.
*Joseph Ellman, President*
*Andrew O'Grady, Executive Director*

1661 **Mental Health Association in Orange County**
Mental Health Association of Orange County
73 James P. Kelly Way 845-342-2400
Middletown, NY 10940-1906 800-832-1200
Fax: 845-343-9665
mha@mhaorangeny.com
www.mhaorangeny.com/
Mental Health Association of Orange County/MHA is a private, not-for-profit organization seeking to promote the mental health and emotional well being of Orange County residents. Under the leadership of a volunteer Board of Directors, MHA's staff members, consultants and volunteers provide free mental health services to thousands of Orange County residents each year. Several volunteers answer several hotlines, provide companionship, public education, direct services and assist with fundraisers.
*David Goggins, President*
*Nadia Allen, Executive Director*

1662 **NAMI Indiana - National Alliance on Mental Illness**
PO Box 22697 317-925-9399
Indianapolis, IN 46222-0697 800-677-6442
Fax: 317-925-9398
info@namiindiana.org
www.namiindiana.org
NAMI Indiana is a non-profit grassroots organization dedicated to improving the lives of people afflicted by serious and persistent mental illness. NAMI Indiana consists of families, consumers, and professionals that are dedicated to helping families through a network of support, education, advocacy, and promotion of research. NAMI Indiana is affiliated with the National Alliance on Mental Illness (NAMI), which is located in Arlington, Virginia.
*Joshua G Sprunger, Executive Director*
*Joanne Abbott, Program Director*

1663 **National Alliance for the Mentally Ill (NA MI) Alaska**
144 West 15th Avenue 907-227-1300
Anchorage, AK 99501-5106 800-478-4462
Fax: 907-227-1400
NAMI Alaska is a grassroots, 501(c)(3) nonprofit, support, educational and advocacy organization of consumers, families, and friends of people with severe brain disorders such as schizophrenia, schizo-affective disorder, bipolar disorder, major depressive disorder, obsessive-compulsive disorder, panic and anxiety disorders, and attention deficit/hyperactivity disorder. In addition, NAMI provides information and referral services and works with local media on stories about mental illness.
*Scott Owens, Co-President*
*Pat Dobbins, Co-President*

1664 **National Alliance for the Mentally Ill: New Hampshire**
85 North State Street 603-225-5359
Concord, NH 03301 800-242-6264
Fax: 603-228-8848
info@naminh.org
www.naminh.org
Family support and advocacy for consumers and family members.
*Michele Grennon, President*
*Ken Norton, Executive Director*

1665 **National Health Information Center**
Office of Disease Prevention & Health Promotion
1101 Wootton Pkwy Fax: 240-453-8281
Rockville, MD 20852 odphpinfo@hhs.gov
www.health.gov/nhic
Supports public health education by maintaining a calendar of National Health Observances; helps connect consumers and health professionals to organizations that can best answer questions and provide up-to-date contact information from reliable sources; up-

dates on a yearly basis toll-free numbers for health information, Federal health clearinghouses and info centers.
*Don Wright, MD, MPH, Director*

1666 **Navajo Nation Office Special Education & Rehabilitation Services**
IHS PO Box 1337 505-722-1454
Gallup, NM 87301 Fax: 505-722-1554
osers@navajo.org
www.osers.navajo-nsn.gov/
Navajo OSERS is a program within the Division of DINE Education, which offers vocational rehabilitation to people with disabilities. Vocational Rehabilitation includes an array of services, which are funded by a grant to the Navajo Nation from the U.S. Department of Education. The goal of vocational rehabilitation is to assist people with disabilities to obtain or maintain employment.
*Treva M Roanhorse, Director*
*Paula S Seanez, Assistant Director*

1667 **Navajo Nation Office of Special Education & Rehabilitation Services (OSERS)**
PO Box 1420 928-871-6338
Window Rock, AZ 86515 866-341-9918
Fax: 928-871-7865
osers@navajo.org
www.osers.navajo-nsn.gov/
Navajo OSERS is a program within the Division of DINE Education, which offers vocational rehabilitation to people with disabilities. Vocational Rehabilitation includes an array of services, which are funded by a grant to the Navajo Nation from the U.S. Department of Education. The goal of vocational rehabilitation is to assist people with disabilities to obtain or maintain employment.
*Treva M Roanhorse, Director*
*Paula S Seanez, Assistant Director*

1668 **PACCT**
8032 Mechanicsville Turnpike 804-559-6833
Mechanesville, VA 23111 Fax: 804-559-6835
*Joyce Scheibe*

1669 **PACCT of Roanoke Valley**
PO Box 21112 703-989-5042
Roanoke, VA 24018 Fax: 703-989-5675
*Sue Critchlow, Director*
*Sandra Spencer, Executive Director Corporate Office (MD)*

1670 **PACER Center**
8161 Normandale Boulevard 952-838-9000
Bloomington, MN 55437-1044 800-537-2237
Fax: 952-838-0199
TTY: 952-838-0190
pacer@pacer.org
www.pacer.org
*Paula F Goldberg, Executive Director*
*Mary Schrock, Chief Operating and Development Officer*

1671 **Uplift**
200 W 17th Street 307-778-8686
Cheyenne, WY 82003 888-875-4383
Fax: 307-778-8681
uplift@upliftwy.org
www.upliftwy.org
*Peggy Logan, President*
*Richard Yep, Executive Director*

## Magazines

1672 **AJMR**
American Association on Mental Retardation
444 N Capitol Street NW 202-387-1968
Washington, DC 20001-1508 800-424-3688
Fax: 202-387-2193
AAMR@access.digex.net
www.aamr.org
Provides information on the latest program advances, current research, and information on products and services in the developmental disabilities field.
*BiMonthly*

1673 **American Journal of Psychiatry**
American Psychiatric Association
1000 Wilson Boulevard 703-907-7322
Arlington, VA 22209-2492 800-368-5777
Fax: 703-907-1091
ajp.psychiatryonline.org
Professional papers on topics in psychiatry.
*Monthly*
*Public Affairs, Division*

1674 **American Psychologist**
American Psychological Association
750 First Street NE 202-336-5510
Washington, DC 20002-4242 800-374-2721
Fax: 202-336-5502
TDD: 202-336-6123
www.apa.org
Articles on current issues in psychology as well as empirical, theoretical and practical articles on broad aspects of psychology.
*9x a year*

1675 **Journal of Clinical Psychology**
Clinical Psychology Publishing Company
4 Conant Square 802-247-6877
Brandon, VT 05733-1018
Scholarly research reports in the field of psychology.

1676 **Mental Retardation**
American Association on Mental Retardation
444 N Capitol Street NW 202-387-1968
Washington, DC 20001-1508 800-424-3688
Fax: 202-387-2193
AAMR@access.digex.net
www.aamr.org
Provides information on the latest program advances, current research, and information on products and services in the developmental disabilities field.
*BiMonthly*
*James R. Patton, Author*

1677 **Psychopharmacology Bulletin**
Superintendent of Documents/NIMH Journal
PO Box 371954 202-512-2250
Pittsburgh, PA 15250-7954
Emphasizes rapid, informal dissemination of recent research findings that have not previously appeared in the more formal literature.
*Quarterly*

1678 **Psychosocial Rehabilitation Journal**
Int'l Assoc. of Psychosocial Rehab. Services
730 Commonwealth Avenue 617-353-3549
Boston, MA 02215-1209
Discusses issues, programs and research on psychiatric rehabilitation.

## Web Sites

1679 **American Psychological Association**
www.apa.org
Mission is to advance psychology as a science and professional organization that represents psychology in the United States.

1680 **Coalition of Voluntary Mental Health Agencies**
www.cvmha.org/
An umbrella advocacy organization of New York's mental health community, representing over 100 non-profit community based mental health agencies that serve more than 300,000 clients in the five boroughs of New York City and its environs.

1681 **Community Access**
www.cairn.org/
A nonprofit agency providing housing and advocacy for people with psychiatric disabilities.

1682 **Healing Well**
www.healingwell.com
An online health resource guide to medical news, chat, information and articles, newsgroups and message boards, books, dis-

ease-related web sites, medical directories, and more for patients, friends, and family coping with disabling diseases, disorders, or chronic illnesses.

**1683 Health Finder**

www.healthfinder.gov

Searchable, carefully developed web site offering information on over 1000 topics. Developed by the US Department of Health and Human Services, the site can be used in both English and Spanish.

**1684 Healthlink USA**

www.healthlinkusa.com

Health information concerning treatment, cures, prevention, diagnosis, risk factors, research, support groups, email lists, personal stories and much more. Updated regularly.

**1685 Internet Mental Health**

www.mentalhealth.com

A site whose goal is to improve understanding, diagnosis, and treatment of mental illness throughout the world. Includes information on specific disorders, medications, diagnosis, research, news, and other internet links.

**1686 MedicineNet**

www.medicinenet.com

An online resource for consumers providing easy-to-read, authoritative medical and health information.

**1687 Medscape**

www.medscape.com

Medscape offers specialists, primary care physicians, and other health professionals the Web's most robust and integrated medical information and educational tools.

**1688 Mental Health America (formerly NMHA) Information Center**

www.mentalhealthamerica.net

Provides informational materials, lobbies for Federal mental health legislation, stimulates funding of research on the causes and treatment of mental illnesses.

**1689 National Alliance for the Mentally Ill**

www.nami.org

Over 900 affiliate groups nationwide offer support to members, advocate better lives for their loved ones, support research efforts and educate the public to reduce the stigma attached to serious mental illnesses.

**1690 National Mental Health Services Knowledge Exchange Network**

www.mentalhealth.org

Leading the national system that delivers mental health services. Provides the treatment and support services neede by adults with mental disorders and children with serious emotional problems.

**1691 WebMD**

www.webmd.com

Provides credible information, supportive communities, and in-depth reference material about health subjects. A source for original and timely health information as well as material from well known content providers.

**1692 World Federation for Mental Health**

www.wfmh.com

Mission is to promote, among all people and nations, the highest possible level of mental health in its broadest biological, medical, educational, and social aspects.

# ENVIRONMENTAL CAUSES

*Although a very high percentage of dementia cases—some studies put the number above 50 percent—are genetically inherited, as many as a third can be attributed to modifiable risk factors such as smoking, depression, diabetes, and cognitive inactivity. This leaves a substantial number of cases that cannot be explained by either cause and there is mounting evidence to suggest that evironmental factors may play a key role in the onset of these dementia cases.*

Recent research suggests that toxic environmental causes pose a significant threat to cognitive function and may, in fact, lead to dementia. While lead exposure has long been known to cause cognitive impairment, particularly in the developmental (childhood) stages, it is now believed that early exposure can lead to the increased production of amyloid-beta in later years, triggering the onset of Alzheimer's. The role of aluminum, as transmitted via drinking water and electromagnetic fields, in causing Alzheimer's has been debated since 1965 and, while no definitive conclusion has been reached, the link between the two remains a subject for further study. Evidence suggests that there may also be a link between iron, copper, and zinc and dementia.

In addition to metallic pollution, air pollution is believed to cause brain inflammation, increasing the risk of neurodegenerative disease. Postmortem comparisons of the brains of people living in polluted versus clean-air cities have suggested a correspondence between pollution and Alzheimer's-type brain tissue. Similarly, pesticides, many of which have long been known to have toxic effects on humans, may, according to recent studies, play a factor in dementia, as examinations of people with long-term occupational exposure have indicated. Although the evidence for the role of environmental factors in triggering dementia remains provisional, it promises to be a fruitful area for further scientific inquiry.

## National Agencies & Associations

1694 **Infectious Diseases Society of America**
4040 Wilson Boulevard 703-299-0200
Arlington, VA 22203 kcortez@idsociety.org
www.idsociety.org
Organization of physicians, scientists and public health experts who specialize in infectious diseases. Affiliated with the HIV Medicine Association and the Emerging Infections Network.
*12,000 members*
*Barbara D. Alexander, MD, President*
*Kathy Cortez, Staff Liaison*

## Magazines

1695 **Clinical Infectious Diseases**
Oxford University Press
2001 Evans Road 919-677-0977
Cary, NC 27513 800-852-7323
Fax: 919-677-1714
academic.oup.com/cid
Leading journal on infectious diseases, with original research, reviews, viewpoints, editorials, invited commentaries, photo quizzes, practice guidelines, correspondence and supplements. The journal has a broad focus, encompassing clinical descriptions, public health, microbiology, immunology, prevention of infection, evaluation of current and novel treatments and promotion of optimal practices for diagnosis and treatment.
*Robert T. Schooley, Editor-in-Chief*
*Ferric C. Fang, Deputy Editor*

1696 **Journal of Infectious Diseases**
Oxford University Press
2001 Evans Road 919-677-0977
Cary, NC 27513 800-852-7323
Fax: 919-677-1714
academic.oup.com/jid
Official publication of the Infectious Diseases Society of America, with original research on infectious diseases.
*Martin S. Hirsch, MD, Editor-in-Chief*
*David C. Hooper, Deputy Editor*

1697 **Journal of Neurodevelopmental Disorders**
Springer Nature
One New York Plaza 800-777-4643
New York, NY 10004-1562 info@biomedcentral.com
jneurodevdisorders.biomedcentral.com
An open-access journal devoted to integrating research from neurobiology, genetics, cognitive neuroscience, psychiatry and psychology.
*Joseph Piven, Editor-in-Chief*

1698 **Journal of Neuroinflammation**
Springer Nature
One New York Plaza 800-777-4643
New York, NY 10004-1562 info@biomedcentral.com
jneuroinflammation.biomedcentral.com
A peer-reviewed, open-access journal focusing on the interactions of the immune system with the nervous system as a means of expanding understanding of chronic neurological diseases.
*Monica J. Carson, Editor-in-Chief*
*Sue T. Griffin, Editor-in-Chief*

1699 **Open Forum Infectious Diseases**
Oxford University Press
2001 Evans Road 919-677-0977
Cary, NC 27513 800-852-7323
Fax: 919-677-1714
academic.oup.com/ofid
Open-access journal featuring clinical, translational and basic research on biomedical science and clinical practice.
*Paul E. Sax, MD, Editor-in-Chief*
*Jonathan Z. Li, MD, Deputy Editor*

# FRONTOTEMPORAL DISORDERS

*Differing from other forms of dementia in that it primarily affects younger patients, Frontotemporal dementia (FTD) is typically diagnosed in people between 45 and 65, and is an umbrella term that refers to a series of disorders characterized by the degeneration of the frontal and temporal lobes of the brain. These areas regulate behavior, problem-solving, speech, the control of emotions, the understanding of words, and the recognition of faces and familiar objects, and FTD is characterized by the deterioration of these functions.*

There are three principal types of frontotemporal dementia: behavioral variant frontotemporal dementia; semantic variant primary progressive aphasia; and non-fluent/agrammatic variant primary progressive aphasia. Although all three represent a different cluster of symptoms, they are all closely related. Typically, an FTD patient first presents with behavioral changes, language dysfunction, or weakness and slowness of movement, with the conditions gradual worsening. FTD is often misdiagnosed as Alzheimer's disease, psychiatric illness, vascular dementia, or Parkinson's disease.

Frontotemporal dementia results from the atrophy and death of nerve cells in the frontal and temporal lobes ,which has been linked to the formation of clumps of abnormal proteins inside the cells, particularly tau proteins. Compared with other forms of dementia, FTD is more likely to run in families, particularly in cases involving behavioral changes and less so in semantic dementia. Children or siblings of people that have the mutation known to cause FTD have a 50 percent chance of carrying that same mutation.

As with other forms of dementia, there is no cure. Treatment of FTD is confined to alleviating the symptoms of the disease and caring for the patient as best as possible. Caring for a person with FTD can be particularly challenging given the frequent behavioral changes and language problems that are usually exhibited. In addition to medical professionals, speech and language therapists are often helpful to those with FTD. Drugs that have been shown to slow Alzheimer's disease have not been effective in treating FTD, but antidepressants and antipsychotics are sometimes prescribed to treat specific symptoms.

## National Agencies & Associations

1701 **American Academy of Neurology**
201 Chicago Avenue
Minneapolis, MN 55415
612-928-6000
800-879-1960
Fax: 612-454-2746
memberservices@aan.com
www.aan.com
Professional society of medical doctors specializing in brain and nervous system diseases. Maintains placement service. Sponsors research and educational programs. Compiles statistics. Publishes scientific journal, Continuum: Lifelong Learning in Neurology.
*Mary E. Post, MBA, CAE, CEO*

1702 **American Society for Investigative Pathology**
1801 Rockville Pike
Rockville, MD 20852
240-283-9700
Fax: 301-984-4047
www.asip.org
The Society seeks to promote experimental pathology and related disciplines through meetings, publications, and educational activities.
*William B. Coleman, PhD, Executive Officer*
*Gina LaBorde, Manager, Marketing & Communications*

1703 **American Society for Neurochemistry**
9037 Ron Den Lane
Windermere, FL 34786
407-909-9064
Fax: 407-876-0750
asnmanager@asneurochem.org
asneurochem.org
The Society aims to advance and promote cellular and molecular neuroscience knowledge, and to facilitate communication and the dissemination of information within the field and with related disciplines.
*Sheilah Jewart, Executive Director*
*Karen Gottlieb, Conference Coordinator*

1704 **Association for Frontotemporal Degeneration**
2700 Horizon Drive
King of Prussia, PA 19406
866-507-7222
info@theaftd.org
www.theaftd.org
Dedicated to improving the quality of life of people with Frontotemporal Degeneration (FTD) and their caregivers. FTD is the most common dementia for people under 60 years of age. The association aims to education and promote awareness.
*Susan L-J Dickinson, CEO*
*Sharon S. Denny, Sr. Director of Programs*

1705 **Frontotemporal Dementia Advocacy Resource Network (FTDARN)**
info@ftdarn.org
www.ftdarn.org
FTDARN is dedicated to raising awareness of Frontotemporal Dementia and improving the quality of life of people diagnosed with FTD through compassion and support.
*Teresa Webb, Founder & Chair*
*Bob Meddaugh, Vice Chair*

1706 **Society for Neuroscience**
1121 14th Street NW
Washginton, DC 20005
202-962-4000
marty@sfn.org
sfn.org
Large international organization of scientists and physicians devoted to the study of the brain and the nervous system.
*37,000 members*
*Marty Saggese, Executive Director*
*Melissa Garcia, Associate Executive Director*

1707 **Society of Nuclear Medicine and Molecular Imaging**
1850 Samuel Morse Drive
Reston, VA 20190
703-708-9000
Fax: 703-708-9015
feedback@snmmi.org
www.snmmi.org
The mission of this nonprofit scientific and professional organization is to promote the science, technology and application of nuclear medicine and molecular imaging. Molecular imaging techniques are used to diagnose and manage the treatment of brain disorders such as Alzheimer's and Parkinson's disease, among other conditions.
*15,000 members*
*Virginia Pappas, CEO*
*Rebecca Maxey, Director, Communications*

## Libraries & Resource Centers

1708 **Frontotemporal Dementia Advocacy Resource Network (FTDARN)**
info@ftdarn.org
www.ftdarn.org
FTDARN is dedicated to raising awareness of Frontotemporal Dementia and improving the quality of life of people diagnosed with FTD through compassion and support.
*Teresa Webb, Founder & Chair*
*Bob Meddaugh, Vice Chair*

## Foundations & Research Centers

1709 **Brain Support Network**
P.O. Box 7264
Menlo Park, CA 94026
650-814-0848
Fax: 650-233-9278
www.brainsupportnetwork.org
Non-profit dedicated to facilitate brain donation for scientific study in the U.S. and Canada, to provide education on neurological conditions worldwide, and run support groups in Northern California.

1710 **Center for Brain Activity Mapping**
UC San Diego
9500 Gilman Drive
La Jolla, CA 92093
858-534-2230
cbam.ucsd.edu
The Center seeks to develop new technologies for detecting neuronal activity, for reporting it out of deep brain tissue, and for processing and analyzing the resulting data, by organizing and supporting research teams and projects.
*Ralph J. Greenspan, PhD, Director*

1711 **Connecticut Frontotemporal Dementia Foundation Inc.**
PO Box 462
Marion, CT 06444
www.ctftdfoundation.org
A local non-profit focused on promoting funding for research, educating health professionals, advocating with public officials, and supporting those diagnosed with FTD and their families.
*Esther Harvey, Founder*

1712 **Kavli Foundation**
5715 Mesmer Avenue
Los Angeles, CA
424-353-8800
info@kavlifoundation.org
www.kavlifoundation.org
The Foundation supports scientific research into the human brain, in the following scientific fields: Astrophysics, Nanoscience, Neuroscience and Theoretical Physics. Within Neuroscience, the study of aging and brain diseases and disorders is supported.
*Robert W. Conn, PhD, President & CEO*
*Eric Marshall, VP, Public Engagement & Prizes*

1713 **Kavli Institute for Brain Science at Columbia University**
Columbia University
3227 Broadway
New York, NY 10027
212-853-1016
Fax: 212-665-9699
kavli@columbia.edu
www.kavli.columbia.edu
The Institute's primary are of study is how signaling in neural circuits controls cognitive function and behavior, and the development of novel experimental and computational strategies for analyzing these signals.
*Eric R. Kandel, MD, Director*
*Rafael Yuste, MD, PhD, Co-Director*

1714 **Kavli Institute for Brain and Mind**
UC San Diego
9500 Gilman Drive
La Jolla, CA 92093-0115
kibm@ucsd.edu
kibm.ucsd.edu

The Institute supports research that furthers the understanding of the origins, evolution and mechanisms of human cognition. Of particular interest is Traumatic Brain Injury.
*Fred H. Gage, Co-Director*
*Nicholas C. Spitzer, Co-Director*

1715 **Neuroscience Research Institute**
UC Santa Barbara
6129 Biology II 805-893-4621
Santa Barbara, CA 93106 www.nri.ucsb.edu
The Institute seeks to allow scientists from different fields to collaborate for the betterment of neurological research. Areas of interest include: Alzheimer's Disease & Related Dementias; Behavioral Neuroscience & Neuroethology; Cell Biology, Biochemistry & Biophysics of the Nervous System; Computational & Theoretical Neuroscience; Development of the Nervous System; and Stem Cells.
*Stuart Feinstein, Co-Director*
*Kenneth Kosik, Co-Director*

1716 **Salk Institute for Biological Studies**
10010 N Torrey Pines Road 858-453-4100
La Jolla, CA 92037 www.salk.edu
Conducts groundbreaking research into cancer, aging, Alzheimer's diabetes and infectious diseases.
*Rusty Gage, PhD, President*
*Martin Hetzer, PhD, VP & Chief Science Officer*

1717 **Sanford Consortium for Regenerative Medicine**
2880 Torrey Pines Scenic Drive 858-246-1071
La Jolla, CA 92037 www.sanfordconsortium.com
The Consortium works to achieve breakthrough discoveries in stem cell research with regards to diagnoses, treatments, and cures for degenerative diseases and injuries.
*Edward W. Holmes, MD, President & CEO*
*Jeffrey Steindorf, PhD, VP & COO*

## Magazines

1718 **ASN NEURO**
Sage Journals
2455 Teller Road 805-499-9774
Thousand Oaks, CA 91320 journals@sagepub.com
journals.sagepub.com/home/asn
Peer-reviewed open access journal focusing on recent advances in the cellular and molecular neurosciences. It is the official publication of the American Society for Neurochemistry.
*Douglas L. Feinstein, Editor-in-Chief*
*Sandra J. Hewitt, Deputy Editor-in-Chief*

1719 **American Journal of Pathology**
Elsevier
1600 John F Kennedy Boulevard 301-634-7959
Philadelphia, PA 19103 Fax: 301-634-7961
ajp@asip.org
ajp.amjpathol.org
Official journal of the American Society for Investigative Pathology, publishing original research reports, reviews, and commentaries related to the molecular and cellular basis of disease.
*Martha Furie, Editor-in-Chief*

1720 **BMC Neuroscience**
Springer Nature
One New York Plaza 800-777-4643
New York, NY 10004-1562 info@biomedcentral.com
bmcneurosci.biomedcentral.com
A peer-reviewed, open-access journal devoted to all aspects of the nervous system (including molecular, cellular, developmental and animal model studies), as well as cognitive and behavioral research, and computational modeling.
*Darren Byrne, Editor*
*Ana Donnelly, Manuscript Editor*

1721 **Brain & Life**
American Academy of Neurology
201 Chicago Avenue 612-928-6000
Minneapolis, MN 55415 800-879-1960
Fax: 612-454-2748
BrainandLife@wolterskluwer.com
www.brainandlife.org
Official magazine of the American Academy of Neurology, aimed at parents and home-caregivers interested in neurology in everyday life.
*Orly Avitzur, MD, MBA, FAAN, Editor-in-Chief*
*Mary Bolster, Managing Editor*

1722 **Brain: A Journal of Neurology**
Oxford University Press
2001 Evans Road 919-677-0977
Cary, NC 27513 800-852-7323
Fax: 919-677-1714
brain@ucl.ac.uk
academic.oup.com/brain
Focus is clinical neurology and translational neuroscience.
*Dimitri M. Kullmann, Editor*
*Joanne Bell, Managing Editor*

1723 **Continuum: Lifelong Learning in Neurology**
American Academy of Neurology
201 Chicago Avenue 612-928-6000
Minneapolis, MN 55415 800-879-1960
continuumcme@aan.com
journals.lww.com/continuum
Official journal of the American Academy of Neurology, aiding professionals in patient care and continuing education.
*Bimonthly*
*Steven L. Lewis, MD, FAAN*
*Andrea J. Weiss, MA, Executive Editor*

1724 **Dementia and Geriatric Cognitive Disorders**
S. Karger Publishers, Inc.
26 W Avon Road 860-675-7834
Unionville, CT 06085 800-828-5479
Fax: 860-675-7302
www.karger.com/DEM
Open-access journal devoted to the study of cognitive dysfunction in preclinical and clinical studies, concentrating on Alzheimer's and Parkinson's disease, Huntington's chorea and other neurodegenerative diseases.
*Victoria Chan-Pilay, Editor-in-Chief*

1725 **JNeurosci**
Society for Neuroscience
1121 14th Street NW 202-962-4000
Washginton, DC 20005 jn@sfn.org
www.jneurosci.org
Official peer-reviewed journal of the Society for Neuroscience, publishing research on a broad range of topics of interest to those working on the nervous system.
*Marina R. Picciotto, Editor-in-Chief*
*Teresa Esch, Features Editor*

1726 **Journal of Molecular Diagnostics**
Elsevier
1600 John F Kennedy Boulevard 301-634-7959
Philadelphia, PA 19103 Fax: 301-634-7961
jmd@asip.org
jmd.amjpathol.org
Official journal of the American Society for Investigative Pathology and the Association for Molecular Pathology, focusing on molecular discoveries in medicine translating into the clinical diagnostic setting, as well as the description and application of technological advances in the field of molecular diagnostic medicine.
*Monthly*
*Barbara Zehnbauer, PhD, Editor-in-Chief*

1727 **Journal of NeuroEngineering and Rehabilitation**
Springer Nature
One New York Plaza 800-777-4643
New York, NY 10004-1562 info@biomedcentral.com
jneuroengrehab.biomedcentral.com

An open-access journal devoted to integrated research from the fields of neuroscience, biomedical engineering, and physical medicine and rehabilitation.
*David J. Reinkensmeyer, Editor-in-Chief*

1728 **Journal of Neuroinflammation**
Springer Nature
One New York Plaza 800-777-4643
New York, NY 10004-1562 info@biomedcentral.com
jneuroinflammation.biomedcentral.com
A peer-reviewed, open-access journal focusing on the interactions of the immune system with the nervous system as a means of expanding understanding of chronic neurological diseases.
*Monica J. Carson, Editor-in-Chief*
*Sue T. Griffin, Editor-in-Chief*

1729 **Journal of Nuclear Medicine**
Society of Nuclear Medicine and Molecular Imaging
1850 Samuel Morse Drive 703-708-9000
Reston, VA 20190 800-513-6853
Fax: 703-708-9015
subscriptions@snm.org
jnm.snmjournals.org
Peer-reviewed journal with clinical investigations, science reports, articles benefitting continuing education, book reviews, employment opportunities, and updates on practice and research.
*Monthly*
*Johannes Czernin, MD, Editor-in-Chief*
*Susan Alexander, Associate Director, Publications*

1730 **Journal of Nuclear Medicine Technology**
Society of Nuclear Medicine and Molecular Imaging
1850 Samuel Morse Drive 703-708-9000
Reston, VA 20190 800-513-6853
Fax: 703-708-9015
subscriptions@snm.org
tech.snmjournals.org
Peer-reviewed journal dedicated to nuclear medicine technology, with information on credentialing, continuing education and licensure requirements, as well as current news and updates on the field.
*Quarterly*
*Kathy S. Thomas, MHA, CNMT, PET, Editor-in-Chief*
*Susan Alexander, Associate Director, Publications*

1731 **Journal of the Neurological Sciences**
Elsevier
LSU Health Sciences Center JNS_England@lsuhsc.edu
New Orleans, LA 70112 www.jns-journal.com
Original articles in neurology and neuroscience from around the world.
*Monthly*
*John D. England, Editor-in-Chief*

1732 **Molecular Imaging**
Sage Journals
2455 Teller Road 805-499-9774
Thousand Oaks, CA 91320 journals@sagepub.com
journals.sagepub.com/home/mix
Peer-reviewed open access journal focusing on molecular imaging research, including basic science, preclinical studies and human applications. Published in association with the Society of Nuclear Medicine and Molecular Imaging.
*Bimonthly*
*Henry F. VanBrocklin, PhD, Editor-in-Chief*

1733 **Molecular Neurodegeneration**
Springer Nature
One New York Plaza 800-777-4643
New York, NY 10004-1562 info@biomedcentral.com
www.biomedcentral.com
A peer-reviewed, open-access journal devoted to all aspects of neurodegeneration research at the molecular and cellular levels.
*Guojun Bu, Editor-in-Chief*
*Huaxi Xu, Editor-in-Chief*

1734 **Neurocase: The Neural Basis of Cognition**
Taylor & Francis Group
530 Walnut Street www.tandfonline.com/toc/nncs20/current
Philadelphia, PA 19106
Rapid response journal featuring case and group studies in neuropsychology, neuropsychiatry and behavioral neurology, with a focus on the neural basis of cognition.
*Bruce L. Miller, Editor*
*Hans J. Markowitsch, Editor*

1735 **Neurology**
American Academy of Neurology
201 Chicago Avenue 612-928-6000
Minneapolis, MN 55415 800-879-1960
Fax: 612-454-2748
journal@neurology.org
n.neurology.org
Official journal of the American Academy of Neurology, peer-reviewed, highlighting clinical neurology research.
*Jose G. Merino, MD, MPhil, FAAN, Editor-in-Chief*
*Patricia K. Baskin, MS, Executive Editor*

1736 **Neurology Clinical Practice**
American Academy of Neurology
201 Chicago Avenue 612-928-6000
Minneapolis, MN 55415 800-879-1960
Fax: 612-454-2748
journal@neurology.org
cp.neurology.org
Official peer-reviewed journal of the American Academy of Neurology for practicing neurologists.
*John R. Corboy, MD, FAAN, Editor*
*Patricia K. Baskin, MS, Executive Editor*

1737 **Neurology: Genetics**
American Academy of Neurology
201 Chicago Avenue 612-928-6000
Minneapolis, MN 55415 800-879-1960
Fax: 612-454-2748
journal@neurology.org
ng.neurology.org
Official journal of the American Academy of Neurology, publishing online open-access peer-reviewed reports in the field of neurogenetics.
*Stefan M. Pulst, MD, FAAN, Editor*
*Patricia K. Baskin, MS, Executive Editor*

1738 **Neurology: Neuroimmunology & Neuroinflammation**
American Academy of Neurology
201 Chicago Avenue 612-928-6000
Minneapolis, MN 55415 800-879-1960
Fax: 612-454-2748
journal@neurology.org
nn.neurology.org
Official journal of the American Academy of Neurology, publishing online open-access peer-reviewed reports of original research and in-depth reviews of topics in neuroimmunology & neuroinflammation.
*Josep O. Dalmau, MD, PhD, Editor*
*Patricia K. Baskin, MS, Executive Editor*

1739 **Translational Neurodegeneration**
Springer Nature
One New York Plaza 800-777-4643
New York, NY 10004-1562 info@biomedcentral.com
www.biomedcentral.com
A peer-reviewed, open-access journal covering research, therapeutics and education for all areas of neurodegenerative diseases.
*Shengdi Chen, Editor-in-Chief*

1740 **Ultrasonic Imaging**
Sage Journals
2455 Teller Road 805-499-9774
Thousand Oaks, CA 91320 journals@sagepub.com
journals.sagepub.com/home/uix
The journal focuses on the rapid publication of original papers on the development and application of ultrasonic techniques, with emphasis on medical diagnosis. Also published are research notes, comments on papers appearing in the journal, book reviews, and occasional review articles.
*Ernest J. Feleppa, Editor-in-Chief*
*Roslyn Raskin, Managing Editor*

1741 **eNeuro**
Society for Neuroscience
1121 14th Street NW
Washginton, DC 20005
202-312-7305
eNeuro@sfn.org
www.eneuro.org

Open-access journal of the Society for Neuroscience.
*Christophe Bernard, Editor-in-Chief*
*Kelly Newton, Director, Scientific Publications*

## Web Sites

1742 **Neuronline**
Society for Neuroscience
1121 14th Street NW
Washginton, DC 20005
202-962-4000
neuronline@sfn.org
neuronline.sfn.org

Online portal for professional development and training resources for individuals in the field of neuroscience, hosted by the Society for Neuroscience.
*Amanda Kimball, Director, Digital Learning*

# HIV-ASSOCIATED DEMENTIA (HAD)

*Typically seen in advanced cases of HIV/AIDS, HIV-associated dementia occurs when the disease spreads to the brain. Purely HIV-associated dementia directly results from neuron damage caused by the virus, but often dementia in HIV patients is also brought about by related infections such as encephalopathy, lymphoma, and various forms of meningitis. Somewhere between 7 and 27 percent of late-stage HIV patients experience dementia.*

The various forms of HIV-associated dementia are known as the AIDS dementia complex (ADC) and typically represent a deterioration of cognitive, motor, and behavioral functions. Among the typical symptoms are memory and concentration problems, behavioral changes, loss of fine motor skills, and progressive loss of mobility. HIV-associated dementia is closely tied to a patient's CD4 (or T-cell) count and typically occurs when this is below 200 and the virus is particularly virulent. The condition is not caused by HIV directly but results from HIV-infected white blood cells (macrophages) and nerve cells (microglia) secreting neurotoxins that affect the nervous tissue. This leads to the degeneration of the ability of neurons to transmit information and, eventually, to cell death. Patients who abuse alcohol or drugs are more likely to have severe dementia symptoms than those that do not. Patients with HAD have a life expectancy of 6 months less than HIV patients without dementia.

Diagnosis of HIV-associated dementia is made using a variety of factors, including medical history, neurological and sensory tests, blood and spinal fluid tests, physical examination, and MRI or CAT scans. Treatment of HAD is similar to treatment of HIV/AIDS and can include antiretroviral therapy, the use of other prescription medications, and lifestyle changes. HIV patients who are taking highly-active antiretroviral therapy (HAART) are less likely to develop HIV-associated dementia and HAART is recommended as a preventative in non-dementia-suffering HIV patients. However, patients using HAART may still develop a lesser form of HAD known as HIV-associated neurocognitive disorder. Supportive measures for HAD patients are similar to those used for other dementia patients, such as creating a bright, cheerful environment and placing clocks and calendars in the patient's room to aid with orientation.

## National Agencies & Associations

1744 **AIDS Coalition of Cape Breton**
150 Bentinck Street 902-567-1766
Sydney, Nova Scotia, B1P-4W4 Fax: 902-567-1766
christine.porter@bellaliant.com
www.aidscoalitionofcapebreton.ca
Provides support and advocacy services for PLW HIV/AIDS (people living with HIV/AIDS). Services provided deal with social, legal, ethical and spiritual issues.
*Christine Porter, Executive Director*
*Jo-Anne Rolls, PHA Program Coordinator*

1745 **AIDS Committee of Durham Region**
115 Simcoe Street South 905-576-1445
Oshawa, Ontario, L1H-4G7 www.aidsdurham.com
To provide HIV/AIDS related services to the infected or affected and the general community in the region of Durham.
*Adrian Betts, Executive Director*
*Michael Morgan, Manager of Operations*

1746 **AIDS Committee of North Bay & Area**
269 Main Street W 705-497-3560
North Bay, Ontario, P1B-2T8 800-387-3701
Fax: 705-497-7850
oaacnba@vianet.ca
www.aidsnorthbay.com
To assist and support all persons infected or affected by HIV/AIDS and to limit the spread of the virus through education and outreach strategies.
*Stacey Mayhall, PhD, Executive Director*
*Steve Lamb, Support Services Coordinator*

1747 **AIDS Committee of Ottawa**
19 Main Street 613-238-5014
Ottawa, Ontario, K1S-1A9 Fax: 613-238-3425
info@aco-cso.ca
www.aco-cso.ca
Works to empower people living with HIV/AIDS and the PLWHA (persons living with HIV/AID) community in Ottawa through promoting the well being and quality of life of those living with, or close affected by HIV/AIDS.
*Khaled Salam, Executive Director*
*Cory Wong, Manager, Support Services*

1748 **AIDS Committee of Toronto**
543 Yonge Street 416-340-2437
Toronto, Ontario, M4Y-1Y5 Fax: 416-340-8224
ask@actoronto.org
www.actoronto.org
Delivers responsive, effective, and valued community-based HIV support services and education, prevention, outreach and fundraising programs that promote health, well-being, worth and rights of individuals and communities living with, affected by and at risk for HIV/AIDS, and increase awareness of HIV/AIDS.
*John Maxwell, Executive Director*
*Jocelyn Watchorn, Director, Support Services*

1749 **AIDS Committee of York Region**
10909 Yonges Street 905-884-0613
Richmond Hill, Ontario, L4C-3E3 800-243-7717
Fax: 905-884-7215
info@acyr.org
www.acyr.org
The AIDS Committee of York Region envisions an informed and compassionate society, which is supportive of people living with HIV/AIDS who are striving to overcome social and service challenges, working with them towards a healthy and empowered lifestyle.
*Vibhuti Mehra, Executive Director*
*Monica Meza-Opazo, Manager, Support Services*

1750 **AIDS Community Resources**
ACR Health
627 W Genesee Street 315-475-2430
Syracuse, NY 13204 800-475-2430
Fax: 315-472-6515
information@ACRhealth.org
acrhealth.org
ACR Health is a not-for-profit, community-based organization providing a range of support services to individuals with chronic diseases, including HIV/AIDS, diabetes, heart disease, obesity, asthma, substance use disorders, and serious mental illnesses, with the goal of positive health outcomes. ACR Health provides a wide variety of targeted prevention and sexual health services to individuals, from youth through adulthood.
*Millicent Davis, Chair*
*Anthony Adornato, Vice Chair*

1751 **AIDS New Brunswick**
65 Brunswick Street 800-561-4009
Fredericton, NB, E3B-1G5 Fax: 888-501-6301
info@aidsnb.com
www.aidsnb.com
A provincial organization committed to facilitating community-based responses to the issues of HIV/AIDS. The aim is to promote and support the health and well-being of persons living with and affected by HIV/AIDS and to reduce the spread of HIV/AIDS in New Brunswick.
*Matthew Smith, Executive Director*
*Keri-Ann Scott, Operation Coordinator*

1752 **AIDS United**
1101 14th Street NW 202-408-4848
Washington, DC 20005 Fax: 202-408-1818
www.aidsunited.org
National organization dedicated to the development, analysis, cultivation, and encouragement of sound policies and programs through the dissemination of information and the building and use of advocacy.
*Jesse Milan, Jr., President & CEO*
*John E. Roane, Jr., Vice President, Operations*

1753 **AIDSinfo**
PO Box 4780 800-448-0440
Rockville, MD 20849-6303 Fax: 301-315-2818
TTY: 888-480-3739
contactus@aidsinfo.nih.gov
www.aidsinfo.nih.gov
A call-in service where trained staff offers quick access to federally approved HIV/AIDS treatment and prevention guidelines, clinical trials, and other research-related information. AIDSinfo is a U.S. Department of Health and Human Services (DHHS) project that offers the latest federally approved information on HIV/AIDS clinical research, treatment and prevention, and medical practice guidelines for those with HIV/AIDS and their families.

1754 **ANKORS: Kootenay & Boundary HIV/AIDS and Hepatitis C Support Services**
101 Baker Street 250-505-5506
Nelson, BC, V1L-4H1 800-421-2437
Fax: 250-505-5507
frontdesk@gmail.com
www.ankors.bc.ca
ANKORS' mission is to respond to the evolving needs of those living with and affected by HIV/AIDS and Hepatitis C.
*Cheryl Dowden, Executive Director*
*Laura Buchanan, Support Services*

1755 **Act Against AIDS**
Centers for Disease Control
1600 Clifton Road 800-232-4636
Atlanta, GA 30333 877-242-9760
Fax: 301-562-1050
TTY: 888-232-6348
www.cdc.gov/actagainstaids
A program of the Centers for Disease Control and Prevention and the White House, aimed at raising awareness about HIV/AIDS among all Americans, and particularly among hardest-hit groups, such as gay and bisexual men, African Americans, Latinos, and other at-risk communities.

1756 **Alberta Reappraising AIDS Society**
Box 61037 403-289-6609
Calgary, Alberta, T2N-4S6 Fax: 403-206-7717
aras@aras.ab.ca
www.aras.ab.ca

Promote critical discussion of the HIV/AIDS dogma.
*David R. Crowe, President*
*Roger Swan, Treasurer*

1757 **American Academy of Neurology**
201 Chicago Avenue 612-928-6000
Minneapolis, MN 55415 800-879-1960
Fax: 612-454-2746
memberservices@aan.com
www.aan.com
Professional society of medical doctors specializing in brain and nervous system diseases. Maintains placement service. Sponsors research and educational programs. Compiles statistics. Publishes scientific journal, Continuum: Lifelong Learning in Neurology.
*Mary E. Post, MBA, CAE, CEO*

1758 **American Autoimmune Related Diseases Association**
22100 Gratiot Avenue 586-776-3900
Eastpointe, MI 48021 800-598-4668
Fax: 586-776-3903
aarda@aarda.org
www.aarda.org
Awareness, education, referrals for patients with any type of autoimmune disease.
*Virginia T. Ladd, President & Executive Director*
*Laura Simpson, Assistant Director*

1759 **American Chronic Pain Association**
PO Box 850 800-533-3231
Rocklin, CA 95677 ACPA@theacpa.org
www.theacpa.org
The ACPA facilitates peer support and education for individuals with chronic pain in its many forms, in order to increase quality of life. Also raises awareness among the healthcare community, and with policy makers.
*Penney Cowan, Founder & CEO*
*Daniel Galia, Director, Global Support*

1760 **American Civil Liberties Union LGBT & AIDS Project**
125 Broad Street 212-549-2500
New York, NY 10004 www.aclu.org/other
Offers legislative and employment information public awareness materials and support for persons with HIV/AIDS and their families, as well as laws and rights specializing in gender identity and sexual orientation.
*Susan Herman, President*
*Anthony D. Romero, Executive Director*

1761 **American Society for Neurochemistry**
9037 Ron Den Lane 407-909-9064
Windermere, FL 34786 Fax: 407-876-0750
asnmanager@asneurochem.org
asneurochem.org
The Society aims to advance and promote cellular and molecular neuroscience knowledge, and to facilitate communication and the dissemination of information within the field and with related disciplines.
*Sheilah Jewart, Executive Director*
*Karen Gottlieb, Conference Coordinator*

1762 **Black Coalition for AIDS Prevention**
20 Victoria Street 416-977-9955
Toronto, M5C-2N8 Fax: 416-977-7664
info@black-cap.com
www.blackcap.ca
A volunteer-driven, charitable, not-for-profit, community-based organization. Works in partnership with organizations and individuals who support in principle and practice our mission, philosophy and activities.
*Andrew B. Campbell, PhD, Chair*
*Alexander Joseph, MSc, BEd, CertEd, Treasurer*

1763 **CDC National Prevention Information Network**
1600 Clifton Road 800-232-4636
Atlanta, GA 30329 TTY: 888-232-6348
NPIN-info@cdc.gov
npin.cdc.gov
The CDC National Prevention Information Network (NPIN) is the U.S. reference, referral, and distribution service for information on HIV/AIDS, sexually transmitted diseases (STDs), and tuberculosis (TB). NPIN produces, collects, catalogs, processes, stocks, and disseminates materials and information on HIV/AIDS, STD's, and TB to organizations and people working in those disease fields in international, national, state, and local settings.

1764 **Committee of Ten Thousand**
71 Winfield Street info@cott1.org
Needham, MA 02492 www.cott1.org
The Committee of Ten Thousand is an education, advocacy and support organization for persons with hemophilia who contracted HIV/AIDS from tainted blood products.

1765 **Elevate NWO**
102-106 Cumberland Street N. 807-345-1516
Thunder Bay, Ontario, P7A-4M2 Fax: 807-345-2505
info@elevatenwo.org
www.elevatenwo.org
Provides support, education and advocacy around HIV and AIDS, and related issues.
*Shawn Hebert, Chair*

1766 **HIV Medicine Association**
4040 Wilson Boulevard 703-299-1215
Arlington, VA 22203 Fax: 703-299-8766
info@hivma.org
www.hivma.org
Organization of medical professionals in HIV medicine, representing health care providers and researchers and their patients by promoting quality in care and advocacy. Affiliated with the Infectious Diseases Society of America.
*Rajesh T. Gandhi, MD, FIDSA, Chair*

1767 **HIV West Yellowhead Services**
152 Athabasca Avenue 780-740-0066
Hinton, Alberta, T7V-1X3 877-291-8811
director@hivwestyellowhead.com
www.hivwestyellowhead.com
Services include harm reduction, needle exchange, overdose prevention, free safe sex supplies, care and support, prevention, and education.
*Lori Phillips, Executive Director*
*Lisa Schwing, Outreach/Support*

1768 **HIV Wisdom for Older Women**
340 Southwest Blvd 913-722-3100
Kansas City, KS 66103 Fax: 913-722-2542
www.hivwisdom.org
HIV prevention in older women and support for those who are infected.
*Jane P. Fowler, Director*

1769 **Health Information Network**
206-784-5655
information@healthinfonetwork.org
www.healthinfonetwork.org
Offers information, public awareness and support for women with HIV/AIDS and the public in general.

1770 **Heart Touch Project™**
3400 Airport Avenue 310-391-2558
Santa Monica, CA 90405 Fax: 310-391-2168
executive@hearttouch.org
www.hearttouch.org
Non-profit, educational and service organization devoted to the delivery of compassionate and healing touch to home or hospital-bound men, women, and children.
*Shawnee Isaac Smith, Co-Founder*
*Rene Russo, Co-Founder*

1771 **Housing Works**
57 Willoughby St. 347-473-7400
Brooklyn, New York, NY 11201 877-296-9264
TTY: 212-925-9560
info@housingworks.org
www.housingworks.org
Housing Works provides advocacy services for those living with HIV/AIDS, as well as housing, healthcare, nutrition, counseling, mental health and substance abuse treatment, job training, and le-

gal assistance. Also runs thrift shops and bookstores that raise money for the organization's services.
*Charles King, Chief Executive Officer*
*Matthew Bernardo, Executive Director*

1772 **Infectious Diseases Society of America**
4040 Wilson Boulevard 703-299-0200
Arlington, VA 22203 kcortez@idsociety.org
www.idsociety.org
Organization of physicians, scientists and public health experts who specialize in infectious diseases. Affiliated with the HIV Medicine Association and the Emerging Infections Network.
*12,000 members*
*Barbara D. Alexander, MD, President*
*Kathy Cortez, Staff Liaison*

1773 **International Council of AIDS Service Organization**
120 Carlton Street 416-921-0018
Toronto, Ontario, M5A-4K2 Fax: 416-921-9979
icaso@icaso.org
www.icaso.org
A global network of non-governmental and community-based organizations.
*Mary Ann Torres, Executive Director*
*Galina Godovanny, Financial Manager*

1774 **Living Positive**
9912-106 Street NW 780-424-2214
Edmonton, Alberta, T5K-1C5 Fax: 780-424-2215
living-positive@telus.net
living-positive.net
Dedicated to providing emotional, spiritual and psychological support to all those living with HIV.

1775 **NMAC**
1000 Vermont Avenue NW 202-815-3129
Washington, DC 20005 communications@nmac.org
nmac.org
Mission is to develop leadership in communitites of color to end the HIV/AIDS epidemic. Formerly the National Minority AIDS Council, its new official name is NMAC.
*Paul Kawata, Executive Director*
*Kim Ferrell, Director, Operations*

1776 **National AIDS Housing Coalition**
1000 Vermont Avenue NW 202-347-0333
Washington, DC 20005 nahc@nationalaidshousing.org
nationalaidshousing.org
Works to end the HIV/AIDS epidemic by ensuring that persons living with the condition have quality, affordable, and appropriate housing.
*Russell Bennett, Executive Director*
*Christine Campbell, Program Consultant*

1777 **National AIDS Memorial**
info@aidsmemorial.org
aidsmemorial.org
To preserve, care for, and use the AIDS Memorial Quilt to foster healing, heighten awareness, and inspire action in the struggle against HIV and AIDS.
*John Cunningham, Executive Director*

1778 **National AIDS Treatment Advocacy Project**
580 Broadway 212-219-0106
New York, NY 10012 888-266-2827
Fax: 212-219-8473
info@natap.org
www.natap.org
Seeks to eudcate by sending out literature, e-mail lists, and host forums on how to prevent HIV, or how to live with it.
*Jules Levin, Executive Director*
*Jessica Gibson Schilling, Chief Operating Officer*

1779 **National Hospice & Palliative Care Organization (NHPCO)**
1731 King Street 703-837-1500
Alexandria, VA 22314 800-646-6460
Fax: 703-837-1233
www.nhpco.org
The organization seeks to improve end-of-life care, widen access to hospice care, and improve quality of life for the dying and their loved ones.
*Edo Banach, JD, President & CEO*
*Hannah Yang Moore, MPH, Chief Advocacy Officer*

1780 **National Native American AIDS Prevention Center**
1031 33rd Street 720-382-2244
Denver, CO 80205 todd@nnaapc.org
Sole mission of this organization is to promote AIDS education, prevention and cures for Native Americans suffering from the illness.
*Todd Theringer, Executive Director*

1781 **Ontario HIV Treatment Network**
1300 Yonge Street 416-642-6486
Toronto, Ontario, M4T-1X3 877-743-6486
Fax: 416-640-4245
info@ohtn.on.ca
www.ohtn.on.ca
To optimize the quality of life of people living with HIV in Ontario and to promote excellence and innovation in treatment, research, education and prevention through a collaborative network of excellence representing consumers, providers, researchers and other stakeholders.
*Jean Bacon, Executive Director*
*Barry Adam, Senior Scientist, Prevention Research*

1782 **PEERS Alliance**
161 St. Peters Road 902-566-2437
Charlottetown, PE, C1A-5P7 Fax: 902-626-3400
info@peersalliance.ca
www.peersalliance.ca
Previously known as AIDS PEI, the organization aims to create a supportive environment for Persons Living with AIDS/HIV, to increase public understanding of the impact of HIV/AIDS, and to reduce the incidence of HIV/AIDS in Prince Edward Island.
*Cybelle Rieber, Executive Director*
*Angela DesRoches, Program Coordinator*

1783 **Peel HIV/AIDS Network**
7700 Hurontario Street 905-361-0523
Brampton, Ontario, L6Y-4M3 866-896-8700
Fax: 905-595-1443
info@phan.ca
www.phan.ca
Committed to serving people living with and affected by HIV/AIDS and to limit the spread of the virus through support, education, advocacy, and volunteerism.
*Nilda Patey, Executive Director*
*Adam Chalcraft, Supervisor, Harm Reduction Program*

1784 **Positive Living British Columbia**
1101 Seymour Street 604-893-2200
Vancouver, BC, V6B-0R1 800-994-2437
Fax: 604-893-2251
info@positivelivingbc.org
www.positivelivingbc.org
Exists to enable persons living with HIV/AIDS to empower themselves through mutual support and collective action. Its board of directors is composed of HIV-positive individuals.
*Victor Elkins, Executive Director*
*Mike Hedges, Director, Operations*

1785 **Positive Living Niagara**
120 Queenston Street 905-984-8684
St. Catharines, Ontario, L2R-2Z3 800-773-9843
Fax: 905-988-1921
info@positivelivingniagara.com
positivelivingniagara.com
AIDS Niagara is dedicated to improving the quality of life for those infected and/or affected by HIV/AIDS.
*Glen Walker, BA, BSW, RSW, Executive Director*
*Cathie Rogers, Chair*

1786 **Positive Women's Network - USA**
436 14th Street 510-698-3811
Oakland, CA 94612 info@pwn-usa.org
www.pwn-usa.org

Aims to empower women living with HIV through social justice and human rights.
*Naina Khanna, Executive Director*
*Jennie Smith-Camejo, Communications Director*

**1787 Project Inform**
25 Taylor Street 415-558-8669
San Francisco, CA 94102 877-435-7443
Fax: 415-558-0684
www.projectinform.org
Runs an HIV Infoline, as well as a Hepatitis C helpline, while engaging in advocacy on behalf of individuals living with HIV/AIDS.
*David Evans, Interim Executive Director*

**1788 Regional HIV/AIDS Connection**
186 King Street 519-434-1601
London, Ontario, N6A-1C7 866-920-1601
Fax: 519-434-1843
info@hivaidsconnection.ca
www.hivaidsconnection.ca
A community-based, charitable organization providing HIV-related services to people living with and concerned about HIV/AIDS in London and the surrounding area.
*Brian Lester, Executive Director*
*Kelly Wright, Director, HIV/HCV Support Services*

**1789 Reseau ACCESS Network**
111 Larch Street 705-688-0500
Sudbury, Ontario, P3C-4T5 800-465-2437
Fax: 705-688-0423
www.reseauaccessnetwork.com
A non-profit, community-based charitable organization, promoting wellness, education, harm and risk reduction.
*Richard Rainville, Executive Director*

**1790 The AIDS Network**
140 King Street East 905-528-0854
Hamilton, ON, L8N-1B2 866-563-0563
Fax: 905-528-6311
info@aidsnetwork.ca
www.aidsnetwork.ca
Providing services and education to Hamilton and the surrounding areas.
*Tim McClemont, Executive Director*
*Karyn Cooper, Director, Programs & Services*

**1791 The Well Project**
update@thewellproject.org
www.thewellproject.org
The Well Project is a not for profit corporation and an initiative conceived, developed, and administered by HIV+ women and those who are affected by the disease.
*Krista Martel, Executive Director*
*Juliana Hawawini Johnson, Director, Operations & Online Resources*

**1792 Turning Point Society of Central Alberta**
4611-50th Avenue 403-346-8858
Red Deer, T4N-3Z9 877-346-8858
Fax: 403-346-2352
info@turningpoint-ca.org
www.turningpoint-ca.org
Turning Point (formerly Central Alberta AIDS Network Society) is a local charity and agency offering support to individuals who are infected or affected by HIV/AIDS, and also provides prevention and education throughout Central Alberta.
*Stacey Carmichael, Executive Director*

**1793 Women Alive**
1301 N. Willowbrook Avenue 310-605-1365
Compton, CA 90222 info@women-alive.org
www.women-alive.org
Coalition of, by and for women living with HIV/AIDS. Created ways to help women connect with each other, bring others out of isolation, exchange information about HIV treatments, and take charge of their lives.

## State Agencies & Associations

**1794 AIDS Outreach Center (AOC)**
400 North Beach Street 817-335-1994
Fort Worth, TX 76111 info@aoc.org
www.aoc.org
The staff and volunteers of the AIDS Outreach Center (AOC) provide a wide range of social services, outreach activities, testing and counseling, prevention education programs and public policy advocacy for men, women and children living with HIV, and their loved ones.
*Shannon Hilgart, Executive Director*
*Mel LeRoy, Associate Executive Director*

**1795 AIDS Resource Center of Wisconsin**
600 Williamson Street 608-252-6540
Madison, WI 53703 800-359-9272
Fax: 608-252-6559
feedback@arcw.org
www.arcw.org
Provides critical AIDS care and prevention services. Sustained in these efforts by the resources, expertise and passion of hundreds of volunteers and donors.
*Mike Gifford, President & CEO*
*Debra J. Endean, PhD, Vice President & COO*

**1796 Alabama Department of Public Health**
201 Monroe Street 334-206-5364
Montgomery, AL 36104-3000 800-228-0469
Fax: 334-206-2092
www.adph.org/aids
Offers health education and risk education activities, including a mobile app called Know Your Status, Manage Your Health, and Live Your Best Life (KML AL), intended to inform, prevent HIV/AIDS transmission, and assist those who have the disease.
*Sharon Jordan, MPH, Director*
*Jora T. White, MA, Program Dir., Prevention & Development*

**1797 Alaska Department of Health and Social Services: HIV/STD Program**
Section Of Epidemiology
3601 C Street 907-269-8000
Anchorage, AK 99503-0249 800-478-0084
Fax: 907-561-4239
hiv-std@alaska.gov
dhss.alaska.gov/dph/Epi/hivstd
The HIV/STD Program addresses public health issues and activities with the goal of preventing sexually transmitted diseases (STDs) and HIV infection in Alaska as well as their impact on health. AIDS program offers education to providers and organizations.
*Merry Carlson, Director, Public Health*
*Joe McLaughlin, MD, State Epidemiologist*

**1798 Arizona Department of Health Services: HIV Prevention Program**
150 N 18th Avenue 602-542-1025
Phoenix, AZ 85007 Fax: 602-542-0883
www.azdhs.gov
Provides HIV and AIDS seropositive surveillance, case investigation, and analysis, as well as AIDS health education and training for the public.
*John Sapero, Office Chief*
*Alyssa Guido, MPH, Program Director*

**1799 Arkansas Department of Health: HIV Prevention Program**
AIDS Prevention Program
4815 West Markham Street 501-661-2408
Little Rock, AR 72205-3867 800-462-0599
Fax: 501-661-2082
www.healthyarkansas.com
Engages in policy development, grants, training, and collaboration with community organizations and state agencies to prevent and control the spread of HIV, as well as monitoring cases across the state.
*Nathaniel Smith, MD, MPH, Director & State Health Officer*

**1800 California Collaborative Treatment Group**
AntiViral Research Center

220 Dickinson Street 619-543-8080
San Diego, CA 92103-8208 avrc.ucsd.edu/programs/cctg
The CCTG is a multi-center clinical trials organization whose primary mission is to improve the scientific basis for HIV patient care and HIV prevention. CCTG develops treatment protocols and drug therapies.
*Jill Kunkel, RN, Director, Operations*
*Adiba Hassan, Data Manager*

1801 **California Department of Public Health: Office of AIDS**
Office of AIDS
PO Box 997426 916-558-1784
Sacramento, CA 95899-7426 www.cdph.ca.gov
Works to develop strategies and implement programs for education and prevention, testing and counseling, supportive care and treatment and research to control the spread of HIV infection.
*Karen Smith, MD, MPH, Director*

1802 **Chicago Department of Public Health**
333 S State Street 312-747-9884
Chicago, IL 60604 Fax: 312-747-9765
TTY: 312-747-2374
www.chicago.gov/city/en/depts/cdph.html
Offers core medical and support services via funding from the federal Ryan White HIV/AIDS Program.
*Julie Morita, MD, Commissioner*
*David Kern, Deputy Commissioner, HIV/STI Bureau*

1803 **Connecticut Department of Health Services AIDS Programs**
410 Capitol Avenue 860-509-7806
Hartford, CT 06134 webmaster.dph@ct.gov
portal.ct.gov/DPH
Operates a speakers bureau, provides training, workshops, seminars, and counseling services, and conducts meetings and offers information and referral services.
*Kate McEvoy, Director*

1804 **County of Los Angeles Public Health: Division of HIV And STD Programs**
AIDS Programs
600 S Commonwealth Avenue 213-351-8000
Los Angeles, CA 90005 800-243-7889
Fax: 213-387-0912
dhsp@ph.lacounty.org
publichealth.lacounty.gov/dhsp
Responsible for planning, coordinating, and implementing county wide HIV/AIDS and sTD efforts.
*Mario J. Perez, Director*

1805 **Delaware Department of Health and Social: Services HIV Prevention Program**
Division of Public Health
540 S DuPont Highway 302-744-1050
Dover, DE 19901 Fax: 302-739-2548
www.dhss.delaware.gov/dhss/dph/index.htm
Provides HIV counseling and testing prevention education and AIDS surveillance and studies.
*Kara Odom Walker, Secretary*

1806 **Florida Department of Health: HIV/AIDS Section**
4052 Bald Cypress Way 850-245-4422
Tallahassee, FL 32399 DiseaseControl@flhealth.gov
www.floridahealth.gov
Seeks to eliminate HIV transmission by making voluntary HIV testing a routine part of medical care, implementing new models for diagnosing HIV infections outside medical settings, and preventing new infections by working with persons diagnosed with HIV and their partners.
*Tom Liberti, Bureau Chief*
*Janell Clemons, Administrative Assistant*

1807 **Georgia Department of Public Health: Office Of HIV/AIDS**
AIDS Section
2 Peachtree Street NW 404-657-3100
Atlanta, GA 30303 dph.georgia.gov
Partners with local health districts, hospitals, colleges/universities, community-based organizations, and other stakeholders to provide prevention and care services.
*Kathleen E. Toomey, MD, MPH, Commissioner*
*L. William Lyons, Director*

1808 **Hawaii Department of Health: Harm Reduction Services Branch**
728 Sunset Avenue 808-733-8443
Honolulu, HI 96816 health.hawaii.gov/harmreduction/hiv-aids
Offers research, education, surveillance and testing components. AIDS information and guidelines about the placement of infants, children and adolescents who test positive for HIV in nursery or school settings are also available.
*Peter Whiticar, Branch Chief*

1809 **Houston Health Department: HIV-STD Viral Hepatitis Prevention**
Houston HIV Prevention Community Planning Group
190 Heights Blvd. 832-393-4675
Houston, TX 77007 Chanda.Phanhphongsane@houstontx.gov
www.houstontx.gov/health/HIV-STD
Plans and implements public health strategies to reduce the spread of HIV and other STDs in Houston.
*Stephen L. Williams, Director*
*David Persse, Health Authority*

1810 **Idaho Department of Health and Welfare: The STD/AIDS Program**
The STD/AIDS Program
450 W State Street 1st Floor 208-334-6527
Boise, ID 83720-0036 Fax: 208-332-7346
DPHinquiries@dhw.idaho.gov
www.healthandwelfare.idaho.gov
Program receives federal funding to support testing treatment and prevention services for Idaho's reportable sexually transmitted infections.

1811 **Illinois Department of Public Health: Division of Infectious Diseases**
525-535 W Jefferson Street 217-782-4977
Springfield, IL 62761 800-243-2437
TTY: 800-547-0466
www.dph.illinois.gov
Provides HIV/AIDS initiatives, surveillance, training, and care services.
*Ngozi O. Ezike, MD, Director*

1812 **Kansas Department of Health & Environment: STI/HIV Section**
1000 SW Jackson 785-296-6174
Topeka, KS 66612 kdhe.info@ks.gov
www.kdheks.gov
Conducts surveillance of HIV/AIDS in Kansas. Conducts Prevention Program with training for counselors and educators, partial funding of counseling test sites and distribution of educational materials. Provides medications and primary care.
*Laura Kelly, Governer*
*Lee A. Norman, MD, Secretary*

1813 **Legal Council for Health Justice**
17 N State Street 312-427-8990
Chicago, IL 60602 Fax: 312-427-8419
legalcouncil.org
Provides legal advice and services for persons who are HIV positive or have AIDS, as well as their families. Also serves individuals with disabilities and chronic illnesses, senior citizens, and the homeless.
*Tom Yates, Executive Director*
*Ruth Edwards, Senior Director, Program Services*

1814 **Louisiana Department of Health: STD/HIV Program**
1450 Poydras Street 504-568-7474
New Orleans, LA 70112 Fax: 504-568-7044
DeAnn.Gruber@la.gov
ldh.la.gov/index.cfm/page/919
The SHP runs statewide programs intended to prevent the transmission of STDs and HIV, track current cases, and provide medical services to those who have STDs and HIV.
*DeAnn Gruber, Program Director*
*Chaquetta Johnson, Program Deputy Director*

1815 **Maine Dept. of Health & Human Services: HIV, STD, & Viral Hepatitis Program**
Division of Disease Surveillance

221 State Street
Augusta, ME 04333
207-287-3747
Fax: 207-287-3498
TTY: 711
Sheila.Krouse@maine.gov
www.maine.gov/dhhs/mecdc

The program seeks to stop the spread of STDs, viral hepatitis, and HIV, and by doing so reduce the prevalence of illness and death. The proigram also promotes the health and well-being of individuals who have, or are at risk of contracting, these diseases.

*Ann Farmer, Division Director*
*Sheila Krouse, Program Support*

**1816 Massachusetts Department of Public Health: Office Of HIV/AIDS**
250 Washington Street
Boston, MA 02108
617-624-6000
Fax: 617-624-6001
TTY: 617-624-5206
www.mass.gov/hiv

The Massachusetts Department of Public Health coordinates HIV/AIDS response with the Bureau of Infectious Disease and Laboratory Services. Resources are provided for the public and healthcare professionals, including treatment guidelines, epidemiologic profiles, educational materials, and other resources.

*Monica Bharel, MD, MPH, Commissioner*
*Lindsey Tucker, Associate Commissioner*

**1817 Michigan Department of Health & Human Services: Division of HIV & STD Programs**
333 S Grand Avenue
Lansing, MI 48909
517-241-0855
www.michigan.gov/mdch

The divison focuses on prevention, care, and treatment of HIV and STDs. It also administers the Ryan White HIV/Aids Program in the state.

*Mary-Grace Brandt, Acting Division Director*
*Dawn Lukomski, Section Manager*

**1818 MidAtlantic AIDS Education and Training Center (MAAETC)**
University of Pittsburgh
130 DeSoto Street
Pittsburgh, PA 15261
412-624-1895
Fax: 412-624-4767
www.maaetc.org

Provides educational programs about HIV infection for healthcare providers to Delaware, District of Columbia, Maryland, Pennsylvania, Virginia, and West Virgina.

*Linda Rose Frank, PhD, Principal Investigator & Exec. Dir.*

**1819 Midwest AIDS Education and Training Center (MATEC)**
1919 West Taylor
Chicago, IL 60612
312-996-1373
312-413-4184
matec@uic.edu
www.matec.info

Provides educational programs about HIV infection for healthcare providers.

*Ricardo A. Rivero, MD, MPH, Executive Director*
*Renslow Sherer, MD, Regional Clinical Director*

**1820 Minnesota Department of Health**
PO Box 64975
St. Paul, MN 55164-0975
612-373-2437
800-248-2437
www.health.state.mn.us/diseases/hiv

The Infectious Disease Epidemiology, Prevention and Control Division oversees HIV/AIDS response in the state. The focus is on prevention and care, with resources offered to the public and to healthcare professionals.

*Stefani Kloiber, Director, Communications & Operations*

**1821 Mississippi State Department of Health: STD/HIV Office**
570 E Woodrow Wilson Drive
Jackson, MS 39216
601-576-7723
800-826-2961
msdh.ms.gov

The STD/HIV Program aims to reduce incidents of death as a result of STDs and HIV through services for disease prevention and control.

*Thomas Dobbs, State Health Officer*
*Melody M. Winston, Communicable Diseases*

**1822 Missouri Department of Health & Senior Services: Bureau of HIV, STD & Hepatitis**
PO Box 570
Jefferson City, MO 65102
573-751-6439
Fax: 573-751-6447
info@health.mo.gov
health.mo.gov

The department offers a range of programs and services for individuals and communities affected by HIV/AIDS, with a focus on prevention, counseling and testing, and healthcare for those living with the disease.

*Randall W. Williams, MD, FACOG, Director*
*D. Adam Crumbliss, Chief Dir., Community & Public Health*

**1823 Montana Deptartment of Public Health & Human Services: HIV/STD/HepC Program**
1400 Broadway
Helena, MT 59620
406-444-3565
dfejes@mt.gov
dphhs.mt.gov/publichealth/hivstd

Provides services and resources for the prevention and treatment of HIV, STDs, and Hepatitis C.

*Sheila Hogan, Director*
*Dana Fejes, Section Supervisor*

**1824 Mountain West AIDS Education and Training Center (MWAETC)**
325 9th Avenue
Seattle, WA 98104
206-543-2704
aetcinfo@uw.edu
mwaetc.org

Provides educational programs about HIV infection for healthcare providers to Alaska, Colorado, Idaho, Montana, Oregon, North and South Dakota, Utah, Washington, and Wyoming.

*David Spach, MD, Principal Investigator/Clinical Director*
*Laurie Sylla, MHSA, Director*

**1825 Nevada Department of Health & Human Services: Office Of HIV Prevention**
Division of Public & Behavioral Health
4126 Technology Way
Carson City, NV 89706
775-684-4200
Fax: 775-684-4056
dpbh@health.nv.gov
dhhs.nv.gov

Works to promote health and reduce the impact of HIV/AIDS, through the lens of public health and social justice.

*Richard Whitley, Director*
*Tory Johnson, MMgt, Section Manager*

**1826 New England AIDS Education and Training Center**
Center for Health Policy and Research
333 South Street
Shrewsbury, MA 01545
617-262-5657
Fax: 617-502-1701
aidsed@neaetc.org
www.neaetc.org

NEAETC serves health care professionals in New England with consultation, technical assistance, and resource materials.

*Philip Bolduc, MD, Clinical Director*
*Jennifer Daly, MD, Co-Clinical Director*

**1827 New Hampshire Department of Health and Human Services**
29 Hazen Drive
Concord, NH 03301
603-271-4502
800-852-3345
Fax: 603-271-0545
TTY: 800-735-2964
nhbidc@dhhs.nh.gov
www.dhhs.nh.gov/dphs/bchs/std

The Infectious Disease Prevention, Investigation and Care Services Section focuses on HIV and STD prevention, including Ryan White Care for the state, as well as viral hepatitis, tuberculosis prevention and control, and more.

*Jeffrey A. Meyers, Commissioner*
*Lisa M. Morris, Director, Public Health*

**1828 New Jersey AIDS Services**
44 South Street
Morristown, NJ 07960
973-285-0006
Fax: 973-285-0067
www.njas-inc.org

Provides support services, housing, prevention techniques, and community education to counter the HIV/AIDS crisis in New Jersey.

*Laurie Litt, Chief Executive Officer*
*Joann McEniry, Chief Operating Officer*

1829 **New Jersey Department of Health: Division of HIV, STD And TB Services**
PO Box 360 800-624-2377
Trenton, NJ 08625-0360 www.nj.gov/health/hivstdtb
Focuses on pevention and care for those affected by HIV, STDs, and tuberculosis.
*Shereef Elnahal, MD, MBA, Commissioner*

1830 **New Mexico Department of Health: HIV Services Program**
1190 S St. Francis Drive 505-476-3628
Santa Fe, NM 87505 nmhealth.org/about/phd/idb/hats
Provides a range of resources for those living with HIV/AIDS, as well as promoting professional development for healthcare providers, and coordinating with community-based organizations.
*Kathy Kunkel, Secretary*
*Laine Snow, Program Manager*

1831 **New York Department of Health: AIDS Institute**
AIDS Institute
Empire State Plaza 800-541-2437
Albany, NY 12237 dohweb@health.ny.gov
www.health.ny.gov/diseases/aids
Awards grants and maintains relationships with regional AIDS service groups, crisis intervention, psychosocial counseling and legal, financial and housing assistance. The Institute also offers preventive education, risk reduction education, HIV counseling and testing and patient care.
*Johanne Morne, Director*
*S. Scully, Dep. Dir., Health Care, Grants & Data*

1832 **North Carolina Department of Health and Human Services**
Communicable Disease Branch
1902 Mail Service Center 919-733-3419
Raleigh, NC 27699-1902 Fax: 919-733-0490
epi.dph.ncdhhs.gov/cd/diseases/aids.html
Oversees the AIDS surveillance program, HIV counseling, testing, partner notification, health education, risk reduction, and public information efforts in North Carolina.
*Mandy Cohen, Secretary*
*Mark Benton, Deputy Secretary, Health Services*

1833 **Northeast/Caribbean AIDS Education and Training Center (NECAAETC)**
Columbia University, HIV Center
601 West 168th Street 646-774-6978
New York, NY 10032 Fax: 212-568-3060
nynjaetc@columbia.edu
necaaetc.org
Provides educational programs about HIV infection for healthcare providers to New Jersey, New York, Puerto Rico and the U.S. Virgin Islands.
*Francine Cournos, MD, Principal Investigator*
*Daria Boccher-Lattimore, DrPH, Director & Co-Investigator*

1834 **Ohio Department of Health: HIV/AIDS Surveillance Program**
246 N High Street 614-387-2722
Columbus, OH 43215-0118 odh.ohio.gov
Consists of AIDS surveillance, seroprevalence programs, health care worker education, health education and risk reduction projects.
*Amy Acton, MD, MPH, Director, Health*
*William McHugh, Assistant Director, Health*

1835 **Oklahoma Department of Health: HIV/STD Service**
Office of The State Epidemiologist
1000 NE 10th 405-271-4636
Oklahoma City, OK 73117 www.ok.gov/health
Services include prevention and intervention, care delivery, and surveillance and analysis.
*Tom Bates, Commissioner of Health*
*Laurence Burnsed, MPH, State Epidemiologist*

1836 **Oregon Health Authority: HIV Prevention Program**
Health Division, HIV Program
800 NE Oregon Street 971-673-0153
Portland, OR 97232 Fax: 971-673-0178
TTY: 711
joshua.s.ferrer@state.or.us
www.oregon.gov/DHS/ph
The program focuses on prevention, training, and resources for the public and healthcare providers.
*Patrick Allen, Director*
*Josh Ferrer, HIV/STD Prevention Manager*

1837 **Pacific AIDS Education and Training Center (PAETC)**
University Of California San Francisco
550 16th Street, 3rd Floor 415-476-6153
San Francisco, CA 94158-2549 paetcmail@ucsf.edu
paetc.org
Provides educational programs about HIV infection for healthcare providers to Arizona, California, Hawaii, Nevada, and the 6 U.S.-affiliated Pacific Jurisdictions.
*E. Michael Reyes, MD, MPH, Principal Investigator*
*Monica Hahn, MD, Regional Clinical Director*

1838 **Pennsylvania Department of Health: Division Of HIV Disease**
Bureau of Communicable Diseases
625 Forster Street 717-783-0572
Harrisburg, PA 17120 Fax: 717-772-6975
www.health.pa.gov
The division seeks to develop and implement a multi-dimensional, coordinated strategy to prevent disease and change high-risk behaviors, as well as provide resources and direction for sustaining preventive behavior and avoiding infection. HIV/AIDS Surveillance and Epidemiology is also run by the Bureau of Epidemiology.
*Rachel Levine, Secretary*
*Loren Robinson, Deputy Secretary, Health Promotion*

1839 **Philadelphia Department of Public Health: STD Control Program**
AIDS Activities Coordinating Office (AACO)
1101 Market Street 215-685-5600
Philadelphia, PA 19107 www.phila.gov/health
Works to stop the spread of STDs, including HIV, in Philadelphia. Other city programs include: Club 1509, providing resources for men and transpeople of color; Take Control Philly, offering free condoms; and Do You, Philly, providing sexual information and resources to young men.
*Thomas Farley, MD, Health Commissioner*
*Raynard Washington, Chief Epidemiologist*

1840 **Pridelines**
6360 NE 4th Court 305-571-9601
Miami, FL 33138 info@pridelines.org
pridelines.org
The organization seeks to support, educate, and empower LGBTQ youth and the community as a whole in South Florida, including providing HIV/AIDS-related health services and support.
*Victor Diaz Herman, Chief Executive Officer*
*Lisa Hayeem Carver, MPH, Director, HIV Services*

1841 **Rhode Island Department of Health**
3 Capitol Hill 401-222-5960
Providence, RI 02908 www.health.ri.gov/diseases/hivaids
The Division of Preparedness, Response, Infectious Disease and Emergency Medical Services oversees a number of programs related to controlling the spread of STDs, including HIV.
*Nicole Alexander-Scott, MD, MPH, Director*
*Steven Boudreau, Chief Administrative Officer*

1842 **San Francisco AIDS Foundation (SFAF)**
1035 Market Street 415-487-3000
San Francisco, CA 94103 info@sfaf.org
www.sfaf.org
SFAF provides confidential array of services-including financial benefits counseling, client advocacy, housing assistance, HIV prevention efforts, and needle exchange.
*Joe Hollendoner, MSW, Chief Executive Officer*
*Lara Brooks, Chief Program Officer*

1843 **San Francisco Community Health Center: HHOME/GTZ-ICM**
730 Polk Street 415-292-3400
San Francisco, CA 94109 Fax: 415-292-3404
TTY: 415-292-3410
sfcommunityhealth.org
HIV Homeless Outreach and Mobile Engagement (HHOME) is a mobile program operating throughout San Francisco, serving homeless people living with HIV/AIDS. Getting to Zero Intensive

Case Management (GTZ-ICM) aims to end new HIV infections across the city by 2020.
*Lance Toma, Chief Executive Officer*
*Ruby Koger, Senior Medical Case Manager*

1844 **South Carolina Department of Health & Environmental Control**
Bureau of Preventive Health Services
2600 Bull Street 803-898-3432
Columbia, SC 29201 info@dhec.sc.gov
www.scdhec.gov
Provides services to prevent the spread of sexually transmitted diseases (STD's) and HIV infection, to reduce associated illness and death, and to provide care and support resources for persons with HIV.
*Rick Toomey, Director*

1845 **South Central AIDS Education and Training Center (SCAETC)**
Parkland Health and Hospital System
8435 North Stemmons Freeway 214-590-2181
Dallas, TX 75247 877-275-2382
Fax: 214-590-2184
sc.aetc@phhs.org
aidseducation.org
Provides educational programs about HIV infection for healthcare providers to Arkansas, Louisiana, New Mexico, Oklahoma, and Texa.
*Henry Pacheco, MD, Project Director*
*Amneris Luqye, MD, Regional Clinical Director*

1846 **Southeast AIDS Education and Training Center (SEAETC)**
Vanderbilt Health
719 Thompson Lane 615-875-7873
Nashville, TN 37204 Fax: 615-936-1583
www.seaetc.com
Provides educational programs about HIV infection for healthcare providers to Alabama, Florida, Georgia, Kentucky, Mississippi, North Carolina, South Carolina, and Tennessee.
*Stephen P. Raffanto, MD, MPH, Principal Investigator*
*Anna Person, MD, Clinical Director*

1847 **Southwest Center For HIV/AIDS**
1101 North Central Avenue 602-307-5330
Phoenix, AZ 85004 Fax: 602-307-5021
swhiv.org
Formerly The Phoenix Body Positive, the organization is a non-profit created by and for people infected and affected by HIV/AIDS, that provides the community with the knowledge, resources and collective strength necessary for individuals to live long and well with HIV and to prevent the spread of the disease.
*Dolph Goldenburg, Interim Executive Director*
*Lisa M. Fontes, PhD, Director, Development*

1848 **Tennessee Department of Health: HIV Prevention Services**
710 James Robertson Parkway 615-741-7500
Nashville, TN 37243 www.tn.gov/health
Provides HIV/STD education and information, as well as collecting monitoring and distributing data. Provides assistance to individuals, and intervention and treatment services.
*Lisa Piercey, MD, MBA, FAAP, Commissioner*
*David R. Reagan, MD, PhD, Chief Medical Officer*

1849 **Test Positive Aware Network (TPAN)**
5537 N Broadway Street 773-989-9400
Chicago, IL 60640-1405 Fax: 773-989-9494
tpan@tpan.com
www.tpan.com
Empowers people living with HIV through peer-led programming support services, information dissemination, and advocacy. Provides services to the broader community to increase HIV knowledge and sensitivity and to reduce the risk of infection.
*Christopher Clark, Chief Executive Officer*
*Julie Supple, MA, LCSW, Director, Client Services*

1850 **Texas Department of State Health Services: HIV-STD Program**
PO Box 149347 512-533-3000
Austin, TX 78714 800-255-1090
Fax: 512-533-3171
hivstd@dshs.texas.gov
www.dshs.state.tx.us
Mission is to prevent, treat, and/or control the spread of HIV, STD, and other communicable diseases to protect the health of the citizens of Texas.
*John Hellerstedt, MD, Commissioner*
*Felipe Rocha, TB/HIV/STD Contact*

1851 **Tucson Interfaith HIV/AIDS Network (TIHAN)**
2660 North 1st Avenue 520-299-6647
Tucson, AZ 85719 www.tihan.org
Serving interfaith communities of Tucson through compassionate care education training and spiritual support so that we can make more people aware of the health crisis which affects all of us. Also provide non-medical in-home help.
*Scott Blades, Executive Director*
*Deidre Demers, Program Manager*

1852 **Utah Department of Health: Bureau of Epidemiology**
Division of Epidemiology & Laboratory Services
288 N 1460 W 801-538-6191
Salt Lake City, UT 84114-2104 888-374-8824
Fax: 801-538-9913
epi@utah.gov
health.utah.gov/epi/diseases/hivaids
Secures and distributes funds for HIV/AIDS prevention services, provides educational programs and counseling to the general public, HIV/AIDS service organizations, health workers and groups at risk.
*Joseph Miner, MD, Executive Director*
*Heather Borski, Director, Disease Control & Prevention*

1853 **Vermont Department of Health: Health Surveillance Division**
PO Box 70 802-863-7240
Burlington, VT 05402 Fax: 802-865-7701
healthvermont.gov/disease-control/hiv
Focuses on HIV prevention, care, and surveillance, as well as providing resources for healthcare providers and the public.
*Mark Levine, MD, Commissioner*
*Tracy Dolan, Deputy Health Commissioner*

1854 **Virginia Department of Health: Division of Disease Prevention**
109 Governor Street 804-864-7964
Richmond, VA 23219 800-533-4148
TTY: 888-232-6348
hiv-stdhotline@vdh.virginia.gov
www.vdh.virginia.gov
Supports local health departments and community-based organizations in the prevention, surveillance and treatment of HIV and other STDs, including their complications, through provision of education, information, and health care services.
*Laurie Forlano, DO, MPH, Director, Office of Epidemiology*

1855 **Washington DC Department of Health: HIV/AIDS, Hepatitis, STD and TB Admin.**
899 North Capitol Street NE 202-442-5955
Washington, DC 20002 Fax: 202-442-4796
TTY: 711
doh@dc.gov
dchealth.dc.gov/service/hivaids
Mission is to reduce the incidence of HIV/AIDS and number of deaths related to HIV/AIDS in the District of Columbia by the application of sound public health practices and initiatives through HIV disease surveillance, tracking, monitoring, and intervention.
*LaQuandra Nesbitt, Director*
*Michael Kharfen, Senior Deputy, HIV/AIDS*

1856 **Washington Department of Health: HIV Program**
PO Box 47840 360-236-3444
Olympia, WA 98504-7840 800-272-2437
Fax: 360-236-3470
Emalie.Huriaux@doh.wa.gov
www.doh.wa.gov
Provides information and referrals to local, state and national resources relating to HIV/AIDS, provides informational and educational materials to individuals, agencies and organizations and actively works with print and broadcast media to promote HIV/AIDS awareness.
*Emalie Huriaux, STD Program Manager*
*Zandt Bryan, Coordinator, Infectious Diseases*

1857 **West Virginia Department of Health & Human Resources: Division of STD and HIV**
350 Capitol Street 800-642-8244
Charleston, WV 25301 oeps.wv.gov
A division of the West Virginia Office of Epidemiology and Prevention Services, it seeks to prevent and control the spread of disease through surveillance, intervention, testing, education, and care.
*Bill J. Crouch, Secretary*

1858 **Whitman-Walker Health**
Washington, DC 202-797-3523
agibbs@whiteman-walker.org
www.whitman-walker.org
Community health centers in Washington with expertise in LGBTQ & HIV care.
*Don Blanchon, CEO*
*Abbie Gibbs, Chief Development Officer*

1859 **Wisconsin Department of Health Services: Wisconsin HIV Program**
1 W Wilson Street 608-267-9005
Madison, WI 53703 877-865-3432
dhswebmaster@dhs.wisconsin.gov
www.dhs.wisconsin.gov/hiv
Coordinates counseling and testing sites activities and services to HIV-infected persons, produces a report that contains information and recommendations for health care workers, emergency medical technicians and food service workers.
*Timothy Pilcher, Supervisor, HIV Prevention Unit*
*Ryan Rohde, Project Development Coordinator*

1860 **Wyoming Department of Health: Communicable Disease Unit**
401 Hathaway Building 307-777-7529
Cheyenne, WY 82002 debi.anderson@wyo.gov
health.wyo.gov/publichealth
Provides services for individuals living with HIV and their loved ones, plus healthcare providers and case managers.
*Debi Anderson, Unit Manager*
*Shelley Hood, Treatment Manager*

## Libraries & Resource Centers

1861 **AIDS Library of Philadelphia**
1233 Locust Street 215-985-4851
Philadelphia, PA 19107 Fax: 215-985-4492
library@aidslibrary.org
www.aidslibrary.org
Improving access to health and support services, preventing HIV transmission, and raising the public awareness of HIV/AIDS related issues.
*Allie Frase, Collection Management Librarian*
*Ben Remsen, Public Services*

1862 **Asian AIDS Project**
730 Polk Street 415-292-3400
San Francisco, CA 94109 Fax: 415-292-3404
Offers support and information for Asian Americans with HIV/AIDS.
*Lance Toma, LCSW, Executive Director*
*Yvonne Watson, CPA, Director of Finance & Administra*

1863 **Medical Library Association**
65 E Wacker Place 312-419-9094
Chicago, IL 60601-7246 Fax: 312-419-8950
websupport@mail.mlahq.org
www.mlanet.org
Non-profit, educational organization comprised of more than 400 institutions and 3,000 individual members in the health sciences information field, committed to educating health information professionals, supporting health information research and promoting access to information.
*Barry Grant, Director, Education*
*Kevin Baliozian, Executive Director*

1864 **National Library of Medicine**
8600 Rockville Pike 301-594-5983
Bethesda, MD 20894 888-346-3656
Fax: 301-402-1384
TDD: 800-735-2258
custserv@nlm.nih.gov
www.nlm.nih.gov/
The National Library of Medicine (NLM), on the campus of the National Institutes of Health in Bethesda, Maryland, is the world's largest medical library. The Library collects materials in all areas of biomedicine and health care, as well as works on biomedical aspects of technology, the humanities, and the physical, life, and social sciences.
*Dr Donald Lindberg, Director*
*Betsy L Humphreys, Deputy Director*

## Foundations & Research Centers

1865 **AIDS Clinical Trials Unit CARES Clinic**
CARES Clinic
2315 Stocktown blvd. 916-734-2011
Sacramento, CA 95817 800-2 U- DAV
Fax: 916-325-1955
actu@ucdavis.edu
www.ucdmc.ucdavis.edu/actu
The ACTU at Davis Medical Center is dedicated to offering the latest in research clinical trials to HIV/AIDS patients throughout Northern Central California.
*Thomas S. Nesbitt, Vice Chancellor*
*david A Acosta, Associate Vice Chancellor*

1866 **AIDS Healthcare Foundation**
6255 Sunset Blvd. 323-860-5200
Los Angeles, CA 90028 www.aidshealth.org
The AHF is a non-profit organization that provides state-of-the-art medicine and advocacy services to over 1,177,000 people in 43 countries. Funding is derived from a network of organization-run pharmacies, thrift stores, healthcare agreements, and other partnerships.
*Michael Weinstein, President*
*Peter Reis, Senior Vice President*

1867 **AIDS School Health Education Database Centers for Disease Control**
Centers for Disease Control
1600 Clifton Road 404-639-3534
Atlanta, GA 30333 800-232-4636
TTY: 888-232-6348
cdcinfo@cdc.gov
www.cdc.gov
An information awareness resource produced by the Division of Adolescent and School Health. The database offers descriptions of various educational resources for professionals relevant to the education of children and youth about HIV infection and AIDS.
*Thomas R. Frieden, Director*
*Ileana Arias, Principal Deputy Director*

1868 **Aaron Diamond AIDS Research Center**
455 1st Avenue 212-448-5000
New York, NY 10016 Fax: 212-725-1126
www.adarc.org
AIDS research.
*David D Ho MD, Director*

1869 **Adult Research Opportunities**
220 Dickinson Street 619-543-8080
San Diego, CA 92103-8208 Fax: 619-543-5066
www.avrctrials.org
A university-based nonprofit clinical trials unit. Conduct's patient-oriented research and educational programs on HIV and other chronic infections. Studies have pioneered the development of treatments that continue to change the course of the HIV epidemic.
*Constance Benson, Director*
*Richard S Garfein, Professor and Chairman*

1870 **Agency for Health Care Research and Quality**
540 Gaither Road 301- 42- 136
Rockville, MD 20850 www.ahcpr.gov

Operated by a branch of the US Department of Health and Human Services, this site provides recommendations (in layman's lingo) on the prevention and treatment of common illnesses and conditions. Just click on Clinical Information, then on Clinical Practice Guidelines Online, then on Consumer's Guides.

1871 **American Foundation for AIDS Research**
120 Wall Street 212-806-1600
New York, NY 10005 Fax: 212-806-1601
www.amfar.org
Supports research in basic, clinical, prevention and public policy and publishes the AIDS/HIV Experimental Treatment Directory.
*Kenneth Cole, Chairman of the Board*
*Kevin Robert Frost, Chief Executive Officer*

1872 **Arizona State University: School of Health Administration & Policy**
300 E. University Drive 480-965-7774
Tempe, AZ 85287 www.asu.edu
Offers research into healthcare delivery issues in the US including program evaluation, rural health and swing beds, new systems and AIDS in managed care systems.
*Eugene S Schneller PhD, Director*

1873 **Asian AIDS Project**
730 Polk Street 415-292-3400
San Francisco, CA 94109 Fax: 415-292-3404
Offers support and information for Asian Americans with HIV/AIDS.
*Lance Toma, LCSW, Executive Director*
*Yvonne Watson, CPA, Director of Finance*

1874 **CDC National Prevention Information Network**
1600 Clifton Road 800-232-4636
Atlanta, GA 30329 TTY: 888-232-6348
NPIN-info@cdc.gov
npin.cdc.gov
The CDC National Prevention Information Network (NPIN) is the U.S. reference, referral, and distribution service for information on HIV/AIDS, sexually transmitted diseases (STDs), and tuberculosis (TB). NPIN produces, collects, catalogs, processes, stocks, and disseminates materials and information on HIV/AIDS, STD's, and TB to organizations and people working in those disease fields in international, national, state, and local settings.

1875 **Canadian Foundation for AIDS Research**
2200 Yonge Street 416-361-6281
Toronto, Ontario, M4S-2C6 844-422-6327
info@canfar.com
canfar.ca
CANFAR is a national charitable foundation whose goal is to raise awareness in order to generate funds for research into all aspects of HIV infection and AIDS.
*Alex Filiatrault, Chief Executive Officer*
*Logan Thayalan, Senior Manager, Development*

1876 **Cascade AIDS Project: Women's Phone Network**
208 SW 5th Avenue 503-223-5907
Portland, OR 97204 Fax: 503-223-6437
info@cascadeaids.org
cascadeaids.org
*Charles Washington, President*
*Warren Jimenez, Vice President*

1877 **Center for AIDS Prevention Studies AIDS Research Institute**
AIDS Research Institute, University of California
50 Beale Street 415-597-9100
San Francisco, CA 94105 Fax: 415-597-9213
CAPS.Web@ucsf.edu
www.caps.ucsf.edu
The mission of the Center for AIDS Prevention Studies is to conduct domestic and international research to prevent the acquisition of HIV and to optimize health outcomes among HIV-infected individuals.
*Stephen F Morin, Director*
*Susan Kegeles, Co-Director*

1878 **Center for AIDS Research: Emory University Rollins School of Public Health**
1518 Clifton Road NE 404-727-2924
Atlanta, GA 30322-4201 Fax: 404-727-9853
cfar@emory.edu
www.cfar.emory.edu
Provides expertise resources and services not otherwise readily obtained through more traditional funding mechanisms.
*James W Curran, Director*
*Carlos del Rio, Co-Director for Clinical Science*

1879 **Center for AIDS Research: Harvard Medical School, Division of AIDS**
The Landmark Buiding
104 Mt. Auburn Street 617-384-9039
Cambridge, MA 02138 Fax: 617-495-8231
aids@hms.harvard.edu
aids.med.harvard.edu/cfar.htm
Provides expertise resources and services not otherwise readily obtained through traditional funding mechanisms.
*Bruce Walker, Director*
*Myron Essex, Associate Director*

1880 **Center for AIDS Research: Johns Hopkins University School of Medicine**
733 N. Broadway 410-955-3182
Baltimore, MD 21205-2196
Provides expertise resources and services not otherwise readily obtained through more traditional funding mechanisms.
*Ronald R Peterson, ,President, JHH/HS*
*Edward D Miller, MD, Dean, CEO*

1881 **Center for Blood Research Harvard Medical School/CBR**
Harvard Medical School/CBR
200 Longwood Avenue 617-278-3140
Boston, MA 02115 Fax: 617-278-3131
kirchhausen@crystal.harvard.edu
Offers research into blood disorders including multidisciplinary studies on AIDS and hemophilia cancer and diabetes research as well.
*Fredrick Alt, President/ Director*
*Stephen Carriuolo, Financial Manager*

1882 **Center for Disease Control**
1600 Clifton Road NE 404-639-3311
Atlanta, GA 30333 www.cdc.gov
Offers reprints, reports, public awareness and educational materials, research grants, and support for persons with HIV/AIDS.
*Elizabeth R Unger PhD*

1883 **Center for Interdisciplinary Research in Immunology and Diseases at UCLA**
UCLA School of Medicine
924 Westwood Blvd. #545 310-825-6373
Los Angeles, CA 90095
Research into immunology and blood disorders with special focus on AIDS and HIV infections.
*Albert Glover, Director, Academic Affairs*

1884 **Centers for AIDS Research: Albert Einstein College of Medicine**
Albert Einstein College of Medicine
Jack and Pearl Resnick Campus 718-430-2000
Bronx, NY 10461 Fax: 718-430-2374
information@einstein.yu.edu
www.aecom.yu.edu/cfar
Provides consultation and support to the medical and research community in the scientific evaluation of CAM therapies.
*Allen M Spiegel MD, Dean*
*Matthew Scharff MD, CFAR Investigator*

1885 **Centers for AIDS Research: Baylor College of Medicine**
Department of Molecular Virology & Microbiology
One Baylor Plaza 713-798-3006
Houston, TX 77030 Fax: 713-798-5019
jbutel@bcm.edu
www.bcm.edu/cfar
A research center that is a branch of the Centers for AIDS Research.
*Janet S Butel, Director*
*William T Shearer, Co-Director*

**1886 Centers for AIDS Research: Brown University**
The Miriam Hospital
CFAR/RISE Building 401-793-4068
Providence, RI 02906 Fax: 401-793-4704
vgodleski@lifespan.org
Provides expertise resources and services not otherwise readily obtained through traditional funding mechanisms.
*Charles C J Carpenter, Director*
*Susan Cu-Uvin, HIV and Women Core Co-Director*

**1887 Centers for AIDS Research: Case Western University**
Department of Medicine
Division of Infectious Diseases 216-368-0271
Cleveland, OH 44106-5029 Fax: 216-368-3055
mxl6@case.edu
www.clevelandactu.org
Provides administrative and shared research support to enhance and coordinate high quality AIDS research projects.
*Michael M Lederman, Co-Director*
*Jonathan Karn, Associate Director*

**1888 Centers for AIDS Research: Columbia University College of Physicians**
Center for AIDS Research
630 W 168th Street 212-305-1296
New York, NY 10032 jka8@columbia.edu
www.cumc.columbia.edu
Provides a comprehensive framework for training educational programs and research which addresses health promotion disease prevention symptom management and quality of life for individuals with HIV. The goal of the Center is to create innovative research and service approaches for the prevention and management of HIV. This objective is fulfilled through research program development and program evaluations.
*Lee Goldman MD, Executive Vice President*
*Lee Bollinger, JD, President of the University*

**1889 Centers for AIDS Research: NYU School of Medicine**
522 First Avenue 212-263-8527
New York, NY 10016 www.hivinfosource.org/hivis/cfar
Provides expertise resources and services not otherwise readily obtained through traditional funding mechanisms.
*Derya Unutmanz MD, Director*
*David levy, Associate Dean*

**1890 Centers for AIDS Research: North-Central California**
UC Davis, Division of Infectious Diseases
4150 V Street 916-734-8033
Sacramento, CA 95817 Fax: 916-734-7766
nccfar@ucdavis.edu
www.ucdmc.ucdavis.edu/nccfar
Provides expertise resources and services not otherwise readily obtained through more traditional funding mechanisms.
*Richard B Pollard, Division Chief*
*Krystin E Cheung, Director*

**1891 Centers for AIDS Research: USCD Center for AIDS Research**
Center for AIDS Research
9500 Gilman Drive 858-534-5545
La Jolla, CA 92093-0716 Fax: 858-822-5840
cfar@ucsd.edu
cfar.ucsd.edu
Provides expertise resources and services and services not otherwise readily obtained through traditional funding mechanisms.
*Douglas Richman, Director*
*Kim Schafer, Administrative Director*

**1892 Centers for AIDS Research: Univeristy of North Carolina at Chapel Hill**
UNC Center For AIDS Research
Lineberger Cancer Center 919-966-8645
Chapel Hill, NC 27599 cfar@med.unc.edu
cfar.med.unc.edu
Administrative and shared research support to synergistically enhance and coordinate high quality AIDS research projects.
*Ronald Swanstrom, Director*
*Myron S Cohen, Associate Director*

**1893 Centers for AIDS Research: University of Alabama at Birmingham**
BBRB 256 205-934-4011
Birmingham, AL 35294-1150 http://www.uab.edu
Provides expertise, resources, and services not otherwise readily obtained through traditional funding mechanisms.
*Robert P. Kimberly, Director*
*Cheryl A. Perry, Deputy Director*

**1894 Centers for AIDS Research: Vanderbilt University Medical Center**
Division of Infectious Disease
1161 21st Avenue S 615-322-8972
Nashville, TN 37232-2582 richard.daquila@vanderbilt.edu
www.mc.vanderbilt.edu/cfar
Provides expertise resources and services not otherwise readily obtained through more traditional funding mechanisms.
*Richard D' Aquila, Director*
*G Fatima Lima Ph.D., Associate Director*

**1895 City of Hope National Medical Center Drug Discover/AIDS Group**
City of Hope
1500 E Duarte Road 626-256-4673
Duarte, CA 91010 www.cityofhope.org
Developmental research into the treatment of AIDS.
*Michael A Friedman MD, CEO*
*Robert Stone, President*

**1896 City of Hope National Medical Center: Beckman Research**
Virology & Infectious Diseases
1500 Duarte Road 626-256-4673
Duarte, CA 91010 www.cityofhope.org
Developmental research into the treatment of AIDS.
*Dr. John A Zaia, Chair and Professor*
*Michael Barish, Chair and Professor, Neuroscienc*

**1897 Clinical Focus on Primary Immune Deficiency Diseases**
Immune Deficiency Foundation
110 West Rd, Ste 300 410-321-6647
Towson, MD 21204 800-296-4433
Fax: 410-321-9165
info@primaryimmune.org
primaryimmune.org
Educational monograph is designed specifically for health care professionals and focuses on topics relevant to primary immune deficiency diseases.
*Marcia Boyle, President & Founder*
*Christine Belser, Senior VP, Programs & Communications*

**1898 Clinical Research Center**
Northwestern Center for Clinical Research
680 N Lake Shore Drive 312-503-6227
Chicago, IL 60611 www.ocrt@northwestern.edu
Offers research into complications and effects of AIDS and HIV infection on the human body.
*Dr. Tom Schnitzer, Program Director*

**1899 Dana Farber Cancer Institute National Drug Discovery Group for AIDS Treatment**
Dana-Farber Cancer Institute
450 Brookline Avenue 617-632-3000
Boston, MA 02215-5450 800-408-3324
TTY: 617-632-5330
TDD: 617-632-5330
dana-farbercontactus@dfci.harvard.edu
www.dana-farber.org
*Edward Benz, President and CEO*
*Dorthy E Puhy, Executive Vice President and COO*

**1900 Department of Epidemiology and Health Policy Research: University of Florida**
1329 SW 16th Street 352-265-8035
Gainesville, FL 32608 Fax: 352-265-8047
www.ehpr.ufl.edu
Studies into child and adolescent health financing and organization of health care delivery systems community health chronic conditions transition from pediatric to adult health care access to

health care for vulnerable populations quality of life and outcomes research.
*Clifford J Crook, Chair*
*John C Bierly, Program Assistant*

1901 **Developmental Evaluation Center**
Children's Hospital
300 Longwood Avenue 617-355-6000
Boston, MA 02115 800-355-7944
www.childrenshospital.org
Studies developmental effects of infants at risk and development effects of congenital HIV infection.
*Sandra L. Fenwick, President , CEO*

1902 **Dwight David Eisenhower Army Medical Center**
Department of Clinical Investigation
300 E Hospital Road 706-787-5811
Fort Gordon, GA 30905
Focuses research on cardiac disorders, immune deficiencies and AIDS.
*Col. Kent M Plowman MC, Chief*

1903 **Educational Materials Database Centers for Disease Control**
Centers for Disease Control
1600 Clifton Road 404-639-3534
Atlanta, GA 30333-4201 800-232-4636
TTY: 888-232-6348
cdcinfo@cdc.gov
www.cdc.gov
An information awareness resource produced by the Division of Adolescent and School Health. The database offers descriptions of various educational resources for professionals relevant to the education of children and youth about HIV infection and AIDS.
*Thomas R. Frieden, Director*
*Ileana Arias, Principal Deputy Director*

1904 **Emory University: National Cooperative Drug Discovery for AIDS Treatment**
Department of Pediatrics
2015 Uppergrate Road 404-712-8356
Atlanta, GA 30322 www.pedsresearch.org
*Dr. Raymond F Schanzi, Principal*
*Thomas Abshire, MD*

1905 **Emory University: Yerkes Regional Primate Research Center**
201 Dowman Drive 404-727-6123
Atlanta, GA 30322 www.emory.edu
Immune research.
*Dr. Thomas R Insel MD, Director*
*Thomas Emory, Owner*

1906 **Funding Database Centers for Disease Control**
Centers for Disease Control
1600 Clifton Road 404-639-3534
Atlanta, GA 30329 800-232-4636
TTY: 888-232-6348
cdcinfo@cdc.gov
www.cdc.gov
A listing of HIV and AIDS related funding opportunities for community-based and HIV and AIDS service organizations.
*Thomas Friedman MD, Director*
*Harold Jaffe, MD, MA, Associate Director of Science*

1907 **General Clinical Research Center Mount Sinai School of Medicine**
Mount Sinai School of Medicine
One Gustave L Levy Place 212-241-6500
New York, NY 10029-6574 Fax: 212-348-5811
hugh.sampson@mssm.edu
www.mssm.edu/gcrc
Focuses on AIDS education and prevention.
*Dennis S Charney, Executive Vice President*
*Kennith Davis, President*

1908 **General Clinical Research Center: UAB**
Room 907 Medical Education Building 205-934-4852
Birmingham, AL 35294 ccts@uab.edu
AIDS and genetics research.
*Burt Nabors, MD, Director*
*Stuart Frank, Co-Principal Investigator*

1909 **George Washington National Cooperative: Drug Discovery/AIDS Treatment**
Department of Pharmacology & Physiology
2300 Eye Street NW 202-994-3541
Washington, DC 20037-2336 Fax: 202-994-2870
www.gwumc.edu/pharm
Studies and researches natural products and synthetic anti-AIDS agents.
*Susan Ceryak, Associate Research Professor*
*Jian-Zhong Guo, Associate Research Professor*

1910 **HIV Center for Clinical and Behavioral Studies**
1051 Riverside Drive 212-543-5969
New York, NY 10032 Fax: 212-543-6003
www.hivcenternyc.org
Interdisciplinary research center that investigates the behavioral causes and consequences of HIV/AIDS. Focusing on the intersections of HIV infection gender and sexuality; treatment strategies for infected populations; and innovative dissemination of scientific findings.
*Anke A Ehrhardt, Director*
*Heino F L Meyer-Bahlbur, Associate Director*

1911 **HIV Prevention Trials Unit University of Washington/Seattle**
University of Washington/Seattle HPTU Site
Cabrini Medical Tower 901 Boren Av 206-520-3800
Seattle, WA 98104 Fax: 206-520-3801
www.depts.washington.edu
A worldwide collaborative clinical trials network established by the National Institutes of Health (NIH) to evaluate the safety and efficacy of non-vaccine prevention interventions alone or in combination using HIV incidence as the primary endpoint.
*Connie Celum, Principal Investigator*

1912 **Immune Deficiency Foundation**
110 West Road 800-296-4433
Towson, MD 21204-4841 Fax: 410-321-9165
info@primaryimmune.org
www.primaryimmune.org
A national charitable organization aimed at fighting the primary immune deficiency diseases. The founders included parents of children with primary immune deficiency, immunologists who treat immune deficient patients, and other individuals with an immune deficiency.
*John G. Boyle, President & CEO*
*Kara Moran, Vice President, Communications*

1913 **Indiana University Bloomington: Center for the Study and Promotion of AIDS**
801 E 7th Street 812- 85- 797
Bloomington, IN 47405 Fax: 812-855-3936
aids@indiana.edu
www.indiana.edu/~aids
AIDS research.
*William L Yarber, Director*
*Suzanne Thorin, Manager*

1914 **Institute for Clinical Research Weill Cornell Medical College**
Weill Cornell Medical College
1300 York Avenue 212-746-5454
New York, NY 10065 Fax: 212-746-8970
cto@med.cornell.edu
www.med.cornell.edu
The mission of the ICR is to support, advance and promote clinical and translational research enterprises at WCMC. As part of Research and Sponsored Programs (RASP) the ICR streamlines the clinical research process and offers a wide range of services, resources and training.
*David J Skorton MD, President of the University*
*Michelle A Lewis, MS, Director (Research and Sponsored Program*

1915 **Johns Hopkins University: Center for Communication Programs**
Johns Hopkins Bloomberg School of Public Health
111 Market Place 410-659-6300
Baltimore, MD 21202 Fax: 410-659-6266
info@jhuccp.org
www.jhuccp.org

Health communications family planning and AIDS prevention research.
*Susan Krenn, Director*
*James bon tempo, Associate Director of Communican Science*

**1916 Kaiser Foundation Research Institute**
3505 Broadway 510-450-2000
Oakland, CA 94611 Fax: 510-873-5130
*Paul Lairson MD, Director*

**1917 Kavli Foundation**
5715 Mesmer Avenue 424-353-8800
Los Angeles, CA info@kavlifoundation.org
www.kavlifoundation.org
The Foundation supports scientific research into the human brain, in the following scientific fields: Astrophysics, Nanoscience, Neuroscience and Theoretical Physics. Within Neuroscience, the study of aging and brain diseases and disorders is supported.
*Robert W. Conn, PhD, President & CEO*
*Eric Marshall, VP, Public Engagement & Prizes*

**1918 Mariposa Education and Research Foundation**
3123 Schweitzer Drive www.wysk.com
Topanga, CA 90290
Research involving the prevention of AIDS.
*Bruce Voeller PhD, President*

**1919 Medical University of South Carolina Health Services Administration**
Medical University of South Carolina
171 Ashley Avenue 843-792-1414
Charleston, SC 29425 800-424-6872
Fax: 843-792-2601
www.musc.edu
Devoted to public health policy and health care management including AIDS research.
*Raymond S Greenburg, President*
*Dr. Mark Sothman, Vice President*

**1920 Medical University of South Carolina: Health Services Administration**
College of Health 843-792-2300
Charleston, SC 29425 academicdepartments.musc.edu
Devoted to public health policy and health care management including AIDS research.
*Mark S. Sothmann, President*

**1921 Midwest AIDS Education and Training Center (MATEC)**
1919 West Taylor 312-996-1373
Chicago, IL 60612 312-413-4184
matec@uic.edu
www.matec.info
Provides educational programs about HIV infection for healthcare providers.
*Ricardo A. Rivero, MD, MPH, Executive Director*
*Renslow Sherer, MD, Regional Clinical Director*

**1922 NAMES Project Foundation AIDS Memorial Quilt**
AIDS Memorial Quilt
117 Luckie Street NW 404-688-5500
Atlanta, GA 30303 Fax: 404-688-5552
info@aidsquilt.org
www.aidsquilt.org
International, non-governmental, non-profit organization that is the custodian of the AIDS Memorial Quilt, a poignant memorial and powerful tool for use in preventing new HIV infections.
*Julie Rhoad, President & CEO*
*Roddy Williams, Director, Operations*

**1923 National Hemophilia Foundation: Hemophilia and AIDS/HIV Network (HANDI)**
110 Greene Street 212-328-3700
New York, NY 10012 Fax: 212-328-3777
handi@hemophilia.org
www.hemophilia.org
Dedicated to the treatment and the cure of hemophilia, AIDS and other blood related disorders. This foundation wishes to improve the quality of life of all those affected through promotion and support of research, education and other services.
*Alan Kinniburgh, CEO*

**1924 Neuroscience Research Institute**
UC Santa Barbara
6129 Biology II 805-893-4621
Santa Barbara, CA 93106 www.nri.ucsb.edu
The Institute seeks to allow scientists from different fields to collaborate for the betterment of neurological research. Areas of interest include: Alzheimer's Disease & Related Dementias; Behavioral Neuroscience & Neuroethology; Cell Biology, Biochemistry & Biophysics of the Nervous System; Computational & Theoretical Neuroscience; Development of the Nervous System; and Stem Cells.
*Stuart Feinstein, Co-Director*
*Kenneth Kosik, Co-Director*

**1925 Purdue University Center for AIDS Research**
School of Pharmacy and Pharmaceutical Sciences
575 Stadium Mall Drive 765-494-1361
W Lafayette, IN 47907-2091 Fax: 765-494-7880
oss@pharmacy.purdue.edu
www.pharmacy.purdue.edu
*Steve Byrn, Department Head*
*Stanley L Hem, Associate Department Head*

**1926 SUNY at Buffalo National Cooperative Drug Discovery Group for AIDS Treatment**
Department of Biochemistry
140 Farber Hall 716-829-2727
Buffalo, NY 14214-3000 Fax: 716-829-2725
jluck@buffalo.edu
www.buffalo.edu
*Kenneth M Blumenthal, Professor and Chairman*
*Elizabeth O'Brocta, Assistant to the Chairman*

**1927 Salk Institute for Biological Studies**
10010 N Torrey Pines Road 858-453-4100
La Jolla, CA 92037 www.salk.edu
Conducts groundbreaking research into cancer, aging, Alzheimer's diabetes and infectious diseases.
*Rusty Gage, PhD, President*
*Martin Hetzer, PhD, VP & Chief Science Officer*

**1928 Sansum Diabetes Research Institute**
2219 Bath Street 805-682-7638
Santa Barbara, CA 93105 Fax: 805-682-3332
info@sansum.org
www.sansum.org
*Rem Laan, Executive Director*

**1929 Scripps Research Institute**
10550 North Torrey Pines Road 858-784-1000
La Jolla, CA www.scripps.edu
The institute seeks to improve human wellbeing through the advancement of bioscience, including research into aging & healthspan, autoimmune diseases, cancer, infectious diseases, neurological disorders, and more.
*Peter Schultz, PhD, President & CEO*
*Eric Topol, MD, EVP, Scripps Research*

**1930 Spellman Center for HIV Related Disease The Spellman Center**
The Spellman Center
415 W Fifty-First Street 212-459-8130
New York, NY 10019
*David Kaufman, Director*

**1931 Stanford University General Clinical Research Center**
GCRC Administration
300 Pasteur Drive 650-723-4000
Stanford, CA 94305-5251 Fax: 650-725-6698
gcrcstanford@stanford.edu
The Stanford General Clinical Research Center (GCRC) is the major clinical research facility for Stanford University School of Medicine. With patient care units in Stanford University Hospital and Lucile Packard Children's Hospital the center plays a crucial role in the school's bench-to-bedside research mission.
*Ellen Jo Baron, Director*
*Branimir I Sikic, Program Director*

**1932 Stanford University National Cooperative Drug Discovery/AIDS Group**
School of Medicine

300 Pasteur Drive
Stanford, CA 94305
650-723-4000
Fax: 650-725-6698
www.med.stanford.edu

*Ellen Jo Baron, Director*
*Branimir I Sikic, Program Director*

1933 **Stanford University: General Clinical Research Center**
300 Pasteur Drive
Palo Alto, CA 94305
650-723-6073
Fax: 650-725-6698
*Dr. David Stevenson, Director*
*Howard Sussman, MD*

1934 **State University of New York: SUNY Stony HIV Treatment Development Center**
Center for Infectious Diseases
101 Nicolls Road
Stony Brook, NY 11794-5120
631-444-4000
Fax: 631-444-2493
rsteigbigel@notes.cc.sunysb.edu
www.stonybrookmedicalcenter.org
Human immunodeficiency virus research.
*Joyce Klien, Director*
*Laura Coppola, Assistant Director*

1935 **Tampa Bay Research Institute**
10900 Roosevelt Boulevard N
Saint Petersburg, FL 33716-2308
727-576-6675
Fax: 727-577-9862
development@tampabayresearch.org
www.tampabayresearch.org
TBRI is the first independent biomedical research organization of its kind in Florida. Our scientists dedicate their lives work to conquering chronic and infectious diseases while gaining a better understanding of the immune system.
*Clifford J Crook, Chair*
*John C Bierly, Program Assistant*

1936 **Thomas Jefferson University: Center for Research in Medical Education**
Jefferson Medical College
1020 Walnut Street
Philadelphia, PA 19107
215-955-6000
Fax: 215-923-7583
Joseph.Gonnella@jefferson.edu
www.jefferson.edu/jmc

*Joseph Gonne MD, Director*
*Robert L Barchi MD, President*

1937 **Toronto People with AIDS Foundation**
200 Gerrard Street E
Toronto, Ontario, M5A-2E6
416-506-1400
Fax: 416-506-1404
info@pwatoronto.org
www.pwatoronto.org
Promotes the health and well-being of all people living with HIV/AIDS by providing accessible, direct, and practical support services.
*Suzanne Paddock, Executive Director*
*Gareth Henry, Director, Programs & Services*

1938 **UCLA AIDS Clinical Research Center**
10940 Wilshire Blvd.
Los Angeles, CA 90024
310-794-4419
Fax: 310- 79- 395
aidsinstitute.ucla.edu

*Irvin S.Y. Chen, PhD, Director*
*Ora Yadin, MD*

1939 **UCSD Antiviral Research Center**
220 Dickinson Street
San Diego, CA 92103-8208
619-543-8080
Fax: 619-543-5066
Develops treatment protocols and drug therapies and recruits research volunteers for AIDS studies and HIV related disorders.
*Jill Kunkel, Director*
*Michael Giancola, Screening Co-ordinator*

1940 **USC Internal Medicine**
1520 San Pablo Street
Los Angeles, CA 90033-1034
800-872-2273
Fax: 213-224-6687
www.usc.edu/health/internal
Research into internal medicine with specialties in cardiovascular endocrinology and diabetes gastrointestinal and liver disease geriatric medicine hematology infectious diseases nephrology oncology pulmonary and critical care and rheumatology and immunology.
*Alexandra Levine, Head*

1941 **University of Alabama at Birmingham: National Cooperative Drug/AIDS**
UAB Center for AIDS Research
BBRB 256
Birmingham, AL 35294-1150
205-934-4011
http://www.uab.edu
*Robert P. Kimberly, Director*
*Cheryl A. Perry, Deputy Director*

1942 **University of California San Francisco Center for AIDS Prevention**
Center for AIDS Prevention Studies (CAPS)
50 Beale Street
San Francisco, CA 94105-3411
415-597-9100
Fax: 415-597-9213
CAPS.web@ucsf.edu
www.caps.ucsf.edu
The mission of the Center for AIDS Prevention Studies is to conduct domestic and international research to prevent the acquisition of HIV and to optimize health outcomes among HIV- infected individuals.
*Stephen F Morin, Director*
*Susan Kegeles, Co-Director*

1943 **University of California: Institute of Health Policy Studies**
333 California Street
San Francisco, CA 94104
415-476-4921
Fax: 415-476-0705
healthpolicy.ucsf.edu
Health policy and AIDS research.
*Philip R Lee, Director*
*Harold Luft, Executive Director*

1944 **University of California: Los Angeles Clinical AIDS Research & Education**
10833 Le Conte Avenue
Los Angeles, CA 90095
310-794-1456
Fax: 310-206-3311
AIDS research
*Alan Fogelman, M.D., Executive Chair*

1945 **University of California: San Diego Center for AIDS Research**
9500 Gilman Drive
La Jolla, CA 92093
858-534-8805
Fax: 619-822-1934
csussman@ucsd.edu
ari.ucsd.edu

AIDS research
*Flossie Wong-Staal PhD, Director*
*Gerry R Boss, MD*

1946 **University of California: San Francisco Center for AIDS Prevention Studies**
Prevention Science Group
50 Beale Street
San Francisco, CA 94105
415-597-9100
fcoates@psg.ucsf.edu
www.caps.ucsf.edu/capsweb

1947 **University of Hawaii: Hawaii AIDS Clinical Research Program**
3675 Kilauea Avenue
Honolulu, HI 96816
808-441-1573
Fax: 808-735-7047
gerschen@hawaii.edu
AIDS research

1948 **University of Maryland: Center for Research, Grants & Contracts**
655 W Lombard Street
Baltimore, MD 21201
410-706-3100
www.nursing.umaryland.edu
Focuses research on public and health policy laws, including AIDS research.

1949 **University of Maryland: Division of Infectious Diseases**
10 S Pine Street
Baltimore, MD 21201
410-706-7070
Fax: 410-706-8414
medschool.umaryland.edu
Focuses research on elderly studies including drug use, treatments and infectious diseases of the aged.

1950 **University of Maryland: Medical Biotechnology Center**
701 E. PRATT ST,ÿ
Baltimore, MD 21202-1513
410-706-8802
Fax: 410-706-8184
ÿhill@UMCES.edu
www.umbi.umd.edu

Offers research into AIDS and HIV infection including vaccine development.
*W Jonathan Lederer, Director*
*Kadir Aslan, Assistant Professor*

1951 **University of Michigan: National Cooperative Drug/AIDS Group**
School of Dentistry
1011 N University Avenue 734-763-6933
Ann Arbor, MI 48109-1078 Fax: 734-763-3453
paulk@umich.edu
www.dent.umich.edu
Focuses on the design of new drugs to fight AIDS.
*John C Drach PhD, Director*
*Paul H Krebsbach, Department Chair*

1952 **University of North Carolina: General Clinical Research Center**
Cb 7600 919-962-2211
Chapel Hill, NC 27599 www.med.unc.edu
Focuses on public policy and health research pertaining to the AIDS community and sexually transmitted disease studies.
*William L. Roper MD, MPH, Dean*

1953 **University of South Florida: Center for HIV Education & Research**
13301 Bruce B Downs Boulevard 813-974-4430
Tampa, FL 33612 Fax: 831-974-8451
contact@usfcenter.org
usfcenter.org
Treatment of persons affected and infected with HIV, provides current AIDS information to physicians and operates a resource center to provide educational materials as well as consultations.
*Jeffrey Beal, MD, AAHIVS, Director*

1954 **University of Vermont: Office of Health Promotion Research**
1 S Prospect Street 802-656-4187
Burlington, VT 05401 Fax: 802-656-8826
www.uvm.edu/~ohpr
Research done into public policy and human health including AIDS information and evaluation.
*Thomas Sullivan, President*

1955 **Utah Department of Health: Division of Community Health Services**
PO Box 141010 801-538-6003
Salt Lake City, UT 84114 health.utah.gov/
Secures and distributes funds for AIDS prevention services, provides educational programs and counseling to the general public, AIDS service organizations, health workers and groups at risk.
*W. David Patton PhD, Executive Director*

1956 **Wayne State University Center for Health Research**
College of Nursing
Center for Health Research 313-577-4082
Detroit, MI 48202 888-837- 08
Fax: 313-577-6949
nursinginfo@wayne.edu
www.nursing.wayne.edu/CHR
Facilitates interdisciplinary health research across diverse settings where nursing is practiced and healthcare is provided.
*Nancy T Artinian, Director*
*Barbara K Redman, Dean*

1957 **Wayne State University: Center for Health Research**
College of Nursing
5557 Cass Avenue 313-577-4082
Detroit, MI 48202 Fax: 313-577-5777
AIDS and HIV infection research and studies.
*Dr. Ada Jacox, Associate Dean*
*Janet Harden, Executive Director*

## Support Groups & Hotlines

1958 **AEGIS AIDS Education Global Information System**
PO Box 184 949-495-1952
San Juan Capistrano, CA 92693 Fax: 949-443-1755
www.aegis.org
A not-for-profit, tax-exempt, educational corpoation that adds more than 3000 documents each month. Reach more than 10 million users annually, including: the US Federal Government, US Educational Institutions, and Nonprofit organizations both here and abroad.
*Vanessa Robison, President*
*Sister Mary Elizabeth, Assistant Operations Director*

1959 **AIDS Alabama**
3521 7th Avenue S 205-324-9822
Birmingham, AL 35222 800-592-2437
Fax: 205-324-9311
maryanne@aidsalabama.org
www.aidsalabama.org
Devotes its energy and resources statewide to helping people with HIV/AIDS live healthy, independent lives and works to prevent the spread of HIV. It is our goal to provide housing for those with HIV in the Birmingham area, secure and administer grants for care of persons with HIV statewide, and specialize in targeted prevention education programs.
*Elaine Cottle, Executive Director*

1960 **AIDS Hotline of Central New York**
AIDS Community Resources
627 W Genesee Street 315-475-2430
Syracuse, NY 13204 800-475-2430
Fax: 315-472-6515
information@aidscommunityresources.com
www.aidscommunityresources.com
A not-for-profit, community-based organization providing prevention, education and support services to those infected with and affected by HIV/AIDS Serves Cayuga, Herkimer, Jefferson, Lewis, Madison, Oneida, Onondaga, Oswego and St. Lawrences counties in New York State.
*Michael Crinnin, Executive Director*

1961 **AIDS Support Group of Cape Cod**
428 S Street 508-778-1957
Hyannis, MA 02610 866-990-2437
Fax: 508-778-4501
info@asgcc.org
www.asgcc.org
Our mission is to provide services that maintain and enhance the quality of life for persons living with HIV and AIDS on Cape Cod and Martha's Vineyard and to provide health education, prevention and harm reduction outreach via timely and accurate information about HIV/AIDS, STIs and viral hepatitis.
*Krystin St. Onge, Interim Director*

1962 **AIDSinfo**
US Department of Health and Human Services
PO Box 6303 301-315-2816
Rockville, MD 20849-6303 800-448-0440
Fax: 301-315-2818
TTY: 888-480-3739
contactus@aidsinfo.nih.gov
www.aidsinfo.nih.gov
Offers the latest federally approved information on HIV/AIDS clinical research, treatment and prevention, and medical practice guidelines for people living with HIV/AIDS, their families and friends, health care providers, scientists, and researchers.

1963 **Alaskan Statewide AIDS Helpline**
1057 W Fireweed 907-263-2050
Anchorage, AK 99503 800-478-AIDS
Fax: 907-263-2051
www.alaskanaids.org
A key collaborator within the state of Alaska in the provision of supportive services to persons living with HIV/AIDS and their families and in the elimination of the transmission of HIV infection and its stigma.
*Heather Davis, Executive Director*
*Maureen Suttman, Client Resource Services*

1964 **BABES Network-YWCA**
1118 Fifth Ave 206-720-5566
Seattle, WA 98101 888-292-1912
Fax: 206-720-5901
the_staff@babesnetwork.org
www.babesnetwork.org
A peer-based program, a sisterhood of women facing HIV together. Reduces isolation, promotes self-empowerment, enhances quality

of life and serves the needs of women facing HIV and their families through peer support, advocacy, education and outreach.
*Rhonda Kimm, Advocacy Coordinator*
*Amelia Vader, Program Manager*

1965 **COMPASS Program**
c/o Institute for Urban Family Health
16 East 16th Street 212-924-7744
New York, NY 10003 Fax: 212-691-4610
info@institute2000.org
Medical services include HIV testing and specialized HIV medical care for adults in addition to women's health services including gynecology, PAP tests, family planning and birth control methods. Mental health services includes individual, couples, and family counseling and psychiatric evaluations and monitoring.
*Neil Calman MD/ABFP/FAAFP, President/Chief Executive Officer*
*Weston Willett, Chief Information Officer*

1966 **Cascade AIDS Project Hotline**
200 SW Fifth Avenue 503-223-5907
Portland, OR 97204 Fax: 503-223-6437
info@cascadeaids.org
www.cascadeaids.org
Provides HIV prevention and services information by phone and internet to youth and adults across Orgeon and the Northwest.
*Charles Washington, President*
*warren Jimanez, Vice President*

1967 **Dunshee House**
303-17th Avenue East 206-322-2437
Seattle, WA 98112 Fax: 206-322-1779
josh@dunsheehouse.org
A non-profit organization, builds community and cultivates powerful, healthy lives by providing emotional support and personal development services to those affected by HIV/AIDS, the Queer communities, and those who love them.
*Michael Kann, President*
*Adrienne Miller, Vice President*

1968 **HEAL**
Sidney Hillman Family Pracitce
16 E 16th Street 212-924-7744
New York, NY 10003-3105 healweb@thorup.com
The Health Education AIDS Liaison provides alternative and holistic support groups and resources for people with HIV.

1969 **King County Crisis Clinic**
9725 3rdÿAvenue NE 206-461-3210
Seattle, WA 98115 866-427-4747
Fax: 206-461-8368
TDD: 206-461-3219
info@crisisclinic.org
www.crisisclinic.org
A non-profit organization, we offer an array of support services available to everyone in King County, Washington.
*Kathleen Southwick, Executive Director*
*Susan Gemmel, Director*

1970 **Life Force: Women Fighting AIDS**
NYC Service
175 Remsen Street 718-797-0937
Brooklyn, NY 11201 www.nycservice.org/organizations/138
A support network offering legislative information, educational awareness and support for women with HIV/AIDS.
*Nur Ibrahim, Treasurer*

1971 **Minnesota AIDS Project AIDSLine**
1400 Park Avenue 612-341-2060
Minneapolis, MN 55404 800-248-7321
Fax: 612-341-4057
TTY: 888-820-2437
mapaidsline@mnaidsproject.org
www.mnaidsproject.org
A statewide, toll-free information and referral service that can answer your questions about HIV and connect you to resources that can help.
*Bill Tiedmann, Executive Director*

1972 **National Health Information Center**
Office of Disease Prevention & Health Promotion
1101 Wootton Pkwy Fax: 240-453-8281
Rockville, MD 20852 odphpinfo@hhs.gov
www.health.gov/nhic
Supports public health education by maintaining a calendar of National Health Observances; helps connect consumers and health professionals to organizations that can best answer questions and provide up-to-date contact information from reliable sources; updates on a yearly basis toll-free numbers for health information, Federal health clearinghouses and info centers.
*Don Wright, MD, MPH, Director*

1973 **Northwestern Connecticut AIDS Project**
100 Migeon Avenue 860-482-1596
Torrington, CT 06790 Fax: 860-482-3606
A nonprofit organization offering support and a variety of services to people with AIDS and their loved ones. Provides education to all segments of the public about AIDS prevention and treatment.
*Patricia Lafayette, Executive Director*

1974 **Project Inform HIV Health InfoLine**
273 Ninth Street 415-558-8669
San Francisco, CA 94103-2621 800-822-7422
Fax: 415-558-0684
web@projectinform.org
www.projectinform.org
Runs an HIV Infoline, as well as a Hepatitis C helpline, while engaging in advocacy on behalf of individuals living with HIV/AIDS.
*Ferdinand Garcia, President*
*Dana Van Gorder, Executive Director*

1975 **Project Inform HIv Health InfoLine**
273 Ninth Street 415-558-8669
San Francisco, CA 94103-2621 800-822-7422
Fax: 415-558-0684
web@projectinform.org
www.projectinform.org
Runs an HIV Infoline, as well as a Hepatitis C helpline, while engaging in advocacy on behalf of individuals living with HIV/AIDS.
*Ferdinand Garcia, President*
*Dana Van Gorder, Executive Director*

## Magazines

1976 **AIDS Alert**
American Health Consultants
3525 Piedmont Road 404-262-5476
Atlanta, GA 30355 800-688-2421
Fax: 404-262-5560
www.ahcmedia.com
Covers up-to-the-minute developments and guidance on the entire spectrum of AIDS challenges, including treatment, education, precautions, screening, diagnosis and policy.

1977 **AIDS Clinical Care**
New England Journal of Medicine
860 Winter Street 781-893-4610
Waltham, MA 02451-1413 800-322-2303
Fax: 781-893-3800
www.massmed.org
Up to date information specifically targeted at physicians with AIDS patients.
*Monthly*

1978 **AIDS: A Year In Review**
Lippincott Williams & Wilkins
16522 Hunters Green Pkwy 301-223-2300
Hagerstown, MD 21740 800-638-3030
Fax: 301-223-2400
orders@lww.com
www.lww.com
An interdisciplinary journal providing a synthesis of AIDS-related information from all relevant clinical and basic sciences.

1979 **AIDS: International Monthly Journal**
Lippincott Williams & Wilkins

16522 Hunters Green Pkwy
Hagerstown, MD 21740
301-223-2300
800-638-3030
Fax: 301-223-2400
orders@lww.com
www.lww.com

An interdisciplinary journal providing a synthesis of AIDS-related information from all relevant clinical and basic sciences.

1980 **AIDS: The Disease State Management Resource**
American Health Consultants
PO Box 550669
Atlanta, GA 30355
404-262-5476
800-688-2421
Fax: 800-284-3291
www.ahcmedia.com

Covers up-to-the-minute developments and guidance on the entire spectrum of AIDS challenges, including treatment, education, precautions, screening, diagnosis and policy.

1981 **ASN NEURO**
Sage Journals
2455 Teller Road
Thousand Oaks, CA 91320
805-499-9774
journals@sagepub.com
journals.sagepub.com/home/asn

Peer-reviewed open access journal focusing on recent advances in the cellular and molecular neurosciences. It is the official publication of the American Society for Neurochemistry.
*Douglas L. Feinstein, Editor-in-Chief*
*Sandra J. Hewitt, Deputy Editor-in-Chief*

1982 **BMC Neuroscience**
Springer Nature
One New York Plaza
New York, NY 10004-1562
800-777-4643
info@biomedcentral.com
bmcneurosci.biomedcentral.com

A peer-reviewed, open-access journal devoted to all aspects of the nervous system (including molecular, cellular, developmental and animal model studies), as well as cognitive and behavioral research, and computational modeling.
*Darren Byrne, Editor*
*Ana Donnelly, Manuscript Editor*

1983 **Clinical Infectious Diseases**
Oxford University Press
2001 Evans Road
Cary, NC 27513
919-677-0977
800-852-7323
Fax: 919-677-1714
academic.oup.com/cid

Leading journal on infectious diseases, with original research, reviews, viewpoints, editorials, invited commentaries, photo quizzes, practice guidelines, correspondence and supplements. The journal has a broad focus, encompassing clinical descriptions, public health, microbiology, immunology, prevention of infection, evaluation of current and novel treatments and promotion of optimal practices for diagnosis and treatment.
*Robert T. Schooley, Editor-in-Chief*
*Ferric C. Fang, Deputy Editor*

1984 **Continuum: Lifelong Learning in Neurology**
American Academy of Neurology
201 Chicago Avenue
Minneapolis, MN 55415
612-928-6000
800-879-1960
continuumcme@aan.com
journals.lww.com/continuum

Official journal of the American Academy of Neurology, aiding professionals in patient care and continuing education.
*Bimonthly*
*Steven L. Lewis, MD, FAAN*
*Andrea J. Weiss, MA, Executive Editor*

1985 **Critical Path AIDS Project**
2062 Lombard Street
Philadelphia, PA 19146-1315
215-545-2212
www.critpath.org

Articles and reprints on experimental treatments and alternative therapies, and a listing of Philadelphia-area resources.
*Monthly*

1986 **Institute on Health Care for the Poor and Underserved at Meharry Medical College**
Sage Publications
1005 DB Todd Boulevard
Nashville, TN 37208
615-327-6819
800-669-1269
Fax: 615-327-6362
vbrennan@mmc.edu

Offers health care and public health policy research focusing on poor and underserved populations.
*100pages 4x a year*
*Dr. Amy Cato, Director*
*Dr. Virginia Brennan, Editor*

1987 **Journal of Acquired Immune Deficiency Syndrome**
Lippincott Williams & Wilkins
16522 Hunters Green Pkwy
Hagerstown, MD 21740-2601
301-223-2300
800-638-3030
Fax: 301-223-2400
orders@lww.com
www.lww.com

An interdisciplinary journal providing a synthesis of AIDS-related information from all relevant clinical and basic sciences.
*Monthly*
*ISBN: 0-894925-5 -*
*William A Hazeltine, Editor*

1988 **Journal of Infectious Diseases**
Oxford University Press
2001 Evans Road
Cary, NC 27513
919-677-0977
800-852-7323
Fax: 919-677-1714
academic.oup.com/jid

Official publication of the Infectious Diseases Society of America, with original research on infectious diseases.
*Martin S. Hirsch, MD, Editor-in-Chief*
*David C. Hooper, Deputy Editor*

1989 **Journal of Neuroinflammation**
Springer Nature
One New York Plaza
New York, NY 10004-1562
800-777-4643
info@biomedcentral.com
jneuroinflammation.biomedcentral.com

A peer-reviewed, open-access journal focusing on the interactions of the immune system with the nervous system as a means of expanding understanding of chronic neurological diseases.
*Monica J. Carson, Editor-in-Chief*
*Sue T. Griffin, Editor-in-Chief*

1990 **Journal of Nuclear Medicine**
Society of Nuclear Medicine and Molecular Imaging
1850 Samuel Morse Drive
Reston, VA 20190
703-708-9000
800-513-6853
Fax: 703-708-9015
subscriptions@snm.org
jnm.snmjournals.org

Peer-reviewed journal with clinical investigations, science reports, articles benefitting continuing education, book reviews, employment opportunities, and updates on practice and research.
*Monthly*
*Johannes Czernin, MD, Editor-in-Chief*
*Susan Alexander, Associate Director, Publications*

1991 **Journal of the Medical Library Association**
Medical Library Association
65 E Wacker Place
Chicago, IL 60601-7246
312-419-9094
Fax: 312-419-8950
info@mlahq.org

An international, peer-reviewed journal that aims to advance the practice and research knowledgebase of health science librarianship.
*Quarterly*
*Kevin Baliozian, Executive Director*
*Susan C.T. Talmage, Managing Editor, Publications*

1992 **Journal of the Neurological Sciences**
Elsevier
LSU Health Sciences Center
New Orleans, LA 70112
JNS_England@lsuhsc.edu
www.jns-journal.com

Original articles in neurology and neuroscience from around the world.
*Monthly*
*John D. England, Editor-in-Chief*

1993 **Molecular Imaging**
Sage Journals
2455 Teller Road
Thousand Oaks, CA 91320
805-499-9774
journals@sagepub.com
journals.sagepub.com/home/mix
Peer-reviewed open access journal focusing on molecular imaging research, including basic science, preclinical studies and human applications. Published in association with the Society of Nuclear Medicine and Molecular Imaging.
*Bimonthly*
*Henry F. VanBrocklin, PhD, Editor-in-Chief*

1994 **Molecular Neurodegeneration**
Springer Nature
One New York Plaza
New York, NY 10004-1562
800-777-4643
info@biomedcentral.com
www.biomedcentral.com
A peer-reviewed, open-access journal devoted to all aspects of neurodegeneration research at the molecular and cellular levels.
*Guojun Bu, Editor-in-Chief*
*Huaxi Xu, Editor-in-Chief*

1995 **Neurocase: The Neural Basis of Cognition**
Taylor & Francis Group
530 Walnut Street
Philadelphia, PA 19106
www.tandfonline.com/toc/nncs20/current
Rapid response journal featuring case and group studies in neuropsychology, neuropsychiatry and behavioral neurology, with a focus on the neural basis of cognition.
*Bruce L. Miller, Editor*
*Hans J. Markowitsch, Editor*

1996 **Neurology**
American Academy of Neurology
201 Chicago Avenue
Minneapolis, MN 55415
612-928-6000
800-879-1960
Fax: 612-454-2748
journal@neurology.org
n.neurology.org
Official journal of the American Academy of Neurology, peer-reviewed, highlighting clinical neurology research.
*Jose G. Merino, MD, MPhil, FAAN, Editor-in-Chief*
*Patricia K. Baskin, MS, Executive Editor*

1997 **Neurology Clinical Practice**
American Academy of Neurology
201 Chicago Avenue
Minneapolis, MN 55415
612-928-6000
800-879-1960
Fax: 612-454-2748
journal@neurology.org
cp.neurology.org
Official peer-reviewed journal of the American Academy of Neurology for practicing neurologists.
*John R. Corboy, MD, FAAN, Editor*
*Patricia K. Baskin, MS, Executive Editor*

1998 **Neurology: Genetics**
American Academy of Neurology
201 Chicago Avenue
Minneapolis, MN 55415
612-928-6000
800-879-1960
Fax: 612-454-2748
journal@neurology.org
ng.neurology.org
Official journal of the American Academy of Neurology, publishing online open-access peer-reviewed reports in the field of neurogenetics.
*Stefan M. Pulst, MD, FAAN, Editor*
*Patricia K. Baskin, MS, Executive Editor*

1999 **Neurology: Neuroimmunology & Neuroinflammation**
American Academy of Neurology
201 Chicago Avenue
Minneapolis, MN 55415
612-928-6000
800-879-1960
Fax: 612-454-2748
journal@neurology.org
nn.neurology.org
Official journal of the American Academy of Neurology, publishing online open-access peer-reviewed reports of original research and in-depth reviews of topics in neuroimmunology & neuroinflammation.
*Josep O. Dalmau, MD, PhD, Editor*
*Patricia K. Baskin, MS, Executive Editor*

2000 **Open Forum Infectious Diseases**
Oxford University Press
2001 Evans Road
Cary, NC 27513
919-677-0977
800-852-7323
Fax: 919-677-1714
academic.oup.com/ofid
Open-access journal featuring clinical, translational and basic research on biomedical science and clinical practice.
*Paul E. Sax, MD, Editor-in-Chief*
*Jonathan Z. Li, MD, Deputy Editor*

2001 **POZ Magazine**
POZ Publishing
462 Seventh Avenue
New York, NY 10018-7424
212-242-2163
Fax: 212-675-8505
www.poz.com
A magazine for people living with, and affected by, HIV/AIDS.
*60 pages BiMonthly*
*Regan Hofmann, Editor in Chief*
*Jennifer Morton, Managing Editor*

2002 **Risky Business**
San Francisco AIDS Foundation Materials Dept.
333 Valencia Street
San Francisco, CA 94103-3547
415-861-3397
A comic book style magazine providing accurate information about AIDS using humor and real-life situations. Contains stories that stress the importance of knowing how AIDS is transmitted and prevented.

2003 **Ultrasonic Imaging**
Sage Journals
2455 Teller Road
Thousand Oaks, CA 91320
805-499-9774
journals@sagepub.com
journals.sagepub.com/home/uix
The journal focuses on the rapid publication of original papers on the development and application of ultrasonic techniques, with emphasis on medical diagnosis. Also published are research notes, comments on papers appearing in the journal, book reviews, and occasional review articles.
*Ernest J. Feleppa, Editor-in-Chief*
*Roslyn Raskin, Managing Editor*

2004 **Washington Update**
Committee of Ten Thousand
500 Belmont Street
Brockton, MA 02301
508-587-2512
cott-dc@earthlink.net
www.cott1.org
Is a primer on government related issues of importance to COTT's constituency. From health care legislation, to regulatory affairs to Administration policy for chronic diseases. A hands-on journal for grass roots health care advocacy in our Nation's capital.
*Bi-Monthly*
*John Rider, Contact*

## Web Sites

2005 **AIDS Education and Training Center National Multicultural Center**
www.aetcnmc.org
Located at Howard University College of Medicine, AETC-NMC acted as an HIV/AIDS training and technical resource for providers of minority HIV-infected patients throughout the country. Today, lack of funding allows the Center to maintain its website only, as an archive of information.

2006 **AIDS United**
www.aidsunited.org
To end the AIDS epidemic in the United States. We will achieve this goal through national, regional and local policy/advocacy, strategic grantmaking, and organizational capacity building. With partners throughout the country, we will work to ensure that people living with and affected by HIV/AIDS have access to the prevention and care services they need and deserve.

**2007 AIDS.ORG**

www.aids.org

The mission of AIDS.ORG is to help prevent HIV infections and to improve the lives of those affected by HIV and AIDS by providing education and facilitating the free and open exchange of knowledge at any easy-to-find centralized website.

**2008 AIDSInfo**

PO Box 4780
Rockville, MD 20849
800-448-0440
Fax: 301-315-2818
TTY: 888-480-3739
contactus@aidsinfo.nih.gov
www.aidsinfo.nih.gov

A call in service where trained staff offers quick access to federally approved HIV/AIDS treatment and prevention guidelines, clinical trials, and other research-related information.

**2009 AIDSVu**

aidsvu.org

Interactive maps of the AIDS epidemic across the states, including downloadable data sets and a services directory.

**2010 Arkansas Department of Health**

4815 W Markham Street
Little Rock, AR 72205
501-661-2000
www.healthy.state.ar

Provides educational materials such as pamphlets and films, conducts HIV and AIDS research and operates a speakers bureau.

**2011 Committee of Ten Thousand**

www.cott1.org

Represents people with hemophilia who contracted HIV/AIDS and Hepatitis C from tainted factory concentrates in the 1970s and 1980s. The only national advocacy, and support agency for this seriously disabled community. Website includes a digital archive of photos, gatherings, and events.

*Carl Weixler, President*
*Ray Dattoli, Vice President*

**2012 HIV.gov**

www.hiv.gov

Online portal for HIV/AIDS-related resources, managed by the U.S. Department of Health & Human Services and supported by the Secretary's Minority AIDS Initiative Fund (SMAIF).

**2013 HIV/Hepatitis C in Prison (HIP) Committee**

www.prisons.org/hivin.htm

Fighting for consistent access to quality medical care including access to all new HIV and Hepatitis C medications, diagnostic testing and combination therapies.

**2014 Healing Well**

www.healingwell.com

A social network and support community for patients, caregivers, and families coping with the daily struggles of diseases, disorders and chronic illness.

**2015 Health Finder**

www.healthfinder.gov

Searchable, carefully developed web site offering information on over 1000 topics. Developed by the US Department of Health and Human Services, the site can be used in both English and Spanish.

**2016 Healthlink USA**

www.healthlinkusa.com

Health information concerning treatment, cures, prevention, diagnosis, risk factors, research, support groups, email lists, personal stories and much more. Updated regularly.

**2017 Immune Deficiency Foundation**

www.primaryimmune.org

The national patient organization dedicated to improving the diagnosis, treatment and quality of life of persons with primary immunodeficiency diseases through advocacy, education and research.

**2018 MedicineNet**

www.medicinenet.com

An online resource for consumers providing easy-to-read, authoritative medical and health information.

**2019 Medscape**

www.medscape.com

Medscape offers specialists, primary care physicians, and other health professionals the Web's most robust and integrated medical information and educational tools.

**2020 National AIDS Information Clearinghouse**

www.cdcnac.org

Provides information and materials for employers on national, state and local resources related to HIV/AIDS in the workplace.

**2021 National Hospice & Palliative Care Organization (NHPCO)**

www.nhpco.org

The organization seeks to improve end-of-life care, widen access to hospice care, and improve quality of life for the dying and their loved ones. NHPCO's website offers information on regulations, advocacy, quality and performance, education, and a variety of other resources.

**2022 Pennsylvania Department of Health: Bureau of HIV/AIDS**

625 Forster Street
Harrisburg, PA 17120
877-724-3258

Offers various community health education presentations, counseling and testing sites. Also offers practical support services, counseling, HIV testing, a hotline and referrals.

*Tom Corbett, Governor*
*Michael Wolf, Secretary*

**2023 People with AIDS Health Group**

www.Aidsinfonyc.org

PWA is a non-profit buyers club organized to assist people with AIDS in obtaining medications — as well as provide support groups committed to the self-empowerment of people living with AIDS. They offer three programs: Treatment Education and Support, Advocacy and Public Policy, and Early Treatment Access.

**2024 Project Inform Hotline**

273 Ninth Street
San Francisco, CA 94103
415-558-8669
877-435-7443
Fax: 415-558-0684

HIV/AIDS treatment information.

*Christopher Esposito, President*
*Ferdinand Garcia, Vice President*

**2025 Smart & Strong**

www.smartstrong.com

A healthcare education company that supports providers and empowers HIV positive patients through publications, seminars and innovative educational programs.

**2026 The Body: The Complete HIV/AIDS Resource**

Remedy Health Media
750 3rd Avenue
New York, NY 10017
www.thebody.com

*Myles Helfand, Editorial Director*
*J.D. Davids, Managing Editor*

**2027 Vermont Department of Healt: HIV/AIDS Program**

www.state.vt.us

We provide riask reduction and health education services, Anonymous HIV counseling and testing sites through Vermont, HIV/AIDS educational materials.

**2028 Virginia Department of Health: Division HIV/STD**

www.vdh.state.va.us/std

The division provides a toll free hotline for HIV/STD and viral Hepatitis information, education, confidentiality and anoymous testing. Tghe division provides referrals for AIDS medication assistance and outpatient care services for income eligible persons with HIV.

**2029 WebMD**

www.webmd.com

Provides credible information, supportive communities, and in-depth reference material about health subjects. A source for original and timely health information as well as material from well known content providers.

# HUNTINGTON'S DISEASE

*Huntington's disease is a progressive neurological disease that leads to the steady breakdown of nerve cells in the brain. Although rare, Huntington's is a notable cause of dementia, resulting in a wide array of movement, cognitive, and psychiatric disorders. Unlike most other dementia-causing diseases, Huntington's typically affects younger patients, with symptoms often first appearing in a patient's 30s or 40s. In rare cases, the disease's onset can occur in a patient's teen years, in a variation known as juvenile Huntington's disease.*

Symptoms of Huntington's disease can vary greatly from patient to patient, but they generally fall into three categories. Movement disorders can consist of jerking, muscle rigidity or contracture, impaired gait, and difficulty with speech or swallowing. Cognitive disorders may include difficulty focusing, lack of impulse control, and slowness of thinking. These symptoms eventually progress to dementia. Finally, a number of psychiatric disorders are linked to Huntington's disease. The most common of these is depression, but obsessive-compulsive disorder and bipolar disorder are also linked to Huntington's, as are more generalized feelings of irritability or apathy and social withdrawal. The dominant symptoms of juvenile Huntington's are slightly different and generally include difficulty paying attention, behavioral problems, tremors, and clumsiness. Patients generally live between 10 to 30 years after diagnosis. This number shortens to about 10 years for juvenile Huntington's.

Huntington's is a genetic disorder caused by a defective gene. Although the disease was first described by Dr. George Huntington in the late 19th century, the gene was not discovered until 1993 and scientists are still learning more about the disease every day. The genetic defect is dominant, so that anyone who inherits the gene will eventually develop the disease. The defective gene leads to the production of a protein known as 'huntingtin' which in turn results in the brain changes that cause Huntington's disease.

Because the gene has been identified, a diagnostic genetic test is available which can confirm whether or not the patient has the defective gene. However, there is no cure for Huntington's disease and treatment is focused on managing the symptoms. In order to treat the involuntary movements that are characteristic of the disease, doctors may prescribe either a drug like tetrabenazine, specifically designed for Huntington's, or a more generalized antipsychotic drug. Antipsychotic drugs may also be prescribed for extreme cases of irritability and anger, although for less severe cases, an antidepressant is generally chosen. Antidepressants may also be prescribed to treat patients who develop obsessive-compulsive disorder. Psychotherapy is also indicated in many of these instances.

## National Agencies & Associations

2031 **American Academy of Neurology**
201 Chicago Avenue
Minneapolis, MN 55415
612-928-6000
800-879-1960
Fax: 612-454-2746
memberservices@aan.com
www.aan.com
Professional society of medical doctors specializing in brain and nervous system diseases. Maintains placement service. Sponsors research and educational programs. Compiles statistics. Publishes scientific journal, Continuum: Lifelong Learning in Neurology.
*Mary E. Post, MBA, CAE, CEO*

2032 **American Society for Investigative Pathology**
1801 Rockville Pike
Rockville, MD 20852
240-283-9700
Fax: 301-984-4047
www.asip.org
The Society seeks to promote experimental pathology and related disciplines through meetings, publications, and educational activities.
*William B. Coleman, PhD, Executive Officer*
*Gina LaBorde, Manager, Marketing & Communications*

2033 **American Society for Neurochemistry**
9037 Ron Den Lane
Windermere, FL 34786
407-909-9064
Fax: 407-876-0750
asnmanager@asneurochem.org
asneurochem.org
The Society aims to advance and promote cellular and molecular neuroscience knowledge, and to facilitate communication and the dissemination of information within the field and with related disciplines.
*Sheilah Jewart, Executive Director*
*Karen Gottlieb, Conference Coordinator*

## Foundations & Research Centers

2034 **Center for Brain Activity Mapping**
UC San Diego
9500 Gilman Drive
La Jolla, CA 92093
858-534-2230
cbam.ucsd.edu
The Center seeks to develop new technologies for detecting neuronal activity, for reporting it out of deep brain tissue, and for processing and analyzing the resulting data, by organizing and supporting research teams and projects.
*Ralph J. Greenspan, PhD, Director*

2035 **Kavli Foundation**
5715 Mesmer Avenue
Los Angeles, CA
424-353-8800
info@kavlifoundation.org
www.kavlifoundation.org
The Foundation supports scientific research into the human brain, in the following scientific fields: Astrophysics, Nanoscience, Neuroscience and Theoretical Physics. Within Neuroscience, the study of aging and brain diseases and disorders is supported.
*Robert W. Conn, PhD, President & CEO*
*Eric Marshall, VP, Public Engagement & Prizes*

2036 **Kavli Institute for Brain Science at Columbia University**
Columbia University
3227 Broadway
New York, NY 10027
212-853-1016
Fax: 212-665-9699
kavli@columbia.edu
www.kavli.columbia.edu
The Institute's primary are of study is how signaling in neural circuits controls cognitive function and behavior, and the development of novel experimental and computational strategies for analyzing these signals.
*Eric R. Kandel, MD, Director*
*Rafael Yuste, MD, PhD, Co-Director*

2037 **Kavli Institute for Fundamental Neuroscience**
UCSF, Sandler Neurosciences Center
675 Nelson Rising Lane
San Francisco, CA 94158
415-476-2018
Fax: 415-502-7332
kavliifn@ucsf.edu
kavliifn.ucsf.edu
The Institute is the central organization for neuroscience research at UCSF and partner institutions, establishing cross-disciplinary teams of scientists and engineers devoted to advancing neuroscience in all its forms.
*Loren Frank, Co-Director*
*Roger Nicoll, Co-Director*

2038 **Kavli Institute for Neuroscience at Yale University**
Yale School of Medicine
295 Congress Avenue
New Haven, CT 06510
203-737-4461
203-737-4467
pietro.decamilli@yale.edu
medicine.yale.edu/neuroscience/kavli
The institute studies nervous system development and function.
*Pietro De Camilli, MD, Director*
*Marina Picciotto, PhD, Deputy Director*

2039 **Kavli Neural Systems Institute**
The Rockefeller University
1230 York Avenue
New York, NY 10065
212-327-8081
lcole@rockefeller.edu
www.rockefeller.edu/research
The Institute unites scientists at The Rockefeller University in the goal of a comprehensive look at the human brain.
*Leslie Vosshall, PhD, Director*
*Lindsey Cole, Administrator*

2040 **Kavli Neuroscience Discovery Institute**
Johns Hopkins University, School of Medicine
725 N Wolfe Street
Baltimore, MD 21205
410-955-4089
Fax: 410-614-6249
KavliNDI@jhu.edu
kavlijhu.org
The Institute looks to advance neuroscience by integrating neuroscience, engineering and computational data science.
*Dwight Bergles, PhD, Director*
*Natasha Hussain, PhD, Scientific Director*

2041 **Neuroscience Research Institute**
UC Santa Barbara
6129 Biology II
Santa Barbara, CA 93106
805-893-4621
www.nri.ucsb.edu
The Institute seeks to allow scientists from different fields to collaborate for the betterment of neurological research. Areas of interest include: Alzheimer's Disease & Related Dementias; Behavioral Neuroscience & Neuroethology; Cell Biology, Biochemistry & Biophysics of the Nervous System; Computational & Theoretical Neuroscience; Development of the Nervous System; and Stem Cells.
*Stuart Feinstein, Co-Director*
*Kenneth Kosik, Co-Director*

2042 **Salk Institute for Biological Studies**
10010 N Torrey Pines Road
La Jolla, CA 92037
858-453-4100
www.salk.edu
Conducts groundbreaking research into cancer, aging, Alzheimer's diabetes and infectious diseases.
*Rusty Gage, PhD, President*
*Martin Hetzer, PhD, VP & Chief Science Officer*

2043 **Sanford Consortium for Regenerative Medicine**
2880 Torrey Pines Scenic Drive
La Jolla, CA 92037
858-246-1071
www.sanfordconsortium.com
The Consortium works to achieve breakthrough discoveries in stem cell research with regards to diagnoses, treatments, and cures for degenerative diseases and injuries.
*Edward W. Holmes, MD, President & CEO*
*Jeffrey Steindorf, PhD, VP & COO*

2044 **Scripps Research Institute**
10550 North Torrey Pines Road
La Jolla, CA
858-784-1000
www.scripps.edu
The institute seeks to improve human wellbeing through the advancement of bioscience, including research into aging & healthspan, autoimmune diseases, cancer, infectious diseases, neurological disorders, and more.
*Peter Schultz, PhD, President & CEO*
*Eric Topol, MD, EVP, Scripps Research*

## Magazines

**2045 ASN NEURO**
Sage Journals
2455 Teller Road 805-499-9774
Thousand Oaks, CA 91320 journals@sagepub.com
journals.sagepub.com/home/asn

Peer-reviewed open access journal focusing on recent advances in the cellular and molecular neurosciences. It is the official publication of the American Society for Neurochemistry.
*Douglas L. Feinstein, Editor-in-Chief*
*Sandra J. Hewitt, Deputy Editor-in-Chief*

**2046 American Journal of Pathology**
Elsevier
1600 John F Kennedy Boulevard 301-634-7959
Philadelphia, PA 19103 Fax: 301-634-7961
ajp@asip.org
ajp.amjpathol.org

Official journal of the American Society for Investigative Pathology, publishing original research reports, reviews, and commentaries related to the molecular and cellular basis of disease.
*Martha Furie, Editor-in-Chief*

**2047 BMC Neuroscience**
Springer Nature
One New York Plaza 800-777-4643
New York, NY 10004-1562 info@biomedcentral.com
bmcneurosci.biomedcentral.com

A peer-reviewed, open-access journal devoted to all aspects of the nervous system (including molecular, cellular, developmental and animal model studies), as well as cognitive and behavioral research, and computational modeling.
*Darren Byrne, Editor*
*Ana Donnelly, Manuscript Editor*

**2048 Brain & Life**
American Academy of Neurology
201 Chicago Avenue 612-928-6000
Minneapolis, MN 55415 800-879-1960
Fax: 612-454-2748
BrainandLife@wolterskluwer.com
www.brainandlife.org

Official magazine of the American Academy of Neurology, aimed at parents and home-caregivers interested in neurology in everyday life.
*Orly Avitzur, MD, MBA, FAAN, Editor-in-Chief*
*Mary Bolster, Managing Editor*

**2049 Brain: A Journal of Neurology**
Oxford University Press
2001 Evans Road 919-677-0977
Cary, NC 27513 800-852-7323
Fax: 919-677-1714
brain@ucl.ac.uk
academic.oup.com/brain

Focus is clinical neurology and translational neuroscience.
*Dimitri M. Kullmann, Editor*
*Joanne Bell, Managing Editor*

**2050 Continuum: Lifelong Learning in Neurology**
American Academy of Neurology
201 Chicago Avenue 612-928-6000
Minneapolis, MN 55415 800-879-1960
continuumcme@aan.com
journals.lww.com/continuum

Official journal of the American Academy of Neurology, aiding professionals in patient care and continuing education.
*Bimonthly*
*Steven L. Lewis, MD, FAAN*
*Andrea J. Weiss, MA, Executive Editor*

**2051 Dementia and Geriatric Cognitive Disorders**
S. Karger Publishers, Inc.
26 W Avon Road 860-675-7834
Unionville, CT 06085 800-828-5479
Fax: 860-675-7302
www.karger.com/DEM

Open-access journal devoted to the study of cognitive dysfunction in preclinical and clinical studies, concentrating on Alzheimer's and Parkinson's disease, Huntington's chorea and other neurodegenerative diseases.
*Victoria Chan-Pilay, Editor-in-Chief*

**2052 Journal of Alzheimer's Disease**
IOS Press
6751 Tepper Drive 703-830-6300
Clifton, VA 20124 Fax: 703-830-2300
editorial@j-alz.com
www.j-alz.com

Research into the etiology, pathogenesis, epidemiology, genetics, behavior, treatment and psychology of Alzheimer's disease.
*George Perry, PhD, Editor-in-Chief*
*Beth Kumar, Managing Editor*

**2053 Journal of Molecular Diagnostics**
Elsevier
1600 John F Kennedy Boulevard 301-634-7959
Philadelphia, PA 19103 Fax: 301-634-7961
jmd@asip.org
jmd.amjpathol.org

Official journal of the American Society for Investigative Pathology and the Association for Molecular Pathology, focusing on molecular discoveries in medicine translating into the clinical diagnostic setting, as well as the description and application of technological advances in the field of molecular diagnostic medicine.
*Monthly*
*Barbara Zehnbauer, PhD, Editor-in-Chief*

**2054 Journal of NeuroEngineering and Rehabilitation**
Springer Nature
One New York Plaza 800-777-4643
New York, NY 10004-1562 info@biomedcentral.com
jneuroengrehab.biomedcentral.com

An open-access journal devoted to integrated research from the fields of neuroscience, biomedical engineering, and physical medicine and rehabilitation.
*David J. Reinkensmeyer, Editor-in-Chief*

**2055 Journal of Neuroinflammation**
Springer Nature
One New York Plaza 800-777-4643
New York, NY 10004-1562 info@biomedcentral.com
jneuroinflammation.biomedcentral.com

A peer-reviewed, open-access journal focusing on the interactions of the immune system with the nervous system as a means of expanding understanding of chronic neurological diseases.
*Monica J. Carson, Editor-in-Chief*
*Sue T. Griffin, Editor-in-Chief*

**2056 Journal of Nuclear Medicine**
Society of Nuclear Medicine and Molecular Imaging
1850 Samuel Morse Drive 703-708-9000
Reston, VA 20190 800-513-6853
Fax: 703-708-9015
subscriptions@snm.org
jnm.snmjournals.org

Peer-reviewed journal with clinical investigations, science reports, articles benefitting continuing education, book reviews, employment opportunities, and updates on practice and research.
*Monthly*
*Johannes Czernin, MD, Editor-in-Chief*
*Susan Alexander, Associate Director, Publications*

**2057 Journal of Nuclear Medicine Technology**
Society of Nuclear Medicine and Molecular Imaging
1850 Samuel Morse Drive 703-708-9000
Reston, VA 20190 800-513-6853
Fax: 703-708-9015
subscriptions@snm.org
tech.snmjournals.org

Peer-reviewed journal dedicated to nuclear medicine technology, with information on credentialing, continuing education and licensure requirements, as well as current news and updates on the field.
*Quarterly*
*Kathy S. Thomas, MHA, CNMT, PET, Editor-in-Chief*
*Susan Alexander, Associate Director, Publications*

2058 **Journal of the Neurological Sciences**
Elsevier
LSU Health Sciences Center JNS_England@lsuhsc.edu
New Orleans, LA 70112 www.jns-journal.com
Original articles in neurology and neuroscience from around the world.
*Monthly*
*John D. England, Editor-in-Chief*

2059 **Molecular Imaging**
Sage Journals
2455 Teller Road 805-499-9774
Thousand Oaks, CA 91320 journals@sagepub.com
journals.sagepub.com/home/mix
Peer-reviewed open access journal focusing on molecular imaging research, including basic science, preclinical studies and human applications. Published in association with the Society of Nuclear Medicine and Molecular Imaging.
*Bimonthly*
*Henry F. VanBrocklin, PhD, Editor-in-Chief*

2060 **Molecular Neurodegeneration**
Springer Nature
One New York Plaza 800-777-4643
New York, NY 10004-1562 info@biomedcentral.com
www.biomedcentral.com
A peer-reviewed, open-access journal devoted to all aspects of neurodegeneration research at the molecular and cellular levels.
*Guojun Bu, Editor-in-Chief*
*Huaxi Xu, Editor-in-Chief*

2061 **Neurocase: The Neural Basis of Cognition**
Taylor & Francis Group
530 Walnut Street www.tandfonline.com/toc/nncs20/current
Philadelphia, PA 19106
Rapid response journal featuring case and group studies in neuropsychology, neuropsychiatry and behavioral neurology, with a focus on the neural basis of cognition.
*Bruce L. Miller, Editor*
*Hans J. Markowitsch, Editor*

2062 **Neurology**
American Academy of Neurology
201 Chicago Avenue 612-928-6000
Minneapolis, MN 55415 800-879-1960
Fax: 612-454-2748
journal@neurology.org
n.neurology.org
Official journal of the American Academy of Neurology, peer-reviewed, highlighting clinical neurology research.
*Jose G. Merino, MD, MPhil, FAAN, Editor-in-Chief*
*Patricia K. Baskin, MS, Executive Editor*

2063 **Neurology Clinical Practice**
American Academy of Neurology
201 Chicago Avenue 612-928-6000
Minneapolis, MN 55415 800-879-1960
Fax: 612-454-2748
journal@neurology.org
cp.neurology.org
Official peer-reviewed journal of the American Academy of Neurology for practicing neurologists.
*John R. Corboy, MD, FAAN, Editor*
*Patricia K. Baskin, MS, Executive Editor*

2064 **Neurology: Genetics**
American Academy of Neurology
201 Chicago Avenue 612-928-6000
Minneapolis, MN 55415 800-879-1960
Fax: 612-454-2748
journal@neurology.org
ng.neurology.org
Official journal of the American Academy of Neurology, publishing online open-access peer-reviewed reports in the field of neurogenetics.
*Stefan M. Pulst, MD, FAAN, Editor*
*Patricia K. Baskin, MS, Executive Editor*

2065 **Neurology: Neuroimmunology & Neuroinflammation**
American Academy of Neurology
201 Chicago Avenue 612-928-6000
Minneapolis, MN 55415 800-879-1960
Fax: 612-454-2748
journal@neurology.org
nn.neurology.org
Official journal of the American Academy of Neurology, publishing online open-access peer-reviewed reports of original research and in-depth reviews of topics in neuroimmunology & neuroinflammation.
*Josep O. Dalmau, MD, PhD, Editor*
*Patricia K. Baskin, MS, Executive Editor*

2066 **Society of Nuclear Medicine and Molecular Imaging**
1850 Samuel Morse Drive 703-708-9000
Reston, VA 20190 Fax: 703-708-9015
feedback@snmmi.org
www.snmmi.org
The mission of this nonprofit scientific and professional organization is to promote the science, technology and application of nuclear medicine and molecular imaging. Molecular imaging techniques are used to diagnose and manage the treatment of brain disorders such as Alzheimer's and Parkinson's disease, among other conditions.
*15,000 members*
*Virginia Pappas, CEO*
*Rebecca Maxey, Director, Communications*

2067 **Translational Neurodegeneration**
Springer Nature
One New York Plaza 800-777-4643
New York, NY 10004-1562 info@biomedcentral.com
www.biomedcentral.com
A peer-reviewed, open-access journal covering research, therapeutics and education for all areas of neurodegenerative diseases.
*Shengdi Chen, Editor-in-Chief*

2068 **Ultrasonic Imaging**
Sage Journals
2455 Teller Road 805-499-9774
Thousand Oaks, CA 91320 journals@sagepub.com
journals.sagepub.com/home/uix
The journal focuses on the rapid publication of original papers on the development and application of ultrasonic techniques, with emphasis on medical diagnosis. Also published are research notes, comments on papers appearing in the journal, book reviews, and occasional review articles.
*Ernest J. Feleppa, Editor-in-Chief*
*Roslyn Raskin, Managing Editor*

## Web Sites

2069 **BrainFacts.org**
Society for Neuroscience
1121 14th Street NW brainfactsinfo@sfn.org
Washington, DC 20005 brainfacts.org
Online public information portal founded by the Kavli Foundation, the Gatsby Charitable Foundation and the Society for Neuroscience, with topics on brain function and anatomy, diseases and disorders, and more.
*Richard Wingate, DPhil, Editor-in-Chief*
*Charles Yokoyama, PhD, Associate Editor*

# MILD COGNITIVE IMPAIRMENT

*Mild cognitive impairment is neither as mild as the normal cognitive decline that comes with aging nor as severe as out-and-out dementia. Although people suffering from mild cognitive impairment experience notable decline in memory or mental function, the condition does not significantly interfere with the patient's daily life. MCI may increase a patient's risk of later developing dementia, but many individuals who suffer from the condition do not get any worse and some even eventually recover.*

Although it can be difficult to differentiate mild cognitive impairment from the general mental decline and forgetfulness that come with aging, MCI patients do experience more severe forms of forgetfulness than their age-equivalent peers. They may find themselves frequently losing their train or thought or unable to follow conversations or movies. They may also find themselves overwhelmed by decision making or have difficulty making their way around familiar environments. In addition, MCI patients may experience depression and anxiety, apathy, or irritability and aggression.

As with the various forms of dementia, there is no single cause of mild cognitive disorder, but it is believed to result from many of the same causes as Alzheimer's and other forms of dementia, albeit in lesser measure. Some of these possible causes include the development of clumps of irregular proteins, small strokes, and reduced blood flow through brain vessels. Although the strongest risk factor for MCI is increasing age, other medical conditions and lifestyle factors can contribute as well. These may include diabetes, smoking, high blood pressure or cholesterol, obesity, and depression.

Diagnosis of mild cognitive impairment is made using a combination of the patient's medical history, an in-office mental exam, and a series of tests such as lab work or brain imaging. The input of friends or family members who are intimate with the patient's behavior is also strongly considered. There is no medical treatment approved for MCI as no drugs have been proven effective in preventing the progression of MCI to dementia. Patients are advised to adhere to a healthy lifestyle and monitor any changes. About 10 to 15 percent of patients with MCI can be expected to develop dementia.

## National Agencies & Associations

2071 **American Academy of Neurology**
201 Chicago Avenue 612-928-6000
Minneapolis, MN 55415 800-879-1960
Fax: 612-454-2746
memberservices@aan.com
www.aan.com
Professional society of medical doctors specializing in brain and nervous system diseases. Maintains placement service. Sponsors research and educational programs. Compiles statistics. Publishes scientific journal, Continuum: Lifelong Learning in Neurology.
*Mary E. Post, MBA, CAE, CEO*

2072 **American Society for Neurochemistry**
9037 Ron Den Lane 407-909-9064
Windermere, FL 34786 Fax: 407-876-0750
asnmanager@asneurochem.org
asneurochem.org
The Society aims to advance and promote cellular and molecular neuroscience knowledge, and to facilitate communication and the dissemination of information within the field and with related disciplines.
*Sheilah Jewart, Executive Director*
*Karen Gottlieb, Conference Coordinator*

2073 **Society for Neuroscience**
1121 14th Street NW 202-962-4000
Washginton, DC 20005 marty@sfn.org
sfn.org
Large international organization of scientists and physicians devoted to the study of the brain and the nervous system.
*37,000 members*
*Marty Saggese, Executive Director*
*Melissa Garcia, Associate Executive Director*

## Magazines

2074 **ASN NEURO**
Sage Journals
2455 Teller Road 805-499-9774
Thousand Oaks, CA 91320 journals@sagepub.com
journals.sagepub.com/home/asn
Peer-reviewed open access journal focusing on recent advances in the cellular and molecular neurosciences. It is the official publication of the American Society for Neurochemistry.
*Douglas L. Feinstein, Editor-in-Chief*
*Sandra J. Hewitt, Deputy Editor-in-Chief*

2075 **American Journal of Geriatric Psychiatry**
Elsevier
1600 John F Kennedy Boulevard www.journals.elsevier.com
Philadelphia, PA 19103
Peer-reviewed articles on the rapidly developing field of geriatric psychiatry, including areas such as the diagnosis and classification of psychiatric disorders, epidemiological and biological correlates of mental health of older adults, and psychopharmacology and other somatic treatments.
*Monthly*
*Charles F. Reynolds III, MD, Editor-in-Chief*

2076 **BMC Neuroscience**
Springer Nature
One New York Plaza 800-777-4643
New York, NY 10004-1562 info@biomedcentral.com
bmcneurosci.biomedcentral.com
A peer-reviewed, open-access journal devoted to all aspects of the nervous system (including molecular, cellular, developmental and animal model studies), as well as cognitive and behavioral research, and computational modeling.
*Darren Byrne, Editor*
*Ana Donnelly, Manuscript Editor*

2077 **Brain & Life**
American Academy of Neurology
201 Chicago Avenue 612-928-6000
Minneapolis, MN 55415 800-879-1960
Fax: 612-454-2748
BrainandLife@wolterskluwer.com
www.brainandlife.org
Official magazine of the American Academy of Neurology, aimed at parents and home-caregivers interested in neurology in everyday life.
*Orly Avitzur, MD, MBA, FAAN, Editor-in-Chief*
*Mary Bolster, Managing Editor*

2078 **Brain: A Journal of Neurology**
Oxford University Press
2001 Evans Road 919-677-0977
Cary, NC 27513 800-852-7323
Fax: 919-677-1714
brain@ucl.ac.uk
academic.oup.com/brain
Focus is clinical neurology and translational neuroscience.
*Dimitri M. Kullmann, Editor*
*Joanne Bell, Managing Editor*

2079 **Continuum: Lifelong Learning in Neurology**
American Academy of Neurology
201 Chicago Avenue 612-928-6000
Minneapolis, MN 55415 800-879-1960
continuumcme@aan.com
journals.lww.com/continuum
Official journal of the American Academy of Neurology, aiding professionals in patient care and continuing education.
*Bimonthly*
*Steven L. Lewis, MD, FAAN*
*Andrea J. Weiss, MA, Executive Editor*

2080 **JNeurosci**
Society for Neuroscience
1121 14th Street NW 202-962-4000
Washginton, DC 20005 jn@sfn.org
www.jneurosci.org
Official peer-reviewed journal of the Society for Neuroscience, publishing research on a broad range of topics of interest to those working on the nervous system.
*Marina R. Picciotto, Editor-in-Chief*
*Teresa Esch, Features Editor*

2081 **Journal of Neuroinflammation**
Springer Nature
One New York Plaza 800-777-4643
New York, NY 10004-1562 info@biomedcentral.com
jneuroinflammation.biomedcentral.com
A peer-reviewed, open-access journal focusing on the interactions of the immune system with the nervous system as a means of expanding understanding of chronic neurological diseases.
*Monica J. Carson, Editor-in-Chief*
*Sue T. Griffin, Editor-in-Chief*

2082 **Journal of Nuclear Medicine**
Society of Nuclear Medicine and Molecular Imaging
1850 Samuel Morse Drive 703-708-9000
Reston, VA 20190 800-513-6853
Fax: 703-708-9015
subscriptions@snm.org
jnm.snmjournals.org
Peer-reviewed journal with clinical investigations, science reports, articles benefitting continuing education, book reviews, employment opportunities, and updates on practice and research.
*Monthly*
*Johannes Czernin, MD, Editor-in-Chief*
*Susan Alexander, Associate Director, Publications*

2083 **Journal of Nuclear Medicine Technology**
Society of Nuclear Medicine and Molecular Imaging
1850 Samuel Morse Drive 703-708-9000
Reston, VA 20190 800-513-6853
Fax: 703-708-9015
subscriptions@snm.org
tech.snmjournals.org
Peer-reviewed journal dedicated to nuclear medicine technology, with information on credentialing, continuing education and

licensure requirements, as well as current news and updates on the field.
*Quarterly*
*Kathy S. Thomas, MHA, CNMT, PET, Editor-in-Chief*
*Susan Alexander, Associate Director, Publications*

2084 **Journal of the Neurological Sciences**
Elsevier
LSU Health Sciences Center JNS_England@lsuhsc.edu
New Orleans, LA 70112 www.jns-journal.com
Original articles in neurology and neuroscience from around the world.
*Monthly*
*John D. England, Editor-in-Chief*

2085 **Molecular Imaging**
Sage Journals
2455 Teller Road 805-499-9774
Thousand Oaks, CA 91320 journals@sagepub.com
journals.sagepub.com/home/mix
Peer-reviewed open access journal focusing on molecular imaging research, including basic science, preclinical studies and human applications. Published in association with the Society of Nuclear Medicine and Molecular Imaging.
*Bimonthly*
*Henry F. VanBrocklin, PhD, Editor-in-Chief*

2086 **Molecular Neurodegeneration**
Springer Nature
One New York Plaza 800-777-4643
New York, NY 10004-1562 info@biomedcentral.com
www.biomedcentral.com
A peer-reviewed, open-access journal devoted to all aspects of neurodegeneration research at the molecular and cellular levels.
*Guojun Bu, Editor-in-Chief*
*Huaxi Xu, Editor-in-Chief*

2087 **Neurocase: The Neural Basis of Cognition**
Taylor & Francis Group
530 Walnut Street www.tandfonline.com/toc/nncs20/current
Philadelphia, PA 19106
Rapid response journal featuring case and group studies in neuropsychology, neuropsychiatry and behavioral neurology, with a focus on the neural basis of cognition.
*Bruce L. Miller, Editor*
*Hans J. Markowitsch, Editor*

2088 **Neurology**
American Academy of Neurology
201 Chicago Avenue 612-928-6000
Minneapolis, MN 55415 800-879-1960
Fax: 612-454-2748
journal@neurology.org
n.neurology.org
Official journal of the American Academy of Neurology, peer-reviewed, highlighting clinical neurology research.
*Jose G. Merino, MD, MPhil, FAAN, Editor-in-Chief*
*Patricia K. Baskin, MS, Executive Editor*

2089 **Neurology Clinical Practice**
American Academy of Neurology
201 Chicago Avenue 612-928-6000
Minneapolis, MN 55415 800-879-1960
Fax: 612-454-2748
journal@neurology.org
cp.neurology.org
Official peer-reviewed journal of the American Academy of Neurology for practicing neurologists.
*John R. Corboy, MD, FAAN, Editor*
*Patricia K. Baskin, MS, Executive Editor*

2090 **Neurology: Genetics**
American Academy of Neurology
201 Chicago Avenue 612-928-6000
Minneapolis, MN 55415 800-879-1960
Fax: 612-454-2748
journal@neurology.org
ng.neurology.org
Official journal of the American Academy of Neurology, publishing online open-access peer-reviewed reports in the field of neurogenetics.
*Stefan M. Pulst, MD, FAAN, Editor*
*Patricia K. Baskin, MS, Executive Editor*

2091 **Neurology: Neuroimmunology & Neuroinflammation**
American Academy of Neurology
201 Chicago Avenue 612-928-6000
Minneapolis, MN 55415 800-879-1960
Fax: 612-454-2748
journal@neurology.org
nn.neurology.org
Official journal of the American Academy of Neurology, publishing online open-access peer-reviewed reports of original research and in-depth reviews of topics in neuroimmunology & neuroinflammation.
*Josep O. Dalmau, MD, PhD, Editor*
*Patricia K. Baskin, MS, Executive Editor*

2092 **Society of Nuclear Medicine and Molecular Imaging**
1850 Samuel Morse Drive 703-708-9000
Reston, VA 20190 Fax: 703-708-9015
feedback@snmmi.org
www.snmmi.org
The mission of this nonprofit scientific and professional organization is to promote the science, technology and application of nuclear medicine and molecular imaging. Molecular imaging techniques are used to diagnose and manage the treatment of brain disorders such as Alzheimer's and Parkinson's disease, among other conditions.
*15,000 members*
*Virginia Pappas, CEO*
*Rebecca Maxey, Director, Communications*

2093 **Translational Neurodegeneration**
Springer Nature
One New York Plaza 800-777-4643
New York, NY 10004-1562 info@biomedcentral.com
www.biomedcentral.com
A peer-reviewed, open-access journal covering research, therapeutics and education for all areas of neurodegenerative diseases.
*Shengdi Chen, Editor-in-Chief*

2094 **Ultrasonic Imaging**
Sage Journals
2455 Teller Road 805-499-9774
Thousand Oaks, CA 91320 journals@sagepub.com
journals.sagepub.com/home/uix
The journal focuses on the rapid publication of original papers on the development and application of ultrasonic techniques, with emphasis on medical diagnosis. Also published are research notes, comments on papers appearing in the journal, book reviews, and occasional review articles.
*Ernest J. Feleppa, Editor-in-Chief*
*Roslyn Raskin, Managing Editor*

2095 **eNeuro**
Society for Neuroscience
1121 14th Street NW 202-312-7305
Washginton, DC 20005 eNeuro@sfn.org
www.eneuro.org
Open-access journal of the Society for Neuroscience.
*Christophe Bernard, Editor-in-Chief*
*Kelly Newton, Director, Scientific Publications*

## Web Sites

2096 **Neuronline**
Society for Neuroscience
1121 14th Street NW 202-962-4000
Washginton, DC 20005 neuronline@sfn.org
neuronline.sfn.org
Online portal for professional development and training resources for individuals in the field of neuroscience, hosted by the Society for Neuroscience.
*Amanda Kimball, Director, Digital Learning*

# MIXED DEMENTIA

*Mixed dementia is a condition in which more than one form of dementia is present in the patient's brain at the same time. Most commonly, this mixed condition consists of the presence of the plaques and tangles associated with Alzheimer's co-existing with the blood vessel changes present in vascular dementia. In other instances, the Alzheimer's changes can co-exist with Lewy bodies, the protein deposits responsible for Lewy body dementia and Parkinson's. In rare cases, all three changes may be present simultaneously.*

Mixed dementia is very common in the elderly, with autopsy studies suggesting that the majority of patients age 80 and older autopsied probably had some form of mixed dementia. It is difficult to diagnose mixed dementia since many patients believed to have just Alzheimer's disease are posthumously revealed to also have a cerebrovascular involvement. The symptoms of mixed dementia vary, depending on the types of dementia experienced but adhere to the usual symptoms associated with Alzheimer's, vascular dementia, or Lewy body dementia, particularly Alzheimer's. These include memory loss, confusion, difficulty completing familiar tasks, and problems speaking and writing.

Mixed dementia is most often diagnosed after death. In cases where a patient displays Alzheimer's symptoms but has also suffered a stroke or other cardiovascular problem, the doctor may diagnosis mixed dementia as well. While there are no approved medications that specifically treat mixed dementia, the use of drugs designed to treat Alzheimer's disease have proven effective with patients suffering mixed dementia. Because of the vascular involvement common to mixed dementia, blood pressure treatment and cholesterol management are frequently undertaken as well.

## National Agencies & Associations

**2098 American Academy of Neurology**
201 Chicago Avenue
Minneapolis, MN 55415
612-928-6000
800-879-1960
Fax: 612-454-2746
memberservices@aan.com
www.aan.com
Professional society of medical doctors specializing in brain and nervous system diseases. Maintains placement service. Sponsors research and educational programs. Compiles statistics. Publishes scientific journal, Continuum: Lifelong Learning in Neurology.
*Mary E. Post, MBA, CAE, CEO*

**2099 American Society for Investigative Pathology**
1801 Rockville Pike
Rockville, MD 20852
240-283-9700
Fax: 301-984-4047
www.asip.org
The Society seeks to promote experimental pathology and related disciplines through meetings, publications, and educational activities.
*William B. Coleman, PhD, Executive Officer*
*Gina LaBorde, Manager, Marketing & Communications*

**2100 American Society for Neurochemistry**
9037 Ron Den Lane
Windermere, FL 34786
407-909-9064
Fax: 407-876-0750
asnmanager@asneurochem.org
asneurochem.org
The Society aims to advance and promote cellular and molecular neuroscience knowledge, and to facilitate communication and the dissemination of information within the field and with related disciplines.
*Sheilah Jewart, Executive Director*
*Karen Gottlieb, Conference Coordinator*

**2101 Society for Neuroscience**
1121 14th Street NW
Washginton, DC 20005
202-962-4000
marty@sfn.org
sfn.org
Large international organization of scientists and physicians devoted to the study of the brain and the nervous system.
*37,000 members*
*Marty Saggese, Executive Director*
*Melissa Garcia, Associate Executive Director*

## Foundations & Research Centers

**2102 Center for Brain Activity Mapping**
UC San Diego
9500 Gilman Drive
La Jolla, CA 92093
858-534-2230
cbam.ucsd.edu
The Center seeks to develop new technologies for detecting neuronal activity, for reporting it out of deep brain tissue, and for processing and analyzing the resulting data, by organizing and supporting research teams and projects.
*Ralph J. Greenspan, PhD, Director*

**2103 Kavli Foundation**
5715 Mesmer Avenue
Los Angeles, CA
424-353-8800
info@kavlifoundation.org
www.kavlifoundation.org
The Foundation supports scientific research into the human brain, in the following scientific fields: Astrophysics, Nanoscience, Neuroscience and Theoretical Physics. Within Neuroscience, the study of aging and brain diseases and disorders is supported.
*Robert W. Conn, PhD, President & CEO*
*Eric Marshall, VP, Public Engagement & Prizes*

**2104 Kavli Institute for Brain Science at Columbia University**
Columbia University
3227 Broadway
New York, NY 10027
212-853-1016
Fax: 212-665-9699
kavli@columbia.edu
www.kavli.columbia.edu
The Institute's primary are of study is how signaling in neural circuits controls cognitive function and behavior, and the development of novel experimental and computational strategies for analyzing these signals.
*Eric R. Kandel, MD, Director*
*Rafael Yuste, MD, PhD, Co-Director*

**2105 Neuroscience Research Institute**
UC Santa Barbara
6129 Biology II
Santa Barbara, CA 93106
805-893-4621
www.nri.ucsb.edu
The Institute seeks to allow scientists from different fields to collaborate for the betterment of neurological research. Areas of interest include: Alzheimer's Disease & Related Dementias; Behavioral Neuroscience & Neuroethology; Cell Biology, Biochemistry & Biophysics of the Nervous System; Computational & Theoretical Neuroscience; Development of the Nervous System; and Stem Cells.
*Stuart Feinstein, Co-Director*
*Kenneth Kosik, Co-Director*

**2106 Salk Institute for Biological Studies**
10010 N Torrey Pines Road
La Jolla, CA 92037
858-453-4100
www.salk.edu
Conducts groundbreaking research into cancer, aging, Alzheimer's diabetes and infectious diseases.
*Rusty Gage, PhD, President*
*Martin Hetzer, PhD, VP & Chief Science Officer*

**2107 Sanford Consortium for Regenerative Medicine**
2880 Torrey Pines Scenic Drive
La Jolla, CA 92037
858-246-1071
www.sanfordconsortium.com
The Consortium works to achieve breakthrough discoveries in stem cell research with regards to diagnoses, treatments, and cures for degenerative diseases and injuries.
*Edward W. Holmes, MD, President & CEO*
*Jeffrey Steindorf, PhD, VP & COO*

**2108 Scripps Research Institute**
10550 North Torrey Pines Road
La Jolla, CA
858-784-1000
www.scripps.edu
The institute seeks to improve human wellbeing through the advancement of bioscience, including research into aging & healthspan, autoimmune diseases, cancer, infectious diseases, neurological disorders, and more.
*Peter Schultz, PhD, President & CEO*
*Eric Topol, MD, EVP, Scripps Research*

## Magazines

**2109 ASN NEURO**
Sage Journals
2455 Teller Road
Thousand Oaks, CA 91320
805-499-9774
journals@sagepub.com
journals.sagepub.com/home/asn
Peer-reviewed open access journal focusing on recent advances in the cellular and molecular neurosciences. It is the official publication of the American Society for Neurochemistry.
*Douglas L. Feinstein, Editor-in-Chief*
*Sandra J. Hewitt, Deputy Editor-in-Chief*

**2110 American Journal of Geriatric Psychiatry**
Elsevier
1600 John F Kennedy Boulevard
Philadelphia, PA 19103
www.journals.elsevier.com
Peer-reviewed articles on the rapidly developing field of geriatric psychiatry, including areas such as the diagnosis and classification of psychiatric disorders, epidemiological and biological correlates of mental health of older adults, and psychopharmacology and other somatic treatments.
*Monthly*
*Charles F. Reynolds III, MD, Editor-in-Chief*

**2111 American Journal of Pathology**
Elsevier
1600 John F Kennedy Boulevard
Philadelphia, PA 19103
301-634-7959
Fax: 301-634-7961
ajp@asip.org
ajp.amjpathol.org

Official journal of the American Society for Investigative Pathology, publishing original research reports, reviews, and commentaries related to the molecular and cellular basis of disease.
*Martha Furie, Editor-in-Chief*

2112 **BMC Neuroscience**
Springer Nature
One New York Plaza 800-777-4643
New York, NY 10004-1562 info@biomedcentral.com
bmcneurosci.biomedcentral.com
A peer-reviewed, open-access journal devoted to all aspects of the nervous system (including molecular, cellular, developmental and animal model studies), as well as cognitive and behavioral research, and computational modeling.
*Darren Byrne, Editor*
*Ana Donnelly, Manuscript Editor*

2113 **Brain & Life**
American Academy of Neurology
201 Chicago Avenue 612-928-6000
Minneapolis, MN 55415 800-879-1960
Fax: 612-454-2748
BrainandLife@wolterskluwer.com
www.brainandlife.org
Official magazine of the American Academy of Neurology, aimed at parents and home-caregivers interested in neurology in everyday life.
*Orly Avitzur, MD, MBA, FAAN, Editor-in-Chief*
*Mary Bolster, Managing Editor*

2114 **Brain: A Journal of Neurology**
Oxford University Press
2001 Evans Road 919-677-0977
Cary, NC 27513 800-852-7323
Fax: 919-677-1714
brain@ucl.ac.uk
academic.oup.com/brain
Focus is clinical neurology and translational neuroscience.
*Dimitri M. Kullmann, Editor*
*Joanne Bell, Managing Editor*

2115 **Continuum: Lifelong Learning in Neurology**
American Academy of Neurology
201 Chicago Avenue 612-928-6000
Minneapolis, MN 55415 800-879-1960
continuumcme@aan.com
journals.lww.com/continuum
Official journal of the American Academy of Neurology, aiding professionals in patient care and continuing education.
*Bimonthly*
*Steven L. Lewis, MD, FAAN*
*Andrea J. Weiss, MA, Executive Editor*

2116 **Dementia and Geriatric Cognitive Disorders**
S. Karger Publishers, Inc.
26 W Avon Road 860-675-7834
Unionville, CT 06085 800-828-5479
Fax: 860-675-7302
www.karger.com/DEM
Open-access journal devoted to the study of cognitive dysfunction in preclinical and clinical studies, concentrating on Alzheimer's and Parkinson's disease, Huntington's chorea and other neurodegenerative diseases.
*Victoria Chan-Pilay, Editor-in-Chief*

2117 **JNeurosci**
Society for Neuroscience
1121 14th Street NW 202-962-4000
Washginton, DC 20005 jn@sfn.org
www.jneurosci.org
Official peer-reviewed journal of the Society for Neuroscience, publishing research on a broad range of topics of interest to those working on the nervous system.
*Marina R. Picciotto, Editor-in-Chief*
*Teresa Esch, Features Editor*

2118 **Journal of Alzheimer's Disease**
IOS Press
6751 Tepper Drive 703-830-6300
Clifton, VA 20124 Fax: 703-830-2300
editorial@j-alz.com
www.j-alz.com
Research into the etiology, pathogenesis, epidemiology, genetics, behavior, treatment and psychology of Alzheimer's disease.
*George Perry, PhD, Editor-in-Chief*
*Beth Kumar, Managing Editor*

2119 **Journal of Molecular Diagnostics**
Elsevier
1600 John F Kennedy Boulevard 301-634-7959
Philadelphia, PA 19103 Fax: 301-634-7961
jmd@asip.org
jmd.amjpathol.org
Official journal of the American Society for Investigative Pathology and the Association for Molecular Pathology, focusing on molecular discoveries in medicine translating into the clinical diagnostic setting, as well as the description and application of technological advances in the field of molecular diagnostic medicine.
*Monthly*
*Barbara Zehnbauer, PhD, Editor-in-Chief*

2120 **Journal of NeuroEngineering and Rehabilitation**
Springer Nature
One New York Plaza 800-777-4643
New York, NY 10004-1562 info@biomedcentral.com
jneuroengrehab.biomedcentral.com
An open-access journal devoted to integrated research from the fields of neuroscience, biomedical engineering, and physical medicine and rehabilitation.
*David J. Reinkensmeyer, Editor-in-Chief*

2121 **Journal of Neurodevelopmental Disorders**
Springer Nature
One New York Plaza 800-777-4643
New York, NY 10004-1562 info@biomedcentral.com
jneurodevdisorders.biomedcentral.com
An open-access journal devoted to integrating research from neurobiology, genetics, cognitive neuroscience, psychiatry and psychology.
*Joseph Piven, Editor-in-Chief*

2122 **Journal of Neuroinflammation**
Springer Nature
One New York Plaza 800-777-4643
New York, NY 10004-1562 info@biomedcentral.com
jneuroinflammation.biomedcentral.com
A peer-reviewed, open-access journal focusing on the interactions of the immune system with the nervous system as a means of expanding understanding of chronic neurological diseases.
*Monica J. Carson, Editor-in-Chief*
*Sue T. Griffin, Editor-in-Chief*

2123 **Journal of Nuclear Medicine**
Society of Nuclear Medicine and Molecular Imaging
1850 Samuel Morse Drive 703-708-9000
Reston, VA 20190 800-513-6853
Fax: 703-708-9015
subscriptions@snm.org
jnm.snmjournals.org
Peer-reviewed journal with clinical investigations, science reports, articles benefitting continuing education, book reviews, employment opportunities, and updates on practice and research.
*Monthly*
*Johannes Czernin, MD, Editor-in-Chief*
*Susan Alexander, Associate Director, Publications*

2124 **Journal of Nuclear Medicine Technology**
Society of Nuclear Medicine and Molecular Imaging
1850 Samuel Morse Drive 703-708-9000
Reston, VA 20190 800-513-6853
Fax: 703-708-9015
subscriptions@snm.org
tech.snmjournals.org
Peer-reviewed journal dedicated to nuclear medicine technology, with information on credentialing, continuing education and

licensure requirements, as well as current news and updates on the field.
*Quarterly*
*Kathy S. Thomas, MHA, CNMT, PET, Editor-in-Chief*
*Susan Alexander, Associate Director, Publications*

2125 **Journal of the Neurological Sciences**
Elsevier
LSU Health Sciences Center JNS_England@lsuhsc.edu
New Orleans, LA 70112 www.jns-journal.com
Original articles in neurology and neuroscience from around the world.
*Monthly*
*John D. England, Editor-in-Chief*

2126 **Molecular Imaging**
Sage Journals
2455 Teller Road 805-499-9774
Thousand Oaks, CA 91320 journals@sagepub.com
journals.sagepub.com/home/mix
Peer-reviewed open access journal focusing on molecular imaging research, including basic science, preclinical studies and human applications. Published in association with the Society of Nuclear Medicine and Molecular Imaging.
*Bimonthly*
*Henry F. VanBrocklin, PhD, Editor-in-Chief*

2127 **Molecular Neurodegeneration**
Springer Nature
One New York Plaza 800-777-4643
New York, NY 10004-1562 info@biomedcentral.com
www.biomedcentral.com
A peer-reviewed, open-access journal devoted to all aspects of neurodegeneration research at the molecular and cellular levels.
*Guojun Bu, Editor-in-Chief*
*Huaxi Xu, Editor-in-Chief*

2128 **Neurocase: The Neural Basis of Cognition**
Taylor & Francis Group
530 Walnut Street www.tandfonline.com/toc/nncs20/current
Philadelphia, PA 19106
Rapid response journal featuring case and group studies in neuropsychology, neuropsychiatry and behavioral neurology, with a focus on the neural basis of cognition.
*Bruce L. Miller, Editor*
*Hans J. Markowitsch, Editor*

2129 **Neurology**
American Academy of Neurology
201 Chicago Avenue 612-928-6000
Minneapolis, MN 55415 800-879-1960
Fax: 612-454-2748
journal@neurology.org
n.neurology.org
Official journal of the American Academy of Neurology, peer-reviewed, highlighting clinical neurology research.
*Jose G. Merino, MD, MPhil, FAAN, Editor-in-Chief*
*Patricia K. Baskin, MS, Executive Editor*

2130 **Neurology Clinical Practice**
American Academy of Neurology
201 Chicago Avenue 612-928-6000
Minneapolis, MN 55415 800-879-1960
Fax: 612-454-2748
journal@neurology.org
cp.neurology.org
Official peer-reviewed journal of the American Academy of Neurology for practicing neurologists.
*John R. Corboy, MD, FAAN, Editor*
*Patricia K. Baskin, MS, Executive Editor*

2131 **Neurology: Genetics**
American Academy of Neurology
201 Chicago Avenue 612-928-6000
Minneapolis, MN 55415 800-879-1960
Fax: 612-454-2748
journal@neurology.org
ng.neurology.org
Official journal of the American Academy of Neurology, publishing online open-access peer-reviewed reports in the field of neurogenetics.
*Stefan M. Pulst, MD, FAAN, Editor*
*Patricia K. Baskin, MS, Executive Editor*

2132 **Neurology: Neuroimmunology & Neuroinflammation**
American Academy of Neurology
201 Chicago Avenue 612-928-6000
Minneapolis, MN 55415 800-879-1960
Fax: 612-454-2748
journal@neurology.org
nn.neurology.org
Official journal of the American Academy of Neurology, publishing online open-access peer-reviewed reports of original research and in-depth reviews of topics in neuroimmunology & neuroinflammation.
*Josep O. Dalmau, MD, PhD, Editor*
*Patricia K. Baskin, MS, Executive Editor*

2133 **Society of Nuclear Medicine and Molecular Imaging**
1850 Samuel Morse Drive 703-708-9000
Reston, VA 20190 Fax: 703-708-9015
feedback@snmmi.org
www.snmmi.org
The mission of this nonprofit scientific and professional organization is to promote the science, technology and application of nuclear medicine and molecular imaging. Molecular imaging techniques are used to diagnose and manage the treatment of brain disorders such as Alzheimer's and Parkinson's disease, among other conditions.
*15,000 members*
*Virginia Pappas, CEO*
*Rebecca Maxey, Director, Communications*

2134 **Translational Neurodegeneration**
Springer Nature
One New York Plaza 800-777-4643
New York, NY 10004-1562 info@biomedcentral.com
www.biomedcentral.com
A peer-reviewed, open-access journal covering research, therapeutics and education for all areas of neurodegenerative diseases.
*Shengdi Chen, Editor-in-Chief*

2135 **Ultrasonic Imaging**
Sage Journals
2455 Teller Road 805-499-9774
Thousand Oaks, CA 91320 journals@sagepub.com
journals.sagepub.com/home/uix
The journal focuses on the rapid publication of original papers on the development and application of ultrasonic techniques, with emphasis on medical diagnosis. Also published are research notes, comments on papers appearing in the journal, book reviews, and occasional review articles.
*Ernest J. Feleppa, Editor-in-Chief*
*Roslyn Raskin, Managing Editor*

2136 **eNeuro**
Society for Neuroscience
1121 14th Street NW 202-312-7305
Washginton, DC 20005 eNeuro@sfn.org
www.eneuro.org
Open-access journal of the Society for Neuroscience.
*Christophe Bernard, Editor-in-Chief*
*Kelly Newton, Director, Scientific Publications*

## Web Sites

2137 **BrainFacts.org**
Society for Neuroscience
1121 14th Street NW brainfactsinfo@sfn.org
Washington, DC 20005 brainfacts.org
Online public information portal founded by the Kavli Foundation, the Gatsby Charitable Foundation and the Society for Neuroscience, with topics on brain function and anatomy, diseases and disorders, and more.
*Richard Wingate, DPhil, Editor-in-Chief*
*Charles Yokoyama, PhD, Associate Editor*

2138 **Neuronline**
Society for Neuroscience
1121 14th Street NW
Washginton, DC 20005
202-962-4000
neuronline@sfn.org
neuronline.sfn.org

Online portal for professional development and training resources for individuals in the field of neuroscience, hosted by the Society for Neuroscience.
*Amanda Kimball, Director, Digital Learning*

# NEUROSYPHILIS

*Neurosyphilis is a condition that results when syphilis, a sexually transmitted infection (STI), spreads to the central nervous system, specifically the brain and the spinal cord. There are several different types of neurosyphilis, all with different symptoms, but patients who develop the general paresis form of the disease experience symptoms similar to other cognitive impairment disorders, including paranoia, personality changes, mood swings, and difficulty with language. The condition can also progress to full-on dementia. Because of the development of antibiotics, neurosyphilis cases, particularly general paresis cases, are rare and are most often found in HIV-infected patients.*

A slow-developing condition, neurosyphilis, in many cases, presents 10 to 20 years after the patient is initially infected with Treponema pallidum, the bacterium that causes syphilis. The most common form of the disease is asymptomatic neurosyphilis which means that a large number of patients never develop any symptoms. For those patients who do experience a neurological symptoms, the most common form this takes in the early stages is meningitis, which causes nausea, headache, and a loss of hearing or vision. Meningeal neurosyphilis, though, may advance to the more serious meningovascular neurosyphilis, which usually involves the patient suffering a stroke. Ten to 12 percent of neurosyphilis patients develop meningovascular neurosyphilis.

The more rare forms of neurosyphilis include general paresis and tabes dorsalis. General paresis is caused by chronic meningoencephalitis that leads to cerebral atrophy. Its symptoms usually appear 10 to 30 years after the initial syphilis infection. Early symptoms include fatigue, headaches, and dizziness which give way to delusions, dysarthria, seizures, confusion, and dementia. After the development of antibiotics, general paresis became increasingly rare. Tabes dorsalis also has a later development, typically presenting about 20 years after the initial infection. Symptoms include loss of coordination, incontinence, and vision problems.

Neurosyphilis is diagnosed by several tests, including a blood test to determine whether or not the patient has syphilis, a spinal tap, and imaging tests. The primary treatment for neurosyphilis is penicillin and other antibiotics. Antibiotics are highly effective in curing syphilis and preventing further damage, but they will not reverse the damage already suffered by later-stage neurosyphilis patients. For neurosyphilis patients who also have HIV, a stronger dose of penicillin treatment is generally needed and the chances for a fuller recovery are lower.

## National Agencies & Associations

2140 **American Academy of Neurology**
201 Chicago Avenue
Minneapolis, MN 55415
612-928-6000
800-879-1960
Fax: 612-454-2746
memberservices@aan.com
www.aan.com
Professional society of medical doctors specializing in brain and nervous system diseases. Maintains placement service. Sponsors research and educational programs. Compiles statistics. Publishes scientific journal, Continuum: Lifelong Learning in Neurology.
*Mary E. Post, MBA, CAE, CEO*

2141 **American Society for Neurochemistry**
9037 Ron Den Lane
Windermere, FL 34786
407-909-9064
Fax: 407-876-0750
asnmanager@asneurochem.org
asneurochem.org
The Society aims to advance and promote cellular and molecular neuroscience knowledge, and to facilitate communication and the dissemination of information within the field and with related disciplines.
*Sheilah Jewart, Executive Director*
*Karen Gottlieb, Conference Coordinator*

2142 **Infectious Diseases Society of America**
4040 Wilson Boulevard
Arlington, VA 22203
703-299-0200
kcortez@idsociety.org
www.idsociety.org
Organization of physicians, scientists and public health experts who specialize in infectious diseases. Affiliated with the HIV Medicine Association and the Emerging Infections Network.
*12,000 members*
*Barbara D. Alexander, MD, President*
*Kathy Cortez, Staff Liaison*

## Foundations & Research Centers

2143 **Neuroscience Research Institute**
UC Santa Barbara
6129 Biology II
Santa Barbara, CA 93106
805-893-4621
www.nri.ucsb.edu
The Institute seeks to allow scientists from different fields to collaborate for the betterment of neurological research. Areas of interest include: Alzheimer's Disease & Related Dementias; Behavioral Neuroscience & Neuroethology; Cell Biology, Biochemistry & Biophysics of the Nervous System; Computational & Theoretical Neuroscience; Development of the Nervous System; and Stem Cells.
*Stuart Feinstein, Co-Director*
*Kenneth Kosik, Co-Director*

2144 **Salk Institute for Biological Studies**
10010 N Torrey Pines Road
La Jolla, CA 92037
858-453-4100
www.salk.edu
Conducts groundbreaking research into cancer, aging, Alzheimer's diabetes and infectious diseases.
*Rusty Gage, PhD, President*
*Martin Hetzer, PhD, VP & Chief Science Officer*

2145 **Scripps Research Institute**
10550 North Torrey Pines Road
La Jolla, CA
858-784-1000
www.scripps.edu
The institute seeks to improve human wellbeing through the advancement of bioscience, including research into aging & healthspan, autoimmune diseases, cancer, infectious diseases, neurological disorders, and more.
*Peter Schultz, PhD, President & CEO*
*Eric Topol, MD, EVP, Scripps Research*

## Magazines

2146 **ASN NEURO**
Sage Journals
2455 Teller Road
Thousand Oaks, CA 91320
805-499-9774
journals@sagepub.com
journals.sagepub.com/home/asn
Peer-reviewed open access journal focusing on recent advances in the cellular and molecular neurosciences. It is the official publication of the American Society for Neurochemistry.
*Douglas L. Feinstein, Editor-in-Chief*
*Sandra J. Hewitt, Deputy Editor-in-Chief*

2147 **BMC Neuroscience**
Springer Nature
One New York Plaza
New York, NY 10004-1562
800-777-4643
info@biomedcentral.com
bmcneurosci.biomedcentral.com
A peer-reviewed, open-access journal devoted to all aspects of the nervous system (including molecular, cellular, developmental and animal model studies), as well as cognitive and behavioral research, and computational modeling.
*Darren Byrne, Editor*
*Ana Donnelly, Manuscript Editor*

2148 **Brain & Life**
American Academy of Neurology
201 Chicago Avenue
Minneapolis, MN 55415
612-928-6000
800-879-1960
Fax: 612-454-2748
BrainandLife@wolterskluwer.com
www.brainandlife.org
Official magazine of the American Academy of Neurology, aimed at parents and home-caregivers interested in neurology in everyday life.
*Orly Avitzur, MD, MBA, FAAN, Editor-in-Chief*
*Mary Bolster, Managing Editor*

2149 **Brain: A Journal of Neurology**
Oxford University Press
2001 Evans Road
Cary, NC 27513
919-677-0977
800-852-7323
Fax: 919-677-1714
brain@ucl.ac.uk
academic.oup.com/brain
Focus is clinical neurology and translational neuroscience.
*Dimitri M. Kullmann, Editor*
*Joanne Bell, Managing Editor*

2150 **Clinical Infectious Diseases**
Oxford University Press
2001 Evans Road
Cary, NC 27513
919-677-0977
800-852-7323
Fax: 919-677-1714
academic.oup.com/cid
Leading journal on infectious diseases, with original research, reviews, viewpoints, editorials, invited commentaries, photo quizzes, practice guidelines, correspondence and supplements. The journal has a broad focus, encompassing clinical descriptions, public health, microbiology, immunology, prevention of infection, evaluation of current and novel treatments and promotion of optimal practices for diagnosis and treatment.
*Robert T. Schooley, Editor-in-Chief*
*Ferric C. Fang, Deputy Editor*

2151 **Continuum: Lifelong Learning in Neurology**
American Academy of Neurology
201 Chicago Avenue
Minneapolis, MN 55415
612-928-6000
800-879-1960
continuumcme@aan.com
journals.lww.com/continuum
Official journal of the American Academy of Neurology, aiding professionals in patient care and continuing education.
*Bimonthly*
*Steven L. Lewis, MD, FAAN*
*Andrea J. Weiss, MA, Executive Editor*

2152 **Journal of Infectious Diseases**
Oxford University Press
2001 Evans Road
Cary, NC 27513
919-677-0977
800-852-7323
Fax: 919-677-1714
academic.oup.com/jid

Official publication of the Infectious Diseases Society of America, with original research on infectious diseases.
*Martin S. Hirsch, MD, Editor-in-Chief*
*David C. Hooper, Deputy Editor*

**2153 Journal of Nuclear Medicine Technology**
Society of Nuclear Medicine and Molecular Imaging
1850 Samuel Morse Drive 703-708-9000
Reston, VA 20190 800-513-6853
Fax: 703-708-9015
subscriptions@snm.org
tech.snmjournals.org
Peer-reviewed journal dedicated to nuclear medicine technology, with information on credentialing, continuing education and licensure requirements, as well as current news and updates on the field.
*Quarterly*
*Kathy S. Thomas, MHA, CNMT, PET, Editor-in-Chief*
*Susan Alexander, Associate Director, Publications*

**2154 Journal of the Neurological Sciences**
Elsevier
LSU Health Sciences Center JNS_England@lsuhsc.edu
New Orleans, LA 70112 www.jns-journal.com
Original articles in neurology and neuroscience from around the world.
*Monthly*
*John D. England, Editor-in-Chief*

**2155 Molecular Imaging**
Sage Journals
2455 Teller Road 805-499-9774
Thousand Oaks, CA 91320 journals@sagepub.com
journals.sagepub.com/home/mix
Peer-reviewed open access journal focusing on molecular imaging research, including basic science, preclinical studies and human applications. Published in association with the Society of Nuclear Medicine and Molecular Imaging.
*Bimonthly*
*Henry F. VanBrocklin, PhD, Editor-in-Chief*

**2156 Molecular Neurodegeneration**
Springer Nature
One New York Plaza 800-777-4643
New York, NY 10004-1562 info@biomedcentral.com
www.biomedcentral.com
A peer-reviewed, open-access journal devoted to all aspects of neurodegeneration research at the molecular and cellular levels.
*Guojun Bu, Editor-in-Chief*
*Huaxi Xu, Editor-in-Chief*

**2157 Neurocase: The Neural Basis of Cognition**
Taylor & Francis Group
530 Walnut Street www.tandfonline.com/toc/nncs20/current
Philadelphia, PA 19106
Rapid response journal featuring case and group studies in neuropsychology, neuropsychiatry and behavioral neurology, with a focus on the neural basis of cognition.
*Bruce L. Miller, Editor*
*Hans J. Markowitsch, Editor*

**2158 Neurology**
American Academy of Neurology
201 Chicago Avenue 612-928-6000
Minneapolis, MN 55415 800-879-1960
Fax: 612-454-2748
journal@neurology.org
n.neurology.org
Official journal of the American Academy of Neurology, peer-reviewed, highlighting clinical neurology research.
*Jose G. Merino, MD, MPhil, FAAN, Editor-in-Chief*
*Patricia K. Baskin, MS, Executive Editor*

**2159 Neurology Clinical Practice**
American Academy of Neurology
201 Chicago Avenue 612-928-6000
Minneapolis, MN 55415 800-879-1960
Fax: 612-454-2748
journal@neurology.org
cp.neurology.org
Official peer-reviewed journal of the American Academy of Neurology for practicing neurologists.
*John R. Corboy, MD, FAAN, Editor*
*Patricia K. Baskin, MS, Executive Editor*

**2160 Neurology: Genetics**
American Academy of Neurology
201 Chicago Avenue 612-928-6000
Minneapolis, MN 55415 800-879-1960
Fax: 612-454-2748
journal@neurology.org
ng.neurology.org
Official journal of the American Academy of Neurology, publishing online open-access peer-reviewed reports in the field of neurogenetics.
*Stefan M. Pulst, MD, FAAN, Editor*
*Patricia K. Baskin, MS, Executive Editor*

**2161 Neurology: Neuroimmunology & Neuroinflammation**
American Academy of Neurology
201 Chicago Avenue 612-928-6000
Minneapolis, MN 55415 800-879-1960
Fax: 612-454-2748
journal@neurology.org
nn.neurology.org
Official journal of the American Academy of Neurology, publishing online open-access peer-reviewed reports of original research and in-depth reviews of topics in neuroimmunology & neuroinflammation.
*Josep O. Dalmau, MD, PhD, Editor*
*Patricia K. Baskin, MS, Executive Editor*

**2162 Open Forum Infectious Diseases**
Oxford University Press
2001 Evans Road 919-677-0977
Cary, NC 27513 800-852-7323
Fax: 919-677-1714
academic.oup.com/ofid
Open-access journal featuring clinical, translational and basic research on biomedical science and clinical practice.
*Paul E. Sax, MD, Editor-in-Chief*
*Jonathan Z. Li, MD, Deputy Editor*

**2163 Society of Nuclear Medicine and Molecular Imaging**
1850 Samuel Morse Drive 703-708-9000
Reston, VA 20190 Fax: 703-708-9015
feedback@snmmi.org
www.snmmi.org
The mission of this nonprofit scientific and professional organization is to promote the science, technology and application of nuclear medicine and molecular imaging. Molecular imaging techniques are used to diagnose and manage the treatment of brain disorders such as Alzheimer's and Parkinson's disease, among other conditions.
*15,000 members*
*Virginia Pappas, CEO*
*Rebecca Maxey, Director, Communications*

**2164 Ultrasonic Imaging**
Sage Journals
2455 Teller Road 805-499-9774
Thousand Oaks, CA 91320 journals@sagepub.com
journals.sagepub.com/home/uix
The journal focuses on the rapid publication of original papers on the development and application of ultrasonic techniques, with emphasis on medical diagnosis. Also published are research notes, comments on papers appearing in the journal, book reviews, and occasional review articles.
*Ernest J. Feleppa, Editor-in-Chief*
*Roslyn Raskin, Managing Editor*

# NORMAL PRESSURE HYDROCEPHALUS

*Normal pressure hydrocephalus is a neurological disorder that results from the abnormal buildup of cerebrospinal fluid in the brain's ventricles. This leads to progressive mental impairment, difficulty walking, decreased bladder control, slowing of movement, and eventually dementia. Typically afflicting patients in their 60s and 70s, NPH is treatable, although it is frequently misdiagnosed as it shares many symptoms with Alzheimer's and other dementia-causing diseases.*

Although normal pressure hydrocephalus can result from other brain disorders such as a tumor or head injury, in most cases the cause remains unknown. Patients that suffer NPH often report a sensation of feeling "stuck," in which they have difficulty moving their body when walking. They also notice a decline in thinking skills, a loss of interest in daily activities, and forgetfulness. Generally, a mild form of dementia accompanies NPH, although it can progress to a more severe form. In later stages of the disease, patients may become incontinent.

Because its symptoms are similar to those of Alzheimer's, Parkinson's, and Creutzfeldt-Jakob patients, NPH is frequently misdiagnosed. When NPH is suspected, often due to the patient's difficulty walking, brain imaging, clinical examination, and cerebrospinal fluid tests are undertaken. This last test is unique to NPH because the condition results from the accumulation of cerebrospinal fluid in the brain's ventricles.

Normal pressure hydrocephalus is one of the only causes of dementia that can be successfully treated. This treatment takes the form of the insertion of a shunt in the brain to drain the excess cerebrospinal fluid into the abdomen where it can be safely absorbed. Nonetheless, this surgery is not effective in all patients and some studies have found a high rate of post-surgical complications and that the benefits of the surgery may decline over time.

## National Agencies & Associations

2166 **American Academy of Neurology**
201 Chicago Avenue 612-928-6000
Minneapolis, MN 55415 800-879-1960
Fax: 612-454-2746
memberservices@aan.com
www.aan.com
Professional society of medical doctors specializing in brain and nervous system diseases. Maintains placement service. Sponsors research and educational programs. Compiles statistics. Publishes scientific journal, Continuum: Lifelong Learning in Neurology.
*Mary E. Post, MBA, CAE, CEO*

2167 **American Society for Neurochemistry**
9037 Ron Den Lane 407-909-9064
Windermere, FL 34786 Fax: 407-876-0750
asnmanager@asneurochem.org
asneurochem.org
The Society aims to advance and promote cellular and molecular neuroscience knowledge, and to facilitate communication and the dissemination of information within the field and with related disciplines.
*Sheilah Jewart, Executive Director*
*Karen Gottlieb, Conference Coordinator*

2168 **Hydrocephalus Association**
4340 East West Highway 301-202-3811
Bethesda, MD 20814-4447 888-598-3789
Fax: 301-202-3813
info@hydroassoc.org
www.hydroassoc.org
Provides support, education and advocacy for families affected by hdrocephalus and professionals.
*Brett Weitz, Chair*
*Susan Fiorella, Vice Chair*

2169 **National Hydrocephalus Foundation**
12413 Centralia Road 562-924-6666
Lakewood, CA 90715-1653 info@nhfonline.org
www.nhfonline.org
A national organization providing information and education, along with peer-to-peer support, physician referrals and more.
*Michael Fields, President & Treasurer*
*Debbi Fields, Executive Director*

2170 **Spina Bifida & Hydrocephalus Association of Nova Scotia**
15 Laura Drive 902-679-1124
Nova Scotia, B3G-1K3 800-304-0450
Fax: 902-679-1433
info@sbhans.ca
www.sbhans.ca
A non-profit, registered charitable organization affiliated with the Spina Bifida and Hydrocephalus Association of Canada.

2171 **The Kidney Foundation of Canada**
310-5160 Decarie Boulevard 514-369-4806
Montreal, Quebec, H3X-2H9 800-361-7494
Fax: 514-369-2472
info@kidney.ca
www.kidney.ca
A national volunteer organization committed to reducing the burden of kidney disease through funding research, providing education and support, and increasing public awareness and commitment to advancing kidney health and organ donation.
*Greg Robbins, President*
*Terry Tomkins, Treasurer*

2172 **World Hypertension League**
ceo@whleague.org
whleague.org
Devoted to the advancement of hypertension prevention and control through joint efforts of all national leagues and societies.

## Foundations & Research Centers

2173 **Neuroscience Research Institute**
UC Santa Barbara
6129 Biology II 805-893-4621
Santa Barbara, CA 93106 www.nri.ucsb.edu
The Institute seeks to allow scientists from different fields to collaborate for the betterment of neurological research. Areas of interest include: Alzheimer's Disease & Related Dementias; Behavioral Neuroscience & Neuroethology; Cell Biology, Biochemistry & Biophysics of the Nervous System; Computational & Theoretical Neuroscience; Development of the Nervous System; and Stem Cells.
*Stuart Feinstein, Co-Director*
*Kenneth Kosik, Co-Director*

2174 **New York University Medical Center Auxiliary of Tisch Hospital**
560 1st Avenue 212-263-5040
New York, NY 10016
Conducts national symposiums on hydrocephalus.

2175 **Sanford Consortium for Regenerative Medicine**
2880 Torrey Pines Scenic Drive 858-246-1071
La Jolla, CA 92037 www.sanfordconsortium.com
The Consortium works to achieve breakthrough discoveries in stem cell research with regards to diagnoses, treatments, and cures for degenerative diseases and injuries.
*Edward W. Holmes, MD, President & CEO*
*Jeffrey Steindorf, PhD, VP & COO*

## Support Groups & Hotlines

2176 **Alliance of Genetic Support Groups**
4301 Connecticut Ave NW 202-966-5557
Washington, DC 20008 800-336-4363
Fax: 202-966-8553
info@geneticalliance.org
www.geneticalliance.org
A coalition of voluntary genetic support groups, consumers and professionals addressing the needs of individuals and families affected by genetic disorders from a national perspective.
*Sharon Terry, President and CEO*
*Jeffrey Giorgi, Communications & Operations Assistant*

2177 **Hydrocephalus Association of North Texas**
PO Box 670552 214-528-2877
Dallas, TX 74637-0552 http://nhfonline.org/treatment.php?id=or
Founded in 1987 the mission is to provide information and support to parents of children with hydrocephalus in the state of Texas and neighboring states.
*Beverly Pozzi*

2178 **Hydrocephalus Association of Philadelphia**
PO Box 2099 610-497-0375
Boothwyn, PA 19061-8099 Fax: 610-497-2836
Founded in 1992 the Association provides support information advocacy and telephone support to families in Pennsylvania New Jersey and Delaware.
*Halmi, Director*

2179 **Hydrocephalus Association of Rhode Island**
PO Box 343 401-723-6065
Valley Falls, RI 02864-0343
Founded in 1993 the mission of this Association is to provide information support and advocacy for individuals with hydrocephalus and for friends and family members.
*Gabriella Pike, President*

2180 **Hydrocephalus Parents Support Group**
1325 Louis Street 908-722-4691
Manville, NJ 08835
Founded in 1993, the group provides support for parents of children with hydrocephalus.

2181 **National Health Information Center**
Office of Disease Prevention & Health Promotion
1101 Wootton Pkwy Fax: 240-453-8281
Rockville, MD 20852 odphpinfo@hhs.gov
www.health.gov/nhic
Supports public health education by maintaining a calendar of National Health Observances; helps connect consumers and health professionals to organizations that can best answer questions and provide up-to-date contact information from reliable sources; up-

dates on a yearly basis toll-free numbers for health information, Federal health clearinghouses and info centers.
*Don Wright, MD, MPH, Director*

## Magazines

2182 **ASN NEURO**
Sage Journals
2455 Teller Road 805-499-9774
Thousand Oaks, CA 91320 journals@sagepub.com
journals.sagepub.com/home/asn
Peer-reviewed open access journal focusing on recent advances in the cellular and molecular neurosciences. It is the official publication of the American Society for Neurochemistry.
*Douglas L. Feinstein, Editor-in-Chief*
*Sandra J. Hewitt, Deputy Editor-in-Chief*

2183 **BMC Neuroscience**
Springer Nature
One New York Plaza 800-777-4643
New York, NY 10004-1562 info@biomedcentral.com
bmcneurosci.biomedcentral.com
A peer-reviewed, open-access journal devoted to all aspects of the nervous system (including molecular, cellular, developmental and animal model studies), as well as cognitive and behavioral research, and computational modeling.
*Darren Byrne, Editor*
*Ana Donnelly, Manuscript Editor*

2184 **Brain & Life**
American Academy of Neurology
201 Chicago Avenue 612-928-6000
Minneapolis, MN 55415 800-879-1960
Fax: 612-454-2748
BrainandLife@wolterskluwer.com
www.brainandlife.org
Official magazine of the American Academy of Neurology, aimed at parents and home-caregivers interested in neurology in everyday life.
*Orly Avitzur, MD, MBA, FAAN, Editor-in-Chief*
*Mary Bolster, Managing Editor*

2185 **Brain: A Journal of Neurology**
Oxford University Press
2001 Evans Road 919-677-0977
Cary, NC 27513 800-852-7323
Fax: 919-677-1714
brain@ucl.ac.uk
academic.oup.com/brain
Focus is clinical neurology and translational neuroscience.
*Dimitri M. Kullmann, Editor*
*Joanne Bell, Managing Editor*

2186 **Continuum: Lifelong Learning in Neurology**
American Academy of Neurology
201 Chicago Avenue 612-928-6000
Minneapolis, MN 55415 800-879-1960
continuumcme@aan.com
journals.lww.com/continuum
Official journal of the American Academy of Neurology, aiding professionals in patient care and continuing education.
*Bimonthly*
*Steven L. Lewis, MD, FAAN*
*Andrea J. Weiss, MA, Executive Editor*

2187 **Journal of NeuroEngineering and Rehabilitation**
Springer Nature
One New York Plaza 800-777-4643
New York, NY 10004-1562 info@biomedcentral.com
jneuroengrehab.biomedcentral.com
An open-access journal devoted to integrated research from the fields of neuroscience, biomedical engineering, and physical medicine and rehabilitation.
*David J. Reinkensmeyer, Editor-in-Chief*

2188 **Journal of Nuclear Medicine**
Society of Nuclear Medicine and Molecular Imaging
1850 Samuel Morse Drive 703-708-9000
Reston, VA 20190 800-513-6853
Fax: 703-708-9015
subscriptions@snm.org
jnm.snmjournals.org
Peer-reviewed journal with clinical investigations, science reports, articles benefitting continuing education, book reviews, employment opportunities, and updates on practice and research.
*Monthly*
*Johannes Czernin, MD, Editor-in-Chief*
*Susan Alexander, Associate Director, Publications*

2189 **Journal of Nuclear Medicine Technology**
Society of Nuclear Medicine and Molecular Imaging
1850 Samuel Morse Drive 703-708-9000
Reston, VA 20190 800-513-6853
Fax: 703-708-9015
subscriptions@snm.org
tech.snmjournals.org
Peer-reviewed journal dedicated to nuclear medicine technology, with information on credentialing, continuing education and licensure requirements, as well as current news and updates on the field.
*Quarterly*
*Kathy S. Thomas, MHA, CNMT, PET, Editor-in-Chief*
*Susan Alexander, Associate Director, Publications*

2190 **Journal of the Neurological Sciences**
Elsevier
LSU Health Sciences Center JNS_England@lsuhsc.edu
New Orleans, LA 70112 www.jns-journal.com
Original articles in neurology and neuroscience from around the world.
*Monthly*
*John D. England, Editor-in-Chief*

2191 **Molecular Imaging**
Sage Journals
2455 Teller Road 805-499-9774
Thousand Oaks, CA 91320 journals@sagepub.com
journals.sagepub.com/home/mix
Peer-reviewed open access journal focusing on molecular imaging research, including basic science, preclinical studies and human applications. Published in association with the Society of Nuclear Medicine and Molecular Imaging.
*Bimonthly*
*Henry F. VanBrocklin, PhD, Editor-in-Chief*

2192 **Molecular Neurodegeneration**
Springer Nature
One New York Plaza 800-777-4643
New York, NY 10004-1562 info@biomedcentral.com
www.biomedcentral.com
A peer-reviewed, open-access journal devoted to all aspects of neurodegeneration research at the molecular and cellular levels.
*Guojun Bu, Editor-in-Chief*
*Huaxi Xu, Editor-in-Chief*

2193 **Neurocase: The Neural Basis of Cognition**
Taylor & Francis Group
530 Walnut Street www.tandfonline.com/toc/nncs20/current
Philadelphia, PA 19106
Rapid response journal featuring case and group studies in neuropsychology, neuropsychiatry and behavioral neurology, with a focus on the neural basis of cognition.
*Bruce L. Miller, Editor*
*Hans J. Markowitsch, Editor*

2194 **Neurology**
American Academy of Neurology
201 Chicago Avenue 612-928-6000
Minneapolis, MN 55415 800-879-1960
Fax: 612-454-2748
journal@neurology.org
n.neurology.org
Official journal of the American Academy of Neurology, peer-reviewed, highlighting clinical neurology research.
*Jose G. Merino, MD, MPhil, FAAN, Editor-in-Chief*
*Patricia K. Baskin, MS, Executive Editor*

2195 **Neurology Clinical Practice**
American Academy of Neurology
201 Chicago Avenue
Minneapolis, MN 55415
612-928-6000
800-879-1960
Fax: 612-454-2748
journal@neurology.org
cp.neurology.org
Official peer-reviewed journal of the American Academy of Neurology for practicing neurologists.
*John R. Corboy, MD, FAAN, Editor*
*Patricia K. Baskin, MS, Executive Editor*

2196 **Neurology: Genetics**
American Academy of Neurology
201 Chicago Avenue
Minneapolis, MN 55415
612-928-6000
800-879-1960
Fax: 612-454-2748
journal@neurology.org
ng.neurology.org
Official journal of the American Academy of Neurology, publishing online open-access peer-reviewed reports in the field of neurogenetics.
*Stefan M. Pulst, MD, FAAN, Editor*
*Patricia K. Baskin, MS, Executive Editor*

2197 **Neurology: Neuroimmunology & Neuroinflammation**
American Academy of Neurology
201 Chicago Avenue
Minneapolis, MN 55415
612-928-6000
800-879-1960
Fax: 612-454-2748
journal@neurology.org
nn.neurology.org
Official journal of the American Academy of Neurology, publishing online open-access peer-reviewed reports of original research and in-depth reviews of topics in neuroimmunology & neuroinflammation.
*Josep O. Dalmau, MD, PhD, Editor*
*Patricia K. Baskin, MS, Executive Editor*

2198 **Society of Nuclear Medicine and Molecular Imaging**
1850 Samuel Morse Drive
Reston, VA 20190
703-708-9000
Fax: 703-708-9015
feedback@snmmi.org
www.snmmi.org
The mission of this nonprofit scientific and professional organization is to promote the science, technology and application of nuclear medicine and molecular imaging. Molecular imaging techniques are used to diagnose and manage the treatment of brain disorders such as Alzheimer's and Parkinson's disease, among other conditions.
*15,000 members*
*Virginia Pappas, CEO*
*Rebecca Maxey, Director, Communications*

2199 **Ultrasonic Imaging**
Sage Journals
2455 Teller Road
Thousand Oaks, CA 91320
805-499-9774
journals@sagepub.com
journals.sagepub.com/home/uix
The journal focuses on the rapid publication of original papers on the development and application of ultrasonic techniques, with emphasis on medical diagnosis. Also published are research notes, comments on papers appearing in the journal, book reviews, and occasional review articles.
*Ernest J. Feleppa, Editor-in-Chief*
*Roslyn Raskin, Managing Editor*

## Web Sites

2200 **Healing Well**
www.healingwell.com
An online health resource guide to medical news, chat, information and articles, newsgroups and message boards, books, disease-related web sites, medical directories, and more for patients, friends, and family coping with disabling diseases, disorders, or chronic illnesses.

2201 **Health Finder**
www.healthfinder.gov
Searchable, carefully developed web site offering information on over 1000 topics. Developed by the US Department of Health and Human Services, the site can be used in both English and Spanish.

2202 **Healthlink USA**
www.healthlinkusa.com
Health information concerning treatment, cures, prevention, diagnosis, risk factors, research, support groups, email lists, personal stories and much more. Updated regularly.

2203 **Hydrocephalus Association**
www.hydroassoc.org
Provides support, education and advocacy for families and professionals. The goal is to insure that families and individuals dealing with the complexities of hydrocephalus receive personal support, comprehensive educational materials and on-going medical care.

2204 **Hydrocephalus Center**
www.patientcenters.com/hydrocephalus
An online reference that was created especially as a resource for those with hydrocephalus and their families.

2205 **MedicineNet**
www.medicinenet.com
An online resource for consumers providing easy-to-read, authoritative medical and health information.

2206 **Medscape**
www.medscape.com
Medscape offers specialists, primary care physicians, and other health professionals the Web's most robust and integrated medical information and educational tools.

2207 **Neurology Channel**
www.healthcommunities.com
Find clearly explained, medically accurate information regarding conditions, including an overview, symptoms, causes, diagnostic procedures and treatment options. On this site it is possible to ask questions and get information from a neurologist and connect to people who have similar health interests.

2208 **WebMD**
www.webmd.com
Provides credible information, supportive communities, and in-depth reference material about health subjects. A source for original and timely health information as well as material from well known content providers.

# PARKINSON'S DISEASE

*Parkinson's disease is a neurological condition characterized by slow and decreased movement. It affects about 1 percent of those over age 65. The cause of Parkinson's disease is unknown, but both genetic and environmental factors may play a role. In a minority of cases, Parkinson's disease develops after repeated head trauma, carbon monoxide poisoning, drug use, or viral infections that affect the brain. Between 50 and 80 percent of Parkinson's patients develop dementia over the course of their illness. Parkinson's dementia is caused by the buildup of abnormal deposits made of alpha-synuclein protein. These deposits are known as Lewy bodies and also appear in the form of dementia known as Lewy body dementia. Patients with Parkinson's dementia may experience changes in memory, trouble interpreting visual information, hallucinations and delusions, and sleep disturbances.*

In about 50 to 80 percent of patients, Parkinson's disease begins with a slight tremor in the hands, resembling "pill-rolling" when at rest. With fatigue and stress, the tremor becomes more pronounced. As the disease progresses, voluntary movements, such as walking and eating, become more and more difficult. Rigidity and postural instability (difficulty standing up) develop. Because Parkinson's disease is characterized by reduced levels of neurotransmitter chemicals, notably dopamine, in certain parts of the brain, therapy has focused on restoring dopamine levels to normal. Monoamine oxidase type B inhibitors given early in the disease's progression, may protect the cells that secrete these chemicals, and thus delay the need for other therapy. When it is necessary to directly manipulate the chemical levels because of progression of the disease, levodopa, related to dopamine, is the mainstay of treatment and is associated with improvement of all Parkinson's symptoms. Levodopa is given with carbidopa, which inhibits the enzyme (peripheral decarboxylase) that degrades levodopa. This combination medication is marketed under the trade name Sinemet. This medication works well for the first 2-5 years, after which symptoms begin to return. The addition of further inhibitors of levodopa degradation (COMT inhibitors and MAO-B inhibitors) can augment the efficacy of levodopa for many more years. Anticholinergic medications are especially helpful in treating tremor and drooling. Dopamine agonists are often used as adjunct treatments with levodopa, particularly early in the course of the disease. These drugs decrease fluctuations in treatment efficacy.

Parkinson's disease is the subject of intense research, and experimental surgical or drug treatments are frequently available to patients whose response to standard therapy has been unsatisfactory. General supportive care should not be neglected and includes physical therapy and an exercise program to help optimize mobility. Stem cell treatments have proven their efficacy in animal models and human clinical trials are in process.

## National Agencies & Associations

2210 **American Academy of Neurology**
201 Chicago Avenue 612-928-6000
Minneapolis, MN 55415 800-879-1960
Fax: 612-454-2746
memberservices@aan.com
www.aan.com
Professional society of medical doctors specializing in brain and nervous system diseases. Maintains placement service. Sponsors research and educational programs. Compiles statistics. Publishes scientific journal, Continuum: Lifelong Learning in Neurology.
*Mary E. Post, MBA, CAE, CEO*

2211 **American Parkinson Disease Association**
135 Parkinson Avenue 800-223-2732
Staten Island, NY 10305 Fax: 718-981-4399
apda@apdaparkinson.org
www.apdaparkinson.org
Works to find the cure for Parkinson's disease and to alleviate the suffering of its victims by subsidizing information and referral centers and providing funds for research. Offers counseling services to patients and their families. Maintains 43 information and referral centers. Conducts symposia.
*Leslie A. Chambers, President & CEO*

2212 **American Society for Investigative Pathology**
1801 Rockville Pike 240-283-9700
Rockville, MD 20852 Fax: 301-984-4047
www.asip.org
The Society seeks to promote experimental pathology and related disciplines through meetings, publications, and educational activities.
*William B. Coleman, PhD, Executive Officer*
*Gina LaBorde, Manager, Marketing & Communications*

2213 **American Society for Neurochemistry**
9037 Ron Den Lane 407-909-9064
Windermere, FL 34786 Fax: 407-876-0750
asnmanager@asneurochem.org
asneurochem.org
The Society aims to advance and promote cellular and molecular neuroscience knowledge, and to facilitate communication and the dissemination of information within the field and with related disciplines.
*Sheilah Jewart, Executive Director*
*Karen Gottlieb, Conference Coordinator*

2214 **Baylor College of Medicine Parkinson's Disease Center & Movement Disorders**
McNair Campus 713-798-2273
Houston, TX 77030 pdcmdc@bcm.edu
www.bcm.edu/healthcare/care-centers

2215 **Davis Phinney Foundation**
357 S McCaslin Boulevard 866-358-0285
Louisville, CO 80027 contact@dpf.com
www.davisphinneyfoundation.org
A non-profit providing essential information, practical tools and inspiration to people living with Parkinson's. Funds early-phase, innovative research that focuses on exercise, speech, movement and other factors that affect quality of life.
*Polly Dawkins, Executive Director*

2216 **International Parkinson and Movement Disorder Society**
555 East Wells Street 414-276-2145
Milwaukee, WI 53202-3823 Fax: 414-276-3349
info@movementdisorders.org
www.movementdisorders.org
The MDS is comprised of clinicians, scientists, and other healthcare professionals interested in Parkinson's disease, as well as related neurodegenerative and neurodevelopmental disorders, hyperkinetic movement disorders, and abnormalities in muscle tone and motor control.
*Jennie Socha, Executive Director*
*Erin Weileder, Director, Membership & Communications*

2217 **Johns Hopkins Parkinson's Disease & Movement Disorders Center**
601 N Caroline Street 410-955-8795
Baltimore, MD 21287 www.hopkinsmedicine.org
Excellence in treating, researching and teaching about movement disorders.

2218 **Massachusetts General Hospital Movement Disorders Unit**
Massachusetts General Hospital, WAC 866-211-6588
Boston, MA 02114 855-644-6387
www.massgeneral.org/neurology
Recognized as a Center of Excellence by the National Parkinson Foundation, Mass General treats patients from around the world for movement disorders.

2219 **Michael J. Fox Foundation for Parkinson's Research**
Grand Central Station 800-708-7644
New York, NY 10163-4777 www.michaeljfox.org
The Michael J. Fox Foundation is dedicated to ensuring the development of a cure for Parkinson's disease through funding for research.
*Deborah W. Brooks, Co-Founder & Executive Vice Chairman*
*Todd Sherer, CEO*

2220 **Mount Sinai Beth Israel Department of Neurology**
281 First Avenue 212-420-2000
New York, NY 10003 www.mountsinai.org/locations/beth-israel
*Barbara Barnett, MD, MHCDS, Chief Medical Officer*

2221 **National Institute of Neurological Disorders and Stroke**
NIH Neurological Institute 301-496-5751
Bethesda, MD 20824 800-352-9424
www.ninds.nih.gov
Seeks to reduce the burden of neurological disease affecting individuals from all walks of life.
*Walter J. Koroshetz, MD, Director*
*Amy B. Adams, Director, Office of Scientific Liaison*

2222 **National Parkinson Foundation**
200 SE 1st Street 800-473-4636
Miami, FL 33131 contact@parkinson.org
www.parkinson.org
A nonprofit organization dedicated to research, diagnosis, treatment and care for men and women suffering from Parkinson's and other related neurological diseases. The Foundation also supports the Bob Hope research and rehabilitation center, which is the leading institute of its kind in the world, donating their time to Parkinson's research.
*John L. Lehr, President & CEO*

2223 **Northwestern University Parkinson's Disease & Movement Disorders Center**
710 N Lake Shore Drive 312-503-4397
Chicago, IL 60611 www.parkinsons.northwestern.edu
Recognized by the National Parkinson Foundation as a Center for Excellence, Northwestern University Parkinson's Disease and Movement Disorders Center conducts research to extend the knowledge and treatment of PD and other movement disorders.
*Tanya Simuni, Director*

2224 **Parkinson Canada**
4211 Yonge Street 416-227-9700
Toronto, Ontario, M2P-2A9 800-565-3000
Fax: 844-440-8963
info@parkinson.ca
www.parkinson.ca
A non-profit, national charity raising money to find a cure for Parkinson's disease through corporate sponsorships, and public donations.
*Judi Richardson, Chair*
*Lindsay Abbey, Director*

2225 **Parkinson's Foundation**
200 SE 1st Street 800-473-4636
Miami, FL 33131-1407 contact@parkinson.org
www.parkinson.org

A non-profit organization dedicated to research, diagnosis, treatment and care for individuals suffering from Parkinson's and other related neurological diseases.
*Howard D. Morgan, Chair*
*Andrew B. Albert, Vice Chair*

2226 **Parkinson's Institute and Clinical Center**
2500 Hospital Drive 408-734-2800
Mountain View, CA 94040 800-655-2273
Fax: 650-770-0204
www.thepi.org
Working for a cure for Parkinson's Disease and providing treatment to those afflicted with the disease.
*Thomas D. Follett, BSE, MSE, MBA, Chair*
*Carrolee Barlow, MD, PhD, CEO*

2227 **Society for Neuroscience**
1121 14th Street NW 202-962-4000
Washginton, DC 20005 marty@sfn.org
sfn.org
Large international organization of scientists and physicians devoted to the study of the brain and the nervous system.
*37,000 members*
*Marty Saggese, Executive Director*
*Melissa Garcia, Associate Executive Director*

2228 **The Parkinson Alliance**
PO Box 308 609-688-0870
Kingston, NJ 08528 800-579-8440
Fax: 609-688-0875
contact@parkinsonalliance.org
www.parkinsonalliance.org
Raising awareness and funds for Parkinson's research.
*Carol J. Walton, President & CEO*

2229 **The Parkinson Council**
555 City Avenue 610-668-4292
Bala Cynwyd, PA 19004 info@theparkinsoncouncil.org
theparkinsoncouncil.org
The Parkinson Council is dedicated to helping those affected by Parkinson's. Funds research, education and programs at various institutions in the Greater Philadelphia area.
*Wendy R. Lewis, Executive Director*

2230 **The Parkinson Disease & Movement Disorders Center**
Penn Medicine Neuroscience Center,
Philadelphia, PA 19107
www.pennmedicine.org/neurology
The Penn Parkinson Disease & Movement Disorders Center is recognized as a Center of Excellence by the National Parkinson Foundation.

## State Agencies & Associations

2231 **Alzheimer/Parkinson Association of Indian River County**
2300 5th Avenue 772-563-0505
Vero Beach, FL 32960 alzsupport@fastmail.fm
www.parkinson.org
*Toni Teresi, Chairperson*

2232 **Arizona Chapter of the National Parkinson Foundation**
20280 N 59th Avenue 480-607-1960
Glendale, AZ 85308-6182 866-637-8772
Fax: 480-607-1957
Affiliate chapter of The National Parkinson Foundation Inc.
*Alan Marks, President*
*Kenneth Larkin, Vice President*

2233 **Cape Cod Chapter National Parkinson Foundation**
33 Ships Way 508-385-2333
Buzzards Bay, MA 02532-0584 meacapecod@yahoo.com
www.parkinson.org
Affiliate of The National Parkinson Foundation.
*Joseph Wimbrow, President*

2234 **Colorado Parkinson Foundation**
1155 Kelly Johnson Boulevard 719-884-0103
Colorado Springs, CO 90920-1494 800-327-4545
Fax: 719-495-909
rpfarrer@msn.com
The mission of the National Parkinson Foundation if to find the cause of the cure for Parkinson disease through research. To improve the quality if life for persons with Parkinson and their caregivers. To also educate persons with Parkinson their carecar
*Ric Pfarrer, Chairperson*

2235 **Eljay Foundation for Parkinson Syndrome Awareness**
715 Ryan Street 337-310-0083
Lake Charles, LA 70601 info@eljayfd.org
www.eljayfd.org
*Eligha Guillory, President*
*Anna C. Drake, Secretary*

2236 **Hawaii Parkinson Association Gwendolyn A Montibon President**
Gwendolyn A Montibon, President
3375 Koapaka St., 808-734-9398
Honolulu, HI 96817 Fax: 808-528-1897
kekim@hawaii.edu
www.parkinson.org
Affiliate of The National Parkinson Foundation.

2237 **Los Angeles Alliance Against Parkinson's Disease**
3251 Oakley Drive 323-851-3230
Los Angeles, CA 90068-1315 www.parkinson.org/chapters.htm#
Affiliate of the National Parkinson Foundation.

2238 **National Parkinson Foundation: California Office**
4929 Wilshire Boulevard 323-442-8434
Los Angeles, CA 90010-3899

2239 **National Parkinson Foundation: Central Savannah River Area**
116 Lottie Lane 706-364-1662
Grovetown, GA 30813 800-473-4636
info@parkinsoncsra.org
www.parkinsoncsra.org
*Joe Kelley, Research Coordinator*

2240 **National Parkinson Foundation: Great Lakes**
ATTN: Great Lakes
200 SE 1st Street 866-920-6673
Miami, FL 33131 greatlakes@parkinson.org
www.parkinson.org/greatlakes
*Lori Gum, Development Manager*

2241 **National Parkinson Foundation: New York Office**
122 E 42nd Street 800-457-6676
New York, NY 10017-5622 www.parkinson.org/

2242 **National Parkinson Foundation: Orange County Chapter**
PO Box 2207 949-945-6200
Newport Beach, CA 92659 Fax: 949-548-4624
info@yahoo.com
www.npfocc.org
Affiliate of The National Parkinson Foundation.
*George Strickland, President*
*Janet Buell, Vice president*

2243 **National Parkinson Foundation:Cape Cod Chapter**
33 Ships Way 508-385-2333
Buzzards Bay, MA 02532-0584 meacapecod@yahoo.com
www.parkinson.org
*Garland Smith, Chairperson*

2244 **Northeast Kansas Parkinson Association**
PO Box 251 785-228-1337
Topeka, KS 66601 www.parkinson.org
*Mary Hatke, Chairperson*

2245 **Northeast Parkinson's and Caregivers**
27 Sutcliffe Road 508-756-7721
Brimfield, MA 01010
*Richard Stake, Chairperson*

2246 **Northstate Parkinson's Chapter**
1003 Yuba Street 530-229-0878
Redding, CA 96001 www.parkinson.org

Affiliate of The National Parkinson Foundation, Inc.
*Craig Boyer*

2247 **Northwest Georgia Parkinson Disease Association**
708 Glen Milner Boulevard 706-235-3164
Rome, GA 30161 webmaster@gaparkinsons.org
*James Trussel, Chairperson*

2248 **Parkinson Alliance**
PO Box 308 609-688-0870
Kingston, NJ 08528 800-579-8440
Fax: 609-688-0875
admin@parkinsonalliance.net
www.parkinsonalliance.net
The Princeton-New Jersey based Parkinson Alliance is a National nonprofit organization dedicated to raising funds to help finance the most promising research to find the cause and curefor Parkinson's disease.
*Martin Tuchman, Chairman*
*Margaret Tuchman, President*

2249 **Parkinson Association of Greater Daytona Beach**
111 North Frederick Avenue 386-252-8959
Daytona Beach, FL 32114 goatie@cfl.rr.com
www.parkinson.org
*Nancy Dawson, Chairperson*

2250 **Parkinson Association of Greater Kansas City**
8900 State Line Road 913-341-8828
Leawood, KS 66206 Fax: 913-341-8885
www.parkinsonheartland.org
Affiliate of The National Parkinson Foundation.
*Kirk Gutekunst, President*
*Mary Lee Shucart, Secretary*

2251 **Parkinson Association of Minnesota**
5905 Golden Valley Road, 763-545-1272
Golden Valley, MN 55422-4602 800-327-4545
info@parkinsonmn.org
www.parkinsonmn.org
Affiliate of The National Parkinson Foundation.
*Paul Blom, President*
*Collen Crane, Therapy Representative*

2252 **Parkinson Association of Northern California**
1024 Iron Point Road 916-357-6641
Folsom, CA 95630 panc@panctoday.org
www.panctoday.org
*Sean Tracy, President*
*Cody O'Keefe, Treasurer*

2253 **Parkinson Association of South Dakota**
PO Box 87952 605-328-4227
Sioux Falls, SD 57109-9938 Fax: 605-328-7150
Affiliate of The National Parkinson Foundation.
*Elaine Spader, President*
*Lori Jones, Vice President*

2254 **Parkinson Association of Southwest Florida**
1048 Goodlette-Frank Road 239-417-3465
Naples, FL 34102 Fax: 239-417-3469
pasfi@aol.com
www.pasfi.org
Affiliate of the National Parkinson Foundation.
*Scott Leamon, Chair*
*Chris Spine, Executive Director*

2255 **Parkinson Association of Southwest Florida**
5926 Premier Way 239-417-3465
Naples, FL 34109 office@parkinsonassociationswfl.org
parkinsonassociationswfl.org
The Parkinson Association of Southwest Flordia is a not-for-profit organization. The mission is to promote quality of life for persons with Parkinson's Disease and their care partners. This is accomplished by providing educational, physical and social programs. The organization also provides education for the community regarding Parkinson's Disease and its effects.
*Linda Goldfield, Executive Director*

2256 **Parkinson Association of the Sacramento Valley**
900 Fulton Avenue 916-534-7279
Sacramento, CA 96825-4502 800-473-4636
Fax: 916-489-0241
parkanc@sbcglobal.net
www.parkinsonsacramento.org
*Bernardine Ford, President*
*George Johnston, 2nd Vice President*

2257 **Parkinson Chapter of Greater Pittsburgh**
6507 Wilkins Avenue 412-365-2086
Pittsburgh, PA 15217
*Doreen Grasso, Chairperson*
*Maggie Schmidt, Executive Director*

2258 **Parkinson Foundation of Western Pennsylvania**
575 Lincoln Avenue 412-837-2542
Pittsburgh, PA 15202 info@pfwpa.org
pfwpa.org
Provides services, education, and support for those with Parkinson's disease and their families. Offers quarterly Lunch and Learns, educational seminars and classes, staff trainings, email newsletters, its website, and social media channels.
*Christine Haythorn, Executive Director*

2259 **Parkinson Foundation of the Heartland Oklahoma Branch**
1000 W Wilshire 405-810-0695
Oklahoma City, OK 73116 www.parkinson.org
Satellite office of the Kansas Chapter
*Jim Keating, Chairperson*

2260 **Parkinson Foundation of the National Capitol Area**
7700 Leesburg Pike, 703-734-1017
Falls church, VA 22043-4201 Fax: 703-734-1241
pfnca@parkinsonfoundation.org
www.parkinsonfoundation.org
*Daniel M Lewis, Chairperson*
*Donna Schena, Vice Chairman*

2261 **Parkinson Network of Mount Diablo**
Po Box 3127 925-284-2189
Walnut Creek, CA 94598-0127 mmhansell@hotmail.com
www.parkinson.org
Affiliate of the National Parkinson Foundation.
*Mary Hansell*

2262 **Parkinsons Resources of Oregon**
3975 Mercantile Drive 503-594-0901
Lake Oswego, OR 97035 800-426-6806
Fax: 503-594-0547
info@parkinsonsresources.org
www.parkinsonsresources.org
*Holly Chaimov, Executive Director*

2263 **Parkinsons Wellness Group of Western New York**
5140 Main Street 716-218-1027
Depew, NY 14221 coach71395@aol.com
http://www.npfwny.org/
Site changed
*Robert J Plunket, President*
*Gary Kurdziel, Vice President*

2264 **South Palm Beach County Chapter of NFP**
PO Box 880145 561-482-2867
Boca Raton, FL 33433-0145 www.parkinson.org
*Irving Layton, Chairperson*

2265 **Southeast Parkinson Disease Association**
6530 Metrowest Boulevard 407-489-4124
Orlando, FL 32835-6520 srh_pres@sepda.org
www.sepda.org
*Steve Hochberger, Chairperson*

2266 **Wisconsin Parkinson Association**
945 N 12th Street 414-219-7061
Milwaukee, WI 53233 800-972-5455
Fax: 414-219-6564
www.wiparkinson.org
Chapter of The National Parkinson Foundation.
*Keith Brewer, President*

## Libraries & Resource Centers

2267 **Parkinson's Resource Organization**
74090 El Paseo
Palm Desert, CA 92260-4135
760-773-5628
877-775-4111
Fax: 760-773-9803
info@parkinsonsresource.org
www.parkinsonsresource.org
Our mission is to help families affected by Parkinson's forge through the journey of the disease's progression with as much quality as life can provide, assuring patients aren't isolated.
*Jo Rosen, Visionary, President, Founder*
*William R Remery, Treasurer*

## Foundations & Research Centers

2268 **APDA Center for Advanced Parkinson Disease Research**
Washington University School of Medicine
660 South Euclid
St Louis, MO 63110
314-362-6909
Fax: 314-362-0168
joel@npg.wustl.edu
www.neuro.wustl.edu/parkinson/
Information and referral research center for Parkinson's disease patients and their families.
*David m Holtzman, Chairman*
*Brad a Racette, Vice Chairman*

2269 **Baylor College of Medicine Parkinson's Disease Center & Movement Disorders**
McNair Campus
Houston, TX 77030
713-798-2273
pdcmdc@bcm.edu
www.bcm.edu/healthcare/care-centers

2270 **California Institute for Medical Research**
2260 Clove Drive
San Jose, CA 95128
408-998-4554
Fax: 408-998-2723
www.cimr.org
Medical research including infectious diseases stroke and cancer specializing in Parkinson's Disease related studies.
*David A Stevens, President*
*John Hotson, Vice President*

2271 **Center for Brain Activity Mapping**
UC San Diego
9500 Gilman Drive
La Jolla, CA 92093
858-534-2230
cbam.ucsd.edu
The Center seeks to develop new technologies for detecting neuronal activity, for reporting it out of deep brain tissue, and for processing and analyzing the resulting data, by organizing and supporting research teams and projects.
*Ralph J. Greenspan, PhD, Director*

2272 **Duke Neurological Disorders Clinic**
Duke Health Center at Morreene Road
Durham, NC 27705
855-855-6484
www.dukemedicine.org/treatments
A National Parkinson's Foundation Center of Excellence.

2273 **Henry Ford Hospital Movement Disorder Center**
Henry Ford Hospital Department of Neurology
2799 W Grand Boulevard
Detroit, MI 48202
www.henryford.com
The team at the Parkinson's Disease and Movement Disorders Center at Henry Ford has decades of experience diagnosing and treating Parkinson's disease, tremor, dystonia and other movement disorders.

2274 **International Parkinson and Movement Disoorder Society**
555 E Wells Street
Milwaukee, WI 53202
414-276-2145
Fax: 414-276-3349
info@movementdisorders.org
www.movementdisorders.org
A professional society of clinicians, scientists, and other healthcare professionals who are interested in Parkinson's disease, related neurodegenerative and neurodevelopmental disorders, hyperkinetic movement disorders, and abnormalities in muscle tone and motor control.
*Claudia Trenwalder, MD, President*

2275 **Kavli Foundation**
5715 Mesmer Avenue
Los Angeles, CA
424-353-8800
info@kavlifoundation.org
www.kavlifoundation.org
The Foundation supports scientific research into the human brain, in the following scientific fields: Astrophysics, Nanoscience, Neuroscience and Theoretical Physics. Within Neuroscience, the study of aging and brain diseases and disorders is supported.
*Robert W. Conn, PhD, President & CEO*
*Eric Marshall, VP, Public Engagement & Prizes*

2276 **Kavli Institute for Brain Science at Columbia University**
Columbia University
3227 Broadway
New York, NY 10027
212-853-1016
Fax: 212-665-9699
kavli@columbia.edu
www.kavli.columbia.edu
The Institute's primary arc of study is how signaling in neural circuits controls cognitive function and behavior, and the development of novel experimental and computational strategies for analyzing these signals.
*Eric R. Kandel, MD, Director*
*Rafael Yuste, MD, PhD, Co-Director*

2277 **Kavli Institute for Brain and Mind**
UC San Diego
9500 Gilman Drive
La Jolla, CA 92093-0115
kibm@ucsd.edu
kibm.ucsd.edu
The Institute supports research that furthers the understanding of the origins, evolution and mechanisms of human cognition. Of particular interest is Traumatic Brain Injury.
*Fred H. Gage, Co-Director*
*Nicholas C. Spitzer, Co-Director*

2278 **Kavli Institute for Fundamental Neuroscience**
UCSF, Sandler Neurosciences Center
675 Nelson Rising Lane
San Francisco, CA 94158
415-476-2018
Fax: 415-502-7332
kavliifn@ucsf.edu
kavliifn.ucsf.edu
The Institute is the central organization for neuroscience research at UCSF and partner institutions, establishing cross-disciplinary teams of scientists and engineers devoted to advancing neuroscience in all its forms.
*Loren Frank, Co-Director*
*Roger Nicoll, Co-Director*

2279 **Kavli Institute for Neuroscience at Yale University**
Yale School of Medicine
295 Congress Avenue
New Haven, CT 06510
203-737-4461
203-737-4467
pietro.decamilli@yale.edu
medicine.yale.edu/neuroscience/kavli
The institute studies nervous system development and function.
*Pietro De Camilli, MD, Director*
*Marina Picciotto, PhD, Deputy Director*

2280 **Kavli Neural Systems Institute**
The Rockefeller University
1230 York Avenue
New York, NY 10065
212-327-8081
lcole@rockefeller.edu
www.rockefeller.edu/research
The Institute unites scientists at The Rockefeller University in the goal of a comprehensive look at the human brain.
*Leslie Vosshall, PhD, Director*
*Lindsey Cole, Administrator*

2281 **Kavli Neuroscience Discovery Institute**
Johns Hopkins University, School of Medicine
725 N Wolfe Street
Baltimore, MD 21205
410-955-4089
Fax: 410-614-6249
KavliNDI@jhu.edu
kavlijhu.org
The Institute looks to advance neuroscience by integrating neuroscience, engineering and computational data science.
*Dwight Bergles, PhD, Director*
*Natasha Hussain, PhD, Scientific Director*

2282 **Michael J. Fox Foundation for Parkinson's**
Grand Central Station 800-708-7644
New York, NY 10163 www.michaeljfox.org
The largest nonprofit funder of Parkinson's research worldwide.
*Todd Sherer, CEO*
*Deborah W. Brooks, Co-Founder & Exec. Vice Chairman*

2283 **Michigan Parkinson Foundation**
30400 Telegraph Road 248-433-1011
Bingham Farms, MI 48025 800-852-9781
info@parkinsonsmi.org
www.parkinsonsmi.org
To educate and provide direct patient support to people affected by Parkinson's disease and related movement disorders, their loved ones and care partners as well as the physicians and other allied health professionals who diagnose and treat those individuals with the disease.
*Mary Sue Lanigan, CEO*
*Diane Kraft, Program Manager*

2284 **NYIT College of Osteopathic Medicine**
New York Institute of Technology
Serota Academic Center, Admissions 516-686-3997
Old Westbury, NY 11568 Fax: 516-686-3831
comadm@nyit.edu
www.nyit.edu/medicine
Information and referral research center for Parkinson's disease patients and their families.
*Sheldon Yao, Chair*

2285 **National Institute of Neurological Disorders & Stroke**
NIH Neurological Institute
PO Box 5801 800-352-9424
Bethesda, MD 20824 www.ninds.nih.gov
Mission: to reduce the burden of neurological disease.
*Codrin Lungu, MD, Director, Movement Disorders*

2286 **Neuroscience Research Institute**
UC Santa Barbara
6129 Biology II 805-893-4621
Santa Barbara, CA 93106 www.nri.ucsb.edu
The Institute seeks to allow scientists from different fields to collaborate for the betterment of neurological research. Areas of interest include: Alzheimer's Disease & Related Dementias; Behavioral Neuroscience & Neuroethology; Cell Biology, Biochemistry & Biophysics of the Nervous System; Computational & Theoretical Neuroscience; Development of the Nervous System; and Stem Cells.
*Stuart Feinstein, Co-Director*
*Kenneth Kosik, Co-Director*

2287 **Northwestern University Parkinson's Disease & Movement Disorders Center**
710 N Lake Shore Drive 312-503-4397
Chicago, IL 60611 www.parkinsons.northwestern.edu
Recognized by the National Parkinson Foundation as a Center for Excellence, Northwestern University Parkinson's Disease and Movement Disorders Center conducts research to extend the knowledge and treatment of PD and other movement disorders.
*Tanya Simuni, Director*

2288 **Oregon Health Sciences University**
3181 SW Sam Jackson Park Road 503-494-8311
Portland, OR 97239 www.ohsu.edu
Information and referral research center for Parkinson's disease patients and their families.
*Danny Jacobs, President*

2289 **Parkinson Disease & Movement Disorders Center**
Penn Neuroscience Center www.pennmedicine.org/neurology
Philadelphia, PA 19107
Raises funds for support of scientific research into causes, prevention, and cure of Parkinson's disease. Supports its own laboratories for research in Parkinsonism. Prepares and distributes information on patient care and rehabilitation including list of clinics where treatment is available, and a list of patient selfhelp groups. Supports a brain bank to permit anatomical and chemical studies. Sponsors scientific symposia.

2290 **Parkinson's Institute & Clinical Center**
2500 Hospital Drive 650-770-0201
Mountain View, CA 94040 Fax: 650-770-0204
www.parkinsonsinstitute.org
Research into new treatment options while providing comprehensive patient care.
*Brian Coulter, CEO*

2291 **Parkinsons Disease Foundation**
1359 Broadway 212-923-4700
New York, NY 10018 800-457-6676
Fax: 212-923-4778
info@pdf.org
www.pdf.org
The foundation has been one of the leaders in subsidizing research into Parkinson's Disease. Offers many services including The Summer Fellowship Program, The Postdoctoral Fellowship Program, support groups nationwide, grants for clinical and laboratory studies, public awareness and government promotion of the disease.
*Howard D. Morgan, Chair/Co President*
*Constance Woodruff Atwell, Vice Chair*

2292 **Presbyterian Hospital of Dallas**
Texas Health Resources
8200 Walnut Hill Lane 214-345-6789
Dallas, TX 75231 www.texashealth.org
Information and referral research center for Parkinson's disease patients and their families.
*Jim Parobek, President*

2293 **Robert Wood Johnson University Hospital**
1 Robert Wood Johnson Place 732-828-3000
New Brunswick, NJ 08901 www.rwjbh.org
Information and referral research center for Parkinson's disease patients and their families.
*John J. Ganther, President & CEO*

2294 **Salk Institute for Biological Studies**
10010 N Torrey Pines Road 858-453-4100
La Jolla, CA 92037 www.salk.edu
Conducts groundbreaking research into cancer, aging, Alzheimer's diabetes and infectious diseases.
*Rusty Gage, PhD, President*
*Martin Hetzer, PhD, VP & Chief Science Officer*

2295 **Sanford Consortium for Regenerative Medicine**
2880 Torrey Pines Scenic Drive 858-246-1071
La Jolla, CA 92037 www.sanfordconsortium.com
The Consortium works to achieve breakthrough discoveries in stem cell research with regards to diagnoses, treatments, and cures for degenerative diseases and injuries.
*Edward W. Holmes, MD, President & CEO*
*Jeffrey Steindorf, PhD, VP & COO*

2296 **Scripps Research Institute**
10550 North Torrey Pines Road 858-784-1000
La Jolla, CA www.scripps.edu
The institute seeks to improve human wellbeing through the advancement of bioscience, including research into aging & healthspan, autoimmune diseases, cancer, infectious diseases, neurological disorders, and more.
*Peter Schultz, PhD, President & CEO*
*Eric Topol, MD, EVP, Scripps Research*

2297 **St. John's Episcopal Hospital**
327 Beach 19th street 718-869-7000
Smithtown, NY 11691 www.ehs.org
Information and referral research center for Parkinson's disease patients and their families.
*Nelson toebbe, Chief Executive Officer*
*Richard A Brown, Chief Operating Officer*

2298 **Texas Tech University: Tarbox Parkinson's Disease Institute**
Texas Tech Physicians Medical Pavilion
3601 4th Street 806-743-2669
Lubbock, TX 79430 patientservices@ttuhsc.edu
www.texastechphysicians.com
Research center dedicated to Parkinson's Disease.

2299 **UCSD National Parkinson Disease Center of Excellence**
UC San Diego Health 858-657-8540
San Diego, CA 92103 health.ucsd.edu/specialties/neuro
A National Parkinson's Foundation Center of Excellence.
*Irene Litvan, Director*

2300 **UCSF Parkinson's Disease Clinic & Research Center**
University of California, San Francisco
350 Parnassus Avenue 415-476-9276
San Francisco, CA 94117 Fax: 415-476-3289
aaron.daley@ucsf.edu
pdcenter.neurology.ucsf.edu
One of the leading neuroscience centers in the United States and a National Parkinson's Foundation Center of Excellence.
*Michael J. Aminoff, Director*

2301 **University of Alabama at Birmingham Parkinsons Disease Center**
1720 7th Avenue S 205-934-4011
Birmingham, AL 35294 Fax: 205-346-78
TDD: 205-934-4642
apda@uab.edu
www.uab.edu
Offers educational emotional and political support to Parkinson disease patients and their families.
*Ray Watts, Interim CEO*
*David G Standaert, Director*

2302 **University of Pittsburgh**
4200 Fifth avenue 412-624-4141
Pittsburgh, PA 15260 Fax: 412-383-2264
webmaster@pitt.edu
www.pitt.edu
Information and referral research center for Parkinson's disease patients and their families.
*Patricia E. Beeson, Vice Chancellor*
*John P Elliott, Director of Internal Affairs*

2303 **University of Rochester**
500 Wilson Boulevard 585-275-3221
Rochester, NY 14627 888-822-2256
www.rochester.edu/
Information and referral research center for Parkinson's disease patients and their families.

2304 **University of Texas HSC at San Antonio**
UT Health Center
7703 Floyd Curl Drive 210-567-7000
San Antonio, TX 78229 uthscsa.edu
Information and referral research center for Parkinson's disease patients and their families.
*William Henrich, President*

2305 **University of Washington**
Box 355840 206-543-5369
Seattle, WA 98195-5840 uwvic@u.washington.edu
www.washington.edu/
Information and referral research center for Parkinson's disease patients and their families.

2306 **Vanderbilt University Medical Center**
1211 Medical Center Drive 615-322-5000
Nashville, TN 37232 www.vanderbilthealth.com
Dedicated to patient care, research, and biomedical education.
*Jeff Balsers, President & CEO*

2307 **William T Gossett Parkinson's Disease Center**
Henry Ford Hospital
Department of Neurology 313-972-1693
Detroit, MI 48202
*Jay M Gorell MD, Director*

## Support Groups & Hotlines

2308 **American Parkinson Disease Association Hotline**
1250 Hylan Boulevard 800-908-2732
Staten Island, NY 10305 Fax: 718-981-4399
Offers information and physician referrals to patients and their families.
*Joel Gerstel, Director*

2309 **Brain Support Network**
P.O. Box 7264 650-814-0848
Menlo Park, CA 94026 Fax: 650-233-9278
www.brainsupportnetwork.org
Non-profit dedicated to facilitate brain donation for scientific study in the U.S. and Canada, to provide education on neurological conditions worldwide, and run support groups in Northern California.

2310 **Dallas Area Parkinsonism Society**
6370 LBJ Freeway 972-620-7600
Dallas, TX 75240 daps.us
DAPS serves as a resource for the Parkinson's community by providing education; speech and exercise classes; and support groups.
*Michael L. Miles, Executive Director*

2311 **Greater Daytona Area Parkinson Support Group**
Bishop's Glen Retirement Center 904-322-4748
Daytona, FL www.parkinson.org
Affiliate of the National Parkinson Foundation.

2312 **Hawai'i Parkinson Association**
PO Box 1312 808-219-8874
Kailua, HI 96734 info@parkinsonshawaii.org
www.parkinsonshawaii.org
*Jerry Boster, President*
*Lindsey Sutton, Secretary*

2313 **Houston Area Parkinson Society**
2700 Southwest Freeway 713-626-7114
Houston, TX 77098 www.hapsonline.org
Offers support to people diagnosed with Parkinson's Disease and their loved ones.
*Kathleen Crist, LMSW, Executive Director*

2314 **Kuakini Parkinson Disease (PD) Information & Referral**
Kuakini Medical Center
347 North Kuakini Street 808-536-2236
Honolulu, HI 96817 800-570-1101
Fax: 808-528-1897
pr@kuakini.org
The Kuakini Parkinson Disease (PD) Information & Referral Office provides referrals to neurologists and other special services for Parkinson disease patients; provides information about community services to assist PD patients and their caregivers in finding optimal care; distributes educational materials; conducts educational conferences and other activities; and assists with support groups for PD patients and caregivers.
*Gary K Kajiwara, President/Chief Executive Officer*
*Gregg Oishi, SVP/Chief Operating Officer*

2315 **Maine Parkinson Society**
146 Parkway S 800-832-4116
Brewer, ME 04412 Fax: 207-573-1031
info@maineparkinson.org
www.maineparkinsonsociety.org
Spreading awareness and improving quality of life for people in Maine with Parkinson's.
*Karen Marsters, President*
*Paul Soucy, Secretary*

2316 **National Parkinson Foundation Hotline**
National Parkinson Foundation
1501 NW 9th Avenue Bob Hope Road 305-243-6666
Miami, FL 33136 800-327-4545
Fax: 305-243-5595
www.parkinson.org
Offers support and emergency information for persons with Parkinson's and their families.
*Jose Garcia Pebrosa, Director*

2317 **National Parkinson Foundation: Central Savannah River Area**
116 Lottie Lane 706-364-1662
Grovetown, GA 30813 800-473-4636
info@parkinsoncsra.org
www.parkinsoncsra.org
*Joe Kelley, Research Coordinator*

2318 **National Parkinson Foundation: Florida**
200 SE 1st Street 305-537-9960
Miami, FL 33131 800-473-4636
florida@parkinson.org
www.parkinson.org/florida
*Amanda Spiehler, Southeast Regional Director*

2319 **National Parkinson Foundation: Great Lakes**
ATTN: Great Lakes
200 SE 1st Street 866-920-6673
Miami, FL 33131 greatlakes@parkinson.org
www.parkinson.org/greatlakes
*Lori Gum, Development Manager*

2320 **National Parkinson Foundation: Heartland**
8900 State Line Road 913-416-4116
Leawood, KS 66206 800-473-4636
heartland@parkinson.org
www.parkinson.org/heartland
Affiliate of the National Parkinson Foundation.
*Abby LacKamp, Regional Director*

2321 **National Parkinson Foundation: Minnesota -Dakotas**
8085 Wayzata Boulevard 763-545-1272
Golden Valley, MN 55426 800-473-4636
minnesotadakotas@parkinson.org
www.parkinson.org/minnesotadakotas
*Jennifer Hendrickson, Development Manager*

2322 **National Parkinson Foundation: New York- New Jersey**
2805 Wehrle Drive 716-449-3795
Williamsville, NY 14221 800-473-4636
NYNJ@parkinson.org
www.parkinson.org/NYN
*Adrienne Casano, Northeast Regional Director*

2323 **New Jersey Parkinson's Disease Information Center**
Robert Wood Johnson University Hospital
One Robert Wood Johnson Place 732-828-3000
New Brunswick, NJ 08901 Fax: 732-745-3114
elizabeth.schaaf@rwjuh.edu
www.rwjuh.edu/medical_services/
The New Jersey Parkinson's Disease Information and Referral Center reaches out to persons affected by Parkinson's disease, including patients, families and healthcare professionals. This Information and Referral Center is committed to providing community education and information as well as support groups for caregivers and persons with Parkinson's disease.
*Elizabeth Schaaf, Parkinson's Disease Center Coordinator*

2324 **New York College of Osteopathic Medicine**
PO Box 8000 516-686-3747
Old Westbury, NY 11568-8000 800-345-6948
Fax: 516-686-7613
http://www.nyit.edu/medicine/
Information and referral research center for Parkinson's disease patients and their families.
*Rosslee , Vice President*

2325 **Northwest Parkinson's Foundation**
7525 SE 24th Street 206-748-9481
Mercer Island, WA 98040 877-980-7500
info@nwpf.org
nwpf.org
Improving the quality of life for the Northwest Parkinson's disease community.
*Melissa Tribelhorn, Executive Director*

2326 **Ozarks Parkinson Support Group**
Po Box 50595 417-885-9595
Springfield, MO 65805
Affiliate of the National Parkinson Foundation.
*Monty Montgomery, Contact*

2327 **Parkinson Association of Northern California**
1024 Iron Point Road 916-357-6641
Folsom, CA 95630 panc@panctoday.org
www.panctoday.org
*Sean Tracy, President*
*Cody O'Keefe, Treasurer*

2328 **Parkinson Association of Southwest Florida**
5926 Premier Way 239-417-3465
Naples, FL 34109 office@parkinsonassociationswfl.org
parkinsonassociationswfl.org
The Parkinson Association of Southwest Flordia is a not-for-profit organization. The mission is to promote quality of life for persons with Parkinson's Disease and their care partners. This is accomplished by providing educational, physical and social programs. The organization also provides education for the community regarding Parkinson's Disease and its effects.
*Linda Goldfield, Executive Director*

2329 **Parkinson Association of the Carolinas**
2101 Sardis Road N 980-245-2786
Charlotte, NC 28227 866-903-7275
pac@parkinsonassociation.org
www.parkinsonassociation.org
The Parkinson Association of the Carolinas (PAC) was established in 2002 to serve as a resource for individuals and their families living in the Carolinas who are affected by Parkinson's disease. PAC seeks to empower these individuals and families through education, outreach and direct support.
*Ann Marie Obrikat, Executive Director*

2330 **Parkinson Association of the Rockies**
1325 S Colorado Boulevard 303-830-1839
Denver, CO 80222 info@parkinsonrockies.org
www.parkinsonrockies.org
Services the Colorado Parkinson's community, providing direct care services including support groups, exercise programs, in-home case assessments, educational programs, informative newsletters and an information hotline to individuals living with Parkinson's, their families and caregivers.
*Jodi Brown, Executive Director*
*Karen Crumback, Director of Development*

2331 **Parkinson Foundation of Oklahoma**
720 W Wilshire Boulevard 405-810-0695
Oklahoma City, OK 73116 info@parkinsonoklahoma.com
parkinsonoklahoma.com
Offers educational programs and support services to individuals in Oklahoma with Parkinson's Disease and related movement disorders.
*Bruce McIntyre, Executive Director*

2332 **Parkinson Support Groups of America**
11376 Cherry Hill Road 301-937-1545
Beltsville, MD 20705
Offers support networks and groups for persons with Parkinson's disease, families, friends and professionals.

2333 **Parkinson's Association of Orange County**
7700 Irvine Drive 949-788-2933
Irvine, CA 92618 Board_Secretary@PAOCinc.org
paocinc.org
*Sam Torres, President*

2334 **Parkinson's Association of San Diego**
PO Box 1633 858-999-5671
Solana Beach, CA 92075 info@parkinsonsassociation.org
www.parkinsonsassociation.org
A leading Parkinson's resource in San Diego county, setting a standard for education, support groups, information and referral, evidence based exercise programs, community events, social opportunities, compassion and encouragement.
*Chris Buscher, Executive Director*

2335 **Parkinson's Association of West Michigan**
260 Jefferson Avenue SE 616-954-8077
Grand Rapids, MI 49503 info@parkinsonswm.org
www.parkinsonswm.org
The Mission of the Parkinson's Association of West Michigan (PAWM) is to provide the best information on opportunities, treatment, research, and care to people with Parkinson's and their families. PAWM is a source for Parkinson's information. Our meetings feature programs on physical and speech therapy, relaxation training, and other measures which are important in learning to live with Parkinson's.
*Kimn Cousineau, President*

2336 **Parkinson's Disease Association of San Diego (PDASD)**
8555 Areo Drive 858-273-6763
San Diego, CA 92123-1746 877-737-7576
Fax: 858-273-6764
info@pdasd.org
www.pdasd.org
Information and referral research center for Parkinson's disease patients and their families.
*Jerry Henberger, Executive Director*
*Rick Brydges, President*

2337 **Parkinson's Resources of Oregon**
8880 SW Nimbus Avenue 503-594-0901
Beaverton, OR 97008 800-426-6806
Fax: 503-594-0547
info@parkinsonsresources.org
www.parkinsonsresources.org
Nationally recognized non-profit dedicated to improving the quality of life for people with Parkinson's in the Pacific Northwest.
*Holly Chaimov, Executive Director*

2338 **Parkinson's Support Group of Upstate New York**
PO Box 23204 716-377-6718
Rochester, NY 14692-3204
Affiliate of The National Parkinson Foundation, Inc.
*David Look, President*

2339 **Pembroke Pines Parkinson Support Group**
Century Village, Club House 954-433-0947
Pembroke Pines, FL 33027 www.parkinson.org
Affiliate of the National Parkinson Foundation.

2340 **Rockford Parkinson's Support Group**
5415 Watson Road 815-654-0614
Rockford, IL 61108 800-972-5455
Affiliate of The National Parkinson Foundation, Inc.

2341 **Texas Tech University Tarbox Parkinson's Disease Institute**
3601 4th Street 806-743-1000
Lubbock, TX 79430 www.ttuhsc.edu
The objectives of the Tarbox Institute are to provide services for Parkinson's disease patients and their families in the underserved West Texas area; to maintain a Parkinson's Disease Information and Referral Center to enable both healthcare professionals and affected families to obtain the latest information on services available.
*Tedd L Mitchell, President*
*Pureza Martinez, Chief of Staff*

2342 **Wisconsin Parkinson Association**
16655 W Bluemound Road 414-312-6990
Brookfield, WI 53005 mail@wiparkinson.org
www.wiparkinson.org
Wisconsin Parkinson Association provides hope, community, support, and resources for people with Parkinson's and their loved ones.
*Gary Garland, Executive Director*

2343 **Parkinson Foundation of Western Pennsylvania**
575 Lincoln Avenue 412-837-2542
Pittsburgh, PA 15202 info@pfwpa.org
pfwpa.org
Provides services, education, and support for those with Parkinson's disease and their families. Offers quarterly Lunch and Learns, educational seminars and classes, staff trainings, email newsletters, its website, and social media channels.
*Christine Haythorn, Executive Director*

## Magazines

2344 **ASN NEURO**
Sage Journals
2455 Teller Road 805-499-9774
Thousand Oaks, CA 91320 journals@sagepub.com
journals.sagepub.com/home/asn
Peer-reviewed open access journal focusing on recent advances in the cellular and molecular neurosciences. It is the official publication of the American Society for Neurochemistry.
*Douglas L. Feinstein, Editor-in-Chief*
*Sandra J. Hewitt, Deputy Editor-in-Chief*

2345 **American Journal of Pathology**
Elsevier
1600 John F Kennedy Boulevard 301-634-7959
Philadelphia, PA 19103 Fax: 301-634-7961
ajp@asip.org
ajp.amjpathol.org
Official journal of the American Society for Investigative Pathology, publishing original research reports, reviews, and commentaries related to the molecular and cellular basis of disease.
*Martha Furie, Editor-in-Chief*

2346 **BMC Neuroscience**
Springer Nature
One New York Plaza 800-777-4643
New York, NY 10004-1562 info@biomedcentral.com
bmcneurosci.biomedcentral.com
A peer-reviewed, open-access journal devoted to all aspects of the nervous system (including molecular, cellular, developmental and animal model studies), as well as cognitive and behavioral research, and computational modeling.
*Darren Byrne, Editor*
*Ana Donnelly, Manuscript Editor*

2347 **Brain & Life**
American Academy of Neurology
201 Chicago Avenue 612-928-6000
Minneapolis, MN 55415 800-879-1960
Fax: 612-454-2748
BrainandLife@wolterskluwer.com
www.brainandlife.org
Official magazine of the American Academy of Neurology, aimed at parents and home-caregivers interested in neurology in everyday life.
*Orly Avitzur, MD, MBA, FAAN, Editor-in-Chief*
*Mary Bolster, Managing Editor*

2348 **Brain: A Journal of Neurology**
Oxford University Press
2001 Evans Road 919-677-0977
Cary, NC 27513 800-852-7323
Fax: 919-677-1714
brain@ucl.ac.uk
academic.oup.com/brain
Focus is clinical neurology and translational neuroscience.
*Dimitri M. Kullmann, Editor*
*Joanne Bell, Managing Editor*

2349 **Continuum: Lifelong Learning in Neurology**
American Academy of Neurology
201 Chicago Avenue 612-928-6000
Minneapolis, MN 55415 800-879-1960
continuumcme@aan.com
journals.lww.com/continuum
Official journal of the American Academy of Neurology, aiding professionals in patient care and continuing education.
*Bimonthly*
*Steven L. Lewis, MD, FAAN*
*Andrea J. Weiss, MA, Executive Editor*

2350 **Dementia and Geriatric Cognitive Disorders**
S. Karger Publishers, Inc.
26 W Avon Road 860-675-7834
Unionville, CT 06085 800-828-5479
Fax: 860-675-7302
www.karger.com/DEM
Open-access journal devoted to the study of cognitive dysfunction in preclinical and clinical studies, concentrating on Alzheimer's and Parkinson's disease, Huntington's chorea and other neurodegenerative diseases.
*Victoria Chan-Pilay, Editor-in-Chief*

2351 **JNeurosci**
Society for Neuroscience

1121 14th Street NW
Washginton, DC 20005
202-962-4000
jn@sfn.org
www.jneurosci.org

Official peer-reviewed journal of the Society for Neuroscience, publishing research on a broad range of topics of interest to those working on the nervous system.
*Marina R. Picciotto, Editor-in-Chief*
*Teresa Esch, Features Editor*

2352 **Journal of Alzheimer's Disease**
IOS Press
6751 Tepper Drive
Clifton, VA 20124
703-830-6300
Fax: 703-830-2300
editorial@j-alz.com
www.j-alz.com

Research into the etiology, pathogenesis, epidemiology, genetics, behavior, treatment and psychology of Alzheimer's disease.
*George Perry, PhD, Editor-in-Chief*
*Beth Kumar, Managing Editor*

2353 **Journal of Molecular Diagnostics**
Elsevier
1600 John F Kennedy Boulevard
Philadelphia, PA 19103
301-634-7959
Fax: 301-634-7961
jmd@asip.org
jmd.amjpathol.org

Official journal of the American Society for Investigative Pathology and the Association for Molecular Pathology, focusing on molecular discoveries in medicine translating into the clinical diagnostic setting, as well as the description and application of technological advances in the field of molecular diagnostic medicine.
*Monthly*
*Barbara Zehnbauer, PhD, Editor-in-Chief*

2354 **Journal of NeuroEngineering and Rehabilitation**
Springer Nature
One New York Plaza
New York, NY 10004-1562
800-777-4643
info@biomedcentral.com
jneuroengrehab.biomedcentral.com

An open-access journal devoted to integrated research from the fields of neuroscience, biomedical engineering, and physical medicine and rehabilitation.
*David J. Reinkensmeyer, Editor-in-Chief*

2355 **Journal of Neurodevelopmental Disorders**
Springer Nature
One New York Plaza
New York, NY 10004-1562
800-777-4643
info@biomedcentral.com
jneurodevdisorders.biomedcentral.com

An open-access journal devoted to integrating research from neurobiology, genetics, cognitive neuroscience, psychiatry and psychology.
*Joseph Piven, Editor-in-Chief*

2356 **Journal of Neuroinflammation**
Springer Nature
One New York Plaza
New York, NY 10004-1562
800-777-4643
info@biomedcentral.com
jneuroinflammation.biomedcentral.com

A peer-reviewed, open-access journal focusing on the interactions of the immune system with the nervous system as a means of expanding understanding of chronic neurological diseases.
*Monica J. Carson, Editor-in-Chief*
*Sue T. Griffin, Editor-in-Chief*

2357 **Journal of Nuclear Medicine**
Society of Nuclear Medicine and Molecular Imaging
1850 Samuel Morse Drive
Reston, VA 20190
703-708-9000
800-513-6853
Fax: 703-708-9015
subscriptions@snm.org
jnm.snmjournals.org

Peer-reviewed journal with clinical investigations, science reports, articles benefitting continuing education, book reviews, employment opportunities, and updates on practice and research.
*Monthly*
*Johannes Czernin, MD, Editor-in-Chief*
*Susan Alexander, Associate Director, Publications*

2358 **Journal of Nuclear Medicine Technology**
Society of Nuclear Medicine and Molecular Imaging
1850 Samuel Morse Drive
Reston, VA 20190
703-708-9000
800-513-6853
Fax: 703-708-9015
subscriptions@snm.org
tech.snmjournals.org

Peer-reviewed journal dedicated to nuclear medicine technology, with information on credentialing, continuing education and licensure requirements, as well as current news and updates on the field.
*Quarterly*
*Kathy S. Thomas, MHA, CNMT, PET, Editor-in-Chief*
*Susan Alexander, Associate Director, Publications*

2359 **Journal of the Neurological Sciences**
Elsevier
LSU Health Sciences Center
New Orleans, LA 70112
JNS_England@lsuhsc.edu
www.jns-journal.com

Original articles in neurology and neuroscience from around the world.
*Monthly*
*John D. England, Editor-in-Chief*

2360 **Molecular Imaging**
Sage Journals
2455 Teller Road
Thousand Oaks, CA 91320
805-499-9774
journals@sagepub.com
journals.sagepub.com/home/mix

Peer-reviewed open access journal focusing on molecular imaging research, including basic science, preclinical studies and human applications. Published in association with the Society of Nuclear Medicine and Molecular Imaging.
*Bimonthly*
*Henry F. VanBrocklin, PhD, Editor-in-Chief*

2361 **Molecular Neurodegeneration**
Springer Nature
One New York Plaza
New York, NY 10004-1562
800-777-4643
info@biomedcentral.com
www.biomedcentral.com

A peer-reviewed, open-access journal devoted to all aspects of neurodegeneration research at the molecular and cellular levels.
*Guojun Bu, Editor-in-Chief*
*Huaxi Xu, Editor-in-Chief*

2362 **Neurocase: The Neural Basis of Cognition**
Taylor & Francis Group
530 Walnut Street
Philadelphia, PA 19106
www.tandfonline.com/toc/nncs20/current

Rapid response journal featuring case and group studies in neuropsychology, neuropsychiatry and behavioral neurology, with a focus on the neural basis of cognition.
*Bruce L. Miller, Editor*
*Hans J. Markowitsch, Editor*

2363 **Neurology**
American Academy of Neurology
201 Chicago Avenue
Minneapolis, MN 55415
612-928-6000
800-879-1960
Fax: 612-454-2748
journal@neurology.org
n.neurology.org

Official journal of the American Academy of Neurology, peer-reviewed, highlighting clinical neurology research.
*Jose G. Merino, MD, MPhil, FAAN, Editor-in-Chief*
*Patricia K. Baskin, MS, Executive Editor*

2364 **Neurology Clinical Practice**
American Academy of Neurology
201 Chicago Avenue
Minneapolis, MN 55415
612-928-6000
800-879-1960
Fax: 612-454-2748
journal@neurology.org
cp.neurology.org

Official peer-reviewed journal of the American Academy of Neurology for practicing neurologists.
*John R. Corboy, MD, FAAN, Editor*
*Patricia K. Baskin, MS, Executive Editor*

2365 **Neurology: Genetics**
American Academy of Neurology
201 Chicago Avenue 612-928-6000
Minneapolis, MN 55415 800-879-1960
Fax: 612-454-2748
journal@neurology.org
ng.neurology.org
Official journal of the American Academy of Neurology, publishing online open-access peer-reviewed reports in the field of neurogenetics.
*Stefan M. Pulst, MD, FAAN, Editor*
*Patricia K. Baskin, MS, Executive Editor*

2366 **Neurology: Neuroimmunology & Neuroinflammation**
American Academy of Neurology
201 Chicago Avenue 612-928-6000
Minneapolis, MN 55415 800-879-1960
Fax: 612-454-2748
journal@neurology.org
nn.neurology.org
Official journal of the American Academy of Neurology, publishing online open-access peer-reviewed reports of original research and in-depth reviews of topics in neuroimmunology & neuroinflammation.
*Josep O. Dalmau, MD, PhD, Editor*
*Patricia K. Baskin, MS, Executive Editor*

2367 **Society of Nuclear Medicine and Molecular Imaging**
1850 Samuel Morse Drive 703-708-9000
Reston, VA 20190 Fax: 703-708-9015
feedback@snmmi.org
www.snmmi.org
The mission of this nonprofit scientific and professional organization is to promote the science, technology and application of nuclear medicine and molecular imaging. Molecular imaging techniques are used to diagnose and manage the treatment of brain disorders such as Alzheimer's and Parkinson's disease, among other conditions.
*15,000 members*
*Virginia Pappas, CEO*
*Rebecca Maxey, Director, Communications*

2368 **Translational Neurodegeneration**
Springer Nature
One New York Plaza 800-777-4643
New York, NY 10004-1562 info@biomedcentral.com
www.biomedcentral.com
A peer-reviewed, open-access journal covering research, therapeutics and education for all areas of neurodegenerative diseases.
*Shengdi Chen, Editor-in-Chief*

2369 **Ultrasonic Imaging**
Sage Journals
2455 Teller Road 805-499-9774
Thousand Oaks, CA 91320 journals@sagepub.com
journals.sagepub.com/home/uix
The journal focuses on the rapid publication of original papers on the development and application of ultrasonic techniques, with emphasis on medical diagnosis. Also published are research notes, comments on papers appearing in the journal, book reviews, and occasional review articles.
*Ernest J. Feleppa, Editor-in-Chief*
*Roslyn Raskin, Managing Editor*

2370 **eNeuro**
Society for Neuroscience
1121 14th Street NW 202-312-7305
Washginton, DC 20005 eNeuro@sfn.org
www.eneuro.org
Open-access journal of the Society for Neuroscience.
*Christophe Bernard, Editor-in-Chief*
*Kelly Newton, Director, Scientific Publications*

## Web Sites

2371 **BrainFacts.org**
Society for Neuroscience
1121 14th Street NW brainfactsinfo@sfn.org
Washington, DC 20005 brainfacts.org
Online public information portal founded by the Kavli Foundation, the Gatsby Charitable Foundation and the Society for Neuroscience, with topics on brain function and anatomy, diseases and disorders, and more.
*Richard Wingate, DPhil, Editor-in-Chief*
*Charles Yokoyama, PhD, Associate Editor*

2372 **Healing Well**
www.healingwell.com
An online health resource guide to medical news, chat, information and articles, newsgroups and message boards, books, disease-related web sites, medical directories, and more for patients, friends, and family coping with disabling diseases, disorders, or chronic illnesses.

2373 **Health Finder**
www.healthfinder.gov
Searchable, carefully developed web site offering information on over 1000 topics. Developed by the US Department of Health and Human Services, the site can be used in both English and Spanish.

2374 **Healthlink USA**
www.healthlinkusa.com
Health information concerning treatment, cures, prevention, diagnosis, risk factors, research, support groups, email lists, personal stories and much more. Updated regularly.

2375 **MedicineNet**
www.medicinenet.com
An online resource for consumers providing easy-to-read, authoritative medical and health information.

2376 **Medscape**
www.medscape.com
Medscape offers specialists, primary care physicians, and other health professionals the Web's most robust and integrated medical information and educational tools.

2377 **National Parkinson Foundation**
www.parkinson.org
Information on research, diagnosis, treatment and care for men and women suffering from parkinson's and other related neurological diseases.

2378 **Neurology Channel**
www.healthcommunities.com
Find clearly explained, medically accurate information regarding conditions, including an overview, symptoms, causes, diagnostic procedures and treatment options. On this site it is possible to ask questions and get information from a neurologist and connect to people who have similar health interests.

2379 **Neuronline**
Society for Neuroscience
1121 14th Street NW 202-962-4000
Washginton, DC 20005 neuronline@sfn.org
neuronline.sfn.org
Online portal for professional development and training resources for individuals in the field of neuroscience, hosted by the Society for Neuroscience.
*Amanda Kimball, Director, Digital Learning*

2380 **WebMD**
www.webmd.com
Provides credible information, supportive communities, and in-depth reference material about health subjects. A source for original and timely health information as well as material from well known content providers.

# PROGRESSIVE SUPRANUCLEAR PALSY

*Progressive supranuclear palsy is a degenerative disease that results from the deterioration and ultimate death of cells in the areas of the brain that control body movement, coordination, cognition, and other important functions. The typical onset of PSP is around ages 60-70 and it affects six people per 100,000. The symptoms of the disease are similar to other dementia-causing diseases such as Parkinson's and Alzheimer's and PSP is often mistaken for them.*

The distinctive symptoms of progressive supranuclear palsy include a loss of balance while walking, particularly a tendency to fall backwards, and an inability to aim the eyes properly, often resulting in blurred and double vision. The disease's other symptoms vary from patient to patient and include impulsive behavior, difficulty with speech and swallowing, awkward movements, and sleep disturbances. Because of these symptoms, a number of complications can result for PSP patients such as choking or inhaling food into the airway, and pneumonia, which is the most common cause of death in people with PSP.

As with most other forms of dementia-causing diseases, the cause of progressive supranuclear palsy is not known but studies have shown that people suffering from the disease have abnormal amounts of a protein called tau in their brain cells. Although PSP has been known to occasionally occur within a family, a genetic link has not been established. Diagnosis of PSP can be difficult because of its similarity to Parkinson's, but a doctor may diagnose PSP if a patient demonstrates Parkinson's symptoms but does not experience shaking or reports difficulty moving their eyes. An MRI or a PET scan can help confirm the diagnosis.

While there is no cure for progressive supranuclear palsy, several treatments have been shown to alleviate the disease's symptoms. Because of its similarity to Parkinson's, medications used to treat that disease, such as levodopa and amantadine, are often prescribed for PSP patients, although the effect of these medications is limited and usually temporary. In addition, OnabotulinumtoxianA (Botox) injections into the muscles around the eyes can help improve eyelid spasms, while a eyeglass prescription with bifocal or prism lenses can aid patients with problems looking downward. In addition, speech and swallowing evaluations can help a patient learn better swallowing techniques. Finally, physical and occupational therapy can help improve the patient's balance.

## National Agencies & Associations

2382 **American Academy of Neurology**
201 Chicago Avenue 612-928-6000
Minneapolis, MN 55415 800-879-1960
Fax: 612-454-2746
memberservices@aan.com
www.aan.com
Professional society of medical doctors specializing in brain and nervous system diseases. Maintains placement service. Sponsors research and educational programs. Compiles statistics. Publishes scientific journal, Continuum: Lifelong Learning in Neurology.
*Mary E. Post, MBA, CAE, CEO*

2383 **American Society for Neurochemistry**
9037 Ron Den Lane 407-909-9064
Windermere, FL 34786 Fax: 407-876-0750
asnmanager@asneurochem.org
asneurochem.org
The Society aims to advance and promote cellular and molecular neuroscience knowledge, and to facilitate communication and the dissemination of information within the field and with related disciplines.
*Sheilah Jewart, Executive Director*
*Karen Gottlieb, Conference Coordinator*

2384 **Brain Support Network**
P.O. Box 7264 650-814-0848
Menlo Park, CA 94026 Fax: 650-233-9278
www.brainsupportnetwork.org
Non-profit dedicated to facilitate brain donation for scientific study in the U.S. and Canada, to provide education on neurological conditions worldwide, and run support groups in Northern California.

## Foundations & Research Centers

2385 **Neuroscience Research Institute**
UC Santa Barbara
6129 Biology II 805-893-4621
Santa Barbara, CA 93106 www.nri.ucsb.edu
The Institute seeks to allow scientists from different fields to collaborate for the betterment of neurological research. Areas of interest include: Alzheimer's Disease & Related Dementias; Behavioral Neuroscience & Neuroethology; Cell Biology, Biochemistry & Biophysics of the Nervous System; Computational & Theoretical Neuroscience; Development of the Nervous System; and Stem Cells.
*Stuart Feinstein, Co-Director*
*Kenneth Kosik, Co-Director*

2386 **Sanford Consortium for Regenerative Medicine**
2880 Torrey Pines Scenic Drive 858-246-1071
La Jolla, CA 92037 www.sanfordconsortium.com
The Consortium works to achieve breakthrough discoveries in stem cell research with regards to diagnoses, treatments, and cures for degenerative diseases and injuries.
*Edward W. Holmes, MD, President & CEO*
*Jeffrey Steindorf, PhD, VP & COO*

## Magazines

2387 **ASN NEURO**
Sage Journals
2455 Teller Road 805-499-9774
Thousand Oaks, CA 91320 journals@sagepub.com
journals.sagepub.com/home/asn
Peer-reviewed open access journal focusing on recent advances in the cellular and molecular neurosciences. It is the official publication of the American Society for Neurochemistry.
*Douglas L. Feinstein, Editor-in-Chief*
*Sandra J. Hewitt, Deputy Editor-in-Chief*

2388 **BMC Neuroscience**
Springer Nature
One New York Plaza 800-777-4643
New York, NY 10004-1562 info@biomedcentral.com
bmcneurosci.biomedcentral.com
A peer-reviewed, open-access journal devoted to all aspects of the nervous system (including molecular, cellular, developmental and animal model studies), as well as cognitive and behavioral research, and computational modeling.
*Darren Byrne, Editor*
*Ana Donnelly, Manuscript Editor*

2389 **Brain & Life**
American Academy of Neurology
201 Chicago Avenue 612-928-6000
Minneapolis, MN 55415 800-879-1960
Fax: 612-454-2748
BrainandLife@wolterskluwer.com
www.brainandlife.org
Official magazine of the American Academy of Neurology, aimed at parents and home-caregivers interested in neurology in everyday life.
*Orly Avitzur, MD, MBA, FAAN, Editor-in-Chief*
*Mary Bolster, Managing Editor*

2390 **Brain: A Journal of Neurology**
Oxford University Press
2001 Evans Road 919-677-0977
Cary, NC 27513 800-852-7323
Fax: 919-677-1714
brain@ucl.ac.uk
academic.oup.com/brain
Focus is clinical neurology and translational neuroscience.
*Dimitri M. Kullmann, Editor*
*Joanne Bell, Managing Editor*

2391 **Continuum: Lifelong Learning in Neurology**
American Academy of Neurology
201 Chicago Avenue 612-928-6000
Minneapolis, MN 55415 800-879-1960
continuumcme@aan.com
journals.lww.com/continuum
Official journal of the American Academy of Neurology, aiding professionals in patient care and continuing education.
*Bimonthly*
*Steven L. Lewis, MD, FAAN*
*Andrea J. Weiss, MA, Executive Editor*

2392 **Dementia and Geriatric Cognitive Disorders**
S. Karger Publishers, Inc.
26 W Avon Road 860-675-7834
Unionville, CT 06085 800-828-5479
Fax: 860-675-7302
www.karger.com/DEM
Open-access journal devoted to the study of cognitive dysfunction in preclinical and clinical studies, concentrating on Alzheimer's and Parkinson's disease, Huntington's chorea and other neurodegenerative diseases.
*Victoria Chan-Pilay, Editor-in-Chief*

2393 **Journal of Alzheimer's Disease**
IOS Press
6751 Tepper Drive 703-830-6300
Clifton, VA 20124 Fax: 703-830-2300
editorial@j-alz.com
www.j-alz.com
Research into the etiology, pathogenesis, epidemiology, genetics, behavior, treatment and psychology of Alzheimer's disease.
*George Perry, PhD, Editor-in-Chief*
*Beth Kumar, Managing Editor*

2394 **Journal of Nuclear Medicine**
Society of Nuclear Medicine and Molecular Imaging
1850 Samuel Morse Drive 703-708-9000
Reston, VA 20190 800-513-6853
Fax: 703-708-9015
subscriptions@snm.org
jnm.snmjournals.org

Peer-reviewed journal with clinical investigations, science reports, articles benefitting continuing education, book reviews, employment opportunities, and updates on practice and research.
*Monthly*
*Johannes Czernin, MD, Editor-in-Chief*
*Susan Alexander, Associate Director, Publications*

2395 **Journal of Nuclear Medicine Technology**
Society of Nuclear Medicine and Molecular Imaging
1850 Samuel Morse Drive 703-708-9000
Reston, VA 20190 800-513-6853
Fax: 703-708-9015
subscriptions@snm.org
tech.snmjournals.org
Peer-reviewed journal dedicated to nuclear medicine technology, with information on credentialing, continuing education and licensure requirements, as well as current news and updates on the field.
*Quarterly*
*Kathy S. Thomas, MHA, CNMT, PET, Editor-in-Chief*
*Susan Alexander, Associate Director, Publications*

2396 **Journal of the Neurological Sciences**
Elsevier
LSU Health Sciences Center JNS_England@lsuhsc.edu
New Orleans, LA 70112 www.jns-journal.com
Original articles in neurology and neuroscience from around the world.
*Monthly*
*John D. England, Editor-in-Chief*

2397 **Molecular Imaging**
Sage Journals
2455 Teller Road 805-499-9774
Thousand Oaks, CA 91320 journals@sagepub.com
journals.sagepub.com/home/mix
Peer-reviewed open access journal focusing on molecular imaging research, including basic science, preclinical studies and human applications. Published in association with the Society of Nuclear Medicine and Molecular Imaging.
*Bimonthly*
*Henry F. VanBrocklin, PhD, Editor-in-Chief*

2398 **Molecular Neurodegeneration**
Springer Nature
One New York Plaza 800-777-4643
New York, NY 10004-1562 info@biomedcentral.com
www.biomedcentral.com
A peer-reviewed, open-access journal devoted to all aspects of neurodegeneration research at the molecular and cellular levels.
*Guojun Bu, Editor-in-Chief*
*Huaxi Xu, Editor-in-Chief*

2399 **Neurocase: The Neural Basis of Cognition**
Taylor & Francis Group
530 Walnut Street www.tandfonline.com/toc/nncs20/current
Philadelphia, PA 19106
Rapid response journal featuring case and group studies in neuropsychology, neuropsychiatry and behavioral neurology, with a focus on the neural basis of cognition.
*Bruce L. Miller, Editor*
*Hans J. Markowitsch, Editor*

2400 **Neurology**
American Academy of Neurology
201 Chicago Avenue 612-928-6000
Minneapolis, MN 55415 800-879-1960
Fax: 612-454-2748
journal@neurology.org
n.neurology.org
Official journal of the American Academy of Neurology, peer-reviewed, highlighting clinical neurology research.
*Jose G. Merino, MD, MPhil, FAAN, Editor-in-Chief*
*Patricia K. Baskin, MS, Executive Editor*

2401 **Neurology Clinical Practice**
American Academy of Neurology
201 Chicago Avenue 612-928-6000
Minneapolis, MN 55415 800-879-1960
Fax: 612-454-2748
journal@neurology.org
cp.neurology.org
Official peer-reviewed journal of the American Academy of Neurology for practicing neurologists.
*John R. Corboy, MD, FAAN, Editor*
*Patricia K. Baskin, MS, Executive Editor*

2402 **Neurology: Genetics**
American Academy of Neurology
201 Chicago Avenue 612-928-6000
Minneapolis, MN 55415 800-879-1960
Fax: 612-454-2748
journal@neurology.org
ng.neurology.org
Official journal of the American Academy of Neurology, publishing online open-access peer-reviewed reports in the field of neurogenetics.
*Stefan M. Pulst, MD, FAAN, Editor*
*Patricia K. Baskin, MS, Executive Editor*

2403 **Neurology: Neuroimmunology & Neuroinflammation**
American Academy of Neurology
201 Chicago Avenue 612-928-6000
Minneapolis, MN 55415 800-879-1960
Fax: 612-454-2748
journal@neurology.org
nn.neurology.org
Official journal of the American Academy of Neurology, publishing online open-access peer-reviewed reports of original research and in-depth reviews of topics in neuroimmunology & neuroinflammation.
*Josep O. Dalmau, MD, PhD, Editor*
*Patricia K. Baskin, MS, Executive Editor*

2404 **Society of Nuclear Medicine and Molecular Imaging**
1850 Samuel Morse Drive 703-708-9000
Reston, VA 20190 Fax: 703-708-9015
feedback@snmmi.org
www.snmmi.org
The mission of this nonprofit scientific and professional organization is to promote the science, technology and application of nuclear medicine and molecular imaging. Molecular imaging techniques are used to diagnose and manage the treatment of brain disorders such as Alzheimer's and Parkinson's disease, among other conditions.
*15,000 members*
*Virginia Pappas, CEO*
*Rebecca Maxey, Director, Communications*

2405 **Translational Neurodegeneration**
Springer Nature
One New York Plaza 800-777-4643
New York, NY 10004-1562 info@biomedcentral.com
www.biomedcentral.com
A peer-reviewed, open-access journal covering research, therapeutics and education for all areas of neurodegenerative diseases.
*Shengdi Chen, Editor-in-Chief*

2406 **Ultrasonic Imaging**
Sage Journals
2455 Teller Road 805-499-9774
Thousand Oaks, CA 91320 journals@sagepub.com
journals.sagepub.com/home/uix
The journal focuses on the rapid publication of original papers on the development and application of ultrasonic techniques, with emphasis on medical diagnosis. Also published are research notes, comments on papers appearing in the journal, book reviews, and occasional review articles.
*Ernest J. Feleppa, Editor-in-Chief*
*Roslyn Raskin, Managing Editor*

# STROKE

*A stroke occurs when the blood supply to the brain is suddenly interrupted. There are two principal types of stroke; the more common, ischemic, stroke results from the blockage of arteries leading to the brain, and hemorrhagic stroke, from a burst blood vessel that bleeds into the brain tissue. The effects of a stroke vary according to severity and which part of the brain is affected but symptoms usually include trouble speaking or understanding what others are saying, headache, trouble walking, and paralysis or numbness of the face, leg, or arm. A stroke sometimes leads to a form of cognitive impairment known as vascular dementia (covered separately) which results in difficulties with thinking, judgment, memory, and other important brain functions.*

When a patient suffers either form of stroke, brain cells die rapidly and prompt medical attention is necessary to prevent death or other lasting complications. Stroke is a highly deadly condition, with more than 140,000 stroke victim dying every year in the U.S. Stroke can largely be prevented by managing common lifestyle and medical risk factors, including obesity, physical inactivity, smoking, heavy drinking or drug use, high blood pressure, diabetes, high cholesterol, or cardiovascular disease. Other non-preventable risk factors include age, sex, and race, with those over 55 or who are male or African American at greater risk. Patients at risk for stroke can reduce their risk by taking anti-platelet drugs or anticoagulants.

Patients that survive a stroke often suffer a number of complications that make their lives considerably more difficult. These conditions include partial paralysis, memory loss, emotional problems, and changes in behavior. In patients suffering from vascular dementia as a result of a stroke, the symptoms are similar to those of Alzheimer's patients, including confusion, decline of cognitive ability, problems with memory, and depression. Vascular dementia often occurs immediately after a stroke, in which case it is known as post-stroke dementia, but in other cases it can develop quite gradually.

Emergency treatment for patients who have suffered a stroke is usually required. In the case of an ischemic stroke, an emergency IV injection of recombinant tissue plasminogen activator (tPA), also known as Activase, is typically administered. This injection works to dissolve the blood clot that caused the stroke and restore blood flow. In addition, emergency endovascular procedures in which the doctor works directly inside the blocked blood vessel to restore flow, are sometimes performed. For a hemorrhagic stroke, options include surgery to remove the blood from the brain and relieve cranial pressure, surgical clipping, in which a clamp is placed at the base of the aneurysm to keep it from bursting, and coiling, where a catheter is inserted in an artery near the groin and guided to the brain, delivering detachable coils to the aneurysm in order fill it. Patients who survive a stroke typically require a long course of rehabilitation, which may include physical, occupational, recreational, and speech therapy, along with consultation with a neurologist, a psychiatrist, or a social worker.

## National Agencies & Associations

**2408 American Academy of Neurology**
201 Chicago Avenue
Minneapolis, MN 55415
612-928-6000
800-879-1960
Fax: 612-454-2746
memberservices@aan.com
www.aan.com
Professional society of medical doctors specializing in brain and nervous system diseases. Maintains placement service. Sponsors research and educational programs. Compiles statistics. Publishes scientific journal, Continuum: Lifelong Learning in Neurology.
*Mary E. Post, MBA, CAE, CEO*

**2409 American Heart Association**
7272 Greenville Avenue
Dallas, TX 75231
888-478-7653
800-242-8721
www.heart.org
The American Heart Association is the nation's oldest, largest voluntary organization devoted to fighting cardiovascular diseases and stroke. Funds research and raises public awareness of heart diseases.
*Nancy Brown, CEO*
*Ivor J. Benjamin, MD, FAHA, President*

**2410 American Society for Neurochemistry**
9037 Ron Den Lane
Windermere, FL 34786
407-909-9064
Fax: 407-876-0750
asnmanager@asneurochem.org
asneurochem.org
The Society aims to advance and promote cellular and molecular neuroscience knowledge, and to facilitate communication and the dissemination of information within the field and with related disciplines.
*Sheilah Jewart, Executive Director*
*Karen Gottlieb, Conference Coordinator*

**2411 American Stroke Association**
7272 Greenville Avenue
Dallas, TX 75231
800-242-9872
888-478-7653
www.heart.org
Dedicated to the prevention, diagnosis, and treatment of stroke. Funds research on stroke and advises the public on how to detect and avoid stroke.
*Nancy Brown, CEO*
*Ivor J. Benjamin, MD, FAHA, President*

**2412 Heart and Stroke Foundation of Canada**
110-1525 Carling Avenue
Ottawa, Ontario, K1Z-8R9
888-473-4636
Fax: 613-727-1895
www.heartandstroke.ca
Leading authority on cardiovascular disease, providing resources for individuals and funding scientific research on heart disease and stroke.
*Yves Savoie, CEO*
*Anne Simard, Chief Mission & Research Officer*

**2413 March of Dimes Canada**
10 Overlea Boulevard
Toronto, Ontario, M4H-1A4
416-425-3463
800-263-3463
Fax: 416-425-1920
www.marchofdimes.ca
A national service offering support, education and community programs for stroke survivors, their caregivers and families.
*Leonard Baker, President & CEO*
*Jerry Lucas, Vice President & COO*

**2414 National Heart, Lung & Blood Institute**
31 Center Drive
Bethesda, MD 20892
nhlbiinfo@nhlbi.nih.gov
www.nhlbi.nih.gov
Trains, conducts research, and educates in order to promote the prevention and treatment of heart, lung, and blood disorders.
*Gary H. Gibbons, MD, Director*
*Nakela Cook, MD, MPH, FACC, Chief of Staff*

**2415 National Institute of Neurological Disorders and Stroke**
NIH Neurological Institute
Bethesda, MD 20824
301-496-5751
800-352-9424
www.ninds.nih.gov
Seeks to reduce the burden of neurological disease affecting individuals from all walks of life.
*Walter J. Koroshetz, MD, Director*
*Amy B. Adams, Director, Office of Scientific Liaison*

**2416 Society for Neuroscience**
1121 14th Street NW
Washginton, DC 20005
202-962-4000
marty@sfn.org
sfn.org
Large international organization of scientists and physicians devoted to the study of the brain and the nervous system.
*37,000 members*
*Marty Saggese, Executive Director*
*Melissa Garcia, Associate Executive Director*

## Foundations & Research Centers

**2417 American Stroke Foundation**
5916 Dearborn
Mission, KS 66202
913-649-1776
866-549-1776
Fax: 913-649-6661
www.americanstroke.org
The vision of the American Stroke Foundation is to reach out to stroke survivors and their families across America and empower them to reclaim hope for life after stroke.
*Joan McDowd, Executive Director*
*Jen Creed, Director of Programs and Outreach*

**2418 Bowman Gray School of Medicine**
Medical Center Boulevard
Winston Salem, NC 27157-0001
919-716-7461
Fax: 919-716-5639
*James Toole MD, Professor*

**2419 Cerebral Blood Flow Laboratories Veterans Administration Medical Center**
Veterans Administration Medical Center
2002 Holcombe Boulevard
Houston, TX 77030-4211
713-795-5807
Fax: 713-957-01
Offers research in cerebrovascular disorders and risk factors for stroke.
*John S Meyer MD, Director*

**2420 Comprehensive Stroke Center of Oregon University of Oregon Health Sciences**
University of Oregon Health Sciences Center
3181 SW Sam Jackson Park Road
Portland, OR 97239-3098
503-494-7225
www.ohsu.edu
The Oregon Stroke Center (OSC) was established to provide comprehensive treatment and prevention services to stroke patients throughout the Northwest. Recognized as a national leader in acute stroke treatment, the OSC mobile stroke team provides novel stroke treatments to multiple Portland hospitals. In addition to clinical care, the OSC is actively involved in clinical and basic research and provides extensive stroke related education to the public and providers.
*Wayne Clark, M.D., Professor*
*Helmi Lutsep, M.D., Professor*

**2421 Departments of Neurology & Neurosurgery: University of California, San Francisco**
UCSF Medical Center
505 Parnassus Avenue
San Francisco, CA 94143
415-476-1537
Fax: 415-476-0616
bill.dillon@radiology.ucsf.edu
www.radiology.ucsf.edu
The Department of Radiology & Biomedical Imaging at the University of California, San Francisco combines clinical excellence, trailblazing research, and outstanding education in a leading academic health sciences institution. Our faculty includes some of the foremost names in diagnostic and interventional radiology today.
*Dr. Ronald Arenson, Chairman*
*Catherine Garzio, Director of Administration*

**2422 Hospital of the University of Pennsylvania**
3400 Spruce Street
Philadelphia, PA 19104
215-662-4000
800-789-PENN
Fax: 215-903-09
www.pennmedicine.org

The Hospital of the University of Pennsylvania (HUP) is world-renowned for its clinical and research excellence, forging the way for newer and better ways to diagnose and treat illnesses and disorders. The world-class faculty and staff of the Hospital of the University of Pennsylvania are dedicated to superior patient care, education and research for a better, healthier future. Their significant and groundbreaking contributions to medicine are recognized both nationally and internationally.
*David E Pleasure MD, Director*

**2423 Kavli Foundation**
5715 Mesmer Avenue 424-353-8800
Los Angeles, CA info@kavlifoundation.org
www.kavlifoundation.org
The Foundation supports scientific research into the human brain, in the following scientific fields: Astrophysics, Nanoscience, Neuroscience and Theoretical Physics. Within Neuroscience, the study of aging and brain diseases and disorders is supported.
*Robert W. Conn, PhD, President & CEO*
*Eric Marshall, VP, Public Engagement & Prizes*

**2424 Kavli Institute for Brain Science at Columbia University**
Columbia University
3227 Broadway 212-853-1016
New York, NY 10027 Fax: 212-665-9699
kavli@columbia.edu
www.kavli.columbia.edu
The Institute's primary are of study is how signaling in neural circuits controls cognitive function and behavior, and the development of novel experimental and computational strategies for analyzing these signals.
*Eric R. Kandel, MD, Director*
*Rafael Yuste, MD, PhD, Co-Director*

**2425 Kavli Institute for Brain and Mind**
UC San Diego
9500 Gilman Drive kibm@ucsd.edu
La Jolla, CA 92093-0115 kibm.ucsd.edu
The Institute supports research that furthers the understanding of the origins, evolution and mechanisms of human cognition. Of particular interest is Traumatic Brain Injury.
*Fred H. Gage, Co-Director*
*Nicholas C. Spitzer, Co-Director*

**2426 Kavli Institute for Fundamental Neuroscience**
UCSF, Sandler Neurosciences Center
675 Nelson Rising Lane 415-476-2018
San Francisco, CA 94158 Fax: 415-502-7332
kavliifn@ucsf.edu
kavliifn.ucsf.edu
The Institute is the central organization for neuroscience research at UCSF and partner institutions, establishing cross-disciplinary teams of scientists and engineers devoted to advancing neuroscience in all its forms.
*Loren Frank, Co-Director*
*Roger Nicoll, Co-Director*

**2427 Kavli Neural Systems Institute**
The Rockefeller University
1230 York Avenue 212-327-8081
New York, NY 10065 lcole@rockefeller.edu
www.rockefeller.edu/research
The Institute unites scientists at The Rockefeller University in the goal of a comprehensive look at the human brain.
*Leslie Vosshall, PhD, Director*
*Lindsey Cole, Administrator*

**2428 Kavli Neuroscience Discovery Institute**
Johns Hopkins University, School of Medicine
725 N Wolfe Street 410-955-4089
Baltimore, MD 21205 Fax: 410-614-6249
KavliNDI@jhu.edu
kavlijhu.org
The Institute looks to advance neuroscience by integrating neuroscience, engineering and computational data science.
*Dwight Bergles, PhD, Director*
*Natasha Hussain, PhD, Scientific Director*

**2429 Massachusetts General Departments of Neurology and Neurosurgery**
Massachusetts General Hospital
55 Fruit Street 617-726-2000
Boston, MA 02114 www.massgeneral.org
Guided by the needs of our patients, our mission is to be the preeminent academic neurology department in the US by: providing outstanding clinical care while rapidly discovering new treatments to reduce and eliminate the devastating impact of neurological disorders; training the very best neurologists and scientists of the future, and improving the health and well-being of the diverse communities we serve.
*Peter Slavin, Director*
*Robert Ackerman, MD*

**2430 Neuroscience Research Institute**
UC Santa Barbara
6129 Biology II 805-893-4621
Santa Barbara, CA 93106 www.nri.ucsb.edu
The Institute seeks to allow scientists from different fields to collaborate for the betterment of neurological research. Areas of interest include: Alzheimer's Disease & Related Dementias; Behavioral Neuroscience & Neuroethology; Cell Biology, Biochemistry & Biophysics of the Nervous System; Computational & Theoretical Neuroscience; Development of the Nervous System; and Stem Cells.
*Stuart Feinstein, Co-Director*
*Kenneth Kosik, Co-Director*

**2431 Sanford Consortium for Regenerative Medicine**
2880 Torrey Pines Scenic Drive 858-246-1071
La Jolla, CA 92037 www.sanfordconsortium.com
The Consortium works to achieve breakthrough discoveries in stem cell research with regards to diagnoses, treatments, and cures for degenerative diseases and injuries.
*Edward W. Holmes, MD, President & CEO*
*Jeffrey Steindorf, PhD, VP & COO*

**2432 Scripps Research Institute**
10550 North Torrey Pines Road 858-784-1000
La Jolla, CA www.scripps.edu
The institute seeks to improve human wellbeing through the advancement of bioscience, including research into aging & healthspan, autoimmune diseases, cancer, infectious diseases, neurological disorders, and more.
*Peter Schultz, PhD, President & CEO*
*Eric Topol, MD, EVP, Scripps Research*

**2433 Stroke Research and Treatment Center UAB Medical Center**
Medical Center
1530 3rd Ave S 205-934-9999
Birmingham, AL 35294-7 800-822-6478
Fax: 205-996-4039
The nationally-ranked UAB Department of Neurology is home to eight comprehensive divisions and seven centers offering an array of clinical activities. Over 26,000 patients are cared for annually through state-of-the-art subspecialty care and innovative treatments. Our residents have the opportunity to work in various neurology fields with 50 clinical and research faculty members.
*Andrei V Alexandrov MD, Director and Professor*
*Andrei V. Alexandrov, M.D., Director, Comprehensive Stroke Research*

**2434 University of Iowa College of Medicine**
451 Newton Road 319-335-6707
Iowa City, IA 52242 www.medicine.uiowa.edu
The Roy J. and Lucille A. Carver College of Medicine is a highly ranked medical school where students learn to become accomplished clinicians and top-flight researchers and educators. Students come to Iowa to study medicine in a program that uses case-based learning as the basis of their education. With its emphasis on problem-solving skills, early exposure to patients, and enhanced community-based experiences, UI medical students typically earn an advantage.
*Debra A. Schwinn, MD, Dean*
*Donna L. Hammond, PhD, Executive Associate Dean*

2435 **University of Maryland Center for Studies of Cerebrovascular Disease & Stroke**
16 S Utah Street 410-328-4323
Baltimore, MD 21201 Fax: 410-328-1149
*Thomas R Price MD, Principal Investor*

2436 **University of Miami School of Medicine Department of Neurology**
1120 NW 14th Street 305-243-6732
Miami, FL 33136 877-243-4340
Fax: 305-243-1632
RSacco@med.miami.edu
www.med.miami.edu
*Ralph L Sacco MD, Chairman-Department of Neurology*
*Myron D Ginsberg MD, Professor*

2437 **Wake Forest University: Cerebrovascular Research Center**
Department of Neurology
300 S Hawthorne Road 336-748-2338
Winston-Salem, NC 27103-2732 Fax: 336-748-5477
Cerebrovascular research.
*Dr James Toole, Director*

2438 **Washington University School of Medicine**
660 S Euclid Avenue 314-362-5000
Saint Louis, MO 63110-1016 www.medicine.wustl.edu
Washington University School of Medicine is a leader in improving human health throughout the world. As noted leaders in patient care, research and education, our outstanding faculty members have contributed many discoveries and innovations to the field of science since the founding of the School of Medicine in 1891. The School of Medicine is one of seven schools of Washington University in St. Louis.
*Larry J. Shapiro, M.D, Executive Vice Chancellor, Medical*

## Support Groups & Hotlines

2439 **Comprehensive Stroke Center of Oregon University of Oregon Health Sciences**
University of Oregon Health Sciences Center
3181 SW Sam Jackson Park Road 503-494-7225
Portland, OR 97239-3098 www.ohsu.edu
The Oregon Stroke Center (OSC) was established to provide comprehensive treatment and prevention services to stroke patients throughout the Northwest. Recognized as a national leader in acute stroke treatment, the OSC mobile stroke team provides novel stroke treatments to multiple Portland hospitals. In addition to clinical care, OSC is actively involved in clinical and basic research.
*Wayne Clark, M.D., Professor*
*Helmi Lutsep, M.D., Professor*

2440 **National Health Information Center**
Office of Disease Prevention & Health Promotion
1101 Wootton Pkwy Fax: 240-453-8281
Rockville, MD 20852 odphpinfo@hhs.gov
www.health.gov/nhic
Supports public health education by maintaining a calendar of National Health Observances; helps connect consumers and health professionals to organizations that can best answer questions and provide up-to-date contact information from reliable sources; updates on a yearly basis toll-free numbers for health information, Federal health clearinghouses and info centers.
*Don Wright, MD, MPH, Director*

2441 **Stroke Clubs International**
805 12th Street 409-762-1022
Galveston, TX 77550 strokeclubs@earthlink.net
www.ninds.nih.gov
Organization of persons who have experienced strokes, their families and friends for the purpose of mutual support, education, social and recreational activities. Provides information and assistance to Stroke Clubs (which are usually sponsored by local organizations).
*Ellis Williamson*

## Magazines

2442 **ASN NEURO**
Sage Journals
2455 Teller Road 805-499-9774
Thousand Oaks, CA 91320 journals@sagepub.com
journals.sagepub.com/home/asn
Peer-reviewed open access journal focusing on recent advances in the cellular and molecular neurosciences. It is the official publication of the American Society for Neurochemistry.
*Douglas L. Feinstein, Editor-in-Chief*
*Sandra J. Hewitt, Deputy Editor-in-Chief*

2443 **BMC Neuroscience**
Springer Nature
One New York Plaza 800-777-4643
New York, NY 10004-1562 info@biomedcentral.com
bmcneurosci.biomedcentral.com
A peer-reviewed, open-access journal devoted to all aspects of the nervous system (including molecular, cellular, developmental and animal model studies), as well as cognitive and behavioral research, and computational modeling.
*Darren Byrne, Editor*
*Ana Donnelly, Manuscript Editor*

2444 **Brain & Life**
American Academy of Neurology
201 Chicago Avenue 612-928-6000
Minneapolis, MN 55415 800-879-1960
Fax: 612-454-2748
BrainandLife@wolterskluwer.com
www.brainandlife.org
Official magazine of the American Academy of Neurology, aimed at parents and home-caregivers interested in neurology in everyday life.
*Orly Avitzur, MD, MBA, FAAN, Editor-in-Chief*
*Mary Bolster, Managing Editor*

2445 **Brain: A Journal of Neurology**
Oxford University Press
2001 Evans Road 919-677-0977
Cary, NC 27513 800-852-7323
Fax: 919-677-1714
brain@ucl.ac.uk
academic.oup.com/brain
Focus is clinical neurology and translational neuroscience.
*Dimitri M. Kullmann, Editor*
*Joanne Bell, Managing Editor*

2446 **Continuum: Lifelong Learning in Neurology**
American Academy of Neurology
201 Chicago Avenue 612-928-6000
Minneapolis, MN 55415 800-879-1960
continuumcme@aan.com
journals.lww.com/continuum
Official journal of the American Academy of Neurology, aiding professionals in patient care and continuing education.
*Bimonthly*
*Steven L. Lewis, MD, FAAN*
*Andrea J. Weiss, MA, Executive Editor*

2447 **JNeurosci**
Society for Neuroscience
1121 14th Street NW 202-962-4000
Washginton, DC 20005 jn@sfn.org
www.jneurosci.org
Official peer-reviewed journal of the Society for Neuroscience, publishing research on a broad range of topics of interest to those working on the nervous system.
*Marina R. Picciotto, Editor-in-Chief*
*Teresa Esch, Features Editor*

2448 **Journal of Alzheimer's Disease**
IOS Press
6751 Tepper Drive 703-830-6300
Clifton, VA 20124 Fax: 703-830-2300
editorial@j-alz.com
www.j-alz.com

Research into the etiology, pathogenesis, epidemiology, genetics, behavior, treatment and psychology of Alzheimer's disease.
*George Perry, PhD, Editor-in-Chief*
*Beth Kumar, Managing Editor*

2449 **Journal of NeuroEngineering and Rehabilitation**
Springer Nature
One New York Plaza 800-777-4643
New York, NY 10004-1562 info@biomedcentral.com
jneuroengrehab.biomedcentral.com
An open-access journal devoted to integrated research from the fields of neuroscience, biomedical engineering, and physical medicine and rehabilitation.
*David J. Reinkensmeyer, Editor-in-Chief*

2450 **Journal of Neuroinflammation**
Springer Nature
One New York Plaza 800-777-4643
New York, NY 10004-1562 info@biomedcentral.com
jneuroinflammation.biomedcentral.com
A peer-reviewed, open-access journal focusing on the interactions of the immune system with the nervous system as a means of expanding understanding of chronic neurological diseases.
*Monica J. Carson, Editor-in-Chief*
*Sue T. Griffin, Editor-in-Chief*

2451 **Journal of Nuclear Medicine**
Society of Nuclear Medicine and Molecular Imaging
1850 Samuel Morse Drive 703-708-9000
Reston, VA 20190 800-513-6853
Fax: 703-708-9015
subscriptions@snm.org
jnm.snmjournals.org
Peer-reviewed journal with clinical investigations, science reports, articles benefitting continuing education, book reviews, employment opportunities, and updates on practice and research.
*Monthly*
*Johannes Czernin, MD, Editor-in-Chief*
*Susan Alexander, Associate Director, Publications*

2452 **Journal of Nuclear Medicine Technology**
Society of Nuclear Medicine and Molecular Imaging
1850 Samuel Morse Drive 703-708-9000
Reston, VA 20190 800-513-6853
Fax: 703-708-9015
subscriptions@snm.org
tech.snmjournals.org
Peer-reviewed journal dedicated to nuclear medicine technology, with information on credentialing, continuing education and licensure requirements, as well as current news and updates on the field.
*Quarterly*
*Kathy S. Thomas, MHA, CNMT, PET, Editor-in-Chief*
*Susan Alexander, Associate Director, Publications*

2453 **Journal of the Neurological Sciences**
Elsevier
LSU Health Sciences Center JNS_England@lsuhsc.edu
New Orleans, LA 70112 www.jns-journal.com
Original articles in neurology and neuroscience from around the world.
*Monthly*
*John D. England, Editor-in-Chief*

2454 **Molecular Imaging**
Sage Journals
2455 Teller Road 805-499-9774
Thousand Oaks, CA 91320 journals@sagepub.com
journals.sagepub.com/home/mix
Peer-reviewed open access journal focusing on molecular imaging research, including basic science, preclinical studies and human applications. Published in association with the Society of Nuclear Medicine and Molecular Imaging.
*Bimonthly*
*Henry F. VanBrocklin, PhD, Editor-in-Chief*

2455 **Molecular Neurodegeneration**
Springer Nature
One New York Plaza 800-777-4643
New York, NY 10004-1562 info@biomedcentral.com
www.biomedcentral.com
A peer-reviewed, open-access journal devoted to all aspects of neurodegeneration research at the molecular and cellular levels.
*Guojun Bu, Editor-in-Chief*
*Huaxi Xu, Editor-in-Chief*

2456 **Neurology**
American Academy of Neurology
201 Chicago Avenue 612-928-6000
Minneapolis, MN 55415 800-879-1960
Fax: 612-454-2748
journal@neurology.org
n.neurology.org
Official journal of the American Academy of Neurology, peer-reviewed, highlighting clinical neurology research.
*Jose G. Merino, MD, MPhil, FAAN, Editor-in-Chief*
*Patricia K. Baskin, MS, Executive Editor*

2457 **Neurology Clinical Practice**
American Academy of Neurology
201 Chicago Avenue 612-928-6000
Minneapolis, MN 55415 800-879-1960
Fax: 612-454-2748
journal@neurology.org
cp.neurology.org
Official peer-reviewed journal of the American Academy of Neurology for practicing neurologists.
*John R. Corboy, MD, FAAN, Editor*
*Patricia K. Baskin, MS, Executive Editor*

2458 **Neurology: Genetics**
American Academy of Neurology
201 Chicago Avenue 612-928-6000
Minneapolis, MN 55415 800-879-1960
Fax: 612-454-2748
journal@neurology.org
ng.neurology.org
Official journal of the American Academy of Neurology, publishing online open-access peer-reviewed reports in the field of neurogenetics.
*Stefan M. Pulst, MD, FAAN, Editor*
*Patricia K. Baskin, MS, Executive Editor*

2459 **Neurology: Neuroimmunology & Neuroinflammation**
American Academy of Neurology
201 Chicago Avenue 612-928-6000
Minneapolis, MN 55415 800-879-1960
Fax: 612-454-2748
journal@neurology.org
nn.neurology.org
Official journal of the American Academy of Neurology, publishing online open-access peer-reviewed reports of original research and in-depth reviews of topics in neuroimmunology & neuroinflammation.
*Josep O. Dalmau, MD, PhD, Editor*
*Patricia K. Baskin, MS, Executive Editor*

2460 **Society of Nuclear Medicine and Molecular Imaging**
1850 Samuel Morse Drive 703-708-9000
Reston, VA 20190 Fax: 703-708-9015
feedback@snmmi.org
www.snmmi.org
The mission of this nonprofit scientific and professional organization is to promote the science, technology and application of nuclear medicine and molecular imaging. Molecular imaging techniques are used to diagnose and manage the treatment of brain disorders such as Alzheimer's and Parkinson's disease, among other conditions.
*15,000 members*
*Virginia Pappas, CEO*
*Rebecca Maxey, Director, Communications*

2461 **Stroke Connection**
American Stroke Foundation
5916 Dearborn St 913-649-1776
Mission, KS 66202 Fax: 913-649-6661
www.americanstroke.org

Official magazine of the American Stroke Foundation. Supports stroke survivors, their families, caregivers and friends by providing resources, services, education and information that improves the quality of life.
*Richard March, Chair*
*David Marshall, Vice Chairman*

**2462 Translational Neurodegeneration**
Springer Nature
One New York Plaza 800-777-4643
New York, NY 10004-1562 info@biomedcentral.com
www.biomedcentral.com
A peer-reviewed, open-access journal covering research, therapeutics and education for all areas of neurodegenerative diseases.
*Shengdi Chen, Editor-in-Chief*

**2463 Ultrasonic Imaging**
Sage Journals
2455 Teller Road 805-499-9774
Thousand Oaks, CA 91320 journals@sagepub.com
journals.sagepub.com/home/uix
The journal focuses on the rapid publication of original papers on the development and application of ultrasonic techniques, with emphasis on medical diagnosis. Also published are research notes, comments on papers appearing in the journal, book reviews, and occasional review articles.
*Ernest J. Feleppa, Editor-in-Chief*
*Roslyn Raskin, Managing Editor*

**2464 eNeuro**
Society for Neuroscience
1121 14th Street NW 202-312-7305
Washginton, DC 20005 eNeuro@sfn.org
www.eneuro.org
Open-access journal of the Society for Neuroscience.
*Christophe Bernard, Editor-in-Chief*
*Kelly Newton, Director, Scientific Publications*

## Web Sites

**2465 American Heart Association**
www.heart.org/HEARTORG
A national organization whose primary concern is the reduction of death and disability due to cardiovascular diseases and stroke.

**2466 BrainFacts.org**
Society for Neuroscience
1121 14th Street NW brainfactsinfo@sfn.org
Washington, DC 20005 brainfacts.org
Online public information portal founded by the Kavli Foundation, the Gatsby Charitable Foundation and the Society for Neuroscience, with topics on brain function and anatomy, diseases and disorders, and more.
*Richard Wingate, DPhil, Editor-in-Chief*
*Charles Yokoyama, PhD, Associate Editor*

**2467 Healing Well**
www.healingwell.com
An online health resource guide to medical news, chat, information and articles, newsgroups and message boards, books, disease-related web sites, medical directories, and more for patients, friends, and family coping with disabling diseases, disorders, or chronic illnesses.

**2468 Health Finder**
www.healthfinder.gov
Searchable, carefully developed web site offering information on over 1000 topics. Developed by the US Department of Health and Human Services, the site can be used in both English and Spanish.

**2469 Healthlink USA**
www.healthlinkusa.com
Health information concerning treatment, cures, prevention, diagnosis, risk factors, research, support groups, email lists, personal stories and much more. Updated regularly.

**2470 MedicineNet**
www.medicinenet.com
An online resource for consumers providing easy-to-read, authoritative medical and health information.

**2471 Medscape**
www.medscape.com
Medscape offers specialists, primary care physicians, and other health professionals the Web's most robust and integrated medical information and educational tools.

**2472 National Heart, Lung & Blood Institute**
www.nhlbi.nih.gov
Primary responsibility of this organization is the scientific investigation of heart, blood vessel, lung and blood disorders. Oversee research, demonstration, prevention, education and training activities in these fields and emphasizes the control of stroke.

**2473 National Stroke Association**
www.stroke.org
A national organization whose sole purpose is to reduce the incidence and impact of stroke through prevention, treatment, rehabilitation and research, and support for stroke survivors and their families. Educational resources on all aspects of stroke available on website.

**2474 Neurology Channel**
www.healthcommunities.com
Find clearly explained, medically accurate information regarding conditions, including an overview, symptoms, causes, diagnostic procedures and treatment options. On this site it is possible to ask questions and get information from a neurologist and connect to people who have similar health interests.

**2475 Neuronline**
Society for Neuroscience
1121 14th Street NW 202-962-4000
Washginton, DC 20005 neuronline@sfn.org
neuronline.sfn.org
Online portal for professional development and training resources for individuals in the field of neuroscience, hosted by the Society for Neuroscience.
*Amanda Kimball, Director, Digital Learning*

**2476 WebMD**
www.webmd.com
Provides credible information, supportive communities, and in-depth reference material about health subjects. A source for original and timely health information as well as material from well known content providers.

# TRAUMATIC BRAIN INJURY

*Traumatic brain injury refers to a wide range of conditions springing from a sudden trauma that causes damage to the brain. This can result from the head violently hitting an object or from an object piercing the skull and entering the brain tissue. The level of severity and list of symptoms of TBI vary widely but often include headache, confusion, dizziness, blurred vision, behavioral and mood changes, and trouble with memory, concentration, or thinking. More severe cases can result in vomiting and nausea, convulsions, slurred speech, increased confusion, or inability to wake from sleep. TBI can both directly cause dementia and increase the patient's risk of developing Alzheimer's and other dementia-causing diseases. A concussion is one of the most common forms of TBI.*

Traumatic brain injury is most often caused by a fall, being struck by an object, or by a car crash. TBI is extremely common, with nearly 3 million new cases each year in the U.S. alone, although the majority of cases are not severe. When the patient suffers TBI from a blow to the head, it usually results in a condition known as a concussion. A concussion is a typically minor condition which generally lasts no longer than a couple of months and is marked by headache, amnesia, nausea, and confusion. In general, TBI is classified into three grades: mild, moderate, and severe. In severe cases, the patient often suffers from ongoing complications. These range from the severe brain death, vegetative state, and coma, to more manageable physical symptoms such as seizures, ongoing headaches, and vertigo. Patients may also experience ongoing cognitive difficulties, behavioral and emotional changes, sensory problems, and symptoms of dementia.

Research in the last 30 years increasingly suggests a link between TBI and Alzheimer's and other dementia-causing diseases. One study suggests that older adults with a history of moderate TBI had 2.3 times greater risk of developing Alzheimer's than seniors with no history of head injury and that, for older adults with a history of severe traumatic brain injury, that number jumps to 4.5 times. Although no evidence exists to show a link between a person suffering a single mild traumatic brain injury and dementia, those suffering repeated mild TBIs may be prone to contracting chronic traumatic encephalopathy (CTE), a newly discovered form of dementia-causing disease.

In recent years, chronic traumatic encephalopathy has been in the news as many ex-football players were revealed post-mortem to suffer from the condition. CTE is a neurodegenerative disease that is caused by repeated head injuries, most commonly the concussions and subconcussive hits from which nearly all athletes who play contact sports suffer. The symptoms typically appear years after the injuries are suffered and consist of behavioral problems, difficulty thinking, and ultimately dementia. Because of recent awareness of the prevalence of CTE in the sport of football, many people have called for either major changes to be made to the sport or for it to be banned altogether.

## National Agencies & Associations

2478 **American Academy of Neurology**
201 Chicago Avenue
Minneapolis, MN 55415
612-928-6000
800-879-1960
Fax: 612-454-2746
memberservices@aan.com
www.aan.com
Professional society of medical doctors specializing in brain and nervous system diseases. Maintains placement service. Sponsors research and educational programs. Compiles statistics. Publishes scientific journal, Continuum: Lifelong Learning in Neurology.
*Mary E. Post, MBA, CAE, CEO*

2479 **American Brain Tumor Association**
8550 W Bryn Mawr Avenue
Chicago, IL 60631
773-577-8750
800-886-2282
Fax: 773-577-8738
info@abta.org
www.abta.org
Services includes over 40 publications which address brain tumors, their treatment and coping with the disease. Materials address brain tumors in all age groups. Provides free social service consultations and a mentorship program for new brain tumor support groups.
*Ralph DeVitto, President & CEO*
*Nicole Willmarth, PhD, Chief Mission Officer*

2480 **American Chronic Pain Association**
PO Box 850
Rocklin, CA 95677
800-533-3231
ACPA@theacpa.org
www.theacpa.org
The ACPA facilitates peer support and education for individuals with chronic pain in its many forms, in order to increase quality of life. Also raises awareness among the healthcare community, and with policy makers.
*Penney Cowan, Founder & CEO*
*Daniel Galia, Director, Global Support*

2481 **American Head and Neck Society**
11300 W Olympic Blvd.
Los Angeles, CA 90064
310-437-0559
310-437-0585
admin@ahns.info
www.ahns.info
The society seeks to advance education, research, and quality of care for hed and neck oncology patients.
*Christina Kasendorf, Executive Director*
*J.J. Jackman, Associate Executive Director*

2482 **Brain Injury Association of America**
1608 Spring Hill Road
Vienna, VA 22182
703-761-0750
Fax: 703-761-0755
info@biausa.org
www.biausa.org
The BIA's mission is to create a better future through brain injury prevention, research, education, and advocacy. Offers information on state and national offices, treatment and rehabilitation, conferences, prevention, financial development and more.
*Susan H. Connors, President & CEO*
*Mary S. Reitter, Executive Vice-President & COO*

2483 **International Brain Injury Association**
5909 Ashby Manor Place
Alexandria, VA 22313
703-960-0027
Fax: 703-960-6603
congress@internationalbrain.org
www.internationalbrain.org
Provides scientific and medical leadership worldwide in the field of brain injury.
*David Arciniegas, Chairman & CEO*
*Nathan Zasler, Vice Chairman & Vice CEO*

2484 **Society for Neuroscience**
1121 14th Street NW
Washginton, DC 20005
202-962-4000
marty@sfn.org
sfn.org
Large international organization of scientists and physicians devoted to the study of the brain and the nervous system.
*37,000 members*
*Marty Saggese, Executive Director*
*Melissa Garcia, Associate Executive Director*

2485 **TBI: Traumatic Brian Injury**
www.tbi.org
The Perspective Network was changed to TBI in 2015; it provides forums and resources for persons with families, caregivers, friends and the professionals who serve them. Their goals are to promote a sense of community and to increase public awareness of brain injury.
*Elaine Jones, Contact*

## State Agencies & Associations

2486 **Alabama Head Injury Foundation**
3100 Lorna Road
Hoover, AL 35216
205-823-3818
800-433-8002
Fax: 205-823-4544
ahifl@bellsouth.net
http://www.ahif.org
Services provided to Alabamians with traumatic brain injury or spinal cord injury include information, housing, respite care, recreation programs, resource coordination.
*Keith Belt, President*
*Charles D Priest, Executive Director*

2487 **Brain Injury Association of Arizona**
5025 E Washington Street
Phoenix, AZ 85034
602-508-8024
888-500-9165
Fax: 602-508-8285
info@biaaz.org
www.biaaz.org
Information and resources for brain injury survivors and their families. Support group listings available. Educational training, conference for families and survivors, neuro-specific resources and helpline.
*Lisa Counters, President*
*Rebecca Armendariz, VicePresident*

2488 **Brain Injury Association of Arkansas**
PO Box 26236
Little Rock, AR 72221-6236
501-374-3585
800-444-6443
Fax: 501-918-6595
info@brainassociation.org
*Dana Austen, President*
*Kortney Coats, Vice President*

2489 **Brain Injury Association of Colorado**
4200 W Conejos Place
Denver, CO 80204
303-355-9969
800-955-2443
Fax: 303-355-9968
www.biacolorado.org
*William Levis, President*
*Gavin Attwood, Executive Director*

2490 **Brain Injury Association of Connecticut**
200 Day Hill Road
Windsor, CT 06095
86 - 2 - 02
800-278-8242
Fax: 86 - 2 - 05
general@biact.org
www.biact.org
*500 Members*
*Paul A Slager, President*
*Julie Peters, Executive Director*

2491 **Brain Injury Association of Delaware**
840 Walker Road
Dover, DE 19904
302-346-2083
800-411-0505
Fax: 888-258-3694
*Devon Dorman, President*
*Esther Curtis, Executive Director*

2492 **Brain Injury Association of Florida**
1637 Metropolitan Boulevard
Tallahassee, FL 32308
850-410-0103
800-992-3442
Fax: 850-410-0105
biaftalla@biaf.org
www.biaf.org
*Valerie E Breen, President/CEO*

2493 **Brain Injury Association of Hawaii**
420 Kuwili Street
Honolulu, HI 96817-1474
808-791-6942
Fax: 808-454-1975
biahi@hawaiiantel.net
www.biausa.org/Hawaii

*Ian Mattoch, President*
*Mary Wilson, Executive Director*

2494 **Brain Injury Association of Idaho**
PO Box 414
Boise, ID 83701-0414
208-342-0999
888-374-3447
Fax: 208-333-0026
info@biaid.org
www.biaid.org

*Michelle Featherston, President*

2495 **Brain Injury Association of Illinois**
PO Box 64420
Chicago, IL 60664-0420
312-726-5699
800-699-6443
Fax: 312-630-4011
info@biail.org
www.biail.org

*Philicia L Deckard, Executive Director*
*Irene Pedersen, Founder*

2496 **Brain Injury Association of Indiana**
9531 Valparaiso Court
Indianapolis, IN 46268
317-356-7722
866-854-4246
Fax: 31 - 8 - 17
info@biai.org

*Anna Garrett, Executive Director*
*Laura C Trexler, TBI Grant Program Director*

2497 **Brain Injury Association of Iowa**
7025 Hickman Road
Urbandale, IA 50322
319-466-7455
800-444-6443
Fax: 800-381-0812
info@biaia.org
www.biaia.org

*Geoffrey Lauer, Executive Director*

2498 **Brain Injury Association of Kansas and Greater Kansas City**
6405 Metcalf Avenue
Overland Park, KS 66202
913-754-8883
800-444-6443
Fax: 816-842-1531
info@biaks.org
www.biaks.org

*Rob Flores, President*
*Betsy Johnson, Executive Director*

2499 **Brain Injury Association of Kentucky**
7410 New Lagrange Roadd
Louisville, KY 40222
502-493-0609
800-592-1117
Fax: 502-426-2993
www.biak.us

*Chell Austin, Executive Director*
*Wes Wilkinson, Development Director*

2500 **Brain Injury Association of Maine**
13 Washington Street
Waterville, ME 04901
207-861-9900
800-275-1233
Fax: 207-861-4617
info@biame.org
www.biame.org

*Mary Lombardo, President*
*Leslie DuVall, Director of Operations*

2501 **Brain Injury Association of Maryland**
2200 Kernan Drive
Baltimore, MD 21207
410-448-2924
800-221-6443
Fax: 410-448-3541
info@biamd.org
www.biamd.org

*Patricia Janus, President*
*Diane Tripplet, Executive Director*

2502 **Brain Injury Association of Massachusetts**
30 Lyman Street
Westborough, MA 01581
508-475-0032
800-242-0030
Fax: 508-475-0400
biama@biama.org
www.biama.org

*Shahriar Khaksari, President*
*Arlene Korab, Executive Director*

2503 **Brain Injury Association of Michigan**
7305 Grand River
Brighton, MI 48114-2334
810-229-5880
800-444-6443
Fax: 810-229-8947
info@biami.org
www.biami.org

Our mission is to enhance the lives of those affected by brain injury through education, advocacy, research and local support groups and to reduce the incidence of brain injury through prevention.
*Katie Knight, Program Coordinator*
*Michael F Dabbs, President*

2504 **Brain Injury Association of Minnesota**
34 13th Avenue NE
Minneapolis, MN 55413
612-378-2742
800-669-6442
Fax: 612-378-2789
info@braininjurymn.org
www.braininjurymn.org

*20-24 pages*
*Andrew Kiragu, Board Chairman*

2505 **Brain Injury Association of Mississippi**
2727 Old Canton
Jackson, MS 39296-5912
601-981-1021
800-444-6443
Fax: 601-981-1039
info@msbia.org
www.msbia.org

*Howard T Katz, Chairman*
*Lee Jenkins, Executive Director*

2506 **Brain Injury Association of Missouri**
10270 Page Avenue
Saint Louis, MO 63132-1322
314-426-4024
800-444-6443
Fax: 314-426-3290
info@biamo.org
www.biamo.org

Information and referral services and support groups through the state of Missouri.
*John Bennett, President of the Board*
*Terrie Price, VP*

2507 **Brain Injury Association of Montana**
1280 S 3rd W
Missoula, MT 59801
406-541-6442
800-241-6442
Fax: 406-541-4360
biam@biamt.org
www.biamt.org

*Bobbi Perkins, President*
*Kristen Morgan, Program Director*

2508 **Brain Injury Association of New Hampshire**
109 N State Street
Concord, NH 03301
603-225-8400
800-773-8400
Fax: 603-228-6749
mail@bianh.org
www.bianh.org

*Brant Elkind, President*
*Steven Wade, Executive Director*

2509 **Brain Injury Association of New Jersey**
825 Georges Road
N Brunswick, NJ 08902
732-745-0200
800-669-4323
Fax: 732-745-0211
info@bianj.org
www.bianj.org

*Barbara Parker, President*

2510 **Brain Injury Association of New Mexico**
3234 Candelaria NE
Albuquerque, NM 87107
505-292-7414
88 - 2 - 74
Fax: 505-271-8983
info@braininjurynm.org
www.braininjurynm.org
*John Tiwald, Board President*
*Mark Pedrotty, VP*

2511 **Brain Injury Association of New York State**
10 Colvin Avenue
Albany, NY 12206-1242
518-459-7911
800-228-8201
Fax: 518-482-5285
info@bianys.org
www.bianys.org
*Marie Cavallo, President*
*Judith Avner, Executive Director*

2512 **Brain Injury Association of North Carolina**
2113 Cameron Street
Raleigh, NC 27605
919-833-9634
800-377-1464
Fax: 919-833-5415
bianc@bianc.net
www.tbicommunity.org
*Cindy Boyd, Board Chairman*
*Sandra Farmer, President*

2513 **Brain Injury Association of Ohio**
855 Grand View Avenue
Columbus, OH 43215-1123
614-481-7100
866-644-6242
Fax: 614-481-7103
help@biaoh.org
www.biaoh.org
*Jon Fishpaw, President*
*Suzanne Minnich, Executive Director*

2514 **Brain Injury Association of Oklahoma**
PO Box 88
Hillsdale, OK 73743-0088
580-233-4363
800-444-6443
Fax: 580-233-4546
brainhelp@braininjuryoklahoma.org
www.braininjuryoklahoma.org
*Tracy Grammer, President*
*Gary Clarke, Chairman*

2515 **Brain Injury Association of Oregon**
PO Box 549
Molalla, OR 97038
503-740-3155
800-544-5243
Fax: 503-961-8730
info@biaoregon.org
www.biaoregon.org
*Tootie Smith, President*
*Sherry Stock, Executive Director*

2516 **Brain Injury Association of Pennsylvania**
950 Walnut Bottom Road
Carlisle, PA 17015
717-657-3601
866-635-7097
Fax: 717-692-5567
info@biapa.org
www.biapa.org
*Drew Nagele, Chairman of Board Development Committee*
*Stewart L Cohen, Chairman*

2517 **Brain Injury Association of Rhode Island**
935 Park Avenue
Cranston, RI 02910-2743
401-461-6599
Fax: 401-461-6561
braininjuryctr@biaofri.org
*Michael Baker, Co-President*
*Colleen McCarthy, Co-President*

2518 **Brain Injury Association of South Carolina**
800 Dutch Square Boulevard
Columbia, SC 29210
803-731-9823
877-TBI-FACT
Fax: 803-731-4804
scbraininjury@bellsouth.net
www.biausa.org/sc
*Elaine Phillips, President*
*Joyce Davis, Executive Director*

2519 **Brain Injury Association of Tennessee**
955 Woodland St
Nashville, TN 37206
615-248-5878
877-757-2428
Fax: 615-383-1176
biaoftn@yahoo.com
www.biaoftn.org
*Guynn Edwards, President*
*Pam Bryan, Executive Director*

2520 **Brain Injury Association of Texas**
316 W 12th Street
Austin, TX 78701
512-326-1212
800-392-0040
Fax: 512-478-3370
www.biatx.org
*Jane Boutte, President*

2521 **Brain Injury Association of Utah**
1800 S W Temple
Salt Lake City, UT 84115
801-484-2240
800-281-8442
Fax: 801-484-5932
biau@sisna.com
www.biau.org
*Teresa Such-Niebar, President*
*Ron S Roskos, Executive Director*

2522 **Brain Injury Association of Vermont**
92 S Main Street
Waterbury, VT 05676
802-244-6850
877-856-1772
Fax: 802-244-4005
support1@biavt.org
www.biavt.org
*Marsha Bancroft, President*
*Trevor Squirrell, Executive Director*

2523 **Brain Injury Association of Virginia**
1506 Willow Lawn Drive
Richmond, VA 23230
804-355-5748
800-444-6443
Fax: 804-355-6381
info@biav.net
www.biav.net
*Anne McDonnell, Executive Director*
*Lynette Scott, Program Director*

2524 **Brain Injury Association of Washington**
800 Jefferson Street
Seattle, WA 98104
206-388-0900
800-523-5438
Fax: 206-388-0901
info@biawa.org
www.biawa.org
*Richard Adler, President*
*Gene van den Bosch, Executive Director*

2525 **Brain Injury Association of West Virginia**
PO Box 574
Institute, WV 25112-0574
304-766-4892
800-356-6443
Fax: 304-766-4940
mdavis@brainman.com
*Michael W Davis, Board of Director*
*Linda Arthur, Board of Director*

2526 **Brain Injury Association of Wisconsin**
21100 W Capitol Drive
Pewaukee, WI 53072
262-790-9660
800-882-9282
Fax: 262-790-9670
admin@execpc.com
www.biaw.org
Advocacy, education, prevention, information, resources, and support groups in regards to traumatic brain injury.
*David Voss, President*
*Mark Warhus, Executive Director*

2527 **Brain Injury Association of Wyoming**
111 W 2nd Street
Casper, WY 82601
307-473-1767
800-643-6457
Fax: 307-237-5222
*Larry Plemmons, President*
*Jack Nokes, Director*

2528 **Choices for Work Program Goodwill Industries-Suncoast**
Goodwill Industries-Suncoast

10596 Gandy Boulevard
St Petersburg, FL 33702
727-523-1512
888-279-1988
Fax: 727-563-9300
TTY: 727-579-1068
gw.marketing@goodwill-suncoast.com
www.goodwill-suncoast.org

A nonprofit community based organization whose purpose is to improve the quality of life for people who are disabled, disadvantaged and/or aged. This mission is accomplished through a staff of over 1,200 employees providing independent living skills, affordable housing, career assessment and job skills training and opportunities.

*Deborah A. Passerini, President*
*Oscar J. Horton, Chair*

**2529 Pensacola Brain Injury TBI/ABI Support Group**
TBI/ABI Support Group
2001 N E Street
Pensacola, FL 32507
850-457-2870
hens8250@bellsouth.net

Survivors and caregivers oriented association. Publishes monthly magazine.

*Peggy Henshall, Support Group Coordinator*

**2530 RRTC on Community Integration of Persons with TBI**
2323 S Shepherd
Houston, TX 77019
713-630-0526
800-732-8124
Fax: 713-630-0529
terri.hudler-hull@memorialhermann.org
www.tbicommunity.org

*Karen A Hart PhD, Director Of Training*
*Sunil Kothari, Medical Director*

## Foundations & Research Centers

**2531 Brady Institute Jamaica Hospital Medical Center**
Jamaica Hospital Medical Center
8900 Van Wyck Expressway
Jamaica, NY 11418-2897
718-206-6000
Fax: 718-206-6559
www.jamaicahospital.org

The James and Sarah Brady Institute for Traumatic Brain Injury.

*David P Rosen, President & CEO*
*Neil Foster Phillips, Chairman*

**2532 Brain Trauma Foundation**
708 Third Avenue
New York, NY 10017-4201
212-772-0608
Fax: 212-772-2035
info@braintrauma.org
www.braintrauma.org

Our goal at the Brain Trauma Foundation is to improve the outcome of TBI patients through Guideline development, clinical research, professional education, and quality improvement programs.

*Quarterly*
*Jamshid Ghajar, MD, President*
*Pamela Drexel, Executive Director*

**2533 Center for Brain Activity Mapping**
UC San Diego
9500 Gilman Drive
La Jolla, CA 92093
858-534-2230
cbam.ucsd.edu

The Center seeks to develop new technologies for detecting neuronal activity, for reporting it out of deep brain tissue, and for processing and analyzing the resulting data, by organizing and supporting research teams and projects.

*Ralph J. Greenspan, PhD, Director*

**2534 Dana Alliance for Brain Initiatives**
745 Fifth Avenue
New York, NY 10151
212-223-4040
Fax: 212-317-8721
danainfo@dana.org
www.dana.org

A non-profit organization of more than 250 neuroscientists which was formed to help provide information about the personal and public benefits of brain research.

*Jane Nevins, Vice President*
*Edward F Rover, President*

**2535 Institute for Rehabilitation and Research**
1333 Moursund Street
Houston, TX 77030
713-799-5000
800-447-3422
Fax: 713-874-1798
tirr.referrals@memorialhermann.org
www.tirr.org

*Carl Josehart, CEO*
*Gerard F. Francisco, Chief Medical Officer*

**2536 Kavli Foundation**
5715 Mesmer Avenue
Los Angeles, CA
424-353-8800
info@kavlifoundation.org
www.kavlifoundation.org

The Foundation supports scientific research into the human brain, in the following scientific fields: Astrophysics, Nanoscience, Neuroscience and Theoretical Physics. Within Neuroscience, the study of aging and brain diseases and disorders is supported.

*Robert W. Conn, PhD, President & CEO*
*Eric Marshall, VP, Public Engagement & Prizes*

**2537 Kavli Institute for Brain Science at Columbia University**
Columbia University
3227 Broadway
New York, NY 10027
212-853-1016
Fax: 212-665-9699
kavli@columbia.edu
www.kavli.columbia.edu

The Institute's primary are of study is how signaling in neural circuits controls cognitive function and behavior, and the development of novel experimental and computational strategies for analyzing these signals.

*Eric R. Kandel, MD, Director*
*Rafael Yuste, MD, PhD, Co-Director*

**2538 Kavli Institute for Brain and Mind**
UC San Diego
9500 Gilman Drive
La Jolla, CA 92093-0115
kibm@ucsd.edu
kibm.ucsd.edu

The Institute supports research that furthers the understanding of the origins, evolution and mechanisms of human cognition. Of particular interest is Traumatic Brain Injury.

*Fred H. Gage, Co-Director*
*Nicholas C. Spitzer, Co-Director*

**2539 Kavli Institute for Fundamental Neuroscience**
UCSF, Sandler Neurosciences Center
675 Nelson Rising Lane
San Francisco, CA 94158
415-476-2018
Fax: 415-502-7332
kavliifn@ucsf.edu
kavliifn.ucsf.edu

The Institute is the central organization for neuroscience research at UCSF and partner institutions, establishing cross-disciplinary teams of scientists and engineers devoted to advancing neuroscience in all its forms.

*Loren Frank, Co-Director*
*Roger Nicoll, Co-Director*

**2540 Kavli Neural Systems Institute**
The Rockefeller University
1230 York Avenue
New York, NY 10065
212-327-8081
lcole@rockefeller.edu
www.rockefeller.edu/research

The Institute unites scientists at The Rockefeller University in the goal of a comprehensive look at the human brain.

*Leslie Vosshall, PhD, Director*
*Lindsey Cole, Administrator*

**2541 Kavli Neuroscience Discovery Institute**
Johns Hopkins University, School of Medicine
725 N Wolfe Street
Baltimore, MD 21205
410-955-4089
Fax: 410-614-6249
KavliNDI@jhu.edu
kavlijhu.org

The Institute looks to advance neuroscience by integrating neuroscience, engineering and computational data science.

*Dwight Bergles, PhD, Director*
*Natasha Hussain, PhD, Scientific Director*

**2542 Neuroscience Research Institute**
UC Santa Barbara

6129 Biology II 805-893-4621
Santa Barbara, CA 93106 www.nri.ucsb.edu
The Institute seeks to allow scientists from different fields to collaborate for the betterment of neurological research. Areas of interest include: Alzheimer's Disease & Related Dementias; Behavioral Neuroscience & Neuroethology; Cell Biology, Biochemistry & Biophysics of the Nervous System; Computational & Theoretical Neuroscience; Development of the Nervous System; and Stem Cells.
*Stuart Feinstein, Co-Director*
*Kenneth Kosik, Co-Director*

2543 **New York University Medical Center Head Trauma Program**
Reet 212-998-9819
New York, NY 10010-4020 Fax: 212-340-7158
Research pertaining to young adults suffering from head injuries.
*Dr Yehuda Ben-Yishay, Coordinator*

2544 **Ohio State University Laboratory of Psychobiology**
1835 Neil Avenue 614-292-8185
Columbus, OH 43210-1222 Fax: 614-292-4537
www.psy.ohio-state.edu/labs
Studies done on recovery of function after brain damage.
*Laura Peterson, Lab Coordinator*
*James Walton, Research Associate*

2545 **Salk Institute for Biological Studies**
10010 N Torrey Pines Road 858-453-4100
La Jolla, CA 92037 www.salk.edu
Conducts groundbreaking research into cancer, aging, Alzheimer's diabetes and infectious diseases.
*Rusty Gage, PhD, President*
*Martin Hetzer, PhD, VP & Chief Science Officer*

2546 **Sanford Consortium for Regenerative Medicine**
2880 Torrey Pines Scenic Drive 858-246-1071
La Jolla, CA 92037 www.sanfordconsortium.com
The Consortium works to achieve breakthrough discoveries in stem cell research with regards to diagnoses, treatments, and cures for degenerative diseases and injuries.
*Edward W. Holmes, MD, President & CEO*
*Jeffrey Steindorf, PhD, VP & COO*

2547 **Scripps Research Institute**
10550 North Torrey Pines Road 858-784-1000
La Jolla, CA www.scripps.edu
The institute seeks to improve human wellbeing through the advancement of bioscience, including research into aging & healthspan, autoimmune diseases, cancer, infectious diseases, neurological disorders, and more.
*Peter Schultz, PhD, President & CEO*
*Eric Topol, MD, EVP, Scripps Research*

2548 **Thomas Jefferson University Ischemia-Shock Research Center**
1020 Locust Street 215-503-4400
Philadelphia, PA 19107-6731 Fax: 215-503-9920
jgsbs-info@jefferson.edu
www.jefferson.edu
Promotes research into head injuries and clinical studies.

2549 **Thomas Jefferson University Ischemia-Shock**
1020 Walnut Street 215-955-6000
Philadelphia, PA 19107 Fax: 215-923-7932
www.jefferson.edu
Promotes research into head injuries and clinical studies.

2550 **Tulane University: US-Japan Biomedical Research Laboratories**
1430 Tulane Avenue 504-988-5187
New Orleans, LA 70112 Fax: 504-394-7169
medsch@tulane.edu
www.tulane.edu/som/
Focuses research efforts on neuroendocrinology and neurosciences.
*Benjamin P Sachs, MB, BS, Senior Vice President, Dean*
*Mary Brown, MBA, Vice President*

2551 **UCLA Neuropsychiatric Institute**
760 Westwood Plaza 310-825-2631
Los Angeles, CA 90095 800-825-9989
Fax: 310-825-9179
pwhybrow@mednet.ucla.edu
www.semel.ucla.edu
Devoted to research and patient care in psychiatry neuroscience and related fields.
*Peter Whybrow, Director*

2552 **University of California: Irvine Brain Imaging Center**
101 The City Drive S 949-824-7872
Irvine, CA 92697-3960 Fax: 949-824-7873
BIC@msx.hsis.uci.edu
Offers PET scan analysis of brain functions focusing on brain damage brain tumors and head injuries.
*Steven L Small, PhD, MD, Director*
*David B Keator, MCS, Technical Director*

2553 **University of California: San Francisco Laboratory for Neurotrauma**
1001 Potrero Avenue 415-206-8313
San Francisco, CA 94110-3518 www.ucsf.edu
Research done into traumatic brain and head injuries.
*Lawrence H Pitts MD*

2554 **University of Memphis: Department of Psychology**
Memphis State University
202 Psychology Building 901-678-2000
Memphis, TN 38152 Fax: 901-678-2579
psycadvise@memphis.edu
www.memphis.edu/psychology/
Evaluation and development of assessment and treatment procedures for neurologically impaired persons.
*Guy Mittleman, Professor Director of CAPR*
*Frank Andrasik, Professor, Chair*

2555 **Virginia Commonwealth University: Rehab Research and Training Center**
1314 W Main Street 804-828-1851
Richmond, VA 23284-2011 Fax: 804-828-2193
TTY: 804-828-2494
www.vcu.edu/rrtcweb/
Focuses research on traumatic brain and head injuries.
*Paul Wehman, Director*
*Jeanne Dalton, Public Relations Assistant Specialist*

2556 **Wayne State University: Gurdjian-Lissner Biomechanics Laboratory**
Department of Neurological Surgery
4160 John R Street 313-831-0777
Detroit, MI 48201 877-486-7978
Fax: 313-966-0368
www.neurosurgery.med.wayne.edu
Head and neck injury research.
*Murali Guthikonda, MD, FACS, Professor (Clinician-Educator) and Chair*
*Patti Bekowies, MBA, Chief Administrative Officer*

## Support Groups & Hotlines

2557 **Alabama Head Injury Foundation Helpline**
3100 Lorna Road 205-823-3818
Hoover, AL 35216-5451 800-433-8002
Fax: 205-823-4544
ahif1@bellsouth.net
www.ahif.org/
The Alabama Head Injury Foundation (AHIF) was founded by professionals and families in 1983 to increase public awareness of Traumatic Brain Injury (TBI) and to stimulate the development of supportive services. AHIF provides accessible resources, services and programs that meet the unique needs of individuals with traumatic brain injury (TBI) as well as spinal cord injury (SCI) in certain programs.
*Charles D Priest, Executive Director*
*Janet Massey, Executive Assistant*

2558 **American Brain Tumor Association**
8550 W Bryn Mawr Avenue 800-886-2282
Chicago, IL 60631 info@abta.org
www.abta.org

CareLine offered for newly diagnosed patients with brain tumors.
*Ralph DeVitto, President & CEO*
*Nicole Willmarth, PhD, Chief Mission Officer*

2559 **Brain Injury Alliance of Iowa Helpline**
Brain Injury Association of America
7025 Hickman Road 319-272-2312
Urbandale, IA 50322 855-444-6443
Fax: 319-272-2109
info@biaia.org
www.biaia.org

*Geoffrey Lauer, Executive Director*
*Natasha Retz, Director of Programs and Services*

2560 **Brain Injury Alliance of Kentucky**
7321 New LaGrange Road 502-493-0609
Louisville, KY 40222 800-592-1117
Fax: 502-426-2993
www.biak.us

Founded in 1980, the Brain Injury Association of America (BIAA) is a national organization serving and representing individuals, families and professionals who are touched by a life-altering, often devastating, traumatic brain injury (TBI). BIAA provides information, education and support through its network of chartered state affiliates, local chapters and support groups across the country to assist the 5.3 million Americans currently living with traumatic brain injury and their families.
*Andrew Horne, President Kentucky State Office*
*Chell Austin, Executive Director*

2561 **Brain Injury Alliance of Minnesota**
34 13th Avenue North East 612-378-2742
Minneapolis, MN 55413 800-669-6442
Fax: 612-378-2789
info@braininjurymn.org
www.braininjurymn.org

*Tom Gode, Executive Director*

2562 **Brain Injury Alliance of Montana**
1280 South 3rd Street West 406-541-6442
Missoula, MT 59801 800-241-6442
Fax: 406-243-2349
kristen@biamt.org
www.biamt.org

*Kristen Morgan, MSW, Program Director*
*Molly Walsh, Outreach Coordinator*

2563 **Brain Injury Alliance of New Jersey**
Brain Injury Association of America
825 Georges Road 732-745-0200
North Brunswick, NJ 08902 800-669-4323
Fax: 732-745-0211
info@bianj.org
www.bianj.org

*Edward Kim, MD, MBA, Chairperson*
*Barbara Geiger-Parker, President/CEO*

2564 **Brain Injury Alliance of New Mexico**
3232 Candelaria NE 505-292-7414
Albuquerque, NM 87107 888-292-7415
Fax: 505-271-8983
www.braininjurynm.org

Founded in 1980, the Brain Injury Association of America (BIAA) is a national organization serving and representing individuals, families and professionals who are touched by a life-altering, often devastating, traumatic brain injury (TBI). BIAA provides information, education and support through its network of chartered state affiliates, local chapters and support groups across the country to assist the 5.3 million Americans currently living with traumatic brain injury and their families.
*John Tiwald, Board President New Mexico State Office*
*Mark Pedrotty, PhD, Vice President*

2565 **Brain Injury Alliance of Oregon**
Brain Injury Association of America
2145 NW Overton Street 503-413-7707
Portland, OR 97210 800-544-5243
Fax: 503-413-6849
biaor@biaoregon.org
www.biaoregon.org

Non-profit providing information and referral, support groups, prevention, education, training, and advocacy for those with brain injury, families, and professionals.
*Ralph Wiser, President*
*Chuck McGilvrary, Vice-President*

2566 **Brain Injury Alliance of Utah**
Brain Injury Association of America
5280 Commerce Dr. 801-716-4993
Murray, UT 84107 800-281-8442
Fax: 801-716-4995
info@biau.org
www.biau.org/

*Antonietta Anna Russo, Ph.D., President*
*Ron S Roskos, Executive Director*

2567 **Brain Injury Alliance of Wisconsin**
21100 W. Capitol Dr. 262-790-9660
Brookfield, WI 53072 800-882-9282
Fax: 262-790-9670
admin@execpc.com
www.biaw.org

Founded in 1980, the Brain Injury Association of America (BIAA) is a national organization serving and representing individuals, families and professionals who are touched by a life-altering, often devastating, traumatic brain injury (TBI). BIAA provides information, education and support through its network of chartered state affiliates, local chapters and support groups across the country to assist the 5.3 million Americans currently living with traumatic brain injury and their families.
*Audrey Nelson, President Wisconsin State Office*
*Lori Schultz, Executive Director*

2568 **Brain Injury Alliance of Wyoming**
111 West 2nd Street 307-473-1767
Casper, WY 82601 800-643-6457
Fax: 307-237-5222
www.wybia.org/

*Dorothy Cronin, Director*

2569 **Brain Injury Association of America's National Family Helpline**
1608 Spring Hill Road 703-761-0750
Vienna, VA 22182 800-444-6443
Fax: 703-761-0755
FamilyHelpline@biausa.org
www.biausa.org

*Greg Oshanick, Chairman*
*Susan Conners, President and CEO*

2570 **Brain Injury Association of Arizona**
5025 E Washington Street 602-508-8024
Phoenix, AZ 85034 888-500-9165
Fax: 602-508-8285
info@biaaz.org
www.biaaz.org

Information and resources for brain injury survivors and their families. Support group listings available. Educational training, conference for families and survivors, neuro-specific resources and helpline.
*Kim Halloran, Executive Director*
*Jeanne Andersen, Information & Referral Manager*

2571 **Brain Injury Association of Arkansas Helpline**
PO Box 26236 501-374-3585
Little Rock, AR 72221-6236 866-610-4841
Fax: 501-918-6595
info@brainassociation.org

Founded in 1980, the Brain Injury Association of America (BIAA) is a national organization serving and representing individuals, families and professionals who are touched by a life-altering, often devastating, traumatic brain injury (TBI). BIAA provides information, education and support through its network of chartered state affiliates, local chapters and support groups across the country to

assist the 5.3 million Americans currently living with traumatic brain injury and their families.
*Dana Austen, President Arkansas State Office*
*Kortney E Gold, Vice President*

2572 **Brain Injury Association of California Helpline**
3501 Mall View Road 661-872-4903
Bakersfield, CA 93306 Fax: 661-873-2508
calbiainfo@yahoo.com
www.biacal.org/
Founded in 1980, the Brain Injury Association of America (BIAA) is a national organization serving and representing individuals, families and professionals who are touched by a life-altering, often devastating, traumatic brain injury (TBI). BIAA provides information, education and support through its network of chartered state affiliates, local chapters and support groups across the country to assist the 5.3 million Americans currently living with traumatic brain injury and their families.
*Paula Daoutis, Administrative Director*
*Ursula Pesta, Project Coordinator*

2573 **Brain Injury Association of Colorado Helpline**
1385 South Colorado Boulevard 303-355-9969
Denver, CO 80222 800-955-2443
Fax: 303-355-9968
biacolo@aol.com
www.BIAColorado.org
*Dannis Schanel, LCSW, CBIST, President*
*Gavin Attwood, Exececutive Director*

2574 **Brain Injury Association of Connecticut Helpline**
200 Day Hill Road 860-219-0291
Windsor, CT 06095-1304 800-278-8242
Fax: 860-219-0568
general@biact.org
www.biact.homestead.com/
Supports persons with brain injuries and their families by promoting services to facilitate full inclusion within their local community and to increase awareness and understanding of brain injury and its prevention through community education.
*500 Members*
*Paul A. Slager, Esq., President*
*Dr. Johnny Magwood, BSME, MBA, DBA, Vice President*

2575 **Brain Injury Association of Delaware Helpline**
32 West Loockerman Street 302-346-2083
Dover, DE 19904 800-411-0505
Fax: 302-678-3183
www.biaofde.org//
Founded in 1980, the Brain Injury Association of America (BIAA) is a national organization serving and representing individuals, families and professionals who are touched by a life-altering, often devastating, traumatic brain injury (TBI). BIAA provides information, education and support through its network of chartered state affiliates, local chapters and support groups across the country to assist the 5.3 million Americans currently living with traumatic brain injury and their families.
*Elizabeth Furber, President Delaware State Office*
*Timothy J Walker, Vice President*

2576 **Brain Injury Association of Florida**
1637 Metropolitan Blvd 850-410-0103
Tallahassee, FL 32308 800-992-3442
Fax: 850-410-0105
admin@biaf.org
www.biaf.org
*Gary Clarke, Chairman*
*Valerie Breen, President/CEO*

2577 **Brain Injury Association of Hawaii**
420 Kuwili Street 808-436-8977
Honolulu, HI 96817 biahi@hawaiiantel.net
Dedicated to serving those affected by brain injury through advocacy, prevention, and support.
*Mary Wilson, Executive Director*
*Ian Mattoch, President*

2578 **Brain Injury Association of Illinois Helpline**
PO Box 64420 312-726-5699
Chicago, IL 60664-420 800-699-6443
Fax: 312-630-4011
info@biail.org
www.biail.org
Works with all people with brain inquiries and their families with professionals who serve them. Provides camp oppurtunities, support groups, educational seminars, information and referrals and a quarterly newsletter.
*Irene Pedersen, Founder*
*Philicia L Deckard, Executive Director*

2579 **Brain Injury Association of Indiana Helpline**
9531 Valparaiso Court 317-356-7722
Indianapolis, IN 46268 866-854-4246
Fax: 317-802-1768
info@biai.org
www.biai.org
Founded in 1980, the Brain Injury Association of America (BIAA) is a national organization serving and representing individuals, families and professionals who are touched by a life-altering, often devastating, traumatic brain injury (TBI). BIAA provides information, education and support through its network of chartered state affiliates, local chapters and support groups across the country to assist the 5.3 million Americans currently living with traumatic brain injury and their families.
*Nancy Ritter, Chairperson*
*Anna Garrett, Executive Director*

2580 **Brain Injury Association of Kansas and Greater Kansas City Helpline**
6701 W. 64th Street 913-754-8883
Overland Park, KS 66202 800-783-1356
Fax: 816-842-1531
rabramowitz@biaks.org
www.biaks.org
*Whitney Sunderland, President*
*Robin Abramowitz, Executive Director*

2581 **Brain Injury Association of Louisiana Helpline**
c/o National Headquarters Office
8325 Oak Street 504-982-0685
New Orleans, LA 70118 800-444-6443
Fax: 703-761-0755
info@biala.org
www.biala.org/
Founded in 1980, the Brain Injury Association of America (BIAA) is a national organization serving and representing individuals, families and professionals who are touched by a life-altering, often devastating, traumatic brain injury (TBI). BIAA provides information, education and support through its network of chartered state affiliates, local chapters and support groups across the country to assist the 5.3 million Americans currently living with traumatic brain injury and their families.
*Janet Clark, Chairman*
*Tommy Lotz, Executive Director*

2582 **Brain Injury Association of Maryland Helpline**
Kernan Hospital
2200 Kernan Drive 410-448-2924
Baltimore, MD 21207 800-221-6443
Fax: 410-448-3541
info@biamd.org
www.biamd.org
Founded in 1980, the Brain Injury Association of America (BIAA) is a national organization serving and representing individuals, families and professionals who are touched by a life-altering, often devastating, traumatic brain injury (TBI). BIAA provides information, education and support through its network of chartered state affiliates, local chapters and support groups across the country to assist the 5.3 million Americans currently living with traumatic brain injury and their families.
*Mark Huslage, President Maryland State Office*
*Bryan Thomas Pugh, Executive Director*

2583 **Brain Injury Association of Massachusetts Helpline**
30 Lyman Street 508-475-0032
Westborough, MA 01581 800-242-0030
Fax: 508-475-0400
TTY: 508-948-0593
biama@biama.org
www.biama.org
Founded in 1980, the Brain Injury Association of America (BIAA) is a national organization serving and representing individuals, families and professionals who are touched by a life-altering, often devastating, traumatic brain injury (TBI). BIAA provides information, education and support through its network of chartered state affiliates, local chapters and support groups across the country to assist the 5.3 million Americans currently living with traumatic brain injury and their families.
*Teresa Hayes, President Massachusetts State Office*
*Mathew Martino, Executive Board*

2584 **Brain Injury Association of Michigan Helpline**
7305 Grand River 810-229-5880
Brighton, MI 48114-2334 800-444-6443
Fax: 810-229-8947
info@biami.org
www.biami.org
*Deborah Newton, Chair*
*Michael F Dabbs, President*

2585 **Brain Injury Association of Mississippi Helpline**
2727 Old Canton Road 601-981-1021
Jackson, MS 39216-5912 800-444-6443
Fax: 601-981-1039
ljenkins@msbia.org
www.msbia.org/
*Howard T Katz, MD, Chair*
*Lee Jenkins, Executive Director*

2586 **Brain Injury Association of Missouri Helpline**
2265 Schuetz Road 314-426-4024
St Louis, MO 63146-1322 800-444-6443
Fax: 314-426-3290
info@biamo.org
www.biamo.org
Information and referral services and support groups throughout the state of Missouri.
*Eric Hart, Psy.D, Board President*
*Stephanie Cooper, Executive Director*

2587 **Brain Injury Association of New Hampshire**
Brain Injury Association of America
109 N State Street 603-225-8400
Concord, NH 03301-4447 800-773-8400
Fax: 603-228-6749
mail@bianh.org
www.bianh.org
*Laura Flashman, PhD, President*
*Steven D Wade, Executive Director*

2588 **Brain Injury Association of New York State Helpline**
10 Colvin Avenue 518-459-7911
Albany, NY 12206-1242 800-228-8201
Fax: 518-482-5285
info@bianys.org
www.bianys.org
*Marie Cavallo, Ph.D, President*
*Judith Avner, Executive Director*

2589 **Brain Injury Association of North Carolina Helpline**
2113 Cameron Street 919-833-9634
Raleigh, NC 27605 800-377-1464
Fax: 919-833-5415
bianc@bianc.net
www.bianc.net/
*Susan Baker, Director of Finance*
*Cindy Boyd, Fundraising Chair*

2590 **Brain Injury Association of North Dakota**
1225 South 12th Street 877-525-2724
Bismarck, ND 58504 Fax: 701-845-1175
www.braininjurynd.com/
Founded in 1980, the Brain Injury Association of America (BIAA) is a national organization serving and representing individuals, families and professionals who are touched by a life-altering, often devastating, traumatic brain injury (TBI). BIAA provides information, education and support through its network of chartered state affiliates, local chapters and support groups across the country to assist the 5.3 million Americans currently living with traumatic brain injury and their families.
*April Fairfield, Executive Director*
*Rebecca Quinn, Eastern Region Contact*

2591 **Brain Injury Association of Ohio**
855 Grandview Avenue 614-481-7100
Columbus, OH 43215-1000 800-444-6443
Fax: 614-481-7103
help@biaoh.org
www.biaoh.org
*Stephanie Ramsey, President*
*Jon Fishpaw, First Vice President*

2592 **Brain Injury Association of Oklahoma Helpline**
3015 E. Skelly Dr. 918-789-0406
Tulsa, OK 74105-0088 800-765-6809
Fax: 918-712-9019
braininjuryoklahoma@gmail.com
www.braininjuryoklahoma.org
Founded in 1980, the Brain Injury Association of America (BIAA) is a national organization serving and representing individuals, families and professionals who are touched by a life-altering, often devastating, traumatic brain injury (TBI). BIAA provides information, education and support through its network of chartered state affiliates, local chapters and support groups across the country to assist the 5.3 million Americans currently living with traumatic brain injury and their families.
*Adam Sherman, PhD, President Oklahoma State Office*
*Mary Dobbs, Vice-President*

2593 **Brain Injury Association of Rhode Island Helpline**
935 Park Avenue 401-461-6599
Cranston, RI 02910-2743 Fax: 401-461-6561
www.biausa.org/RI/
Founded in 1980, the Brain Injury Association of America (BIAA) is a national organization serving and representing individuals, families and professionals who are touched by a life-altering, often devastating, traumatic brain injury (TBI). BIAA provides information, education and support through its network of chartered state affiliates, local chapters and support groups across the country to assist the 5.3 million Americans currently living with traumatic brain injury and their families.
*Michael L. Baker, Co-President*
*Sharon Brinkworth, Executive Director*

2594 **Brain Injury Association of Tennessee Helpline**
955 Woodland Street 615-248-2541
Nashville, TN 37206 800-444-6443
Fax: 615-383-1176
biaoftn@yahoo.com
www.braininjurytn.org/
Founded in 1980, the Brain Injury Association of America (BIAA) is a national organization serving and representing individuals, families and professionals who are touched by a life-altering, often devastating, traumatic brain injury (TBI). BIAA provides information, education and support through its network of chartered state affiliates, local chapters and support groups across the country to assist the 5.3 million Americans currently living with traumatic brain injury and their families.
*Guynn Edwards, President Tennessee State Office*
*Pam Bryan, Executive Director*

2595 **Brain Injury Association of Vermont Helpline**
92 South Main Street 802-244-6850
Waterbury, VT 05676 877-856-1772
Fax: 802-244-4005
support1@biavt.org
www.biavt.org
Founded in 1980, the Brain Injury Association of America (BIAA) is a national organization serving and representing individuals, families and professionals who are touched by a life-altering, often devastating, traumatic brain injury (TBI). BIAA provides information, education and support through its network of chartered state affiliates, local chapters and support groups across the country to

assist the 5.3 million Americans currently living with traumatic brain injury and their families.
*Marsha Bancroft, President Vermont State Office*
*Trevor Squirrell, Executive Director*

2596 **Brain Injury Association of Virginia Helpline**
1506 Willow Lawn Dr
Richmond, VA 23230-5018
804-355-5748
800-444-6443
Fax: 804-355-6381
info@biav.net
www.biav.net
Nonprofit organization providing information and resources related to brain injury to individuals with brain injuries, their families and professionals who deal with brain injury.
*Kimberly Moore, President*
*Anne McDonnell, Executive Director*

2597 **Brain Injury Association of Washington Helpline**
P.O. Box 3044
Seattle, WA 98114
206-467-4800
877-982-4292
Fax: 206-467-4808
info@braininjurywa.org
www.braininjurywa.org/
Founded in 1980, the Brain Injury Association of America (BIAA) is a national organization serving and representing individuals, families and professionals who are touched by a life-altering, often devastating, traumatic brain injury (TBI). BIAA provides information, education and support through its network of chartered state affiliates, local chapters and support groups across the country to assist the 5.3 million Americans currently living with traumatic brain injury and their families.
*Mark T Long, President Washington State Office*
*Deborah Crawley, Executive Director*

2598 **Brain Injury Association of West Virginia Helpline**
Brain Injury Association of America
PO Box 574
Institute, WV 25112-574
304-400-4506
800-356-6443
Fax: 304-766-4940
mdavis@brainman.com
*Michael W Davis, President*

2599 **Brain Injury Resource Center**
Brain Injury Resource Center
PO Box 84151
Seattle, WA 98124-5451
206-621-8558
Fax: 206-329-4355
brain@headinjury.com
www.headinjury.com
Disseminates head injury information and provides referrals to facilitate adjustment to life following head injury. Organizes seminars for professionals, head injury survivors, and their families.
*Constance Miller MA, Founder/President*
*B Parker Lindner MPA, Communications Specialist*

2600 **Cafe Plus**
216 W Manlius Street
East Syracuse, NY 13057
315-446-3124
For people who have survived a head-injury or some type of head trauma.
*David Listowski, Manager*

2601 **Family Caregiver Alliance/National Center on Caregiving**
101 Montgomery Street
San Francisco, CA 94104
415-434-3388
800-445-8106
www.caregiver.org
Caregiver information and assistance via phone or e-mail; fact sheets and publications describing and documenting caregiver needs and services.
*Jacquelyn Kung, PhD, Chief Executive Officer*
*Wyatt Ritchie, MBA, Managing Director*

2602 **Hy Feinstein Clubhouse**
Long Island Head Injury Association
300 Kennedy Drive
Hauppauge, NY 11788
631-543-2245
Fax: 631-543-2261
lgiordano@headinjuryassoc.org
The LIHIA provides a place for people with head injury to participate in meaningful work, to have the opportunity to meet and build friendships and ultimately seek employment within the community.
*Stuart Gleiber, President*
*Leonard Feinstein, Vice President*

2603 **Jodi House**
625 Chapala St.
Santa Barbara, CA 93101
805-563-2882
Fax: 805-563-3982
info@jodihouse.org
www.jodihouse.org
Jodi House is a community-based, post-rehabilitation day program that provides opportunities for social interaction, life skill training, recreation, and support for adults living with acquired brain injury (i.e. from head trauma, tumor, and stroke) and their families.
*Gayle Cummings, Co-President*
*Timothy Morton-Smith, Co-President/Vice President of Finance*

2604 **National Health Information Center**
Office of Disease Prevention & Health Promotion
1101 Wootton Pkwy
Rockville, MD 20852
Fax: 240-453-8281
odphpinfo@hhs.gov
www.health.gov/nhic
Supports public health education by maintaining a calendar of National Health Observances; helps connect consumers and health professionals to organizations that can best answer questions and provide up-to-date contact information from reliable sources; updates on a yearly basis toll-free numbers for health information, Federal health clearinghouses and info centers.
*Don Wright, MD, MPH, Director*

2605 **VALT Support Group (Vital Active Life After Trauma)**
53 Linden Street
Brookline, MA 02149
617-277-6327

## Magazines

2606 **BMC Neuroscience**
Springer Nature
One New York Plaza
New York, NY 10004-1562
800-777-4643
info@biomedcentral.com
bmcneurosci.biomedcentral.com
A peer-reviewed, open-access journal devoted to all aspects of the nervous system (including molecular, cellular, developmental and animal model studies), as well as cognitive and behavioral research, and computational modeling.
*Darren Byrne, Editor*
*Ana Donnelly, Manuscript Editor*

2607 **Brain & Life**
American Academy of Neurology
201 Chicago Avenue
Minneapolis, MN 55415
612-928-6000
800-879-1960
Fax: 612-454-2748
BrainandLife@wolterskluwer.com
www.brainandlife.org
Official magazine of the American Academy of Neurology, aimed at parents and home-caregivers interested in neurology in everyday life.
*Orly Avitzur, MD, MBA, FAAN, Editor-in-Chief*
*Mary Bolster, Managing Editor*

2608 **Brain: A Journal of Neurology**
Oxford University Press
2001 Evans Road
Cary, NC 27513
919-677-0977
800-852-7323
Fax: 919-677-1714
brain@ucl.ac.uk
academic.oup.com/brain
Focus is clinical neurology and translational neuroscience.
*Dimitri M. Kullmann, Editor*
*Joanne Bell, Managing Editor*

2609 **Continuum: Lifelong Learning in Neurology**
American Academy of Neurology
201 Chicago Avenue
Minneapolis, MN 55415
612-928-6000
800-879-1960
continuumcme@aan.com
journals.lww.com/continuum

Official journal of the American Academy of Neurology, aiding professionals in patient care and continuing education.
*Bimonthly*
*Steven L. Lewis, MD, FAAN*
*Andrea J. Weiss, MA, Executive Editor*

2610 **JNeurosci**
Society for Neuroscience
1121 14th Street NW
Washginton, DC 20005
202-962-4000
jn@sfn.org
www.jneurosci.org
Official peer-reviewed journal of the Society for Neuroscience, publishing research on a broad range of topics of interest to those working on the nervous system.
*Marina R. Picciotto, Editor-in-Chief*
*Teresa Esch, Features Editor*

2611 **Journal of Head Trauma Rehabilitation**
Aspen Publishers
2001 Market Street
Philadelphia, PA 19103-3129
215-521-8300
800-638-8437
www.lww.com
Scholarly journal designed to provide information on clinical management and rehabilitation of the head-injured for the practicing professional.

*Jennifer E. Brogan, Vice President*
*Kivmars Bowling, Senior Publisher*

2612 **Journal of NeuroEngineering and Rehabilitation**
Springer Nature
One New York Plaza
New York, NY 10004-1562
800-777-4643
info@biomedcentral.com
jneuroengrehab.biomedcentral.com
An open-access journal devoted to integrated research from the fields of neuroscience, biomedical engineering, and physical medicine and rehabilitation.
*David J. Reinkensmeyer, Editor-in-Chief*

2613 **Journal of Neuroinflammation**
Springer Nature
One New York Plaza
New York, NY 10004-1562
800-777-4643
info@biomedcentral.com
jneuroinflammation.biomedcentral.com
A peer-reviewed, open-access journal focusing on the interactions of the immune system with the nervous system as a means of expanding understanding of chronic neurological diseases.
*Monica J. Carson, Editor-in-Chief*
*Sue T. Griffin, Editor-in-Chief*

2614 **Journal of the Neurological Sciences**
Elsevier
LSU Health Sciences Center
New Orleans, LA 70112
JNS_England@lsuhsc.edu
www.jns-journal.com
Original articles in neurology and neuroscience from around the world.
*Monthly*
*John D. England, Editor-in-Chief*

2615 **Molecular Neurodegeneration**
Springer Nature
One New York Plaza
New York, NY 10004-1562
800-777-4643
info@biomedcentral.com
www.biomedcentral.com
A peer-reviewed, open-access journal devoted to all aspects of neurodegeneration research at the molecular and cellular levels.
*Guojun Bu, Editor-in-Chief*
*Huaxi Xu, Editor-in-Chief*

2616 **Neurology**
American Academy of Neurology
201 Chicago Avenue
Minneapolis, MN 55415
612-928-6000
800-879-1960
Fax: 612-454-2748
journal@neurology.org
n.neurology.org
Official journal of the American Academy of Neurology, peer-reviewed, highlighting clinical neurology research.
*Jose G. Merino, MD, MPhil, FAAN, Editor-in-Chief*
*Patricia K. Baskin, MS, Executive Editor*

2617 **Neurology Clinical Practice**
American Academy of Neurology
201 Chicago Avenue
Minneapolis, MN 55415
612-928-6000
800-879-1960
Fax: 612-454-2748
journal@neurology.org
cp.neurology.org
Official peer-reviewed journal of the American Academy of Neurology for practicing neurologists.
*John R. Corboy, MD, FAAN, Editor*
*Patricia K. Baskin, MS, Executive Editor*

2618 **Neurology: Genetics**
American Academy of Neurology
201 Chicago Avenue
Minneapolis, MN 55415
612-928-6000
800-879-1960
Fax: 612-454-2748
journal@neurology.org
ng.neurology.org
Official journal of the American Academy of Neurology, publishing online open-access peer-reviewed reports in the field of neurogenetics.
*Stefan M. Pulst, MD, FAAN, Editor*
*Patricia K. Baskin, MS, Executive Editor*

2619 **Neurology: Neuroimmunology & Neuroinflammation**
American Academy of Neurology
201 Chicago Avenue
Minneapolis, MN 55415
612-928-6000
800-879-1960
Fax: 612-454-2748
journal@neurology.org
nn.neurology.org
Official journal of the American Academy of Neurology, publishing online open-access peer-reviewed reports of original research and in-depth reviews of topics in neuroimmunology & neuroinflammation.
*Josep O. Dalmau, MD, PhD, Editor*
*Patricia K. Baskin, MS, Executive Editor*

2620 **Translational Neurodegeneration**
Springer Nature
One New York Plaza
New York, NY 10004-1562
800-777-4643
info@biomedcentral.com
www.biomedcentral.com
A peer-reviewed, open-access journal covering research, therapeutics and education for all areas of neurodegenerative diseases.
*Shengdi Chen, Editor-in-Chief*

2621 **eNeuro**
Society for Neuroscience
1121 14th Street NW
Washginton, DC 20005
202-312-7305
eNeuro@sfn.org
www.eneuro.org
Open-access journal of the Society for Neuroscience.
*Christophe Bernard, Editor-in-Chief*
*Kelly Newton, Director, Scientific Publications*

## Web Sites

2622 **Agency for Healthcare: Research Facility**
www.ahcpr.gov
The Agency for Healthcare Research and Quality's (AHRQ) mission is to produce evidence to make health care safer, higher quality, more accessible, equitable, and affordable, and to work within the U.S. Department of Health and Human Services and with other partners to make sure that the evidence is understood and used.

2623 **American Brain Tumor Association**
www.abta.org
Provide free social service consultations; a mentorship program for new brain tumor support group leaders; a nationwide database of established support groups; the Connections pen-pal program; networking with organizations that provide services to patients and families; a resource listing of physicians offering investgative treatments.

2624 **Brain Injury Association of America**
www.biausa.org

Seeking to improve the quality of life for people with brain injuries and their families through information and resource referral, legislative advocacy, prevention awareness, and professional education. BIA's mission is to create a better future through brain injury prevention, research, education and advocacy.

**2625 Brain Research Institute: Medicine School University of California, Los Angeles**

www.bri.ucla.edu

The UCLA Brain Research Institute (BRI) is a catalyst for education, outreach, and research collaborations among current and future scientists, engineers and clinicians who seek to understand the healthy and diseased brain.

**2626 Headinjury.Com**

www.headinjury.com

Maintained by the Head Injury Hotline, a non-profit clearinghouse founded and operated by head injury activist. The primary goal are to empower through education, resources and support. The basic premise is that the medical system is deeply flawed and that the brain injury rehab industry is no exception. The site integrates resources from diverse organizations including support groups, rehabilitation and research sites.

**2627 Healing Well**

www.healingwell.com

An online health resource guide to medical news, chat, information and articles, newsgroups and message boards, books, disease-related web sites, medical directories, and more for patients, friends, and family coping with disabling diseases, disorders, or chronic illnesses.

**2628 Health Finder**

www.healthfinder.gov

Searchable, carefully developed web site offering information on over 1000 topics. Developed by the US Department of Health and Human Services, the site can be used in both English and Spanish.

**2629 Healthlink USA**

www.healthlinkusa.com

Health information concerning treatment, cures, prevention, diagnosis, risk factors, research, support groups, email lists, personal stories and much more. Updated regularly.

**2630 MedicineNet**

www.medicinenet.com

An online resource for consumers providing easy-to-read, authoritative medical and health information.

**2631 Medscape**

www.medscape.com

Medscape offers specialists, primary care physicians, and other health professionals the Web's most robust and integrated medical information and educational tools.

**2632 Neurology Channel**

www.healthcommunities.com

Find clearly explained, medically accurate information regarding conditions, including an overview, symptoms, causes, diagnostic procedures and treatment options. On this site it is possible to ask questions and get information from a neurologist and connect to people who have similar health interests.

**2633 Neuronline**

Society for Neuroscience
1121 14th Street NW
Washginton, DC 20005

202-962-4000
neuronline@sfn.org
neuronline.sfn.org

Online portal for professional development and training resources for individuals in the field of neuroscience, hosted by the Society for Neuroscience.

*Amanda Kimball, Director, Digital Learning*

**2634 Road Less Traveled**

Dedicated to survivors and families of victims of Traumatic Brain Injury.

**2635 TBI Help**

www.tbihelp.com

Information concerning head injury.

**2636 TBI: Traumatic Brian Injury**

www.tbi.org

The Perspective Network was changed to TBI in 2015; it provides forums and resources for persons with families, caregivers, friends and the professionals who serve them. Their goals are to promote a sense of community and to increase public awareness of brain injury.

**2637 Traumatic Brain Injury**

www.traumaticbraininjury.com

Internet resource for education, advocacy, research and support for brain injury survivors, their families, and medical and rehabilitation professionals.

**2638 http://diagnosecte.com**

Information about a 7-year, multi-site research project whose goal is to develop methods of diagnosing cTE during life, and to examine risk factors.

**2639 https://Consussionfoundation.org-resources /what-is-CTE**

Offers information about signs, symptoms and resources for CTE patients and their families. Newletter also available.

**2640 https://www.dementiacarecentral.com/aboutd ementia/cte/**

Offers information on causes, treatments, and support for caregivers.

# VASCULAR DEMENTIA

*Vascular dementia is caused by brain damage from impaired blood flow to the brain, most often as the result of a stroke. It leads to difficulties with reasoning, planning, judgment, and memory. Vascular dementia can present immediately after the patient suffers a stroke or can develop over time as the result of strokes that do not immediately cause cognitive impairment. Other conditions that narrow or restrict brain blood vessels, such as high blood pressure, atherosclerosis, diabetes, and brain hemorrhage, can also lead to the onset of vascular dementia.*

Symptoms of vascular cognitive impairment vary widely depending on both the area of the brain that is affected and the severity of the damage. Memory loss is not always a symptom of the condition but if the damage is experienced in the areas of the brain that are responsible for storing and retrieving information, the symptoms may be quite similar to those who suffer Alzheimer's disease, with memory loss and significant cognitive impairment. Other common symptoms of vascular dementia include confusion, disorientation, trouble with speech, difficulty walking, and numbness or partial paralysis.

Vascular dementia is diagnosed by neurocognitive testing in conjunction with an MRI to confirm that the patient has suffered a stroke or other vascular brain changes. This sort of screening is recommended for anyone who has suffered a stroke or a transient ischemic attack (TIA). No drugs have been specifically approved to treat vascular dementia, although there is some evidence that medication used to treat Alzheimer's disease may offer some benefits. As with stroke, management of vascular dementia largely centers both on controlling risk factors, such as blood pressure, weight, and smoking and alcohol use, to prevent further deterioration, and on physical and occupational therapy. Nonetheless, the prognosis for vascular dementia patients is not promising, with those who suffer the condition following a stroke living an average of three years.

## National Agencies & Associations

2642 **American Academy of Neurology**
201 Chicago Avenue 612-928-6000
Minneapolis, MN 55415 800-879-1960
Fax: 612-454-2746
memberservices@aan.com
www.aan.com
Professional society of medical doctors specializing in brain and nervous system diseases. Maintains placement service. Sponsors research and educational programs. Compiles statistics. Publishes scientific journal, Continuum: Lifelong Learning in Neurology.
*Mary E. Post, MBA, CAE, CEO*

2643 **American Society for Investigative Pathology**
1801 Rockville Pike 240-283-9700
Rockville, MD 20852 Fax: 301-984-4047
www.asip.org
The Society seeks to promote experimental pathology and related disciplines through meetings, publications, and educational activities.
*William B. Coleman, PhD, Executive Officer*
*Gina LaBorde, Manager, Marketing & Communications*

2644 **American Society for Neurochemistry**
9037 Ron Den Lane 407-909-9064
Windermere, FL 34786 Fax: 407-876-0750
asnmanager@asneurochem.org
asneurochem.org
The Society aims to advance and promote cellular and molecular neuroscience knowledge, and to facilitate communication and the dissemination of information within the field and with related disciplines.
*Sheilah Jewart, Executive Director*
*Karen Gottlieb, Conference Coordinator*

2645 **Society for Neuroscience**
1121 14th Street NW 202-962-4000
Washginton, DC 20005 marty@sfn.org
sfn.org
Large international organization of scientists and physicians devoted to the study of the brain and the nervous system.
*37,000 members*
*Marty Saggese, Executive Director*
*Melissa Garcia, Associate Executive Director*

## Foundations & Research Centers

2646 **Center for Brain Activity Mapping**
UC San Diego
9500 Gilman Drive 858-534-2230
La Jolla, CA 92093 cbam.ucsd.edu
The Center seeks to develop new technologies for detecting neuronal activity, for reporting it out of deep brain tissue, and for processing and analyzing the resulting data, by organizing and supporting research teams and projects.
*Ralph J. Greenspan, PhD, Director*

2647 **Kavli Foundation**
5715 Mesmer Avenue 424-353-8800
Los Angeles, CA info@kavlifoundation.org
www.kavlifoundation.org
The Foundation supports scientific research into the human brain, in the following scientific fields: Astrophysics, Nanoscience, Neuroscience and Theoretical Physics. Within Neuroscience, the study of aging and brain diseases and disorders is supported.
*Robert W. Conn, PhD, President & CEO*
*Eric Marshall, VP, Public Engagement & Prizes*

2648 **Kavli Institute for Brain Science at Columbia University**
Columbia University
3227 Broadway 212-853-1016
New York, NY 10027 Fax: 212-665-9699
kavli@columbia.edu
www.kavli.columbia.edu
The Institute's primary arc of study is how signaling in neural circuits controls cognitive function and behavior, and the development of novel experimental and computational strategies for analyzing these signals.
*Eric R. Kandel, MD, Director*
*Rafael Yuste, MD, PhD, Co-Director*

2649 **Neuroscience Research Institute**
UC Santa Barbara
6129 Biology II 805-893-4621
Santa Barbara, CA 93106 www.nri.ucsb.edu
The Institute seeks to allow scientists from different fields to collaborate for the betterment of neurological research. Areas of interest include: Alzheimer's Disease & Related Dementias; Behavioral Neuroscience & Neuroethology; Cell Biology, Biochemistry & Biophysics of the Nervous System; Computational & Theoretical Neuroscience; Development of the Nervous System; and Stem Cells.
*Stuart Feinstein, Co-Director*
*Kenneth Kosik, Co-Director*

2650 **Salk Institute for Biological Studies**
10010 N Torrey Pines Road 858-453-4100
La Jolla, CA 92037 www.salk.edu
Conducts groundbreaking research into cancer, aging, Alzheimer's diabetes and infectious diseases.
*Rusty Gage, PhD, President*
*Martin Hetzer, PhD, VP & Chief Science Officer*

2651 **Sanford Consortium for Regenerative Medicine**
2880 Torrey Pines Scenic Drive 858-246-1071
La Jolla, CA 92037 www.sanfordconsortium.com
The Consortium works to achieve breakthrough discoveries in stem cell research with regards to diagnoses, treatments, and cures for degenerative diseases and injuries.
*Edward W. Holmes, MD, President & CEO*
*Jeffrey Steindorf, PhD, VP & COO*

2652 **Scripps Research Institute**
10550 North Torrey Pines Road 858-784-1000
La Jolla, CA www.scripps.edu
The institute seeks to improve human wellbeing through the advancement of bioscience, including research into aging & healthspan, autoimmune diseases, cancer, infectious diseases, neurological disorders, and more.
*Peter Schultz, PhD, President & CEO*
*Eric Topol, MD, EVP, Scripps Research*

## Magazines

2653 **ASN NEURO**
Sage Journals
2455 Teller Road 805-499-9774
Thousand Oaks, CA 91320 journals@sagepub.com
journals.sagepub.com/home/asn
Peer-reviewed open access journal focusing on recent advances in the cellular and molecular neurosciences. It is the official publication of the American Society for Neurochemistry.
*Douglas L. Feinstein, Editor-in-Chief*
*Sandra J. Hewitt, Deputy Editor-in-Chief*

2654 **American Journal of Pathology**
Elsevier
1600 John F Kennedy Boulevard 301-634-7959
Philadelphia, PA 19103 Fax: 301-634-7961
ajp@asip.org
ajp.amjpathol.org
Official journal of the American Society for Investigative Pathology, publishing original research reports, reviews, and commentaries related to the molecular and cellular basis of disease.
*Martha Furie, Editor-in-Chief*

2655 **BMC Neuroscience**
Springer Nature
One New York Plaza 800-777-4643
New York, NY 10004-1562 info@biomedcentral.com
bmcneurosci.biomedcentral.com
A peer-reviewed, open-access journal devoted to all aspects of the nervous system (including molecular, cellular, developmental and

animal model studies), as well as cognitive and behavioral research, and computational modeling.
*Darren Byrne, Editor*
*Ana Donnelly, Manuscript Editor*

2656 **Brain & Life**
American Academy of Neurology
201 Chicago Avenue 612-928-6000
Minneapolis, MN 55415 800-879-1960
Fax: 612-454-2748
BrainandLife@wolterskluwer.com
www.brainandlife.org
Official magazine of the American Academy of Neurology, aimed at parents and home-caregivers interested in neurology in everyday life.
*Orly Avitzur, MD, MBA, FAAN, Editor-in-Chief*
*Mary Bolster, Managing Editor*

2657 **Brain: A Journal of Neurology**
Oxford University Press
2001 Evans Road 919-677-0977
Cary, NC 27513 800-852-7323
Fax: 919-677-1714
brain@ucl.ac.uk
academic.oup.com/brain
Focus is clinical neurology and translational neuroscience.
*Dimitri M. Kullmann, Editor*
*Joanne Bell, Managing Editor*

2658 **Continuum: Lifelong Learning in Neurology**
American Academy of Neurology
201 Chicago Avenue 612-928-6000
Minneapolis, MN 55415 800-879-1960
continuumcme@aan.com
journals.lww.com/continuum
Official journal of the American Academy of Neurology, aiding professionals in patient care and continuing education.
*Bimonthly*
*Steven L. Lewis, MD, FAAN*
*Andrea J. Weiss, MA, Executive Editor*

2659 **JNeurosci**
Society for Neuroscience
1121 14th Street NW 202-962-4000
Washginton, DC 20005 jn@sfn.org
www.jneurosci.org
Official peer-reviewed journal of the Society for Neuroscience, publishing research on a broad range of topics of interest to those working on the nervous system.
*Marina R. Picciotto, Editor-in-Chief*
*Teresa Esch, Features Editor*

2660 **Journal of Alzheimer's Disease**
IOS Press
6751 Tepper Drive 703-830-6300
Clifton, VA 20124 Fax: 703-830-2300
editorial@j-alz.com
www.j-alz.com
Research into the etiology, pathogenesis, epidemiology, genetics, behavior, treatment and psychology of Alzheimer's disease.
*George Perry, PhD, Editor-in-Chief*
*Beth Kumar, Managing Editor*

2661 **Journal of Molecular Diagnostics**
Elsevier
1600 John F Kennedy Boulevard 301-634-7959
Philadelphia, PA 19103 Fax: 301-634-7961
jmd@asip.org
jmd.amjpathol.org
Official journal of the American Society for Investigative Pathology and the Association for Molecular Pathology, focusing on molecular discoveries in medicine translating into the clinical diagnostic setting, as well as the description and application of technological advances in the field of molecular diagnostic medicine.
*Monthly*
*Barbara Zehnbauer, PhD, Editor-in-Chief*

2662 **Journal of NeuroEngineering and Rehabilitation**
Springer Nature
One New York Plaza 800-777-4643
New York, NY 10004-1562 info@biomedcentral.com
jneuroengrehab.biomedcentral.com
An open-access journal devoted to integrated research from the fields of neuroscience, biomedical engineering, and physical medicine and rehabilitation.
*David J. Reinkensmeyer, Editor-in-Chief*

2663 **Journal of Neurodevelopmental Disorders**
Springer Nature
One New York Plaza 800-777-4643
New York, NY 10004-1562 info@biomedcentral.com
jneurodevdisorders.biomedcentral.com
An open-access journal devoted to integrating research from neurobiology, genetics, cognitive neuroscience, psychiatry and psychology.
*Joseph Piven, Editor-in-Chief*

2664 **Journal of Neuroinflammation**
Springer Nature
One New York Plaza 800-777-4643
New York, NY 10004-1562 info@biomedcentral.com
jneuroinflammation.biomedcentral.com
A peer-reviewed, open-access journal focusing on the interactions of the immune system with the nervous system as a means of expanding understanding of chronic neurological diseases.
*Monica J. Carson, Editor-in-Chief*
*Sue T. Griffin, Editor-in-Chief*

2665 **Journal of Nuclear Medicine**
Society of Nuclear Medicine and Molecular Imaging
1850 Samuel Morse Drive 703-708-9000
Reston, VA 20190 800-513-6853
Fax: 703-708-9015
subscriptions@snm.org
jnm.snmjournals.org
Peer-reviewed journal with clinical investigations, science reports, articles benefitting continuing education, book reviews, employment opportunities, and updates on practice and research.
*Monthly*
*Johannes Czernin, MD, Editor-in-Chief*
*Susan Alexander, Associate Director, Publications*

2666 **Journal of Nuclear Medicine Technology**
Society of Nuclear Medicine and Molecular Imaging
1850 Samuel Morse Drive 703-708-9000
Reston, VA 20190 800-513-6853
Fax: 703-708-9015
subscriptions@snm.org
tech.snmjournals.org
Peer-reviewed journal dedicated to nuclear medicine technology, with information on credentialing, continuing education and licensure requirements, as well as current news and updates on the field.
*Quarterly*
*Kathy S. Thomas, MHA, CNMT, PET, Editor-in-Chief*
*Susan Alexander, Associate Director, Publications*

2667 **Journal of the Neurological Sciences**
Elsevier
LSU Health Sciences Center JNS_England@lsuhsc.edu
New Orleans, LA 70112 www.jns-journal.com
Original articles in neurology and neuroscience from around the world.
*Monthly*
*John D. England, Editor-in-Chief*

2668 **Molecular Imaging**
Sage Journals
2455 Teller Road 805-499-9774
Thousand Oaks, CA 91320 journals@sagepub.com
journals.sagepub.com/home/mix
Peer-reviewed open access journal focusing on molecular imaging research, including basic science, preclinical studies and human applications. Published in association with the Society of Nuclear Medicine and Molecular Imaging.
*Bimonthly*
*Henry F. VanBrocklin, PhD, Editor-in-Chief*

**2669 Molecular Neurodegeneration**
Springer Nature
One New York Plaza 800-777-4643
New York, NY 10004-1562 info@biomedcentral.com
www.biomedcentral.com
A peer-reviewed, open-access journal devoted to all aspects of neurodegeneration research at the molecular and cellular levels.
*Guojun Bu, Editor-in-Chief*
*Huaxi Xu, Editor-in-Chief*

**2670 Neurocase: The Neural Basis of Cognition**
Taylor & Francis Group
530 Walnut Street www.tandfonline.com/toc/nncs20/current
Philadelphia, PA 19106
Rapid response journal featuring case and group studies in neuropsychology, neuropsychiatry and behavioral neurology, with a focus on the neural basis of cognition.
*Bruce L. Miller, Editor*
*Hans J. Markowitsch, Editor*

**2671 Neurology**
American Academy of Neurology
201 Chicago Avenue 612-928-6000
Minneapolis, MN 55415 800-879-1960
Fax: 612-454-2748
journal@neurology.org
n.neurology.org
Official journal of the American Academy of Neurology, peer-reviewed, highlighting clinical neurology research.
*Jose G. Merino, MD, MPhil, FAAN, Editor-in-Chief*
*Patricia K. Baskin, MS, Executive Editor*

**2672 Neurology Clinical Practice**
American Academy of Neurology
201 Chicago Avenue 612-928-6000
Minneapolis, MN 55415 800-879-1960
Fax: 612-454-2748
journal@neurology.org
cp.neurology.org
Official peer-reviewed journal of the American Academy of Neurology for practicing neurologists.
*John R. Corboy, MD, FAAN, Editor*
*Patricia K. Baskin, MS, Executive Editor*

**2673 Neurology: Genetics**
American Academy of Neurology
201 Chicago Avenue 612-928-6000
Minneapolis, MN 55415 800-879-1960
Fax: 612-454-2748
journal@neurology.org
ng.neurology.org
Official journal of the American Academy of Neurology, publishing online open-access peer-reviewed reports in the field of neurogenetics.
*Stefan M. Pulst, MD, FAAN, Editor*
*Patricia K. Baskin, MS, Executive Editor*

**2674 Neurology: Neuroimmunology & Neuroinflammation**
American Academy of Neurology
201 Chicago Avenue 612-928-6000
Minneapolis, MN 55415 800-879-1960
Fax: 612-454-2748
journal@neurology.org
nn.neurology.org
Official journal of the American Academy of Neurology, publishing online open-access peer-reviewed reports of original research and in-depth reviews of topics in neuroimmunology & neuroinflammation.
*Josep O. Dalmau, MD, PhD, Editor*
*Patricia K. Baskin, MS, Executive Editor*

**2675 Society of Nuclear Medicine and Molecular Imaging**
1850 Samuel Morse Drive 703-708-9000
Reston, VA 20190 Fax: 703-708-9015
feedback@snmmi.org
www.snmmi.org
The mission of this nonprofit scientific and professional organization is to promote the science, technology and application of nuclear medicine and molecular imaging. Molecular imaging techniques are used to diagnose and manage the treatment of brain disorders such as Alzheimer's and Parkinson's disease, among other conditions.
*15,000 members*
*Virginia Pappas, CEO*
*Rebecca Maxey, Director, Communications*

**2676 Translational Neurodegeneration**
Springer Nature
One New York Plaza 800-777-4643
New York, NY 10004-1562 info@biomedcentral.com
www.biomedcentral.com
A peer-reviewed, open-access journal covering research, therapeutics and education for all areas of neurodegenerative diseases.
*Shengdi Chen, Editor-in-Chief*

**2677 Ultrasonic Imaging**
Sage Journals
2455 Teller Road 805-499-9774
Thousand Oaks, CA 91320 journals@sagepub.com
journals.sagepub.com/home/uix
The journal focuses on the rapid publication of original papers on the development and application of ultrasonic techniques, with emphasis on medical diagnosis. Also published are research notes, comments on papers appearing in the journal, book reviews, and occasional review articles.
*Ernest J. Feleppa, Editor-in-Chief*
*Roslyn Raskin, Managing Editor*

**2678 eNeuro**
Society for Neuroscience
1121 14th Street NW 202-312-7305
Washginton, DC 20005 eNeuro@sfn.org
www.eneuro.org
Open-access journal of the Society for Neuroscience.
*Christophe Bernard, Editor-in-Chief*
*Kelly Newton, Director, Scientific Publications*

## Web Sites

**2679 BrainFacts.org**
Society for Neuroscience
1121 14th Street NW brainfactsinfo@sfn.org
Washington, DC 20005 brainfacts.org
Online public information portal founded by the Kavli Foundation, the Gatsby Charitable Foundation and the Society for Neuroscience, with topics on brain function and anatomy, diseases and disorders, and more.
*Richard Wingate, DPhil, Editor-in-Chief*
*Charles Yokoyama, PhD, Associate Editor*

**2680 Neuronline**
Society for Neuroscience
1121 14th Street NW 202-962-4000
Washginton, DC 20005 neuronline@sfn.org
neuronline.sfn.org
Online portal for professional development and training resources for individuals in the field of neuroscience, hosted by the Society for Neuroscience.
*Amanda Kimball, Director, Digital Learning*

# WERNICKE-KORSAKOFF SYNDROME

*Wernicke-Korsakoff syndrome is a neurodegenerative disorder that results from a vitamin B1 (thiamine) deficiency. Technically two related conditions that occur together, WKS consists of Wernicke encephalopathy and Korsakoff syndrome. Both result in cognitive malfunction, with Korsakoff syndrome resulting in more serious and lasting conditions such as loss of memory, hallucinations, and dementia. WKS is most commonly the result of alcohol misuse.*

Vitamin B1 (thiamine) helps brain cells convert sugar into energy. When the body does not get enough B1, brain cells cannot function properly and, in extreme cases, can lead to the rare condition known as Wernicke-Korsakoff syndrome. Most WKS patients first develop Wernicke encephalopathy, an acute brain reaction to the lack of B1. A life-threatening condition, Wernicke encephalopathy results in confusion, loss of muscle coordination, and vision changes. If untreated, it can lead to coma and death, and patients who seek medical attention are immediately given an injection of B1. About 85 percent of patients who develop Wernicke encephalopathy then go on to suffer from Korsakoff syndrome, although it is possible to develop Korsakoff syndrome without experiencing Wernicke encephalopathy. The symptoms of Korsakoff syndrome include the inability to form new memories, severe memory loss, confabulation (a tendency to make up stories that are not true but which the patient believes), hallucinations, and dementia.

Wernicke-Korsakoff syndrome is most commonly caused by alcohol misuse, which severely depletes the body's supply of vitamin B1, but it can also be associated with other conditions such as AIDS, cancer, chronic infections, and poor nutrition. Patients who have had bariatric surgery may also be at risk for WKS. Diagnosis of Korsakoff syndrome is difficult as there are no specific tests available to confirm the disorder. In addition, many of the symptoms mirror those of other conditions suffered by people who abuse alcohol, such as withdrawal or memory loss. Typically, any patient admitted to the hospital for an alcohol-related condition will be screened for memory loss and cognitive changes to rule out WKS.

Treatment of Wernicke encephalopathy, an acute condition, requires the immediate injection of vitamin B1 into the patient's vein. This prevents the patient from dying and the symptoms typically improve rapidly. If the patient then develops Korsakoff syndrome, a regimen of oral supplements of B1 and other vitamins is typically prescribed. In addition, if the disease is brought on by alcohol misuse, it is highly recommended that patient refrain from further consumption of alcohol. The prognosis for patients with Korsakoff syndrome is relatively good, with 25 percent of patients recovering fully, 50 percent improving but not completely recovering, and 25 percent remaining unchanged. Studies suggest that a patient with Korsakoff syndrome may experience a normal life expectancy, provided they give up alcohol.

## National Agencies & Associations

2682 **American Academy of Neurology**
201 Chicago Avenue 612-928-6000
Minneapolis, MN 55415 800-879-1960
Fax: 612-454-2746
memberservices@aan.com
www.aan.com
Professional society of medical doctors specializing in brain and nervous system diseases. Maintains placement service. Sponsors research and educational programs. Compiles statistics. Publishes scientific journal, Continuum: Lifelong Learning in Neurology.
*Mary E. Post, MBA, CAE, CEO*

2683 **American Society for Neurochemistry**
9037 Ron Den Lane 407-909-9064
Windermere, FL 34786 Fax: 407-876-0750
asnmanager@asneurochem.org
asneurochem.org
The Society aims to advance and promote cellular and molecular neuroscience knowledge, and to facilitate communication and the dissemination of information within the field and with related disciplines.
*Sheilah Jewart, Executive Director*
*Karen Gottlieb, Conference Coordinator*

## Foundations & Research Centers

2684 **Neuroscience Research Institute**
UC Santa Barbara
6129 Biology II 805-893-4621
Santa Barbara, CA 93106 www.nri.ucsb.edu
The Institute seeks to allow scientists from different fields to collaborate for the betterment of neurological research. Areas of interest include: Alzheimer's Disease & Related Dementias; Behavioral Neuroscience & Neuroethology; Cell Biology, Biochemistry & Biophysics of the Nervous System; Computational & Theoretical Neuroscience; Development of the Nervous System; and Stem Cells.
*Stuart Feinstein, Co-Director*
*Kenneth Kosik, Co-Director*

2685 **Sanford Consortium for Regenerative Medicine**
2880 Torrey Pines Scenic Drive 858-246-1071
La Jolla, CA 92037 www.sanfordconsortium.com
The Consortium works to achieve breakthrough discoveries in stem cell research with regards to diagnoses, treatments, and cures for degenerative diseases and injuries.
*Edward W. Holmes, MD, President & CEO*
*Jeffrey Steindorf, PhD, VP & COO*

## Magazines

2686 **ASN NEURO**
Sage Journals
2455 Teller Road 805-499-9774
Thousand Oaks, CA 91320 journals@sagepub.com
journals.sagepub.com/home/asn
Peer-reviewed open access journal focusing on recent advances in the cellular and molecular neurosciences. It is the official publication of the American Society for Neurochemistry.
*Douglas L. Feinstein, Editor-in-Chief*
*Sandra J. Hewitt, Deputy Editor-in-Chief*

2687 **BMC Neuroscience**
Springer Nature
One New York Plaza 800-777-4643
New York, NY 10004-1562 info@biomedcentral.com
bmcneurosci.biomedcentral.com
A peer-reviewed, open-access journal devoted to all aspects of the nervous system (including molecular, cellular, developmental and animal model studies), as well as cognitive and behavioral research, and computational modeling.
*Darren Byrne, Editor*
*Ana Donnelly, Manuscript Editor*

2688 **Brain & Life**
American Academy of Neurology
201 Chicago Avenue 612-928-6000
Minneapolis, MN 55415 800-879-1960
Fax: 612-454-2748
BrainandLife@wolterskluwer.com
www.brainandlife.org
Official magazine of the American Academy of Neurology, aimed at parents and home-caregivers interested in neurology in everyday life.
*Orly Avitzur, MD, MBA, FAAN, Editor-in-Chief*
*Mary Bolster, Managing Editor*

2689 **Brain: A Journal of Neurology**
Oxford University Press
2001 Evans Road 919-677-0977
Cary, NC 27513 800-852-7323
Fax: 919-677-1714
brain@ucl.ac.uk
academic.oup.com/brain
Focus is clinical neurology and translational neuroscience.
*Dimitri M. Kullmann, Editor*
*Joanne Bell, Managing Editor*

2690 **Continuum: Lifelong Learning in Neurology**
American Academy of Neurology
201 Chicago Avenue 612-928-6000
Minneapolis, MN 55415 800-879-1960
continuumcme@aan.com
journals.lww.com/continuum
Official journal of the American Academy of Neurology, aiding professionals in patient care and continuing education.
*Bimonthly*
*Steven L. Lewis, MD, FAAN*
*Andrea J. Weiss, MA, Executive Editor*

2691 **Dementia and Geriatric Cognitive Disorders**
S. Karger Publishers, Inc.
26 W Avon Road 860-675-7834
Unionville, CT 06085 800-828-5479
Fax: 860-675-7302
www.karger.com/DEM
Open-access journal devoted to the study of cognitive dysfunction in preclinical and clinical studies, concentrating on Alzheimer's and Parkinson's disease, Huntington's chorea and other neurodegenerative diseases.
*Victoria Chan-Pilay, Editor-in-Chief*

2692 **Journal of Nuclear Medicine**
Society of Nuclear Medicine and Molecular Imaging
1850 Samuel Morse Drive 703-708-9000
Reston, VA 20190 800-513-6853
Fax: 703-708-9015
subscriptions@snm.org
jnm.snmjournals.org
Peer-reviewed journal with clinical investigations, science reports, articles benefitting continuing education, book reviews, employment opportunities, and updates on practice and research.
*Monthly*
*Johannes Czernin, MD, Editor-in-Chief*
*Susan Alexander, Associate Director, Publications*

2693 **Journal of Nuclear Medicine Technology**
Society of Nuclear Medicine and Molecular Imaging
1850 Samuel Morse Drive 703-708-9000
Reston, VA 20190 800-513-6853
Fax: 703-708-9015
subscriptions@snm.org
tech.snmjournals.org
Peer-reviewed journal dedicated to nuclear medicine technology, with information on credentialing, continuing education and licensure requirements, as well as current news and updates on the field.
*Quarterly*
*Kathy S. Thomas, MHA, CNMT, PET, Editor-in-Chief*
*Susan Alexander, Associate Director, Publications*

2694 **Journal of the Neurological Sciences**
Elsevier

LSU Health Sciences Center JNS_England@lsuhsc.edu
New Orleans, LA 70112 www.jns-journal.com
Original articles in neurology and neuroscience from around the world.
*Monthly*
*John D. England, Editor-in-Chief*

2695 **Molecular Imaging**
Sage Journals
2455 Teller Road 805-499-9774
Thousand Oaks, CA 91320 journals@sagepub.com
journals.sagepub.com/home/mix
Peer-reviewed open access journal focusing on molecular imaging research, including basic science, preclinical studies and human applications. Published in association with the Society of Nuclear Medicine and Molecular Imaging.
*Bimonthly*
*Henry F. VanBrocklin, PhD, Editor-in-Chief*

2696 **Molecular Neurodegeneration**
Springer Nature
One New York Plaza 800-777-4643
New York, NY 10004-1562 info@biomedcentral.com
www.biomedcentral.com
A peer-reviewed, open-access journal devoted to all aspects of neurodegeneration research at the molecular and cellular levels.
*Guojun Bu, Editor-in-Chief*
*Huaxi Xu, Editor-in-Chief*

2697 **Neurocase: The Neural Basis of Cognition**
Taylor & Francis Group
530 Walnut Street www.tandfonline.com/toc/nncs20/current
Philadelphia, PA 19106
Rapid response journal featuring case and group studies in neuropsychology, neuropsychiatry and behavioral neurology, with a focus on the neural basis of cognition.
*Bruce L. Miller, Editor*
*Hans J. Markowitsch, Editor*

2698 **Neurology**
American Academy of Neurology
201 Chicago Avenue 612-928-6000
Minneapolis, MN 55415 800-879-1960
Fax: 612-454-2748
journal@neurology.org
n.neurology.org
Official journal of the American Academy of Neurology, peer-reviewed, highlighting clinical neurology research.
*Jose G. Merino, MD, MPhil, FAAN, Editor-in-Chief*
*Patricia K. Baskin, MS, Executive Editor*

2699 **Neurology Clinical Practice**
American Academy of Neurology
201 Chicago Avenue 612-928-6000
Minneapolis, MN 55415 800-879-1960
Fax: 612-454-2748
journal@neurology.org
cp.neurology.org
Official peer-reviewed journal of the American Academy of Neurology for practicing neurologists.
*John R. Corboy, MD, FAAN, Editor*
*Patricia K. Baskin, MS, Executive Editor*

2700 **Neurology: Genetics**
American Academy of Neurology
201 Chicago Avenue 612-928-6000
Minneapolis, MN 55415 800-879-1960
Fax: 612-454-2748
journal@neurology.org
ng.neurology.org
Official journal of the American Academy of Neurology, publishing online open-access peer-reviewed reports in the field of neurogenetics.
*Stefan M. Pulst, MD, FAAN, Editor*
*Patricia K. Baskin, MS, Executive Editor*

2701 **Neurology: Neuroimmunology & Neuroinflammation**
American Academy of Neurology
201 Chicago Avenue 612-928-6000
Minneapolis, MN 55415 800-879-1960
Fax: 612-454-2748
journal@neurology.org
nn.neurology.org
Official journal of the American Academy of Neurology, publishing online open-access peer-reviewed reports of original research and in-depth reviews of topics in neuroimmunology & neuroinflammation.
*Josep O. Dalmau, MD, PhD, Editor*
*Patricia K. Baskin, MS, Executive Editor*

2702 **Society of Nuclear Medicine and Molecular Imaging**
1850 Samuel Morse Drive 703-708-9000
Reston, VA 20190 Fax: 703-708-9015
feedback@snmmi.org
www.snmmi.org
The mission of this nonprofit scientific and professional organization is to promote the science, technology and application of nuclear medicine and molecular imaging. Molecular imaging techniques are used to diagnose and manage the treatment of brain disorders such as Alzheimer's and Parkinson's disease, among other conditions.
*15,000 members*
*Virginia Pappas, CEO*
*Rebecca Maxey, Director, Communications*

2703 **Ultrasonic Imaging**
Sage Journals
2455 Teller Road 805-499-9774
Thousand Oaks, CA 91320 journals@sagepub.com
journals.sagepub.com/home/uix
The journal focuses on the rapid publication of original papers on the development and application of ultrasonic techniques, with emphasis on medical diagnosis. Also published are research notes, comments on papers appearing in the journal, book reviews, and occasional review articles.
*Ernest J. Feleppa, Editor-in-Chief*
*Roslyn Raskin, Managing Editor*

# MEDICATION

## Drugs A-Z

2704 **Abilify**
Generic: aripiprazole
Used in the treatment of psychotic disorders and bipolar disorder. This product is manufactured by Bristol-Myers Squibb and Otsuka. See manufacturers section for company information.

2705 **Adderall/Adderall XR**
Generic: amphetamine/dextroamphetamine
Used to manage anxiety disorders and some cases of attention deficit hyperactivity disorder. This product is manufactured by Shire Richwood. See Manufacturers section for company information.

2706 **Antabuse**
Generic: disulfiram
Used in the treatment of alcohol and substance abuse. This product is manufactured by Wyeth-Ayers. See Manufacturers section for company information.

2707 **Aricept**
Generic: donepezil
Used in the treatment of Alzheimer's disease. This product is manufactured by Eisai. See Manufacturers section for company information.

2708 **Asenapine**
Generic: saphris
Sublingual tablets used in the treatment for schizophreina. Manufactured by Schering-Plough. See Manufacturers section for company information.

2709 **Ativan**
Generic: lorazepam
Used in the treatment of anxiety and as a preanesthetic medication in adults. This product is manufactured by Wyeth. See Manufacturers section for company information.

2710 **Celexa**
Generic: citalopram
Used in the treatment of depression. This product is manufactured by Forest Laboratories. See Manufacturers section for company information.

2711 **Clozaril**
Generic: clozapine
Used in the treatment of severe schizophrenia, and also sold as Clozaril and Fazaclo. This product is manufactured by Novartis. See Manufacturers section for company information.

2712 **Cymbalta**
Generic: dulozetine
Used in the treatment of depression. Manufactured by Eli Lilly and Company. See Manufacturers section for company information.

2713 **Daytrana**
Generic: methyphenidate transdermal system
Used in the treatment of ADHD in children 6-17 years old. This product is manufactured by Noven Pharmaceuticals. See Manufacturers section for company information.

2714 **Depakote**
Generic: valproic acid
Used in the treatment of manic episodes associated with bipolar disorder and mania, and also sold as Depakene. This product is manufactured by Abbott Laboratories. See Manufacturers section for company information.

2715 **Desoxyn**
Generic: methamphetamine
Used in the treatment of attention deficit hyperactivity disorder. This product is manufactured by Abbott Laboratories. See Manufacturers section for company information.

2716 **Desyrel**
Generic: trazodone hcl
Used in the treatment of major depressive disorder. This product is manufactured by Labopharm Europe Limited. See manufacturers section for company information.

2717 **Dexedrine**
Generic: dextroamphetamine
Used in the treatment of attention deficit hyperactivity disorder, and also sold as DextroState, Focalin (by Novartis), Metadate, and Methylin. This product is manufactured by Mallinckrodt. See Manufacturers section for company information.

2718 **Effexor**
Generic: venlafazine
Used in the treatment of depression and generalized anxiety disorder. This product is manufactured by Wyeth-Ayerst Laboratories. See Manufacturers section for company information.

2719 **Elavil**
Generic: amitryptiline
Used in the treatment of depression, also sold as Limbitrol (by Valeant). This product is manufactured by Astra Zeneca Pharmaceuticals. See Manufacturers section for company information.

2720 **Emsam**
Generic: selegiline
Used in the treatment of major depressive disorder. This product is manufactured by Bristol-Myers Squibb. See manufacturers section for company information.

2721 **Eskalith**
Generic: lithium
Used in the treatment of bipolar disorder. This product is manufactured by GlaxoSmithKline. See Manufacturers section for company information.

2722 **Exelon**
Generic: rivastigmine
Used in the treatment of Alzheimer's disease. This product is manufactured by Novartis. See Manufacturers section for company information.

2723 **FazaClo**
Generic: clozapine, USP
Used in the treatment of Schizophrenia. This product is manufactured by Jazz Pharmaceuticals plc. See Manufacturers section for company information.

2724 **Fluoxetine Tablets, 60 mg**
Used in the treatment of Major Depressive Disorder, Obsessive Compulsive Disorder in adults and pediatrics and Bulimia Nervosa and Panic Disorder is adults. This product is manufactured by Edgemont Pharmaceuticals. See Manufacturers section for company information.

2725 **Focalin/Focalin XR**
Generic: dexmethylphenidate
Used in the treatment of attention deficit hyperactivity disorder. This product is manufactured by Novartis. See Manufacturers section for company information.

2726 **Haldol**
Generic: haloperidol
Used in the treatment of Schizophrenia. This product is manufactured by Johnson & Johnson. See manufacturers section for company information.

2727 **Intermezzo**
Generic: zolpidem
Used in the treatment of insomnia. This product is manufactured by Purdue/Transcept. See Manufacturers section for company information.

2728 **Invega**
Generic: paliperidone

Used in the treatment of Schizophrenia. This product is manufactured by Janssen. See manufacturers section for company information.

2729 **Klonopin**
Generic: clonazepam
Used in the treatment of panic attacks/anxiety. This product is manufactured by Hoffman-La Roche. See Manufacturers section for company information.

2730 **Lamictal**
Generic: lamotrigine
Used in the treatment of bipolar disorder. This product is manufactured by GlaxoSmithKline. See Manufacturers section for company information.

2731 **Latuda**
Generic: lurasidone hcl
Used in the treatment of schizophrenia. This product is manufactured by Sunovion. See manufacturers section for company information.

2732 **Lexapro**
Generic: escitalopram
Used in the treatment of depression. This product is manufactured by Forest Laboratories. See Manufacturers section for company information.

2733 **Lithobid**
Generic: lithium carbonate
Used in the treatment of bipolar disorder and depression. This product is manufactured by Noven Pharmaceuticals. See Manufacturers section for company information.

2734 **Lunesta**
Generic: eszopiclone
Used in the treatment of insomnia. This product is manufactured by Sunovion Pharmaceuticals. See Manufacturers section for company information.

2735 **Namenda**
Generic: memantine
Used in the treatment of dementia. This product is manufactured by Forest Pharmaceuticals. See Manufacturers section for company information.

2736 **Neurontin**
Generic: gabapentin
Used in the treatment of seizures and neuropathic pais. This product is manufactured by Pfizer. See Manufacturers section for company information.

2737 **Niravam**
Generic: alprazolam
Used in the treatment of anxiety. This product is manufactured by Jazz Pharmaceuticals plc. See Manufacturers section for company information.

2738 **Parnate**
Generic: tranylcypromine
Used to help manage depression. This product is manufactured by GlaxoSmithKline. See Manufacturers section for company information.

2739 **Paxil**
Generic: paroxetine hcl
Used in the treatment of depression, and anxiety disorders. This product is manufactured by GlaxoSmithKline. Sold also as Pexeva by Synthon. See Manufacturers section for company information.

2740 **Pexeva**
Generic: paroxetine mesylate
Used in the treatment of depression, and anxiety disorders. This product is manufactured by Noven Pharmaceuticals. See Manufacturers section for company information.

2741 **Pristiq**
Generic: Desvenlafaxine
Used in the treatment of depression. Manufacturered by Pfizer. See Manufacturers section for company information.

2742 **Prozac**
Generic: fluozetine
Used in the treatment of depression and anxiety disorders. This product is manufactured by Eli Lilly and Company. See Manufacturers section for company information.

2743 **Relpax**
Generic: eletriptan
Used in the treatment of migraines. This product is manufactured by Pfizer. See Manufacturers section for company information.

2744 **Remeron**
Generic: mirtazapine
Used in the treatment of suicidality and depression. This product is manufactured by Merck & Co. See Manufacturers section for company information.

2745 **Restoril**
Generic: temazepam
Used in the treatment of insomnia. This product is manufactured by Mallinckrodt Pharmaceuticals Group. See manufacturers section for company information.

2746 **Risperdal**
Generic: risperidone
Used in the treatment of schizophrenia and other mental illnesses such as psychosis. This product is manufactured by Janssen. See Manufacturers section for company information.

2747 **Ritalin**
Generic: methylphenidate
Used in the treatment of attention deficit hyperactivity disorders and in some forms of narcolepsy. This product is manufactured by Novartis. See Manufacturers section for company information.

2748 **Rozerem**
Generic: ramelteon
Used in the treatment of insomnia. This product is manufactured by Takeda Pharmaceuticals. See Manufacturers section for company information.

2749 **Saphris**
Generic: asenapine
Used in the treatment of Schizophrenia and Bipolar Mania. This product is manufactured by Merck & Co. See Manufacturers section for company information.

2750 **Sarafem**
Generic: fluoxetine
Used in the treatment of premenstrual dysphoric disorder. This product is manufactured by Warner Chilcott. See Manufacturers section for company information.

2751 **Stavzor**
Generic: valproic acid
Used in the treatment of bipolar disorder. This product is manufactured by Noven Pharmaceuticals. See Manufacturers section for company information.

2752 **Strattera**
Generic: atomoxetine
Used in the treatment of attention deficit disorder. This product is manufactured by Eli Lilly & Company. See Manufacturers section for company information.

2753 **Valium**
Generic: diazepam
Used in the treatment of anxiety. This product is manufactured by Hoffman-La Roche. See Manufacturers section for company information.

2754 **Viibryd**
Generic: vilazodone HCI
Used in the treatment of depression. This product is manufactured by Forest Pharmacuecticals. See manufacturers section for company information.

2755 **Vyvanse**
Generic: lixdexamfetamine
Used in the treatment of attention deficit hyperactivity disorder. This product is manufactured by Shire Richwood. See Manufacturers section for company information.

2756 **Wellbutrin, Wellbutrin SR, Wellbutrin XL**
Generic: bupropion
Used in the treatment of depression. This product is manufactured by Sanofi-Aventis. See Manufacturers section for company information.

2757 **Xanax**
Generic: alprazolam
Used in the treatment of anxiety. This product is manufactured by Pfizer. See Manufacturers section for company information.

2758 **Xyrem**
Generic: sodium oxybate
Used in the treatment of narcolepsy. This product is manufactured by Jazz Pharmaceuticals. See Manufacturers section for company information.

2759 **Zoloft**
Generic: sertraline
Used in the treatment of depression and anxiety disorders. This product is manufactured by Pfizer. See Manufacturers section for company information.

# MEDIAGRAPHY

## FILM, FICTION, TELEVISION & MUSIC

The following compiles media portrayals of the complex issues of dementia. Media includes movies, TV, books of fiction, plays, and music. Critical aspects and themes related to dementia are explored in the context of relationships—whether between spouses, parents and children, or grandparents and children—and of memories. This list is by no means comprehensive, but rather meant to be representative of the many portrayals of dementia in popular media.

### FILMS

*Age Old Friends* (1989), directed by Allan Kroeker. This film, starring Hume Cronyn, Vincent Gardenia, Esther Rolle, and Tandy Cronyn, is about a man who turns down a chance to live with his daughter in favor of residing at a retirement home. Once at the home, he enjoys a close friendship with another resident, only to find that his friend is beginning to experience senility. The main character's struggle to decide whether to stay in the home to help his friend or to go to his daughter's home becomes the crux of this film whose primary themes are loyalty, friendship, personal meaning, and the decisions elders make later in life.

*Aurora Borealis* (2005), set in Minneapolis, Minnesota, follows Duncan (Joshua Jackson) as he struggles with the death of his father and his fears of letting go of his past. His grandfather, Ron (Donald Sutherland), is deteriorating with Alzheimer's disease and believes he can see the Northern Lights from his balcony. Duncan begins to help Ron in coping with his condition, eventually falling in love with Ron's home assistant, Kate (Juliette Lewis), finding something to live for.

*Away from Her* (2006), Julie Christie (1940–) plays Fiona who has been happily married for many years to Grant (Gordon Pinsent). When Fiona's Alzheimer's worsens, she goes to a nursing home. When Grant visits her, he finds that she barely knows him and has grown attached to another man, a fellow resident at the home.

*Barney's Version* (2010), directed by Richard J. Lewis, was nominated for the Golden Lion at the 67th Venice International Film Awards. The film spans three decades, focusing on the wild and politically incorrect life of Barney Panofsky (Paul Giamatti). The film follows Barney as he marries three times, has children, and eventually begins to suffer from memory loss and dementia.

*Choke* (2008) is a black comedy film written and directed by Clark Gregg. It tells the story of a man who works in a colonial theme park, attends sexual addiction recovery meetings, and intentionally chokes on food in upscale restaurants so his "rescuers" would give him money out of sympathy and thus cover his mother's Alzheimer's disease hospital bills.

*Coco* (2017) is a Disney-Pixar 3D animated film that follows the lives and deaths of a family living in Mexico. The matriarch of the family is Coco and suffering from old age and dementia. The film shows the importance of remembering those we've lost, and what may happen if we forget. "Remember Me" is the main song from the movie and won Best Original Song at the 90th Academy Awards.

*Glen Campbell…I'll Be Me* (2014) is about country-music legend Glen Campbell and his "Goodbye Tour" in 2011. Recently diagnosed with Alzheimer's, Campbell decided to tour one last time, initially setting out for 5 weeks, but ending up playing 151 sold-out shows over a year and a half. The film documents this extraordinary journey as he and his family attempt to navigate the wildly unpredictable nature of Glen's progressing disease using love, laughter and music as their medicine of choice.

*Iris* (2001) is a biographical drama film that tells the story of Irish-born British novelist Dame Iris Murdoch (Judi Dench) and her relationship with her husband John Bayley (Jim Broadbent), who wrote the book on which the film was based. When Iris begins experiencing forgetfulness and dementia, the devoted John struggles with hopelessness and frustration, and becomes her caretaker, as his wife's mind deteriorates from the ravages of Alzheimer's disease.

*Is Anybody There?* (2008) is a British drama film directed by John Crowley. In 1987 Edward (Bill Milner) is a ten-year-old boy who lives at an old people's home run by his parents. Surrounded by death and dying, he becomes obsessed with finding evidence for the afterlife. He is helped in his search by Clarence (Michael Caine), an elderly ex-magician in the early stages of dementia who has recently entered the home. The film follows their quest and their friendship, which ultimately allows both Edward and Clarence to come to terms with their respective situations.

*The Leisure Seeker* (2017), directed by Paolo Virzi. Traveling in a vintage Winnebago recreational vehicle, John and Ella Spencer (Donald Sutherland and Helen Mirren) take one last road trip from Wellesley, Massachusetts to the Ernest Hemingway House in the Florida Keys before his dementia and her cancer can catch up with them.

*Marjorie Prime* (2017) is a science fiction film written and directed by Michawl Almereyda, starring Jon Hamm, Tim Robbins, Geena Davis, and Lois Smith. Around the year 2050, 85-year-old Marjorie (Smith) is experiencing the first symptoms of Alzheimer's disease. To bring her comfort her daughter Tess (Davis) and son-in-law Jon (Robbins) hire a service called Prime, designed to assist Alzheimer patients by creating holographic projections of deceased family members which are "fed" with the patients' memories so that they can "retell" them back in case they forget them.

*The Notebook* (2004), based on Nicholas Sparks' best-selling novel of the same name, depicts and elderly couple living in a nursing home. Allie (Gena Rowlands) suffers from Alzheimer's disease and often can't remember her husband or their children. Her husband Noah (James Garner) tries to rekindle her memories by reading the story of their romance to her from his notebook every day. Rachel McAdams and Ryan Gosling portray the young Allie and Noah.

*Remember* (2015) stars Christopher Plummer as Zev, a Holocaust survivor currently living in a NYC nursing home with dementia. His family was killed at Auschwitz by a man who later came to America, under the pseudonym of Rudy Kurlander. Zev begins a journey to find and kill this man, using a letter from his friend to help with his confusion. He must investigate the four Rudy Kurlanders in the country, but what he finds is not what he expects.

*Rise of the Planet of the Apes* (2011) is a science fiction action move that continued the Planet of the Apes series from the 1960s. Will Rodman (James Franco), a pharmaceutical chemist at the San Francisco biotech company Gen-Sys, is testing the viral-based drug ALZ-112 on chimpanzees to find a cure for Alzheimer's disease, from which his father suffers. ALZ-112 greatly affects the chimpanzees' intelligence, leading to more independent and dangerous, apes.

*Robot & Frank* (2012) is a science fiction comedy-drama film. Set in the near future, an aging ex-convict and thief named Frank Weld (Frank Langella) lives alone and suffers from increasingly severe dementia. Frank's son Hunter purchases a robot companion, which is programmed to provide Frank with therapeutic care, including a fixed daily routine and activities like gardening. At first, Frank is irritated by the new-fangled help, but when he learns that he can train the robot, he starts to plan a new string of burglaries that get him and Robot into a tight situation.

*Safe House* (1998) is a thriller starring Patrick Stewart as Mace Sowell, an ex-DIA (Defense Intelligence Agency) agent recently diagnosed with Alzheimer's disease. Sowell believes his life is in danger as he has information on his former boss that could incriminate him. His daughter and psychiatrist believe the disease is making him paranoid and insist on a live-in caretaker, Andi (Kimberly Williams). Mace slowly begins to trust and depend upon Andi as his mental faculties continue to deteriorate.

*The Savages* (2007), starring Laura Linney and Philip Seymour Hoffman as siblings caring for their father, played by Philip Bosco, as he rapidly slips into dementia. The siblings must uproot their lives to care for their father, while also dealing with trauma from their childhood which has caused both to seek unhealthy relationships. Their visits to the nursing home and their father's eventual death allow them to gain new perspective on their past and their futures.

*Still Alice* (2014), based on Lisa Genova's 2007 best-selling book of the same name. Julianne Moore stars as Alice Howland, a professor diagnosed with early-onset Alzheimer's disease. Alice attempts to keep her mind sharp with personal questions on her phone that she answers every day. The disease continues to progress and she loses her job and has trouble recognizing her children. Moore was heavily praised for her depiction of Alice, winning the Best Actress Academy Award in 2015.

*What They Had* (2018) stars Blythe Danner as Ruth Everhardt, a woman dealing with Alzheimer's disease. When Ruth wanders into a blizzard on Christmas Eve, her daughter Bridget (Hilary Swank) and son Nicky (Michael Shannon) try to convince their father to put her in a nursing home, which he is resistant to.

**WRITTEN WORKS & DRAMA**

"The Bear Came Over the Mountain" (1999) by Alice Munro interweaves the tale of two couples, their chance meeting, and the consequences of their involvement in each other's lives. Fiona and Grant, a married couple of many years, experience both physical and emotional separation when she is diagnosed with Alzheimer's disease and moves into a medical facility where she can receive round-the-clock care. Grant realizes that the intimacy that they once shared during their marriage is waning as Fiona gradually loses her memory.

*Beyond Forgetting: Poetry and Prose about Alzheimer's Disease* (2009) is an award-winning collection of poetry and short prose about Alzheimer's disease written by 100 contemporary writers—doctors, nurses, social workers, hospice workers, daughters, sons, wives, and husbands—whose lives have been touched by the disease. Through the transformative power of poetry, their words enable the reader to move "beyond forgetting," beyond the stereotypical portrayal of Alzheimer's disease to honor and affirm the dignity of those afflicted.

Connie's Colander (2015) is a play about a mother and daughter. Connie is a retired domestic science teacher. Emily, her daughter, is enjoying hosting her first TV cookery show. Sensitively, with humor and tenderness, this newly written play traces the evolving relationship throughout their lives and the impact of Connie's Alzheimer's.

*The Day We Met* (2015) by Rowan Coleman, follows Claire, who has a loving family and a great career. However, she is losing her memory, including that of the day she met her husband. Claire fills the pages of a blank book Greg gives her with private memories and keepsakes, jotting down beginnings and endings and everything in between. The book becomes the story of Claire—her passions, her sorrows, her joys, her adventures in a life that refuses to surrender to a fate worse than dying: disappearing.

*Death of a Salesman* (1949). Acclaimed Pulitzer Prize and Tony Award winning drama by Arthur Miller, debuted on Broadway in 1949, with actor Lee J. Cobb as Willy Loman, an aging, tired, unsuccessful and unstable travelling salesman and his relationship with his wife and sons, Biff and Happy. It was made into a 1951 movie with Fredric March as Willy Loman, and again in a 1985 made-for-TV version with Dustin Hoffman as Loman. *Death of a Salesman* was revived on Broadway four times; and has been performed across the world. While not mentioned in the script by name, Willy Loman exhibits many notable signs of Alzheimer's disease.

*The Father* (2012) is a play by French playwright Florian Zeller and won the 2014 Molière Award for Best Play. *The Father* is a tragi-comic mystery, a sobering and realistic family story, and an unsentimental, emotionally intense look at the world through the eyes of a man experiencing dementia, a dramatic illustration of the physical losses which occur along with the mental ones.

*Forget Me Not* (2017), by Garrett Davis, is a play that takes the audience into the life of an African American family facing Alzheimer's disease and shows how the disease impacts everyone, from immediate family to friends and the African American community-at-large. The play is part of the Forget Me Not Project, which aims to enhance the capacity and support of caregivers while educating the general public with special emphasis on underserved communities where health disparities exist.

*Forgetting Home: Poems about Alzheimer's* (2013), edited by Anna M. Evans, hits the nail on the head with this collection of poems about Alzheimer's from multiple perspectives. The book is cleverly separated into sections such as "Reverse Parenting", "Nobody's Fault", and "The Un-naming."

*The Gingerbread House* (2017) by Kate Beaufoy takes place in the English countryside at a manor house. Tess believes that the few weeks she must care for her aging mother-in-law will be the perfect time for her to finish the novel she's writing. Narrated by Katia – her only child – who prefers not to speak but observes everything, *The Gingerbread House* is a deeply moving and compassionate story of a family and its tensions and struggles with her grandmother's dementia, as the reclusive teenager describes the effect it has on everyone in a strangely detached but compassionate way.

*Goodbye, Vitamin* (2018) by Rachel Khong. Freshly disengaged from her fiancé and feeling that life has not turned out quite the way she planned, thirty-year-old Ruth quits her job, leaves town and arrives at her parents' home to find that situation more complicated than she'd realized. Her father, a prominent history professor, is losing his memory and is only erratically lucid. Ruth's mother, meanwhile, is lucidly erratic. But as Ruth's father's condition intensifies, the comedy in her situation takes hold, gently transforming all her grief.

*Grandma Forgets* (2017) is a children's book written by Paul Russell to help young children deal with a relative's dementia. The heart-warming story is of a family bound by love as they cope with their grandma's dementia. Over the years, the little girl has built up a treasure trove of memories of time spent with Grandma. The book contends that your grandmother not remembering your name should be sad, but maybe it is also an opportunity to tell her more often how much you love her.

*Honeycomb: Poems by Carol Frost* (2010) was inspired after Frost cared for her mother during her struggle with Alzheimer's disease, forming a deeply moving meditation on memory and its role in the creation and evolution of identity and relationships.

*In Other Words* (2017) is a play by Matthew Seager that journeys through 50 years of Arthur and Jane's relationship, jumping in and out of memories and experiencing, for brief moments, a failing mind as it loses its grip on reality. Connected by the music of Frank Sinatra, this intimate, humorous, moving love story explores the effects of Alzheimer's disease and the transformative power of music in our lives.

"The Jilting of Granny Weatherall" (1930), by Katherine Anne Porter. This short story is about an older woman who is on her death bed, recounting her life and the people in her life. What is most profound about this story is its message of how losses, disappointments, and the emotional trauma attached to unexpected events in life can stay with a person to the end of life and even into the process of dying. See entry in *Aging*.

*King Lear*, by William Shakespeare. "How sharper than a serpent's tooth it is / to have a thankless child" (Act 1, Scene 4). King *Lear* is a tragedy written by William Shakespeare. It tells the tale of a king who bequeaths his power and land to two of his three daughters, after they declare their love for him in an extremely fawning and obsequious manner. His third daughter gets nothing, because she will not flatter him as her sisters had done. When he feels disrespected by the two daughters who now have his wealth and power, he becomes furious to the point of madness. He eventually becomes tenderly reconciled to his third daughter, just before tragedy strikes her and then the king. The play has been widely adapted for the stage and motion pictures, with the title role coveted by many of the world's most accomplished actors.

*Listening to Mozart: Poems of Alzheimer's* (2014) follows author Esther Altshul Helfgott's moving memoir *Dear Alzheimer's,* about living with the gradual loss of her husband. *Listening to Mozart* is a fitting and lovely companion collection that both takes the reader through her grieving and celebrates the husband she's lost. From the new widow's first angry bewilderment (you must be busy/ —what are you doing/that's so important) to her gradual coming to terms, she vividly conveys how alive the dead are after they've left us with their enormous

*Living in the Land of Limbo: Fiction and Poetry about Family Caregiving* (2014) is an anthology, edited by Carol Lewis, comprised of poems and short stories about family caregivers. It is dedicated to the caregiver's experience. Many of the authors are well-known poets and writers and they come from a wide range of cultural backgrounds.

*The Memory Box* (1992) by Mary Bahr. This picture book for middle readers refreshingly features a family that talks about difficult topics. Gramps sometimes forgets to shave, cuts his feet when he accidentally leaves home without shoes on and talks to a daughter who isn't there. The problem is Alzheimer's disease: he knows it, Gram knows it and young Zach, the narrator, knows it. The memory box is a small carved wooden treasure chest of bits of paper recording the good times, filled by the three of them.

*Nora's Lost* (2005) is a play about Nora Blodget, debilitated by Alzheimer's disease. Nora follows the vision of her late husband into the woods on a cold night. Her life flashes before her — revealing her former life as a dynamic teacher, a caring wife, and a loving mother.

*Old Fools* (2018), written by Tristan Bernays, is the story of Tom and Viv and their lives together from their first meeting until final parting. Like all couples, they have their ups and downs but stay together through the good times and the bad. And then their normal lives are shattered as Alzheimer's raises its unwelcome head.

*On Golden Pond* (1979), by Ernest Thompson. This play shows how the experience of a family retreat can quell long-standing disagreements and friction among different generations of family members. It also shows the value of not letting such disagreements get in the way of having a relationship, as well as the value of developing and nurturing family relationships, even in later life. The play was made into a film in 1981. See entry in *Films*.

*The Outgoing Tide* (2012) is a poignant play about illness, death and personal choice. Gunner, a blue-collar guy and former owner of a small trucking company, is suffering from Alzheimer's, and his concerned wife hopes to get him into an assisted living facility. But Gunner, who has stretches of great lucidity, is completely resistant, so Peg turns to their son, Jack, on a visit to the cottage, to help her.

*The Stone Angel* (1964), by Margaret Laurence. In this novel, ninety-year-old Hagar Shipley tells her life story. Her complex narrative focuses on the double nature of most things in life, particularly one's way of handing people and situations. The story does well to show how elders work hard to maintain a cohesive, competent social facade and how most people of age struggle to compose coherent narratives of their experiences. Key life events that occur around the beginnings and ends of relationships are also central to this work, once again emphasizing the importance of memories to everyone, but particularly to the elderly.

*A Story of Forgetting* (2004) by Stefan Merrill Block blends myth, science, and dazzling storytelling as it follows Abel Haggard, a lonely old-man adrift in recollections of those he loved and lost long ago, and Seth Waller, a teenager determined to help his mother when she develops a rare genetic disease. Though neither knows of the other's existence, Abel and Seth are linked by a dual legacy: the disease that destroys the memories of those they love, and the story of Isidora—a land without memory where nothing is ever possessed, so nothing can be lost.

*The Sweetness of Forgetting* (2012) by Kristin Harmel shows the main character, Hope, as she struggles with divorce, poverty, and raising her troubled child. Her beloved French-born grandmother Mamie is drifting away into a haze of Alzheimer's. But in a rare moment of clarity, Mamie realizes that unless she tells Hope about the past, the secrets she has held on to for so many years will soon be lost forever. She sends Hope to France to uncover a seventy-year-old mystery.

*The Things We Keep* (2017) by Sally Hepworth. Anna Forster is only thirty-eight years old, but her mind is slowly slipping away from her. She knows that her family is doing what they believe to be best when they take her to an assisted living facility. But Anna does not plan on staying. She also knows there's just one another resident who is her age, Luke. As her disease steals more and more of her memory, Anna fights to hold on to what she knows, including her relationship with Luke.

*Turn of Mind* (2012) by Alice LaPlante is a literary thriller about a retired orthopedic surgeon suffering from dementia and accused of killing her best friend. With unmatched patience and a pulsating intensity, Alice LaPlante's debut novel brings us deep into a brilliant woman's deteriorating mind, where the impossibility of recognizing reality can be both a blessing and a curse.

*Visitors* (2014) is a play by English playwright Barney Norris. A seventyish couple, Arthur and Edie, are slowly falling into decay. Arthur feigns robustness but is prone to falling down, while Edie shows all the symptoms of dementia. The sedate rhythm of their lives changes only with the arrival of a blue-haired carer, Kate, who has problems of her own, and with the determination of their son, Stephen, to put his mother into a home and sell the family farm.

*The Waverly Gallery* (2000) is a play by Kenneth Lonergan. It is considered a "memory play." The show follows a grandson watching his grandmother slowly die from Alzheimer's disease.

*The Wide Circumference of Love* (2017) by Marita Golden traces the arc of one African American family through the triumphs and tragedies that compose a life. As the well-respected founder of a Washington, D.C., architectural firm, Gregory Tate has formed a career designing buildings, but when he is diagnosed with early-onset dementia at age 68, his world crumbles. Golden takes a frank and authentic approach to dementia's relentless and all-encompassing nature—losing one's dignity, forgetting loved ones' names, bewildering personality changes, disappearing friends—while also calling attention to the increased prevalence of Alzheimer's in the African American community.

*You Are Not Alone: Poems about Alzheimer's* (2013) by Lon Cole speaks to the heart of those in need of healing and hope. Cole was diagnosed with early-onset Alzheimer's disease. That is when the poems began to flow. He meets moments of despair with honest hope and faith.

**SONGS**

Bergman, Alan, Marilyn Bergman, and Marvin Hamlisch. "Way We Were" (1974). The theme song to the popular 1973 film of the same name, and originally recorded by the star of the film, Barbra Streisand. This song dramatically conveys the power of memories and photographs to evoke strong feelings and how, even when strong, memories can be called into question as one struggles to make sense out of how events did or did not happen in life.

Campbell, Ashley. "Remembering" (2015). Campbell wrote this song for her father, Glen Campbell, who suffered from Alzheimer's disease. She started writing the song after her father's farewell tour, for which she played banjo.

Campbell, Glen and Julian Raymond. "I'm Not Going to Miss You" (2014). The song was released on September 30, 2014 for the soundtrack to the documentary *Glen Campbell: I'll Be Me*, which focuses on the singer's diagnosis of Alzheimer's disease and his final tour.

Caretaker, The. *An Empty Bliss Beyond this World* (2011). English musician Leyland Kirby was inspired to create this album because of a 2010 study about the ability of people with Alzheimer's disease to remember music they listened to when they were younger, as well as where they were and how they felt when they listened to it.

Chesney, Kenny. "While He Still Knows Who I Am" (2012). This song is told from the perspective of a son going to visit his father with Alzheimer's disease. It deals with the importance o\ making sure the people in your life know how much you love them while they can still remember you.

Costello, Elvis. "Veronica" (1989). The song focuses on an older woman who has experienced severe memory loss. Costello's inspiration for this song was his grandmother, who suffered from Alzheimer's.

Dixie Chicks. "Silent House" (2006). This song is about the house where Dixie Chick Natalie Maines' grandmother used to live. Her grandmother had Alzheimer's disease, and the song is about memories of her triggered by walking through the house.

Eldredge, Brett. "Raymond" (2010). This song tells the story of a maintenance worker at a nursing home and his relationship with a patient with Alzheimer's disease, who believes that the maintenance worker is her son Raymond, who was killed in action in Vietnam in 1971. Eldredge was inspired to write the song because his grandmother had Alzheimer's disease for several years.

Fastball. "The Way" (1998). Front man Tony Scalzo came up with the lead single from *All the Pain Money Can Buy* after reading articles about the disappearance of an elderly couple in Texas. Scalzo makes the song a romanticized version of the event, imagining the couple going out to have fun like when they first met.

Gilmour, David. "Faces of Stone" (2015). Former Pink Floyd member Gilmour wrote this song about a peculiar time in his life when he was surrounded by birth and death. "Towards the end of my mother's life, when she was suffering from dementia, there was a brief crossover period of about nine months, when she was alive and my daughter was newly born," Gilmour wrote.

Jessie J. "I Miss Her" (2013). From the album *Alive*, Jessie has said this song is '…about somebody in my family who's unwell, and it's the most personal song I've ever written. That person is still here, but they are not their old selves anymore."

Johnson, Tim. "She Misses Him" (2000). The song discusses Alzheimer's disease as seen from the perspective of a woman married to a victim of said illness.

Longley, Liz. "Unraveling" (2010). Longley wrote the song after her grandmother was diagnosed with Alzheimer's disease and Liz watched her suffer as the disease progressed. Her grandmother, an avid antique collector, soon forgot the meaning of each piece and the names of her family members. The lyrics of "Unraveling" tell the story of watching a loved one slip away.

McEntire, Reba. "Moving Oleta" (2003). Barry Dean wrote this song about his Alzheimer's-stricken grandmother having to move to a nursing home. "My grandfather was caring for her," he recalled to Billboard magazine. "I realized that he saw her as she was when he met her. He didn't see her in the condition she was. I was really moved by that and wrote about two-thirds of that song by myself in Kansas."

Mann, Chris and Rudy Tanzi. "Remember Me" (2015). This song is a unique collaboration between artist Chris Mann and neuroscientist Dr. Rudy Tanzi. The two co-wrote the song as an anthem to Alzheimer's. It was part of a grassroots social media campaign designed to raise awareness and funding for Alzheimer's research in partnership with Cure Alzheimer's Fund. Proceeds from sales of the song and direct donations will support innovative research into the causes of the disease and the development of effective therapies to stop it.

Massive Dog. "When You Were Superman" (2014). The song, which raised money for the Alzheimer's Society, was written by Colin Parish, ten years ago when his dad developed the condition. Mr Parish's dad, Sidney Parish, died in 2005 and he was unable to sing the song for years, as it was too upsetting. Mr Parish said: "I was teaching my son to tie his shoes as the man who taught me forgot how to tie his own. Although the realisation was heartbreaking, the song itself contains the hope that a cure for dementia can be found."

Mattea, Kathy. "Where've You Been" (1989). Co-written by Mattea's husband, Jon Vezner, and Don Henry, the song is about two lovers, Edwin and Claire. It uses three interpretations of the phrase "where've you been", all spoken by Claire toward Edwin in various situations. In the first verse, she asks him where he has been all her life; in the second, she asks him where he has been after coming home late one night; and in the third, the two are elderly hospital patients: Claire has "lost her memory" of family and friends, and close to death, asks Edwin upon seeing him, "where've you been".

Sheeran, Ed. "Afire Love" (2014). This song is about Sheeran's late grandfather who suffered from Alzheimer's disease for 20 years. He died of the disease two weeks after Sheeran began writing about it. He finished writing the song at his grandfather's funeral. The lyrics discuss Sheeran's reaction to the disease as a child all the way up until his grandfather's funeral.

Simon, Paul, and Art Garfunkel. "Bookends Theme" (1967). The importance of preserving memories is poignantly conveyed in this song from the album *Bookends.*

———. "A Hazy Shade of Winter" (1967). The sadder side of being old is conveyed in this song of advice offered by an old man who tells the tales of being old and lonely, filled with despair, and in need. The song also touches on the themes of the importance of memory to elders and the value of being remembered by others.

Snow Patrol. "Soon" (2018). From the album *Wildness*, this song is about singer Gary Lightbody's father, who was diagnosed with dementia in 2015. Lightbody wrote the song as a supportive message to him.

Underwood, Carrie."Forever Changed" (2012). Underwood tells the story of a young girl who grows into a woman, gets married and gives birth to a daughter before being struck down by Alzheimer's as she comes to the end of her life.

Williams, Lucinda. "If My Love Could Kill" (2016). Williams wrote this song about her father's struggle with Alzheimer's and how it affected her family. Without mentioning the disease by name, Williams personifies it and expresses deep anger

**TELEVISION PROGRAMS**

*Black Mirror* (Netflix). "Playtest." Cooper is a charismatic American on a gap-year style tour of Europe, who winds up short of cash in England and signs up to trial a revolutionary video game designed around a haunted house. The game taps into players' fears and decorates a virtual landscape that gradually builds the intensity of fear inducing events. Cooper projects his fears of developing dementia onto his mother and himself as he finds terror in the loss of identity and self that can occur with some end-stage dementia diseases.

———. "San Junipero." This episode s set in a future where dying people are able to relive their youth. They can choose a year to visit for a limited length of time per week and live as their younger selves in fictional settings. It is explained by character Kelly that this 'immersive nostalgia' was originally created to help people living with Alzheimer's disease.

*Grey's Anatomy* (ABC) has aired since 2005, becoming massively popular. The first three seasons featured a running subplot of Meredith Grey's (Ellen Pompeo) struggle, first to keep her mother's Alzheimer's a secret, and then to cope with her mother's disease as her state worsened.

*Mad Men* (AMC). "Man With a Plan." In this episode, viewers witnessed the return of primary character Pete Campbell's mother Dorothy after five years. Her situation had become dire, and her sense of the past and present both had been affected by Alzheimer's disease. The episode explores some of the challenges presented to Pete as he deals with his mother moving into his small apartment while still navigating his tumultuous work life.

*The Sopranos* (HBO). Dominic Chianese plays Junior Soprano, a mob boss suffering from Alzheimer's disease. The actor himself had been caregiver to his own mother with dementia, and his sensitive portrayal has resulted in honors from the Alzheimer's Association and recognition by the American Academy of Neurology.

# GLOSSARY OF TERMS

## AS THEY RELATE TO DEMENTIA AND OTHER COGNITIVE DEGENERATIVE DISORDERS

*acetylcholine:* chemical released by motor neuron terminals that causes muscle contraction

*activities of daily living (ADLs):* general personal care activities such as eating, dressing, and bathing

*acute*: disease process of sudden onset and short duration

*acute confusion*: transient condition caused by social and/or biological stressors, including inattention, disorganized thinking, and emotional problems

*agnosia*: inability to interpret sensations or recognize things

*Alzheimer's disease:* progressive disease characterized by a loss of brain cells, causing memory impairment and cognitive deficits

*amygdala*: almond-shaped mass of gray matter inside each cerebral hemisphere, involved with experiencing of emotions

*anomia:* inability to remember names of persons or objects despite recognizing them

*aphasia*: inability to understand or express speech

*apraxia*: inability to perform particular purposive actions

*Argyrophilic grain disease:* form of late-onset dementia, marked by decreased short-term memory, behavioral disturbances, disorientation, and reading and writing disorders

*assessment:* systematic process of collecting, validating, and communicating patient data, including information gathered from the patient's history and the results of physical examination and laboratory tests

*basal ganglia*: group of structures linked to the thalamus in the base of the brain and involved in coordination of movement

*blackout:* memory loss, usually as a result of taking substances known to disrupt memory; the affected person may appear to be aware of what is happening, despite having no memory of it

*brain:* most complex organ in the body, used for thinking, learning, remembering, seeing, hearing, and many other conscious and subconscious functions

*brain tumors:* often lead to cognitive dysfunction that matches the definition of dementia

*cerebellum:* located just above the brain stem and controls balance, coordination, and motion

*cerebrum:* largest and uppermost section of the brain, which integrates memory, speech, writing, and emotional responses

*chronic traumatic encephalopathy (CTE):* neurodegenerative disease caused by repeated head injuries whose symptoms typically appear years after the injuries and include behavioral problems, difficulty thinking, and ultimately dementia

*clinical trial:* research study to compare standard treatment against potentially better treatment

*cognition:* mental processes involved in the acquisition and use of knowledge, such as attention, thinking, problem solving, and perception; cognitive learning emphasizes these processes in the acquisition of new behaviors

*cognitive appraisal:* assessment of the meaningfulness of an event to an individual

*cognitive processes:* processes of thought, including attending to an event, storing information in memory, recalling and making sense of information

*communicative skills*: skills required to express thoughts, desires, and feelings effectively through verbal and nonverbal communication

*continuous care:* services provided for extended periods of time, such as shifts of eight, ten, twelve, or twenty-four hours

*cortex*: surface (outer layer) of the brain, which receives and interprets sensory input, and relates behavior to external stimuli; responsible for perception and conscious thought

*Creutzfeldt-Jakob disease:* deadly degenerative brain disorder that includes memory loss, behavior changes and visual disturbances

*cued recall*: retrieval of memory with the help of cues

*decay*: disappearance of a memory trace

*delirium:* mental state of sudden confusion and disorientation

*delusion*: symptom of psychosis that consists of a strong irrational belief held despite considerable evidence against it; types include delusions of grandeur, reference, and persecution

*dementia*: impairment/loss of intellect and personality due to loss or damage of neurons in the brain

*depression*: psychological disorder characterized by extreme feelings of sadness, hopelessness, or personal unworthiness, as well as loss of energy, withdrawal, and either sleeplessness or excessive sleep

*desynchronization*: relation that exists when things occur at unrelated times

*durable power of attorney*: designation of a person with legal authority to make health care decisions if a patient becomes incapable of making decisions for himself or herself

*dysphasia*: disturbance of such language skills as speaking, reading, writing, and comprehension

*echoic memory*: sensory memory for sound

*episodic memory*: type of long-term memory that involves conscious recollection of earlier experiences together with their context in terms of time, place, and associated emotions

*extended care:* long-term, ongoing medical care for individuals with serious, chronic, or terminal conditions; may be carried out in a medical/hospice facility or in the patient's home

*fluid intelligence*: intelligence that reflects speed of information processing, reasoning, and memory capacity rather than factual knowledge

*forgetting*: loss of information from memory

*free-recall test*: participants study a list of items, then are prompted to recall the items in any order

*frontal lobe:* anterior portion of each cerebral hemisphere of the brain, containing control of motor areas and most of the higher intellectual functions of the brain, including speech

*frontotemporal dementia (FTD)*: group of neurodegenerative disorders that affect the frontal and temporal lobes of the brain

*geriatrics*: branch of medicine that treats the conditions and diseases associated with aging and old age

*globus pallidus*: structure in the brain involved in the regulation of voluntary movement

*HAD* (HIV-associated dementia): occurs in advanced stages of HIV when the disease spreads to the brain

*hallucinations*: perception of sensations without relevant external stimuli

*hippocampus*: elongated ridges on the floor of each lateral ventricle of the brain, thought to be the center of emotion, memory, and the autonomic nervous system

*home care:* outside services provided to a patient living in a home setting

*hospice*: program designed to ease the suffering for terminally ill patients and their families that is provided in the home or in a special hospice setting, with emphasis on palliative care rather than on the extension of life

*Huntington's disease*: genetic disease characterized by uncoordinated movements as a result of neuron degeneration

*hydrocephalus:* excessive collection of cerebrospinal fluid in the brain

*iconic memory*: brief sensory memory for vision

*incompetency*: legally established lack of sufficient knowledge and judgment to maintain a given right or responsibility

*incontinence*: inability to control the expulsion of urine or feces

*informed consent*: process of educating a patient fully about the purpose, benefits, and risks of a clinical trial or procedure and obtaining authorization to proceed

*intelligence*: ability to perform various mental tasks, including reasoning, knowledge, comprehension, memory, applying concepts, and manipulating figures

*Korsakoff's syndrome*: alcohol-induced brain damage that causes disorientation, impaired long-term memory, and production of false memories to fill memory gaps

*Lewy body dementia*: type of dementia that results when protein deposits develop in nerve cells in the regions of the brain that are involved in thinking, movement, and memory

*living will*: legally binding document with instructions concerning whether or not to prolong life by externally administered life-support systems if the patient is unable to express his or her decision

*long-term care*: health care or personal care for a patient who is chronically unable to provide his or her own care

*long-term memory*: memory system of unlimited capacity that consists of more or less permanent knowledge

*Medicare*: U.S. federal program that covers many of the hospital costs and doctor bills for elderly and disabled persons

*memory*: mental processes involved in storing and recalling previously experienced images, information, and events

*mild cognitive dementia:* notable decline of memory or mental function that does not significantly interfere with the patient's daily life

*mixed dementia:* one or more forms of dementia present at the same time, most commonly Alzheimer's and vascular dementia

*neurodegenerative*: resulting in or characterized by degeneration of the nervous system, especially the neurons in the brain

*neurofibrillary tangles*: hallmark lesions of Alzheimer's disease and several other disorders consisting of intracellular aggregates of the structural protein tau

*neurologic*: dealing with the nervous system and its disorders

*neurology*: study of the central nervous system, composed of the brain and spinal cord

*neuroscience*: specialization that deals with mental processes, occurrences, and disturbances in terms of underlying mechanisms in the brain and the nervous system

*neurosyphilis:* results when syphilis spreads to the central nervous system and causes symptoms ranging from mild cognitive impairment to full-on dementia

*normal pressure hydrocephalus*: abnormal buildup of cerebrospinal fluid in the brain's ventricles that leads to progressive mental impairment and eventually dementia

*organic brain syndromes*: clusters of behavioral and psychological symptoms involving impaired brain function, where etiology is unknown; includes delirium, delusions, amnesia, intoxication, and dementias

*Parkinson's disease:* neurological condition characterized by slow and decreased movement; 50 - 80 percent of patients with Parkinson's develop dementia

*paranoia*: pervasive distrust and suspiciousness of others and a tendency to interpret others' motives as malevolent

*perception*: psychological process by which information that comes in through the sense organs is meaningfully interpreted by the brain

*procedural memory*: type of long-term memory involving how to perform different actions and skills

*progressive supranuclear palsy:* degenerative disease that results in the deterioration of cells in the areas of the brain that control movement, coordination and cognition

*recognition memory*: ability to recognize earlier encountered events, objects, or people

*semantic memory*: long-term representation of a person's factual knowledge of the world

*senescence*: condition or process of deterioration with age

*short-term memory*: memory system of limited capacity that uses rehearsal processes either to retain current memories or to pass them on to long-term memory

*source memory*: recalls the source of learned information, such as knowledge of when or where something was learned

*spatial memory*: part of the memory responsible for the recording of information about one's environment and spatial orientation

*stroke*: vascular incident resulting from either the rupture of a vessel or the blocking of blood flow in an artery

*temporal lobe*: lower portion on the side of each of the brain's cerebral hemispheres, containing the sites of sensory interpretation, and memory of visual and auditory patterns

*traumatic brain injury*: sudden trauma to the brain that can both cause dementia and increase the risk of developing dementia-causing diseases

*vascular dementia*: caused by brain damage from impaired blood flow to the brain, most often as the result of a stroke

*Wernicke-Korsakoff syndrome*: neurodegenerative disorder that results from a vitamin B1 deficiency leading to cognitive malfunction and dementia

## A

## B

## C

## D



## E



## F



## G

## O

## P



## Q



## R



## S

## T



## U

## V



## W

## X



## Y



## Z

## Alabama



## Alaska



## Arizona



## Arkansas



## California

## Canada



## Colorado



## Connecticut



## Delaware



## District of Columbia

## Florida



## Georgia



## Hawaii

## Idaho



## Illinois



## Indiana



## Iowa



## Kansas



## Kentucky



## Louisiana



## Maine

## Maryland



## Massachusetts



## Michigan

## Minnesota



## Mississippi



## Missouri



## Montana



## Nebraska



## Nevada



## New Hampshire



## New Jersey

## New Mexico



## New York



## North Carolina

## North Dakota



## Ohio



## Oklahoma



## Oregon



## Pennsylvania



## Rhode Island



## South Carolina

## South Dakota



## Tennessee



## Texas



## Utah



## Vermont



## Virginia

## Washington



## West Virginia



## Wisconsin



## Wyoming

# Grey House Imprints

Visit www.GreyHouse.com for Product Information, Table of Contents, and Sample Pages.

## Statistics & Demographics

America's Top-Rated Cities
America's Top-Rated Smaller Cities
The Comparative Guide to American Suburbs
Profiles of America
Profiles of California
Profiles of Florida
Profiles of Illinois
Profiles of Indiana
Profiles of Massachusetts
Profiles of Michigan
Profiles of New Jersey
Profiles of New York
Profiles of North Carolina & South Carolina
Profiles of Ohio
Profiles of Pennsylvania
Profiles of Texas
Profiles of Virginia
Profiles of Wisconsin

## Canadian Resources

Associations Canada
Canadian Almanac & Directory
Canadian Environmental Resource Guide
Canadian Parliamentary Guide
Canadian Venture Capital & Private Equity Firms
Canadian Who's Who
Cannabis Canada
Careers & Employment Canada
Financial Post: Directory of Directors
Financial Services Canada
FP Bonds: Corporate
FP Bonds: Government
FP Equities: Preferreds & Derivatives
FP Survey: Industrials
FP Survey: Mines & Energy
FP Survey: Predecessor & Defunct
Health Guide Canada
Libraries Canada

## Weiss Financial Ratings

Financial Literacy Basics
Financial Literacy: How to Become an Investor
Financial Literacy: Planning for the Future
Weiss Ratings Consumer Guides
Weiss Ratings Guide to Banks
Weiss Ratings Guide to Credit Unions
Weiss Ratings Guide to Health Insurers
Weiss Ratings Guide to Life & Annuity Insurers
Weiss Ratings Guide to Property & Casualty Insurers
Weiss Ratings Investment Research Guide to Bond & Money Market Mutual Funds
Weiss Ratings Investment Research Guide to Exchange-Traded Funds
Weiss Ratings Investment Research Guide to Stock Mutual Funds
Weiss Ratings Investment Research Guide to Stocks

## Books in Print Series

American Book Publishing Record® Annual
American Book Publishing Record® Monthly
Books In Print®
Books In Print® Supplement
Books Out Loud™
Bowker's Complete Video Directory™
Children's Books In Print®
El-Hi Textbooks & Serials In Print®
Forthcoming Books®
Law Books & Serials In Print™
Medical & Health Care Books In Print™
Publishers, Distributors & Wholesalers of the US™
Subject Guide to Books In Print®
Subject Guide to Children's Books In Print®

SALEM PRESS

# Titles from Salem Press

SALEM PRESS

Visit www.SalemPress.com for Product Information, Table of Contents, and Sample Pages.

## LITERATURE

### Critical Insights: Authors

Louisa May Alcott
Sherman Alexie
Isabel Allende
Maya Angelou
Isaac Asimov
Margaret Atwood
Jane Austen
James Baldwin
Saul Bellow
Roberto Bolano
Ray Bradbury
The Brontë Sisters
Gwendolyn Brooks
Albert Camus
Raymond Carver
Willa Cather
Geoffrey Chaucer
John Cheever
Joseph Conrad
Charles Dickens
Emily Dickinson
Frederick Douglass
T. S. Eliot
George Eliot
Harlan Ellison
Louise Erdrich
William Faulkner
F. Scott Fitzgerald
Gustave Flaubert
Horton Foote
Benjamin Franklin
Robert Frost
Neil Gaiman
Gabriel Garcia Marquez
Thomas Hardy
Nathaniel Hawthorne
Robert A. Heinlein
Lillian Hellman
Ernest Hemingway
Langston Hughes
Zora Neale Hurston
Henry James
Thomas Jefferson
James Joyce
Jamaica Kincaid
Stephen King
Martin Luther King, Jr.
Barbara Kingsolver
Abraham Lincoln
Mario Vargas Llosa
Jack London
James McBride
Cormac McCarthy
Herman Melville
Arthur Miller
Toni Morrison
Alice Munro
Tim O'Brien
Flannery O'Connor
Eugene O'Neill
George Orwell
Sylvia Plath
Edgar Allan Poe
Philip Roth
Salman Rushdie
J.D. Salinger
Mary Shelley
John Steinbeck
Amy Tan
Leo Tolstoy
Mark Twain
John Updike
Kurt Vonnegut
Alice Walker
David Foster Wallace
Edith Wharton
Walt Whitman
Oscar Wilde
Tennessee Williams
Virginia Woolf
Richard Wright
Malcolm X

### Critical Insights: Works

Absalom, Absalom!
Adventures of Huckleberry Finn
Adventures of Tom Sawyer
Aeneid
All Quiet on the Western Front
Animal Farm
Anna Karenina
The Awakening
The Bell Jar
Beloved
Billy Budd, Sailor
The Book Thief
Brave New World
The Canterbury Tales
Catch-22
The Catcher in the Rye
The Color Purple
The Crucible
Death of a Salesman
The Diary of a Young Girl
Dracula
Fahrenheit 451
The Grapes of Wrath
Great Expectations
The Great Gatsby
Hamlet
The Handmaid's Tale
Harry Potter Series
Heart of Darkness
The Hobbit
The House on Mango Street
How the Garcia Girls Lost Their Accents
The Hunger Games Trilogy
I Know Why the Caged Bird Sings
In Cold Blood
The Inferno
Invisible Man
Jane Eyre
The Joy Luck Club
Julius Caesar
King Lear
The Kite Runner
Life of Pi
Little Women
Lolita
Lord of the Flies
The Lord of the Rings
Macbeth
The Metamorphosis
Midnight's Children
A Midsummer Night's Dream
Moby-Dick
Mrs. Dalloway
Nineteen Eighty-Four
The Odyssey
Of Mice and Men
The Old Man and the Sea
On the Road
One Flew Over the Cuckoo's Nest
One Hundred Years of Solitude
Othello
The Outsiders
Paradise Lost
The Pearl
The Poetry of Baudelaire
The Poetry of Edgar Allan Poe
A Portrait of the Artist as a Young Man
Pride and Prejudice
The Red Badge of Courage
Romeo and Juliet
The Scarlet Letter
Short Fiction of Flannery O'Connor
Slaughterhouse-Five
The Sound and the Fury
A Streetcar Named Desire
The Sun Also Rises
A Tale of Two Cities
The Tales of Edgar Allan Poe
Their Eyes Were Watching God
Things Fall Apart
To Kill a Mockingbird
War and Peace
The Woman Warrior

### Critical Insights: Themes

The American Comic Book
American Creative Non-Fiction
The American Dream
American Multicultural Identity
American Road Literature
American Short Story
American Sports Fiction
The American Thriller
American Writers in Exile
Censored & Banned Literature
Civil Rights Literature, Past & Present
Coming of Age
Conspiracies
Contemporary Canadian Fiction
Contemporary Immigrant Short Fiction
Contemporary Latin American Fiction
Contemporary Speculative Fiction
Crime and Detective Fiction
Crisis of Faith
Cultural Encounters
Dystopia
Family
The Fantastic
Feminism

SALEM PRESS

# Titles from Salem Press

SALEM PRESS

Visit www.SalemPress.com for Product Information, Table of Contents, and Sample Pages.

Flash Fiction
Gender, Sex and Sexuality
Good & Evil
The Graphic Novel
Greed
Harlem Renaissance
The Hero's Quest
Historical Fiction
Holocaust Literature
The Immigrant Experience
Inequality
LGBTQ Literature
Literature in Times of Crisis
Literature of Protest
Love
Magical Realism
Midwestern Literature
Modern Japanese Literature
Nature & the Environment
Paranoia, Fear & Alienation
Patriotism
Political Fiction
Postcolonial Literature
Pulp Fiction of the '20s and '30s
Rebellion
Russia's Golden Age
Satire
The Slave Narrative
Social Justice and American Literature
Southern Gothic Literature
Southwestern Literature
Survival
Technology & Humanity
Truth & Lies
Violence in Literature
Virginia Woolf & 20th Century Women Writers
War

## Critical Insights: Film

Bonnie & Clyde
Casablanca
Alfred Hitchcock
Stanley Kubrick

## Critical Approaches to Literature

Critical Approaches to Literature: Feminist
Critical Approaches to Literature: Moral
Critical Approaches to Literature: Multicultural
Critical Approaches to Literature: Psychological

## Critical Surveys of Literature

Critical Survey of American Literature
Critical Survey of Drama
Critical Survey of Graphic Novels: Heroes & Superheroes
Critical Survey of Graphic Novels: History, Theme, and Technique
Critical Survey of Graphic Novels: Independents & Underground Classics
Critical Survey of Graphic Novels: Manga
Critical Survey of Long Fiction
Critical Survey of Mystery and Detective Fiction
Critical Survey of Mythology & Folklore: Gods & Goddesses
Critical Survey of Mythology & Folklore: Heroes and Heroines
Critical Survey of Mythology & Folklore: Love, Sexuality, and Desire
Critical Survey of Mythology & Folklore: World Mythology
Critical Survey of Poetry
Critical Survey of Poetry: Contemporary Poets
Critical Survey of Science Fiction & Fantasy Literature
Critical Survey of Shakespeare's Plays
Critical Survey of Shakespeare's Sonnets
Critical Survey of Short Fiction
Critical Survey of World Literature
Critical Survey of Young Adult Literature

## Cyclopedia of Literary Characters & Places

Cyclopedia of Literary Characters
Cyclopedia of Literary Places

## Introduction to Literary Context

American Poetry of the 20th Century
American Post-Modernist Novels
American Short Fiction
English Literature
Plays
World Literature

## Magill's Literary Annual

Magill's Literary Annual, 2022
Magill's Literary Annual, 2021
Magill's Literary Annual, 2020
Magill's Literary Annual (Backlist Issues 2019-1977)

## Masterplots

Masterplots, Fourth Edition
Masterplots, 2010-2018 Supplement

## Notable Writers

Notable African American Writers
Notable American Women Writers
Notable Mystery & Detective Fiction Writers
Notable Writers of the American West & the Native American Experience
Novels into Film: Adaptations & Interpretation
Recommended Reading: 600 Classics Reviewed

SALEM PRESS

# Titles from Salem Press

SALEM PRESS

Visit www.SalemPress.com for Product Information, Table of Contents, and Sample Pages.

## HISTORY

### The Decades

The 1910s in America
The Twenties in America
The Thirties in America
The Forties in America
The Fifties in America
The Sixties in America
The Seventies in America
The Eighties in America
The Nineties in America
The 2000s in America
The 2010s in America

### Defining Documents in American History

Defining Documents: The 1900s
Defining Documents: The 1910s
Defining Documents: The 1920s
Defining Documents: The 1930s
Defining Documents: The 1950s
Defining Documents: The 1960s
Defining Documents: The 1970s
Defining Documents: The 1980s
Defining Documents: American Citizenship
Defining Documents: The American Economy
Defining Documents: The American Revolution
Defining Documents: The American West
Defining Documents: Business Ethics
Defining Documents: Capital Punishment
Defining Documents: Civil Rights
Defining Documents: Civil War
Defining Documents: The Constitution
Defining Documents: The Cold War
Defining Documents: Dissent & Protest
Defining Documents: Domestic Terrorism
Defining Documents: Drug Policy
Defining Documents: The Emergence of Modern America
Defining Documents: Environment & Conservation
Defining Documents: Espionage & Intrigue
Defining Documents: Exploration and Colonial America
Defining Documents: The First Amendment
Defining Documents: The Free Press
Defining Documents: The Great Depression
Defining Documents: The Great Migration
Defining Documents: The Gun Debate
Defining Documents: Immigration & Immigrant Communities
Defining Documents: The Legacy of 9/11
Defining Documents: LGBTQ+
Defining Documents: Manifest Destiny and the New Nation
Defining Documents: Native Americans
Defining Documents: Political Campaigns, Candidates & Discourse
Defining Documents: Postwar 1940s
Defining Documents: Prison Reform
Defining Documents: Secrets, Leaks & Scandals
Defining Documents: Slavery
Defining Documents: Supreme Court Decisions
Defining Documents: Reconstruction Era
Defining Documents: The Vietnam War
Defining Documents: U.S. Involvement in the Middle East
Defining Documents: World War I
Defining Documents: World War II

### Defining Documents in World History

Defining Documents: The 17th Century
Defining Documents: The 18th Century
Defining Documents: The 19th Century
Defining Documents: The 20th Century (1900-1950)
Defining Documents: The Ancient World
Defining Documents: Asia
Defining Documents: Genocide & the Holocaust
Defining Documents: Nationalism & Populism
Defining Documents: Pandemics, Plagues & Public Health
Defining Documents: Renaissance & Early Modern Era
Defining Documents: The Middle Ages
Defining Documents: The Middle East
Defining Documents: Women's Rights

### Great Events from History

Great Events from History: The Ancient World
Great Events from History: The Middle Ages
Great Events from History: The Renaissance & Early Modern Era
Great Events from History: The 17th Century
Great Events from History: The 18th Century
Great Events from History: The 19th Century
Great Events from History: The 20th Century, 1901-1940
Great Events from History: The 20th Century, 1941-1970
Great Events from History: The 20th Century, 1971-2000
Great Events from History: Modern Scandals
Great Events from History: African American History
Great Events from History: The 21st Century, 2000-2016
Great Events from History: LGBTQ Events
Great Events from History: Human Rights
Great Events from History: Women's History

### Great Lives from History

Computer Technology Innovators
Fashion Innovators
Great Athletes
Great Athletes of the Twenty-First Century
Great Lives from History: African Americans
Great Lives from History: American Heroes
Great Lives from History: American Women
Great Lives from History: Asian and Pacific Islander Americans
Great Lives from History: Inventors & Inventions
Great Lives from History: Jewish Americans
Great Lives from History: Latinos
Great Lives from History: Scientists and Science
Great Lives from History: The 17th Century
Great Lives from History: The 18th Century
Great Lives from History: The 19th Century
Great Lives from History: The 20th Century
Great Lives from History: The 21st Century, 2000-2017
Great Lives from History: The Ancient World
Great Lives from History: The Incredibly Wealthy
Great Lives from History: The Middle Ages
Great Lives from History: The Renaissance & Early Modern Era
Human Rights Innovators
Internet Innovators
Music Innovators
Musicians and Composers of the 20th Century
World Political Innovators

SALEM PRESS

# Titles from Salem Press

SALEM PRESS

Visit www.SalemPress.com for Product Information, Table of Contents, and Sample Pages.

## History & Government

American First Ladies
American Presidents
The 50 States
The Ancient World: Extraordinary People in Extraordinary Societies
The Bill of Rights
The Criminal Justice System
The U.S. Supreme Court

## SOCIAL SCIENCES

Civil Rights Movements: Past & Present
Countries, Peoples and Cultures
Countries: Their Wars & Conflicts: A World Survey
Education Today: Issues, Policies & Practices
Encyclopedia of American Immigration
Ethics: Questions & Morality of Human Actions
Issues in U.S. Immigration
Principles of Sociology: Group Relationships & Behavior
Principles of Sociology: Personal Relationships & Behavior
Principles of Sociology: Societal Issues & Behavior
Racial & Ethnic Relations in America
World Geography

## HEALTH

Addictions, Substance Abuse & Alcoholism
Adolescent Health & Wellness
Aging
Cancer
Community & Family Health Issues
Integrative, Alternative & Complementary Medicine
Genetics and Inherited Conditions
Infectious Diseases and Conditions
Magill's Medical Guide
Nutrition
Parenting: Styles & Strategies
Psychology & Behavioral Health
Women's Health

## Principles of Health

Principles of Health: Allergies & Immune Disorders
Principles of Health: Anxiety & Stress
Principles of Health: Depression
Principles of Health: Diabetes
Principles of Health: Nursing
Principles of Health: Obesity
Principles of Health: Pain Management
Principles of Health: Prescription Drug Abuse

## SCIENCE

Ancient Creatures
Applied Science
Applied Science: Engineering & Mathematics
Applied Science: Science & Medicine
Applied Science: Technology
Biomes and Ecosystems
Earth Science: Earth Materials and Resources
Earth Science: Earth's Surface and History
Earth Science: Earth's Weather, Water and Atmosphere
Earth Science: Physics and Chemistry of the Earth
Encyclopedia of Climate Change
Encyclopedia of Energy
Encyclopedia of Environmental Issues
Encyclopedia of Global Resources
Encyclopedia of Mathematics and Society
Forensic Science
Notable Natural Disasters
The Solar System
USA in Space

## Principles of Science

Principles of Anatomy
Principles of Astronomy
Principles of Behavioral Science
Principles of Biology
Principles of Biotechnology
Principles of Botany
Principles of Chemistry
Principles of Climatology
Principles of Computer-aided Design
Principles of Information Technology
Principles of Computer Science
Principles of Ecology
Principles of Energy
Principles of Fire Science
Principles of Geology
Principles of Marine Science
Principles of Mathematics
Principles of Microbiology
Principles of Modern Agriculture
Principles of Pharmacology
Principles of Physical Science
Principles of Physics
Principles of Programming & Coding
Principles of Robotics & Artificial Intelligence
Principles of Scientific Research
Principles of Sports Medicine & Kinesiology
Principles of Sustainability
Principles of Zoology

SALEM PRESS

# Titles from Salem Press

SALEM PRESS

Visit www.SalemPress.com for Product Information, Table of Contents, and Sample Pages.

## CAREERS

Careers: Paths to Entrepreneurship
Careers in Artificial Intelligence
Careers in the Arts: Fine, Performing & Visual
Careers in the Automotive Industry
Careers in Biology
Careers in Building Construction
Careers in Business
Careers in Chemistry
Careers in Communications & Media
Careers in Education & Training
Careers in Engineering
Careers in Environment & Conservation
Careers in Financial Services
Careers in Forensic Science
Careers in Gaming
Careers in Green Energy
Careers in Healthcare
Careers in Hospitality & Tourism
Careers in Human Services
Careers in Information Technology
Careers in Law, Criminal Justice & Emergency Services
Careers in the Music Industry
Careers in Manufacturing & Production
Careers in Nursing
Careers in Physics
Careers in Protective Services
Careers in Psychology & Behavioral Health
Careers in Public Administration
Careers in Sales, Insurance & Real Estate
Careers in Science & Engineering
Careers in Social Media
Careers in Sports & Fitness
Careers in Sports Medicine & Training
Careers in Technical Services & Equipment Repair
Careers in Transportation
Careers in Writing & Editing
Careers Outdoors
Careers Overseas
Careers Working with Infants & Children
Careers Working with Animals

## BUSINESS

Principles of Business: Accounting
Principles of Business: Economics
Principles of Business: Entrepreneurship
Principles of Business: Finance
Principles of Business: Globalization
Principles of Business: Leadership
Principles of Business: Management
Principles of Business: Marketing

# Titles from H.W. Wilson

Visit www.HWWilsonInPrint.com for Product Information, Table of Contents, and Sample Pages.

## Core Collections

Children's Core Collection
Fiction Core Collection
Graphic Novels Core Collection
Middle & Junior High School Core
Public Library Core Collection: Nonfiction
Senior High Core Collection
Young Adult Fiction Core Collection

## The Reference Shelf

Affordable Housing
Aging in America
Alternative Facts, Post-Truth and the Information War
The American Dream
Artificial Intelligence
The Business of Food
Campaign Trends & Election Law
College Sports
Democracy Evolving
The Digital Age
Embracing New Paradigms in Education
Food Insecurity & Hunger in the United States
Future of U.S. Economic Relations: Mexico, Cuba, & Venezuela
Global Climate Change
Guns in America
Hate Crimes
Immigration
Income Inequality
Internet Abuses & Privacy Rights
Internet Law
LGBTQ in the 21st Century
Marijuana Reform
Mental Health Awareness
National Debate Topic 2014/2015: The Ocean
National Debate Topic 2015/2016: Surveillance
National Debate Topic 2016/2017: US/China Relations
National Debate Topic 2017/2018: Education Reform
National Debate Topic 2018/2019: Immigration
National Debate Topic 2019/2021: Arms Sales
National Debate Topic 2020/2021: Criminal Justice Reform
National Debate Topic 2021/2022: Water Resources
National Debate Topic 2022/2023
New Frontiers in Space
Policing in 2020
Pollution
Prescription Drug Abuse
Propaganda and Misinformation
Racial Tension in a Postracial Age
Reality Television
Representative American Speeches, Annual Editions
Rethinking Work
Revisiting Gender
The South China Sea Conflict
Sports in America
The Supreme Court
The Transformation of American Cities
The Two Koreas
UFOs
Vaccinations
Voters' Rights
Whistleblowers

## Current Biography

Current Biography Cumulative Index 1946-2021
Current Biography Monthly Magazine
Current Biography Yearbook

## Readers' Guide to Periodical Literature

Abridged Readers' Guide to Periodical Literature
Readers' Guide to Periodical Literature

## Indexes

Index to Legal Periodicals & Books
Short Story Index
Book Review Digest

## Sears List

Sears List of Subject Headings
Sears: Lista de Encabezamientos de Materia

## History

American Game Changers: Invention, Innovation & Transformation
American Reformers
Speeches of the American Presidents

## Facts About Series

Facts About the 20th Century
Facts About American Immigration
Facts About China
Facts About the Presidents
Facts About the World's Languages

## Nobel Prize Winners

Nobel Prize Winners: 1901-1986
Nobel Prize Winners: 1987-1991
Nobel Prize Winners: 1992-1996
Nobel Prize Winners: 1997-2001
Nobel Prize Winners: 2002-2018

## Famous First Facts

Famous First Facts
Famous First Facts About American Politics
Famous First Facts About Sports
Famous First Facts About the Environment
Famous First Facts: International Edition

## American Book of Days

The American Book of Days
The International Book of Days